Thieme

Endoscopic Transnasal Anatomy of the Skull Base and Adjacent Areas

A Lab Dissection and Radiological Atlas

Piero Nicolai, MD
Professor
Department of Otorhinolaryngology–Head and Neck Surgery
University of Brescia
Brescia, Italy

Marco Ferrari, MD
Resident
Department of Otorhinolaryngology–Head and Neck Surgery
University of Brescia
Brescia, Italy

Roberto Maroldi, MD
Professor
Department of Radiology
University of Brescia
Brescia, Italy

Marco Maria Fontanella, MD
Professor
Department of Neurosurgery
University of Brescia
Brescia, Italy

Lena Hirtler, MA, MD, PhD
Lecturer
Division of Anatomy
Center for Anatomy and Cell Biology
Medical University of Vienna
Vienna, Austria

Manfred Tschabitscher, MD, PhD
Professor
Division of Anatomy
Center for Anatomy and Cell Biology
Medical University of Vienna
Vienna, Austria;
Section of Anatomy and Physiopathology
Department of Clinical and Experimental Sciences
University of Brescia
Brescia, Italy

Luigi Fabrizio Rodella, MD, MSc
Professor
Section of Anatomy and Physiopathology
Department of Clinical and Experimental Sciences
University of Brescia
Brescia, Italy

1070 illustrations

Thieme
Stuttgart • New York • Delhi • Rio de Janeiro

Library of Congress Cataloging-in-Publication Data is available from the publisher

Important note: Medicine is an ever-changing science undergoing continual development. Research and clinical experience are continually expanding our knowledge, in particular our knowledge of proper treatment and drug therapy. Insofar as this book mentions any dosage or application, readers may rest assured that the authors, editors, and publishers have made every effort to ensure that such references are in accordance with **the state of knowledge at the time of production of the book.**

Nevertheless, this does not involve, imply, or express any guarantee or responsibility on the part of the publishers in respect to any dosage instructions and forms of applications stated in the book. **Every user is requested to examine carefully** the manufacturers' leaflets accompanying each drug and to check, if necessary in consultation with a physician or specialist, whether the dosage schedules mentioned therein or the contraindications stated by the manufacturers differ from the statements made in the present book. Such examination is particularly important with drugs that are either rarely used or have been newly released on the market. Every dosage schedule or every form of application used is entirely at the user's own risk and responsibility. The authors and publishers request every user to report to the publishers any discrepancies or inaccuracies noticed. If errors in this work are found after publication, errata will be posted at www.thieme.com on the product description page.

Some of the product names, patents, and registered designs referred to in this book are in fact registered trademarks or proprietary names even though specific reference to this fact is not always made in the text. Therefore, the appearance of a name without designation as proprietary is not to be construed as a representation by the publisher that it is in the public domain.

Thieme Medical Publishers New York
333 Seventh Avenue
New York, New York 10001 USA
+1 800 782 3488, customerservice@thieme.com

Georg Thieme Verlag KG
Rüdigerstrasse 14, 70469 Stuttgart, Germany
+49 [0]711 8931 421, customerservice@thieme.de

Thieme Publishers Delhi
A-12, Second Floor, Sector-2, Noida-201301
Uttar Pradesh, India
+91 120 45 566 00, customerservice@thieme.in

Thieme Publishers Rio de Janeiro,
Thieme Publicações Ltda.
Edifício Rodolpho de Paoli, 25º andar
Av. Nilo Peçanha, 50 – Sala 2508,
Rio de Janeiro 20020-906 Brasil
+55 21 3172-2297

Cover design: Thieme Publishing Group
Typesetting by DiTech, India

Printed in Germany by CPI Books

5 4 3 2 1

ISBN 978-31-3-241562-1

Also available as an e-book:
eISBN 978-3-13-241563-8

To Wolfgang Draf and Heinz Stammberger, two unforgettable giants. With their leadership, teachings, and vision, they will stand forever in the history of our discipline.

Contents

Foreword ... ix
Fred Gentili

Foreword ... x
Ricardo L. Carrau

Preface ... xi
Piero Nicolai

Preface ... xii
Marco Ferrari

Contributors ... xiii

1 **Classification of Endoscopic Transnasal Approaches to the Skull Base and Adjacent Areas** ... 1
Piero Nicolai, Marco Ferrari, Roberto Maroldi, Alperen Vural, Marco Maria Fontanella, Luigi Fabrizio Rodella, Lena Hirtler, Manfred Tschabitscher

2 **Nasal Corridors** ... 26
Vittorio Rampinelli, Davide Mattavelli, Marco Ravanelli, Alberto Schreiber

3 **Corridor to the Anterior Skull Base and Orbit** ... 38
Davide Mattavelli, Giacomo Bertazzoni, Alberto Schreiber, Marco Ravanelli, Luca Pianta

4 **Corridor to Sella Turcica, Surrounding Areas, Posterior Skull Base, and Cervical Spine** ... 57
Francesco Belotti, Davide Lancini, Marco Ravanelli, Stefano Taboni, Francesco Doglietto

5 **Corridor to Lateral Spaces** ... 75
Alberto Schreiber, Vittorio Rampinelli, Marco Ferrari, Marco Ravanelli

6 **Transfrontal Approach** ... 95
Francesco Belotti, Marco Ravanelli, Marco Angelo Cocchi, Vittorio Rampinelli, Francesco Doglietto

7 **Transcribriform Approach** ... 108
Marco Ferrari, Marco Ravanelli, Davide Lancini, Vittorio Rampinelli, Alberto Schreiber

8 **Transplanum–Transtuberculum Approach** ... 133
Davide Mattavelli, Marco Ravanelli, Davide Lancini, Marco Ferrari, Alberto Schreiber

9 **Transsellar Approach** ... 152
Francesco Doglietto, Marco Ravanelli, Francesco Belotti, Marco Maria Fontanella

10 **Transsellar Transdorsal Approach** ... 166
Marco Ferrari, Marco Ravanelli, Francesco Belotti, Francesco Doglietto

11 **Transclival (Midclivus) Approach** ... 190
Vittorio Rampinelli, Davide Mattavelli, Marco Ravanelli, Davide Lancini, Alberto Schreiber

12 **Transclival (Lower Clivus) Approach** ... 211
Marco Ferrari, Marco Ravanelli, Davide Mattavelli, Alberto Schreiber, Francesco Doglietto

13 **Transodontoid Approach** ... 229
Francesco Doglietto, Francesco Belotti, Andrea Bolzoni Villaret, Marco Ravanelli

14 **Orbital Decompression, Optic Decompression, Supraorbital Approach, and Transorbital Approach** ... 251
Davide Mattavelli, Marco Ravanelli, Andrea Luigi Camillo Carobbio, Davide Lombardi

15 Transpterygomaxillary Approach 271
Piero Nicolai, Alberto Schreiber, Marco Ravanelli, Davide Mattavelli, Alberto Deganello

16 Infratemporal Fossa Approach 289
Alberto Schreiber, Marco Ravanelli, Marco Ferrari, Vittorio Rampinelli

17 Medial Transcavernous Approach 307
Marco Ferrari, Marco Ravanelli, Davide Lancini, Francesco Belotti, Francesco Doglietto

18 Lateral Transcavernous Approach 320
Marco Ferrari, Marco Ravanelli, Francesco Belotti, Alberto Schreiber, Roberto Maroldi

19 Medial Petrous Apex Approach 338
Vittorio Rampinelli, Marco Ravanelli, Andrea Bolzoni Villaret, Francesco Doglietto

20 Infrapetrous Approach 359
Davide Lancini, Marco Ravanelli, Marco Ferrari, Alberto Schreiber

21 The Suprapetrous (Meckel's Cave) Approach 374
Vittorio Rampinelli, Marco Ravanelli, Marco Ferrari, Davide Lancini, Alberto Schreiber

22 Transcondylar/Transjugular Tuberculum ("Far-Medial") Approach 393
Marco Ferrari, Marco Ravanelli, Francesco Belotti, Francesco Doglietto

23 Medial Parapharyngeal Approach 409
Alberto Schreiber, Marco Ferrari, Marco Ravanelli, Vittorio Rampinelli, Davide Lancini

24 Lateral Parapharyngeal Approach 429
Marco Ferrari, Marco Ravanelli, Davide Lancini, Alberto Schreiber, Davide Mattavelli

Index 457

Foreword

It is with great pleasure and honor that I write this foreword to this atlas, a scholarly work that is the result of a truly dedicated and knowledgeable multidisciplinary team. I had the good fortune of meeting Piero Nicolai, an outstanding surgeon, some years ago at a skull base surgery meeting. Since then, I have had the opportunity to get to know him better and the privilege of visiting, on several occasions, the unique center led by himself, Prof. Fontanella (Neurosurgery), Prof. Maroldi (Radiology), and Prof. Rodella (Anatomy) at the University of Brescia, in Brescia, Italy.

Since its foundation, skull base surgery has been a truly multidisciplinary surgical specialty, and endoscopic skull base surgery has evolved and expanded, thanks to a collaboration not only between otolaryngologists and neurosurgeons, but also between surgical anatomists and radiologists. This atlas is an exquisite example of the result of a close collaboration between all these specialties and provides in-depth anatomical data on the skull base with a surgical perspective, supported by high-quality endoscopic and radiological images. Indeed, the meticulous preparations and excellent dissections presented meet the need for understanding the complex anatomy of the region, as seen from multiple operative approaches.

I am certain the knowledge contained here will contribute significantly to improving the skill set not only of neurosurgeons and otolaryngologists dedicated to endoscopic skull base surgery, but also of other surgeons and radiologists who have an interest in the field.

I congratulate the entire team on this outstanding volume and for the significant contribution to the field.

Fred Gentili, MD, MSc, FRCSC, FACS, FAANS
Professor of Neurosurgery
Crean Hotson Chair in Skull Base Surgery
Alan and Susan Hudson Chair in Neuro-oncology
Toronto Western Hospital
University Health Network
University of Toronto
Toronto, Ontario, Canada

Foreword

I received the honor of writing a foreword for this welcome addition to the skull base literature, *Endoscopic Transnasal Anatomy of the Skull Base and Adjacent Areas* by Piero Nicolai, Marco Ferrari, Roberto Maroldi, Marco Maria Fontanella, Lena Hirtler, Manfred Tschabitscher, and Luigi Fabrizio Rodella. Despite its fixed nature, the understanding and recognition of any pertinent surgical anatomy will vary significantly as one changes the surgical perspective. In great part, this is due to the fact that pattern recognition, essential for the identification of anatomical structures, is more dependent on brain processing than on visual pathways. The dictum "your eyes don't see what your brain doesn't know" has a strong physiologic basis. In that regard, these authors have assembled a beautifully illustrated atlas that adds clarity to the anatomy of the skull base as perceived from the ventral perspective afforded by transnasal endoscopy.

Anatomy presents the map that guides our surgeries, adding efficiency, subtracting potential accidental injuries to critical structures, and avoiding complications. To the patient, this translates into optimal outcomes, oncological and functional. Therefore, as a skull base surgeon I consider anatomical mastery a critical component of my craft.

This book offers a correlation of detailed endoscopic and radiological images coupled with their surgical implications and applications, a unique combination of information that will be of interest to multiple members of the skull base team. It will serve as a reference for rhinologists, head and neck surgeons, neurosurgeons, radiologists, and any other specialty interested in the anatomy of this region.

My congratulations to the authors for producing an expert and well-polished opus. The beauty and complexity of the human anatomy is an art, and as such this compendium is a true masterpiece.

Ricardo L. Carrau, MD, MBA
Professor
Lynne Shepard Jones Chair in Head and Neck Oncology
Department of Otolaryngology—Head and Neck Surgery
Department of Neurological Surgery
Director of the Comprehensive Skull Base Surgery Program
The Ohio State University Medical Center
Columbus, Ohio, United States

Preface

As reiterated in the second preface, the idea behind this book is the result of a creative intuition of Dr. Marco Ferrari, who, together with a group of other young talented physicians, came to me with a detailed project to be developed during their residency regarding correlation between the dissection steps of transnasal endoscopic approaches and corresponding CT or MRI images. Although demanding, we knew that we could rely on the cooperation of all the members of the Skull Base Team at the University of Brescia and the supervision of Prof. Manfred Tschabitscher, a worldwide leader in endoscopic anatomy of the sinonasal tract and skull base. Knowledge of anatomy and the ability to interpret radiologic images are the two pillars to safely approach surgery in an anatomic area that is characterized by great complexity and variability. The introduction and rapid expansion of transnasal endoscopic approaches has required that surgeons view anatomy according to perspectives that are frequently different from those of open approaches. This process has been helped by the technological evolutions, which have provided surgeons with new tools (navigation systems, 3D endoscopy, intraoperative Doppler) enhancing the quality of visualization and the safety of dissection. However, none of these tools can replace the confidence with anatomy acquired with appropriate dissection training in the laboratory and a learning curve judiciously progressing from basic to advanced approaches.

I express my deep gratitude to all my co-editor friends for their expert guidance in supervising the different phases of the project, with a special mention for Prof. Roberto Maroldi and his team: their contribution reflects longstanding expertise in the field of head and neck and skull base radiology and the leading position acquired in the international community. Finally, I want to acknowledge all the young colleagues who have been enthusiastically working in the laboratory. Without their tireless commitment, this book could have not been realized.

Piero Nicolai, MD

Preface

The idea to produce the present atlas dates back to early 2012, when a group of "charmed" medical students and residents of the University of Brescia (myself, Francesco Belotti, Davide Lancini, Vittorio Rampinelli, Davide Mattavelli, and Alberto Schreiber) asked Prof. Manfred Tschabitscher, dubbed by Wolfgang Draf as the "founder of endoscopic anatomy," to be guided in the production of a comprehensive atlas of surgical endoscopic anatomy of the skull base and adjacent areas. This request from the "young group" at an early stage was also endorsed by renowned worldwide experts of the skull base such as Prof. Piero Nicolai, Prof. Roberto Maroldi, Prof. Marco Maria Fontanella, and Prof. Francesco Doglietto, who cooperated in creating a multidisciplinary mentorship that is reliably mirrored in the multifaceted nature of the present atlas. Accordingly, a large number of hours have been spent in the dissecting rooms of the medical universities of Brescia and Vienna under the watchful guidance of expert anatomists, namely Prof. Luigi Fabrizio Rodella, Prof. Manfred Tschabitscher, and Dr. Lena Hirtler, with the intent to create a visual step-by-step guide aimed at facilitating the understanding, learning, and practice of endoscopic skull base surgery. Fervent commitment, scrupulous attention to details, and intense teamwork moved the project forward during the following years. Several long-lasting sessions of endoscopic dissection have been progressively rewarded with 24 chapters that provide the reader with a thorough description of surgical transnasal corridors toward the skull base and neighboring areas. Each chapter is structured according to a scheme that includes an anatomical-clinical overview of the surgical corridor, radiologic anatomy, and step-by-step endoscopic anatomy, thus reflecting the anatomical-radiologic-surgical concept behind the atlas. The many years and efforts dedicated to the present atlas led me to spontaneously associate it with the African proverb "if you want to go fast, go alone; if you want to go far, go together," which brings me to acknowledge my sincere gratitude to Vittorio Rampinelli, Alberto Schreiber, Davide Mattavelli, Andrea Carobbio, Alperen Vural, and Marco Ravanelli for their teachings, professionalism, and friendship. On behalf of all the editors and authors of the atlas, we wish the reader a fruitful reading and rewarding dissection!

Marco Ferrari, MD

Contributors

Francesco Belotti, MD
Resident
Department of Neurosurgery
University of Brescia
Brescia, Italy

Giacomo Bertazzoni, MD
Resident
Department of Otorhinolaryngology–Head and Neck Surgery
University of Brescia
Brescia, Italy

Andrea Bolzoni-Villaret, MD
Consultant
Department of Otorhinolaryngology–Head and Neck Surgery
University of Brescia
Brescia, Italy

Andrea Luigi Camillo Carobbio, MD
Resident
Department of Otorhinolaryngology–Head and Neck Surgery;
IRCCS Ospedale Policlinico San Martino
University of Genoa
Genoa, Italy;

Marco Angelo Cocchi, MSc, PhD
Research Assistant
Section of Anatomy and Physiopathology
Department of Clinical and Experimental Sciences
University of Brescia
Brescia, Italy

Alberto Deganello, MD, PhD
Associate Professor
Department of Otorhinolaryngology–Head and Neck Surgery
University of Brescia
Brescia, Italy

Francesco Doglietto, MD, PhD
Associate Professor
Department of Neurosurgery
University of Brescia
Brescia, Italy

Marco Ferrari, MD
Resident
Department of Otorhinolaryngology–Head and Neck Surgery
University of Brescia
Brescia, Italy

Marco Maria Fontanella, MD
Professor
Department of Neurosurgery
University of Brescia
Brescia, Italy

Lena Hirtler, MA, MD, PhD
Lecturer
Division of Anatomy
Center for Anatomy and Cell Biology
Medical University of Vienna
Vienna, Austria

Davide Lancini, MD
Resident
Department of Otorhinolaryngology–Head and Neck Surgery
University of Brescia
Brescia, Italy

Davide Lombardi, MD
Consultant
Department of Otorhinolaryngology–Head and Neck Surgery
University of Brescia
Brescia, Italy

Roberto Maroldi, MD
Professor
Department of Radiology
University of Brescia
Brescia, Italy

Davide Mattavelli, MD
Assistant Professor
Department of Otorhinolaryngology–Head and Neck Surgery
University of Brescia
Brescia, Italy

Piero Nicolai, MD
Professor
Department of Otorhinolaryngology–Head and Neck Surgery
University of Brescia
Brescia, Italy

Luca Pianta, MD
Consultant
Department of Otorhinolaryngology–Head and Neck Surgery
University of Brescia
Brescia, Italy

Vittorio Rampinelli, MD
Resident
Department of Otorhinolaryngology–Head and Neck Surgery
University of Brescia
Brescia, Italy

Marco Ravanelli, MD
Consultant
Department of Radiology
University of Brescia
Brescia, Italy

Luigi Fabrizio Rodella, MD, MSc
Professor
Section of Anatomy and Physiopathology
Department of Clinical and Experimental Sciences
University of Brescia
Brescia, Italy

Alberto Schreiber, MD, PhD
Consultant
Department of Otorhinolaryngology–Head and Neck Surgery
University of Brescia
Brescia, Italy

Stefano Taboni, MD
Resident
Department of Otorhinolaryngology–Head and Neck Surgery
University of Brescia
Brescia, Italy

Manfred Tschabitscher, MD, PhD
Professor
Division of Anatomy
Center for Anatomy and Cell Biology
Medical University of Vienna
Vienna, Austria;
Section of Anatomy and Physiopathology
Department of Clinical and Experimental Sciences
University of Brescia
Brescia, Italy

Alperen Vural, MD
Assistant Professor
Faculty of Medicine
Department of Otorhinolaryngology–Head and Neck Surgery
Erciyes University
Kayseri, Turkey

1 Classification of Endoscopic Transnasal Approaches to the Skull Base and Adjacent Areas

Piero Nicolai, Marco Ferrari, Roberto Maroldi, Alperen Vural, Marco Maria Fontanella, Luigi Fabrizio Rodella, Lena Hirtler, Manfred Tschabitscher

The development of transnasal endoscopic techniques has provided immense perspectives in the field of skull base surgery. Various meticulous anatomical studies have improved the understanding of skull base anatomy from the endoscopic perspective, and endoscopic transnasal surgery has become notably valuable for accessing and treating pathologies of the skull base.[1–3] This significant evolution, which started with pituitary surgery, has progressively provided a myriad of approaches extending from the posterior frontal plate to axis (C2) and laterally to the parasellar area, petrous apex, jugular foramen, infratemporal fossa, and upper parapharyngeal space.[1,4–8]

By using the natural surgical corridor of the sinonasal tract, transnasal approaches give access to a wide range of sites, which can harbor a proportionally wide range of lesions. The ideal approach to a specific lesion should be selected with the intent to provide an exposure that avoids complications and achieves complete surgical resection and adequate reconstruction. Another characteristic should be the potential of being expanded in case unanticipated extension of the lesion is detected, and permit identification and protection of important neurovascular structures.[3,9] Consequently, selection of the surgical approach is mostly based on the type and location of the disease, its relationships with critical structures, and characteristics of the expected defect.[1,6,9] Specifically, critical neurovascular structures must be located around the perimeter of the corridor. This allows for direct manipulation of the lesion, minimizing the need to cross neurovascular structures when coming from a transnasal route.[10] Thus, a thorough understanding of the numerous anatomic relationships is crucial for the surgeon to determine the safest and most effective way of accessing lesions of the ventral skull base. Knowledge of anatomy allows one to minimize morbidity, maximize patient safety, and contribute to the progress of the surgeon throughout the learning curve of transnasal endoscopic surgery.[2]

Anatomic surgical modules, based on their relation to the internal carotid artery (ICA) in the sagittal and coronal planes, provide access to the entire ventral skull base (▸Table 1.1).[6,7,9] The sphenoid sinus is the center at the intersection of these planes and is the starting point for most approaches, in which significant structures such as optic nerves and ICA are identified and then followed through other areas of the skull base.[11] Moreover, a number of additional "doors" can be used to get access to several regions of the skull base, including the frontal sinus, nasoethmoidal complex, maxillary sinus, nasopharynx, orbital walls, and pterygoid process. Sagittal plane modules provide exposure of median structures extending from the posterior plate of frontal sinus to C2 between the two orbits and ICAs.[9,12,13] These consist of transfrontal, transcribriform, transplanum–transtuberculum, transsellar, transclival, and transodontoid approaches.[11] Coronal plane modules comprise the paramedian and lateral skull base, covering areas adjacent or lateral to the ICA. Three progressively deep planes are considered to further classify coronal plane modules. The anterior one corresponds to the anterior cranial fossa and orbits, including approaches to the lamina papyracea, orbital roof, and orbital cavity. The middle one is in relation to the parasellar area, middle cranial fossa, and anterior infracranial spaces, extending from the lateral wall of sphenoid sinus and posterior nasal cavity to the cavernous sinus, superior petrous apex, Meckel's cave, and pterygopalatine and infratemporal fossa. The posterior one corresponds to the posterior fossa and posterior infracranial spaces, providing access to the inferior petrous apex, lateral craniocervical junction, and upper parapharyngeal space.[9,11,13] All these modules are mutually related and partially overlapping. This atlas aims to provide a thorough and schematic knowledge of these modules, which can be variably combined and suited according to actual clinical needs.

The framework of the skull base and adjacent areas is essentially made of bony structures. As a consequence, anatomical orientation mostly relies on bony planes and landmarks, with subperiosteal dissection being probably one of the key abilities to move within this exceedingly complex area. Moreover, some neurovascular structures pass across different modules in a relatively constant fashion, thus serving as valuable guides to get oriented and judiciously pursue dissection.[10,13] The complexity and numerosity of structures forming the skull base and adjacent areas force the surgeon to simplify an extraordinarily intricate geometry into a reliable schematization. Overall, the mental map of skull base anatomy should be built up based on the reciprocal relationships of key structures, namely defined anatomical landmarks (▸Table 1.2, ▸Table 1.3).

Finally, it is worth remembering that each module is associated with idiosyncratic lesions. This concept is of utmost importance when considering that the nature of the lesion substantially dictates the type of resection that is required. Therefore, tumor characteristics should affect the choice of a specific surgical route along with patient comorbidities, general status, and skill and experience of the operating team. Indeed, each case should be evaluated thoroughly, balancing the purpose to be elegant and minimally invasive with the probability of complications.[1,5–7]

The following figures summarize the anatomical structures of skull base and adjacent areas while mapping the approaches described in the atlas on the sagittal.

Table 1.1 Overview of sagittal and coronal endoscopic transnasal approaches to the skull base and adjacent areas

Plane	Approach		
Sagittal	Transfrontal (Chapter 6)		
	Transcribriform (Chapter 7)		
	Transplanum–transtuberculum (Chapter 8)		
	Transsellar (Chapter 9)		
	Transclival	Upper clivus (transdorsal) (Chapters 10 and 11)	
		Middle clivus (midclivus) (Chapter 11)	
		Lower clivus (Chapter 12)	
	Transodontoid (Chapter 13)		
Coronal	Anterior	Orbital decompression (Chapter 14)	
		Supraorbital (Chapter 14)	
		Transorbital (Chapter 14)	
	Middle	Transcavernous	Medial (Chapter 17)
			Lateral (Chapter 18)
		Optic decompression (Chapter 14)	
		Medial petrous apex (Chapter 19)	
		Transpterygomaxillary (Chapter 15)	
		Infratemporal fossa (Chapter 16)	
		Transpterygoid	Upper (Chapter 21)
			Lower (Chapter 23)
		Suprapetrous (Meckel's cave) and transalisphenoid (Chapter 21)	
	Posterior	Infrapetrous (Chapter 20)	
		Transcondylar–transjugular tuberculum (Chapter 22)	
		Parapharyngeal space	Medial (Chapter 23)
			Lateral (Chapter 24)

Table 1.2 Main characteristics of endoscopic transnasal sagittal approaches to the skull base and adjacent areas

Approach	Anatomical boundaries	Key anatomical landmarks	Critical structures	Target(s)	Limitations	Common pathologies
Transfrontal	• Nasal bones anteriorly • Nasal septum and cribriform plate posteriorly • Orbital cavities bilaterally	• First olfactory phyla • Crista galli	• Superior sagittal sinus • Medial orbitofrontal and frontopolar vessels • Bridge veins	• Posterior wall of frontal sinus	• Far-lateral extension (beyond the orbital sagittal midplane) • Involvement of the anterior frontal plate	• Intracranial complications of rhinosinusitis (epidural abscess and subdural empyema)[14] • Mucocele/mucopyocele[15] • Tumors (fibro-osseous tumors and inverted papilloma)[16,17] • Dermoid cyst and other nasofrontal dysembryogenic lesions[18,19] • CSF leaks[20,21]
Transcribriform	• Posterior wall of frontal sinus anteriorly • Planum sphenoidale posteriorly • Lamina papyracea bilaterally	• Ethmoidal arteries • Crista galli • Falx cerebri • Periorbit	• Medial orbitofrontal vessels • Anterior cerebral arteries • Superior sagittal sinus • Gyrus rectus • Medial orbitofrontal gyrus	• Midline anterior skull base above the nasoethmoidal complex	• Far-lateral extension (beyond the orbital sagittal midplane) • Massive cranial extension • Extension to the suprasellar area • Extension to nasal bones and face soft tissues	• Nasoethmoidal malignancies[1,22–24] • Meningiomas[25–27] • Schwannomas[28,29] • Dysembryogenic lesions[30]

Table 1.2 *(Continued)* Main characteristics of endoscopic transnasal sagittal approaches to the skull base and adjacent areas

Approach		Anatomical boundaries	Key anatomical landmarks	Critical structures	Target(s)	Limitations	Common pathologies
Transplanum–transtuberculum		• Fovea ethmoidalis and cribriform plate anteriorly • Sella turcica posteriorly • Optic canals and paraclinoid and intracranial ICAs bilaterally	• Medial optic-carotid recesses • Optic canals • Posterior clinoid processes	• Circle of Willis • Paraclinoid and intracranial ICAs • Optic nerves • Optic chiasm • Optic tracts • Pituitary stalk • Superior hypophyseal arteries • Gyrus rectus • Medial orbitofrontal gyrus	• Midline anterior skull base above the sphenoid sinus • Suprasellar area • Third ventricle	• Extension lateral to ICAs • Extension lateral to optic nerves	• Pituitary adenomas[6,31,32] • Craniopharyngiomas[33–35] • Meningiomas[36] • Aneurysms of the anterior cerebral circulation[37,38] • Tumors of the third ventricle[39,40,41]
Transsellar		• Anterior superior intercavernous sinus superiorly • Anterior inferior intercavernous sinus inferiorly • Cavernous sinuses bilaterally	• Tuberculum sellae • Lateral and medial optic-carotid recesses • Carotid prominences • Sellar floor • "Four blues" (anterior superior intercavernous, anterior inferior intercavernous, and cavernous sinuses)	• Parasellar and paraclinoid ICAs • Pituitary gland • Optic chiasm	• Sella turcica	• Extension lateral to ICA • Extension posterior to dorsum sellae • Suprasellar extension	• Pituitary adenomas/apoplexy[6,42] • Rathke's cleft cysts[43,44] • Craniopharyngiomas[45] • Arachnoid cysts[46]
Transclival	Transdorsal	• Cavernous sinus bilaterally • Midclivus inferiorly • Suprasellar area superiorly	• Sellar floor • Dorsum sellae • Posterior clinoid process • Parasellar ICA	• Oculomotor nerve • Parasellar and paraclinoid ICAs • Pituitary gland and stalk • Basilar artery and its branches • Mesencephalon and pons	• Upper clivus • Inter- and parapeduncular space (retroclival area)	• Extension lateral to ICA • Extension lateral to the oculomotor nerve • Suprasellar extension • Inferior prepontine extension	• Chordomas[47] • Craniopharyngiomas[48] • Meningiomas[49] • Aneurysms[50]
	Midclivus	• Sellar floor superiorly • Paraclival ICAs bilaterally • Plane of the vidian nerves inferiorly	• Vidian nerves • Fibrocartilago basalis	• Abducens nerve • Paraclival ICAs • Basilar artery and its branches • Pons	• Midclivus • Prepontine space	• Extension lateral to ICA • Extension lateral to abducens nerve • Superior prepontine interpeduncular extension • Premedullary extension	• Chordomas[51] • Chondrosarcomas[52,53] • Meningiomas[54] • Aneurysms[50]
	Lower clivus	• Plane of the vidian nerves superiorly • Hypoglossal canals bilaterally • Foramen magnum inferiorly	• Basion • Jugular tubercula • Occipital condyles • Hypoglossal canals	• Abducens nerve • Hypoglossal nerve • Vertebral arteries and their branches • Medulla oblongata	• Lower clivus • Superior premedullary space	• Extension lateral to hypoglossal nerves • Superior prepontine extension • Extension to the craniocervical junction or inferior premedullary space	• Chordomas[55] • Chondrosarcomas[53] • Meningiomas[55] • Aneurysms[50]
Transod-ontoid		• Basion superiorly • Superior border of the axis body inferiorly • Occipital condyles and lateral masses of the atlas bilaterally	• Lower clivus • Basion • Anterior arch of the atlas • Odontoid process	• Vertebral arteries • First and second cervical nerves • Suboccipital cavernous sinuses	• Craniocervical junction • Inferior premedullary space	• Inferior extension to the body of the axis • Lateral extension to occipital condyles or lateral masses of the atlas • Superior premedullary extension	• Inflammatory pannus[56] • Craniovertebral invagination[56] • Chordomas[57]

Abbreviations: CSF, cerebrospinal fluid; ICA, internal carotid artery.

Table 1.3 Main characteristics of endoscopic transnasal coronal approaches to the skull base and adjacent areas

Approach		Anatomical boundary	Key anatomical landmark	Critical structures	Limitations	Common pathologies
Anterior	• Orbital decompression • Supraorbital • Transorbital	• Orbital roof and related dura superiorly • Orbital floor inferiorly • Lacrimal system and eyeball anteriorly • Orbital apex posteriorly	• Lamina papyracea • Ethmoidal arteries • Superior oblique, medial rectus, and inferior rectus muscles	• Optic nerve • Ophthalmic artery • Extrinsic ocular muscles and their nerve supply	• Lateral and/or superior extension with respect to the optic nerve and ophthalmic artery • Extension to lacrimal system • Preseptal extension • Extension to orbital apex	• Graves orbitopathy[58,59] • Hemangiomas[60] • Schwannomas[61] • Meningiomas[61]
Middle	Medial transcavernous	• Sella turcica medially • Parasellar ICA laterally • Petroclival junction inferiorly • Posterior clinoid process and oculomotor triangle posteriorly and superiorly (of note, the corridor can be extended posteriorly and superiorly via interdural hypophysiopexy[62] and transoculomotor approach)[63]	• Medial optic-carotid recess • Carotid prominence • Pituitary ligaments • Medial wall of the cavernous sinus • Posterior clinoid process • Oculomotor triangle	• Parasellar ICA • Meningohypophyseal trunk • Oculomotor nerve • Abducens nerve	• Extension to the lateral and posterior compartments of the cavernous sinus • Extension to the sella turcica	• Pituitary adenomas[64,65] • Meningiomas[66]
	Lateral transcavernous	• Parasellar and paraclival ICA medially • Meckel's cave and dura of the middle cranial fossa laterally • Anterior clinoid process and roof of the cavernous sinus superiorly • Petrolingual ligament inferiorly	• Lateral optic-carotid recess • Carotid prominence • Carotid sulcus • Maxillary strut	• Parasellar and paraclival ICA • Oculomotor nerve • Trochlear nerve • Abducens nerve • Ophthalmic nerve • Maxillary nerve • Inferolateral trunk	• Lateral extension to the Meckel's cave • Extension to the superior compartment of the cavernous sinus • Extension to the petrous apex	• Meningiomas[66,67] • Schwannomas[66,68] • Hemangiomas[66]
	Optic decompression	• Medial optic-carotid recess and tuberculum sellae posteromedially • Lateral optic-carotid recess inferiorly • Planum sphenoidale superiorly • Lamina papyracea anterolaterally	• Medial optic-carotid recess • Lateral optic-carotid recess • Annulus of Zinn	• Optic nerve • Ophthalmic artery • Paraclinoid ICA • Extrinsic ocular muscles	• Extension to the orbital cavity • Extension lateral and/or superior to the optic nerve • Extension to cavernous sinus/ suprasellar space	• Traumatic optic neuropathy[69] • Nontraumatic optic neuropathy[70]
	Medial petrous apex	• Midclivus medially • Paraclival ICA anterolaterally • Abducens nerve superiorly	• Vidian canal and vidian nerve • Carotid sulcus • Fibrocartilago basalis	• Paraclival ICA • Abducens nerve	• Extension to the inferior petrous apex or lateral portion of the superior petrous apex (lateral to the abducens nerve) • Extension to cavernous sinus	• Chordomas[71] • Chondrosarcomas[72,73] • Cholesterol granulomas[74] • Meningiomas[54,75]
	Transpterygomax-illary	• Tails of turbinates medially • Pterygomaxillary fissure laterally • Inferior orbital fissure superiorly • Pterygomaxillary junction inferiorly	• Posterior maxillary wall • Infraorbital canal • Sphenopalatine foramen • Pterygoid process • Pterygomaxillary junction	• Internal maxillary artery and its branches • Maxillary nerve	• Lateral extension to the infratemporal fossa • Superior extension to the orbital cavity • Posterior and/or inferior extension to the masticatory space	• Schwannomas[76] • Angiofibromas[77] • Malignant tumors[77]
	Infratemporal fossa	• Lateral pterygoid plate posteromedially • Orbital floor superiorly • Alveolar process inferiorly • Coronoid process anterolaterally	• Infraorbital canal • Zygomatic recess • Coronoid process • Lateral pterygoid muscle • Temporal muscle	• Internal maxillary artery and its branches • Mandibular nerve	• Extension to the temporal fossa • Extension to the buccal space • Extension to the parapharyngeal space • Extension to the adjacent skull base	• Angiofibromas[78,79] • Schwannomas[80,81] • Meningiomas[82] • Sinonasal or nasopharyngeal tumors[80,83]

(Continued)

Table 1.3 (*Continued*) Main characteristics of endoscopic transnasal coronal approaches to the skull base and adjacent areas

Approach		Anatomical boundary	Key anatomical landmark	Critical structures	Limitations	Common pathologies
	Transpterygoid	*Upper transpterygoid* • Greater wing of the sphenoid bone laterally • Sphenoid floor medially • Superior orbital fissure superiorly • Scaphoid fossa inferiorly *Lower transpterygoid* • Base of the pterygoid process superiorly • Lateral pterygoid muscle laterally • Pterygomaxillary junction inferiorly • Nasopharynx medially	• Descending palatine canal • Vidian nerve and vidian canal • Foramen rotundum • Fibrocartilago basalis • Medial and lateral pterygoid plate • Foramen ovale • Pterygomaxillary junction	• Anterior genu of the internal carotid artery (between the petrous and paraclival tract) • Pterygoid, pharyngeal, and foraminal plexuses • Maxillary nerve	• Depending on the targeted area (see column "Common pathologies")	• The transpterygoid approach is propaedeutic to other approaches (i.e., suprapetrous, infrapetrous, and parapharyngeal) that are characterized by idiosyncratic lesions
	• Suprapetrous (Meckel's cave) • Transalisphenoid	• Abducens nerve superiorly • Paraclival ICA and petrolingual ligament medially • Gasserian ganglion and dura of the middle cranial fossa laterally • Petrous ICA inferiorly	• Vidian nerve • Foramen rotundum • Maxillary strut • Lingual process of the sphenoid and petrolingual ligament • Mandibular strut	• Paraclival and petrous ICA • Abducens nerve • Gasserian ganglion and trigeminal branches	• Extension to the cavernous sinus • Extension to the inferior petrous apex or medial portion of the superior petrous apex • Extension to infratemporal fossa • Far-lateral extension into the middle cranial fossa	• Schwannomas[84] • Meningiomas[84] • Malignant tumors (nasopharyngeal carcinoma and minor salivary gland carcinomas)[84]
Posterior	Infrapetrous	• Petrous ICA superiorly and laterally • Jugular tuberculum and hypoglossal canal inferiorly • Lower clivus medially	• Medial pterygoid plate • Vidian canal • Fibrocartilago basalis • Hypoglossal canal	• Petrous ICA • Hypoglossal nerve	• Extension to the posteroinferior petrous apex or superior petrous apex • Extension to the clivus • Extension to occipital condyle	• Cholesterol granulomas[85] • Chordomas[86] • Chondrosarcomas[87]
	Transcondylar–transjugular tuberculum (far-medial)	• Lower clivus medially • Carotid canal and jugular foramen laterally • Craniocervical junction inferiorly • Inferior petrosal sinus superiorly	• Anterior rectus capitis muscle • Jugular tuberculum • Hypoglossal canal • Occipital condyle	• Vertebral artery • Hypoglossal nerve • Glossopharyngeal, vagus, and accessory nerve • Acoustic-facial bundle • Inferior petrosal sinus	• Extension to the petrous apex • Extension to the vascular compartment of the jugular foramen • Extension to parapharyngeal space • Extension to the atlas	• Chordomas[88,89] • Chondrosarcomas[88,89] • Other malignant tumors[89]
	Medial parapharyngeal space	• Nasopharynx medially • Base of the pterygoid process and fibrocartilago basalis superiorly • Lateral pterygoid plate laterally • Axial plane passing through the pterygomaxillary junction inferiorly	• Medial pterygoid plate • Eustachian tube • Tensor veli palatini muscle • Levator veli palatini muscle • Lateral pterygoid plate	• Parapharyngeal ICA	• Extension to adjacent skull base • Extension to infratemporal fossa • Extension to the jugular foramen • Extension to middle parapharyngeal space	• Malignant nasopharyngeal tumors (nasopharyngeal carcinomas, minor salivary gland carcinomas, and sarcomas)[80,90]
	Lateral parapharyngeal space	• Nasopharynx medially • Base of the pterygoid process and fibrocartilago basalis superiorly • Lateral pterygoid muscle laterally • Axial plane passing through the pterygomaxillary junction inferiorly	• Lateral pterygoid plate • Foramen ovale • Foramen spinosum • Tensor veli palatini muscle • Levator veli palatini muscle	• Parapharyngeal ICA • Internal jugular vein • Glossopharyngeal nerve • Vagus nerve • Spinal accessory nerve • Hypoglossal nerve	• Extension to adjacent skull base • Extension to infratemporal fossa • Extension to middle parapharyngeal space	• Malignant nasopharyngeal tumors (nasopharyngeal carcinomas, minor salivary gland carcinomas, and sarcomas)[80,90]

Abbreviation: ICA, internal carotid artery.

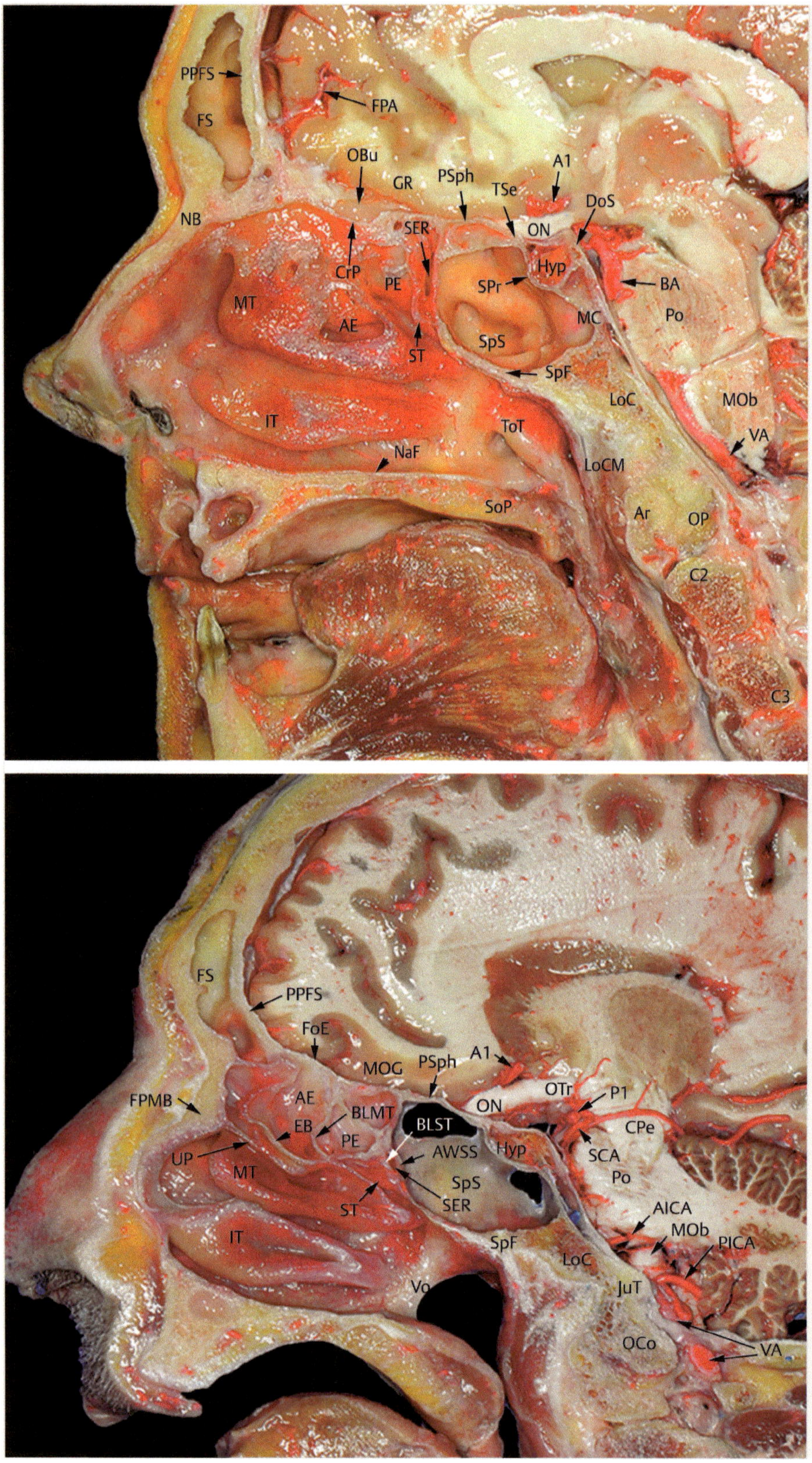

Fig. 1.1 Sagittal view of the skull base and adjacent areas (part 1). Medial-to-lateral view of the right side (upper image) and lateral-to-medial view of the left side (lower image). A1, precommunicating tract of the anterior cerebral artery; AE, anterior ethmoidal compartment; AICA, anterior inferior cerebellar artery; Ar, anterior arch of the atlas; AWSS, anterior wall of the sphenoid sinus; BA, basilar artery; BLMT, basal lamella of the middle turbinate; BLST, basal lamella of the superior turbinate; C2, axis (body); C3, third cervical vertebra (body); CPe, cerebral peduncle; CrP, cribriform plate; DoS, dorsum sellae; EB, ethmoidal bulla; FoE, fovea ethmoidalis; FPA, frontopolar artery; FPMB, frontal process of the maxillary bone; FS, frontal sinus; GR, gyrus rectus; Hyp, hypophysis (pituitary gland); IT, inferior turbinate; JuT, jugular tuberculum; LoC, lower clivus; LoCM, longus capitis muscle; MC, midclivus; MOG, medial orbital gyrus; MOb, medulla oblongata; MT, middle turbinate; NaF, nasal floor; NB, nasal bone; OBu, olfactory bulb; OCo, occipital condyle; ON, optic nerve; OP, odontoid process; OTr, optic tract; P1, precommunicating tract of the posterior cerebral artery; PE, posterior ethmoidal compartment; PICA, posterior inferior cerebellar artery; Po, pons; PPFS, posterior plate of the frontal sinus; PSph, planum sphenoidale; SCA, superior cerebellar artery; SER, sphenoethmoidal recess; SoP, soft palate; SpF, sphenoidal floor; SPr, sellar prominence; SpS, sphenoid sinus; ST, superior turbinate; ToT, torus tubarius; TSe, tuberculum sellae; UP, uncinate process; VA, vertebral artery; Vo, vomer.

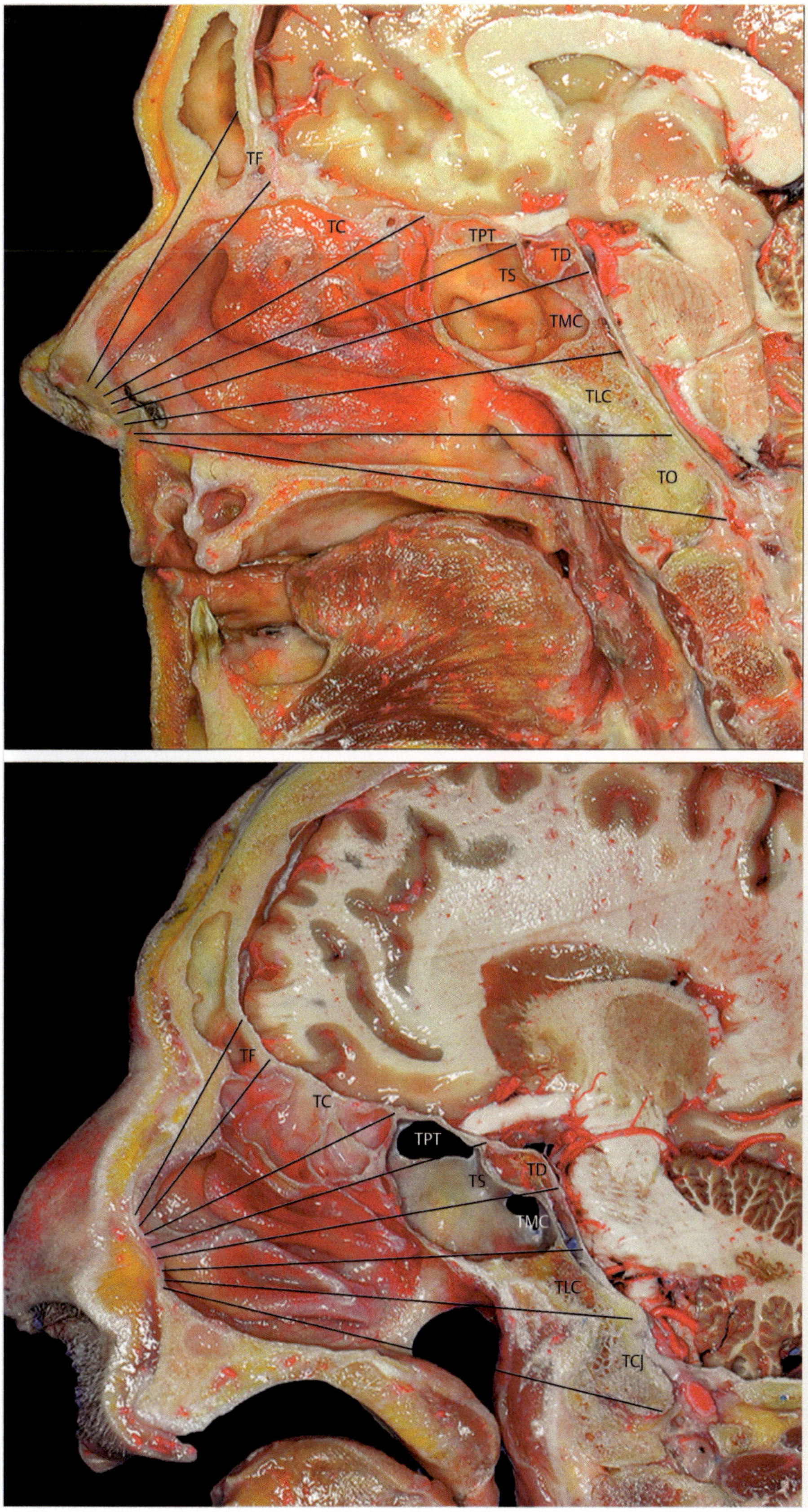

Fig. 1.2 Mapping of endoscopic transnasal approaches on a sagittal section (part 1). Medial-to-medial view of the right side (upper image) and lateral-to-medial view of the left side (lower image). TC, transcribriform approach; TCJ, transcondylar–transjugular tuberculum approach; TD, transdorsal approach; TF, transfrontal approach; TLC, transclival (lower clivus) approach; TMC, transclival (midclivus) approach; TO, transodontoid approach; TPT, transplanum–transtuberculum approach; TS, transsellar approach.

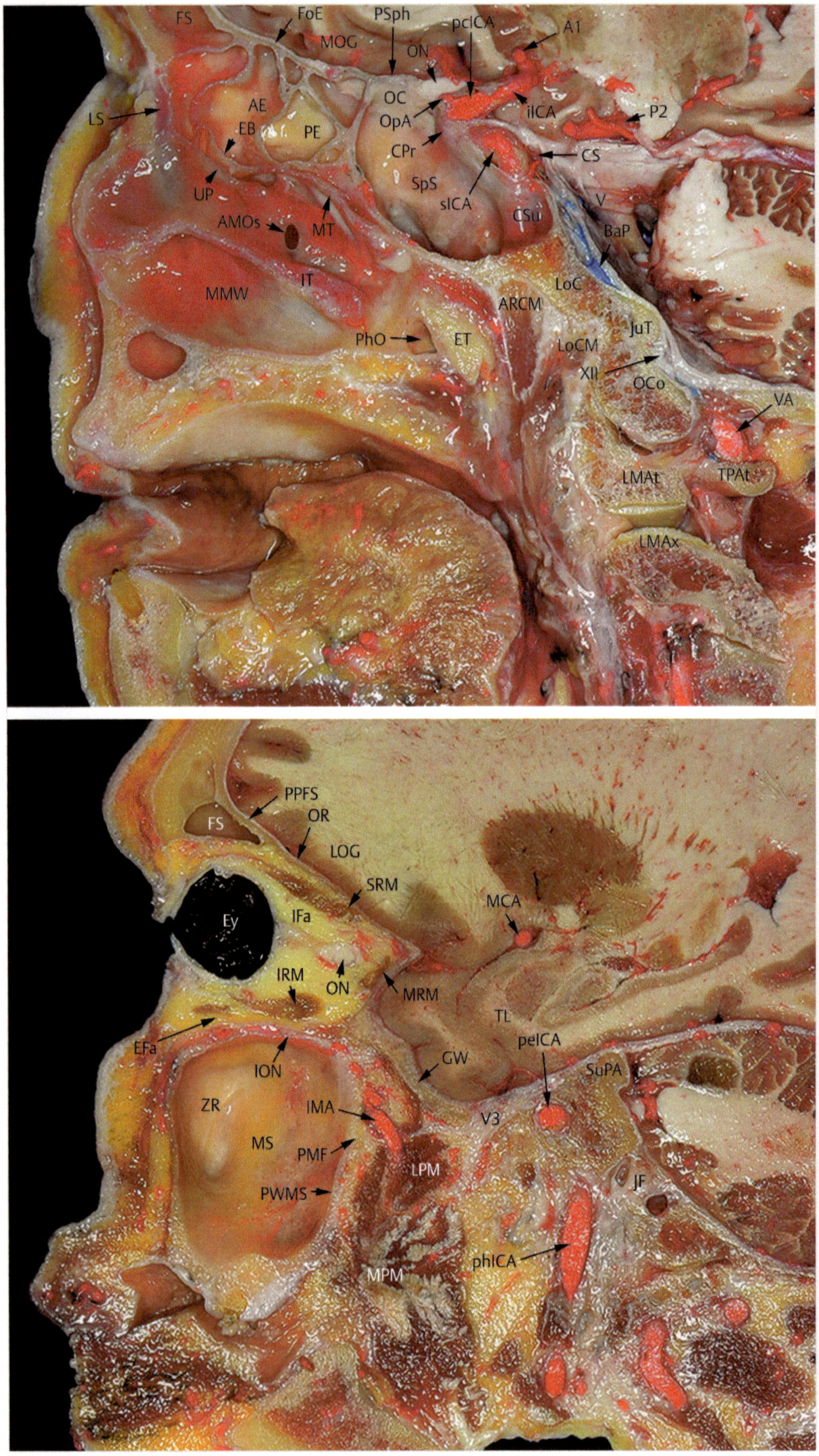

Fig. 1.3 Sagittal view of the skull base and adjacent areas (part 2). Medial-to-lateral view of the right side (both images). V, trigeminal stem; V3, mandibular nerve; XII, hypoglossal nerve; A1, precommunicating tract of the anterior cerebral artery; AE, anterior ethmoidal complex; AIPA, anterior inferior petrous apex; AMOs, accessory maxillary ostium; ARCM, anterior rectus capitis muscle; BaP, basilar plexus; CPr, carotid prominence; CS, cavernous sinus; CSu, carotid sulcus; EB, ethmoidal bulla; EFa, extraconal fat; ET, eustachian tube; Ey, eyeball; FoE, fovea ethmoidalis; FS, frontal sinus; GW, greater wing of the sphenoid bone; IFa, intraconal fat; iICA, intracranial tract of the internal carotid artery; IMA, internal maxillary artery; ION, infraorbital nerve; IRM, inferior rectus muscle; IT, inferior turbinate; JF, jugular foramen; JuT, jugular tuberculum; LMAt, lateral mass of the atlas; LMAx, lateral mass of the axis; LoC, lower clivus; LoCM, longus capitis muscle; LOG, lateral orbital gyrus; LPM, lateral pterygoid muscle; LS, lacrimal sac; MCA, middle cerebral artery; MOG, medial orbital gyrus; MPM, medial pterygoid muscle; MRM, medial rectus muscle; MS, maxillary sinus; MT, middle turbinate; OC, optic canal; OCo, occipital condyle; ON, optic nerve; OpA, ophthalmic artery; OR, orbital roof; P2, postcommunicating tract of the posterior cerebral artery; pcICA, paraclinoid tract of the internal carotid artery; PE, posterior ethmoidal complex; peICA, petrous tract of the internal carotid artery; phICA, parapharyngeal tract of the internal carotid artery; PhO, pharyngeal ostium of the eustachian tube; PMF, pterygomaxillary fissure; PPFS, posterior plate of the frontal sinus; PSph, planum sphenoidale; PWMS, posterior wall of the maxillary sinus; sICA, parasellar tract of the internal carotid artery; SpS, sphenoid sinus; SRM, superior rectus muscle; SuPA, superior petrous apex; TL, temporal lobe; TPAt, transverse process of the atlas; UP, uncinate process; VA, vertebral artery; ZR, zygomatic recess.

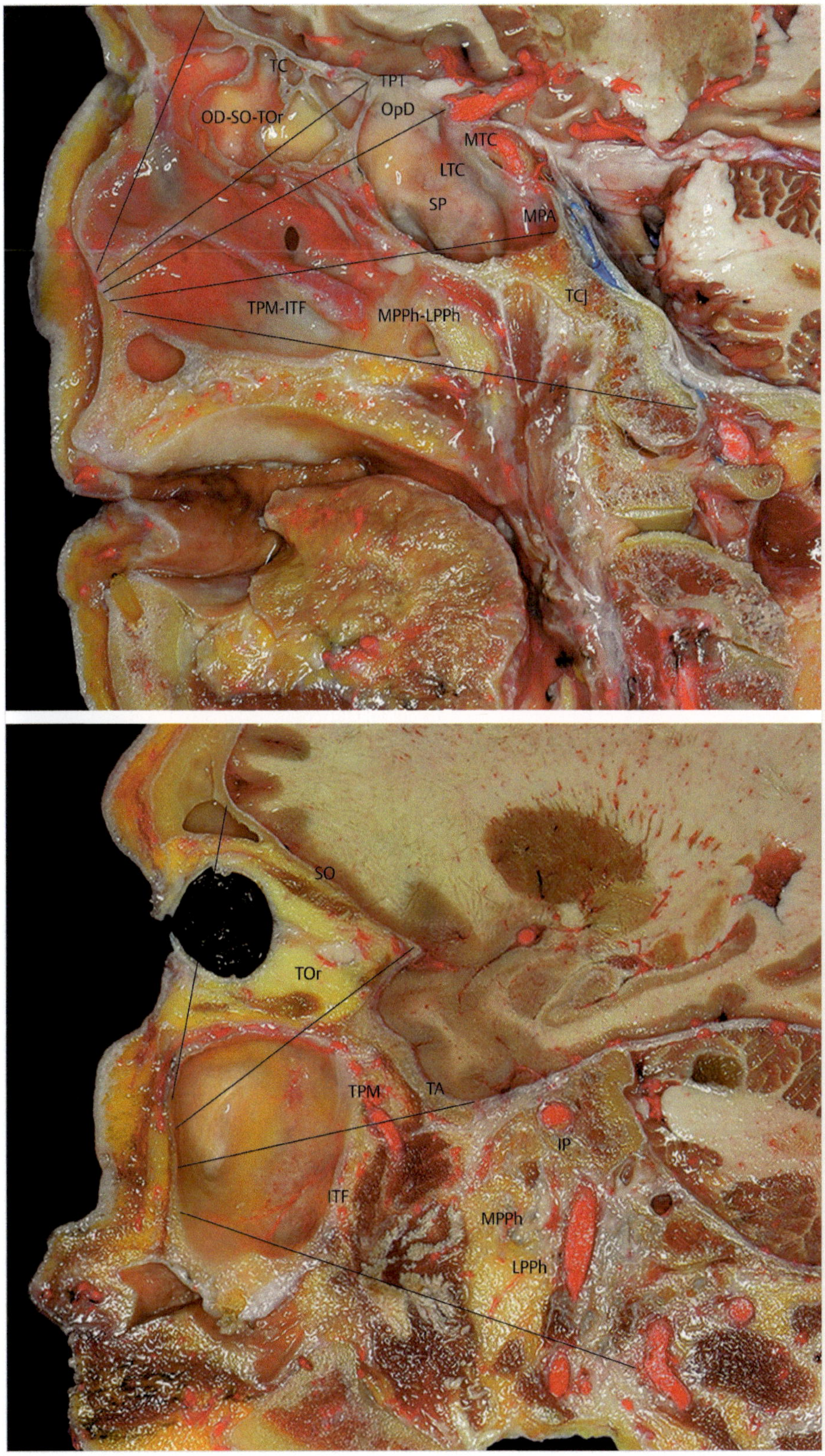

Fig. 1.4 Mapping of endoscopic transnasal approaches on a sagittal section (part 2). Medial-to-lateral view of the right side (both images). IP, infrapetrous approach; ITF, infratemporal fossa approach; LPPh, lateral parapharyngeal space approach; LTC, lateral transcavernous approach; MPA, medial petrous apex approach; MPPh, medial parapharyngeal space approach; MTC, medial transcavernous approach; OD, orbital decompression; OpD, optic decompression; SO, supraorbital approach; SP, suprapetrous (Meckel's cave) approach; TA, transalisphenoid approach; TC, transcribriform approach; TCJ, transcondylar–transjugular tuberculum approach; TOr, transorbital approach; TPM, transpterygomaxillary approach; TPT, transplanum–transtuberculum approach.

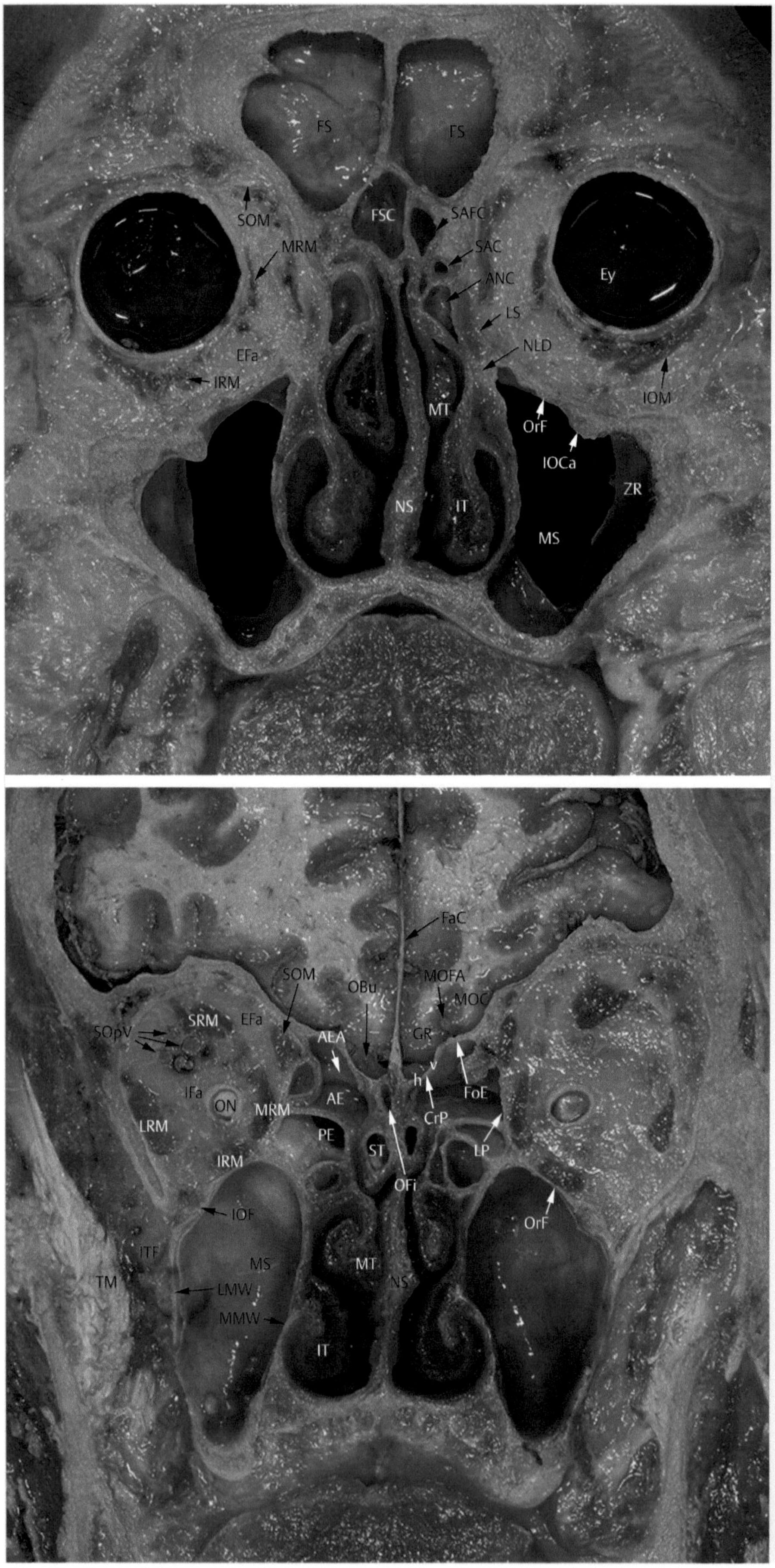

Fig. 1.5 Coronal view of the skull base and adjacent areas (part 1). Anterior-to-posterior view (both images). AE, anterior ethmoidal compartment; AEA, anterior ethmoidal artery; ANC, agger nasi cell; CrP, cribriform plate; EFa, extraconal fat; Ey, eyeball; FaC, falx cerebri; FoE, fovea ethmoidalis; FS, frontal sinus; FSC, frontal septal cell; GR, gyrus rectus; h, horizontal lamella of the cribriform plate; IFa, intraconal fat; IOCa, infraorbital canal; IOF, inferior orbital fissure; IOM, inferior oblique muscle; IRM, inferior rectus muscle; IT, inferior turbinate; ITF, infratemporal fossa; LMW, lateral maxillary wall; LP, lamina papyracea; LRM, lateral rectus muscle; LS, lacrimal sac; MMW, medial maxillary wall; MOFA, medial orbitofrontal artery; MOG, medial orbital gyrus; MRM, medial rectus muscle; MS, maxillary sinus; MT, middle turbinate; NLD, nasolacrimal duct; NS, nasal septum; OBu, olfactory bulb; OFi, olfactory fissure (or cleft); ON, optic nerve; OrF, orbital floor; PE, posterior ethmoidal compartment; SAC, supra-agger cell; SAFC, supra-agger frontal cell; SOM, superior oblique muscle; SOpV, superior ophthalmic vein; SRM, superior rectus muscle; ST, superior turbinate; TM, temporal muscle; v, vertical lamella of the cribriform plate; ZR, zygomatic recess.

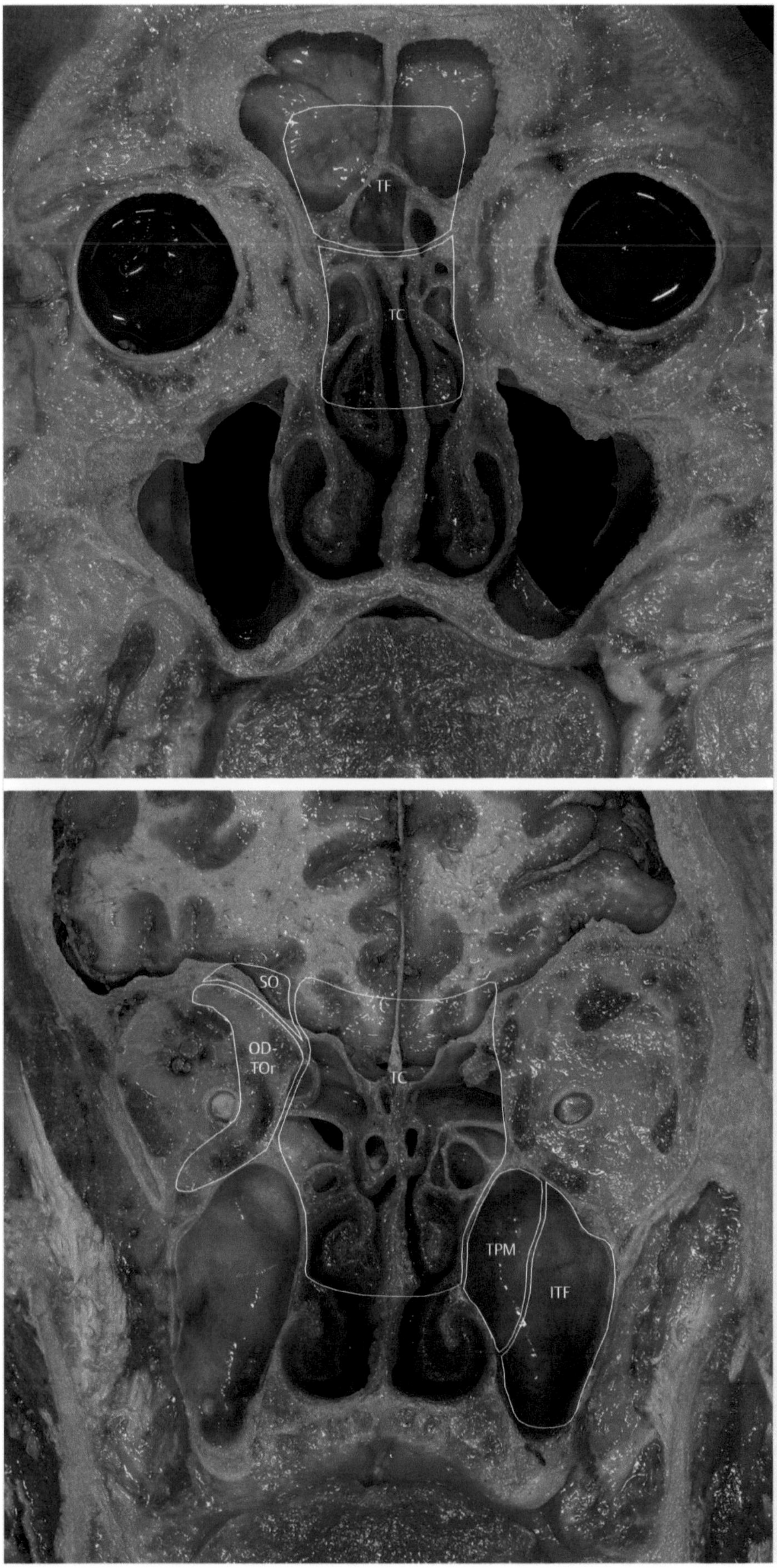

Fig. 1.6 Mapping of endoscopic transnasal approaches on a coronal section (part 1). Anterior-to-posterior view (both images). ITF, infratemporal fossa approach; OD, orbital decompression; SO, supraorbital approach; TC, transcribriform approach; TF, transfrontal approach; TOr, transorbital approach; TPM, transpterygomaxillary approach.

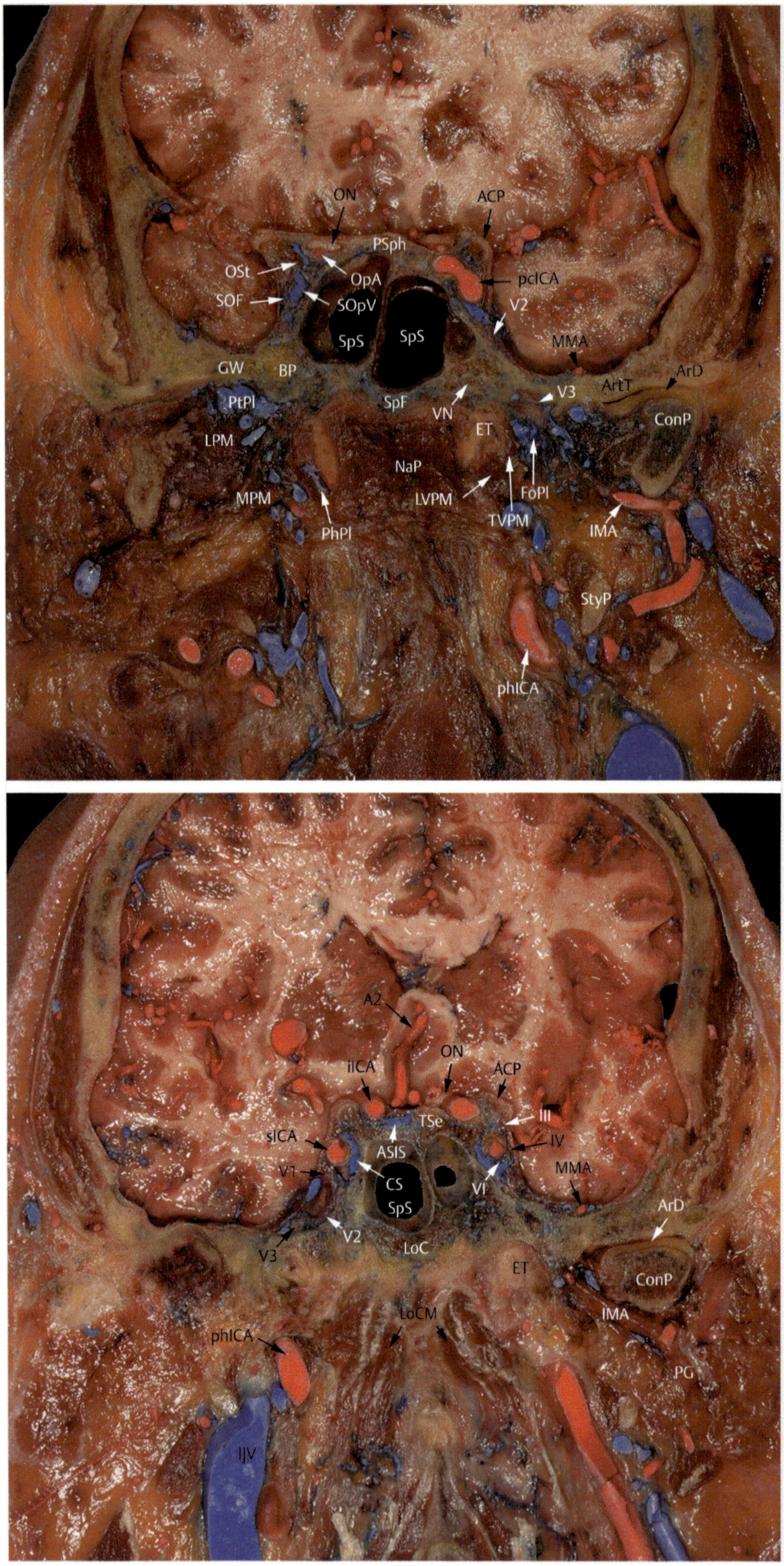

Fig. 1.7 Coronal view of the skull base and adjacent areas (part 2). Anterior-to-posterior view (both images). III, oculomotor nerve; IV, trochlear nerve; VI, abducens nerve; V1, ophthalmic nerve; V2, maxillary nerve; V3, mandibular nerve; A2, postcommunicating tract of the anterior cerebral artery; ACP, anterior clinoid process; ArD, articular disk (temporomandibular joint); ArtT, articular tuberculum; ASIS, anterior superior intercavernous sinus; BP, base of the pterygoid process (or basipterygoid); ConP, condylar process of the mandible; ET, eustachian tube; FoPl, foraminal plexus; GW, greater wing of the sphenoid bone; iICA, intracranial tract of the internal carotid artery; IJV, internal jugular vein; IMA, internal maxillary artery; LoC, lower clivus; LoCM, longus capitis muscle; LPM, lateral pterygoid plexus; LVPM, levator veli palatini muscle; MMA, middle meningeal artery; MPM, medial pterygoid plexus; NaP, nasopharyngeal posterior wall; ON, optic nerve; OpA, ophthalmic artery; OSt, optic strut; pcICA, paraclinoid tract of the internal carotid artery; PG, parotid gland; phICA, parapharyngeal tract of the internal carotid artery; PhPl, pharyngeal plexus; PSph, planum sphenoidale; PtPl, pterygoid plexus; sICA, parasellar tract of the internal carotid artery; SOF, superior orbital fissure; SOpV, superior ophthalmic vein; SpF, sphenoidal floor; SpS, sphenoid sinus; StyP, styloid process; TSe, tuberculum sellae; TVPM, tensor veli palatini muscle; VN, vidian nerve.

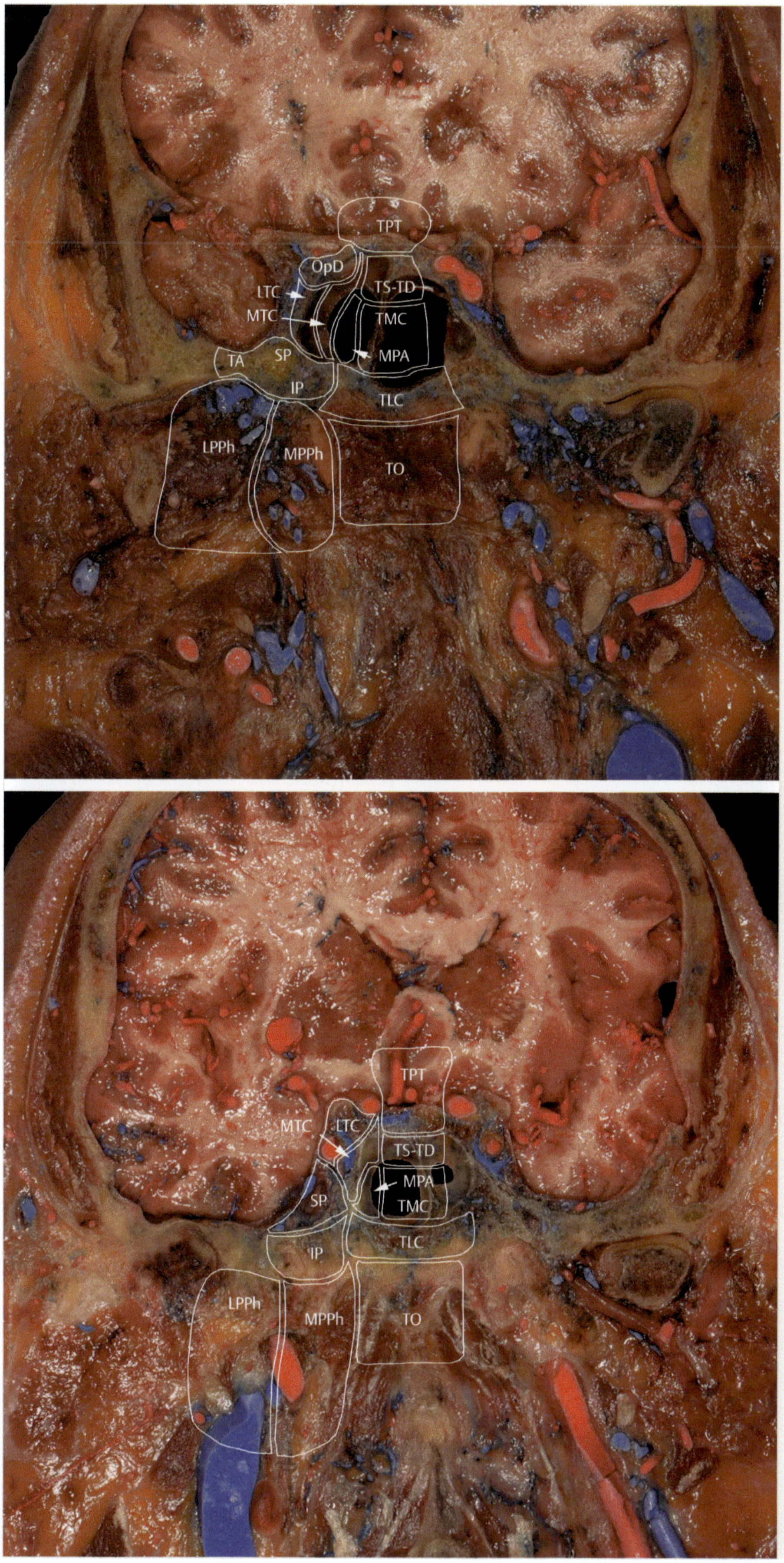

Fig. 1.8 Mapping of endoscopic transnasal approaches on a coronal section (part 2). Anterior-to-posterior view (both images). IP, infrapetrous approach; LPPh, lateral parapharyngeal space approach; LTC, lateral transcavernous approach; MPA, medial petrous apex approach; MPPh, medial parapharyngeal space approach; MTC, medial transcavernous approach; OpD, optic decompression; SP, suprapetrous (Meckel's cave) approach; TA, transalisphenoid approach; TD, transdorsal approach; TLC, transclival (lower clivus) approach; TMC, transclival (middle clivus) approach; TPT, transplanum–transtuberculum approach; TO, transodontoid approach; TS, transsellar approach.

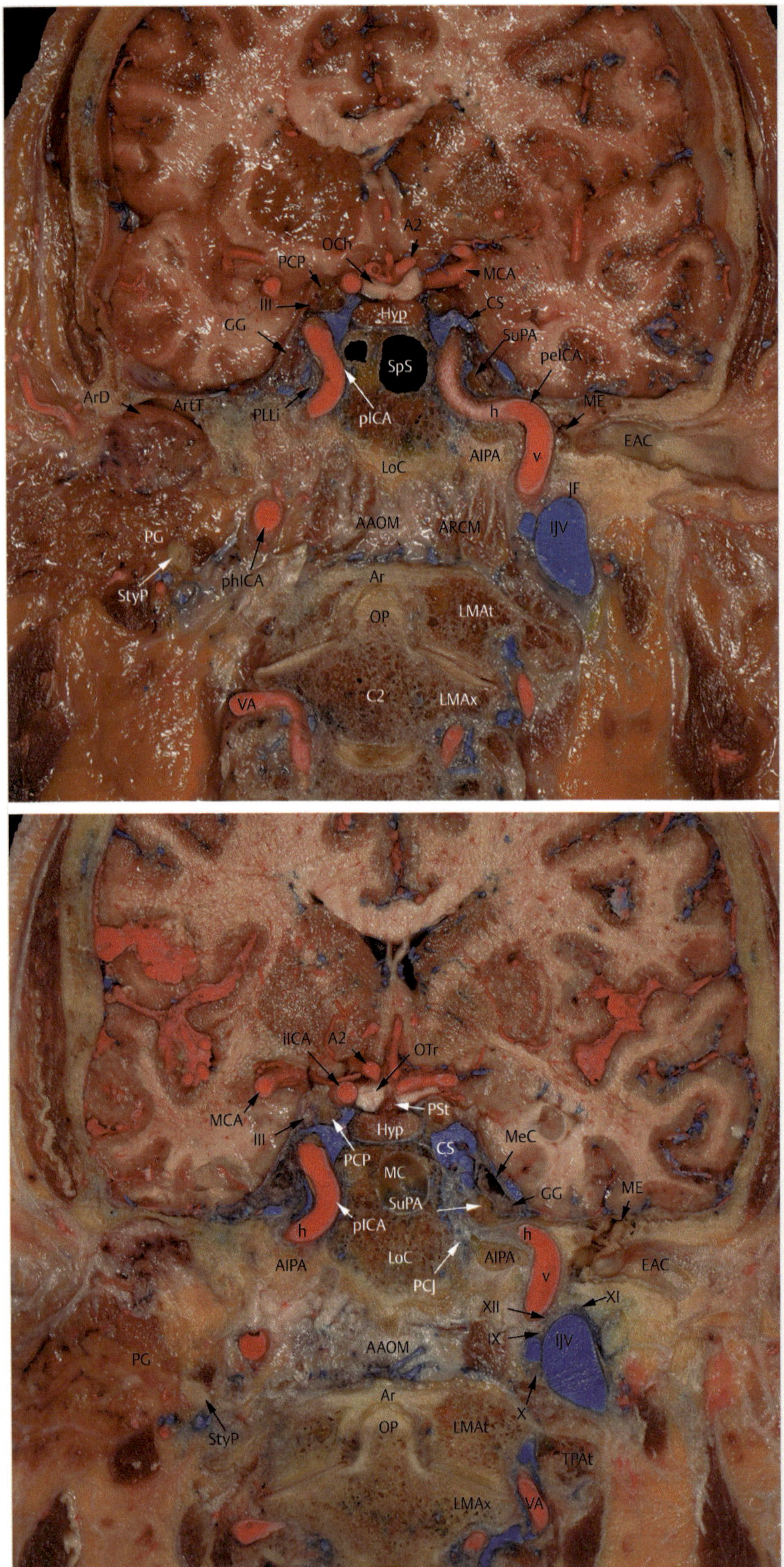

Fig. 1.9 Coronal view of the skull base and adjacent areas (part 3). Posterior-to-anterior view (upper image) and anterior-to-posterior view (lower image). III, oculomotor nerve; IX, glossopharyngeal nerve; X, vagus nerve; XI, spinal accessory nerve; XII, hypoglossal nerve; A2, postcommunicating tract of the anterior cerebral artery; AAOM, anterior atlanto-occipital membrane; AIPA, anterior inferior petrous apex; Ar, anterior arch of the atlas; ARCM, anterior rectus capitis muscle; ArD, articular disk (temporomandibular joint); ArtT, articular tuberculum; C2, axis (body); CS, cavernous sinus; EAC, external auditory canal; GG, gasserian ganglion; h, horizontal portion of the petrous tract of the internal carotid artery; Hyp, hypophysis; iICA, intracranial tract of the internal carotid artery; IJV, internal jugular vein; JF, jugular foramen; LMAt, lateral mass of the atlas; LMAx, lateral mass of the axis; LoC, lower clivus; MC, midclivus; MCA, middle cerebral artery; ME, middle ear; MeC, Meckel's cave; OCh, optic chiasm; OP, odontoid process; OTr, optic tract; PCJ, petroclival junction; PCP, posterior clinoid process; peICA, petrous tract of the internal carotid artery; PG, parotid gland; phICA, parapharyngeal tract of the internal carotid artery; pICA, paraclival tract of the internal carotid artery; PLLi, petrolingual ligament; PSt, pituitary stalk; SpS, sphenoid sinus; StyP, styloid process; SuPA, superior petrous apex; TPAt, transverse process of the atlas; v, vertical portion of the petrous tract of the internal carotid artery; VA, vertebral artery.

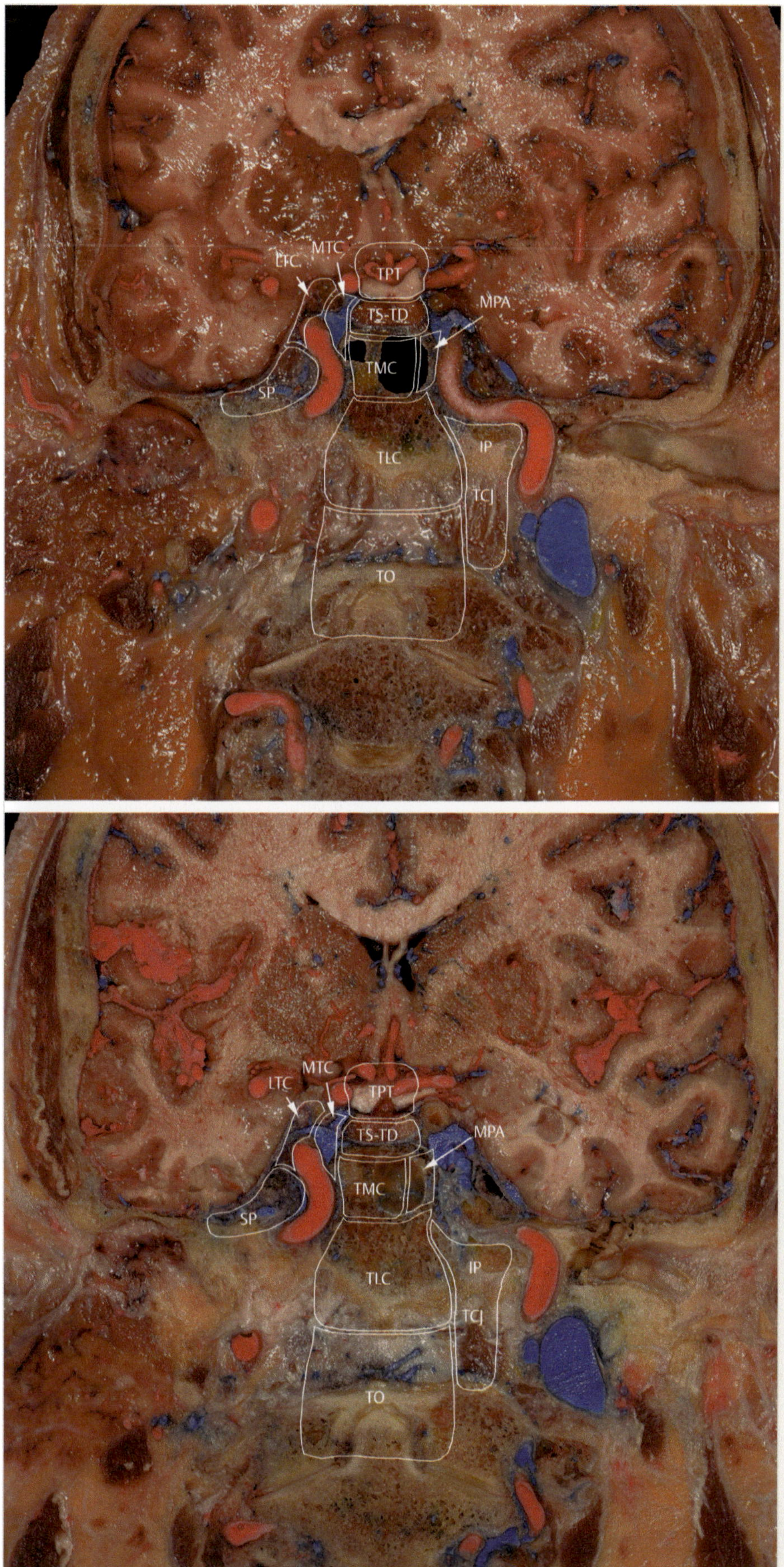

Fig. 1.10 Mapping of endoscopic transnasal approaches on a coronal section (part 3). Posterior-to-anterior view (upper image) and anterior-to-posterior view (lower image). IP, infrapetrous approach; LTC, lateral transcavernous approach; MPA, medial petrous apex approach; MTC, medial transcavernous approach; SP, suprapetrous approach; TCJ, transcondylar–transjugular tuberculum approach; TD, transdorsal approach; TLC, transclival (lower clivus) approach; TMC, transclival (midclivus) approach; TO, transodontoid approach; TPT, transplanum–transtuberculum approach; TS, transsellar approach.

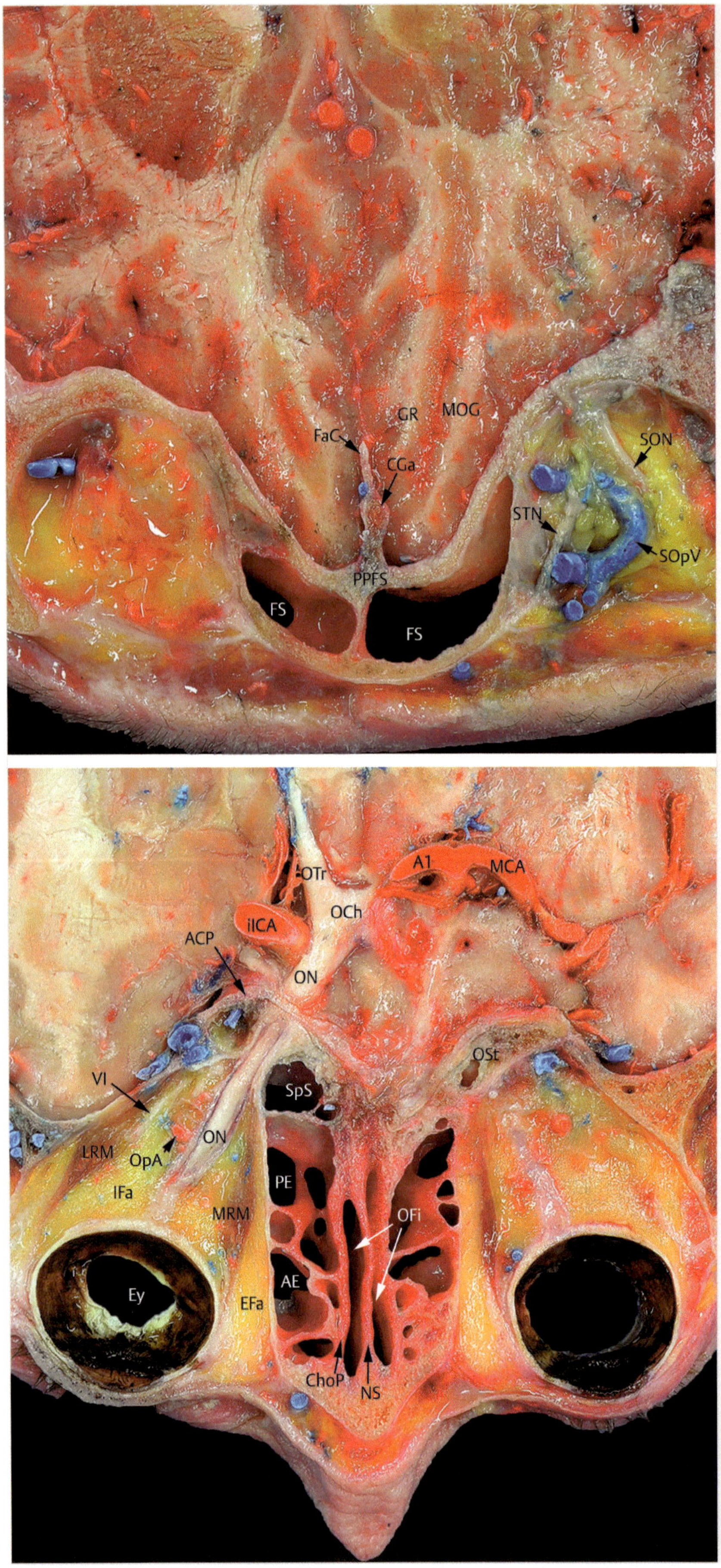

Fig. 1.11 Axial view of the skull base and adjacent areas (part 1). Inferior-to-superior view (upper image) and superior-to-inferior view (lower image). VI, abducens nerve; A1, precommunicating tract of the anterior cerebral artery; ACP, anterior clinoid process; AE, anterior ethmoidal compartment; CGa, crista galli; ChoP, conchal plate; EFa, extraconal fat; Ey, eyeball; FaC, falx cerebri; FS, frontal sinus; GR, gyrus rectus; IFa, intraconal fat; iICA, intracranial tract of the internal carotid artery; LRM, lateral rectus muscle; MCA, middle cerebral artery; MOG, medial orbital gyrus; MRM, medial rectus muscle; NS, nasal septum; OCh, optic chiasm; OFi, olfactory fissure; ON, optic nerve; OpA, ophthalmic artery; OSt, optic strut; OTr, optic tract; PE, posterior ethmoidal compartment; PPFS, posterior plate of the frontal sinus; SON, supraorbital nerve; SOpV, superior ophthalmic vein; SpS, sphenoid sinus; STN, supratrochlear nerve.

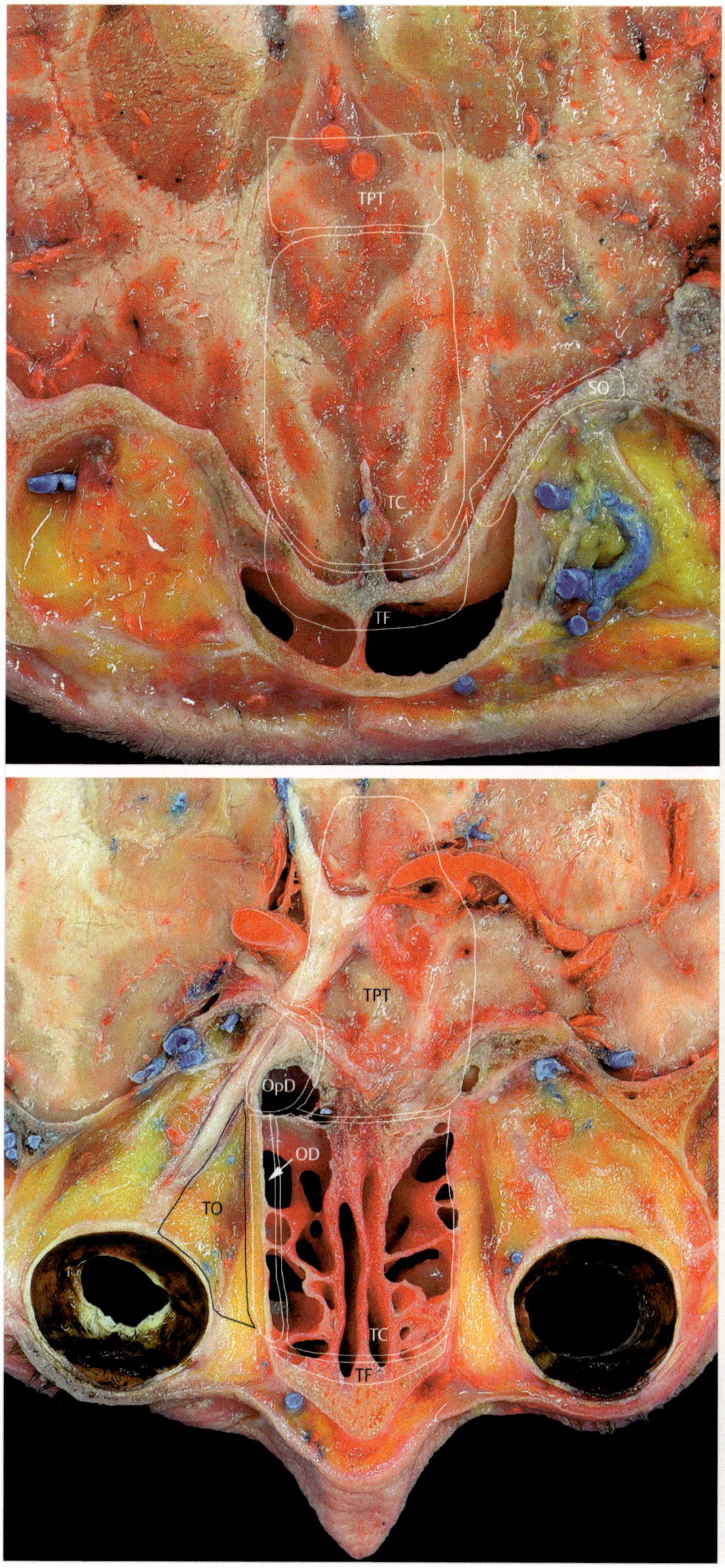

Fig. 1.12 Mapping of endoscopic transnasal approaches on an axial section (part 1). Inferior-to-superior view (upper image) and superior-to-inferior view (lower image). OD, orbital decompression; OpD, optic decompression; SO, supraorbital approach; TC, transcribriform approach; TF, transfrontal approach; TOr, transorbital approach; TPT, transplanum–transtuberculum approach.

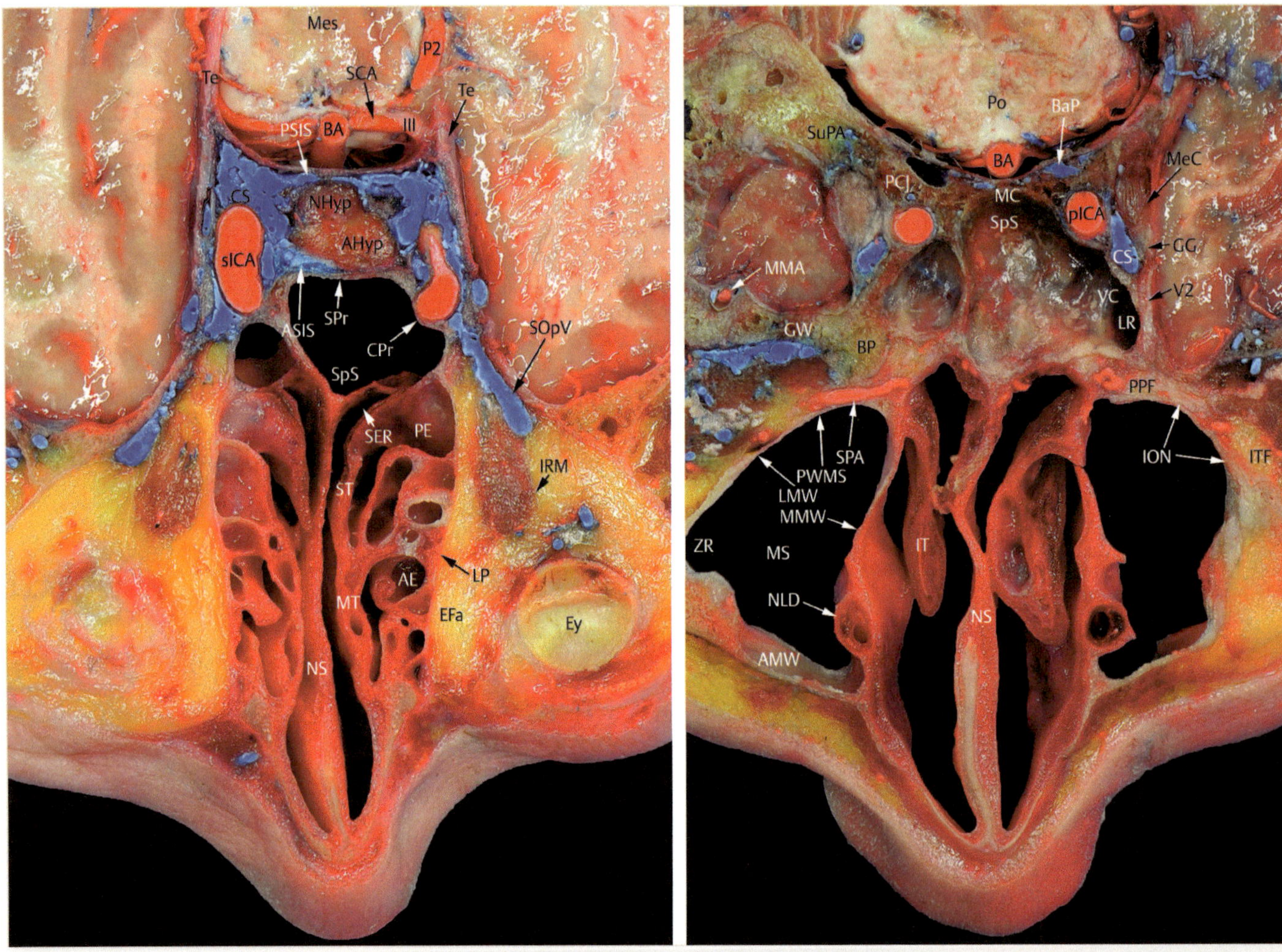

Fig. 1.13 Axial view of the skull base and adjacent areas (part 2). Superior-to-inferior view (both images). III, oculomotor nerve; V2, maxillary nerve; AE, anterior ethmoidal artery; AMW, anterior maxillary wall; ASIS, anterior superior intercavernous sinus; BA, basilar artery; BaP, basilar plexus; BP, base of the pterygoid process; CPr, carotid prominence; CS, cavernous sinus; EFa, extraconal fat; Ey, eyeball; GG, gasserian ganglion; GW, greater wing of the sphenoid sinus; ION, infraorbital nerve; IRM, inferior rectus muscle; IT, inferior turbinate; ITF, infratemporal fossa; LMW, lateral maxillary wall; LP, lamina papyracea; LR, lateral recess of the sphenoid bone; MC, midclivus; MeC, Meckel's cave; Mes, mesencephalon; MMA, middle meningeal artery; MMW, medial maxillary wall; MS, maxillary sinus; MT, middle turbinate; NLD, nasolacrimal duct; NS, nasal septum; P2, postcommunicating tract of the posterior cerebral artery; PCJ, petroclival junction; PE, posterior ethmoidal compartment; pICA, paraclival tract of the internal carotid artery; Po, pons; PPF, pterygopalatine fossa; PSIS, posterior superior intercavernous sinus; PWMS, posterior wall of the maxillary sinus; SCA, superior cerebellar artery; SER, sphenoethmoidal recess; sICA, parasellar tract of the internal carotid artery; SOpV, superior ophthalmic vein; SPA, sphenopalatine artery; SPr, sellar prominence; SpS, sphenoid sinus; ST, superior turbinate; SuPA, superior petrous apex; Te, tentorium cerebri; VC, vidian canal; ZR, zygomatic recess of the maxillary sinus.

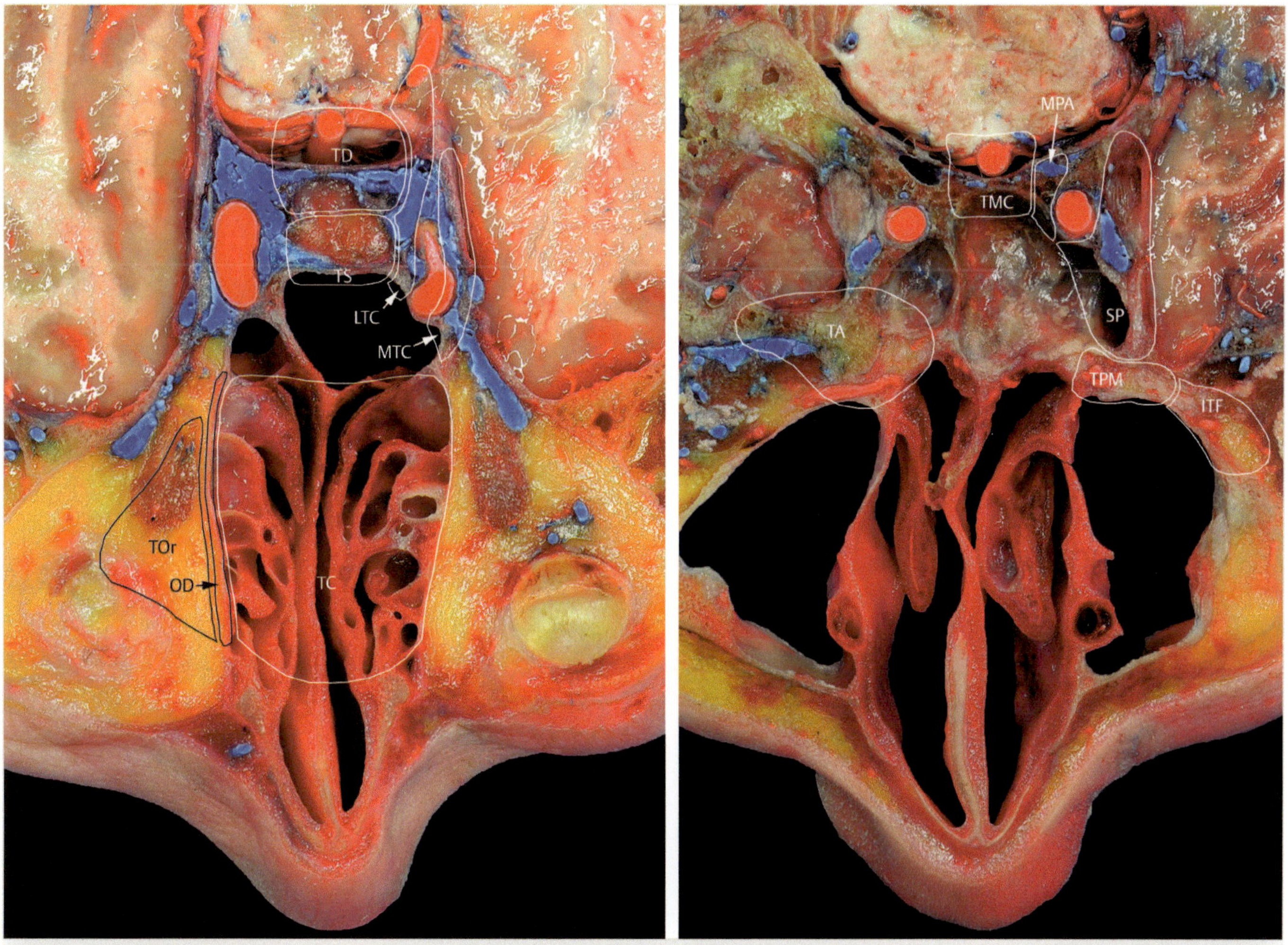

Fig. 1.14 Mapping of endoscopic transnasal approaches on an axial section (part 2). Superior-to-inferior view (both images). ITF, infratemporal fossa approach; LTC, lateral transcavernous approach; MPA, medial petrous apex approach; MTC, medial transcavernous approach; OD, orbital decompression; SP, suprapetrous (Meckel's cave) approach; TA, transalisphenoid approach; TC, transcribriform approach; TD, transdorsal approach; TMC, transclival (midclivus) approach; TOr, transorbital approach; TPM, transpterygomaxillary approach; TS, transsellar approach.

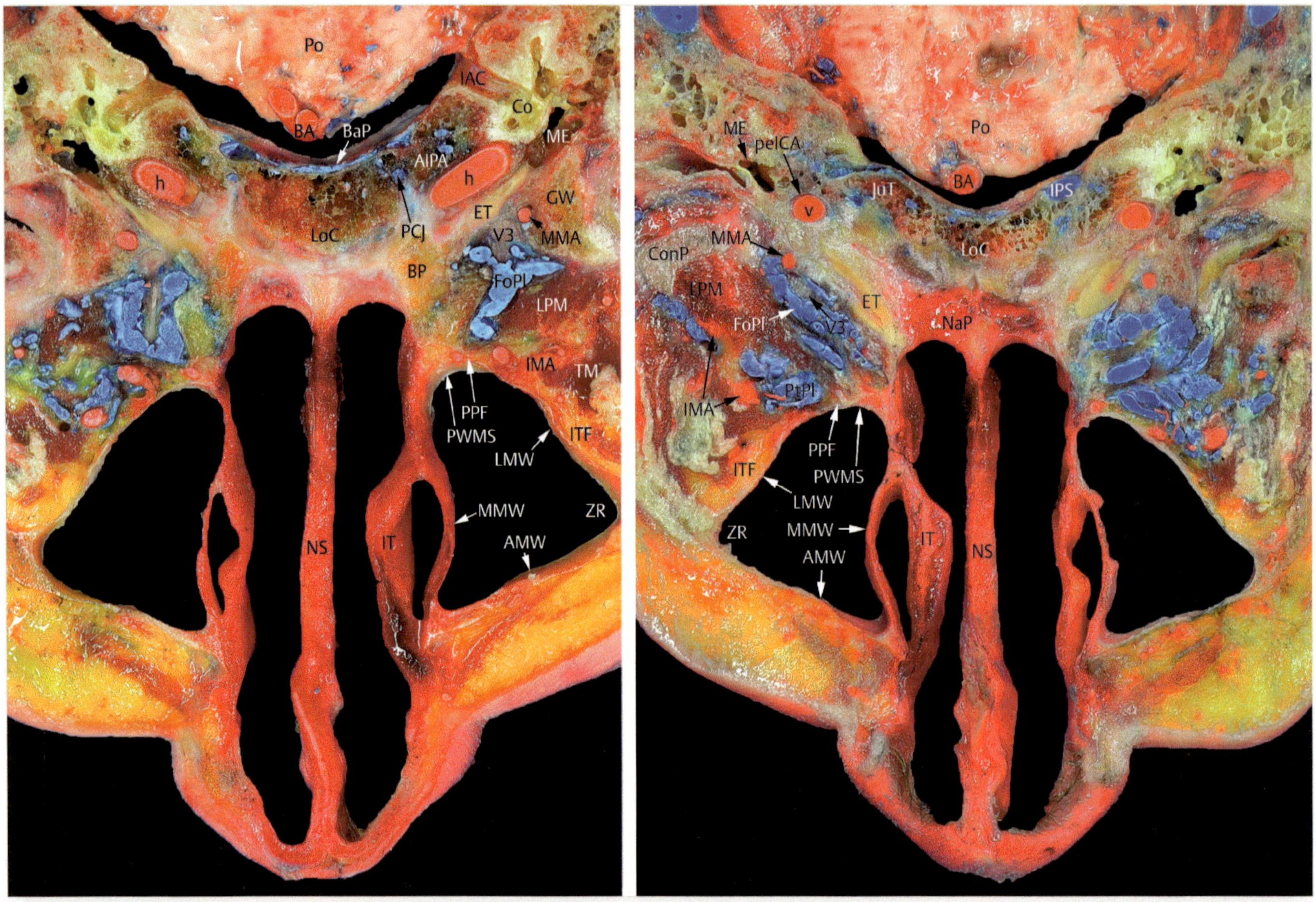

Fig. 1.15 Axial view of the skull base and adjacent areas (part 3). Superior-to-inferior view (both images). V3, mandibular nerve; AIPA, anterior inferior petrous apex; AMW, anterior maxillary wall; BA, basilar artery; BaP, basilar plexus; BP, base of the pterygoid process; Co, cochlea; ConP, condylar process of the mandible; ET, eustachian tube; FoPl, foraminal plexus; GW, greater wing of the sphenoid bone; h, horizontal portion of the petrous tract of the internal carotid artery; IAC, internal auditory canal; IMA, internal maxillary artery; IPS, inferior petrosal sinus; IT, inferior turbinate; ITF, infratemporal fossa; JuT, jugular tuberculum; LoC, lower clivus; LMW, lateral maxillary wall; LPM, lateral pterygoid muscle; ME, middle ear; MMA, middle meningeal artery; MMW, medial maxillary wall; NaP, nasopharyngeal posterior wall; NS, nasal septum; PCJ, petroclival junction; pelCA, petrous tract of the internal carotid artery; Po, pons; PPF, pterygopalatine fossa; PtPl, pterygoid plexus; PWMS, posterior wall of the maxillary sinus; TM, temporal muscle; v, vertical portion of the petrous tract of the internal carotid artery; ZR, zygomatic recess.

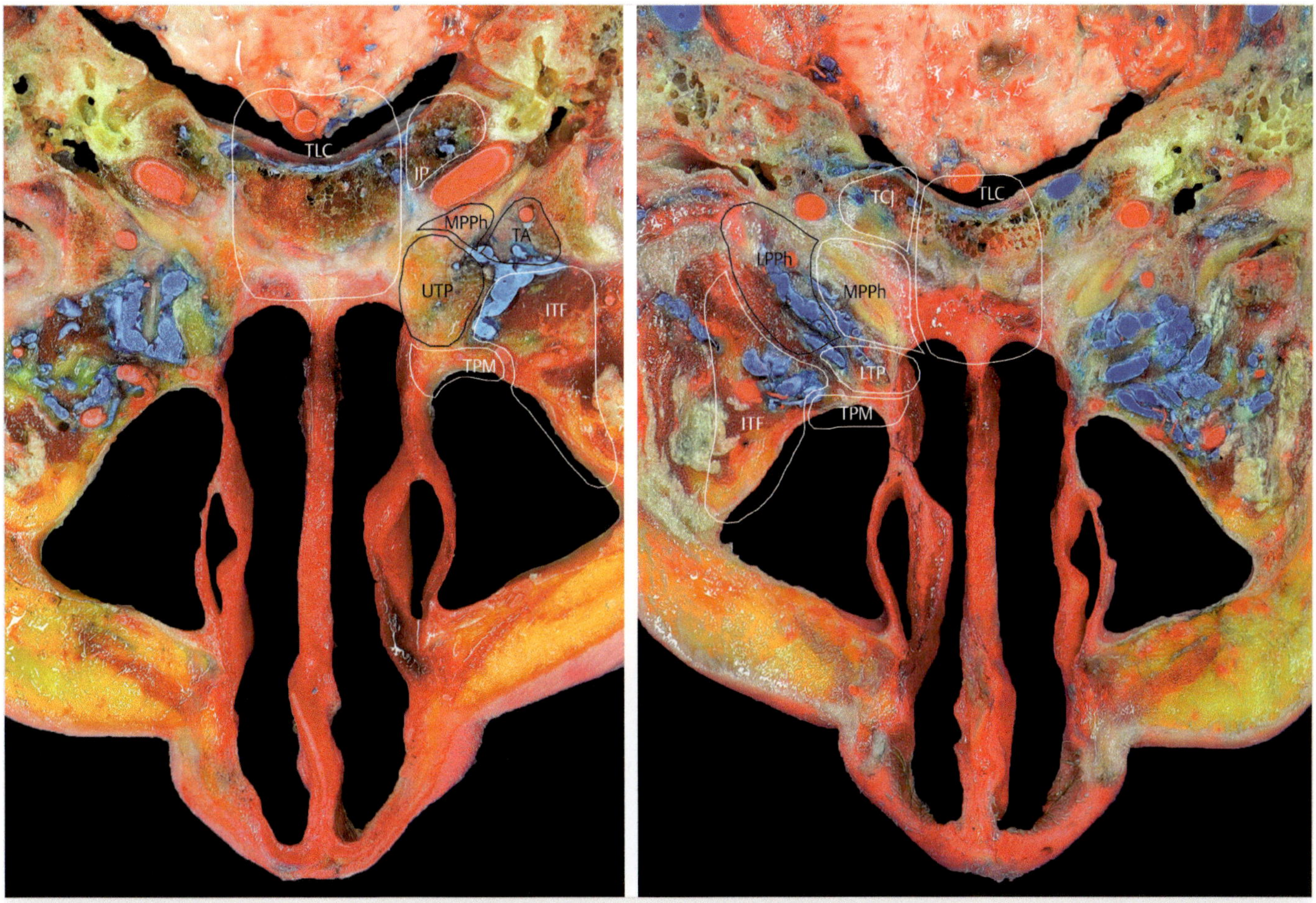

Fig. 1.16 Mapping of endoscopic transnasal approaches on an axial section (part 3). Superior-to-inferior view (both images). IP, infrapetrous approach; ITF, infratemporal fossa approach; LPPh, lateral parapharyngeal space approach; LTP, lower transpterygoid approach; MPPh, medial parapharyngeal space approach; TA, transalisphenoid approach; TCJ, transcondylar–transjugular tuberculum approach; TLC, transclival (lower clivus) approach; TPM, transpterygomaxillary approach; UTP, upper transpterygoid approach.

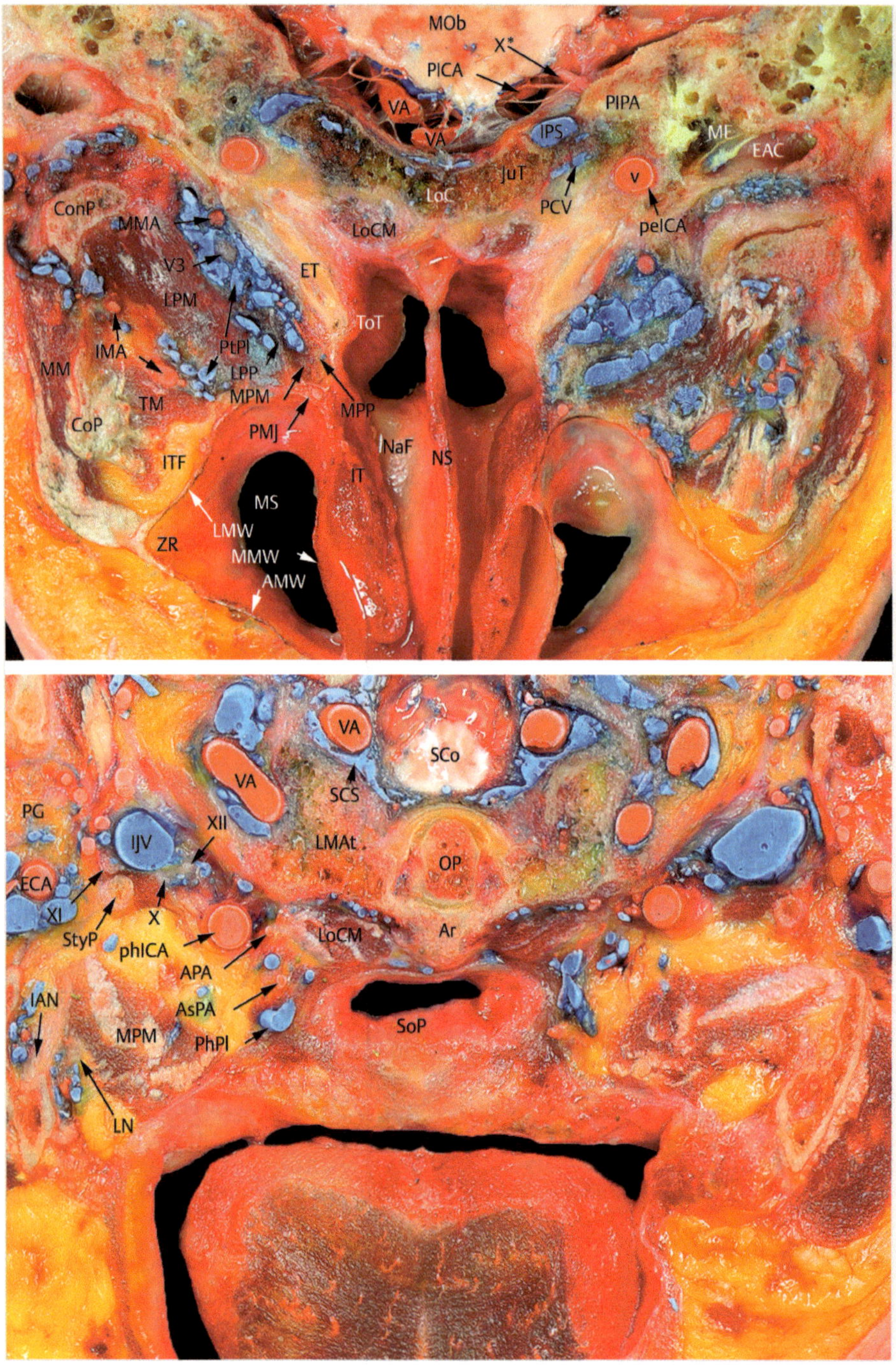

Fig. 1.17 Axial view of the skull base and adjacent areas (part 4). Superior-to-inferior view (both images). V3, mandibular nerve; X, vagus nerve; X*, glossopharyngeal, vagus, and accessory nerve; XI, spinal accessory nerve; XII, hypoglossal nerve; AMW, anterior maxillary wall; APA, ascending pharyngeal artery; Ar, anterior arch of the atlas; AsPA, ascending palatine artery; CoP, coronoid process; EAC, external auditory canal; ECA, external carotid artery; ET, eustachian tube; IAN, inferior alveolar nerve; IMA, internal maxillary artery; IPS, inferior petrosal sinus; IT, inferior turbinate; ITF, infratemporal fossa; IJV, internal jugular vein; JuT, jugular tuberculum; LMAt, lateral mass of the atlas; LMW, lateral maxillary wall; LN, lingual nerve; LoC, lower clivus; LoCM, longus capitis muscle; LPM, lateral pterygoid muscle; LPP, lateral pterygoid plate; ME, middle ear; MM, masseteric muscle; MMA, middle meningeal artery; MMW, medial maxillary wall; MOb, medulla oblongata; MPM, medial pterygoid muscle; MPP, medial pterygoid plate; MS, maxillary sinus; NaF, nasal floor; NS, nasal septum; OP, odontoid process; PCV, petroclival vein; peICA, petrous tract of the internal carotid artery; PG, parotid gland; phICA, parapharyngeal tract of the internal carotid artery; PhPl, pharyngeal plexus; PICA, posterior inferior cerebellar artery; PIPA, posterior inferior petrous apex; PMJ, pterygomaxillary junction; PtPl, pterygoid plexus; SCo, spinal cord; SCS, suboccipital cavernous sinus; SoP, soft palate; StyP, styloid process; TM, temporal muscle; ToT, torus tubarius; v, vertical portion of the petrous tract of the internal carotid artery; VA, vertebral artery; ZR, zygomatic recess.

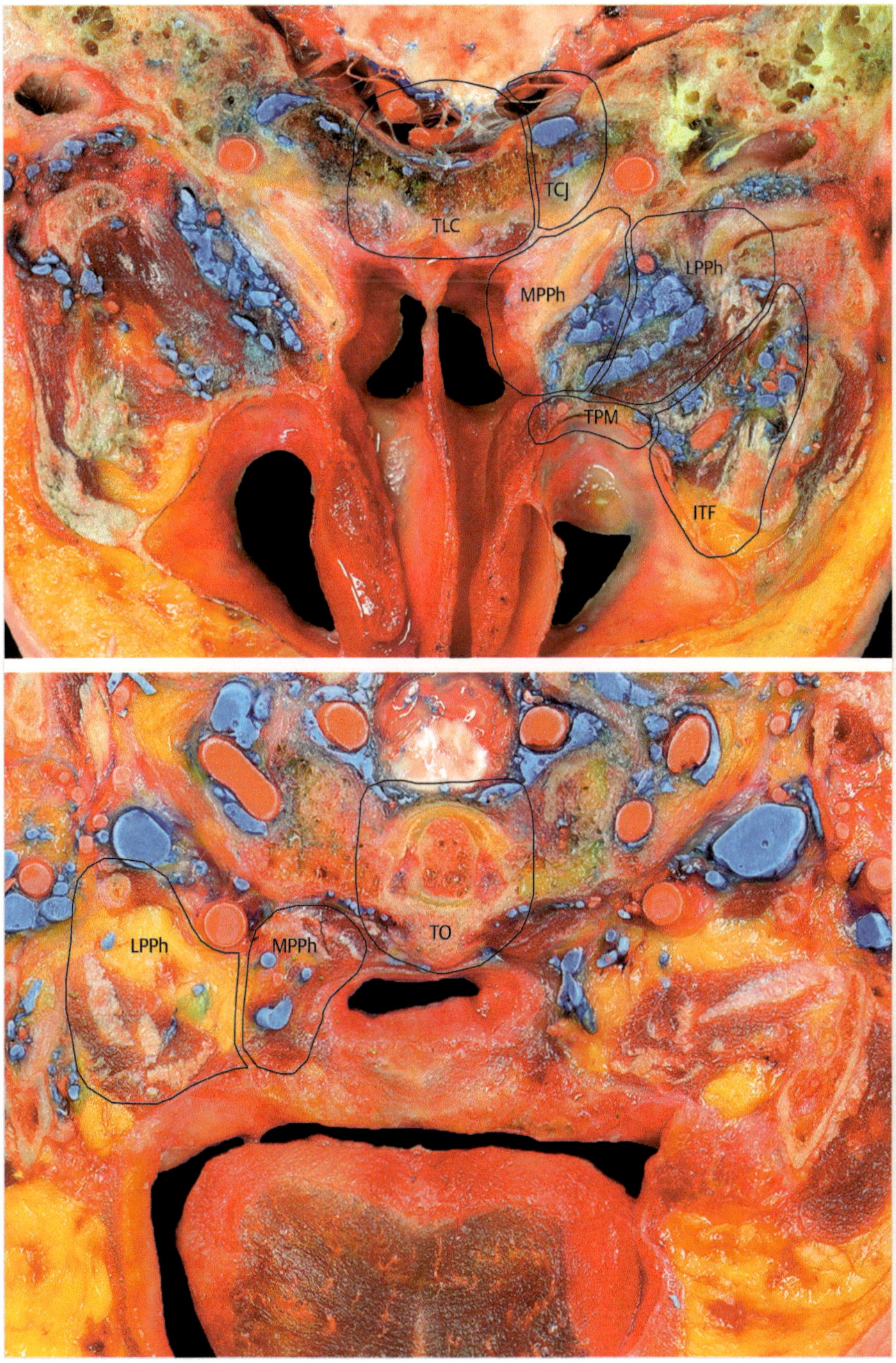

Fig. 1.18 Mapping of endoscopic transnasal approaches on an axial section (part 4). Superior-to-inferior view (both images). ITF, infratemporal fossa approach; LPPh, lateral parapharyngeal space approach; MPPh, medial parapharyngeal space approach; TCJ, transcondylar–transjugular tuberculum approach; TLC, transclival (lower clivus) approach; TO, transodontoid approach; TPM, transpterygomaxillary approach.

References

[1] Lund VJ, Stammberger H, Nicolai P, et al; European Rhinologic Society Advisory Board on Endoscopic Techniques in the Management of Nose, Paranasal Sinus and Skull Base Tumours. European position paper on endoscopic management of tumours of the nose, paranasal sinuses and skull base. Rhinol Suppl 2010;22:1–143

[2] Patel CR, Fernandez-Miranda JC, Wang WH, Wang EW. Skull base anatomy. Otolaryngol Clin North Am 2016;49(1):9–20

[3] Verillaud B, Bresson D, Sauvaget E, et al. Endoscopic endonasal skull base surgery. Eur Ann Otorhinolaryngol Head Neck Dis 2012;129(4):190–196

[4] Emmanuel J, Mahmoud M, Moncef B. Endoscopic endonasal skull base surgery: current state of the art and future trends. In: Iancu C, ed. Advances in Endoscopic Surgery. Rijeka: InTech; 2011:3–38

[5] Kassam AB, Gardner P, Snyderman C, Mintz A, Carrau R. Expanded endonasal approach: fully endoscopic, completely transnasal approach to the middle third of the clivus, petrous bone, middle cranial fossa, and infratemporal fossa. Neurosurg Focus 2005;19(1):E6

[6] Kassam A, Snyderman CH, Mintz A, Gardner P, Carrau RL. Expanded endonasal approach: the rostrocaudal axis. Part I. Crista galli to the sella turcica. Neurosurg Focus 2005;19(1):E3

[7] Kassam A, Snyderman CH, Mintz A, Gardner P, Carrau RL. Expanded endonasal approach: the rostrocaudal axis. Part II. Posterior clinoids to the foramen magnum. Neurosurg Focus 2005;19(1):E4

[8] Schwartz TH, Fraser JF, Brown S, Tabaee A, Kacker A, Anand VK. Endoscopic cranial base surgery: classification of operative approaches. Neurosurgery 2008;62(5):991–1002, discussion 1002–1005

[9] Kasemsiri P, Carrau RL, Ditzel Filho LF, et al. Advantages and limitations of endoscopic endonasal approaches to the skull base. World Neurosurg 2014;82(6, Suppl):S12–S21

[10] Prevedello DM, Kassam AB, Snyderman C, et al. Endoscopic cranial base surgery: ready for prime time? Clin Neurosurg 2007;54:48–57

[11] Snyderman CH, Carrau RL, Kassam AB, et al. Endoscopic skull base surgery: principles of endonasal oncological surgery. J Surg Oncol 2008;97(8):658–664

[12] Carrau RL, Kassam AB, Snyderman CH. Pituitary surgery. Otolaryngol Clin North Am 2001;34(6):1143–1155, ix

[13] Kassam AB, Prevedello DM, Carrau RL, et al. Endoscopic endonasal skull base surgery: analysis of complications in the authors' initial 800 patients. J Neurosurg 2011;114(6):1544–1568

[14] Garin A, Thierry B, Leboulanger N, et al. Pediatric sinogenic epidural and subdural empyema: the role of endoscopic sinus surgery. Int J Pediatr Otorhinolaryngol 2015;79(10):1752–1760

[15] Cervantes SS, Lal D. Crista galli mucocele: endoscopic marsupialization via frontoethmoid approach. Int Forum Allergy Rhinol 2014;4(7):598–602

[16] Selleck AM, Desai D, Thorp BD, Ebert CS, Zanation AM. Management of frontal sinus tumors. Otolaryngol Clin North Am 2016;49(4):1051–1065

[17] Thong JF, Chatterjee D, Hwang SY. Endoscopic modified Lothrop approach for the excision of bilateral frontal sinus tumors. Ear Nose Throat J 2014;93(3):116–119

[18] Pinheiro-Neto CD, Snyderman CH, Fernandez-Miranda J, Gardner PA. Endoscopic endonasal surgery for nasal dermoids. Otolaryngol Clin North Am 2011;44(4):981–987, ix

[19] Re M, Tarchini P, Macrì G, Pasquini E. Endonasal endoscopic approach for intracranial nasal dermoid sinus cysts in children. Int J Pediatr Otorhinolaryngol 2012;76(8):1217–1222

[20] Ma J, Huang Q, Li X, et al. Endoscopic transnasal repair of cerebrospinal fluid leaks with and without an encephalocele in pediatric patients: from infants to children. Childs Nerv Syst 2015;31(9):1493–1498

[21] Nyquist GG, Anand VK, Mehra S, Kacker A, Schwartz TH. Endoscopic endonasal repair of anterior skull base non-traumatic cerebrospinal fluid leaks, meningoceles, and encephaloceles. J Neurosurg 2010;113(5):961–966

[22] Castelnuovo P, Battaglia P, Turri-Zanoni M, et al. Endoscopic endonasal surgery for malignancies of the anterior cranial base. World Neurosurg 2014;82(6, Suppl):S22–S31

[23] Nicolai P, Battaglia P, Bignami M, et al. Endoscopic surgery for malignant tumors of the sinonasal tract and adjacent skull base: a 10-year experience. Am J Rhinol 2008;22(3):308–316

[24] Nicolai P, Castelnuovo P, Bolzoni Villaret A. Endoscopic resection of sinonasal malignancies. Curr Oncol Rep 2011;13(2):138–144

[25] Fernandez-Miranda JC, Gardner PA, Prevedello DM, Kassam AB. Expanded endonasal approach for olfactory groove meningioma. Acta Neurochir (Wien) 2009;151(3):287–288, author reply 289–290

[26] Koutourousiou M, Fernandez-Miranda JC, Wang EW, Snyderman CH, Gardner PA. Endoscopic endonasal surgery for olfactory groove meningiomas: outcomes and limitations in 50 patients. Neurosurg Focus 2014;37(4):E8

[27] Verillaud B, Bresson D, Sauvaget E, et al. Transcribriform and transplanum endoscopic approach for skull-base tumors. Eur Ann Otorhinolaryngol Head Neck Dis 2013;130(4):233–236

[28] Liu JK, Eloy JA. Expanded endoscopic endonasal transcribriform approach for resection of anterior skull base olfactory schwannoma. J Neurosurg 2012;32(Suppl):E3

[29] Blake DM, Husain Q, Kanumuri VV, Svider PF, Eloy JA, Liu JK. Endoscopic endonasal resection of sinonasal and anterior skull base schwannomas. J Clin Neurosci 2014;21(8):1419–1423

[30] Vaz-Guimaraes F, Koutourousiou M, de Almeida JR, et al. Endoscopic endonasal surgery for epidermoid and dermoid cysts: a 10-year experience. J Neurosurg 2018 (e-pub ahead of print). doi:10.3171/2017.7.JNS162783

[31] Barazi SA, Pasquini E, D'Urso PI, et al. Extended endoscopic transplanum-transtuberculum approach for pituitary adenomas. Br J Neurosurg 2013;27(3):374–382

[32] Laufer I, Anand VK, Schwartz TH. Endoscopic, endonasal extended transsphenoidal, transplanum transtuberculum approach for resection of suprasellar lesions. J Neurosurg 2007;106(3):400–406

[33] Cavallo LM, Solari D, Esposito F, Villa A, Minniti G, Cappabianca P. The role of the endoscopic endonasal route in the management of craniopharyngiomas. World Neurosurg 2014;82(6, Suppl):S32–S40

[34] Fomichev D, Kalinin P, Kutin M, Sharipov O. Extended transsphenoidal endoscopic endonasal surgery of suprasellar craniopharyngiomas. World Neurosurg 2016;94:181–187

[35] Nishioka H, Fukuhara N, Yamaguchi-Okada M, Yamada S. Endoscopic endonasal surgery for purely intrathird ventricle craniopharyngioma. World Neurosurg 2016;91:266–271

[36] Liu JK, Christiano LD, Patel SK, Tubbs RS, Eloy JA. Surgical nuances for removal of tuberculum sellae meningiomas with optic canal involvement using the endoscopic endonasal extended transsphenoidal transplanum transtuberculum approach. Neurosurg Focus 2011;30(5):E2

[37] Froelich S, Cebula H, Debry C, Boyer P. Anterior communicating artery aneurysm clipped via an endoscopic endonasal approach: technical note. Neurosurgery 2011;68(2, Suppl Operative):310–316, discussion 315–316

[38] Xiao LM, Tang B, Xie SH, et al. Endoscopic endonasal clipping of anterior circulation aneurysm: surgical techniques and results. World Neurosurg 2018;115:e33–e44

[39] Kulwin C, Chan D, Ting J, Hattab EM, Cohen-Gadol AA. Endoscopic endonasal transplanum transtuberculum resection of a large solid choroid plexus papilloma of the third ventricle. J Clin Neurosci 2014;21(7):1263–1266

[40] Yoneoka Y, Yoshimura J, Sano M, Okada M, Kakita A, Fujii Y. Third ventricle germ cell tumor originating from the infundibulum with rapidly expansive enlargement. Pediatr Neurosurg 2018;53(1):49–54

[41] Zoli M, Mazzatenta D, Valluzzi A, et al. Expanding indications for the extended endoscopic endonasal approach to hypothalamic gliomas: preliminary report. Neurosurg Focus 2014;37(4):E11

[42] Cappabianca P, Cavallo LM, Solari D, Stagno V, Esposito F, de Angelis M. Endoscopic endonasal surgery for pituitary adenomas. World Neurosurg 2014;82(6, Suppl):S3–S11

[43] Ratha V, Patil S, Karmarkar VS, Shah NJ, Deopujari CE. Surgical management of Rathke cleft cysts. World Neurosurg 2017;107:276–284

[44] Zada G, Kelly DF, Cohan P, Wang C, Swerdloff R. Endonasal transsphenoidal approach for pituitary adenomas and other sellar lesions: an assessment of efficacy, safety, and patient impressions. J Neurosurg 2003;98(2):350–358

[45] Tang B, Xiao L, Xie S, et al. Extended endoscopic endonasal approach for recurrent or residual symptomatic craniopharyngiomas. Clin Neurol Neurosurg 2018;168:38–45

[46] Somma T, Solari D, Beer-Furlan A, et al. Endoscopic endonasal management of rare sellar lesions: clinical and surgical experience of 78 cases and review of the literature. World Neurosurg 2017;100:369–380

[47] Fernandez-Miranda JC, Gardner PA, Snyderman CH, et al. Clival chordomas: a pathological, surgical, and radiotherapeutic review. Head Neck 2014;36(6):892–906

[48] Fernandez-Miranda JC, Gardner PA, Snyderman CH, et al. Craniopharyngioma: a pathologic, clinical, and surgical review. Head Neck 2012;34(7):1036–1044

[49] Montaser AS, Revuelta Barbero JM, Todeschini A, et al. Endoscopic endonasal pituitary gland hemi-transposition for resection of a dorsum sellae meningioma. Neurosurg Focus 2017;43(VideoSuppl2):V7

[50] Gardner PA, Vaz-Guimaraes F, Jankowitz B, et al. Endoscopic endonasal clipping of intracranial aneurysms: surgical technique and results. World Neurosurg 2015;84(5):1380–1393

[51] Fraser JF, Nyquist GG, Moore N, Anand VK, Schwartz TH. Endoscopic endonasal transclival resection of chordomas: operative technique, clinical outcome, and review of the literature. J Neurosurg 2010;112(5):1061–1069

[52] Ditzel Filho LF, Prevedello DM, Dolci RL, et al. The endoscopic endonasal approach for removal of petroclival chondrosarcomas. Neurosurg Clin N Am 2015;26(3):453–462

[53] Vaz-Guimaraes F, Fernandez-Miranda JC, Koutourousiou M, et al. Endoscopic endonasal surgery for cranial base chondrosarcomas. Oper Neurosurg (Hagerstown) 2017;13(4):421–434

[54] Beer-Furlan A, Abi-Hachem R, Jamshidi AO, Carrau RL, Prevedello DM. Endoscopic trans-sphenoidal surgery for petroclival and clival meningiomas. J Neurosurg Sci 2016;60(4):495–502

[55] Kooshkabadi A, Choi PA, Koutourousiou M, et al. Atlanto-occipital instability following endoscopic endonasal approach for lower clival lesions: experience with 212 cases. Neurosurgery 2015;77(6):888–897, discussion 897

[56] Morales-Valero SF, Serchi E, Zoli M, Mazzatenta D, Van Gompel JJ. Endoscopic endonasal approach for craniovertebral junction pathology: a review of the literature. Neurosurg Focus 2015;38(4):E15

[57] Shkarubo AN, Andreev DN, Konovalov NA, et al. Surgical treatment of skull base tumors, extending to craniovertebral junction. World Neurosurg 2017;99:47–58

[58] Boboridis KG, Uddin J, Mikropoulos DG, et al. Critical appraisal on orbital decompression for thyroid eye disease: a systematic review and literature search. Adv Ther 2015;32(7):595–611

[59] Di Somma A, Cavallo LM, de Notaris M, et al. Endoscopic endonasal medial-to-lateral and transorbital lateral-to-medial optic nerve decompression: an anatomical study with surgical implications. J Neurosurg 2017;127(1):199–208

[60] Dallan I, Locatelli D, Turri-Zanoni M, et al. Transorbital endoscopic assisted resection of a superior orbital fissure cavernous haemangioma: a technical case report. Eur Arch Otorhinolaryngol 2015;272(12):3851–3856

[61] Kong DS, Young SM, Hong CK, et al. Clinical and ophthalmological outcome of endoscopic transorbital surgery for cranioorbital tumors. J Neurosurg 2018 (e-pub ahead of print). doi:10.3171/2018.3.JNS173233

[62] Fernandez-Miranda JC, Gardner PA, Rastelli MM Jr, et al. Endoscopic endonasal transcavernous posterior clinoidectomy with interdural pituitary transposition. J Neurosurg 2014;121(1):91–99

[63] Ferrareze Nunes C, Lieber S, Truong HQ, et al. Endoscopic endonasal transoculomotor triangle approach for adenomas invading the parapeduncular space: surgical anatomy, technical nuances, and case series. J Neurosurg 2018

[64] Cohen-Cohen S, Gardner PA, Alves-Belo JT, et al. The medial wall of the cavernous sinus. Part 2: selective medial wall resection in 50 pituitary adenoma patients. J Neurosurg 2018 (e-pub ahead of print). doi:10.3171/2018.5.JNS18595

[65] Toda M, Kosugi K, Ozawa H, Ogawa K, Yoshida K. Surgical treatment of cavernous sinus lesion in patients with nonfunctioning pituitary adenomas via the endoscopic endonasal approach. J Neurol Surg B Skull Base 2018;79(Suppl 4):S311–S315

[66] Koutourousiou M, Vaz Guimaraes Filho F, Fernandez-Miranda JC, et al. Endoscopic endonasal surgery for tumors of the cavernous sinus: a series of 234 patients. World Neurosurg 2017;103:713–732

[67] Lobo B, Zhang X, Barkhoudarian G, Griffiths CF, Kelly DF. Endonasal endoscopic management of parasellar and cavernous sinus meningiomas. Neurosurg Clin N Am 2015;26(3):389–401

[68] Patrona A, Patel KS, Bander ED, et al. Endoscopic endonasal surgery for nonadenomatous, nonmeningeal pathology involving the cavernous sinus. J Neurosurg 2017;126(3):880–888

[69] Emanuelli E, Bignami M, Digilio E, Fusetti S, Volo T, Castelnuovo P. Post-traumatic optic neuropathy: our surgical and medical protocol. Eur Arch Otorhinolaryngol 2015;272(11):3301–3309

[70] Berhouma M, Jacquesson T, Abouaf L, Vighetto A, Jouanneau E. Endoscopic endonasal optic nerve and orbital apex decompression for nontraumatic optic neuropathy: surgical nuances and review of the literature. Neurosurg Focus 2014;37(4):E19

[71] Koutourousiou M, Gardner PA, Tormenti MJ, et al. Endoscopic endonasal approach for resection of cranial base chordomas: outcomes and learning curve. Neurosurgery 2012;71(3):614–624, discussion 624–625

[72] Carlson ML, O'Connell BP, Breen JT, et al. Petroclival chondrosarcoma: a multicenter review of 55 cases and new staging system. Otol Neurotol 2016;37(7):940–950

[73] Mesquita Filho PM, Ditzel Filho LF, Prevedello DM, et al. Endoscopic endonasal surgical management of chondrosarcomas with cerebellopontine angle extension. Neurosurg Focus 2014;37(4):E13

[74] Georgalas C, Kania R, Guichard JP, Sauvaget E, Tran Ba Huy P, Herman P. Endoscopic transsphenoidal surgery for cholesterol granulomas involving the petrous apex. Clin Otolaryngol 2008;33(1):38–42

[75] Koutourousiou M, Fernandez-Miranda JC, Vaz-Guimaraes Filho F, et al. Outcomes of endonasal and lateral approaches to petroclival meningiomas. World Neurosurg 2017;99:500–517

[76] Shi J, Chen J, Chen T, et al. Neuroendoscopic resection of trigeminal schwannoma in the pterygopalatine/infratemporal fossa via the transnasal perpendicular plate palatine bone or transnasal maxillary sinus approach. World Neurosurg 2018;120:e1011–e1016

[77] Battaglia P, Turri-Zanoni M, Lepera D, et al. Endoscopic transnasal approaches to pterygopalatine fossa tumors. Head Neck 2016;38(Suppl 1):E214–E220

[78] Langdon C, Herman P, Verillaud B, et al. Expanded endoscopic endonasal surgery for advanced stage juvenile angiofibromas: a retrospective multi-center study. Rhinology 2016;54(3):239–246

[79] Schreiber A, Bertazzoni G, Ferrari M, et al. Management of persistent juvenile angiofibroma after endoscopic resection: analysis of a single institution series of 74 patients. Head Neck 2019;41(5):1297–1303

[80] Battaglia P, Turri-Zanoni M, Dallan I, et al. Endoscopic endonasal transpterygoid transmaxillary approach to the infratemporal and upper parapharyngeal tumors. Otolaryngol Head Neck Surg 2014;150(4):696–702

[81] Raza SM, Amine MA, Anand V, Schwartz TH. Endoscopic endonasal resection of trigeminal schwannomas. Neurosurg Clin N Am 2015;26(3):473–479

[82] Shin M, Shojima M, Kondo K, et al. Endoscopic endonasal craniofacial surgery for recurrent skull base meningiomas involving the pterygopalatine fossa, the infratemporal fossa, the orbit, and the paranasal sinus. World Neurosurg 2018;112:e302–e312

[83] Lee JT, Suh JD, Carrau RL, Chu MW, Chiu AG. Endoscopic Denker's approach for resection of lesions involving the anteroinferior maxillary sinus and infratemporal fossa. Laryngoscope 2017;127(3):556–560

[84] Kassam AB, Prevedello DM, Carrau RL, et al. The front door to Meckel's cave: an anteromedial corridor via expanded endoscopic endonasal approach—technical considerations and clinical series. Neurosurgery 2009;64(3, Suppl):ons71–ons82, discussion ons82–ons83

[85] McLaughlin N, Kelly DF, Prevedello DM, Shahlaie K, Carrau RL, Kassam AB. Endoscopic endonasal management of recurrent petrous apex cholesterol granuloma. J Neurol Surg B Skull Base 2012;73(3):190–196

[86] Taniguchi M, Akutsu N, Mizukawa K, Kohta M, Kimura H, Kohmura E. Endoscopic endonasal translacerum approach to the inferior petrous apex. J Neurosurg 2016;124(4):1032–1038

[87] Maurer AJ, Bonney PA, Iser CR, Ali R, Sanclement JA, Sughrue ME. Endoscopic endonasal infrapetrous transpterygoid approach to the petroclival junction for petrous apex chondrosarcoma: technical report. J Neurol Surg Rep 2015;76(1):e113–e116

[88] Morera VA, Fernandez-Miranda JC, Prevedello DM, et al. "Far-medial" expanded endonasal approach to the inferior third of the clivus: the transcondylar and transjugular tubercle approaches. Neurosurgery 2010;66(6, Suppl Operative):211–219, discussion 219–220

[89] Vaz-Guimaraes F, Nakassa ACI, Gardner PA, Wang EW, Snyderman CH, Fernandez-Miranda JC. Endoscopic endonasal approach to the ventral jugular foramen: anatomical basis, technical considerations, and clinical series. Oper Neurosurg (Hagerstown) 2017;13(4):482–491

[90] Castelnuovo P, Nicolai P, Turri-Zanoni M, et al. Endoscopic endonasal nasopharyngectomy in selected cancers. Otolaryngol Head Neck Surg 2013;149(3):424–430

2 Nasal Corridors

Vittorio Rampinelli, Davide Mattavelli, Marco Ravanelli, Alberto Schreiber

Endoscopic surgery of the skull base and adjacent areas takes advantage of the natural corridor of the sinonasal tract. This concept represents an extension of functional endoscopic sinus surgery, in which natural drainage pathways are followed to open the sinuses.[1-4] Even though employed as corridors toward the skull base, sinonasal cavities should be dissected following the principles of functional surgery as much as possible, aiming at avoiding unnecessary morbidity and minimizing postoperative complications. The first step when starting the surgical procedure is to examine the natural corridors of the nasal cavity in order to get oriented. The lumen of the nasal cavity is irregularly shaped: on the medial side, it takes the shape of the nasal septum and can be accordingly narrowed or enlarged by its deviations and spurs; the lateral side consists of the turbinates and related nasal meati, which can be enlarged by pneumatization (i.e., concha bullosa) or present an everted shape (i.e., paradoxical turbinate); the caudal surface corresponds to the nasal floor and is usually flat and regular; the cranial boundary of the lumen is the olfactory cleft (or fissure), which is a narrow niche enclosed between the highest portions of middle and superior turbinates laterally and nasal septum medially.

Endoscopic skull base surgery is based on the profound knowledge of anatomical landmarks, which provide the surgeon with a mental scheme to depict where neurovascular and musculoskeletal structures are located before exposing them.[4-14] As a consequence, understanding of anatomy in an untouched nasal cavity is indispensable and of paramount importance to plan and proceed with safe and oriented surgery. With the intent to facilitate the identification of sinonasal landmarks, the nasal cavity has been divided into three nasal corridors, as follows:

- Inferior nasal corridor: Between the inferior turbinate and nasal septum.
- Middle nasal corridor: Between the bulbous portions of middle and superior turbinates and nasal septum.
- Superior nasal corridor: Between the common laminar portion of middle and superior turbinates and nasal septum.

The inferior nasal corridor runs from the nasal vestibule to the nasopharynx along the nasal floor. It can be merged with the contralateral one by removing the nasal septum; usually, a posteroinferior septectomy is sufficient when addressing the craniocervical junction and neighboring areas. Laterally, the corridor can be expanded passing through the palatine bone, pterygoid process, and maxillary sinus to access the upper parapharyngeal space, pterygopalatine fossa, and infratemporal fossa.

The middle nasal corridor provides a straight trajectory toward the sphenoid sinus. It can be merged with the contralateral corridor with a posterosuperior septectomy. On the lateral side, the corridor can be expanded through the ethmoid complex, medial

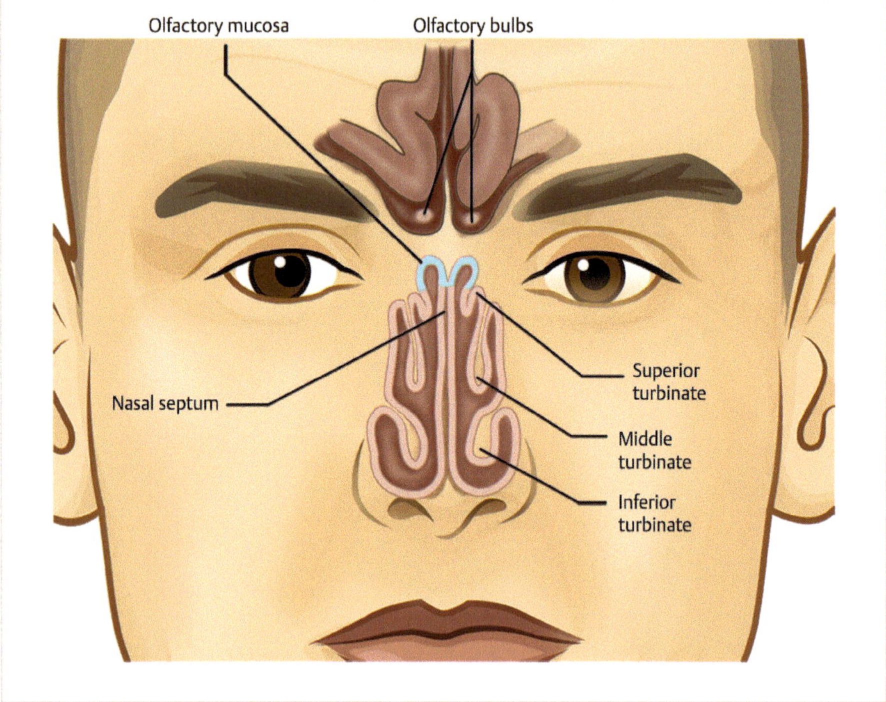

Fig. 2.1 Coronal view of nasal cavity architecture. This illustration shows anatomy of the main components of the nasal cavity: nasal septum and turbinates.

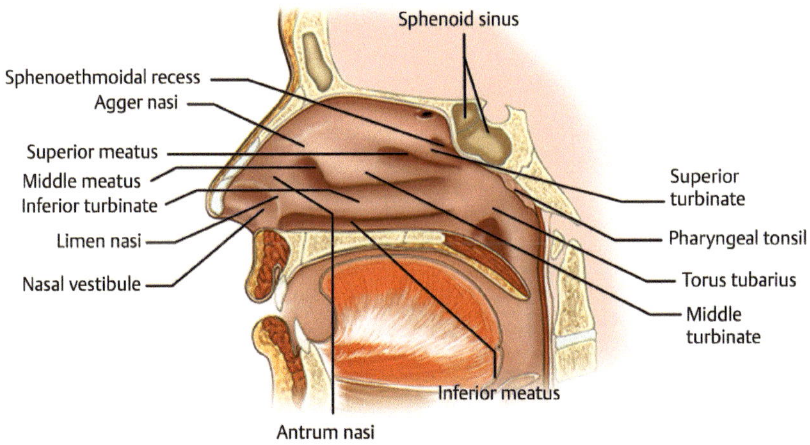

Fig. 2.2 Sagittal view of nasal cavity architecture. This illustration shows the anatomy of the lateral nasal wall.

orbital wall, and lateral sphenoidal wall to reach the orbital cavity, Meckel's cave, and cavernous sinus.

The superior nasal corridor guides toward the midline anterior skull base and can be fused with the contralateral one with removal of the entire nasal septum. This corridor is oriented toward the olfactory grooves and can be extended laterally through the ethmoidal compartments to expose the ethmoidal roof (also called fovea ethmoidalis).

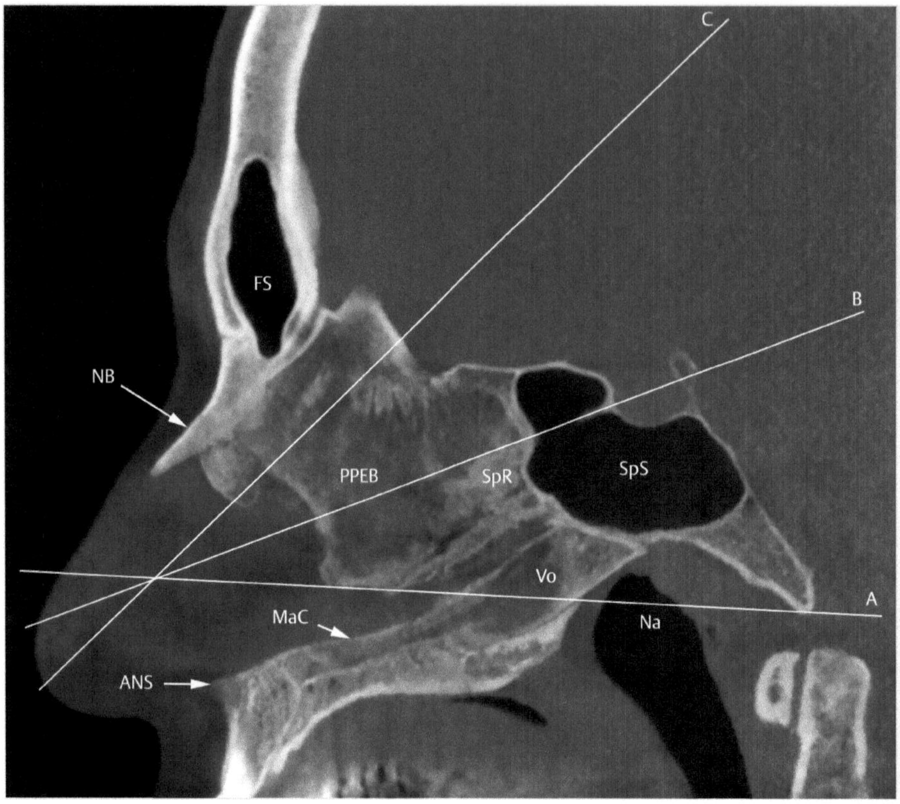

Fig. 2.3 Sagittal CT anatomy of the sinonasal tract. The three natural sinonasal corridors are shown with white lines (A–C), corresponding to the orientation of images composing ▶Fig. 2.4. As seen in the sagittal view, the inferior, middle, and superior nasal corridors are oriented toward the nasopharynx (Na), sphenoid sinus (SpS), and midline anterior skull base. ANS, anterior nasal spine; FS, frontal sinus; MaC, maxillary crest; NB, nasal bone; PPEB, perpendicular plate of the ethmoid bone; SpR, sphenoid rostrum; Vo, vomer.

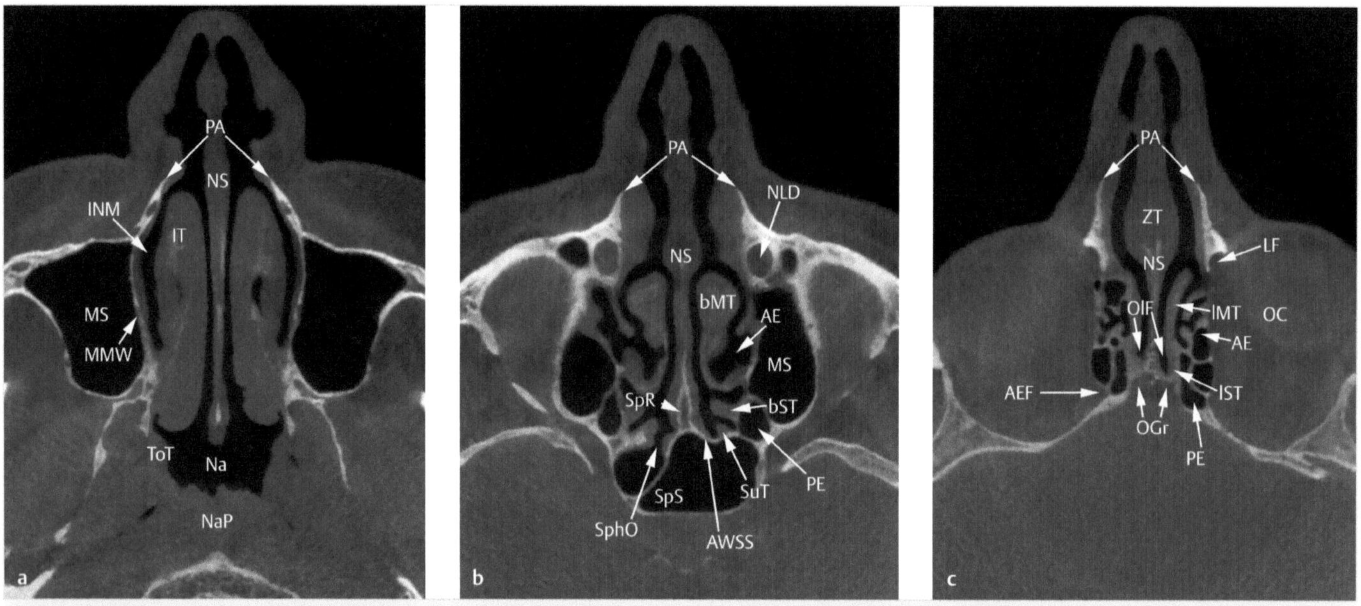

Fig. 2.4 Axial and para-axial CT anatomy of the natural nasal corridors. The panel includes one axial **(a)** and two para-axial images **(b, c)** oriented along the trajectories of the inferior, middle, and superior nasal corridors, respectively. The orientation of images is shown in ▶Fig. 2.3. The inferior nasal corridor is enclosed between the nasal septum (NS) medially and inferior turbinate (IT) laterally. This corridor reaches the nasopharynx (Na) and ends on the nasopharyngeal posterior wall (NaP) posteriorly. At this level, the luminal cavity is delimited by the tori tubarii (ToT) bilaterally. The inferior nasal corridor is at the same craniocaudal level of the inferior nasal meatus (INM) and maxillary sinus (MS), which are separated by the medial maxillary wall (MMW). The middle nasal meatus is bounded by the nasal septum and bulbous portion of the middle (bMT), superior (bST), and supreme turbinate (SuT), when present. This corridor ends on the anterior wall of the sphenoid sinus (AWSS) where the sphenoidal ostium (SphO) is located. This corridor is parallel to several structures of the lateral nasal wall, which are, from anterior to posterior, the nasolacrimal duct (NLD), anterior ethmoidal complex (AE), and posterior ethmoidal complex (PE). Moreover, the middle nasal corridor is located at the same level of the cranial portion of the maxillary sinus and caudal portion of the orbital cavity (OC). The superior nasal corridor is located between the nasal septum and the laminar portion of the middle (lMT) and superior turbinates (lST), which are fused together forming a lamella that is also called the conchal plate. This corridor ends in the ipsilateral olfactory fissure (OlF) and can be remarkably narrowed when the Zuckerkandl tubercle (ZT), which is a thickening of the anterosuperior septal mucosa, is hypertrophic. The superior nasal corridor is parallel to the lacrimal fossa (LF) and to the cranial portion of the ethmoid complex and orbital cavity. AEF, anterior ethmoidal foramen; OGr, olfactory groove; PA, pyriform aperture.

Endoscopic Dissection

- Step 1: Exploration of the inferior nasal corridor.
- Step 2: Lateralization of the inferior turbinate.
- Step 3: Exploration of the inferior nasal meatus.
- Step 4: Exploration of the middle nasal corridor.
- Step 5: Lateralization of the middle and superior turbinates.
- Step 6: Exploration of the middle nasal meatus.
- Step 7: Exposure of the sphenopalatine artery.
- Step 8: Exploration of the superior nasal corridor

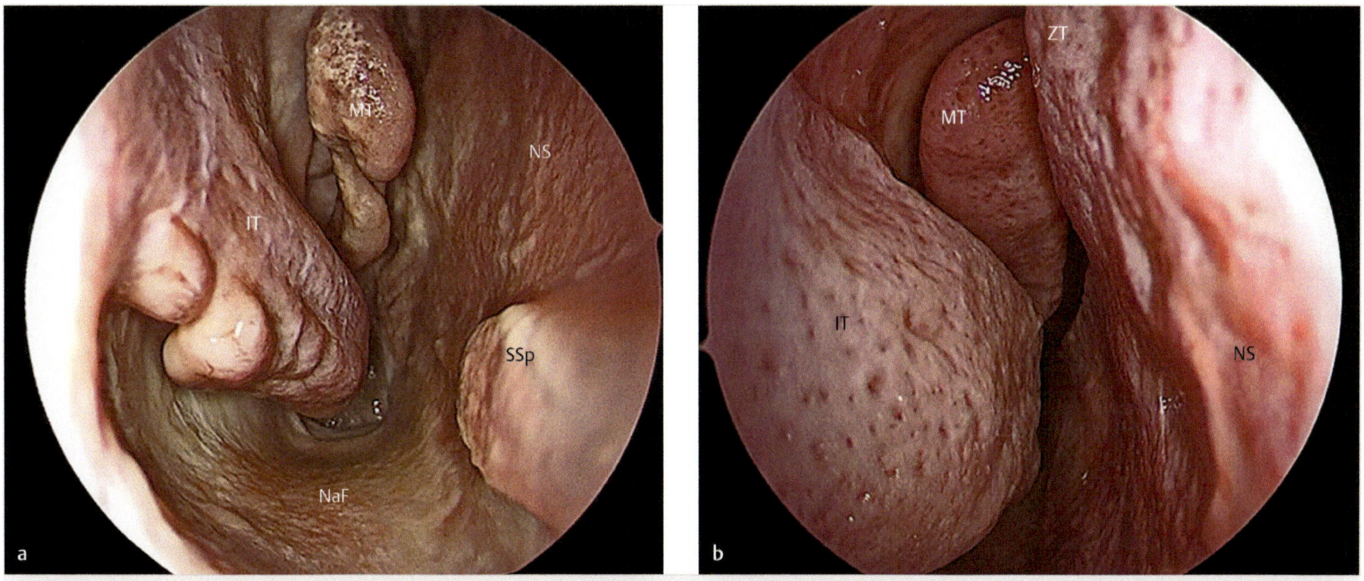

Fig. 2.5 (a, b) Step 1 (part 1). The inferior nasal corridor is bounded by the inferior turbinate (IT) laterally, nasal floor (NaF) inferiorly, and nasal septum (NS) medially. It can be narrowed by septal spur (SSp), septal deviation, hypertrophic inferior turbinate, or Zuckerkandl tubercle (ZT), which is a mucosal thickening in the anterosuperior portion of the nasal septum formed by the same erectile tissue constituting nasal turbinates.

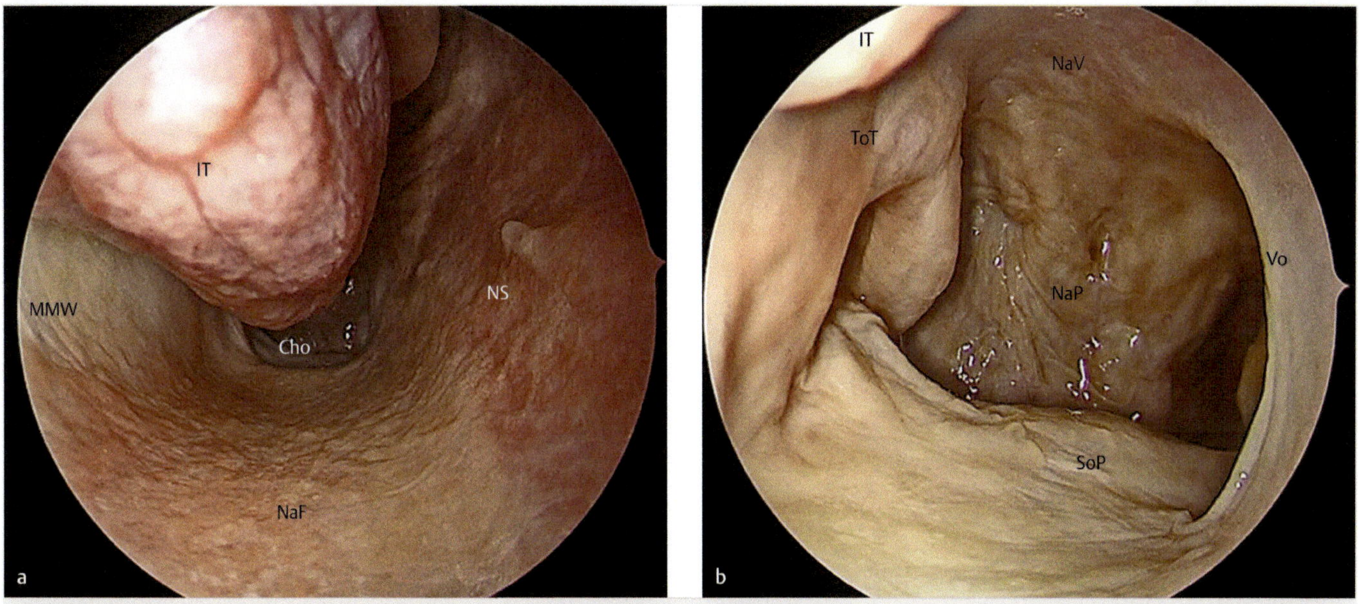

Fig. 2.6 (a, b) Step 1 (part 2). While reaching the nasopharynx through the inferior nasal corridor, the medial maxillary wall (MMW) comes into view laterally to the inferior turbinate (IT). Once in the nasopharynx passing through the choana (Cho), its boundaries can be identified: the torus tubarius (ToT) laterally, nasopharyngeal vault superiorly (NaV), soft palate inferiorly (SoP), and nasopharyngeal posterior wall (NaP) posteriorly. The vomer (Vo) forms the posteroinferior portion of the nasal septum (NS) and divides the two choanae.

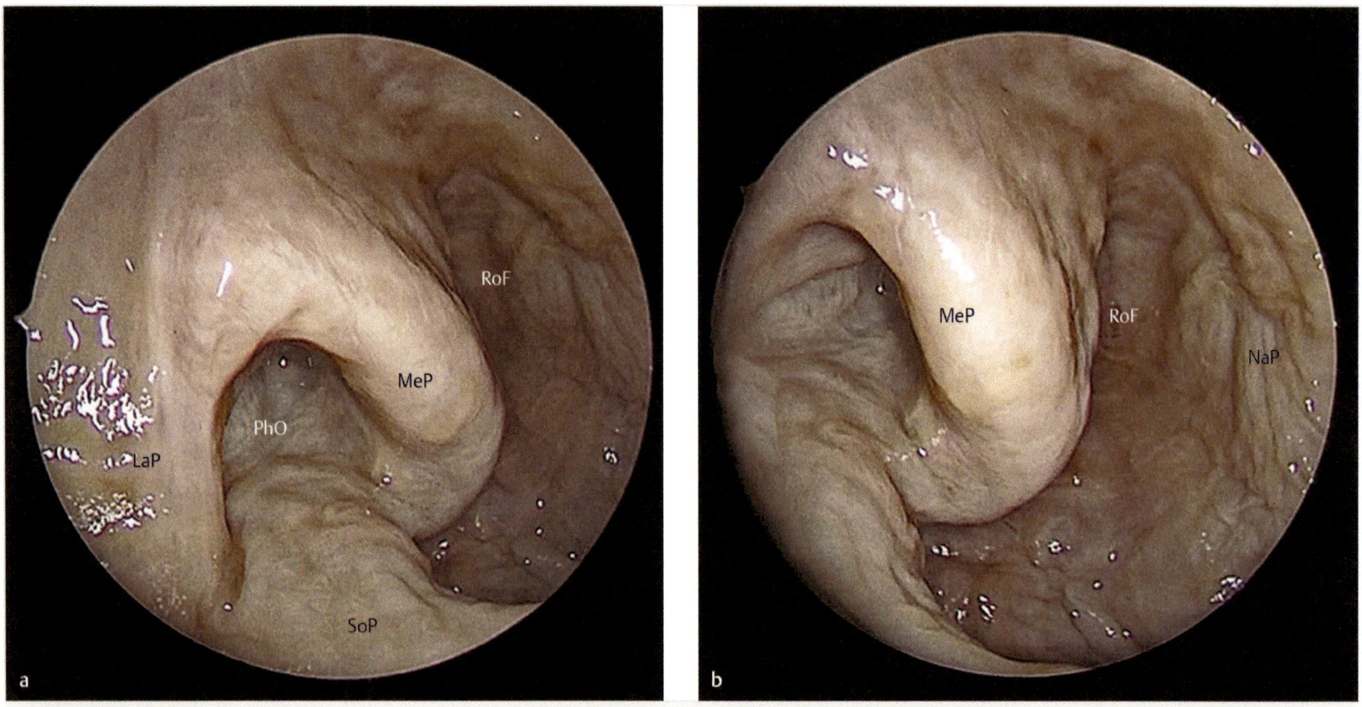

Fig. 2.7 (a, b) The eustachian tube. The eustachian tube can be best analyzed with a 70-degree scope turned laterally. The pharyngeal ostium (Pho) is located between the lateral (LaP) and medial (MeP) cartilaginous plate of the eustachian cartilage, which imprints the mucosa of the nasopharynx forming the torus tubarius. Owing to their diagonal trajectory, these cartilaginous plates can be also called anterior and posterior, respectively. The Rosenmüller fossa (RoF) is found behind the medial plate, in front of the lateral portion of the nasopharyngeal posterior wall (NaP). As seen with a 70-degree scope turned laterally, it is evident that both the floor of the eustachian tube and the posterior portion of the nasopharyngeal face of the soft palate (SoP) are made by the same structure located underneath the mucosa, which is the levator veli palatini muscle.

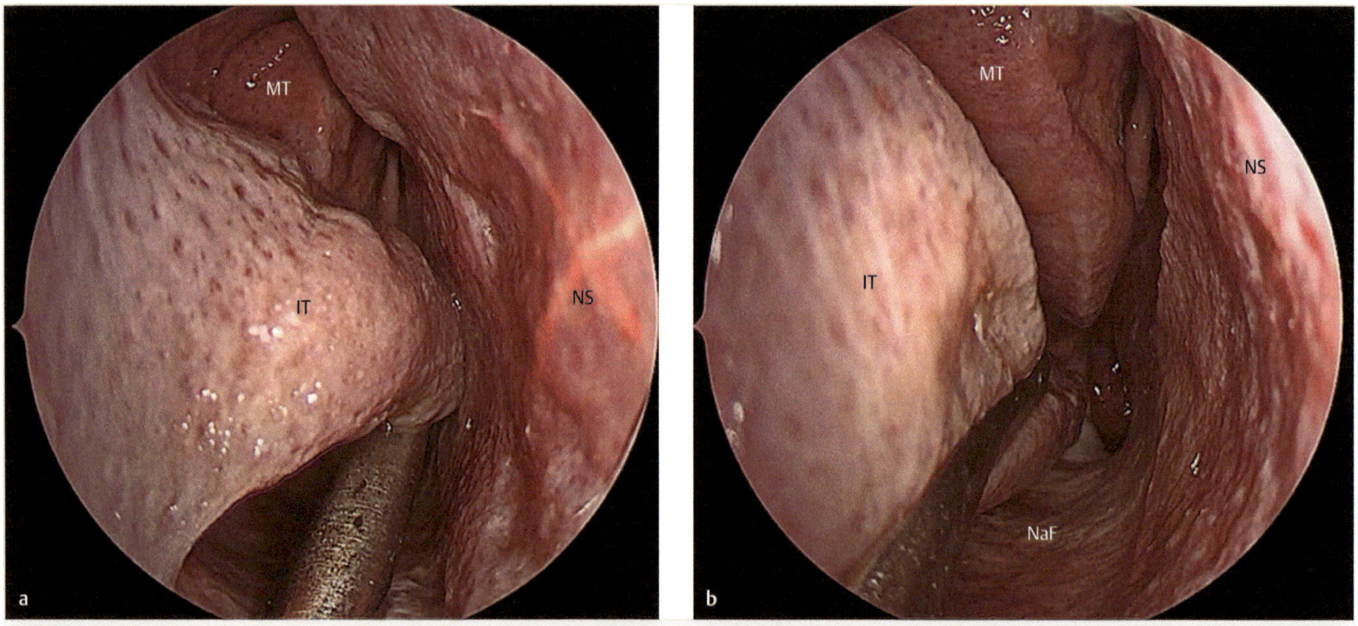

Fig. 2.8 (a, b) Step 2. Using a dissector, the inferior turbinate (IT) is pushed and fractured medially and superiorly, thus widening the exposure of the inferior meatus. Subsequently, the turbinate is pushed laterally proceeding from anterior to posterior. MT, middle turbinate; NaF, nasal floor; NS, nasal septum.

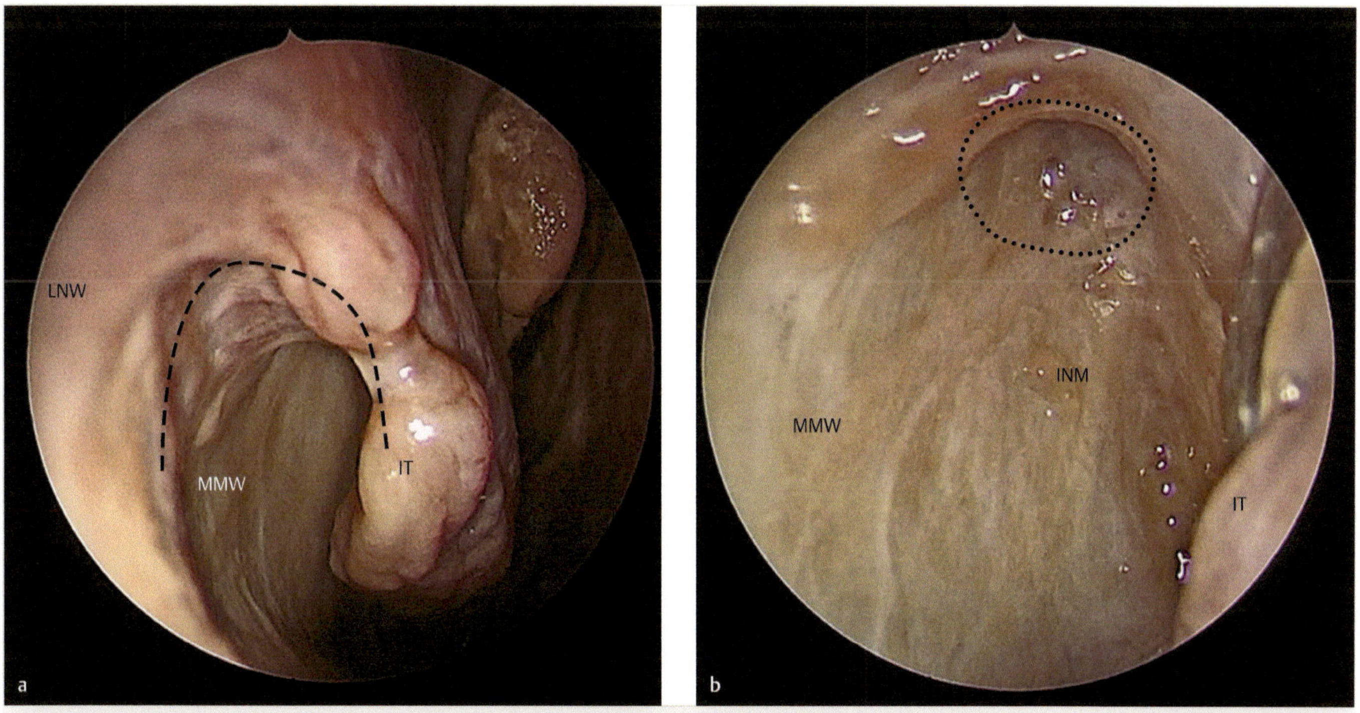

Fig. 2.9 (a, b) Step 3 (part 1). The inferior nasal meatus (INM) is located between the inferior turbinate (IT) and the medial maxillary wall (MMW). Its anterior limit is the axilla of the inferior turbinate (*black dashed line*), which is the connection between the inferior turbinate and the most anterior portion of the lateral nasal wall (LNW). The axilla of the inferior turbinate can be used as a landmark to identify the inferior end of the nasolacrimal duct (*black dotted line*), which can be clearly seen with a 70-degree scope turned upward **(b)** positioned into the anterior portion of the inferior nasal meatus.

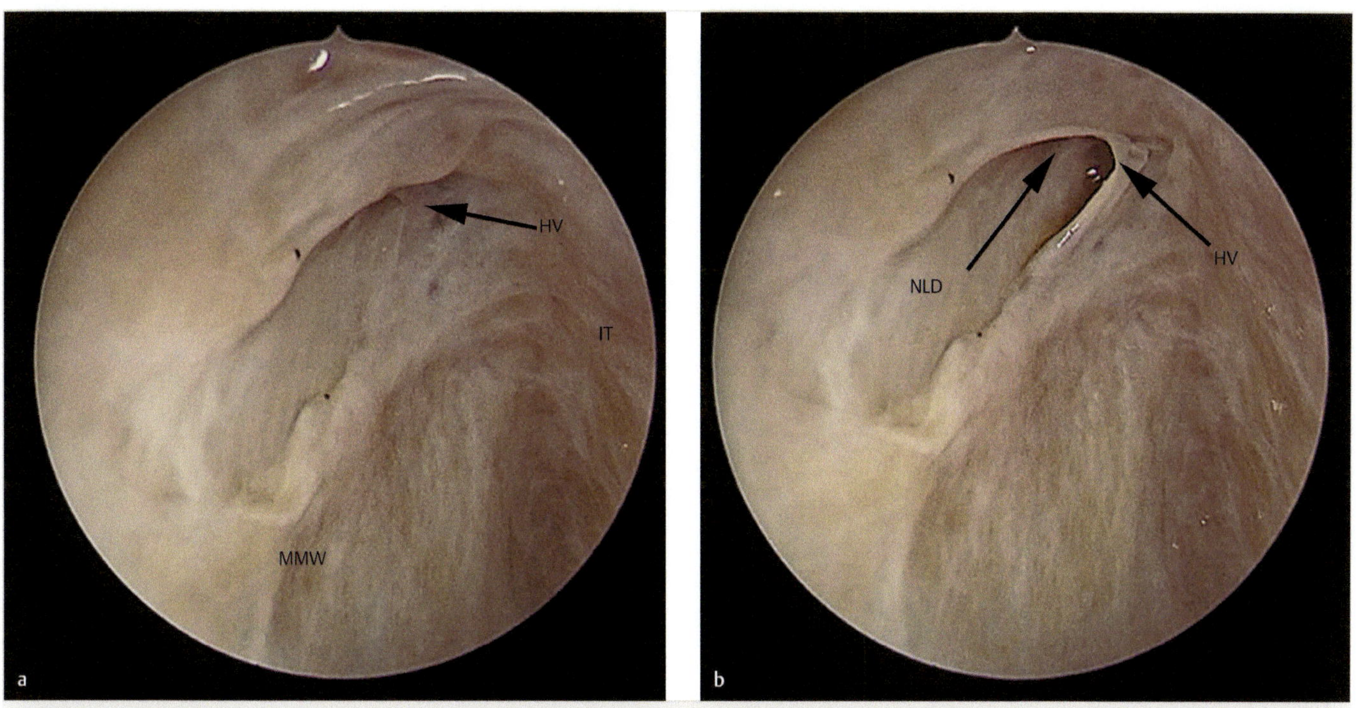

Fig. 2.10 (a, b) Hasner's valve. The mucosa of the inferior turbinate (IT) is folded to create a valve, called Hasner's valve (HV), which allows lacrimal secretion to flow into the inferior nasal meatus but prevents nasal secretion to ascend into the nasolacrimal duct (NLD) while breathing or sneezing. MMW, medial wall of the maxillary sinus.

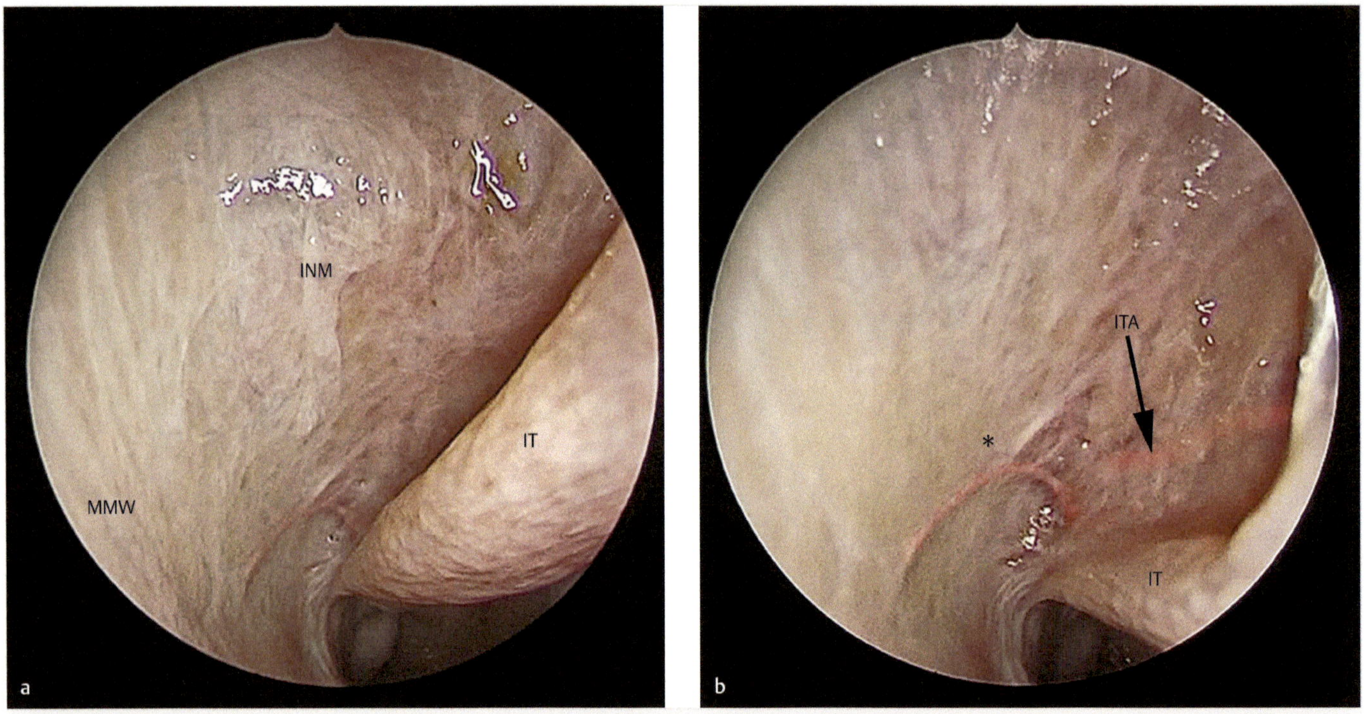

Fig. 2.11 (a, b) Step 3 (part 2). In the inferior nasal meatus (INM), at the level of the tail of the inferior turbinate (IT), some branches of the sphenopalatine artery can be identified: the inferior turbinal artery (ITA) runs in a lateral-to-medial and posterior-to-anterior direction, while a small branch (*black asterisk*) turns laterally to reach the medial maxillary wall (MMW).

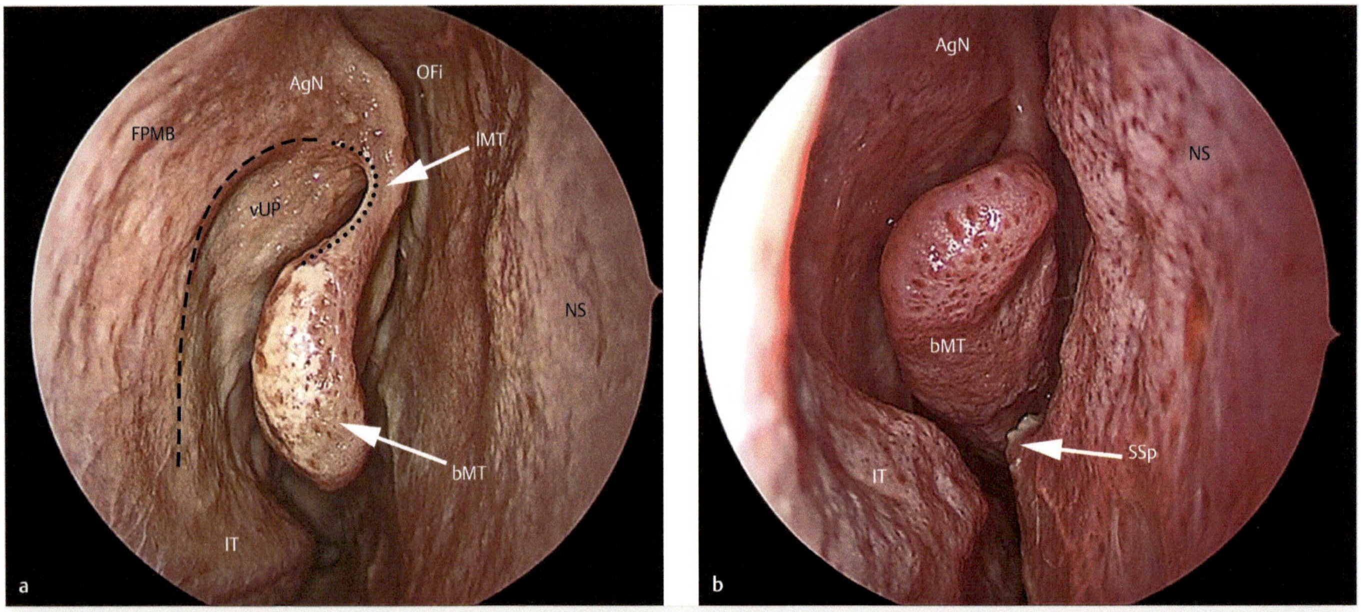

Fig. 2.12 (a, b) Step 4 (part 1). The middle nasal corridor is comprised between the bulbous portion of the middle turbinate (bMT) laterally and nasal septum (NS) medially. It can be narrowed by a hypertrophic or pneumatized middle turbinate, septal spur (SSp), or hypertrophic Zuckerkandl tubercle. The middle turbinate is composed of the bulbous and laminar portion (lMT). The latter structure inserts superiorly on the agger nasi (AgN), which is a lateral-to-medial prominence of the lateral nasal wall. The junction between the frontal process of the maxillary bone (FPMB) and the vertical portion of the uncinate process (vUP) is called maxillary line (*black dashed line*) and almost corresponds to the suture between the maxilla and lacrimal bone. The axilla of the middle turbinate is made up by the maxillary line and the laminar portion of the middle turbinate (*black dotted line*). IT, inferior turbinate; OFi, olfactory fissure.

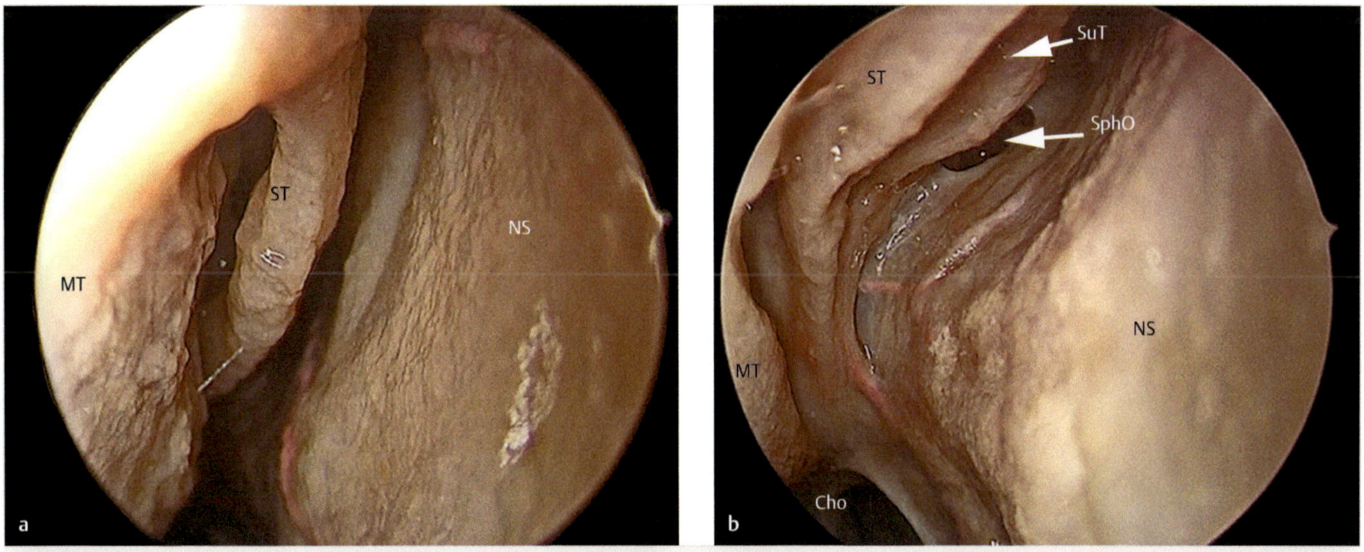

Fig. 2.13 (a, b) Step 4 (part 2). The superior turbinate (ST) is identified by moving the scope posteriorly through the middle nasal corridor. According to the size and pneumatization of the superior turbinate, the sphenoethmoidal recess, which is the space between the superior turbinate and the anterior wall of the sphenoid sinus, can be seen proceeding further posteriorly with the scope. In the posteromedial portion of the sphenoethmoidal recess, it is possible to identify the sphenoidal ostium (SphO) between the superior turbinate and nasal septum. The sphenoethmoidal recess can be partially filled by the supreme turbinate (SuT), when present. Cho, choana; MT, middle turbinate; NS, nasal septum.

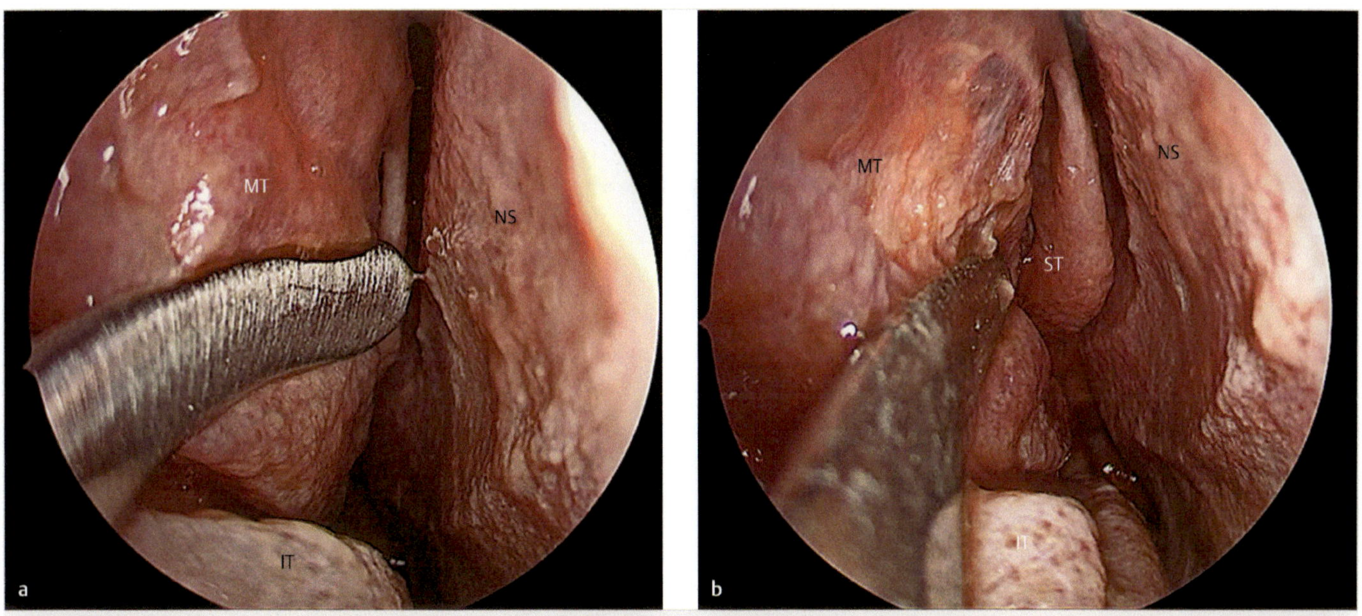

Fig. 2.14 (a, b) Step 5. To widen the middle nasal corridor, a dissector is used to push the bulbous portion of the middle turbinate (MT) laterally. The same maneuver can be repeated for the superior turbinate (ST). It is important to avoid lateralization of the laminar portion of the middle turbinate as this structure is directly connected to the cribriform plate and its manipulation can result in the injury of the skull base. IT, inferior turbinate; NS, nasal septum.

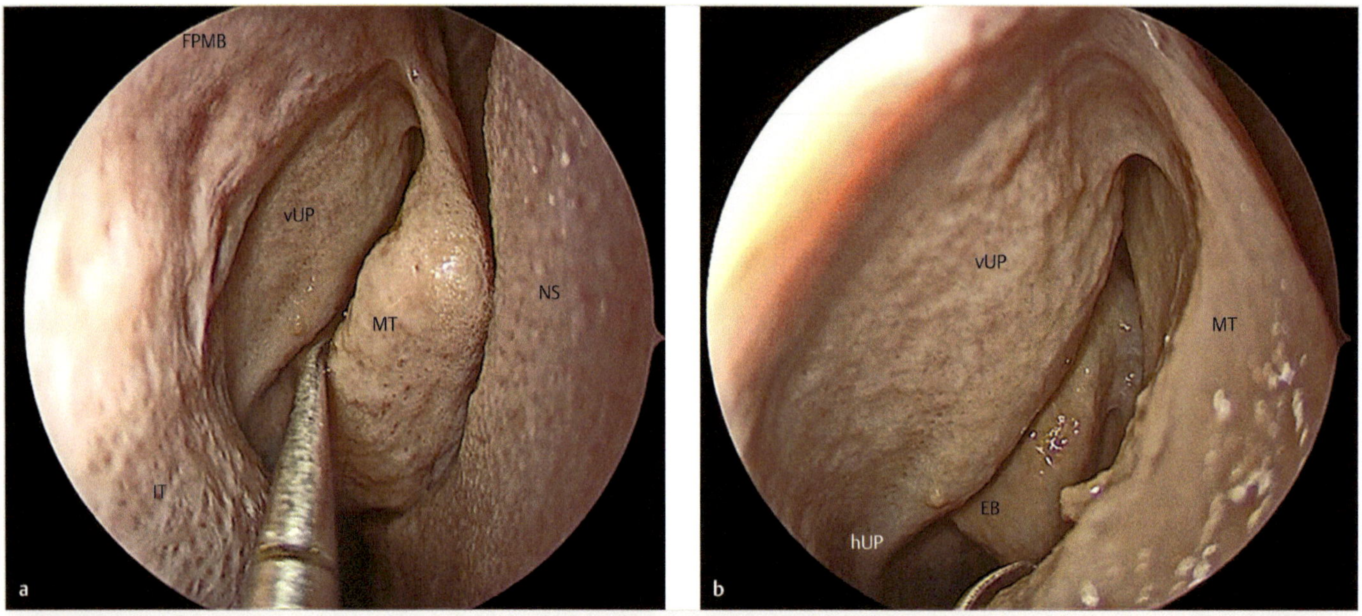

Fig. 2.15 (a, b) Step 6 (part 1). A dissector is used to gently medialize the middle turbinate (MT) and explore the middle meatus. The vertical portion of the uncinate process (vUP) comes firstly into view posterior to the frontal process of the maxillary bone (FPMB). The horizontal portion of the uncinate process (hUP) can be identified more posteriorly. The ethmoid bulla (EB) lies behind the vertical portion and above the horizontal portion of the uncinate process. The vertical portion of the uncinate process and the anterior wall of the ethmoid bulla are the first and second among the five doors of the nasal–ethmoidal–sphenoidal compartment. IT, inferior turbinate; NS, nasal septum.

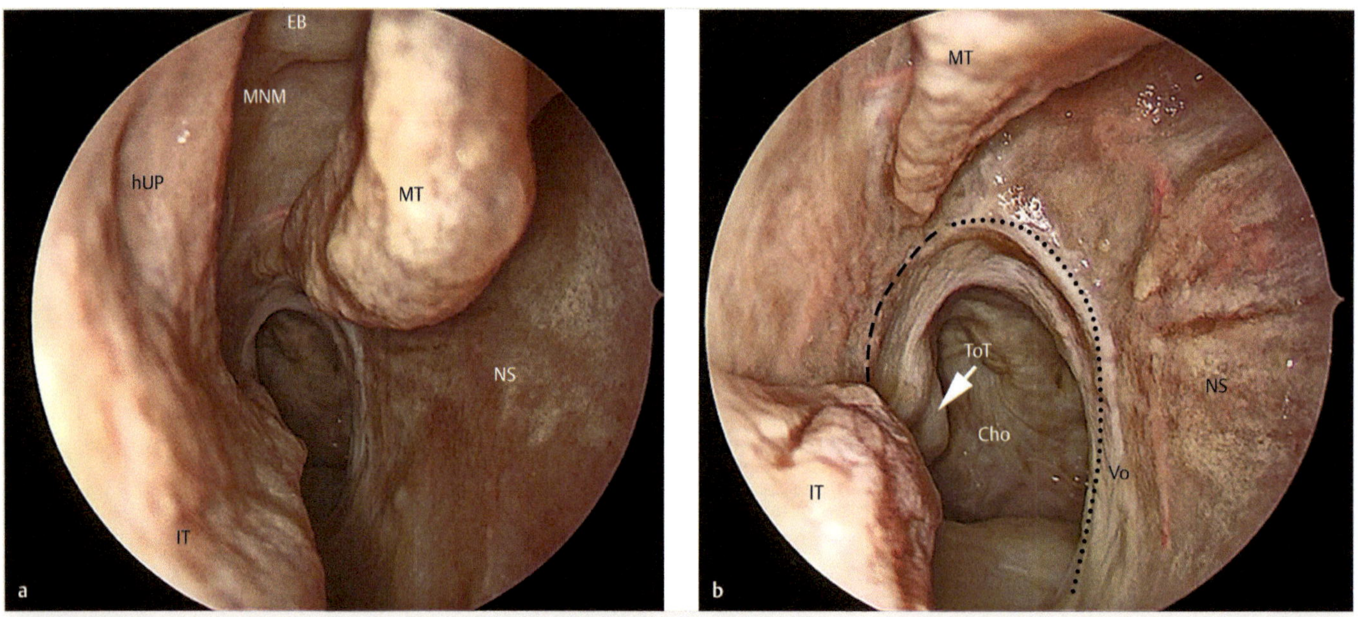

Fig. 2.16 (a, b) Step 6 (part 2). The scope is moved through the middle nasal meatus (MNM) below the ethmoid bulla (EB). The area of the tails of the turbinates is reached proceeding between the horizontal portion of the uncinate process (hUP) and the middle turbinate (MT). The tails of the inferior (IT) and middle turbinate mark the position of the perpendicular process of the palatine bone (*black dashed line*), which forms the choana (Cho) together with the posterolateral margin (*black dotted line*) of the vomer (Vo) and nasal floor. Of note, the tail of the inferior turbinate can be used as a landmark for the torus tubarius (ToT). NS, nasal septum.

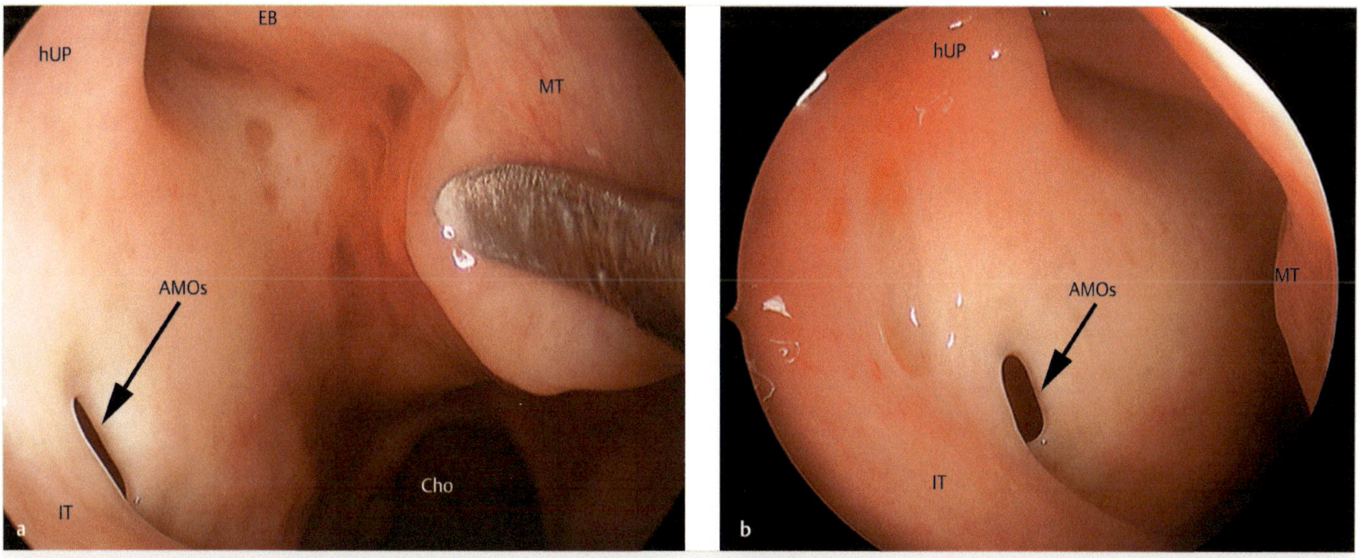

Fig. 2.17 (a, b) Accessory maxillary ostium/ostia. In some cases, a defect along the junction between the horizontal portion of the uncinate process (hUP) and the inferior turbinate (IT) can be identified. This defect(s) is called accessory maxillary ostium (AMOs) and can cause vicious circulation of the mucous coming from the maxillary sinus between the natural and accessory ostia. Cho, choana; EB, ethmoid bulla; MT, middle turbinate.

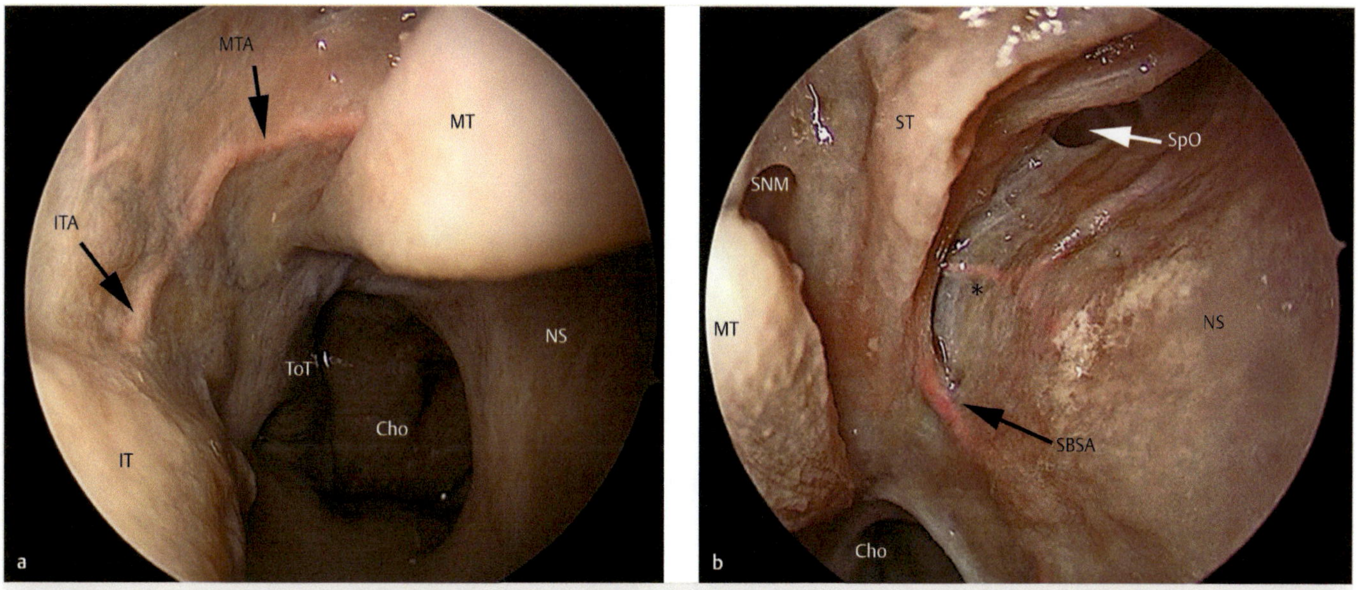

Fig. 2.18 (a, b) Branches of the sphenopalatine artery. Some of the main branches of the sphenopalatine artery can be identified just underneath the mucosa that covers the nasal meati and sphenoethmoidal recess. The inferior (ITA) and middle (MTA) turbinal arteries can be identified in the area of the tails of the turbinates where they run toward the inferior (IT) and middle (MT) turbinates, respectively. The septal branch of the sphenopalatine artery (SBSA) can be identified in the area of the sphenoethmoidal recess and choana (Cho). It runs above the tail of the superior turbinate (ST) toward the nasal septum (NS). Very frequently, a small artery (*black asterisk*) supplying the posterosuperior portion of the nasal septum can be found just inferior to the sphenoid ostium (SpO). This artery can be confused with the septal branch of the sphenopalatine artery. SNM, superior nasal meatus; ToT, torus tubarius.

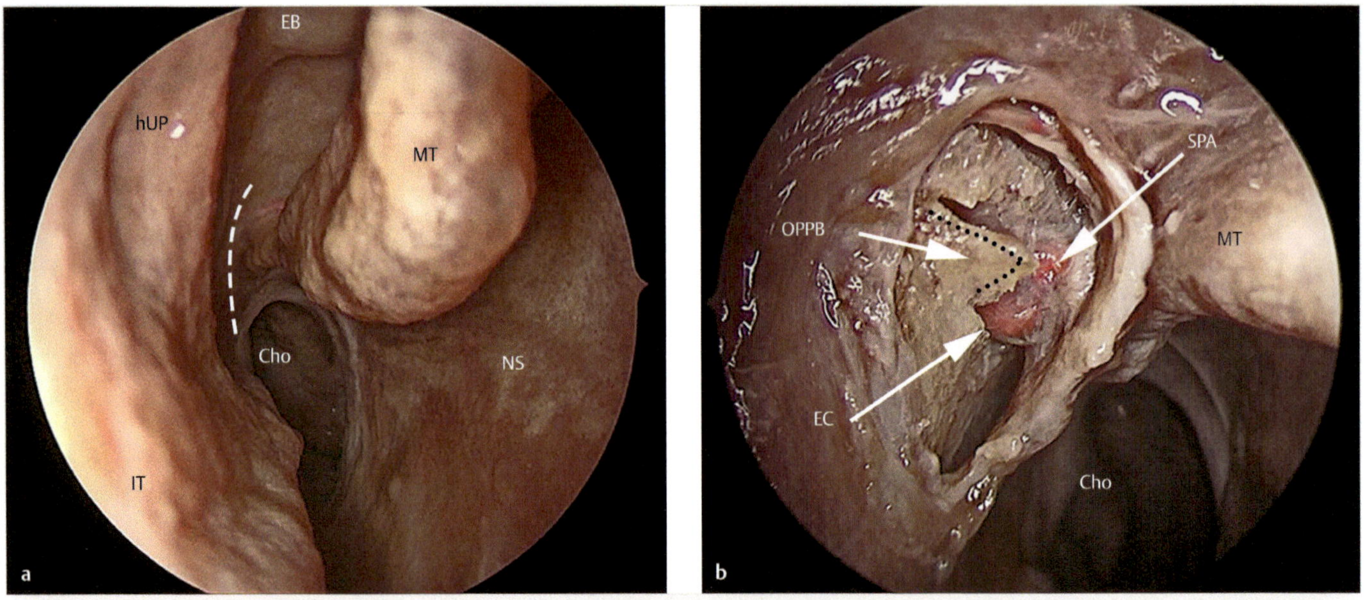

Fig. 2.19 (a, b) Step 7. A small vertical incision (*white dashed line*) is made along the lateral wall of the posterior portion of the middle nasal meatus, in front of the tail of the middle turbinate (MT). By performing a subperiosteal dissection along the orbital process of the palatine bone (OPPB), the anterior portion of the ethmoid crest (EC) is identified. This structure forms a lateral-to-medial pointer (*black dotted line*), which marks the position of the sphenopalatine foramen and the direction of the sphenopalatine artery (SPA). Cho, choana; EB, ethmoid bulla; hUP, horizontal portion of the uncinate process; IT, inferior turbinate; NS, nasal septum.

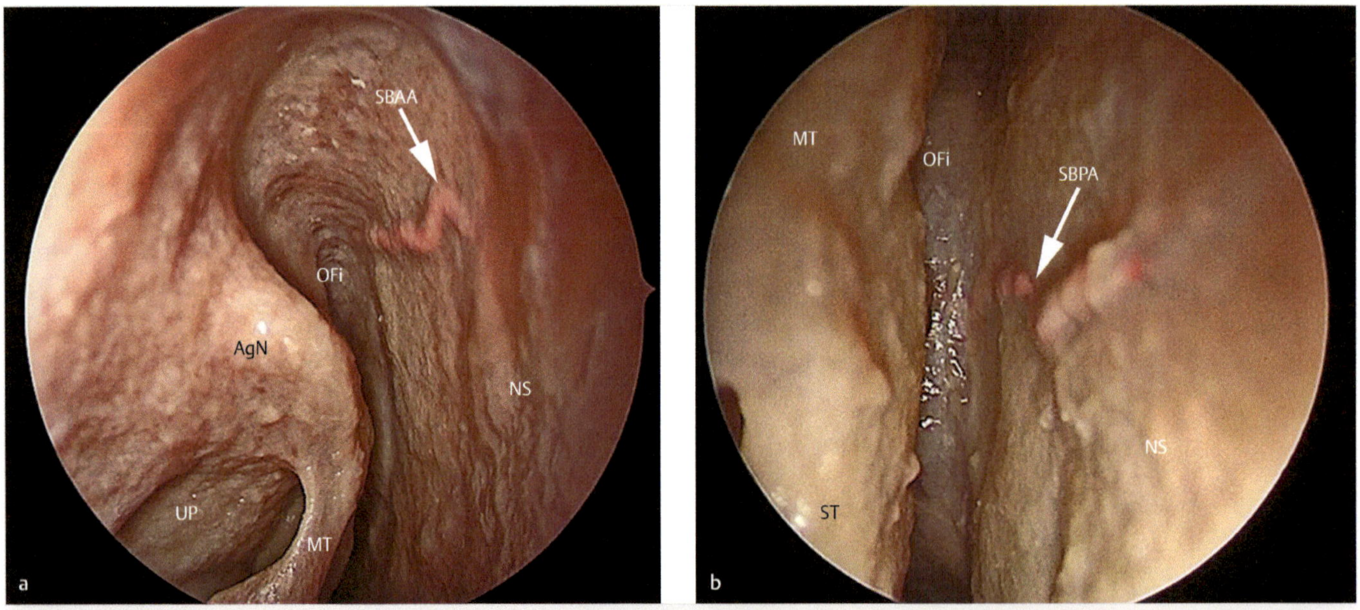

Fig. 2.20 (a, b) Step 8. The superior nasal corridor is limited by the laminar portions of the middle (MT) and superior turbinates (ST) laterally, the superior portion of the nasal septum (NS) medially, and the olfactory fissure (OFi) superiorly. The olfactory fissure houses the olfactory mucosa and lies superior to the level of the axillae of the middle and superior turbinates. The superior nasal corridor can be narrowed by a prominent agger nasi (AgN), deviation of the nasal septum, or hypertrophic Zuckerkandl tubercle. The septal branch of the anterior ethmoidal artery (SBAA) can be identified with a 0-degree scope just underneath the mucosa in the most anterior and superior portion of the nasal septum. The septal branch of the posterior ethmoidal artery (SBPA) is identified with a 70-degree scope turned upward and positioned at the passage between middle and superior turbinates. The former has a diagonal trajectory from posterosuperior to anteroinferior, while the latter runs from cranial to caudal. UP, uncinate process.

References

[1] Stammberger H, Posawetz W. Functional endoscopic sinus surgery. Concept, indications and results of the Messerklinger technique. Eur Arch Otorhinolaryngol 1990;247(2):63–76

[2] Stammberger H. Endoscopic endonasal surgery—concepts in treatment of recurring rhinosinusitis. Part II. Surgical technique. Otolaryngol Head Neck Surg 1986;94(2):147–156

[3] Stammberger H. Endoscopic endonasal surgery—concepts in treatment of recurring rhinosinusitis. Part I. Anatomic and pathophysiologic considerations. Otolaryngol Head Neck Surg 1986;94(2):143–147

[4] Messerklinger W. Background and evolution of endoscopic sinus surgery. Ear Nose Throat J 1994;73(7):449–450

[5] Cavallo LM, de Divitiis O, Aydin S, et al. Extended endoscopic endonasal transsphenoidal approach to the suprasellar area: anatomic considerations—part 1. Neurosurgery 2008;62(6, Suppl 3):1202–1212

[6] Kassam AB, Vescan AD, Carrau RL, et al. Expanded endonasal approach: vidian canal as a landmark to the petrous internal carotid artery. J Neurosurg 2008;108(1):177–183

[7] Kassam A, Snyderman CH, Mintz A, Gardner P, Carrau RL. Expanded endonasal approach: the rostrocaudal axis. Part II. Posterior clinoids to the foramen magnum. Neurosurg Focus 2005;19(1):E4

[8] Kassam A, Snyderman CH, Mintz A, Gardner P, Carrau RL. Expanded endonasal approach: the rostrocaudal axis. Part I. Crista galli to the sella turcica. Neurosurg Focus 2005;19(1):E3

[9] Cavallo LM, Messina A, Cappabianca P, et al. Endoscopic endonasal surgery of the midline skull base: anatomical study and clinical considerations. Neurosurg Focus 2005;19(1):E2

[10] Jho HD, Ha HG. Endoscopic endonasal skull base surgery: part 3—the clivus and posterior fossa. Minim Invasive Neurosurg 2004;47(1):16–23

[11] Jho HD, Ha HG. Endoscopic endonasal skull base surgery: part 2—the cavernous sinus. Minim Invasive Neurosurg 2004;47(1):9–15

[12] Jho HD, Ha HG. Endoscopic endonasal skull base surgery: part 1—the midline anterior fossa skull base. Minim Invasive Neurosurg 2004;47(1):1–8

[13] Magro F, Solari D, Cavallo LM, et al. The endoscopic endonasal approach to the lateral recess of the sphenoid sinus via the pterygopalatine fossa: comparison of endoscopic and radiological landmarks. Neurosurgery 2006;59(4,Suppl 2):ONS237–ONS242, discussion ONS242–ONS243

[14] Sandu K, Monnier P, Pasche P. Anatomical landmarks for transnasal endoscopic skull base surgery. Eur Arch Otorhinolaryngol 2012;269(1):171–178

3 Corridor to the Anterior Skull Base and Orbit

Davide Mattavelli, Giacomo Bertazzoni, Alberto Schreiber, Marco Ravanelli, Luca Pianta

The corridor toward midline anterior skull base and orbit is mostly formed by the ethmoid and frontal sinus. In addition, the sphenoid sinus serves as a natural corridor toward the most posterior portion of the anterior skull base (i.e., planum sphenoidale and tuberculum sellae), but this pathway will be discussed in Chapter 4. The dissection of the ethmoid complex is usually divided into three parts: dissection of the frontal recess, removal of the bullar complex, and dissection of the posterior ethmoid. As in functional endoscopic sinus surgery, these different types of ethmoidectomy can be combined to expose the adjacent skull base based on the specific needs.

The frontal recess consists of the space between the anterior bullar wall posteriorly, frontal process of the maxillary bone anteriorly, middle turbinate medially, and medial orbital wall laterally (mostly by the pars orbitalis ossis frontalis; see below).[1] This space is compartmentalized by insertions of the uncinate process. The air chambers formed by these insertions, which are overall referred to as the agger complex,[2] are intimately adjacent to the drainage pathway of the frontal sinus. The anatomy of the frontal recess is exceedingly variable, including a number of variants that were thoroughly studied and described during the last decades. Since the first attempt of categorizing these air spaces by Kuhn in 1996,[3] it took 20 years to reach a unanimous classification, namely the International Frontal Sinus Anatomy Classification.[4] The different air spaces that can be found result from the variable anatomy of the uncinate process. The agger nasi cell is the most anterior air space of the anterior ethmoid; more precisely, it should be defined as the agger nasi cell only when the air space reaches the *agger nasi*, which is a lateral-to-medial prominence of the frontal process of the maxillary bone where the head of the middle turbinate is inserted. Otherwise, this cell is called the lacrimal cell when it does not extend anteriorly and remains confined nearby the lacrimal fossa. In the same area, a funnel-shaped space with a dead end, called the terminal recess, can be identified instead of agger nasi or lacrimal cell. The supra-agger cell is an air space lying above the agger nasi cell, lacrimal cell, and/or terminal recess. When extended cranially so far that it exceeds the axial plane passing through the floor of the frontal sinus, this cell is defined as the supra-agger frontal cell. An air space extending cranially and pneumatizing the interfrontal sinus septum is called the frontal septal cell. Of note, all these air spaces are formed according to the variable and multiple insertions of the uncinate process, which has been consequently described as a palmlike structure.[5] While getting closer to the frontal ostium (the narrowest area between the frontal recess and frontal sinus), the uncinate process inserts posteriorly onto the anterior bullar wall forming the suprainfundibular plate, which in turn can be used as a landmark to define the drainage pathway of the frontal sinus as medial or lateral to the uncinate process.[6] Supra-agger (frontal) and frontal septal cells are usually associated with a medial and lateral drainage pathway, respectively; these associations can be considered a hallmark of different developmental mechanisms of the frontal recess.[7–9] In addition to these variants, the middle turbinate can be variably pneumatized: when the pneumatization is limited to the laminar portion, the air space is called interlamellar Grunwald cell; when the air extends to the bulbous portion, the turbinate is defined as concha bullosa.

From a surgical perspective, different degrees of clearance of the frontal recess were described by Draf[10]: Draf type I frontal sinusotomy consists of a simple dissection of the frontal recess without enlargement of the frontal ostium. In Draf type II frontal

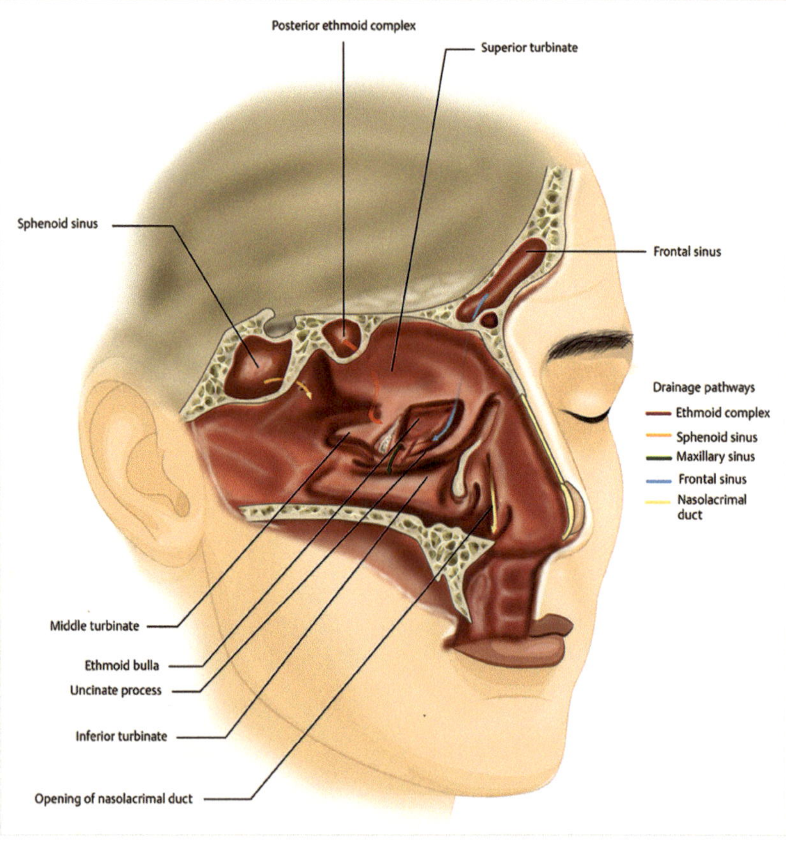

Fig. 3.1 Schematic architecture of the nasal cavity and paranasal sinuses.

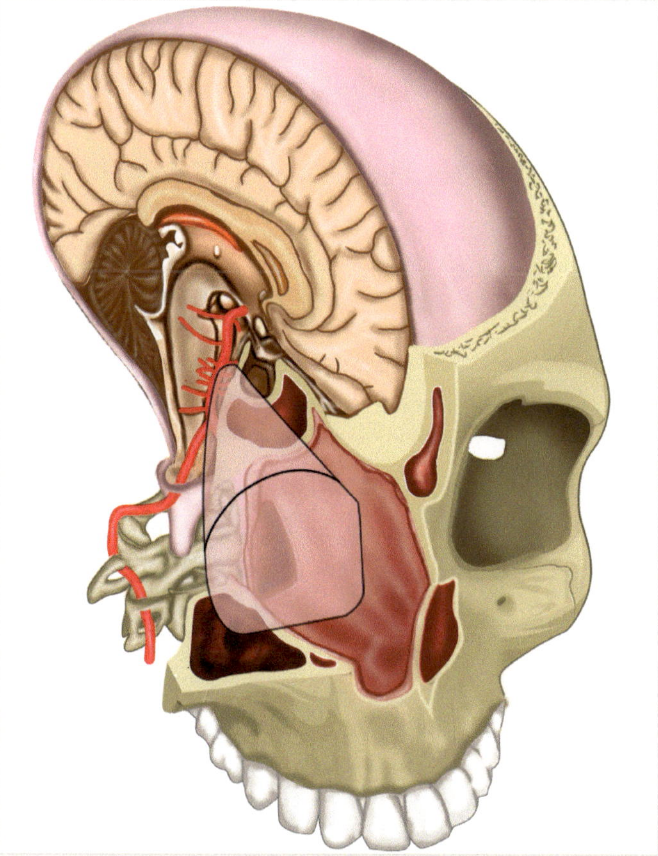

Fig. 3.2 Diagonal view of the transnasal corridor toward anterior skull base and orbit. This drawing shows the position of the transnasal corridor toward anterior skull base and orbit with respect to other sinonasal and skull base structures.

sinusotomy, the frontal ostium is widened by simply removing frontal cells and/or mildly enlarging the frontal ostium with a punch (type IIa) or by entirely removing the medial portion of the floor of the targeted frontal sinus (type IIb), which is called frontal beak due to its peaked shape. Draf type III frontal sinusotomy consists in merging the frontal sinuses through an anterosuperior septal window, with bilateral removal of the frontal beak and interfrontal sinus septum.

The bullar complex is a group of air spaces enclosed between the anterior bullar wall anteriorly, basal lamella of the middle turbinate posteriorly, middle turbinate medially, and medial orbital wall laterally.[2] Frequently, air spaces within the bullar complex are disposed in a cranial–caudal fashion, with the cells that are adjacent to the skull base being called suprabullar cells. The latter can extend within the orbital roof or toward the frontal sinus, thus acquiring the name of supraorbital ethmoid cell or suprabullar frontal cell, respectively. When a suprabullar frontal cell is encountered, the frontal ostium is narrowed and pushed anteriorly. By virtue of its relationship with the medial orbital wall and anterior skull base, the safest area to begin the dissection of the bullar complex is at the inferior–medial corner. In some cases, surgical access to the frontal sinus requires the dissection of this area, especially when the bullar complex, by protruding anteriorly, hampers surgical maneuvers with curved instruments. Otherwise, an intact bulla frontal sinusotomy can be performed.[11]

Given the anatomical variability of the frontoethmoidal area, some information must be collected before dissecting the frontal sinus. In particular, keeping in mind the medial or lateral position of the frontal sinus drainage pathway is of utmost importance. Indeed, the dissection is performed by marsupializing the air spaces that surround the drainage pathway in a centrifugal fashion, proceeding from the middle nasal meatus to the frontal sinus. The total number of air spaces to be opened and the presence of cells extending toward the frontal sinus are also important. The agger-bullar classification is a valuable tool to systematically assess these anatomic features before and during surgery.[2] This classification was aimed at providing a systematic, anatomic approach to perform endoscopic frontal sinusotomy.

The boundaries of the posterior ethmoid are the basal lamella of the middle turbinate anteriorly, basal lamella of the superior turbinate posteriorly, superior turbinate medially, and medial orbital wall laterally. The sphenoethmoidal recess is a narrow space lying between the basal lamella of the superior turbinate and the anterior sphenoidal wall. The widest anatomical variability in the posterior ethmoid is found at its posterior limit. In well-pneumatized posterior ethmoids, the superior turbinate ends posteriorly onto the anterior sphenoidal wall, just lateral to the sphenoidal ostium, and the sphenoethmoidal recess is absent. When the pneumatization of the posterior ethmoid exceeds the anterior wall of the sphenoid sinus in an anterior-to-posterior direction, it forms a sphenoethmoidal cell called the Onodi cell. The latter is formally defined only if the air space is in contact with the optic canal. In poorly pneumatized posterior ethmoids, the basal lamella of the superior turbinate turns laterally toward the medial orbital wall and the sphenoethmoidal recess takes shape. In these cases, an additional turbinate, called supreme turbinate, can be found within the sphenoethmoidal recess.

Particular attention should be taken when dissecting the lateral, superior, and medial boundaries of the ethmoid compartments.

The lateral boundary is the medial orbital wall, which is made up of bones with variable thickness. The anterior portion of the medial orbital wall is formed by the lacrimal bone inferiorly and *pars orbitalis ossis frontalis* superiorly, the former being very thin and the latter thick similar to the ethmoidal and orbital roofs. The posterior portion of the medial orbital wall is the lamina papyracea, which is usually thin as suggested by the name deriving from the Latin term *papyrus*.

The superior boundary of anterior and posterior ethmoids is formed by the ethmoidal roof (also defined fovea ethmoidalis), which is a thick lamina of the frontal bone. The ethmoidal arteries run from the ethmoidal foramina to the olfactory groove parallel to the ethmoidal roof. They are usually two, one per ethmoidal compartment; however, a middle ethmoidal artery can be found in 29 to 38% of cases.[12–14] The cranial–caudal position with respect to the ethmoidal roof and anteroposterior position with respect to ethmoidal lamellae is variable: the anterior ethmoidal artery runs most frequently below the skull base and along the basal lamella of the middle turbinate; consequently, the anterior ethmoidal artery cannot be exposed when the bullar complex is left completely intact; the posterior and middle ethmoidal arteries lie mostly within the skull base and in a variable location between the basal lamella of the middle turbinate and anterior sphenoidal wall.[12]

The medial boundary of the ethmoidal box is formed by the middle turbinate, superior turbinate, their common lamella (also called conchal plate),[15] and the vertical portion of the cribriform plate. The latter structure is so delicate that it is considered the *locus minoris resistentiae* of the entire skull base.[16] Moreover, its cranial–caudal length and grade of tilting are remarkably variable and considerably affect the risk of skull base injury during sinus surgery.

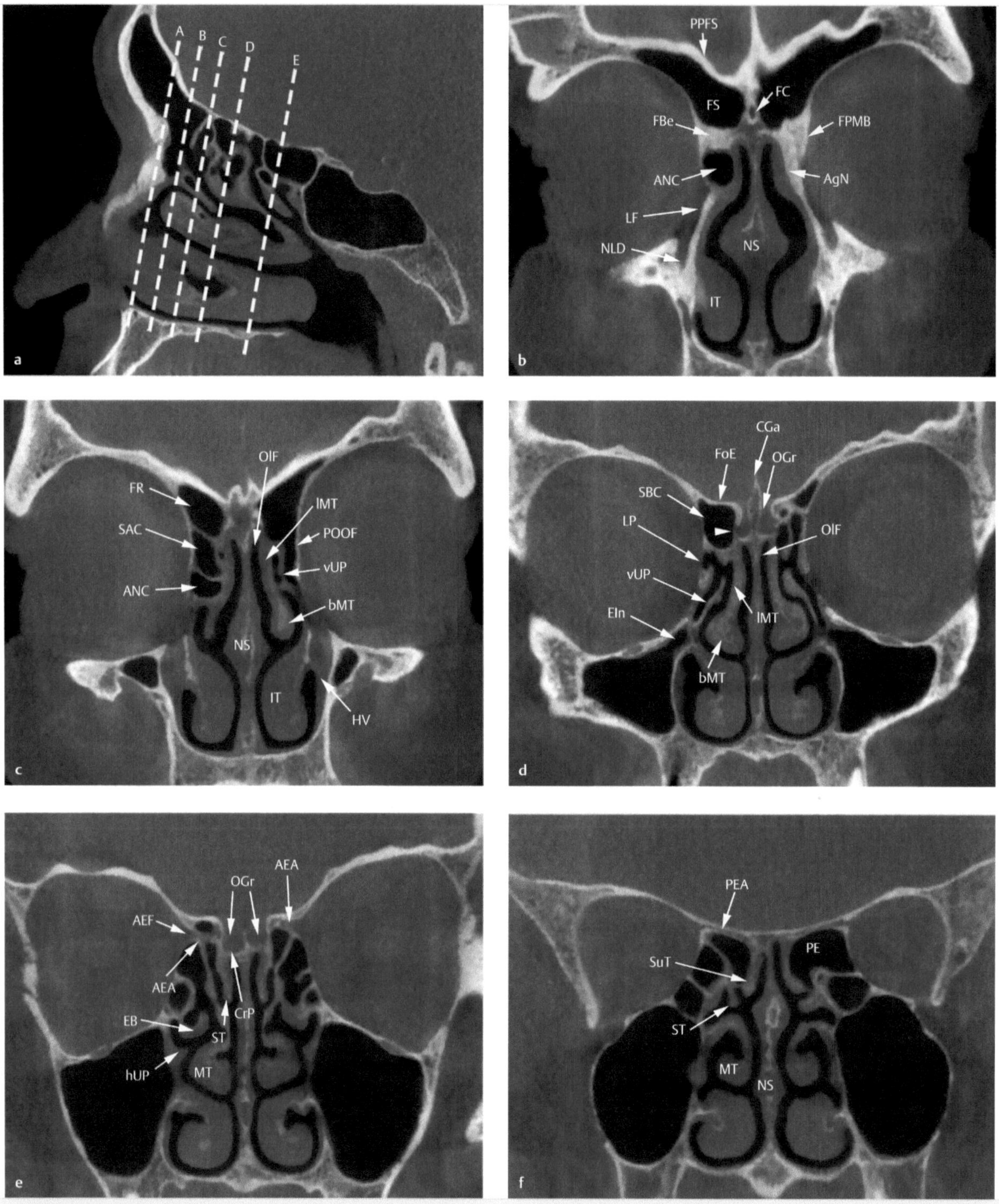

Fig. 3.3 Coronal CT anatomy of the nasoethmoidal box. The panel includes one sagittal scan **(a)** depicting the position of five coronal scans **(b–f)** with *white dashed lines*, which are disposed from anterior to posterior along the nasoethmoidal complex. The agger nasi cell (ANC) is the pneumatization of the agger nasi (AgN), which is a small bony ridge of the frontal process of the maxillary bone (FPMB) that serves as insertion for the middle turbinate (MT). The anterior ethmoidal complex is formed by several air spaces bounded by the palmlike insertions of the vertical portion of the uncinate process (vUP) onto the boundaries of the ethmoidal box, which are the lacrimal fossa (LF) and lamina papyracea (LP) laterally, the laminar portion of the middle turbinate (lMT) medially, and the fovea ethmoidalis (FoE) superiorly (also defined ethmoidal roof). Moreover, the posterior portion of the anterior ethmoidal complex is compartmentalized by the air spaces composing the ethmoidal bulla (EB). The posterior ethmoidal complex (PE) is located posterior and superior to the basal lamella of the middle turbinate and is bounded medially by the superior turbinate (ST). The anterior (AEA) and posterior ethmoidal arteries (PEA) are located in the anterior and posterior ethmoidal compartment, respectively. These vessels run in bony canals that can be variably located with respect to the fovea ethmoidalis. In this case, the right anterior ethmoidal artery runs caudally to the fovea ethmoidalis, whereas the canal of the left artery is included in the skull base. The ethmoidal canals arise from a foramen in the lamina papyracea, which is usually located along the frontoethmoidal suture, and end in a small defect (*white arrowhead*) of the vertical lamella of the cribriform plate (CrP). This defect is also called ethmoidal sulcus. The two olfactory fissures (OlF) are located on the midline and separated by the nasal septum (NS). Laterally, the olfactory fissures are delimited by the laminar portion of the middle and superior turbinate. Superiorly, they face the horizontal lamina of the cribriform plate, which serves as the caudal limit of the olfactory grooves (OGr). AEF, anterior ethmoidal foramen; bMT, bulbous portion of the middle turbinate; CGa, crista galli; Eln, ethmoidal infundibulum; FBe, frontal beak; FC, foramen coecum; FR, frontal recess; FS, frontal sinus; hUP, horizontal portion of the uncinate process; HV, Hasner's valve; IT, inferior turbinate; NLD, nasolacrimal duct; POOF, pars orbitalis ossis frontalis; PPFS, posterior plate of the frontal sinus; SAC, supra-agger cell; SBC, suprabullar cell; SuT, supreme turbinate.

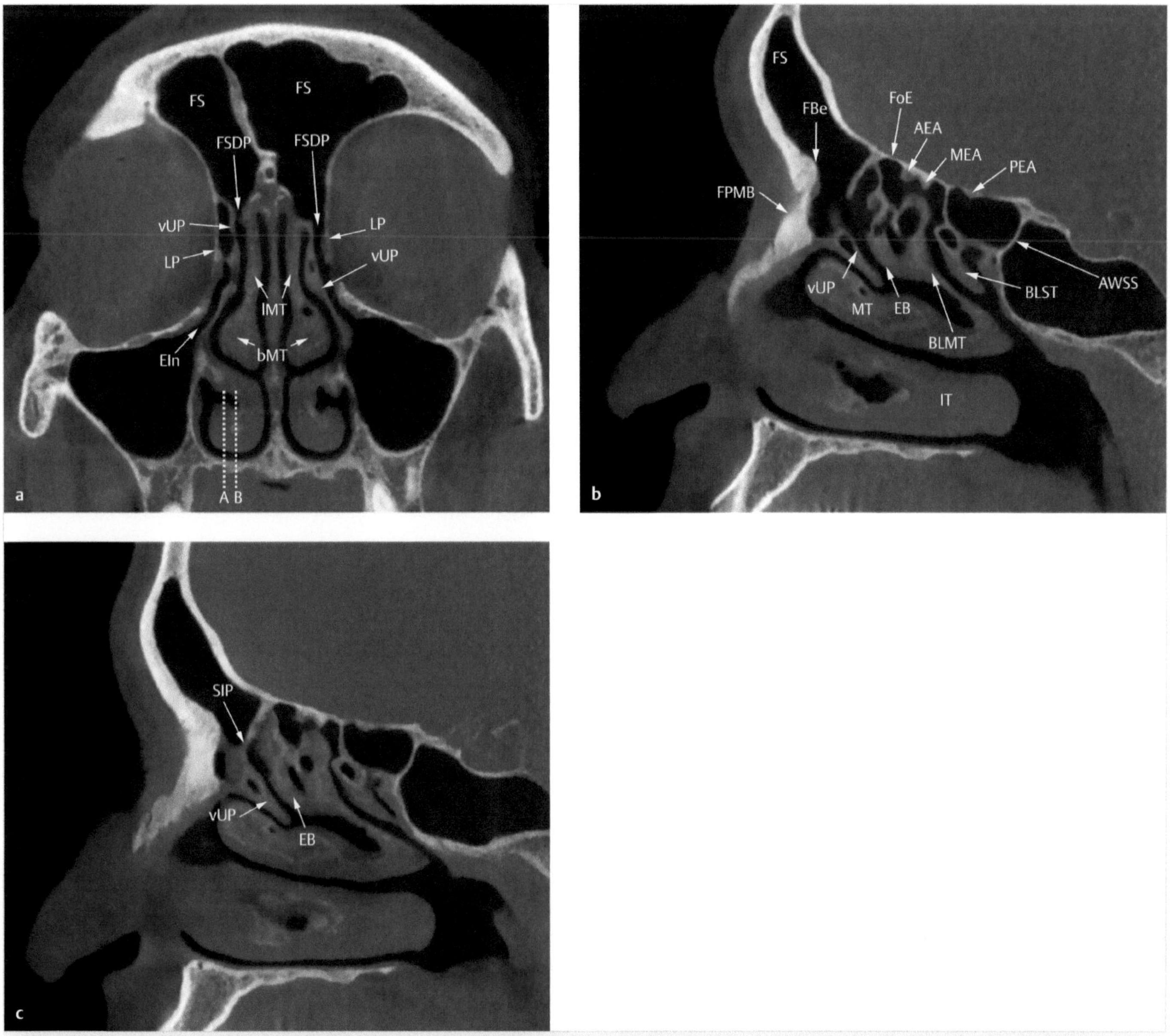

Fig. 3.4 Paracoronal and sagittal CT anatomy of anatomic variants of the nasoethmoidal box (part 1). The panel includes one paracoronal **(a)** scan passing through the frontal sinus drainage pathways (FSDP) and depicting the position (A, B) of two sagittal images **(b, c)** with *white dotted lines*. The frontal sinus drainage pathway can be located either medial (right side of **a**) or lateral (left side of **a**) to the cranial insertion of the vertical portion of the uncinate process (vUP). As seen on a coronal/paracoronal plane, this insertion can be variably located on the lamina papyracea (LP), fovea ethmoidalis (FoE), cribriform plate, and laminar (lMT) or bulbous portion of the middle turbinate (bMT). On a sagittal plane, this insertion, which is also called suprainfundibular plate (SIP) due to its cranial position with respect to the ethmoidal infundibulum (EIn), anchors to the anterior wall of the ethmoidal bulla (EB). As seen on a sagittal scan, the nasoethmoidal complex can be described based on five bony lamellae disposed from anterior to posterior: the uncinate process, anterior wall of the ethmoidal bulla, basal lamella of the middle turbinate (BLMT), basal lamella of the superior turbinate (BLST), and anterior wall of the sphenoid sinus (AWSS). The anterior ethmoid is located between the frontal process of the maxillary bone (FPMB) anteriorly and basal lamella of the middle turbinate posteriorly. The vertical portion of the uncinate process compartmentalizes the most anterior portion of the anterior ethmoid forming several air spaces, whereas the ethmoidal bulla makes up a number of chambers in the posterior portion of the anterior ethmoidal complex. The posterior ethmoidal complex is enclosed between the basal lamellae of the middle turbinate anteriorly and superior turbinate posteriorly. The sphenoethmoidal recess is located between the basal lamella of the superior turbinate and the anterior wall of the sphenoid sinus. In addition to the anterior (AEA) and posterior ethmoidal arteries (PEA), the middle ethmoidal artery (MEA) can be found in around one-third of patients. FBe, frontal beak; FS, frontal sinus; IT, inferior turbinate.

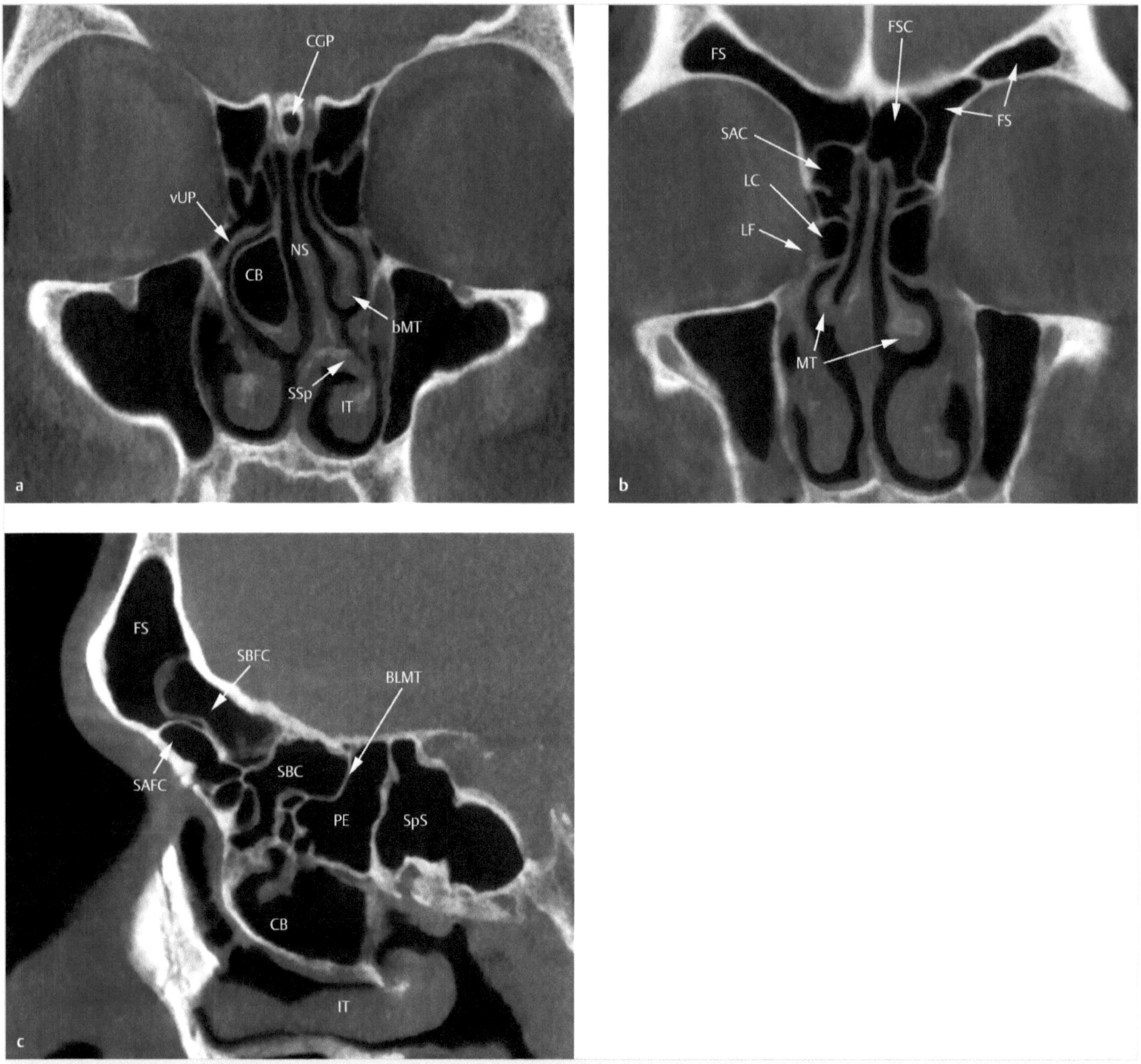

Fig. 3.5 Coronal and sagittal CT anatomy of anatomic variants of the nasoethmoidal box (part 2). The panel includes two coronal **(a, b)** and one sagittal **(c)** CT scans, showing the most relevant anatomic variants of the nasoethmoidal complex. Most of the anatomic variability in this area relies on the pattern of pneumatization of the nasoethmoidal box. The bulbous portion of the middle turbinate (bMT) can be pneumatized to form the concha bullosa (CB), which can remarkably narrow the middle and superior nasal corridors and is frequently associated with a contralateral septal deviation. The most anterior and inferior air space of the anterior ethmoidal complex is defined as lacrimal cell (LC) due to its adjacency to the lacrimal fossa. When this space is sufficiently extended anterior to reach the agger nasi, it is defined as the agger nasi cell. Air spaces located above the lacrimal cell or agger nasi cell are classified according to their craniocaudal extension with respect to the floor of the frontal sinus (FS): simple supra-agger cells (SAC) are limited to the anterior ethmoidal complex, whereas supra-agger frontal cells (SAFC) extend cranially to the floor of frontal sinus. Of note, all the above-mentioned cells are bounded by the multiple insertions of the vertical portion of the uncinate process (vUP). The pneumatization process can also extend to midline structures such as the interfrontal sinus septum and crista galli, forming the frontal septal cell (FSC) and pneumatized crista galli (CGP), respectively. The ethmoidal bulla is formed by a variable number of air spaces. Conventionally, the most inferior, anterior, and medial air space is defined as ethmoidal bullar cell. Air spaces located above this cell are defined as suprabullar cells (SBC) or suprabullar frontal cell (SBFC) when further extended to reach the posterior plate of the frontal sinus. BLMT, basal lamella of the middle turbinate; IT, inferior turbinate; MT, middle turbinate; PE, posterior ethmoidal complex; SpS, sphenoid sinus; SSp, septal spur.

Endoscopic Dissection

- Step 1: Partial middle turbinectomy (a) or concha bullosa plasty (b).
- Step 2: Anterograde (a) or retrograde (b) vertical uncinectomy.
- Step 3: Draf I frontal sinusotomy (partial anterior ethmoidectomy).
- Step 4: Draf IIa frontal sinusotomy.
- Step 5: Draf IIb frontal sinusotomy.
- Step 6: Draf III frontal sinusotomy.
- Step 7: Section of the anterior ethmoidal artery and orbital transposition.
- Step 8: Removal of the ethmoidal bulla (complete anterior ethmoidectomy).
- Step 9: Posterior ethmoidectomy.

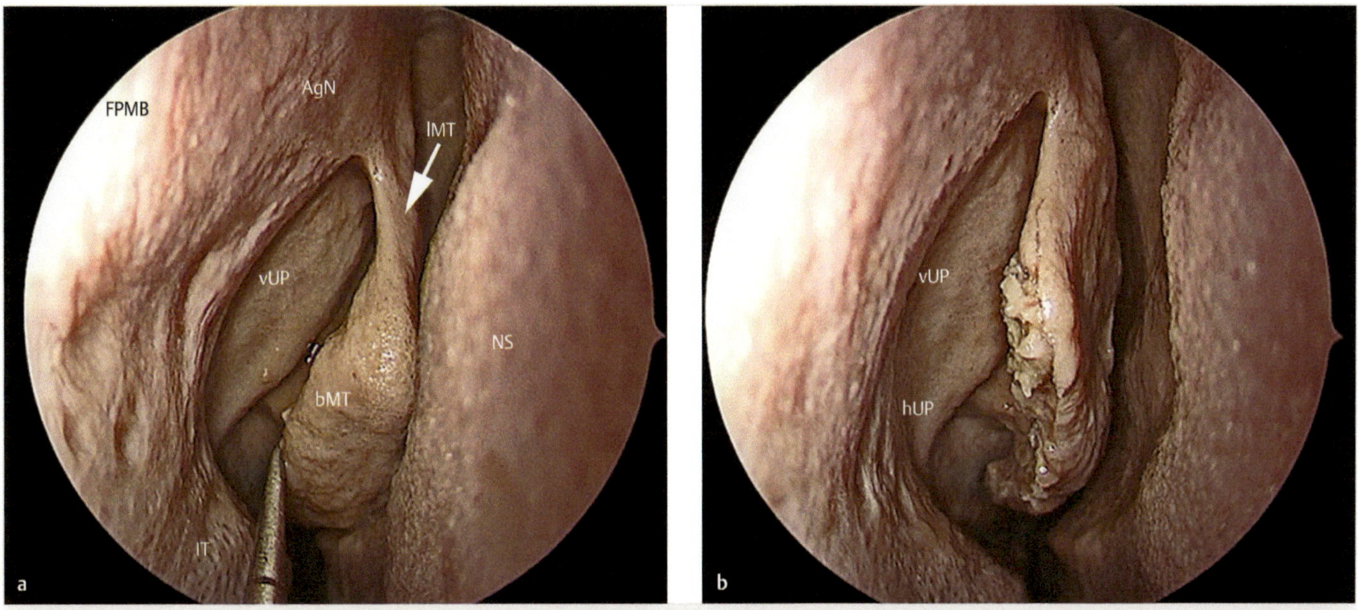

Fig. 3.6 (a, b) Step 1a. The bulbous portion of the middle turbinate (bMT) is gently displaced toward the nasal septum (NS) to expose the vertical portion of the uncinate process (vUP). The access to the middle meatus is bordered by the inferior turbinate (IT) inferiorly, frontal process of the maxillary bone (FPMB) laterally, agger nasi (AgN) superiorly, and laminar (lMT) and bulbous portions of the middle turbinate (bMT) medially. The partial resection of the bulbous portion of the middle turbinate improves the exposure toward the middle meatus. hUP, horizontal portion of the uncinate process.

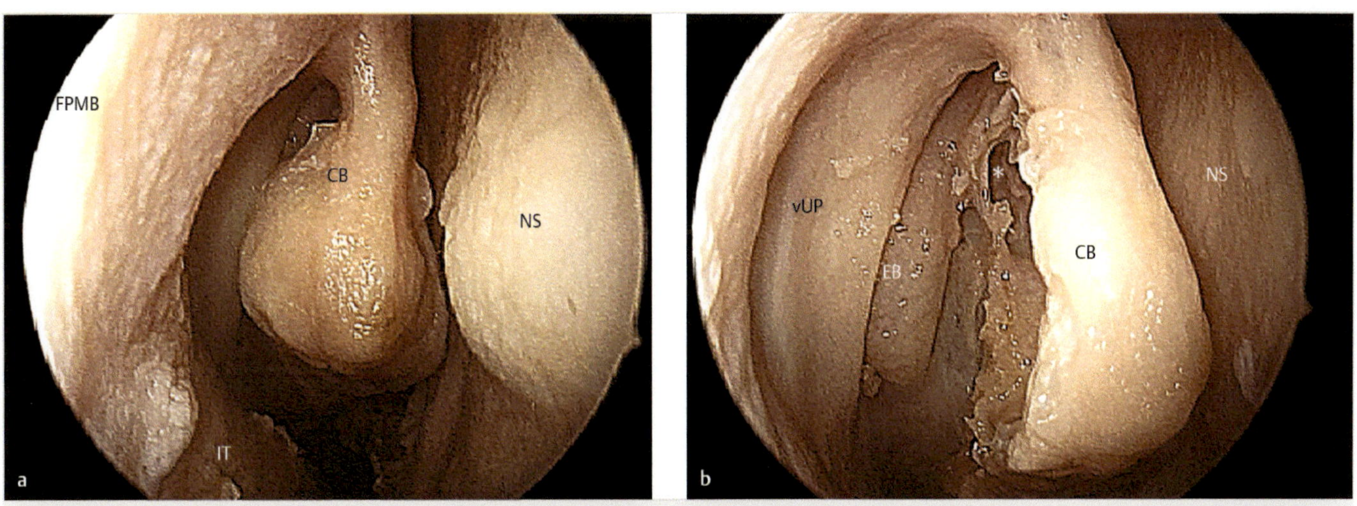

Fig. 3.7 (a, b) Step 1b. The concha bullosa (CB) results from pneumatization of the bulbous portion of the middle turbinate. The removal of the lateral wall of the concha provides optimal exposure of the middle meatus. After this step, the vertical portion of the uncinate process (vUP) and the ethmoid bulla (EB) can be easily identified. Usually, the pneumatization of the middle turbinate originates from the posterior ethmoidal air spaces (*white asterisk*). FPMB, frontal process of the maxillary bone; IT, inferior turbinate; NS, nasal septum.

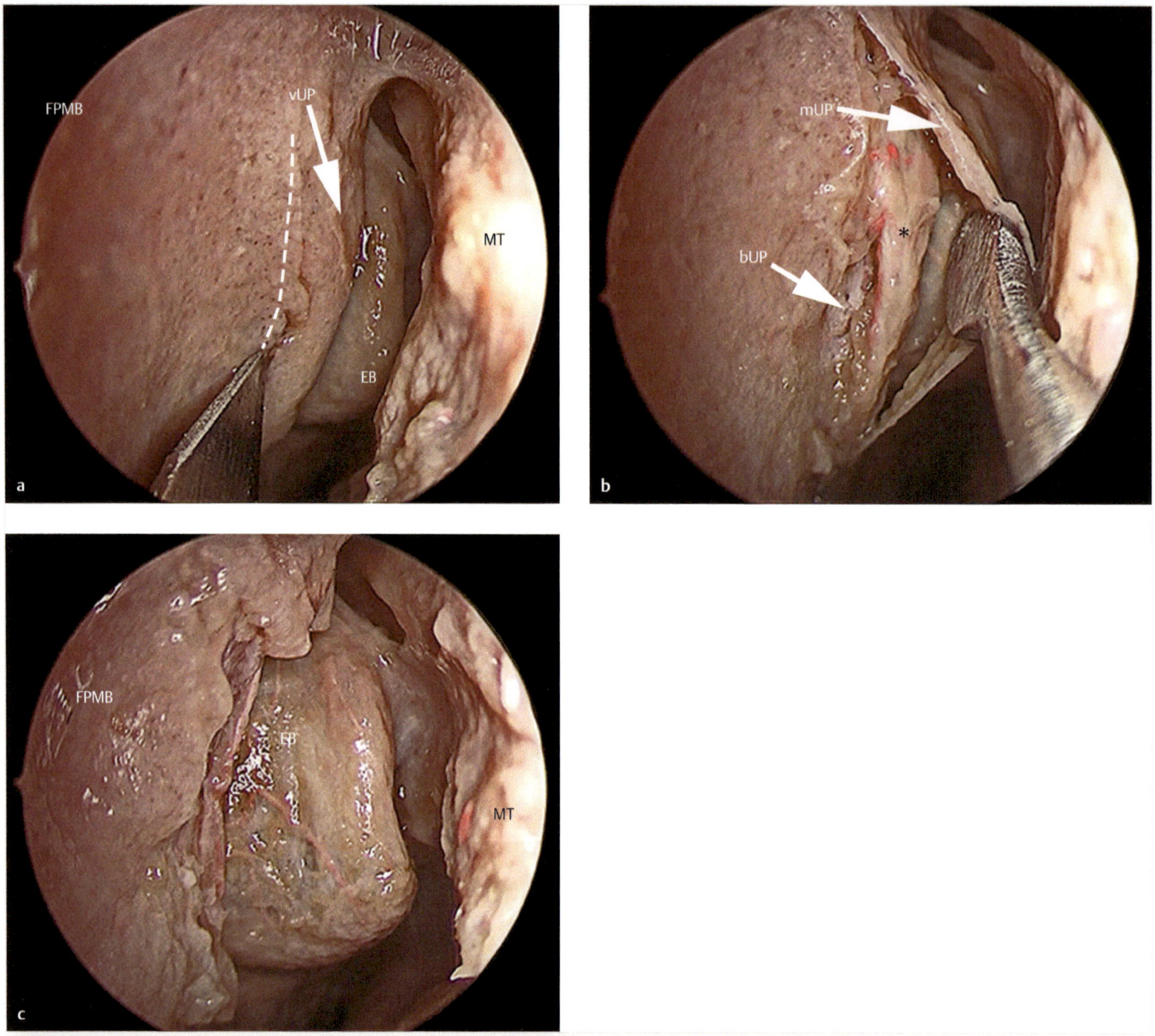

Fig. 3.8 (a–c) Step 2a. The vertical portion of the uncinate process (vUP) is incised along the maxillary line (*white dashed line*). A dissector can be used to elevate the mucosa (mUP) over the bony uncinate process (bUP). With this maneuver, neural and vascular structures running parallel to the uncinate process can be identified (*black asterisk*). Then, the dissector is pushed into the ethmoidal infundibulum and the vertical portion of the uncinate process is removed to fully expose the ethmoid bulla (EB).

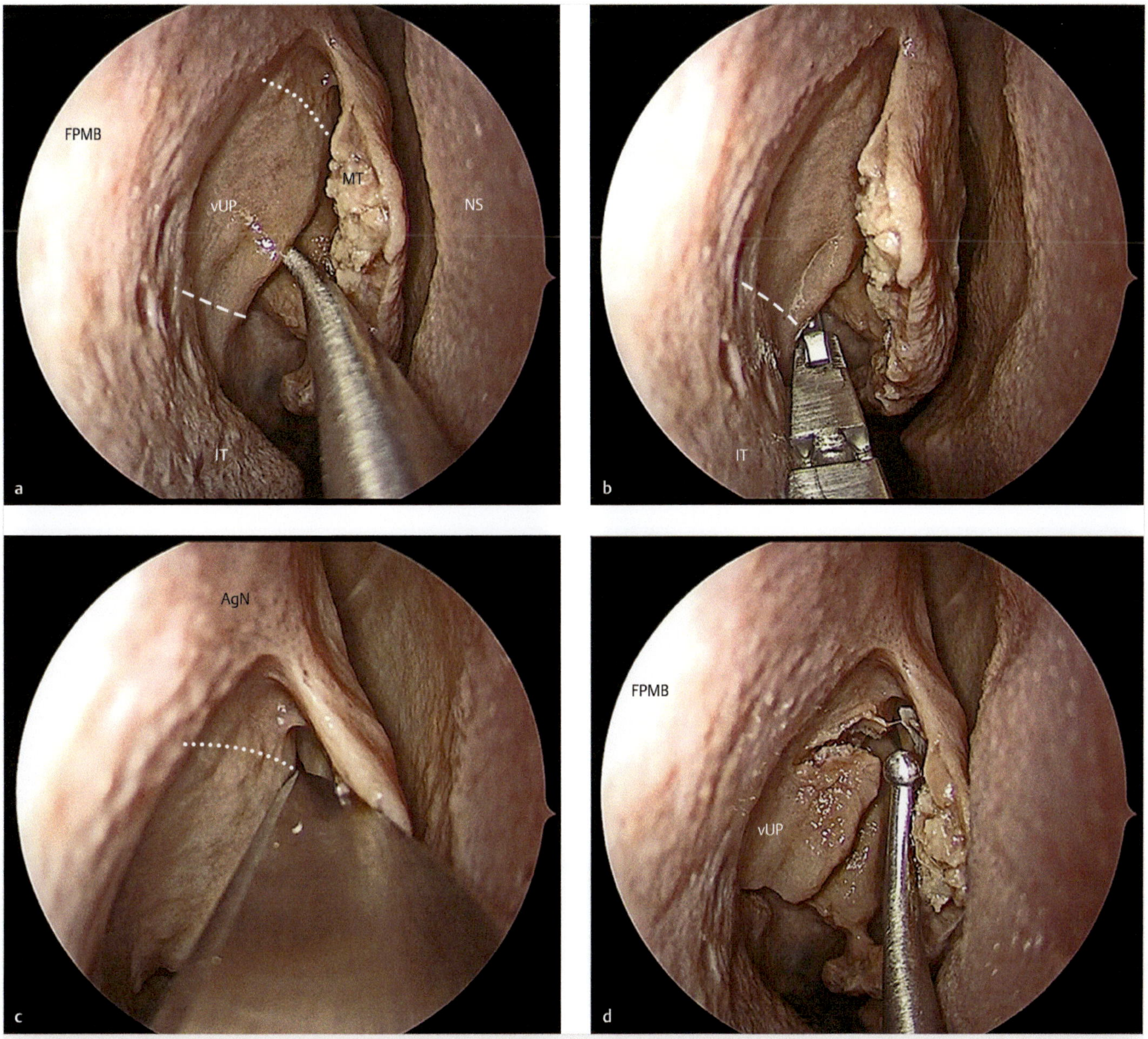

Fig. 3.9 (a–d) Step 2b (part 1). A ball probe is inserted around the free edge of the vertical portion of the uncinate process (vUP) into the ethmoidal infundibulum. The uncinate process is then fractured anteriorly. Superior (*white dotted line*) and inferior (*white dashed line*) uncinotomies are made at the level of the axilla of the middle turbinate and inferior border of the ethmoid bulla, respectively. A backbiting punch is inserted in the ethmoidal infundibulum to perform the inferior uncinotomy. A cutting instrument is then used to make the superior uncinotomy. FPMB, frontal process of the maxillary bone; IT, inferior turbinate; MT, middle turbinate; NS, nasal septum.

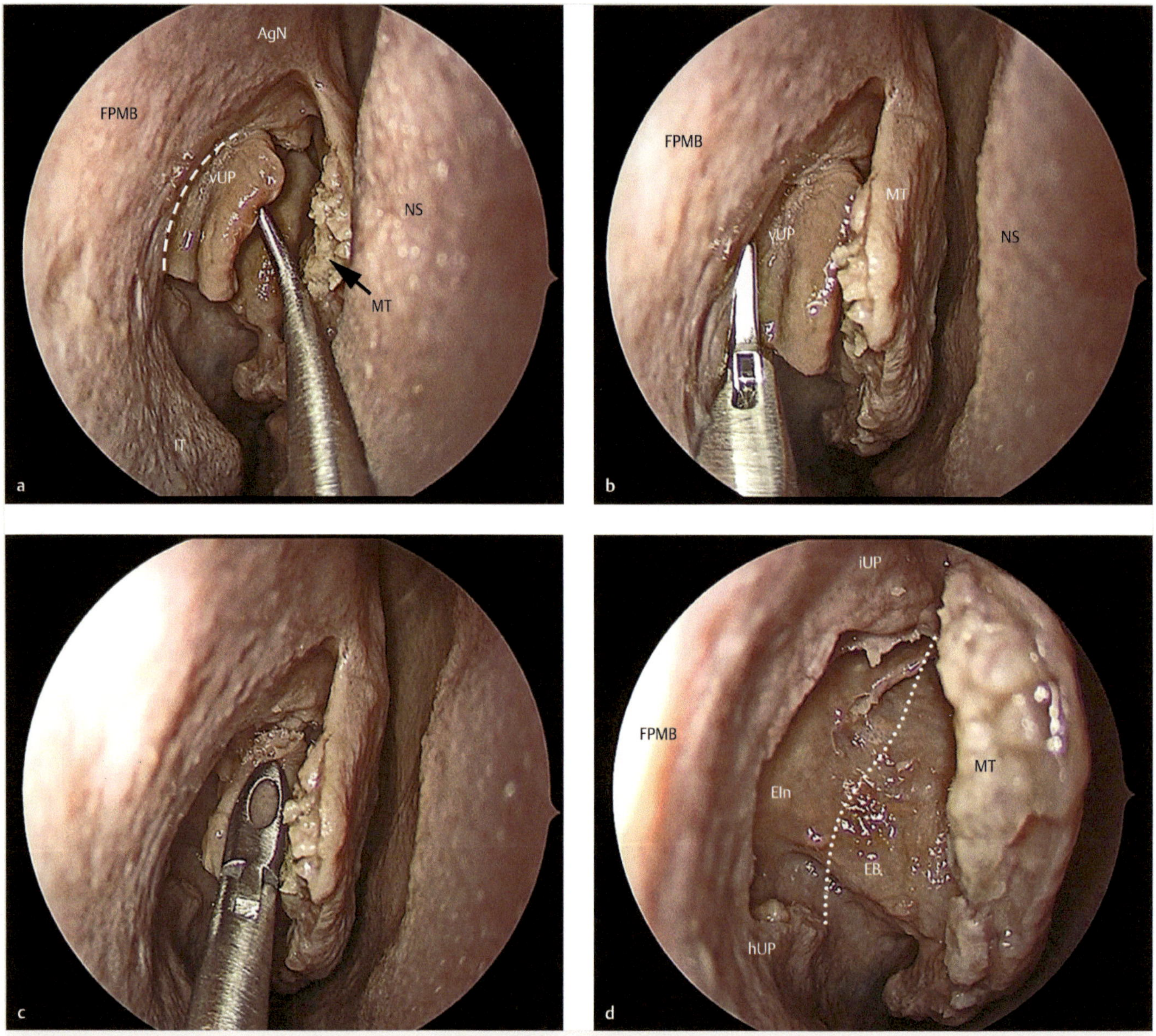

Fig. 3.10 (a–d) Step 2b (part 2). The vertical portion of the uncinate process (vUP) is moved anteriorly to highlight its anterior insertion (*white dashed line*) on the frontal process of the maxillary bone (FPMB) and lacrimal bone. The anterior insertion of the uncinate process is cut with an upward cutting instrument and the vertical uncinectomy is completed. The *white dotted line* outlines the previous position of the free edge of the uncinate process. AgN, agger nasi; EB, ethmoid bulla; EIn, ethmoidal infundibulum; hUP, horizontal portion of the uncinate process; iUP, cranial insertion of the uncinate process; IT, inferior turbinate; MT, middle turbinate; NS, nasal septum.

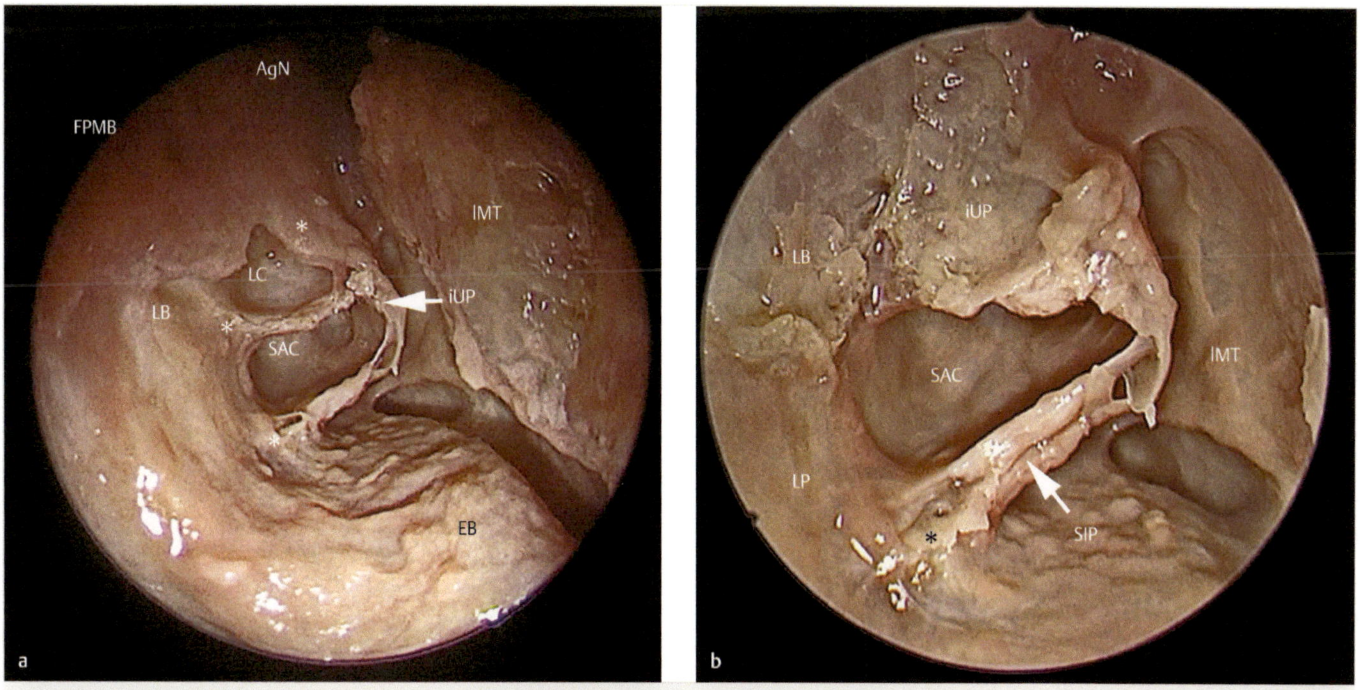

Fig. 3.11 (a, b) The palmlike framework of the uncinate process. A 45-degree scope is inserted in the middle meatus to explore the area of cranial insertion of the uncinate process (iUP). The anatomy of this region is highly variable and several variants are shown in the present and following figures. The cranial insertions (*white asterisks*) of the uncinate process are usually numerous and can attach to the frontal process of the maxillary bone (FPMB), lacrimal bone (LB), lamina papyracea (LP), laminar portion of the middle turbinate (IMT), and/or skull base. These insertions make up the walls of the most anterior air spaces of the anterior ethmoid. An air space close to the lacrimal fossa is called lacrimal cell (LC). A lacrimal cell extending anteriorly up to reach the agger nasi (AgN) is called an agger nasi cell. A cell lying above a lacrimal/agger nasi cell is called a supra-agger cell (SAC). The suprainfundibular plate (SIP) is the cranial insertion of the uncinate process that attaches on the anterior wall of the ethmoid bulla (EB). This structure must be used as a reference to establish whether the frontal sinus drainage pathway is medial or lateral to the uncinate process.

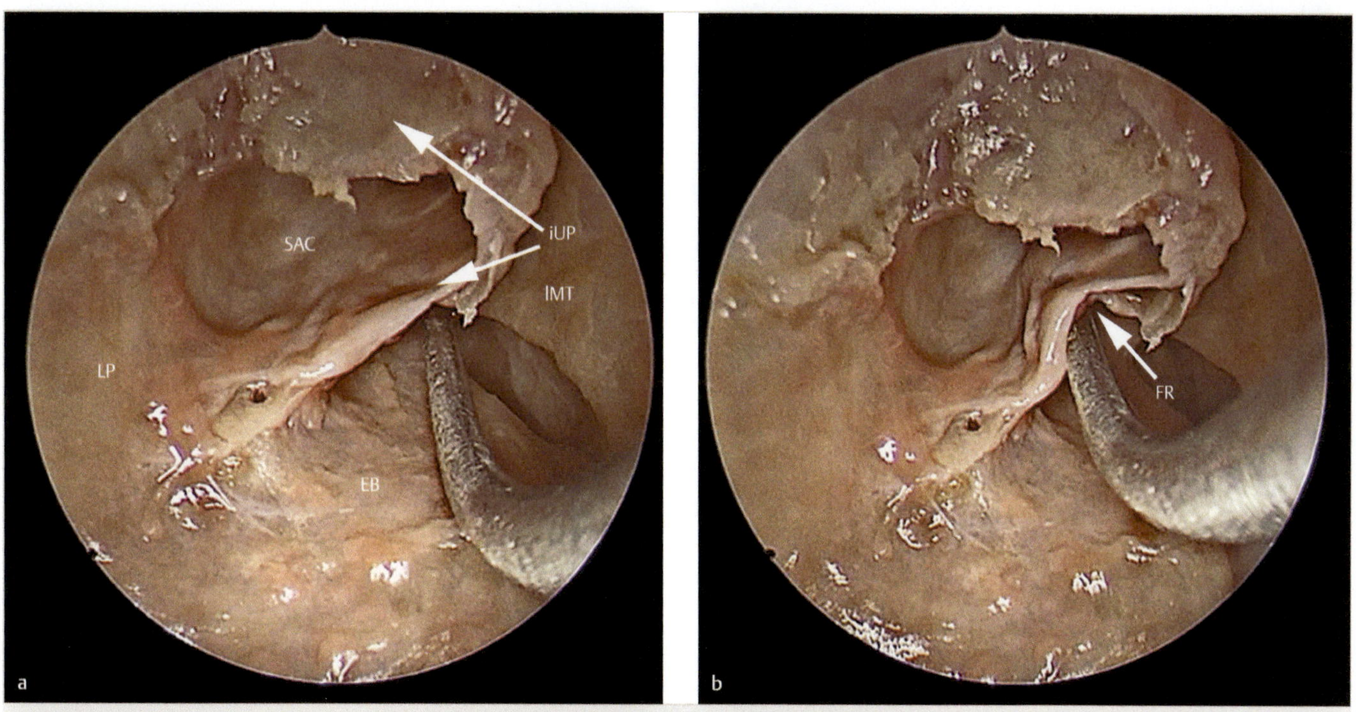

Fig. 3.12 (a, b) Step 3. After identifying the frontal sinus drainage pathway within the complex system delineated by the cranial insertions of the uncinate process (iUP), a curved instrument is placed in the frontal recess (FR) and the walls of lacrimal, agger nasi, and/or supra-agger nasi cells (SAC) are progressively fractured in a centrifugal fashion. This maneuver has been metaphorically defined as “uncapping the egg.” EB, ethmoid bulla; LP, lamina papyracea.

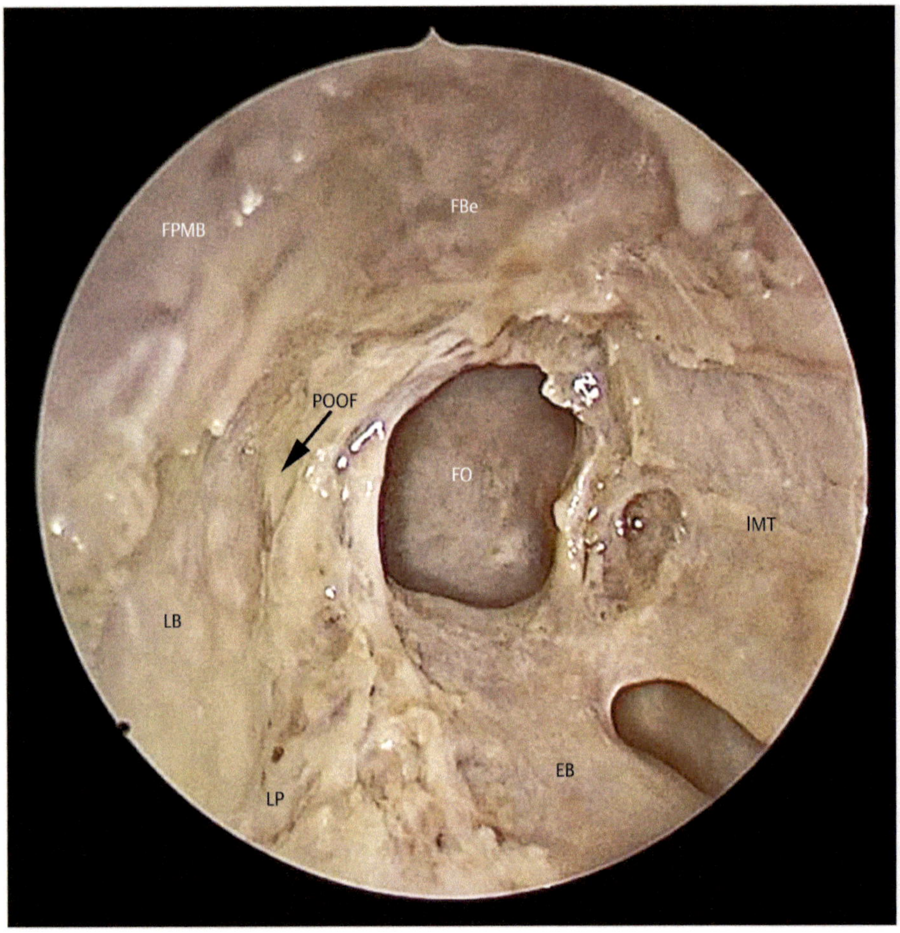

Fig. 3.13 Step 3. Draf I sinusotomy is completed when a complete clearance of the frontal recess from the palmlike cranial insertions of the uncinate process is accomplished. This can be confirmed with a 45-degree scope by checking the boundaries of the frontal recess, which are the frontal process of the maxillary bone (FPMB) and frontal beak (FBe) anteriorly, medial orbital wall laterally, laminar portion of the middle turbinate (lMT) medially, and anterior wall of the ethmoid bulla (EB) posteriorly. The bony architecture of the medial orbital wall is complex at this level: it is composed by the frontal process of the maxillary bone, lacrimal bone (LB), pars orbitalis ossis frontalis (POOF), and lamina papyracea (LP). In the uppermost portion of the frontal recess, the frontal ostium (FO) marks the passage to the frontal sinus.

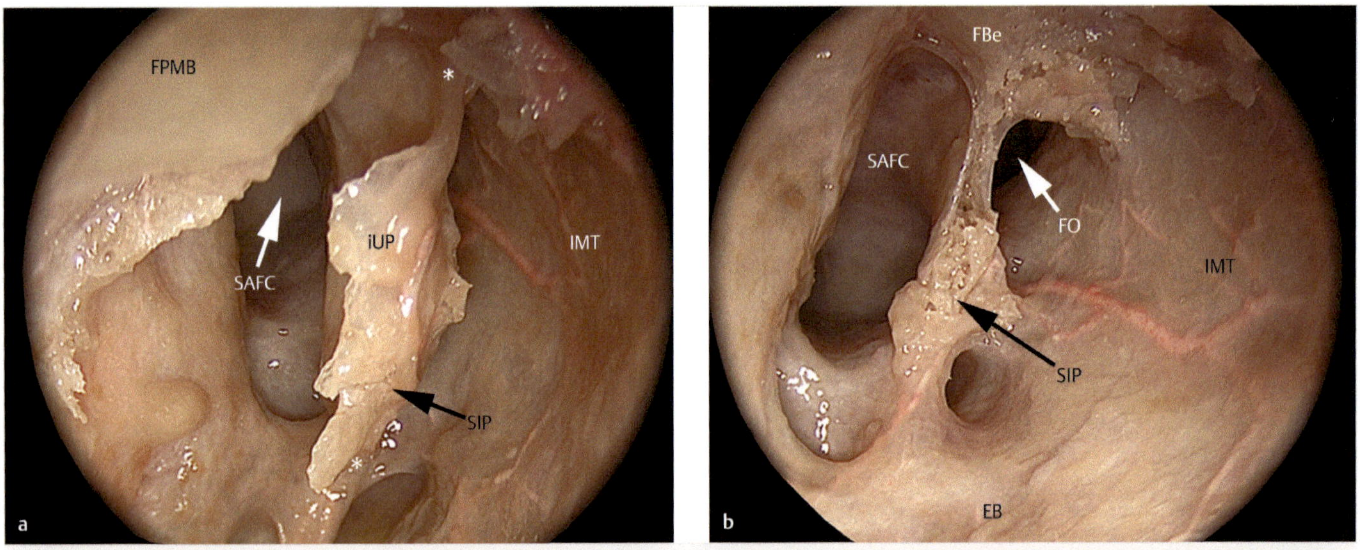

Fig. 3.14 (a, b) The supra-agger frontal cell. When a supra-agger cell pneumatizes the uppermost portion of the frontal process of the maxillary bone (FPMB) and frontal beak (FBe), it grows within the frontal sinus and is called a supra-agger frontal cell (SAFC). The cranial insertions of the uncinate process (iUP) form the medial wall of the supra-agger frontal cell. As seen with a 45-degree scope, the frontal ostium (FO) is narrowed and displaced medially and posteriorly when compared to the anatomy showed in ▶Fig. 3.13. The supra-agger frontal cell is usually associated with a frontal sinus drainage pathway located between the suprainfundibular plate (SIP) and laminar portion of the middle turbinate (lMT). EB, ethmoid bulla.) (*Asterisks*, cranial insertions of the uncinate process).

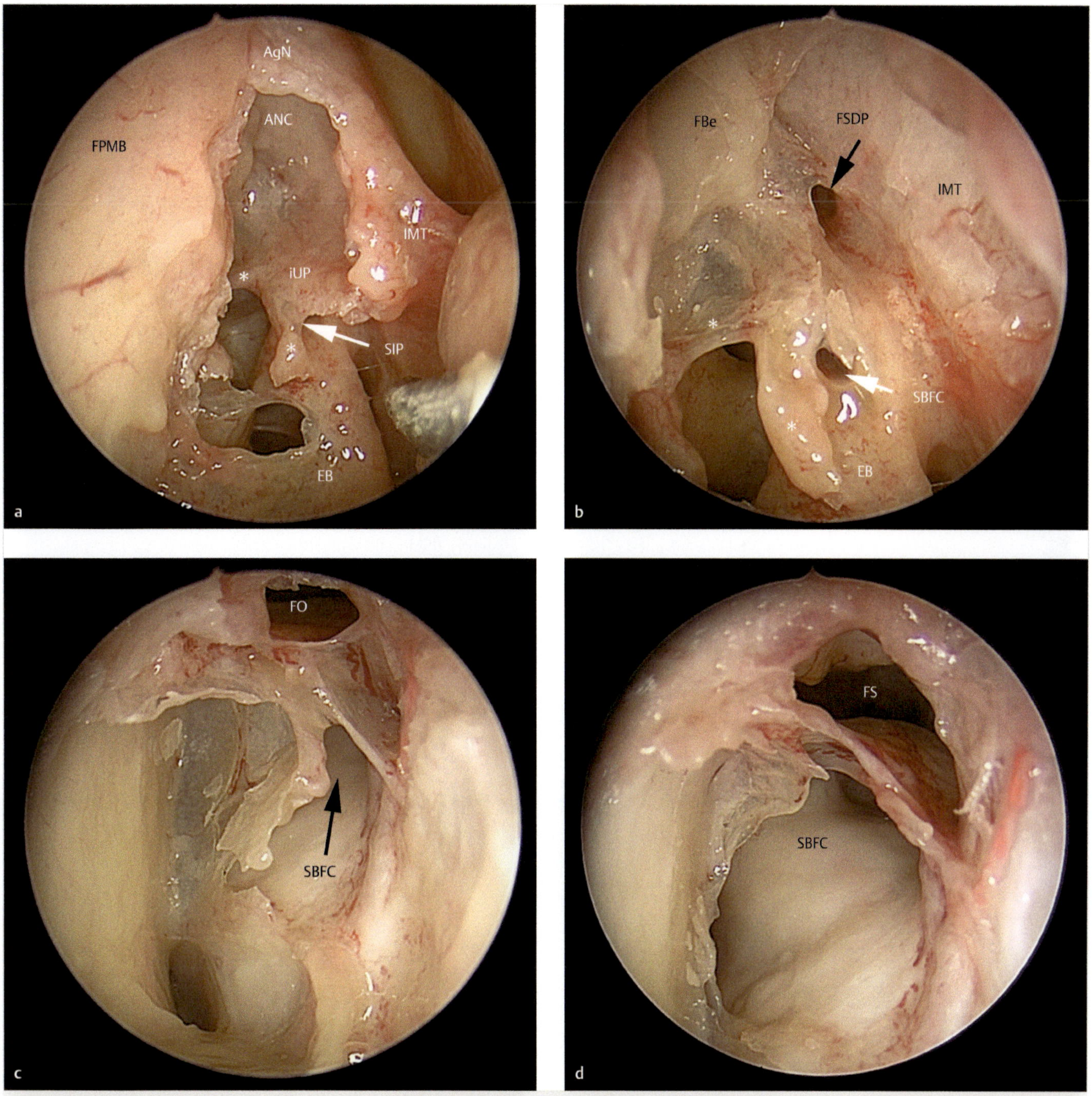

Fig. 3.15 (a–d) The agger nasi cell and suprabullar frontal cell. The panel shows a step-by-step Draf I frontal sinusotomy with a 45-degree scope in a specimen with an agger nasi cell (ANC) and suprabullar frontal cell (SBFC). The agger nasi cell results from the extension of air space of the anterior ethmoid into the agger nasi area (AgN). After removing the walls of the agger nasi cell and partially opening the ethmoidal bulla (EB), two narrow pathways are identified between the remnants (*white asterisks*) of the cranial insertions of the uncinate process (iUP): the more anterior is the frontal sinus drainage pathway (FSDP), running between the suprainfundibular plate (SIP) and laminar portion of the middle turbinate (lMT), and the more posterior leads to the suprabullar frontal cell, which is a suprabullar cell growing within the frontal sinus (FS) along the skull base. In this anatomical configuration, the frontal ostium (FO) is narrowed and pushed anteriorly when compared to ▶Fig. 3.13. FBe, frontal beak; FPMB, frontal process of the maxillary bone.

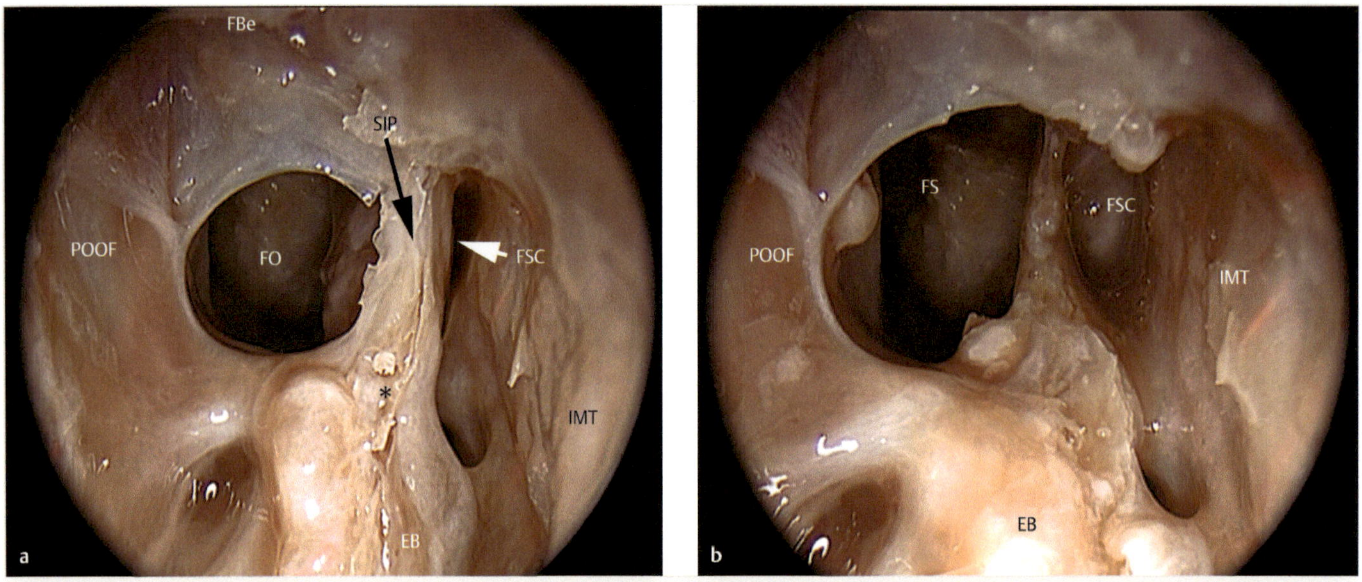

Fig. 3.16 (a, b) The frontal septal cell. The frontal septal cell (FSC) is the cranial extension within the interfrontal sinus septum of the space between the suprainfundibular plate (SIP) and the laminar portion of the middle turbinate (lMT). The lateral walls of the frontal septal cell correspond to the medial walls of frontal sinuses (FS). As seen with a 45-degree scope, the frontal ostium (FO) is displaced laterally, lying between the suprainfundibular plate and the pars orbitalis ossis frontalis (POOF). Consequently, the frontal septal cell is associated with a frontal sinus drainage pathway running laterally to the suprainfundibular plate. EB, ethmoid bulla; FBe, frontal beak. (*Black asterisk*, cranial insertion of the uncinate process.

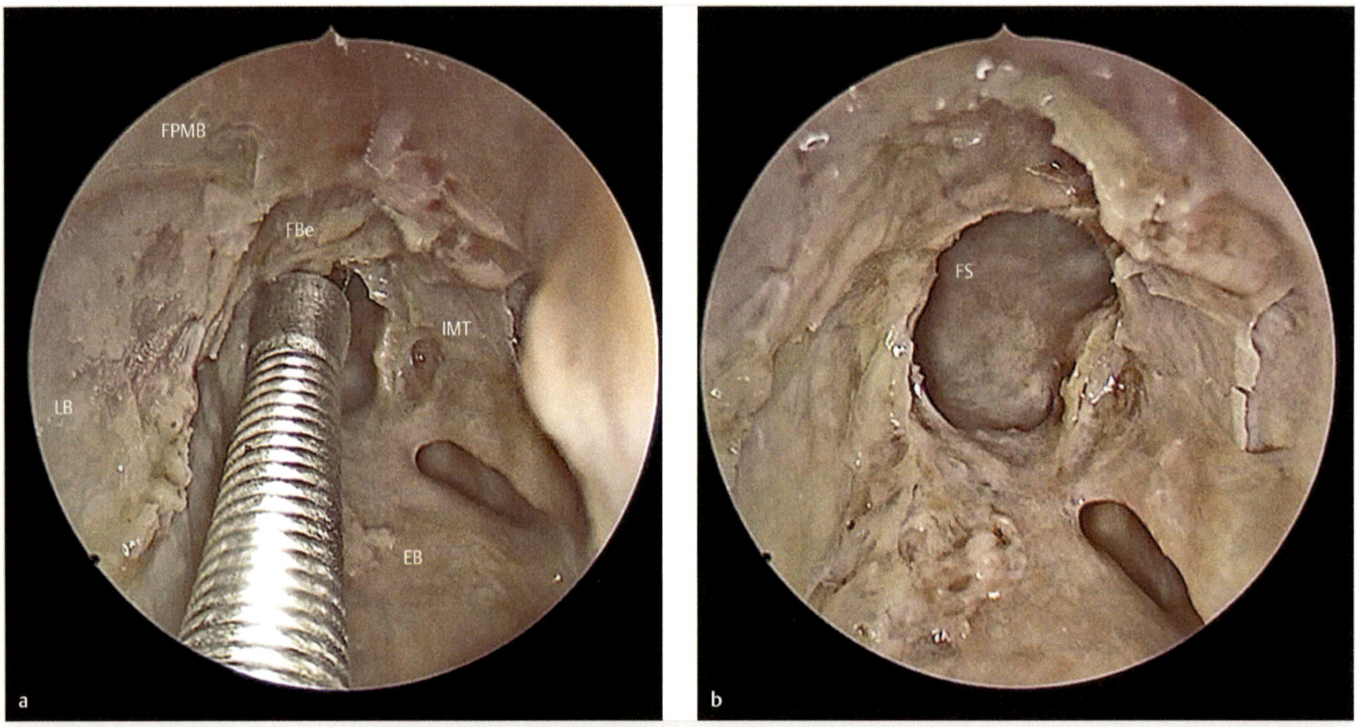

Fig. 3.17 (a, b) Step 4. A frontal punch is placed through the frontal ostium and used to partially remove the frontal beak (FBe). In this way, a Draf IIa frontal sinusotomy is performed by enlarging the ostium of the frontal sinus (FS). When a supra-agg er frontal cell, suprabullar frontal cell, or frontal septal cell is present, it must be completely marsupialized to accomplish a Draf IIa sinusotomy. In case of an ethmoidal bulla (EB) with bulky anterior extension, this procedure cannot be performed without partially removing the ethmoid bulla. FPMB, frontal process of the maxillary bone; LB, lacrimal bone; IMT, laminar portion of the middle turbinate.

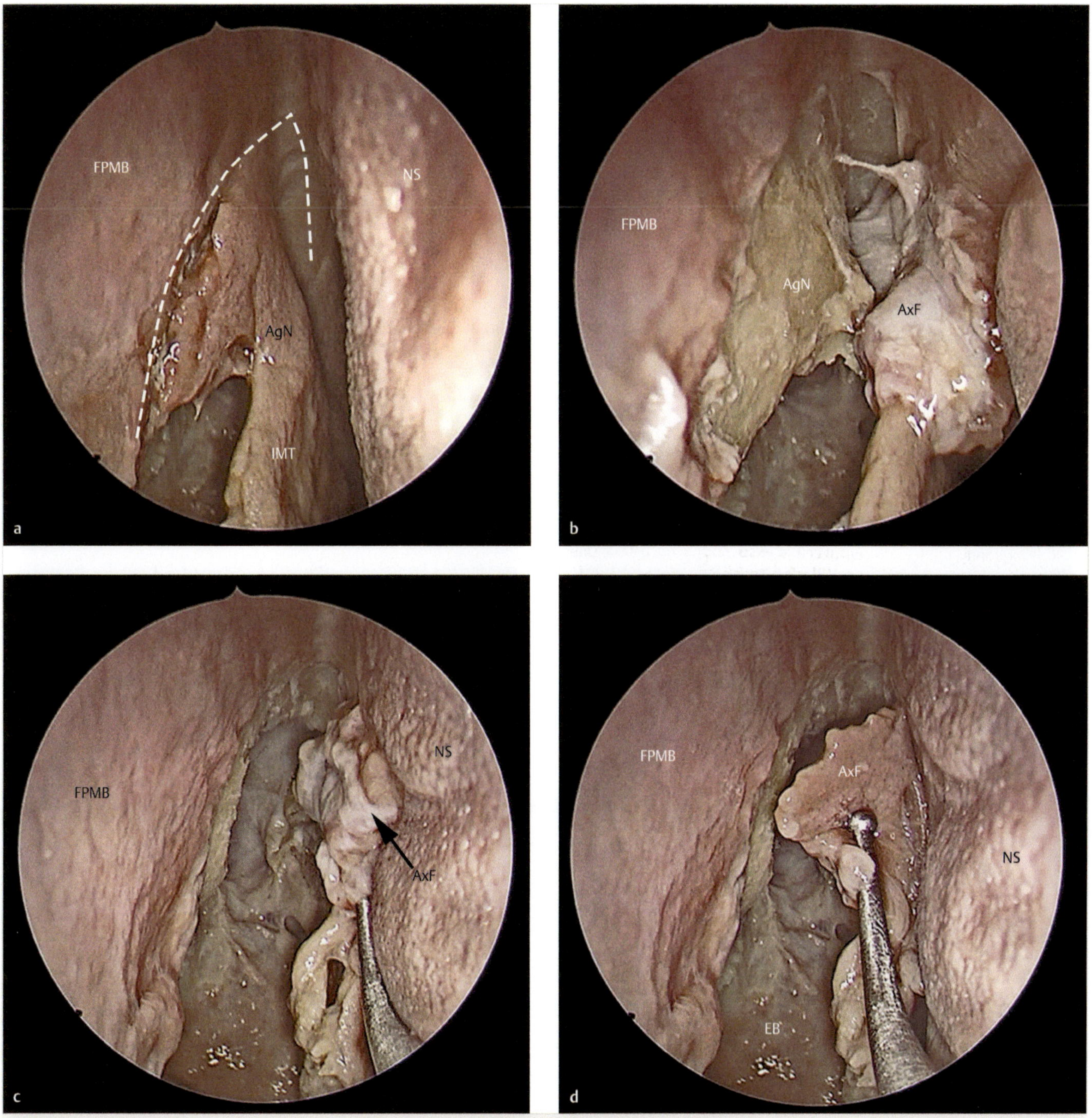

Fig. 3.18 (a–d) Step 5 (part 1). Before performing a Draf IIb frontal sinusotomy, an axillary flap (AxF) is harvested by incising the mucoperiosteum lateral to the agger nasi (AgN) and along the nasal vault (*white dashed line*). Then, the medial portion of the frontal process of the maxillary bone (FPMB), which corresponds to the frontal beak, is removed. The axillary flap is positioned to cover the medial surface of the sinusotomy.
EB, ethmoidal bulla; IMT, laminar portion of the middle turbinate; NS, nasal septum.

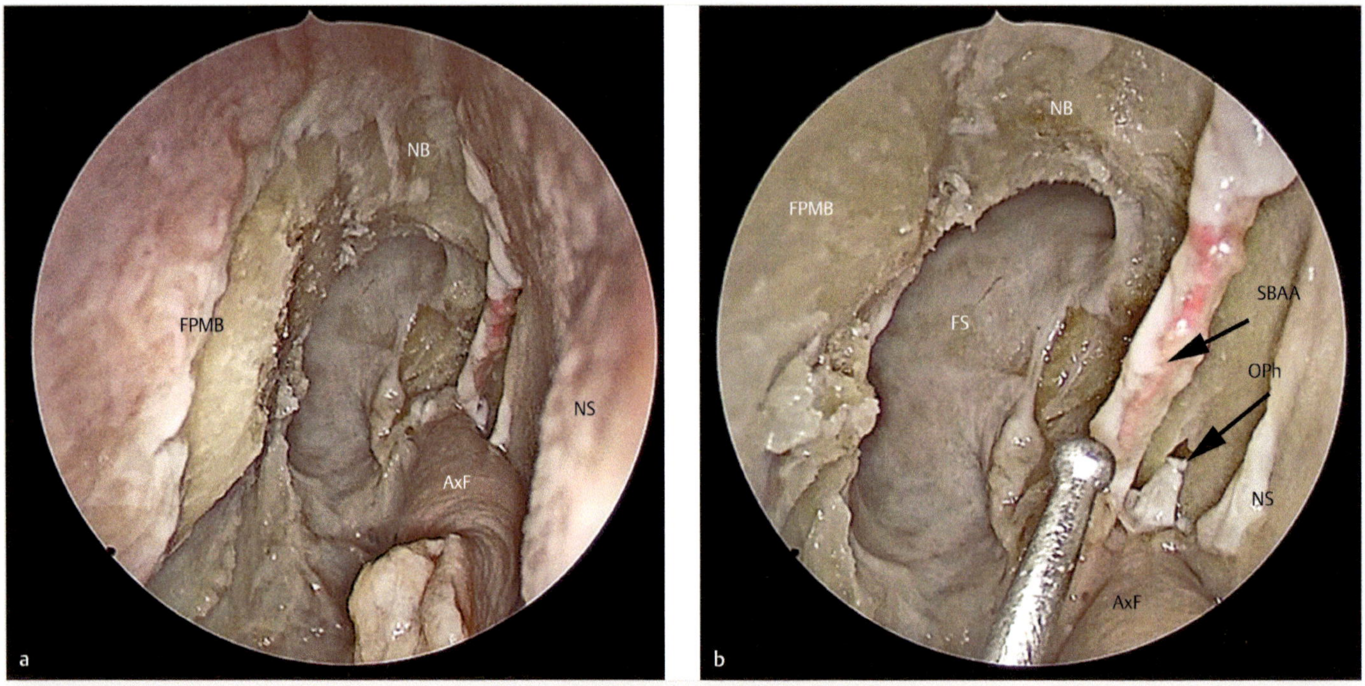

Fig. 3.19 (a, b) Step 5 (part 2). The nasal bone (NB) comes into view after removing the frontal beak. The septal branch of the anterior ethmoidal artery (SBAA) runs at the medial boundary of the sinusotomy. The most anterior olfactory phylum (OPh), which can be found between the middle turbinate and nasal septum (NS), marks the anterior limit of the cribriform plate. AxF, axillary flap; FPMB, frontal process of the maxillary bone; FS, frontal sinus.

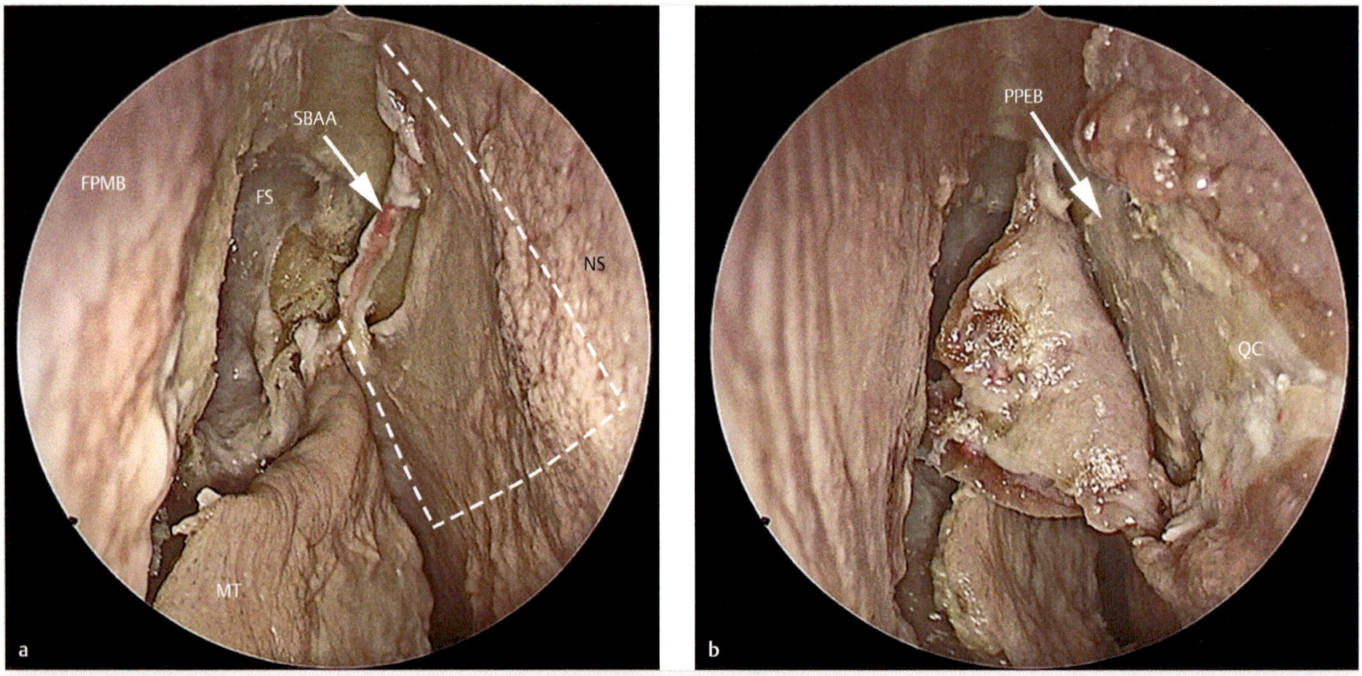

Fig. 3.20 (a, b) Step 6 (part 1). A squared area (*white dashed line*) of the mucosa is incised in the anterosuperior portion of the nasal septum (NS). By performing a subperiosteal dissection, the perpendicular plate of the ethmoid bone (PPEB) and quadrangular cartilage (QC) are exposed. This area of mucosa is mainly supplied by the septal branch of the anterior ethmoidal artery (SBAA). FPMB, frontal process of the maxillary bone; FS, frontal sinus; MT, middle turbinate.

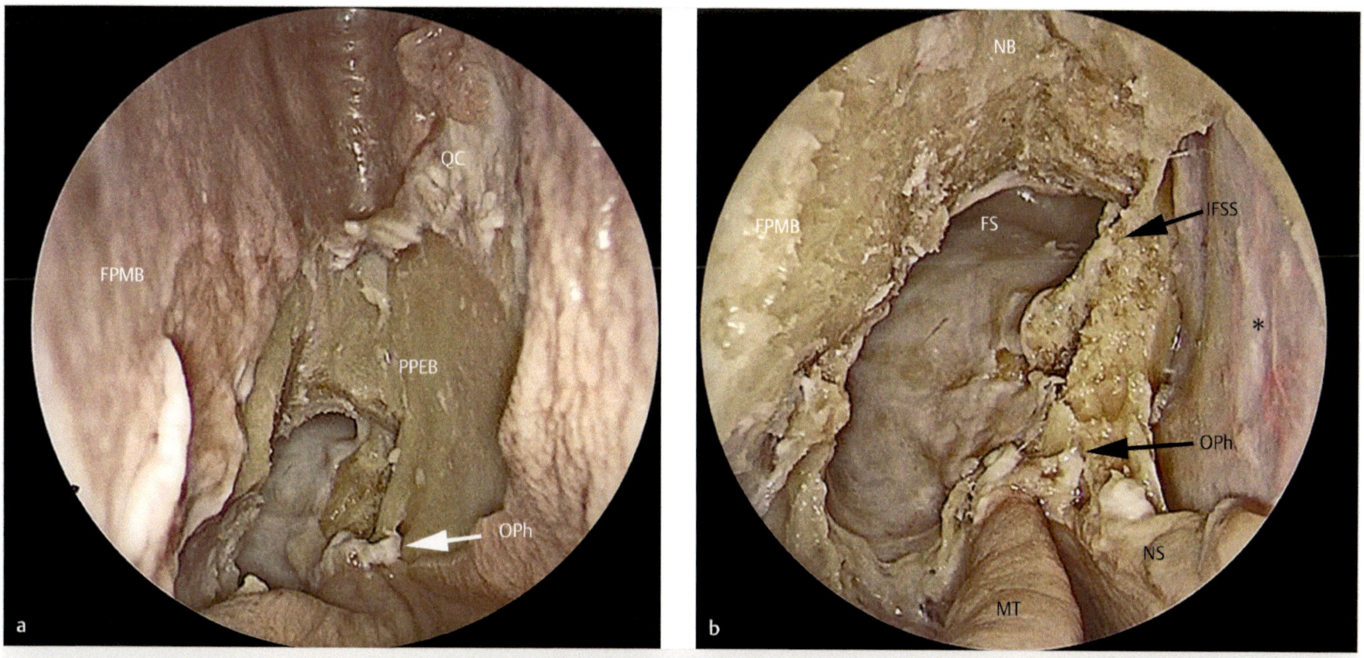

Fig. 3.21 (a, b) Step 6 (part 2). The anterosuperior portion of the nasal septum (NS) is removed to expose the contralateral septal mucoperiosteum (*black asterisk*). The resection should not exceed the first olfactory phylum (OPh) posteriorly and the anterior wall of the frontal sinus (FS) anteriorly, which almost corresponds to the junction between the perpendicular plate of the ethmoid bone (PPEB), quadrangular cartilage (QC), and nasal bone (NB). FPMB, frontal process of the maxillary bone; IFSS, interfrontal sinus septum; MT, middle turbinate.

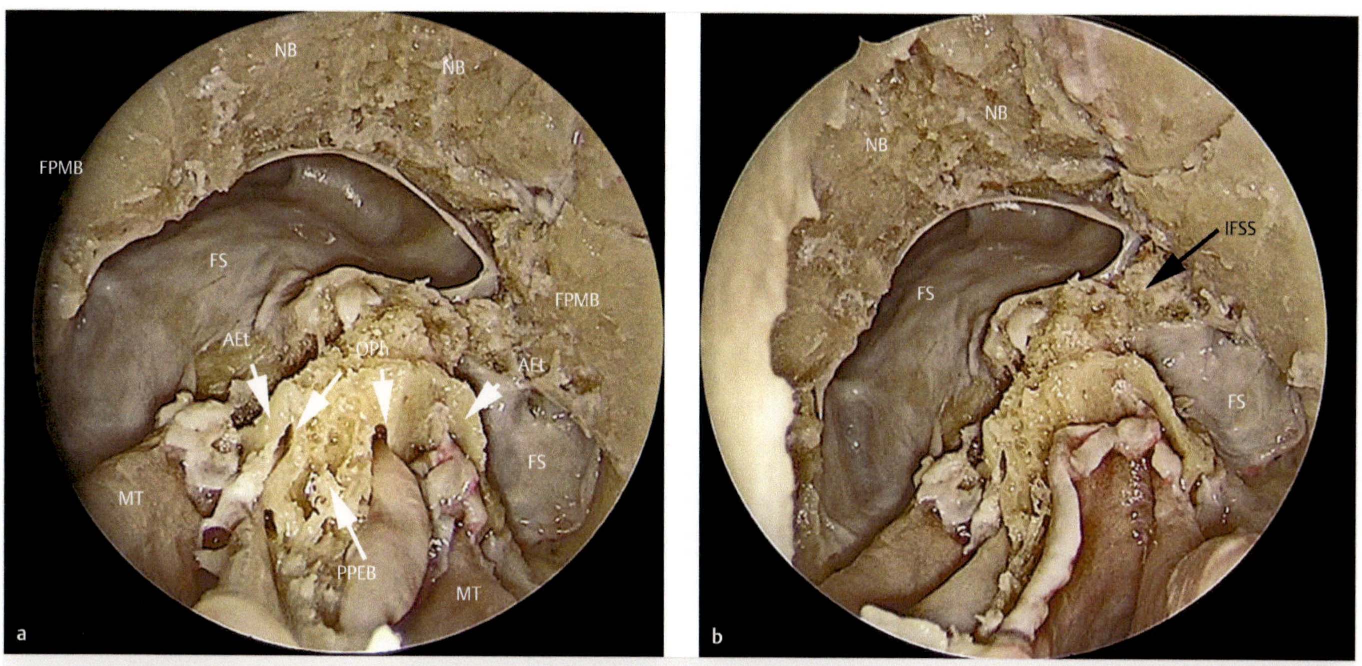

Fig. 3.22 (a, b) Step 6 (part 3). To complete a Draf III frontal sinusotomy, the mucoperiosteum of the contralateral side is removed and the previous steps are repeated on the contralateral side. Finally, the interfrontal sinus septum (IFSS) is drilled out. Placing a 0-degree scope through the anterosuperior septectomy, all the boundaries of the sinusotomy can be seen: the frontal processes of maxillary bones (FPMB) laterally, nasal bones (NB) anteriorly, and the most anterior portion of the ethmoid bone posteriorly. The latter, also called "Draf T," is formed by the perpendicular plate of the ethmoid bone (PPEB) in the midline and by the ala ethmoidalis (AEt) bilaterally. MT, middle turbinate; OPh, olfactory phylum.

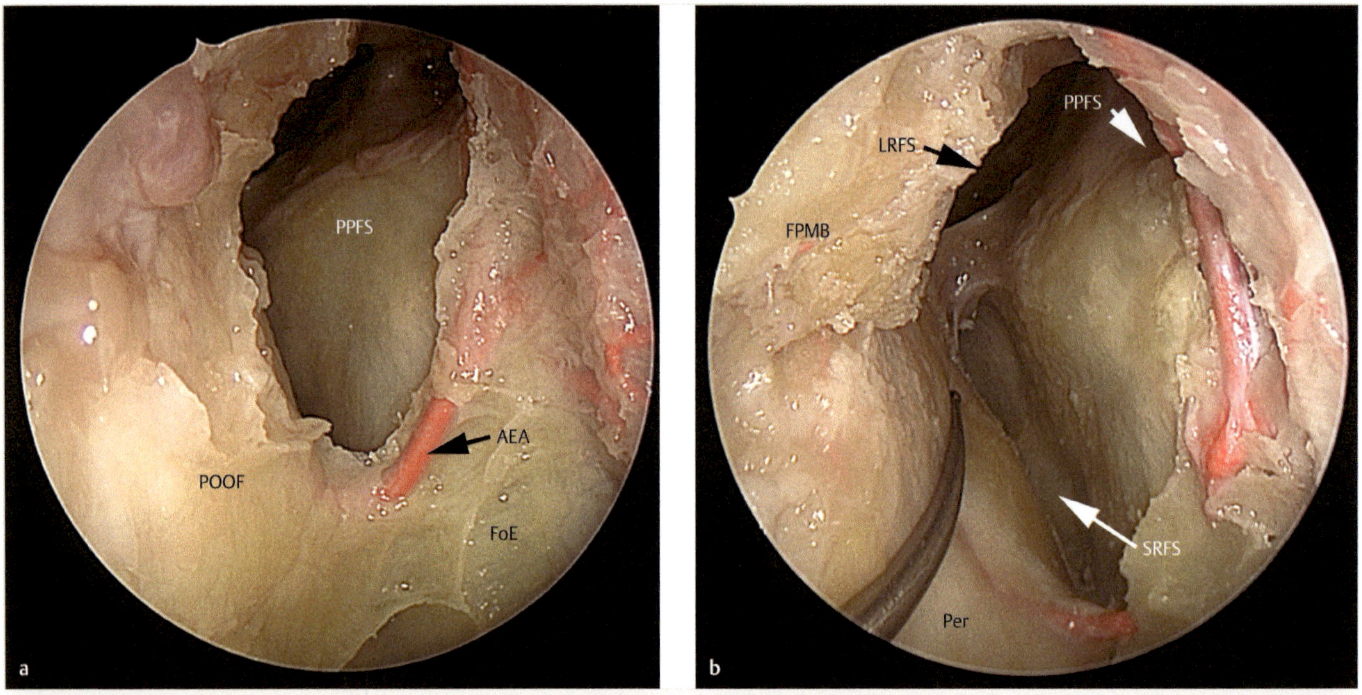

Fig. 3.23 (a, b) Step 7. To maximize the lateral exposure of the frontal sinus and supraorbital air spaces, it is possible to cut the anterior ethmoidal artery (AEA), remove the pars orbitalis ossis frontalis (POOF), and displace the periorbit (Per) laterally and inferiorly. With this maneuver, both the lateral (LRFS) and supraorbital (SRFS) recesses of the frontal sinus (and also the supraorbital ethmoid cell, when present) can be exposed and reached with curved instruments. FoE, fovea ethmoidalis; FPMB, frontal process of the maxillary bone; PPFS, posterior plate of the frontal sinus.

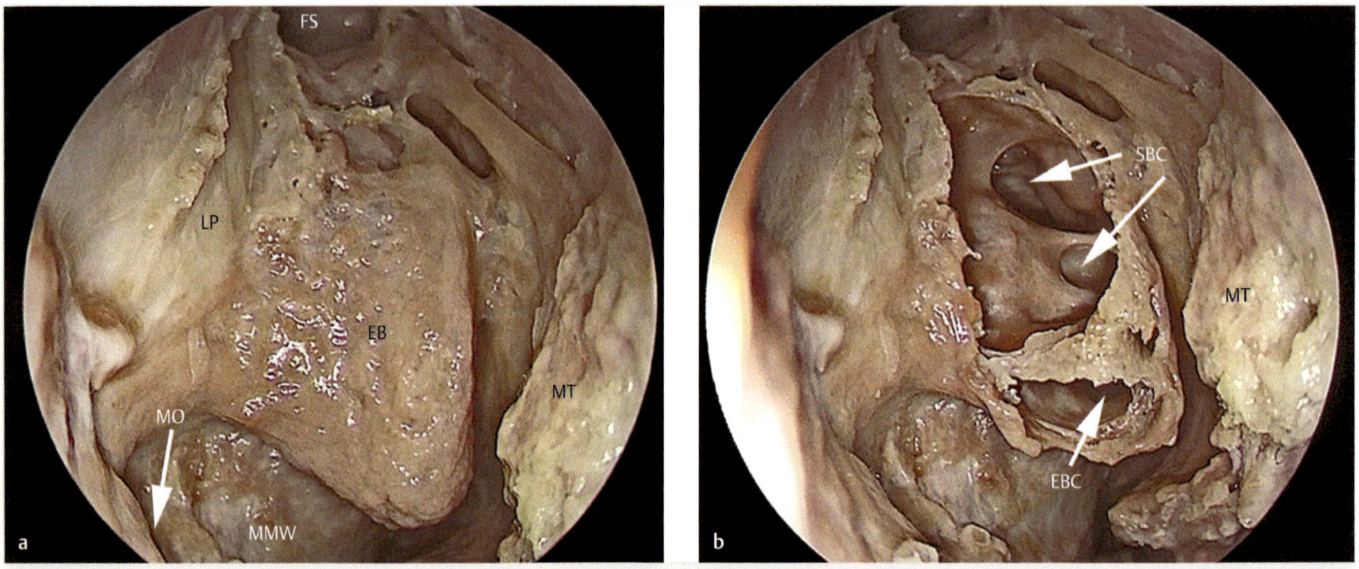

Fig. 3.24 (a, b) Step 8. The ethmoidal bulla (EB) is opened from its inferomedial portion. Commonly, the ethmoidal bulla is made up of an inferior ethmoidal bulla cell (EBC) and several suprabullar cells (SBC). Noteworthy, the axial plane passing through the inferior border of the ethmoidal bulla can be used as a landmark to identify the position of the maxillary sinus and orbital cavity: the orbital cavity is covered by the lamina papyracea (LP) and lies above the plane, whereas the maxillary sinus, which can be accessed through the maxillary ostium (MO), is located inferiorly to it. FS, frontal sinus; MMW, medial maxillary wall [posterior portion]; MT, middle turbinate.

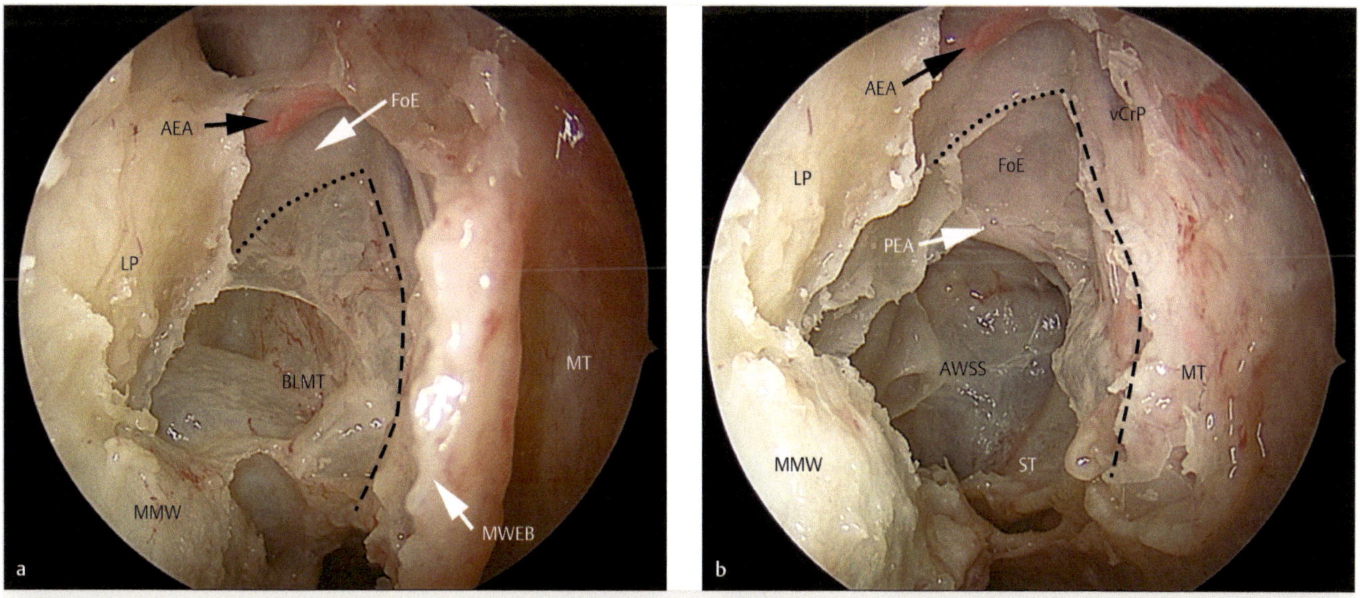

Fig. 3.25 (a, b) Step 9. Bony lamellae of the ethmoidal bulla, which are located between the lamina papyracea (LP) and medial wall of the ethmoidal bulla (MWEB), are progressively removed to identify the basal lamella of the middle turbinate (BLMT). The medial wall of the ethmoidal bulla inserts on the basal lamella of the middle turbinate (*black dashed line*), which is attached to the fovea ethmoidalis (FoE) superiorly (*black dotted line*) and the lamina papyracea (LP) and medial maxillary wall (MMW) laterally. Removing the basal lamella of the middle turbinate, the posterior ethmoid is opened and its bony lamellae can be removed to expose the anterior wall of the sphenoid sinus (AWSS), which can partially or totally correspond to the basal lamella of the superior turbinate according to the extent of the sphenoethmoidal recess. PEA, posterior ethmoidal artery; ST, superior turbinate; vCrP, vertical lamella of the cribriform plate.

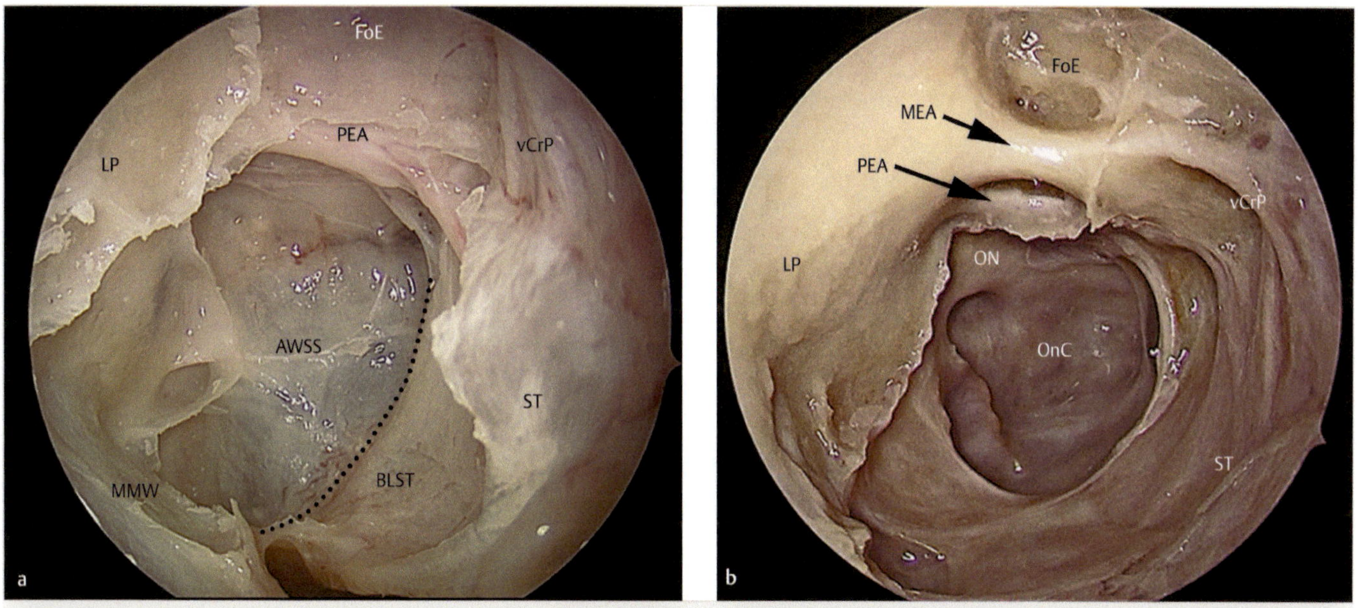

Fig. 3.26 (a, b) Onodi cell. On the left, a 0-degree scope is placed within a posterior ethmoid with standard pneumatization. The basal lamella of the superior turbinate (BLST) can be distinguished from the superior turbinate (ST) based on its orientation: the former is coronal, while the latter is sagittal. The position where the basal lamella of the superior turbinate inserts (*black dotted line*) on the anterior wall of the sphenoid sinus (AWSS) depends on the balance between the pneumatization of the sphenoethmoidal recess and posterior ethmoid. When the posterior ethmoid invades the sphenoid sinus reaching the canal of the optic nerve (ON), this air space is called the Onodi cell (OnC). Compared to the sphenoid sinus, it can be easily recognized due to its flat floor. FoE, fovea ethmoidalis; LP, lamina papyracea; MEA, middle ethmoidal artery; MMW, medial maxillary wall; PEA, posterior ethmoidal artery; vCrP, vertical lamella of the cribriform plate.

References

[1] Schreiber A, Ferrari M, Rodella LF, et al. Anatomy of the frontal sinus and recess. In: Lal D, Hwang PH, eds. Frontal Sinus Surgery—A Systematic Approach. Springer International Publishing; 2019

[2] Pianta L, Ferrari M, Schreiber A, et al. Agger-bullar classification (ABC) of the frontal sinus drainage pathway: validation in a preclinical setting. Int Forum Allergy Rhinol 2016;6(9):981–989

[3] Kuhn F. Chronic frontal sinusitis: the endoscopic frontal recess approach. Oper Tech Otolaryngol Head Neck Surg 1996;7:222–229

[4] Wormald PJ, Hoseman W, Callejas C, et al. The international frontal sinus anatomy classification (IFAC) and classification of the extent of endoscopic frontal sinus surgery (EFSS). Int Forum Allergy Rhinol 2016;6(7):677–696

[5] Márquez S, Tessema B, Clement PA, Schaefer SD. Development of the ethmoid sinus and extramural migration: the anatomical basis of this paranasal sinus. Anat Rec (Hoboken) 2008;291(11):1535–1553

[6] Yoon JH, Moon HJ, Kim CH, Hong SS, Kang SS, Kim K. Endoscopic frontal sinusotomy using the suprainfundibular plate as a key landmark. Laryngoscope 2002;112(9):1703–1707

[7] Terracol J, Ardouin P. [Anatomy of the Nasal Fossae and Associated Cavities]. Paris: Maloine; 1965

[8] Terrier F, Weber W, Ruefenacht D, Porcellini B. Anatomy of the ethmoid: CT, endoscopic, and macroscopic. AJR Am J Roentgenol 1985;144(3):493–500

[9] Ferrari M, Schreiber A, Mattavelli D, et al. The Terracol and Ardouin developmental model of frontal sinus drainage pathway and surrounding spaces: a radiologic validation. Int Forum Allergy Rhinol 2018;8(5):624–630

[10] Draf W. Endonasal micro-endoscopic frontal sinus surgery. The Fulda concept. Oper Tech Otolaryngol Head Neck Surg 1991;2:234–240

[11] Loury MC. Endoscopic frontal recess and frontal sinus ostium dissection. Laryngoscope 1993;103(4 Pt 1):455–458

[12] Ferrari M, Pianta L, Borghesi A, et al. The ethmoidal arteries: a cadaveric study based on cone beam computed tomography and endoscopic dissection. Surg Radiol Anat 2017;39(9):991–998

[13] Wang L, Youseef A, Al Qahtani AA, et al. Endoscopic anatomy of the middle ethmoidal artery. Int Forum Allergy Rhinol 2014;4(2):164–168

[14] Mason E, Solares CA, Carrau RL, Figueroa R. Computed tomographic exploration of the middle ethmoidal artery. J Neurol Surg B Skull Base 2015;76(5):372–378

[15] Kim KS, Kim HU, Chung IH, Lee JG, Park IY, Yoon JH. Surgical anatomy of the nasofrontal duct: anatomical and computed tomographic analysis. Laryngoscope 2001;111(4 Pt 1):603–608

[16] Kainz J, Stammberger H. [The roof of the anterior ethmoid: a locus minoris resistentiae in the skull base] Laryngol Rhinol Otol (Stuttg) 1988;67(4):142–149

4 Corridor to Sella Turcica, Surrounding Areas, Posterior Skull Base, and Cervical Spine

Francesco Belotti, Davide Lancini, Marco Ravanelli, Stefano Taboni, Francesco Doglietto

The corridors illustrated in this chapter pass through the sphenoid sinuses, ethmoidal complex, and nasopharynx, providing a direct trajectory toward the posterior portion of the anterior skull base (i.e., planum sphenoidale and tuberculum sellae), the median/paramedian portions of the middle and posterior skull base, the craniocervical junction, and part of the cervical spine.[1–11] Similarly to the corridor toward the anterior skull base and orbit, the amount of structures to be removed can be modulated according to the need of exposure.[12–15]

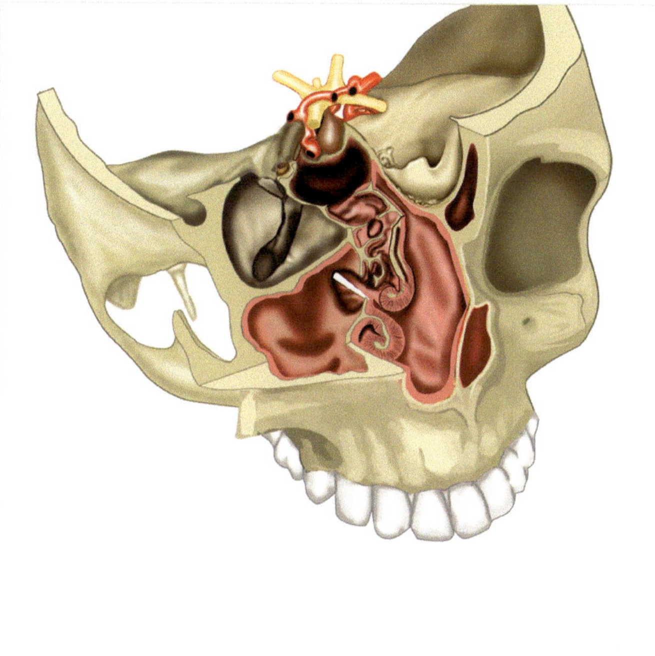

Fig. 4.1 Coronal view of sphenoid sinus and main adjacent structures. This illustration shows anatomy of the sphenoid sinus and neighboring neurovascular structures. III, oculomotor nerve; IV, trochlear nerve; V1, ophthalmic nerve; V2, maxillary nerve; V3, mandibular nerve; VI, abducens nerve; ACA, anterior cerebral artery; ICA, internal carotid artery; MCA, middle cerebral artery.

Being located at the center of the skull, the sphenoid sinus and nasopharynx serve as crossroads toward several subunits of the cranial base. A large number of bony landmarks (discussed in depth in the following chapters) can be identified on the walls of the sphenoid sinus. The roof of the sphenoid sinus is a thick and flat lamina called planum sphenoidale, which further thickens posteriorly forming the tuberculum sellae. The latter corresponds to the cranial limit of the posterior wall of the sphenoid sinus, which ends inferiorly merging with the sphenoidal floor. The midline portion of the posterior wall is formed by the sellar prominence superiorly and clival recess (when present) inferiorly, while the lateral portions are formed by the carotid prominences superiorly and carotid sulci inferiorly, corresponding to the parasellar and paraclival tracts of the internal carotid artery, respectively. The intersphenoid sinus septum is rarely located on the midline; rather, it attaches onto the carotid prominence and/or sulcus of one side. In addition, a number of incomplete septa, frequently inserting on the bony canal of neighboring neurovascular structures, can be found in the sphenoid sinuses. As a consequence, drilling is favored over fracturing bony septa and sepimentations due to the risk to injure the internal carotid artery by creating sharp bony edges along fracture rims. The lateral sphenoidal wall lies anteriorly and laterally to the carotid bony landmarks (i.e., carotid prominence and sulcus). The dihedral angle where the lateral sphenoidal wall joins the planum sphenoidale houses the optic canal, which follows posterior-to-anterior and medial-to-lateral directions to connect the suprasellar area to the orbital cavity.

The possibility to identify sphenoid bony landmarks depends on the degree of pneumatization of the sphenoid sinus, which is

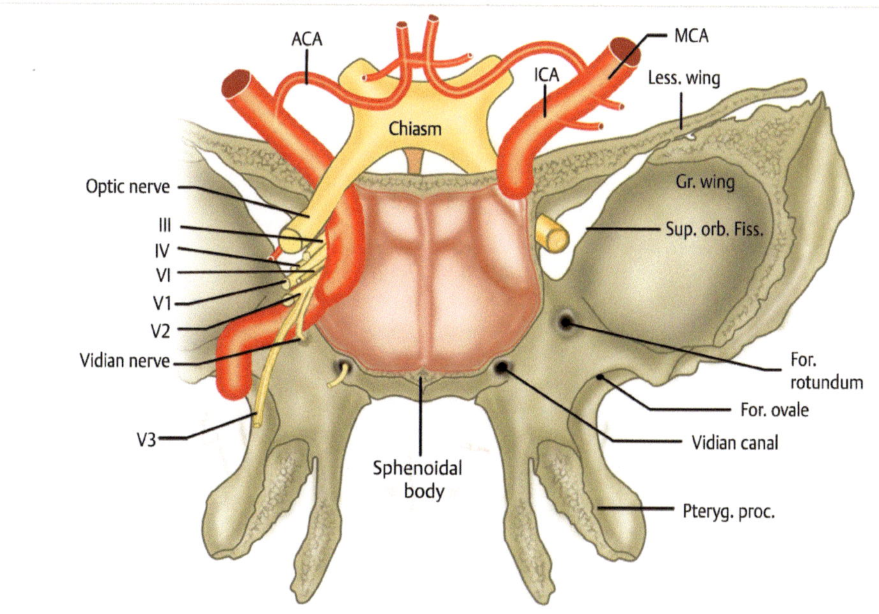

Fig. 4.2 Diagonal view of the transnasal corridor toward sella turcica and adjacent areas. This illustration shows the trajectory toward the sella turcica and adjacent area via the nasal cavity and sphenoid sinus.

variable on both the anterior-to-posterior and medial-to-lateral axes.[16] On the anterior-to-posterior axis, the sphenoid sinus can be classified according to where the air space ends posteriorly: a conchal (agenesis/hypoplasia of the sphenoid sinus), presellar (air space anterior to the plane passing through the anterior sellar wall), sellar (air space below the sella turcica, between the planes passing through anterior sellar wall, anteriorly, and dorsum sellae, posteriorly), or retrosellar/clival type (air space posterior to the plane passing through the dorsum sellae) can be distinguished. On the medial-to-lateral axis, the sphenoid sinus can be classified as body (when pneumatization does not overcome the lateral wall), lesser wing (when an optic-carotid recess takes shape; this variant will be discussed in the following chapters), and lateral type (when the pneumatization overcomes the line connecting the vidian canal to foramen rotundum, forming a space called lateral recess). The lateral recess is, in turn, classified as greater wing, pterygoid, or full type, according to the extent of pneumatization.

The sphenoid sinus is usually opened via the nasal cavity (i.e., paraseptal sphenoidotomy) proceeding centrifugally from the sphenoid ostium, which is found medial to the superior turbinate. Lateralization or partial removal of the superior turbinate can be necessary to gain enough space to handle instruments. The same procedure can be done through the ethmoid after completing a total ethmoidectomy (i.e., functional transethmoidal sphenoidotomy); in such a scenario, it is advantageous to remove the inferior part of the superior turbinate in order to identify the sphenoid ostium rather than blindly pierce the anterior sphenoidal wall. An additional way to open the sphenoid sinus is by harvesting a submucosal corridor along the nasal septum (i.e., subseptal sphenoidotomy). Differently from functional sinus surgery, the opening of the sphenoid sinus should be enlarged as much as possible in order to provide an adequate working volume toward the skull base. As a consequence, the anterior sphenoidal wall between the nasal septum medially, superior turbinate laterally, sphenoidal floor inferiorly, and planum sphenoidale superiorly is completely removed. When further exposure and/or a binostril approach are needed, a posterosuperior septectomy with transrostral sphenoidotomy can be performed. Increasing working volume and skull base exposure can be obtained with expanded transrostral and modular transethmoidal sphenoidotomy: the former consists of removing the superior turbinate and part of the orbital process of the palatine bone, the latter is accomplished adding a posterior or total ethmoidectomy.

The nasopharynx is delimited by the vault (which corresponds to the sphenoidal floor), lateral walls with *tori tubarii* (that are the footprint of eustachian tubes on the nasopharyngeal mucosa), and posterior wall. The limit between the posterior and lateral wall corresponds to the lateral recess of the nasopharynx, which is also called Rosenmüller fossa. As a result of the natural communication with the nasal cavities via the choanae, the nasopharynx is easily accessed through the inferior nasal corridors, which can be merged via a posteroinferior septectomy. When needing a wide corridor, including the transsphenoidal pathway as well, the sphenoidal floor/nasopharyngeal vault is removed to connect the nasopharynx with the sphenoidal lumen. The lateral landmarks used to entirely remove the sphenoidal floor are the vidian canals. The lateral portion of the sphenoidal floor houses several neurovascular structures (palatovaginal and vomerovaginal bundles).[17]

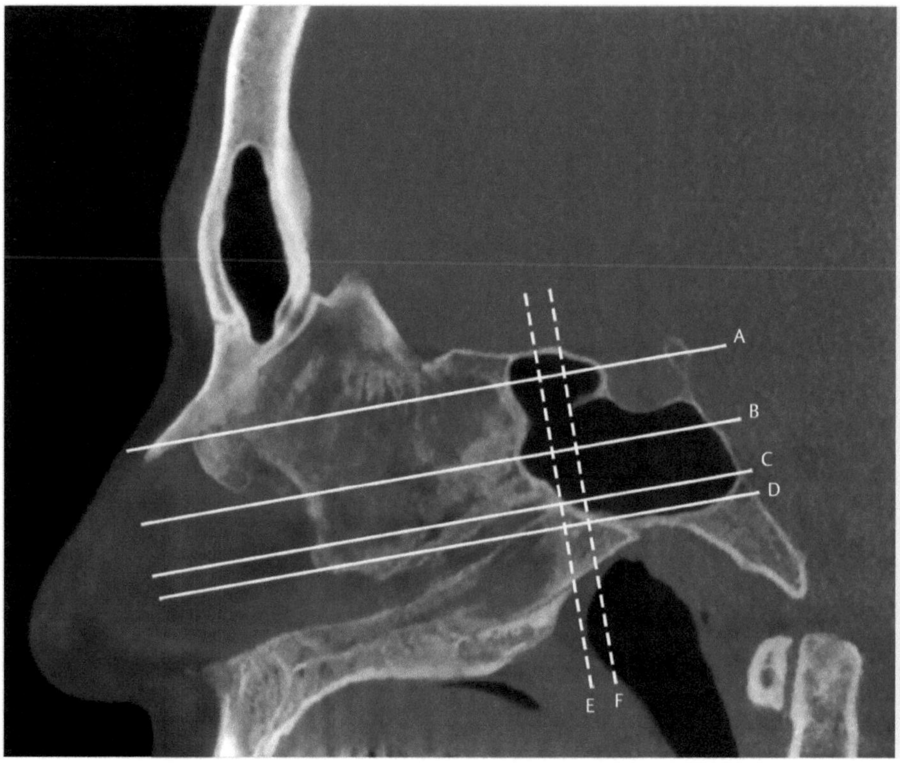

Fig. 4.3 Midline sagittal CT scan. This midline sagittal CT scan depicts the position and orientation of images composing ▶Fig. 4.4 (A–D) and ▶Fig. 4.5 (E, F) through *white continue* and *dashed lines*, respectively.

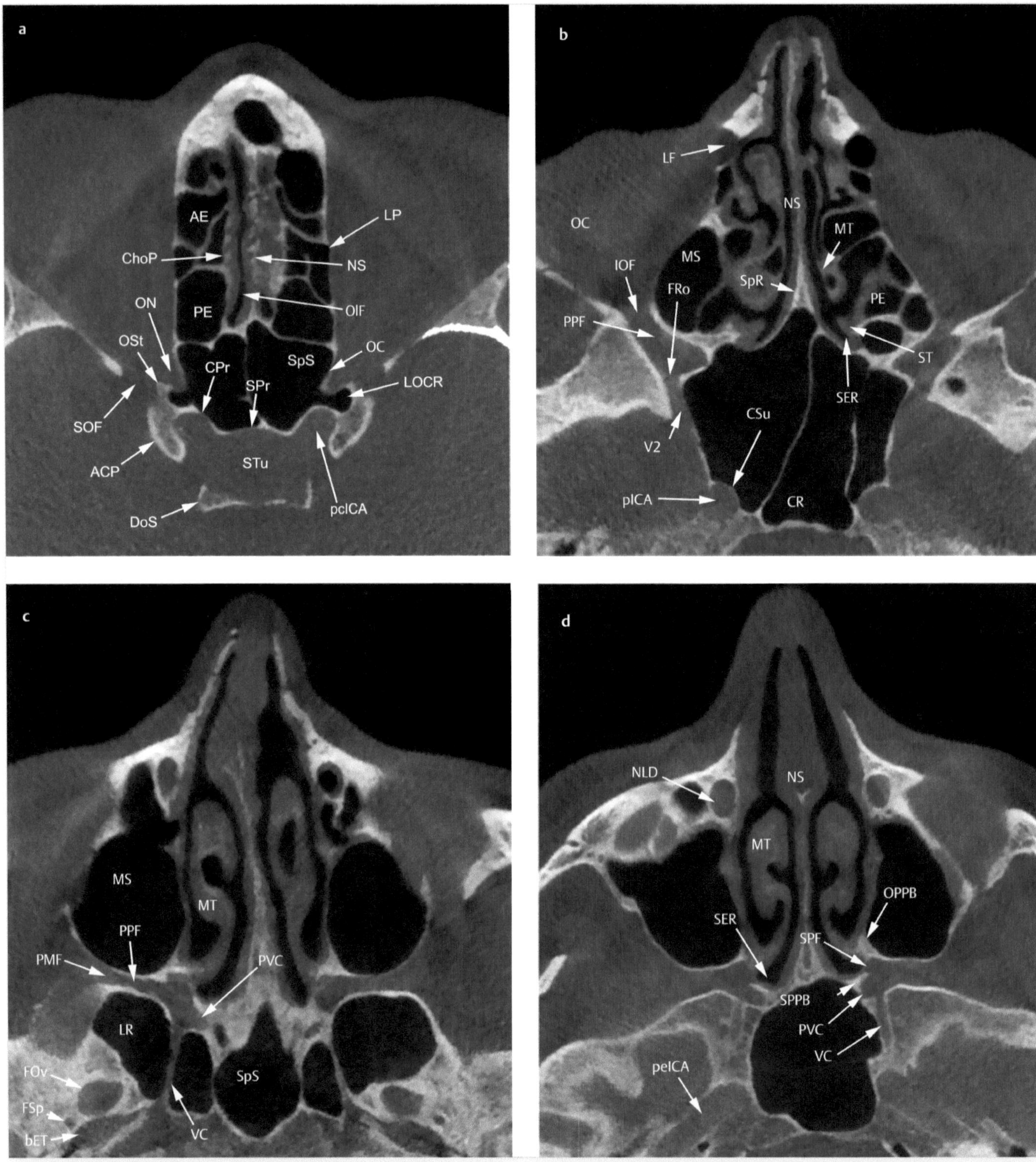

Fig. 4.4 (a–d) Axial anatomy of the sphenoethmoidal complex. The panel includes four axial CT images disposed from cranial **(a)** to caudal **(d)**. The position of each image is depicted in ▶ Fig. 4.3. The sphenoid sinus (SpS) is located at the center of the skull. From a transnasal perspective, it can be reached through a paraseptal trajectory, which includes the nasal cavity and olfactory fissure (OlF) and is located medially to the middle turbinate (MT), superior turbinate (ST), and their common conchal plate (ChoP). The two paraseptal corridors can be merged by removing the sphenoidal rostrum (SpR) and the posterosuperior portion of the nasal septum (NS). From medial to lateral, the anterior wall of the sphenoid sinus is intimately adjacent to the olfactory fissure, sphenoethmoidal recess (SER), and posterior ethmoidal compartment (PE). The posterior wall of the sphenoid sinus includes the sellar prominence (SPr), carotid prominence (CPr), carotid sulcus (CSu), and, when present, the clival recess (CR), which mark the position of the sella turcica (STu), paraclinoid (pclCA), parasellar, and paraclival tracts of the internal carotid artery (pICA), and midclivus, respectively. The lateral wall of the sphenoid sinus and its lateral recess (LR) neighbor a number of relevant bony landmarks, namely the optic canal (OC), superior orbital fissure (SOF), foramen rotundum (FRo), foramen ovale (FOv), and vidian canal (VC). When a direct exposure of these structures is needed, the corridor toward the sphenoid sinus can be enlarged passing through the anterior ethmoidal compartment (AE), posterior ethmoidal compartment, maxillary sinus (MS), and pterygopalatine fossa (PPF). V2, maxillary nerve; ACP, anterior clinoid process; bET, bony portion of the eustachian tube; DoS, dorsum sellae; FPs, foramen spinosum; IOF, inferior orbital fissure; LF, lacrimal fossa; LOCR, lateral optic-carotid recess; LP, lamina papyracea; NLD, nasolacrimal duct; OC, orbital cavity; ON, optic nerve; OPPB, orbital process of the palatine bone; OSt, optic strut; peICA, petrous tract of the internal carotid artery; PMF, pterygomaxillary fissure; PVC, palatovaginal canal; SPF, sphenopalatine foramen; SPPB, sphenoidal process of the palatine bone.

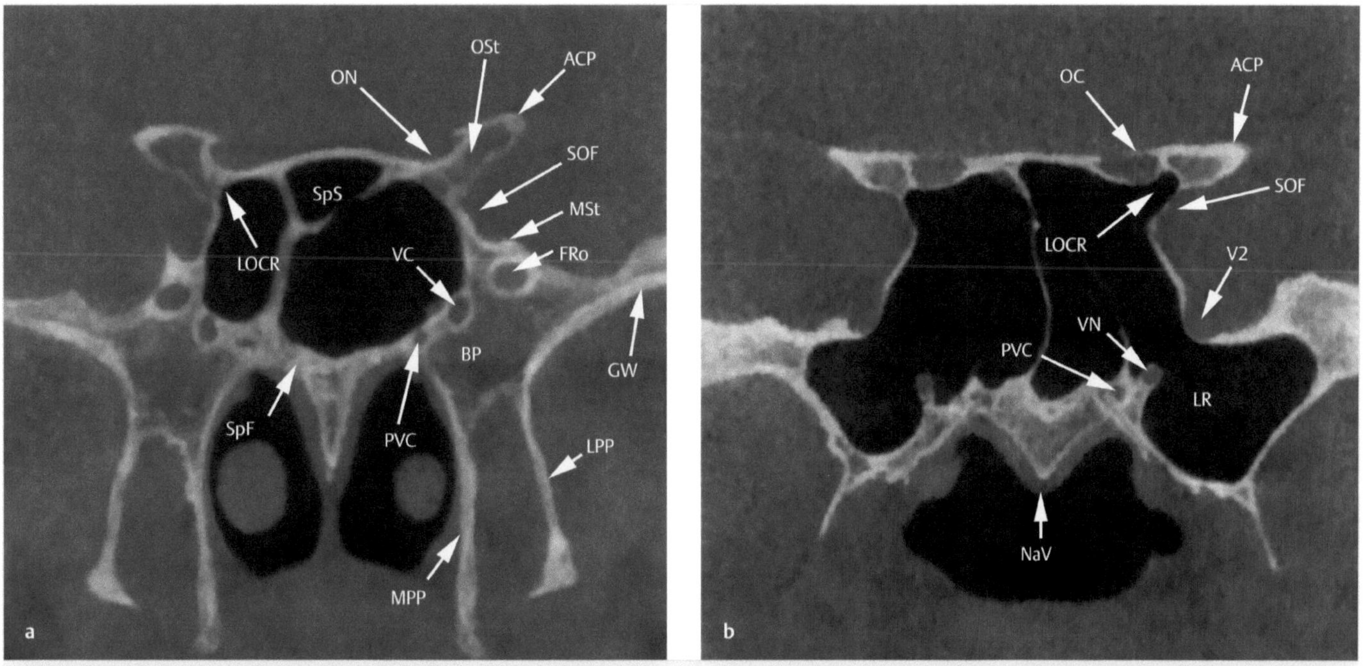

Fig. 4.5 Coronal CT anatomy of the sphenoid sinus and adjacent areas. The panel includes two coronal CT scans passing through the sphenoid sinus in subjects with poor **(a)** and pronounced **(b)** pneumatization of the lateral recess (LR). The lateral recess is the pneumatization of the base of the pterygoid process (BP). The passage between the lumen of the sphenoid sinus (SpS) and the lateral recess is conventionally considered the line connecting the foramen rotundum (FRo) with the vidian canal (VC). When particularly extended, the pneumatization can reach the greater wing of the sphenoid bone (GW) and the foramen ovale. The lateral wall of the sphenoid sinus separates its lumen from several neurovascular structures, including the optic nerve (ON), superior orbital fissure (SOF), and maxillary nerve (V2). The vidian nerve runs along the passage between the sphenoidal floor (SpF) and lateral sphenoidal wall. According to the grade of pneumatization of the sinus, each structure can be identified based on specific bony landmarks. For instance, the lateral optic-carotid recess (LOCR) can be used as a landmark for the optic strut (OSt), which is the inferomedial root of the anterior clinoid process (ACP) and separates the internal carotid artery from the optic canal (OC) and superior orbital fissure. The sphenoidal floor separates the lumen of the sphenoid sinus from the nasopharynx. It is a flat and thick bony floor, which includes canals that house neurovascular structures with variable size. From lateral to medial, these are the vidian, palatovaginal (PVC), lateral vomerovaginal, and medial vomerovaginal canals. LPP, lateral pterygoid plate; MPP, medial pterygoid plate; MSt, maxillary strut; NaV, nasopharyngeal vault; VN, vidian nerve.

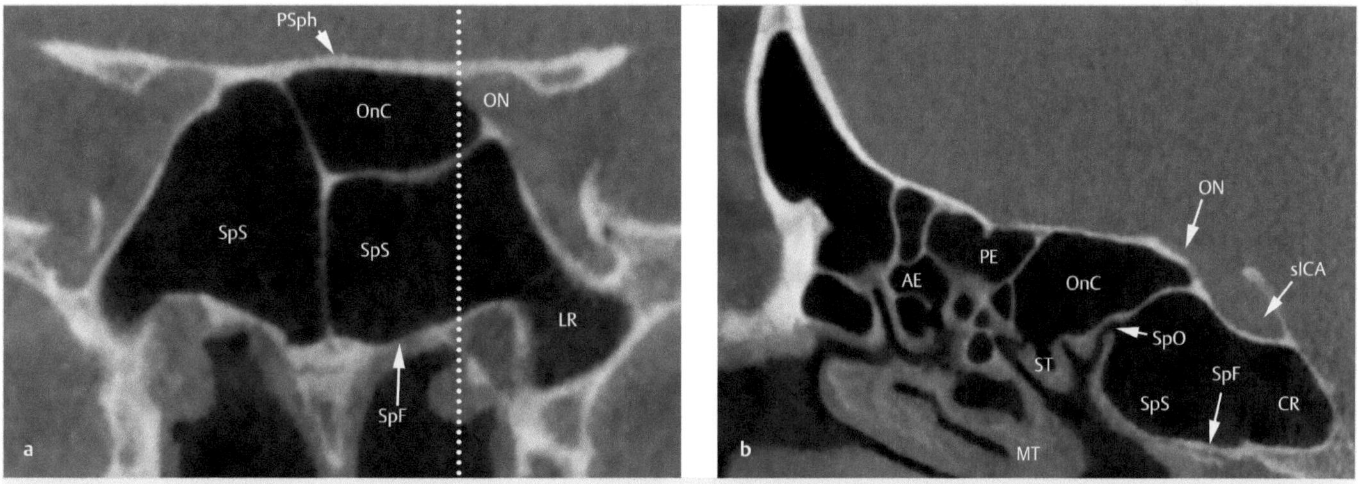

Fig. 4.6 Coronal and sagittal CT anatomy of Onodi cell. The *white dotted* line in the coronal image **(a)** shows the position of the sagittal image **(b)**. Onodi cell (OnC) is an air space of the posterior ethmoidal compartment (PE) that pneumatizes the sphenoid body and reaches the optic canal. The floor of Onodi cell is frequently flat, horizontally oriented, and located cranially to the tails of the middle (MT) and superior turbinates (ST). During endoscopic procedure, these characteristics are used to distinguish Onodi cell from the sphenoidal floor (SpF), which in turn is more irregular due to septations, tilted inferoposteriorly toward the clival recess (CR), and located approximately at the level of the tails of middle and superior turbinates. AE, anterior ethmoidal compartment; LR, lateral recess; ON, optic nerve; PSph, planum sphenoidale; sICA, parasellar tract of the internal carotid artery; SpO, sphenoidal ostium; SpS, sphenoid sinus.

Endoscopic Dissection

- Step 1: Partial superior turbinectomy (if needed).
- Step 2: Paraseptal sphenoidotomy.
- Step 3: Subseptal sphenoidotomy.
- Step 4: Transrostral sphenoidotomy.
- Step 5: Extended transrostral sphenoidotomy.
- Step 6: Modular (a) or functional (b) transethmoidal sphenoidotomy.
- Step 7: Posteroinferior septectomy.
- Step 8: Removal of the floor of the sphenoid sinus.

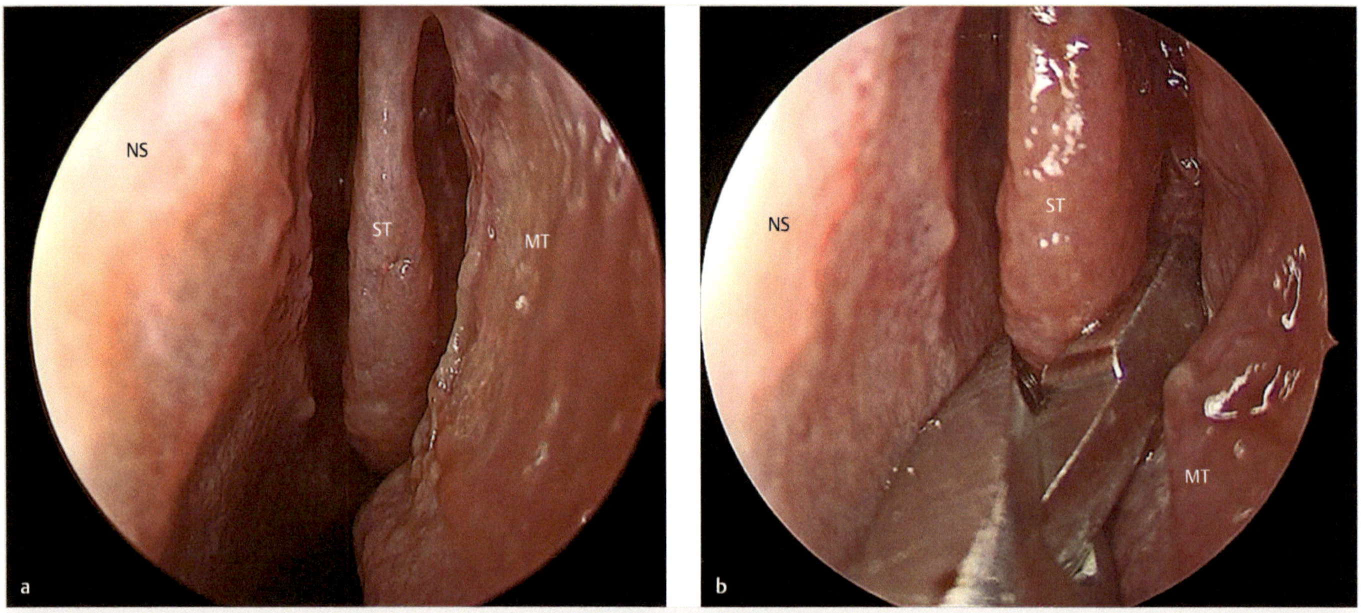

Fig. 4.7 (a, b) Step 1 (part 1). The bulbous portion of the superior turbinate (ST) is removed, whereas the laminar portion is left as a landmark for next steps of the dissection. MT, middle turbinate; NS, nasal septum.

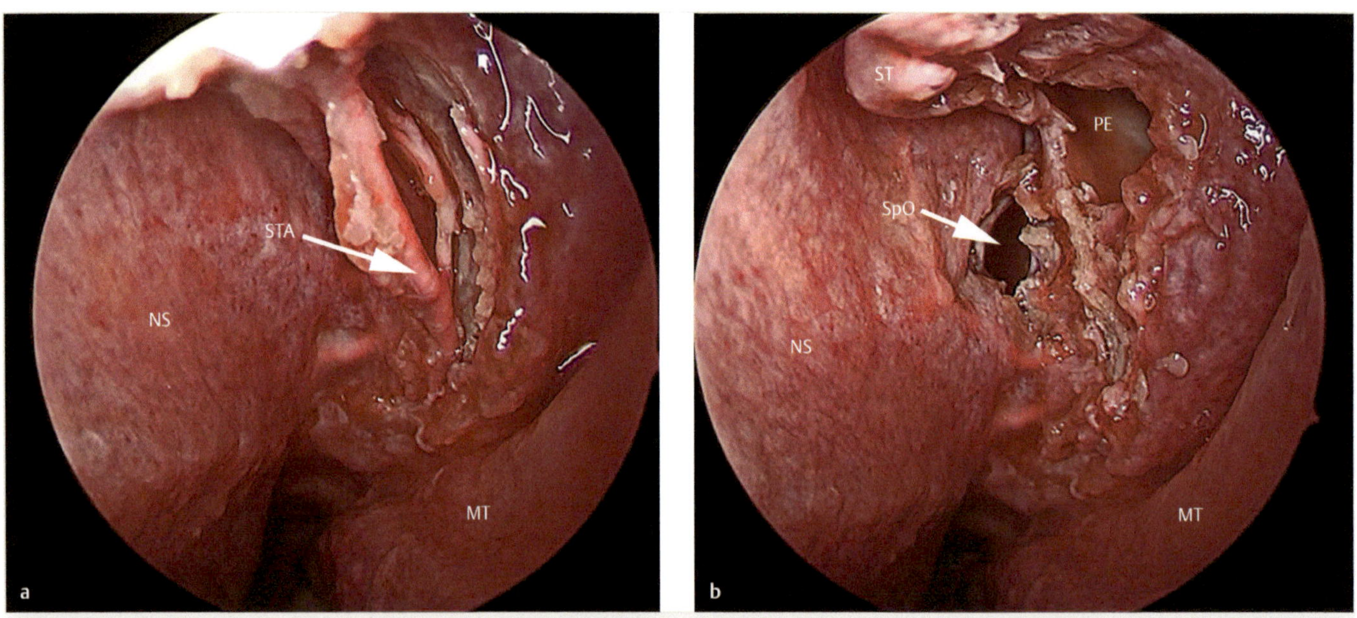

Fig. 4.8 (a, b) Step 1 (part 2). The sphenoid ostium (SpO) and the air spaces of the posterior ethmoid (PE) are identified after removing the superior turbinate (ST) up to its posterior insertion. The superior turbinal artery (STA), a branch of the sphenopalatine artery, can be identified within the superior turbinate. Superior turbinectomy is frequently necessary; however, it can be avoided when the sphenoid ostium can be directly identified through the middle nasal corridor. MT, middle turbinate; NS, nasal septum.

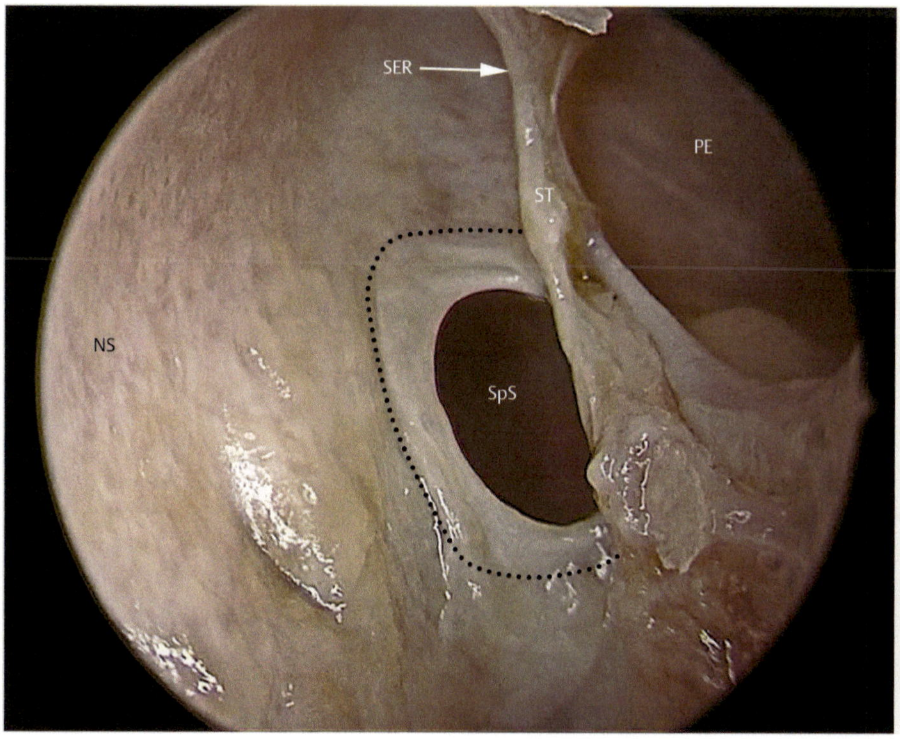

Fig. 4.9 The sphenoid ostium. The sphenoid sinus (SpS) communicates with the nasal cavity through a mucosal ostium, which is usually narrower than its bony counterpart (*black dotted line*). The sphenoethmoidal recess (SER) is the space between the anterior wall of the sphenoid sinus posteromedially and superior turbinate (ST) anterolaterally. NS, nasal septum; PE, posterior ethmoid.

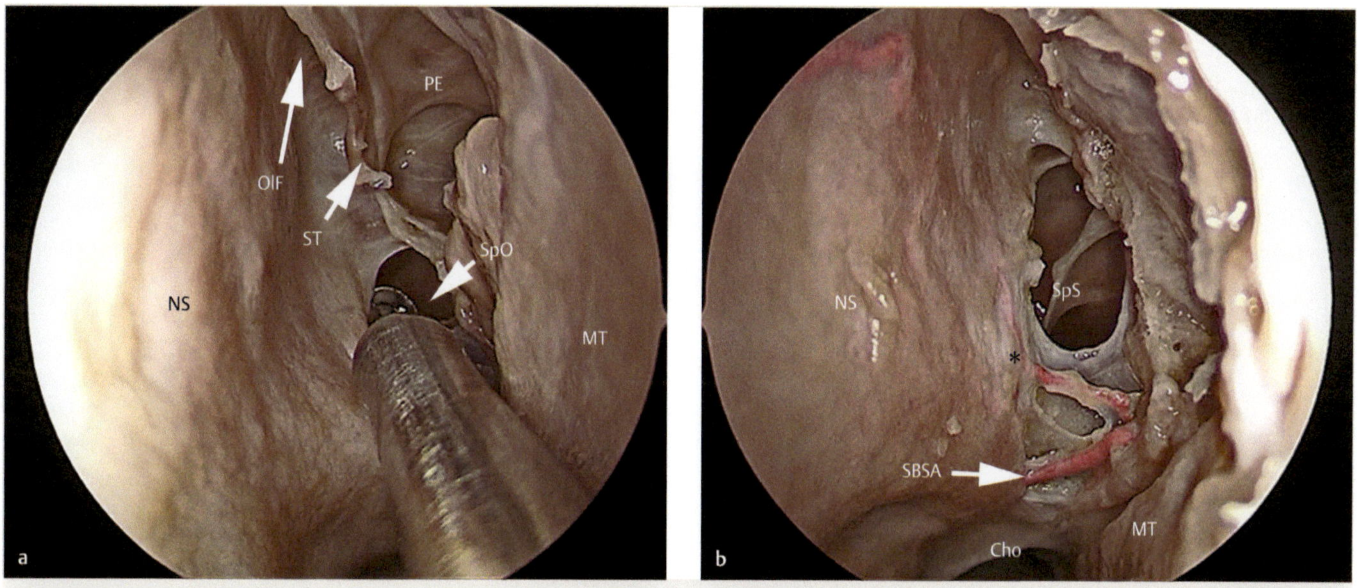

Fig. 4.10 (a, b) Step 2 (part 1). A straight punch is used to enlarge the sphenoid ostium (SpO). While extending inferiorly the aperture of the sphenoid sinus (SpS), a small artery (*black asterisk*) is encountered early; this artery can be misinterpreted as the septal branch of sphenopalatine artery (SBSA), which runs from the sphenopalatine ostium to the nasal septum (NS) in a more caudal plane located almost midway between the bony sphenoid ostium and the superior border of the choana (Cho). MT, middle turbinate; OlF, olfactory fissure; PE, posterior ethmoid; ST, superior turbinate.

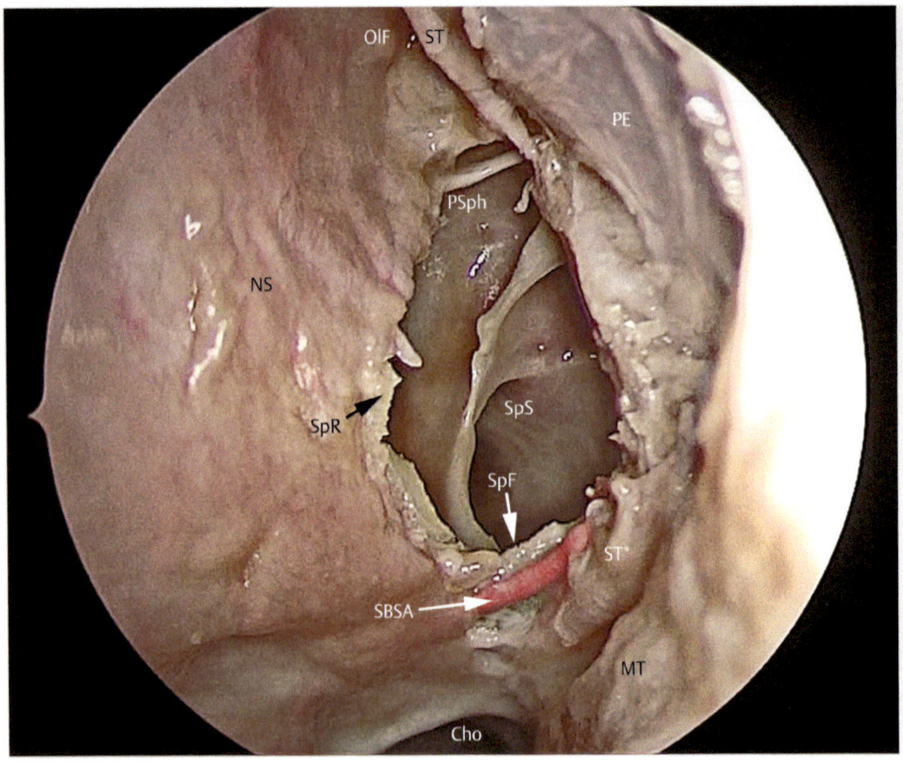

Fig. 4.11 Step 2 (part 2). The paraseptal sphenoidotomy is completed by removing the anterior sphenoidal wall up to the sphenoid rostrum (SpR) medially, posterior ethmoid (PE) and tail of the superior turbinate (ST) laterally, planum sphenoidale (PSph) and laminar portion of the superior turbinate cranially, and the sphenoid floor (SpF) caudally. The septal branch of sphenopalatine artery (SBSA) is preserved. Variable bony septa are identified within the sphenoid sinus (SpS) through the sphenoidotomy. Cho, choana; MT, middle turbinate; NS, nasal septum; OlF, olfactory fissure.

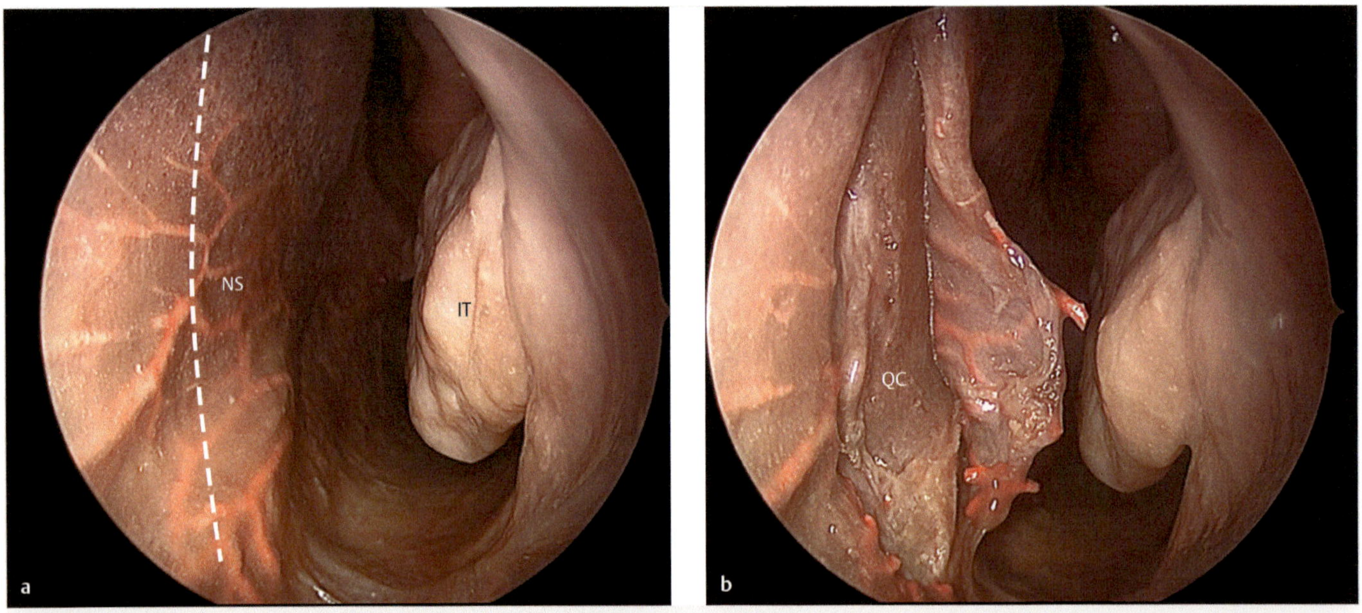

Fig. 4.12 (a, b) Step 3 (part 1). A vertical incision (*white dashed line*) of the nasal septum (NS) is made at the level of the head of the inferior turbinate (IT). The plane between the perichondrium and quadrangular cartilage is found to start the subperichondrial–subperiosteal dissection. This step can be performed on the contralateral side with respect to the paraseptal sphenoidotomy.

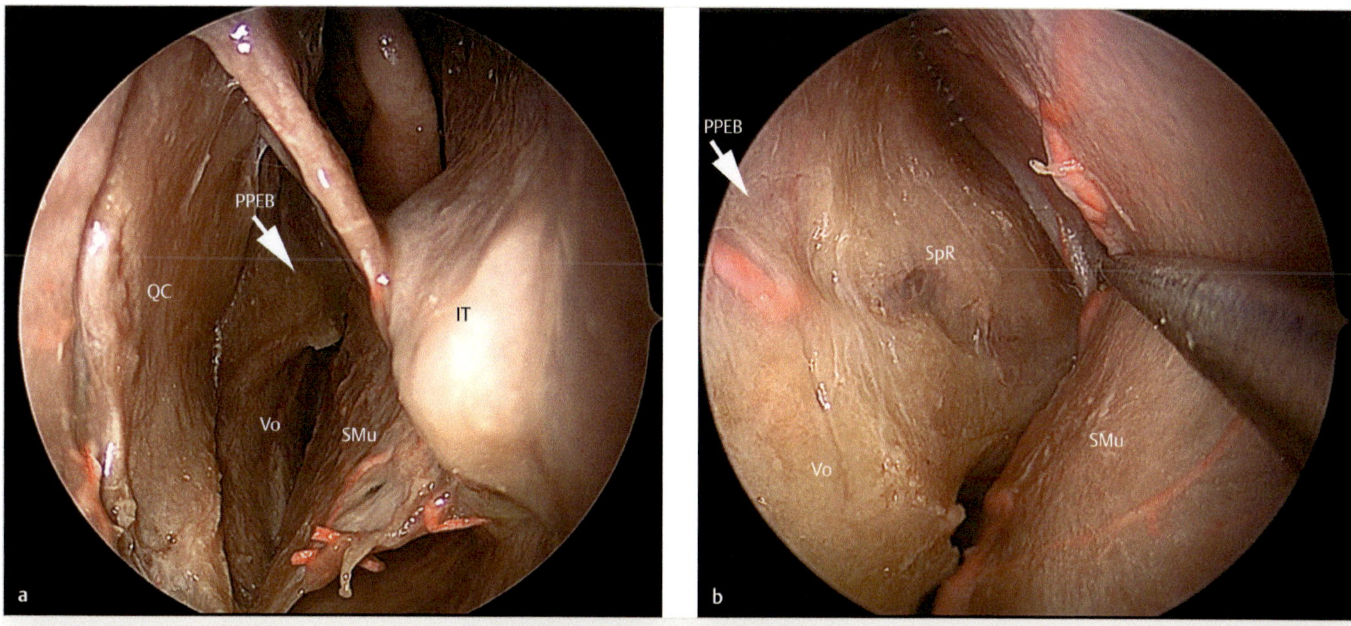

Fig. 4.13 (a, b) Step 3 (part 2). The subperichondrial–subperiosteal dissection is extended posteriorly along the quadrangular cartilage (QC), perpendicular plate of the ethmoid bone (PPEB), and vomer (Vo). The sphenoidal rostrum (SpR) is identified where the bony plane turns from sagittal to coronal above the nasal choana. IT, inferior turbinate; SMu, septal mucosa.

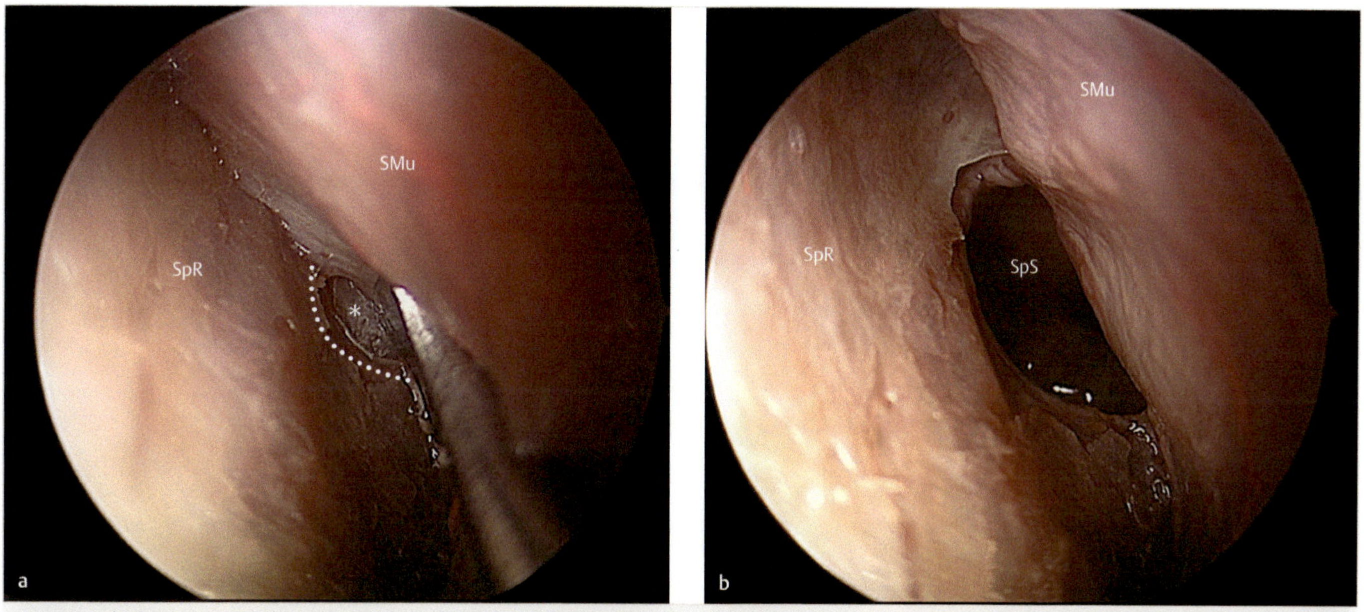

Fig. 4.14 (a, b) Step 3 (part 3). The sphenoidal ostium (*white dotted line*) is identified lateral and posterior to the sphenoidal rostrum (SpR), where the septal mucosa turns medially to line the ostium (*white asterisk*) and merge with the sphenoidal mucosa. The mucosa of the sphenoidal ostium is opened to expose the sphenoid sinus (SpS).

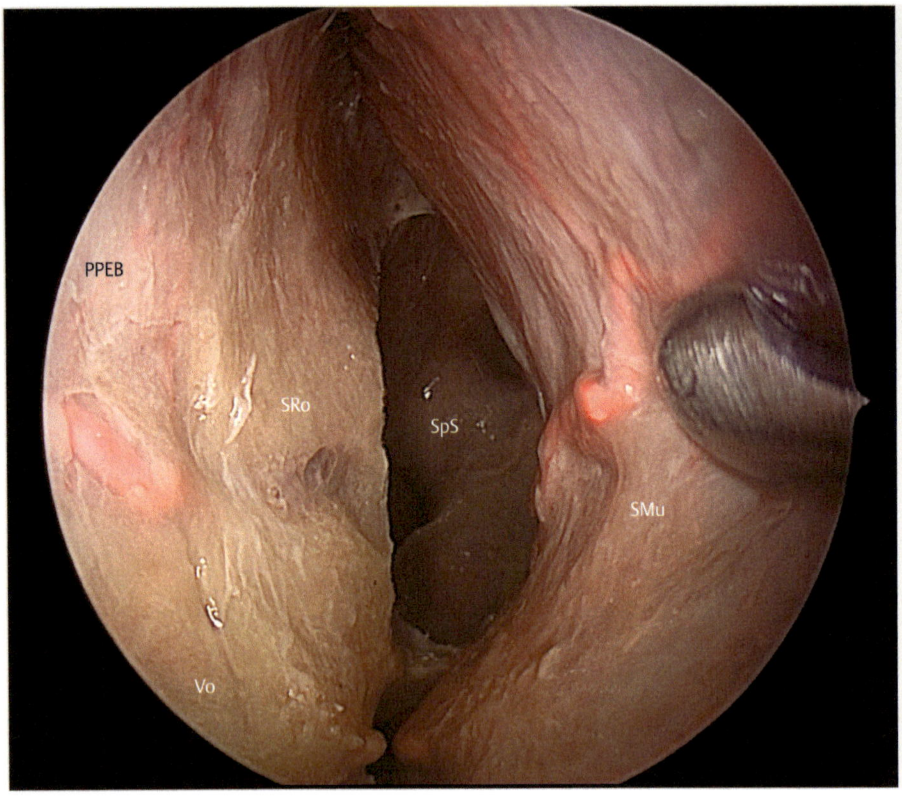

Fig. 4.15 Step 3 (part 4). The sphenoidotomy is completed by exposing the planum sphenoidale superiorly and sphenoidal floor inferiorly. The sphenoidal rostrum (SpR) and septal mucosa (SMu) are the medial and lateral boundaries of the corridor toward the sphenoid sinus (SpS), respectively. PPEB, perpendicular plate of ethmoidal bone; Vo, vomer.

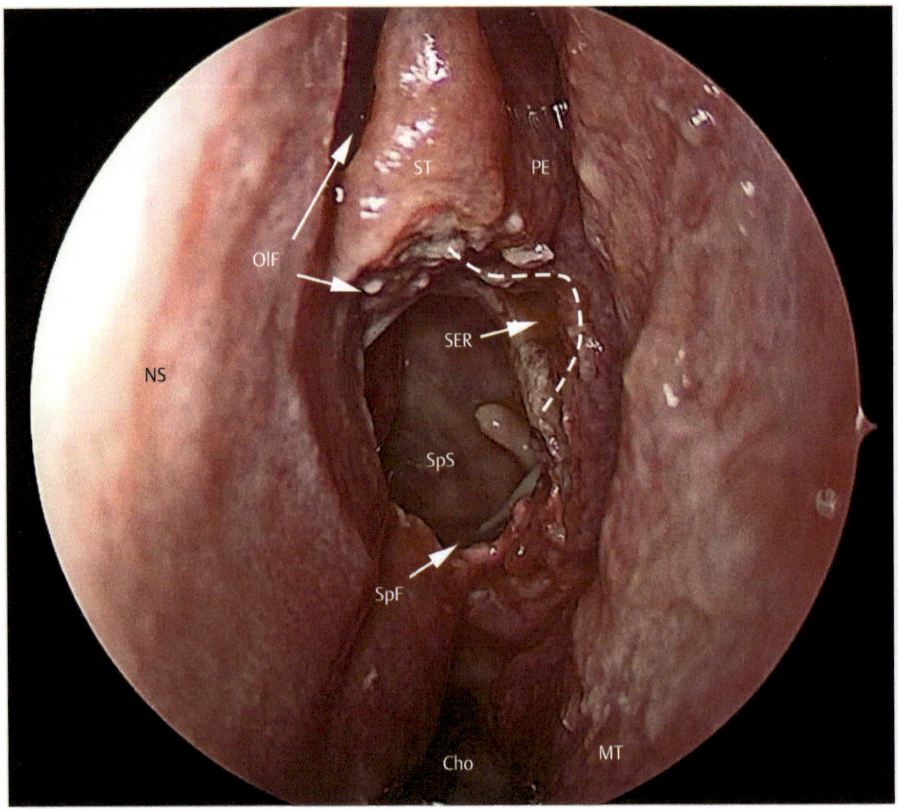

Fig. 4.16 The sphenoethmoidal recess. The sphenoethmoidal recess (SER) is a narrow cleft between the superior turbinate (ST) and the anterior wall of the sphenoid sinus (SpS). This space can have a variable extension according to where the superior turbinate (ST) inserts on the anterior wall of the sphenoid sinus (*white dashed line*). Cho, choana; MT, middle turbinate; NS, nasal septum; OlF, olfactory fissure; PE, posterior ethmoid; SpF, sphenoidal floor.

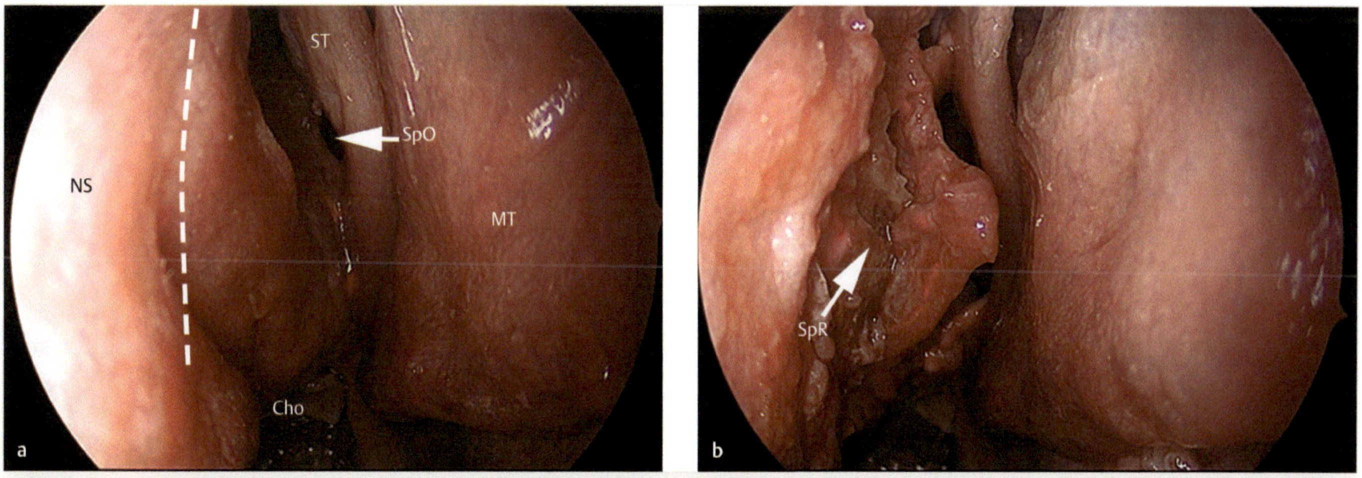

Fig. 4.17 (a, b) Step 4 (part 1). A vertical incision (*white dashed line*) is made on the nasal septum (NS) from the level of the axilla of the superior turbinate (ST) to the level of the inferior edge of the middle turbinate (MT) to expose the sphenoidal rostrum (SpR). Cho, choana; PE, posterior ethmoid; SpO, sphenoidal ostium.

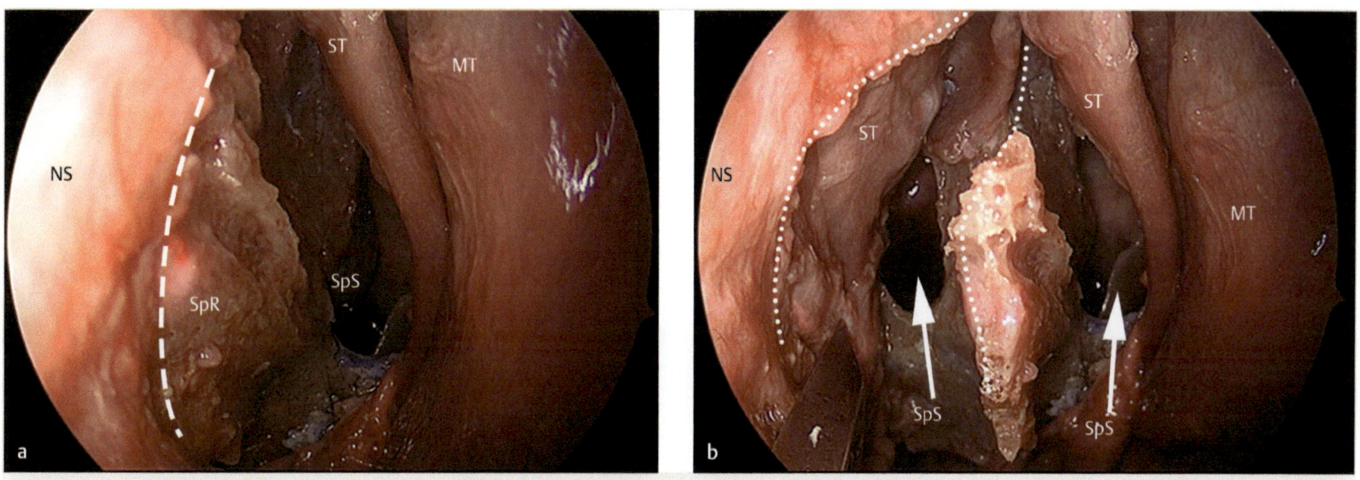

Fig. 4.18 (a, b) Step 4 (part 2). A dissector or chisel is used to fracture the nasal septum (NS) at the junction (*white dashed line* before fracture and *white dotted lines* after fracture) between the sphenoidal rostrum (SpR) and perpendicular plate of the ethmoid bone. After completing this maneuver, both sphenoid sinuses (SpS) are identified through paraseptal sphenoidotomies. MT, middle turbinate; ST, superior turbinate.

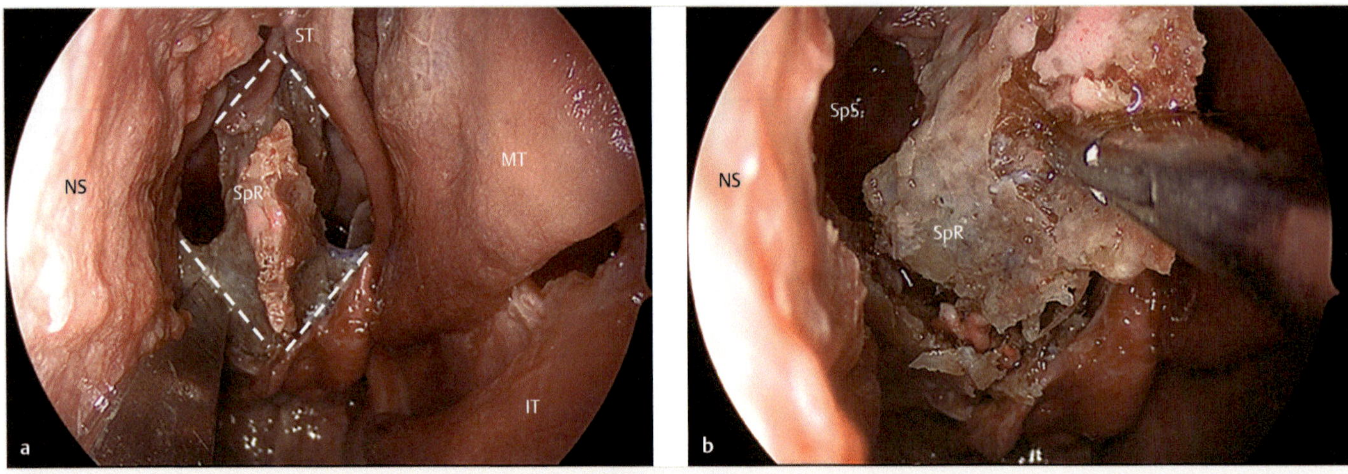

Fig. 4.19 (a, b) Step 4 (part 3). Four diagonal osteotomies (*white dashed lines*) are made to create a rhomboid fracture around the sphenoidal rostrum (SpR), which is subsequently removed. IT, inferior turbinate; MT, middle turbinate; NS, nasal septum; SpS, sphenoid sinus; ST, superior turbinate.

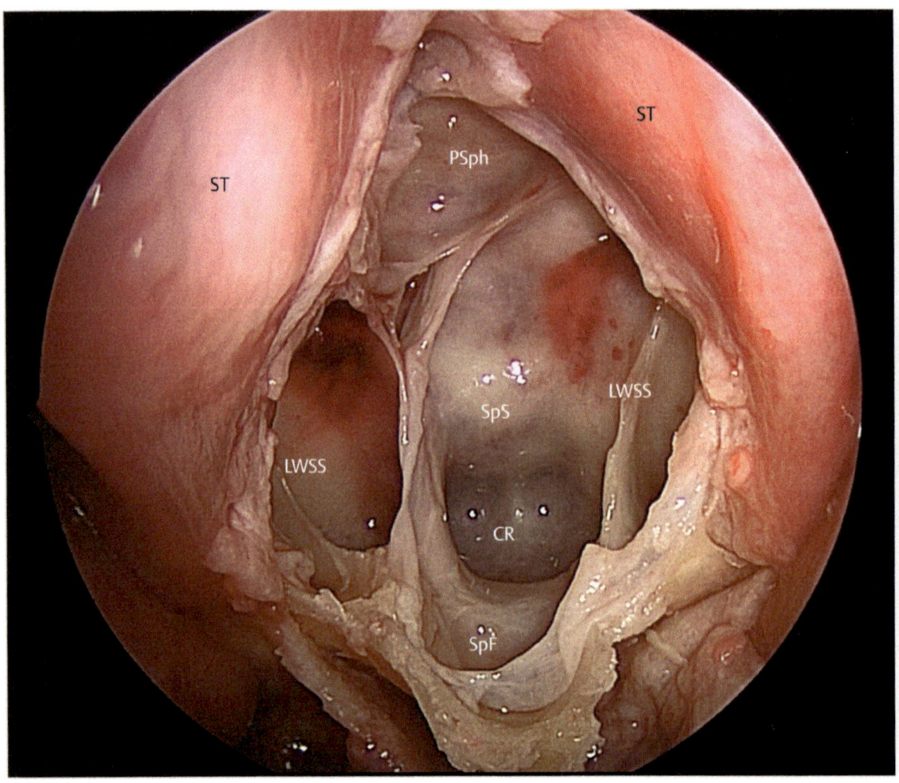

Fig. 4.20 Step 4 (part 4). The transrostral sphenoidotomy has a rhomboid shape, bounded by the superior turbinates (ST) superiorly and the sphenoidal floor (SpF) inferiorly. CR, clival recess; LWSS, lateral wall of sphenoid sinus; PSph, planum sphenoidale; Sps, sphenoid sinus.

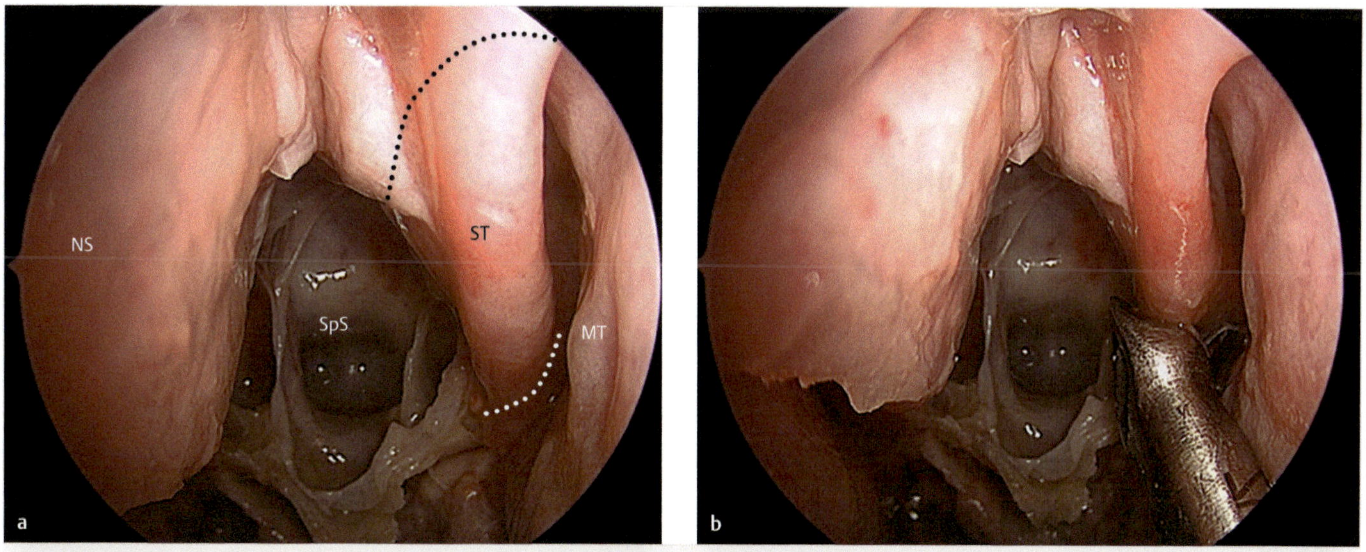

Fig. 4.21 (a, b) Step 5 (part 1). Both laminar and bulbous portions of superior turbinate (ST) are removed with a cutting instrument (*black and white dotted lines*). MT, middle turbinate; NS, nasal septum; SpS, sphenoid sinus.

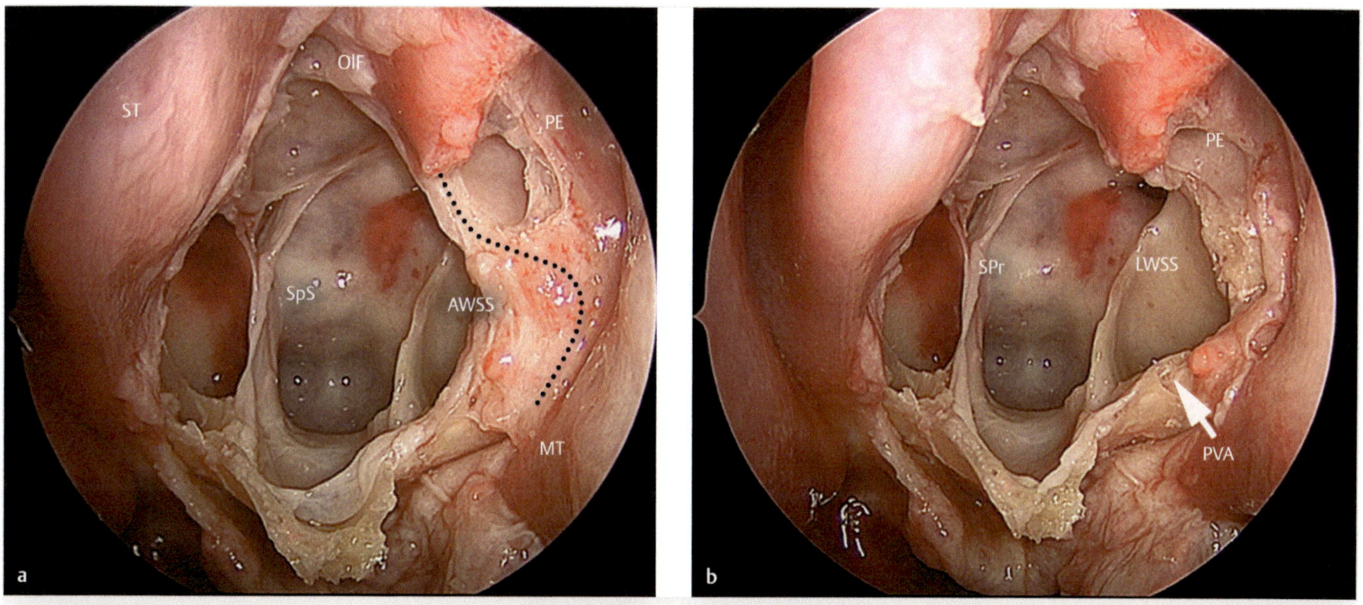

Fig. 4.22 (a, b) Step 5 (part 2). The portion of the anterior wall of sphenoid sinus (AWSS) that lies medial to the posterior insertion of the superior turbinate (*black dotted line*) is removed. The palatovaginal artery (PVA) can be identified in the inferolateral corner of the extended transrostral sphenoidotomy, above the tail of the middle turbinate (MT). LWSS, lateral wall of sphenoid sinus; MT, middle turbinate; OlF, olfactory fissure; PE, posterior ethmoid; SPr, sellar prominence; SpS, sphenoid sinus.

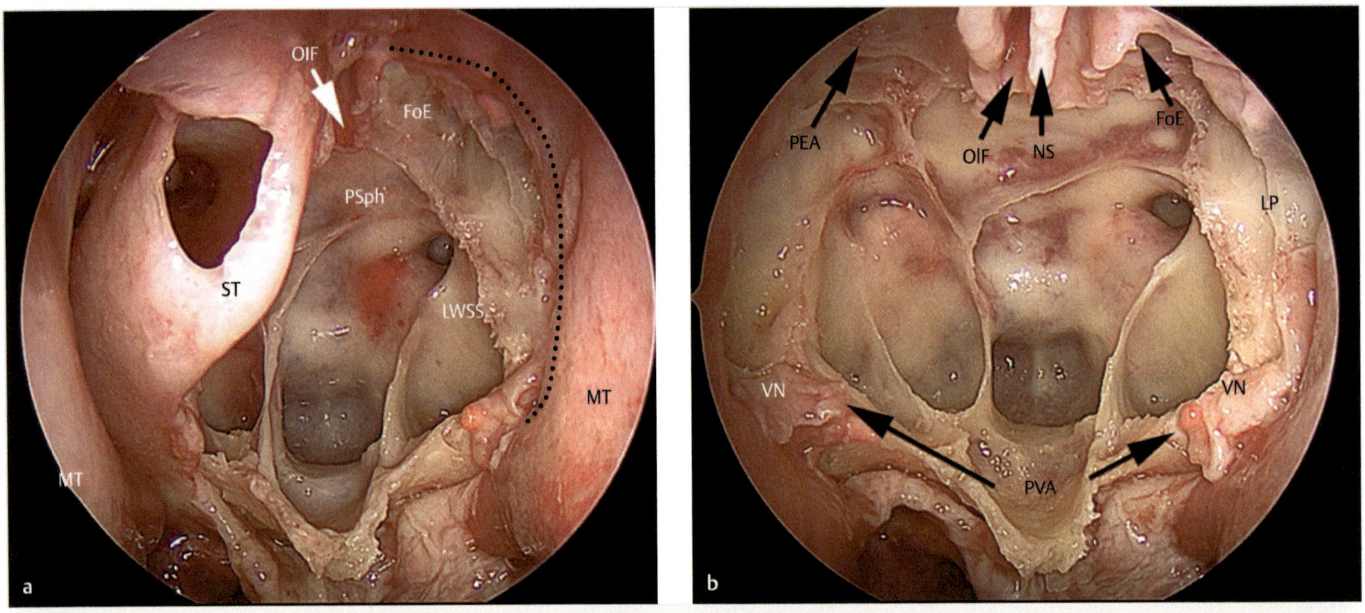

Fig. 4.23 (a, b) Step 6a. The posterior ethmoid is removed until exposing (*black dotted line*) the planum sphenoidale (PSph) and fovea ethmoidalis (FoE) superiorly and the lateral wall of sphenoid sinus (LWSS) and the lamina papyracea (LP) laterally. A rectangular window toward the central skull base is obtained by performing a bilateral modular transethmoidal sphenoidotomy. The vidian nerve (VN) and posterior ethmoidal artery (PEA) run in the inferolateral and superolateral corners of the sphenoidotomy, respectively. NS, nasal septum; OlF, olfactory fissure; ST, superior turbinate.

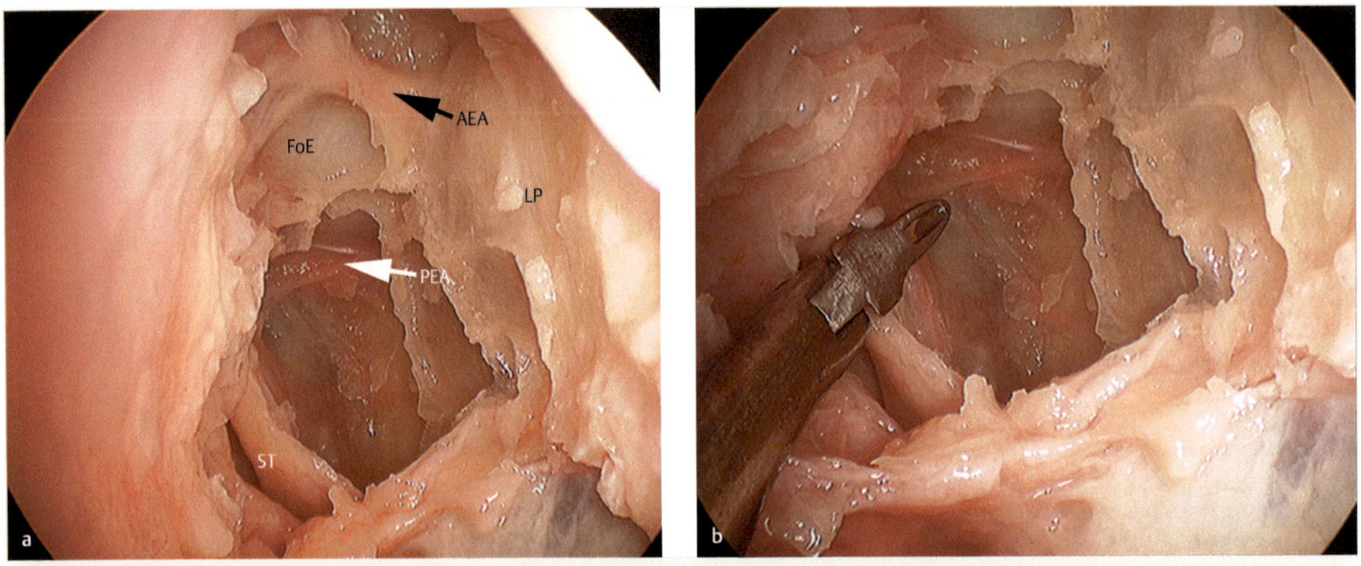

Fig. 4.24 (a, b) Step 6b (part 1). Functional transethmoidal sphenoidotomy is the opening of the sphenoid sinus through the ethmoid after completing anterior and posterior ethmoidectomy. The bulbous portion of the superior turbinate (ST) is identified in the medial border of the posterior ethmoid and is removed with a cutting instrument. AEA, anterior ethmoidal artery; FoE, fovea ethmoidalis; LP, lamina papyracea; PEA, posterior ethmoidal artery.

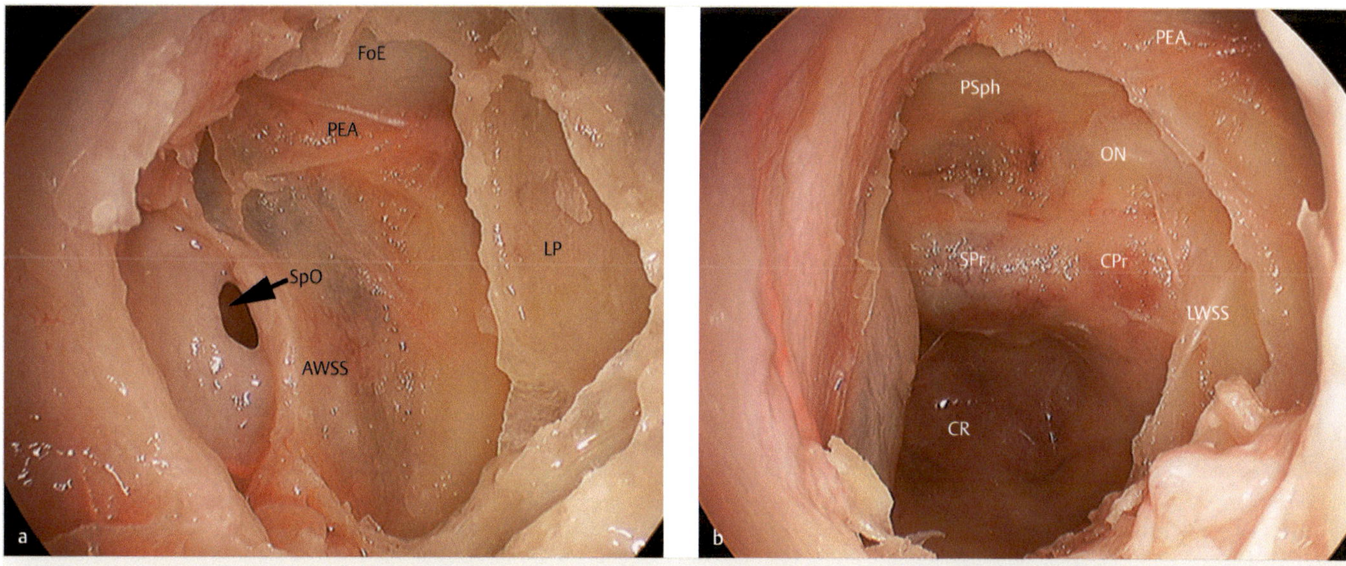

Fig. 4.25 (a, b) Step 6b (part 2). After removing the superior turbinate, the sphenoidal ostium (SpO) can be identified. The anterior wall of the sphenoid sinus (AWSS) is safely removed starting from the sphenoid ostium and proceeding toward the planum sphenoidale superiorly (PSph), lateral wall of the sphenoid sinus (LWSS) laterally, intersphenoid sinus septum medially, and sphenoidal floor inferiorly. CPr, carotid prominence; CR, clival recess; FoE, fovea ethmoidalis; LP, lamina papyracea; ON, optic nerve (within the optic canal); PEA, posterior ethmoidal artery; SPr, sellar prominence.

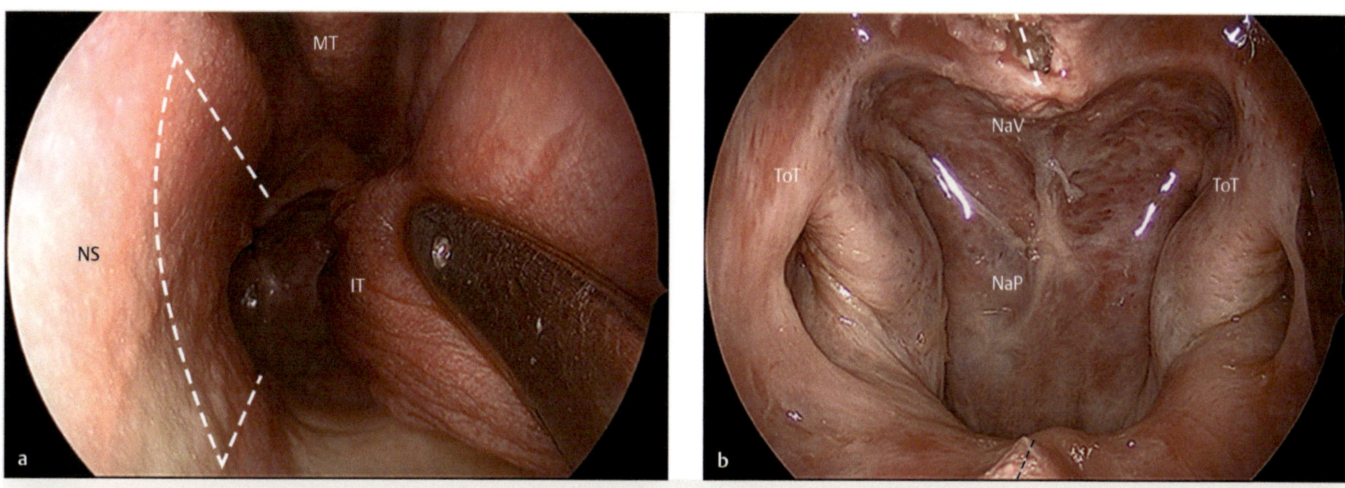

Fig. 4.26 (a, b) Step 7. A posteroinferior septectomy is performed removing the nasal septum (NS) along the nasal floor inferiorly and the plane passing through the upper border of the choana superiorly (*white dashed line*). The anterior incision is made 1.5 to 2 cm anterior to the choana and can be modulated according to the need of contralateral exposure. This approach allows joining the two inferior nasal corridors to work toward the posterior wall of the nasopharynx (NaP), nasopharyngeal vault (NaV), and tori tubarii (ToT). IT, inferior turbinate; MT, middle turbinate.

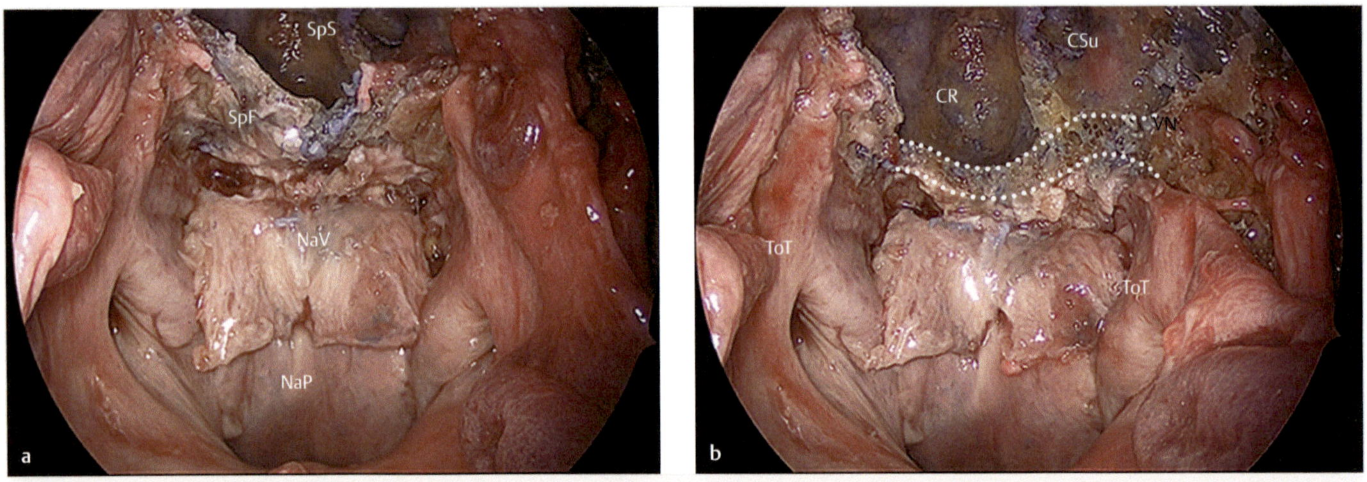

Fig. 4.27 (a, b) Step 8. After performing an extended transrostral or modular transethmoidal sphenoidotomy and posteroinferior septectomy, the mucosal nasopharyngeal vault (NaV) is dissected off the sphenoidal floor (SpF) and folded on the posterior wall of the nasopharynx (NaP). The sphenoidal floor is removed to merge the sphenoid sinuses (SpS) with nasopharynx. The lateral boundary of the removal of the sphenoidal floor is the vidian nerve (VN), while the posterior limit (*white dotted lines*) is the clival recess (CR) on the midline and the inferior end of the carotid sulcus (CSu) laterally. ToT, torus tubarius.

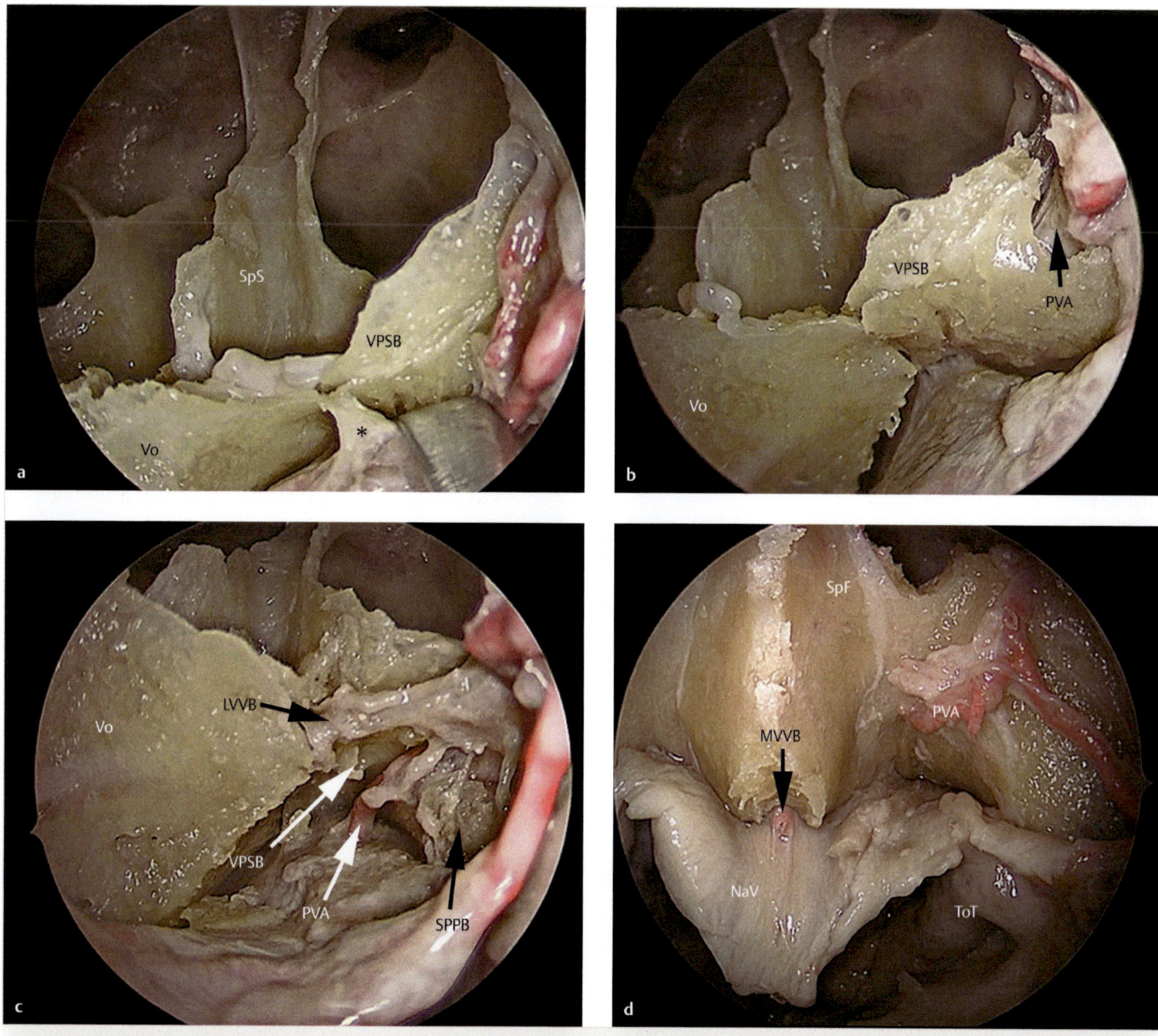

Fig. 4.28 (a–d) Palatovaginal and vomerovaginal bundles. The corner between the vomer, palatine bone, and sphenoidal floor (SpF) has a complex anatomy, including several neurovascular bundles. The ala of the vomer (Vo) joins with the vaginal process of the sphenoid bone (VPSB), forming a narrow canal that houses the lateral vomerovaginal bundle (LVVB). Frequently, other small nerves (*black asterisk*) joins the lateral vomerovaginal bundle passing through the interface between the vomer and sphenoid bone. The palatovaginal artery (PVA) runs in a small canal between the sphenoid process of the palatine bone (SPPB) and the vaginal process of the sphenoid bone. The pharyngeal nerve (also called Bock's nerve) arises from the pterygopalatine ganglion and reaches the nasopharyngeal mucosa passing through either the palatovaginal or lateral vomerovaginal canal or dividing and giving small branches for both the canals. The median vomerovaginal bundle (MVVB) is an anatomical variant that can be identified additionally to the lateral vomerovaginal structures: it can be found on the midline along the junction between the vomer and sphenoidal floor, from where it reaches the nasopharyngeal vault (NaV) by piercing the bone. SpS, sphenoid sinus; ToT, torus tubarius.

References

[1] Jho HD. Endoscopic pituitary surgery. Pituitary 1999;2(2):139–154

[2] Jho HD, Carrau RL. Endoscopic endonasal transsphenoidal surgery: experience with 50 patients. J Neurosurg 1997;87(1):44–51

[3] Dehdashti AR, Ganna A, Karabatsou K, Gentili F. Pure endoscopic endonasal approach for pituitary adenomas: early surgical results in 200 patients and comparison with previous microsurgical series. Neurosurgery 2008;62(5):1006–1015, discussion 1015–1017

[4] Berhouma M, Messerer M, Jouanneau E. Occam's razor in minimally invasive pituitary surgery: tailoring the endoscopic endonasal uninostril trans-sphenoidal approach to sella turcica. Acta Neurochir (Wien) 2012;154(12):2257–2265

[5] Cavallo LM, de Divitiis O, Aydin S, et al. Extended endoscopic endonasal transsphenoidal approach to the suprasellar area: anatomic considerations—part 1. Neurosurgery 2008;62(6, Suppl 3):1202–1212

[6] Kassam A, Snyderman CH, Mintz A, Gardner P, Carrau RL. Expanded endonasal approach: the rostrocaudal axis. Part II. Posterior clinoids to the foramen magnum. Neurosurg Focus 2005;19(1):E4

[7] Kassam A, Snyderman CH, Mintz A, Gardner P, Carrau RL. Expanded endonasal approach: the rostrocaudal axis. Part I. Crista galli to the sella turcica. Neurosurg Focus 2005;19(1):E3

[8] Cavallo LM, Messina A, Cappabianca P, et al. Endoscopic endonasal surgery of the midline skull base: anatomical study and clinical considerations. Neurosurg Focus 2005;19(1):E2

[9] Jho HD, Ha HG. Endoscopic endonasal skull base surgery: part 3—the clivus and posterior fossa. Minim Invasive Neurosurg 2004;47(1):16–23

[10] Jho HD, Ha HG. Endoscopic endonasal skull base surgery: part 2—the cavernous sinus. Minim Invasive Neurosurg 2004;47(1):9–15

[11] Jho HD, Ha HG. Endoscopic endonasal skull base surgery: part 1—the midline anterior fossa skull base. Minim Invasive Neurosurg 2004;47(1):1–8

[12] Belotti F, Doglietto F, Schreiber A, et al. Modular classification of endoscopic endonasal transsphenoidal approaches to sellar region: anatomic quantitative study. World Neurosurg 2018;109:e281–e291

[13] de Divitiis E, Cappabianca P, Cavallo LM. Endoscopic transsphenoidal approach: adaptability of the procedure to different sellar lesions. Neurosurgery 2002;51(3):699–705, discussion 705–707

[14] Linsler S, Gaab MR, Oertel J. Endoscopic endonasal transsphenoidal approach to sellar lesions: a detailed account of our mononostril technique. J Neurol Surg B Skull Base 2013;74(3):146–154

[15] Moreland DB, Diaz-Ordaz E, Czajka GA. Endoscopic endonasal hemisphenoidotomy for resection of pituitary lesions confined to the sella: report of 3 cases and technical note. Minim Invasive Neurosurg 2000;43(2):57–61

[16] Wang J, Bidari S, Inoue K, Yang H, Rhoton A Jr. Extensions of the sphenoid sinus: a new classification. Neurosurgery 2010;66(4):797–816

[17] Karligkiotis A, Volpi L, Abbate V, et al. Palatovaginal (pharyngeal) artery: clinical implication and surgical experience. Eur Arch Otorhinolaryngol 2014;271(10):2839–2843

5 Corridor to Lateral Spaces

Alberto Schreiber, Vittorio Rampinelli, Marco Ferrari, Marco Ravanelli

Lateral exposure is exceedingly important when approaching skull base pathologies with extension along the medial–lateral axis. Some coronal approaches basically consist of the lateral extension of midline corridors across neighboring cranial base areas. Conversely, several pathways along the coronal plane require a complex and specific preparatory phase. In particular, six bony doors can be schematically considered to access lateral portions of the skull base and adjacent areas: the maxillary walls, orbital walls (Chapter 14), pterygoid process (Chapters 21, 23, and 24), lateral sphenoidal wall (Chapters 18 and 21), petrous bone (Chapters 19 and 20), and occipital condyle (Chapter 22). The maxillary sinus, besides being the target in functional procedures and selected sinonasal neoplasms (i.e., schneiderian papillomas), represents a natural corridor toward several infracranial areas (i.e., pterygopalatine fossa, infratemporal fossa, and upper parapharyngeal space). The present chapter focuses on modular types of removal of the medial and anterior walls of the maxillary sinus, referred to as "modular endoscopic medial maxillectomies."[1] Moreover, a brief description of the lacrimal sac anatomy as seen through an endoscopic dacryocystorhinostomy is reported.

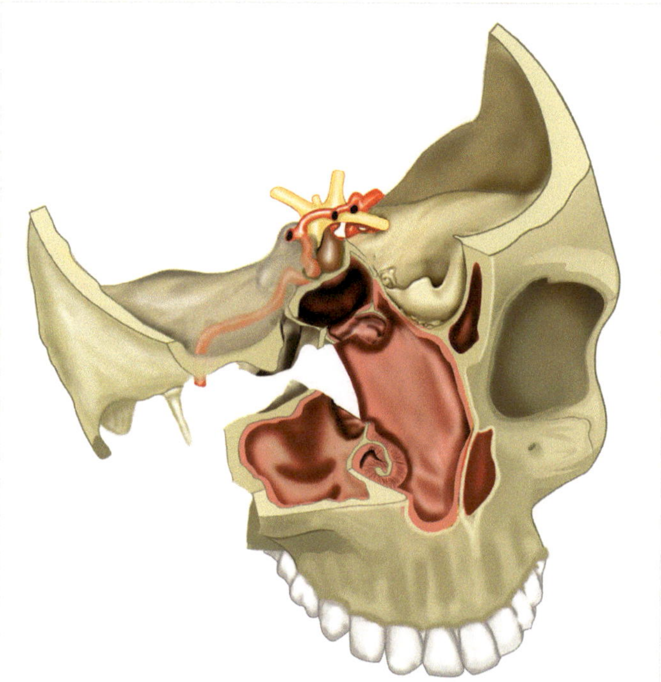

Fig. 5.1 Diagonal view of transnasal routes toward the lateral spaces. This illustration shows anatomy of the maxillary sinus and neighboring spaces.

The medial wall of the maxillary sinus is a complex and heterogeneous structure, composed by the horizontal portion of the uncinate process, inferior turbinate, bony nasolacrimal duct, and a vertical bony lamina going from the nasal floor to the inferomedial orbital corner.[1,2] The maxillary ostium lies in the superior and anterior portion of the medial maxillary wall. It is oriented anteriorly, superiorly, and medially, facing the intermediate third of the uncinate process, between its vertical and horizontal portions. Not infrequently, one or more defects of the medial maxillary wall (called accessory maxillary ostia or fontanelles) can be found along the inferior insertion of the uncinate process. This complex wall can be disassembled in a modular fashion to tailor the entity of bone removal in relation to the need for lateral and inferior exposure.[1] The anterior wall of the maxillary sinus can be divided into two halves with respect to the sagittal plane passing through the

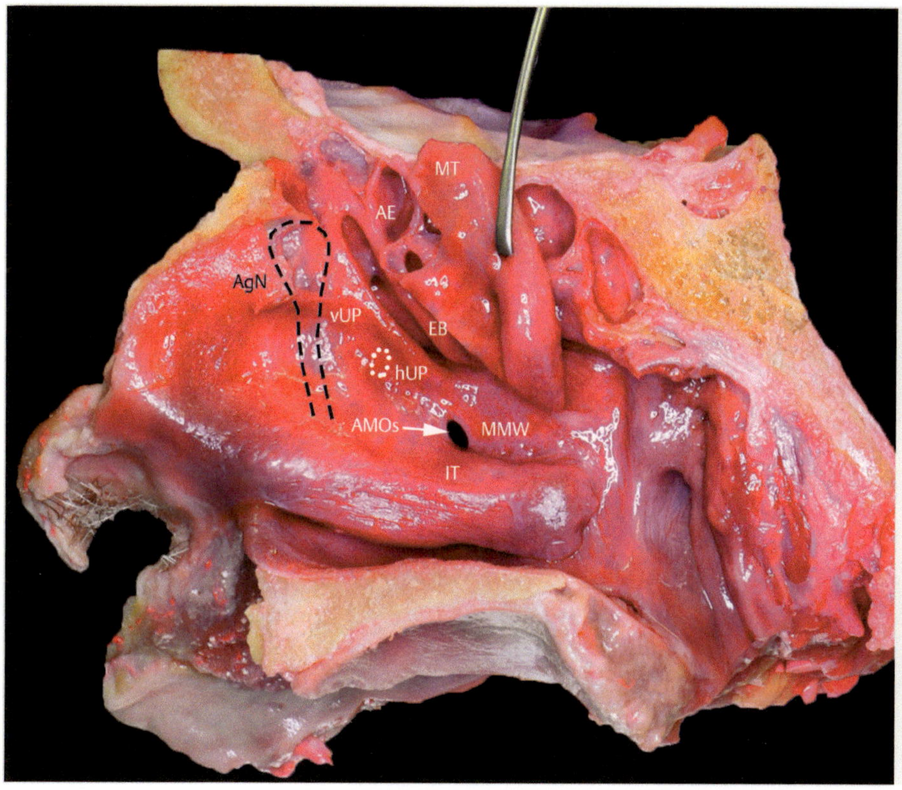

Fig. 5.2 Sagittal view of the lateral nasal wall and medial maxillary wall. This cadaver cut shows anatomy of the medial maxillary wall. AE, anterior ethmoidal compartment; AgN, agger nasi; AMOs, accessory maxillary ostium; EB, ethmoid bulla; hUP, horizontal segment of the uncinate process; IT, inferior turbinate; MMW, medial maxillary wall; MT, middle turbinate; vUP, vertical segment of the uncinate process. (*Black dashed line*, position of the lacrimal sac and nasolacrimal duct; *white dotted line*, position of the maxillary ostium).

infraorbital foramen. The medial half of the anterior wall can be removed to enhance the working space toward maxillary and retromaxillary areas, as formerly described by Denker, Sturmann, and Canfield in the early 20th century.[3–5] The lateral half of the anterior maxillary wall can be partially removed when far-lateral exposure is required.[2–7]

Aiming to standardize the nomenclature and facilitate teaching and learning the surgical technique of endoscopic medial maxillectomies, a modular classification was recently proposed by our group.[1] The distinction among four different types of maxillectomies is based on preclinical evidence of gain in terms of working volume and exposure. Type A endoscopic medial maxillectomy includes an inferior uncinectomy and removal of the medial maxillary wall to the inferior turbinate insertion (inferiorly), orbital floor (superiorly), descending palatine canal (posteriorly), and nasolacrimal duct (anteriorly). Type B maxillectomy corresponds to a type A plus inferior turbinectomy and removal of the maxillary sinus medial wall posterior to the nasolacrimal duct. Type C procedure also includes the resection of the nasolacrimal duct and removal of the residual anterior portion of the medial maxillary wall. Type D endoscopic maxillectomy involves the removal of the anterior wall of the maxillary sinus medial to the infraorbital foramen. The modularity of the classification allows easy extension from a less to a more invasive removal of the maxillary walls, according to intraoperative findings and need for exposure. In terms of medial–lateral exposure, types A to D maxillectomies allow reaching the foramen rotundum, foramen spinosum, mandibular condyle, and coronoid process, respectively. In terms of cranial–caudal exposure, a type A procedure reaches the vidian nerve, types B and C maxillectomies reach the axial plane passing through the root of the styloid process, and type D resection also provides the exposure of the inferior border of the lateral pterygoid plate.[1]

With the intent to minimize surgical morbidity related to endoscopic maxillectomies, some authors have designed variants of traditional approaches. For instance, the prelacrimal approach consists of a surgical corridor that passes lateral to the nasolacrimal duct with the intent to prevent lacrimal stenosis.[8–13] In terms of exposure, this approach is similar to types C and D endoscopic maxillectomies, depending on whether the bony edge of the piriform aperture is spared or removed, respectively. As an alternative, transseptal approaches through the contralateral nostril were developed to optimize lateral exposure while minimizing disassembling of maxillary walls.[1,14,15]

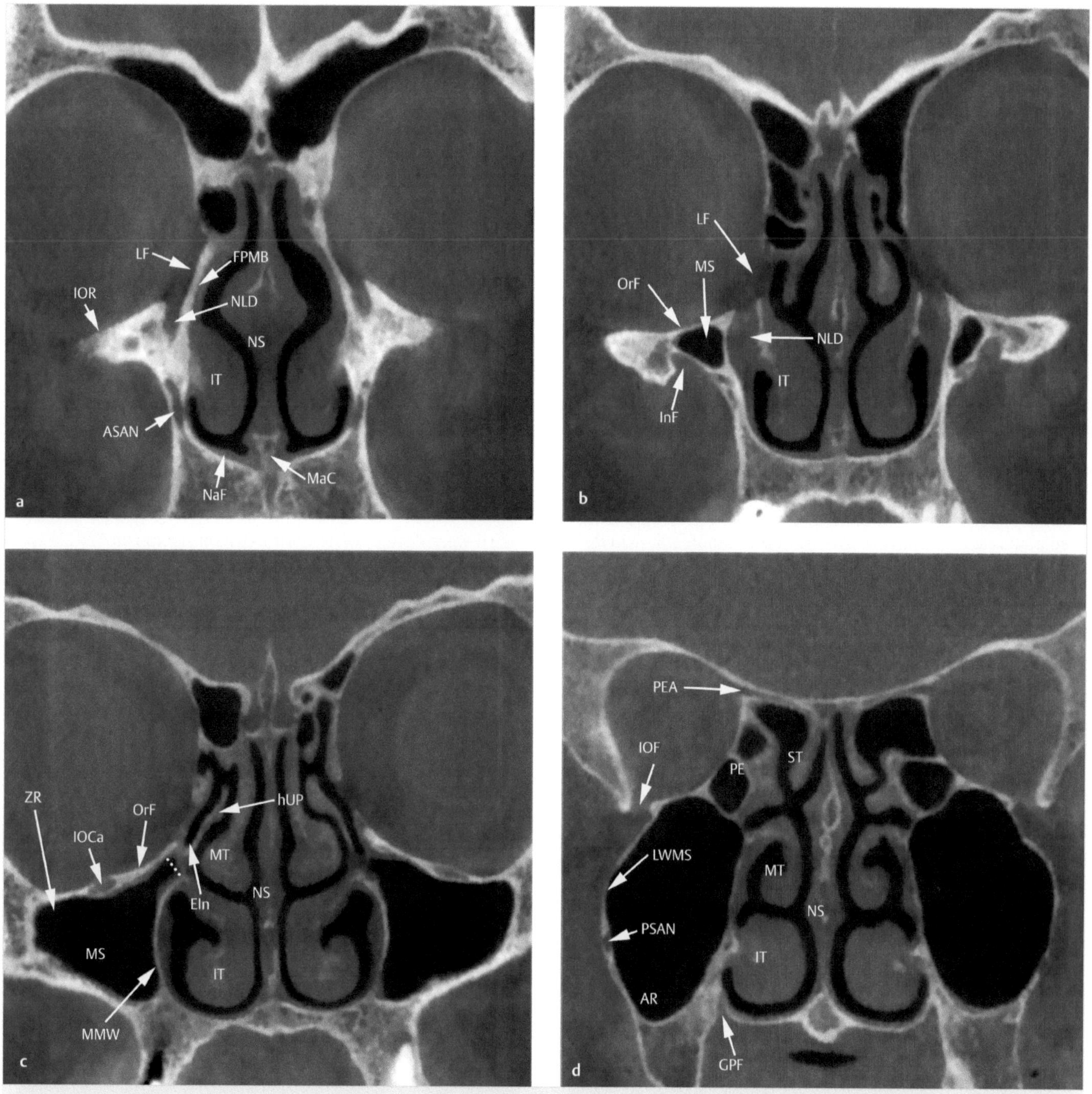

Fig. 5.3 (a–d) Coronal CT anatomy of the maxillary sinus and adjacent structures. The panel includes four coronal CT scans passing through the maxillary sinus (MS) disposed from anterior **(a)** to posterior **(d)**. The maxillary sinus can be described according to its six walls. On a coronal plane, the medial, inferior, lateral, and superior walls can be analyzed. The medial maxillary wall (MMW) separates the maxillary sinus from the inferior nasal meatus and ethmoidal compartment. The maxillary ostium (*white dotted line*) connects the maxillary sinus with the ethmoidal infundibulum (EIn) and is located in the superior and anterior portion of the medial maxillary wall. Anteriorly, the medial maxillary wall enlarges to house the nasolacrimal duct (NLD). The passage between the medial and anterior walls of the maxillary sinus corresponds to the frontal process of the maxillary bone, where the anterior superior alveolar nerve (ASAN) is located. Of note, the posterior ethmoid (PE), horizontal portion of the uncinate process (hUP), and inferior (IT) and middle turbinate (MT) insert onto the medial maxillary wall. The inferior wall is formed by the alveolar process of the maxilla, which can be variably pneumatized by the alveolar recess (AR). The latter can also extend into the hard palate in highly pneumatized maxillary sinuses. The lateral wall of the maxillary sinus (LWMS) is variably deep in the anterior portion, where it forms the zygomatic recess (ZR), and flat in the posterior portion, where it smoothly continues into the posterior wall. The lateral wall houses the posterior superior alveolar nerve (PSAN). The superior wall of the maxillary sinus is the orbital floor (OrF), where the infraorbital canal (IOCa) is located. GPF, greater palatine foramen; InF, infraorbital foramen; IOF, infraorbital fissure; IOR, infraorbital rim; LF, lacrimal fossa; MaC, maxillary crest; NaF, nasal floor; NS, nasal septum; PEA, posterior ethmoidal artery; ST, superior turbinate.

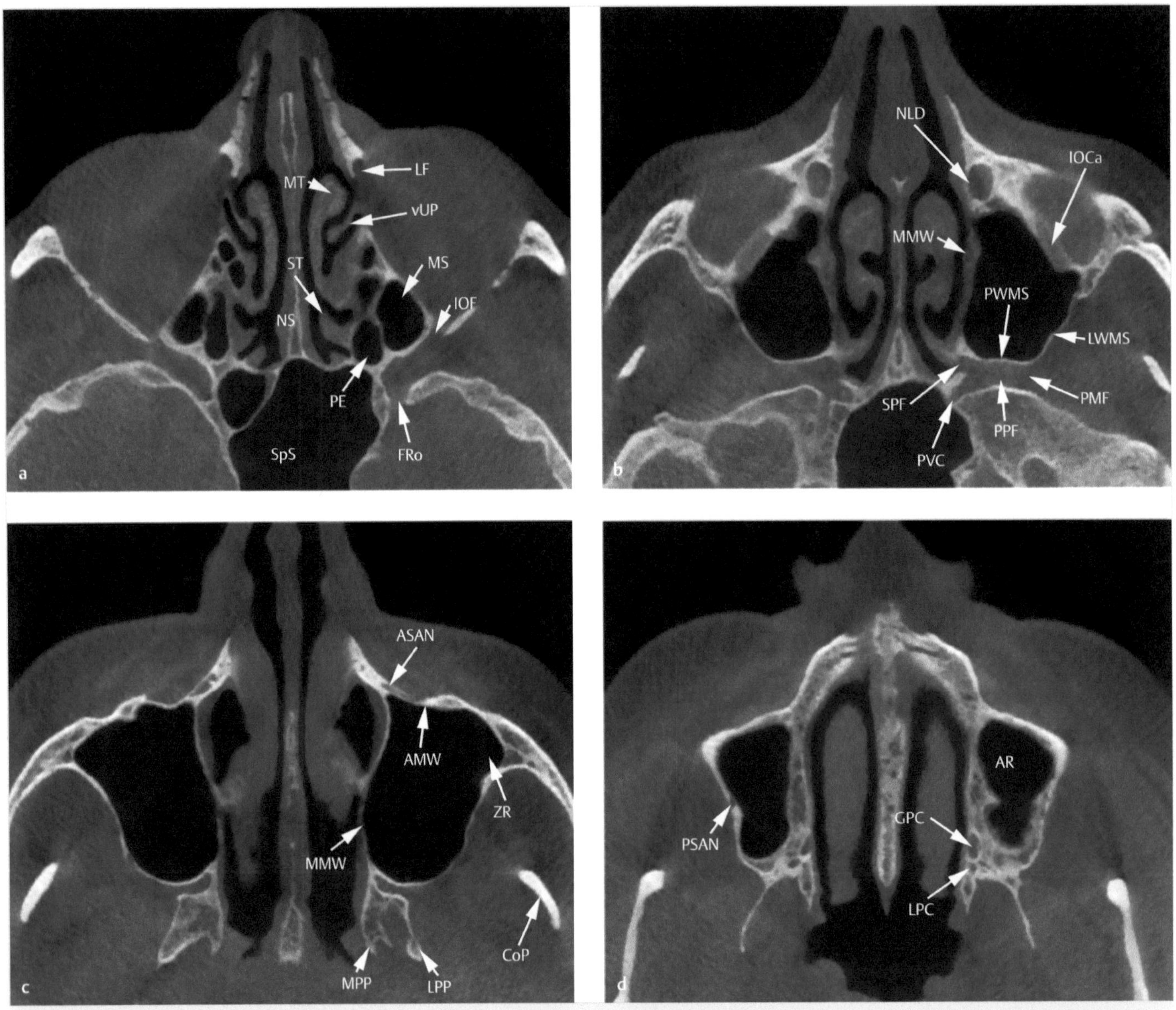

Fig. 5.4 (a–d) Axial CT anatomy of the maxillary sinus and adjacent areas. The panel includes four axial CT scans passing through the maxillary sinus (MS) disposed from cranial **(a)** to caudal **(d)**. The anterior maxillary wall (AMW) separates the maxillary sinus from the premaxillary tissue and houses the anterior superior alveolar nerve (ASAN). The posterior (PWMS) and lateral walls of the maxillary sinus (LWMS) neighbor the pterygopalatine (PPF) and infratemporal fossa, respectively. The lateral wall houses the posterior superior alveolar nerve (PSAN). The angle between the posterior and medial maxillary wall (MMW) represents the pterygomaxillary junction, where the descending, greater (GPC), and lesser palatine canals (LPC) run toward the caudal face of the hard palate. AR, alveolar recess; CoP, coronoid process; FRo, foramen rotundum; IOCa, infraorbital canal; IOF, inferior orbital fissure; LF, lacrimal fossa; LPP, lateral pterygoid plate; MPP, medial pterygoid plate; MT, middle turbinate; NLD, nasolacrimal duct; NS, nasal septum; PE, posterior ethmoidal compartment; PMF, pterygomaxillary fissure; PVC, palatovaginal canal; SPF, sphenopalatine foramen; SpS, sphenoid sinus; ST, superior turbinate; vUP, vertical portion of the uncinate process; ZR, zygomatic recess.

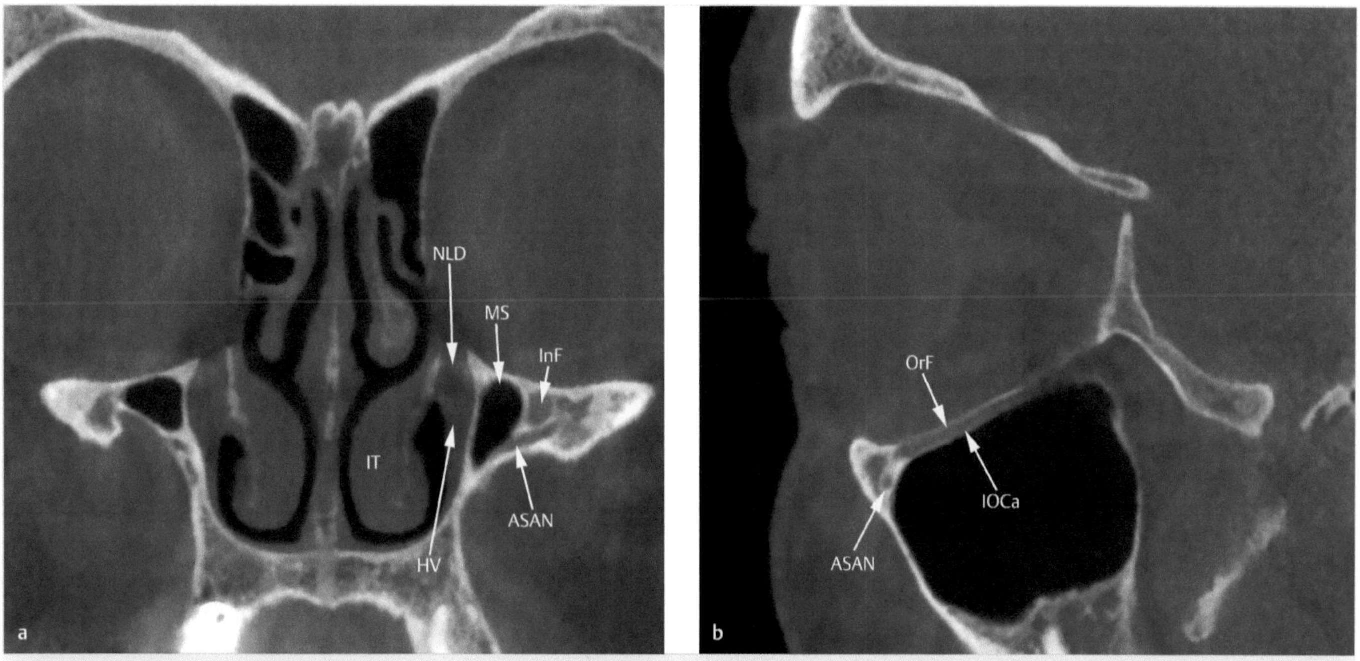

Fig. 5.5 Coronal and parasagittal CT anatomy of the infraorbital canal and adjacent structures. The panel includes one coronal **(a)** and one parasagittal CT scans **(b)** passing through the infraorbital canal (IOCa). The infraorbital canal runs along the orbital floor (OrF). In the most anterior portion, the course of the canal turns anteroinferiorly to reach the anterior maxillary wall and form the infraorbital foramen (InF). At this level, the canal gives off a small secondary canal inferolaterally that houses the anterior superior alveolar nerve (ASAN). The latter canal runs inferiorly to the infraorbital foramen with a lateral-to-medial direction to reach the lateral bony edge of the pyriform aperture, where it turns caudally. As seen in a coronal plane, the most anterior and medial portion of the maxillary sinus (MS) form a niche between the nasolacrimal duct (NLD) and infraorbital foramen. This niche is also called the retrolacrimal recess and can be tricky to expose from a transnasal perspective. HV, Hasner's valve; IT, inferior turbinate.

Endoscopic Dissection

Steps

- Step 1: Horizontal uncinectomy.
- Step 2: Type A endoscopic medial maxillectomy.
- Step 3: Inferior turbinectomy.
- Step 4: Type B endoscopic medial maxillectomy.
- Step 5: Nasolacrimal duct resection.
- Step 6: Type C endoscopic medial maxillectomy.
- Step 7: Exposure of the bone of the piriform aperture.
- Step 8: Premaxillary dissection.
- Step 9: Type D endoscopic medial maxillectomy.
- Step 10: Transposition of the infraorbital nerve.
- Step 11: Prelacrimal type D endoscopic medial maxillectomy.
- Step 12: Transseptal approach.
- Step 13: Dacryocystorhinostomy.

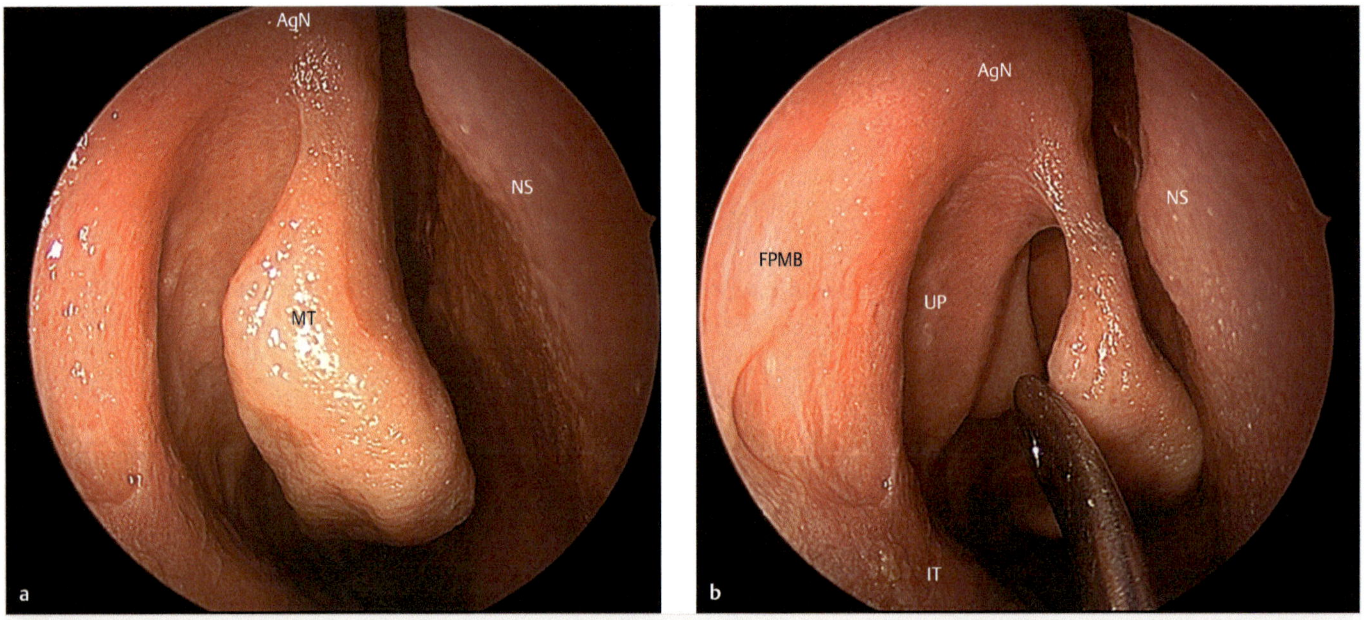

Fig. 5.6 (a, b) Landmarks of the middle nasal meatus. A dissector is used to medialize the middle turbinate (MT) and explore the middle nasal meatus. AgN, agger nasi; FPMB, frontal process of the maxillary bone; IT, inferior turbinate; NS, nasal septum; UP, uncinate process.

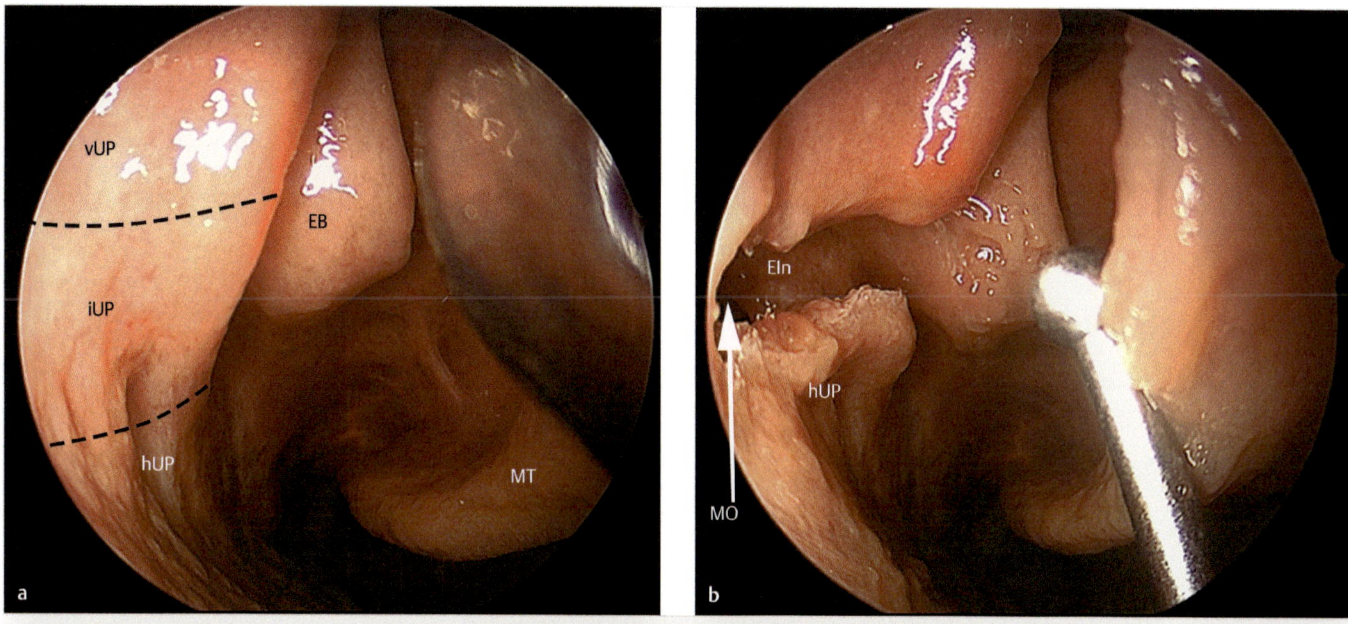

Fig. 5.7 (a, b) Step 1 (part 1). The uncinate process is formed of three segments called vertical (vUP), intermediate (iUP), and horizontal (hUP) portions. A retrograde cutting instrument is used to remove the intermediate portion (*black dashed lines*). The removal of the intermediate portion of the uncinate process is extended anteriorly till the bony portion of the lacrimal duct is reached. This maneuver exposes the ethmoidal infundibulum (EIn) and the natural ostium of the maxillary sinus (MO). EB, ethmoidal bulla; MT, middle turbinate.

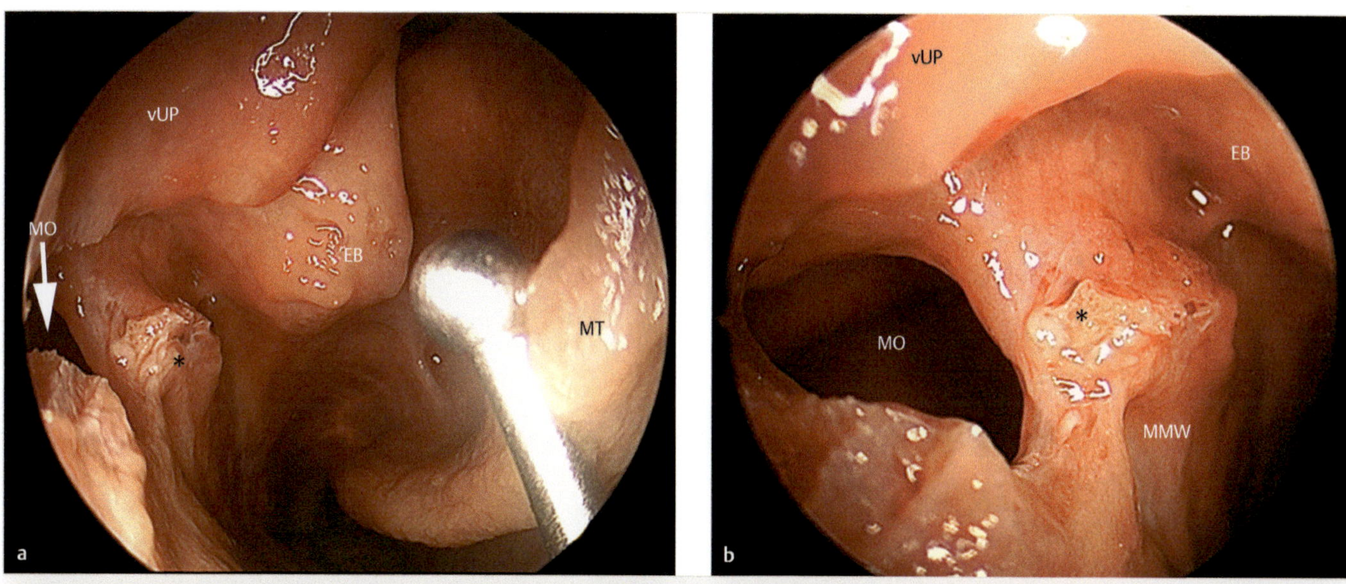

Fig. 5.8 (a, b) Step 1 (part 2). The horizontal portion of the uncinate process is removed up to its posterior insertion (*asterisk*) on the medial maxillary wall (MMW). A 45-degree scope turned laterally is employed to identify the maxillary ostium (MO). The boundaries of the natural ostium of the maxillary sinus (MO) are preserved. The maxillary ostium lies below the plane passing through the inferior border of the ethmoid bulla (EB). MT, middle turbinate; vUP, vertical portion of the uncinate process.

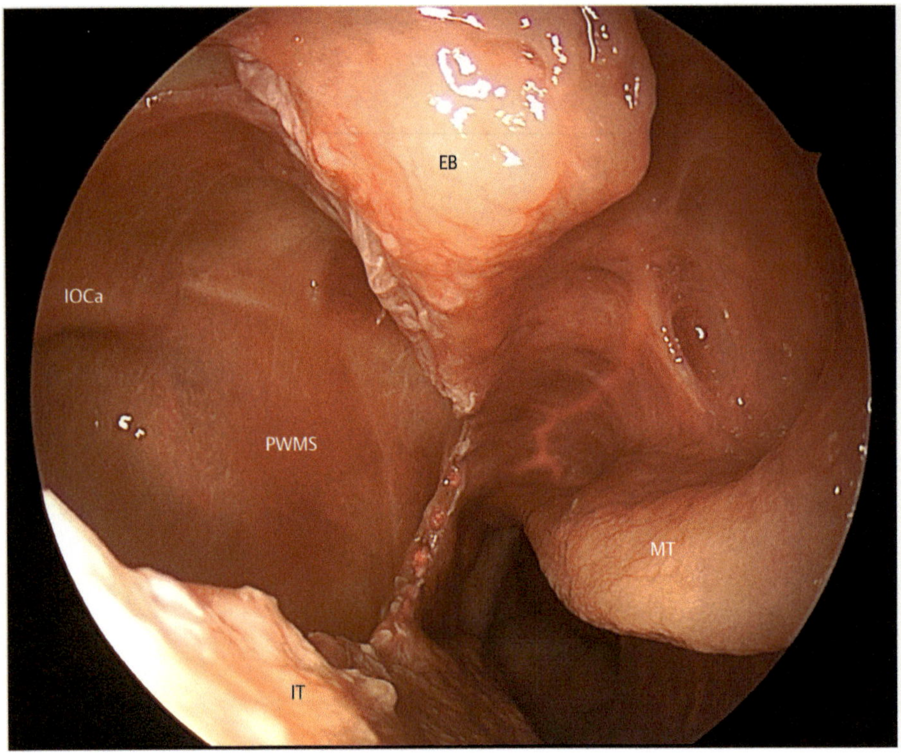

Fig. 5.9 Step 2. Type A medial maxillectomy is started from the maxillary ostium and completed by removing the medial maxillary wall up to the posterior wall of the maxillary sinus (PWMS) posteriorly, insertion of the inferior turbinate (IT) inferiorly, ethmoid bulla (EB) superiorly, and nasolacrimal duct anteriorly. This type of maxillectomy provides adequate exposure of the superomedial quadrant of the posterior wall of the maxillary sinus, medial to the infraorbital canal (IOCa) and superior to the inferior turbinate. MT, middle turbinate.

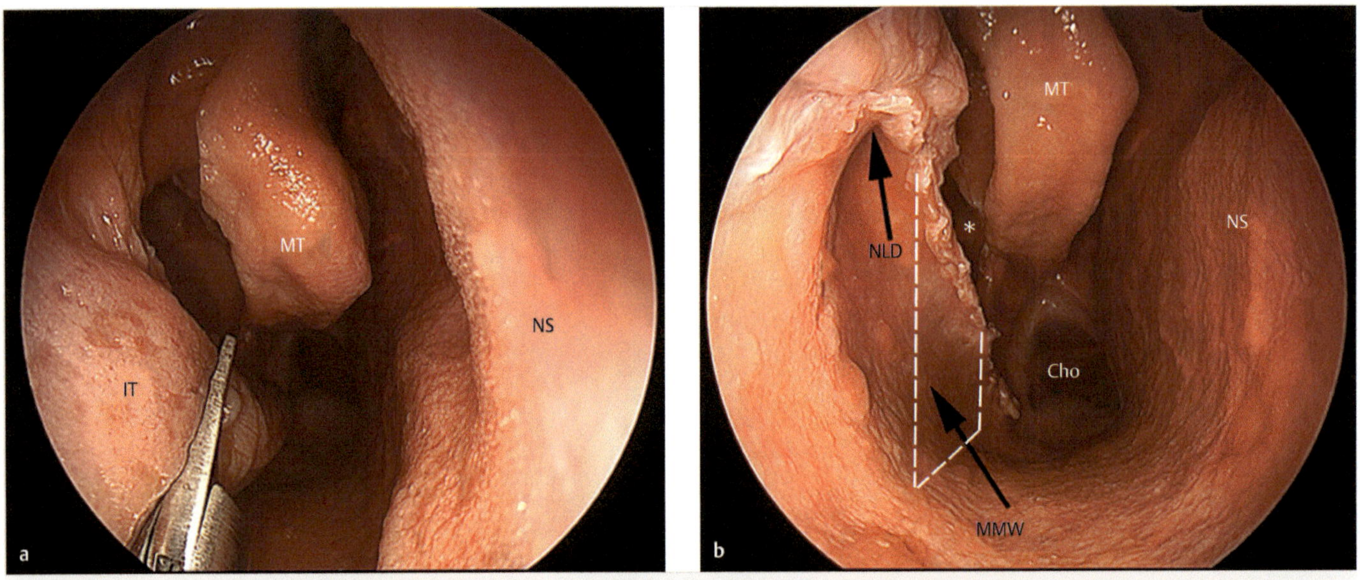

Fig. 5.10 (a, b) Step 3. Removal of the inferior turbinate (IT) is the first step of type B endoscopic medial maxillectomy. The head of the inferior turbinate is left intact to spare the nasolacrimal duct (NLD). The residual medial maxillary wall (MMW) posterior to the nasolacrimal duct (*white dashed line*) is removed to complete type B endoscopic medial maxillectomy. Cho, choana; MT, middle turbinate; NS, nasal septum.) (*White asterisk*, window of the type A endoscopic medial maxillectomy.

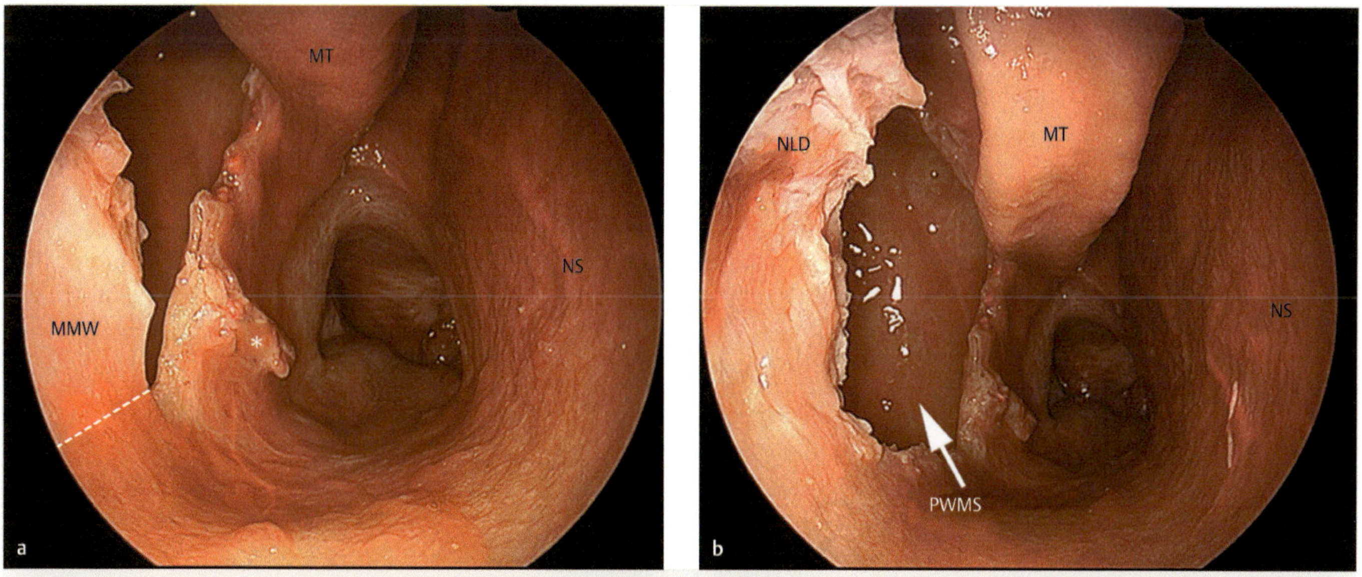

Fig. 5.11 (a, b) Step 4. The removal of the medial maxillary wall (MMW) is started from the posterior border, anteriorly to the tail of the inferior turbinate (*white asterisk*) to spare the descending palatine vessels. Then, the incision is continued inferiorly (*white dashed line*) and superiorly (as shown in ▶ Fig. 5.10). MT, middle turbinate; NLD, nasolacrimal duct; NS, nasal septum; PWMS, posterior wall of the maxillary sinus.

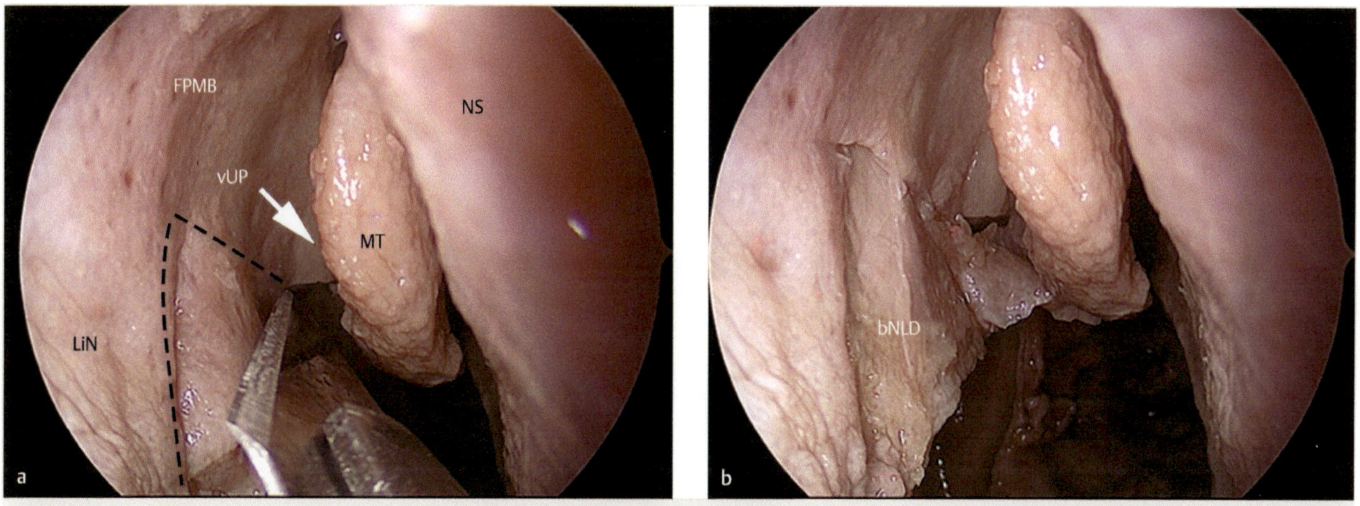

Fig. 5.12 (a, b) Step 5 (part 1). The mucosa covering the frontal process of the maxillary bone (FPMB) is incised (*black dashed line*), from posterior to anterior, along the plane of the orbital floor for about 5 mm and then down to the limen nasi (LiN). Subperiosteal dissection is performed to expose the medial bony wall of the nasolacrimal duct (bNLD). MT, middle turbinate; NS, nasal septum; vUP, vertical portion of the uncinate process.

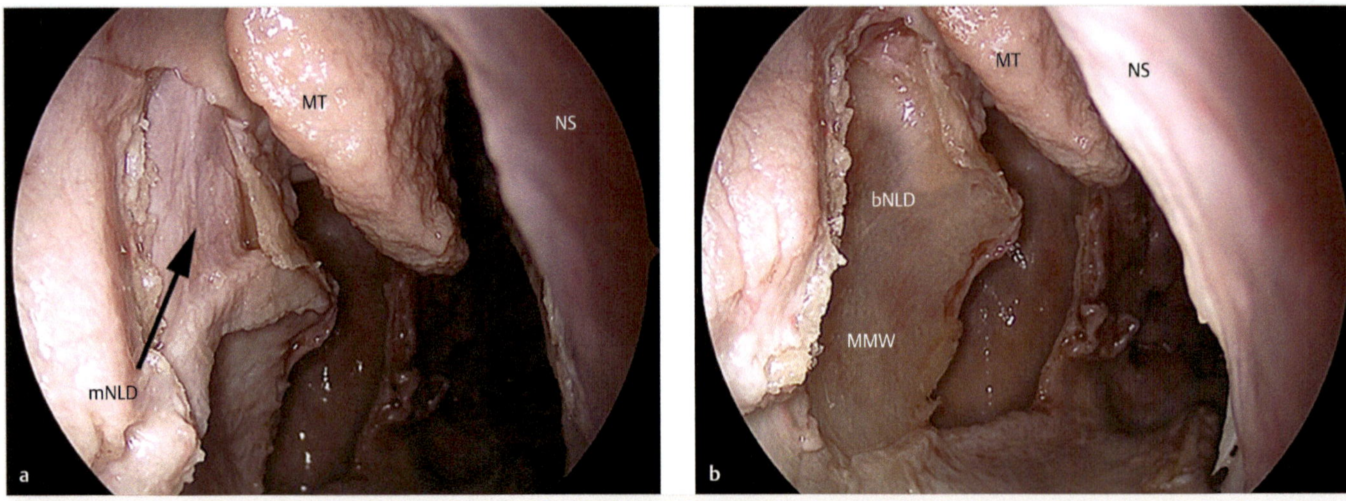

Fig. 5.13 (a, b) Step 5 (part 2). The head of the inferior turbinate and the medial bony wall of the nasolacrimal duct are removed to identify the mucosal nasolacrimal duct (mNLD). The latter is cut at the level of the inferior end of the lacrimal sac to expose the lateral portion of the bony nasolacrimal duct (bNLD) and the residual medial maxillary wall (MMW). MT, middle turbinate; NS, nasal septum.

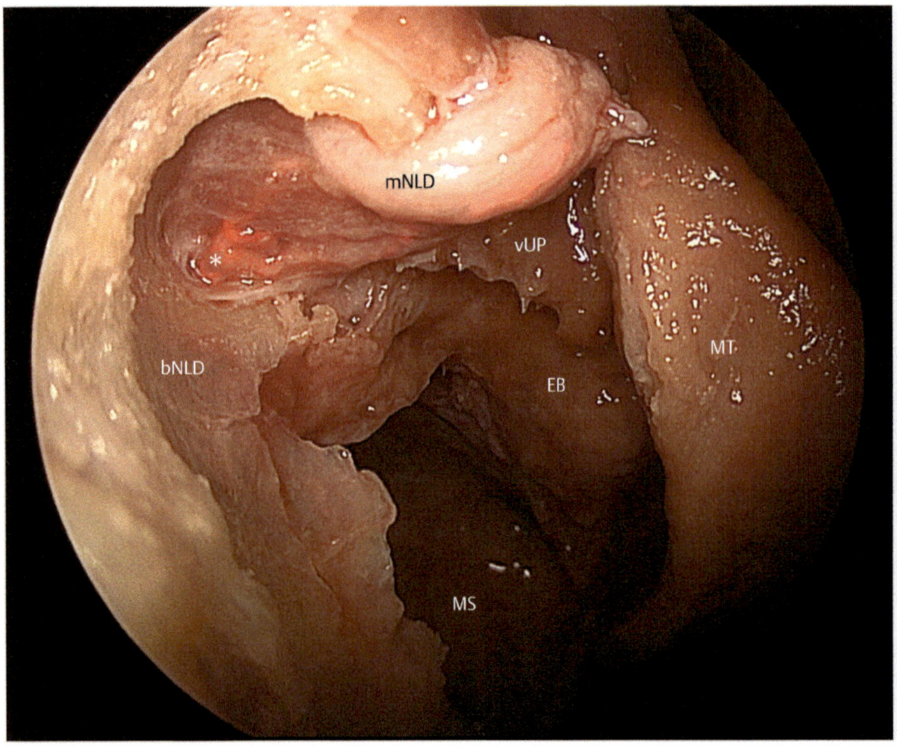

Fig. 5.14 Vascularization of the nasolacrimal duct. With a 45-degree endoscope, a small artery (*white asterisk*) coming from the lacrimal fossa is identified. This artery takes origin from the system of the angular artery and provides vascularization to the nasolacrimal duct. EB, ethmoidal bulla; mNLD, mucosal nasolacrimal duct; bNLD, bony nasolacrimal duct; MS, maxillary sinus; MT, middle turbinate; vUP, vertical portion of the uncinate process.

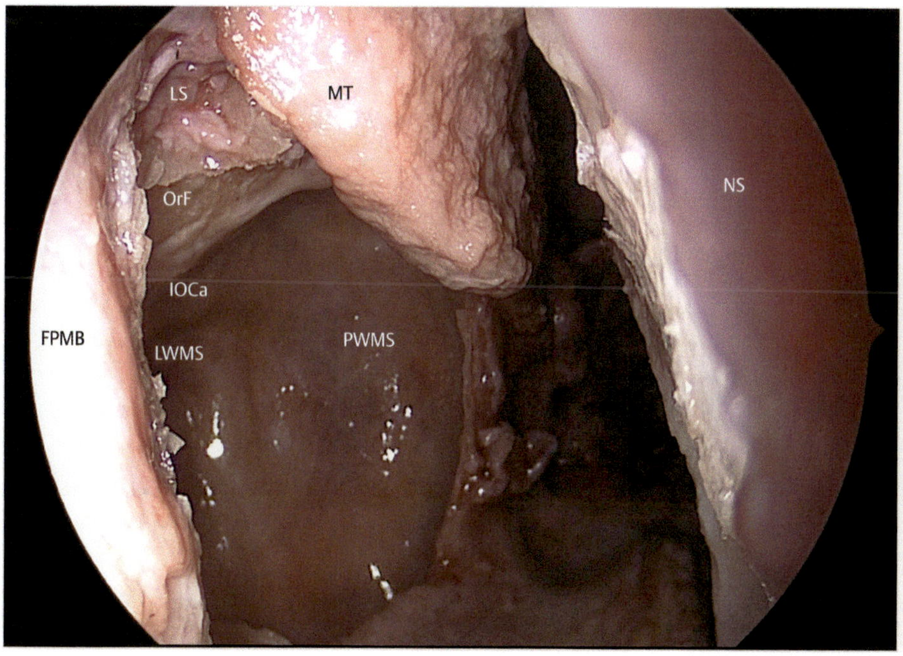

Fig. 5.15 Step 6. Removal of the medial maxillary wall is extended anteriorly up to the frontal process of the maxillary bone (FPMB) to complete type C endoscopic medial maxillectomy. This window provides adequate exposure of both the posterior wall of the maxillary sinus (PWMS) and orbital floor (OrF) medial to the infraorbital canal (IOCa). The nasolacrimal duct must be removed up to the lacrimal sac (LS) to fully expose the orbital floor and retrolacrimal recess. The posterior portion of the lateral wall of the maxillary sinus (LWMS) can be partially seen with this approach. MT, middle turbinate; NS, nasal septum.

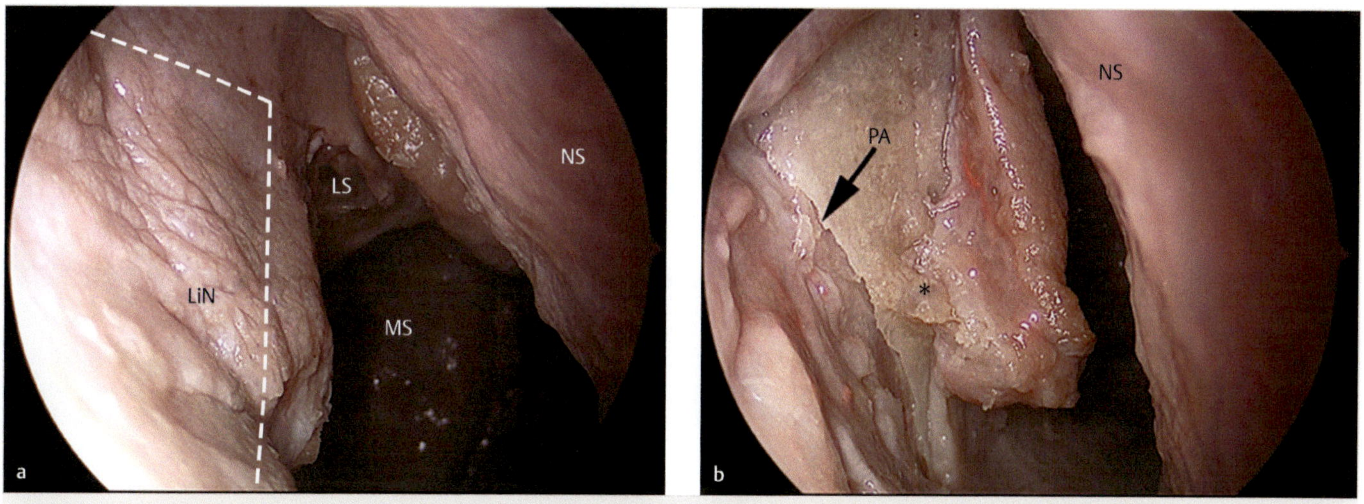

Fig. 5.16 (a, b) Step 7. An incision (*white dashed line*) is made posterior to the limen nasi (LiN) and along the axial plane passing through the inferior border of the lacrimal sac (LS). Subperiosteal dissection is performed in a posterior-to-anterior direction to expose the piriform aperture (PA), which is located in front of the bony head of the inferior turbinate (*black asterisk*). MS, maxillary sinus; NS, nasal septum.

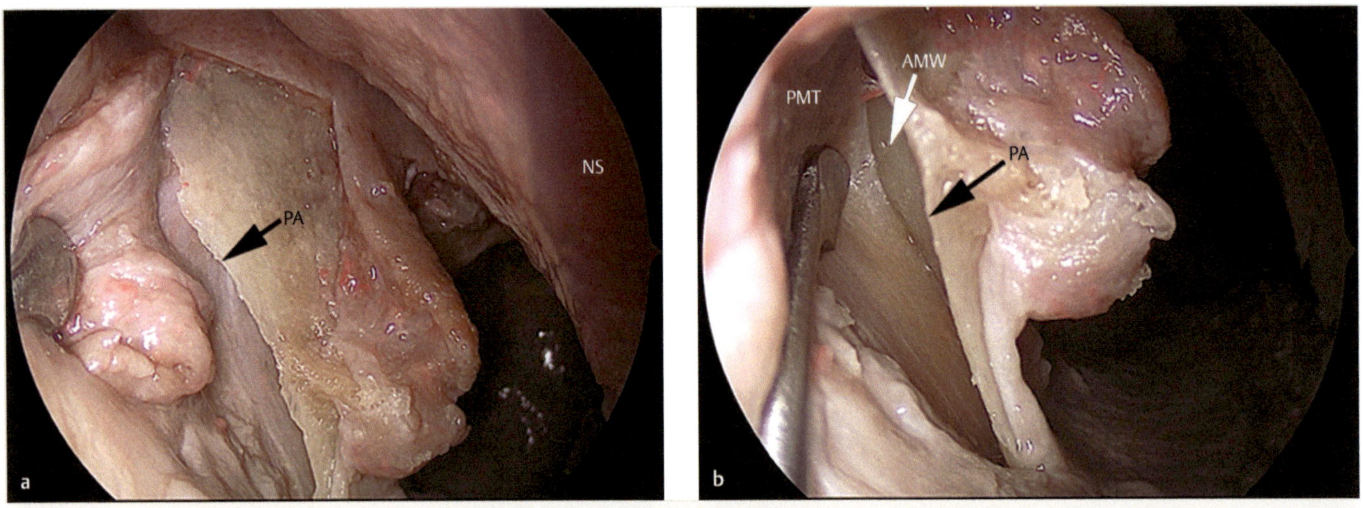

Fig. 5.17 (a, b) Step 8. Starting from the piriform aperture (PA), a subperiosteal dissection is performed along the anterior maxillary wall (AMW), which is exposed by displacing anteriorly and laterally premaxillary soft tissues (PMT). NS, nasal septum.

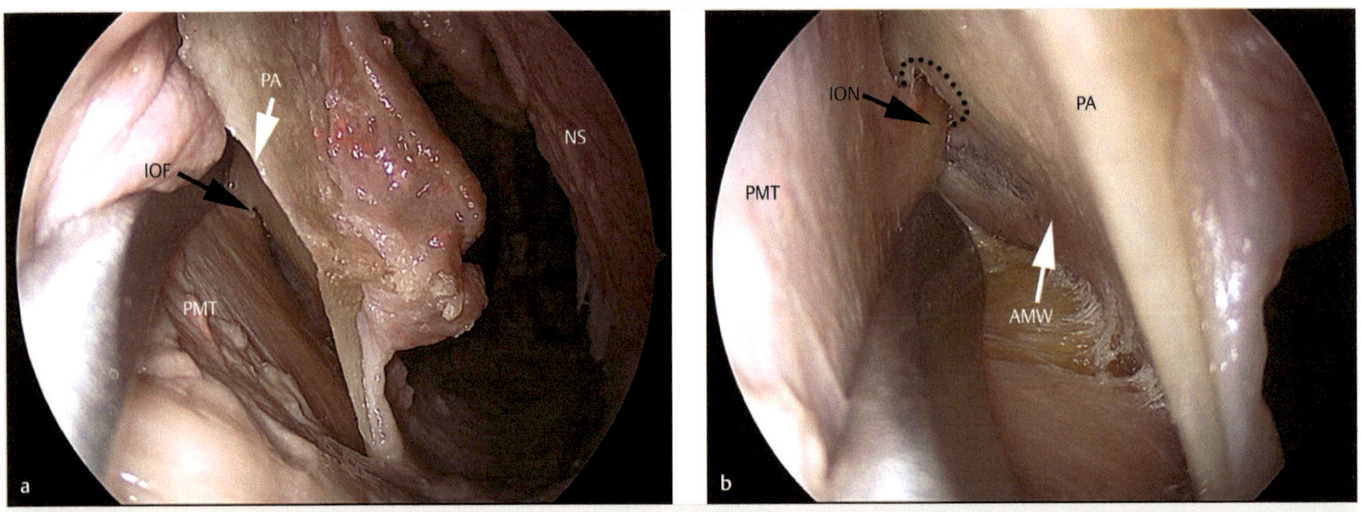

Fig. 5.18 (a, b) The infraorbital foramen. Subperiosteal dissection is extended toward the infraorbital foramen (IOF; *black dotted line*). Attention should be paid to not damage the dissected periosteum that covers premaxillary tissues (PMT) to avoid fat tissue prolapse into the dissection field. AMW, anterior maxillary wall; ION, infraorbital nerve; NS, nasal septum; PA, piriform aperture.

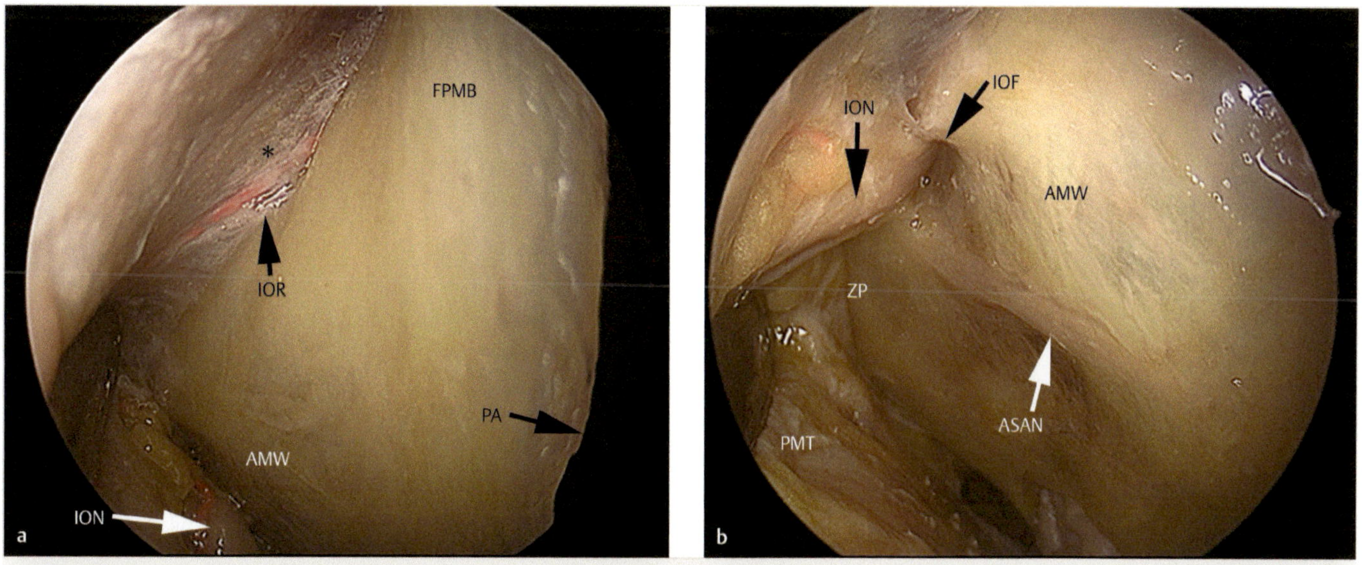

Fig. 5.19 (a, b) Anterior maxillary wall. By extending subperiosteal dissection on the anterior maxillary wall (AMW) in a superior and lateral direction, the frontal process of the maxillary bone (FPMB) and inferior orbital rim (IOR) are exposed. A small branch (*black asterisk*) of the angular artery running toward the lacrimal sac is identified in the medial portion of the inferior orbital rim. When the dissection is carried inferiorly and laterally to the infraorbital foramen (IOF) and nerve (ION), the zygomatic process (ZP) of the maxillary bone is exposed. The anterior superior alveolar nerve (ASAN) can be identified within the anterior maxillary wall. PA, piriform aperture; PMT, premaxillary tissue.

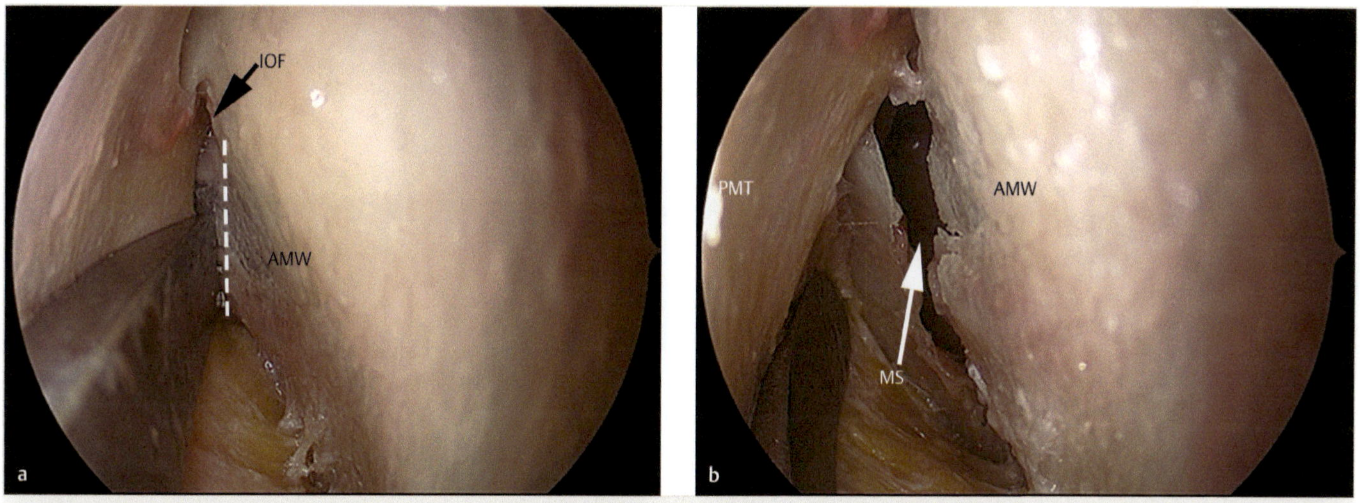

Fig. 5.20 (a, b) Step 9 (part 1). The lateral osteotomy (*white dashed line*) of the anterior maxillary wall (AMW) is performed on a sagittal plane passing through the medial border of the infraorbital foramen (IOF). MS, maxillary sinus; PMT, premaxillary tissues.

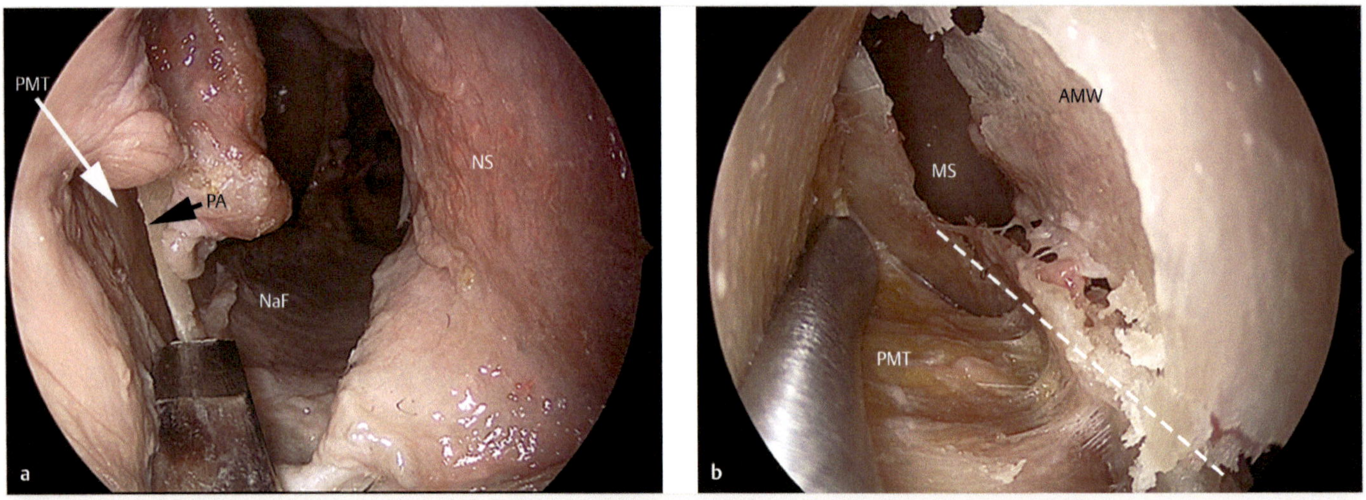

Fig. 5.21 (a, b) Step 9 (step 2). The inferior osteotomy (*white dashed line*) of the anterior maxillary wall (AMW) is performed along the plane of the nasal floor (NaF), from the piriform aperture (PA) to the lateral osteotomy. MS, maxillary sinus; NS, nasal septum; PMT, premaxillary tissue.

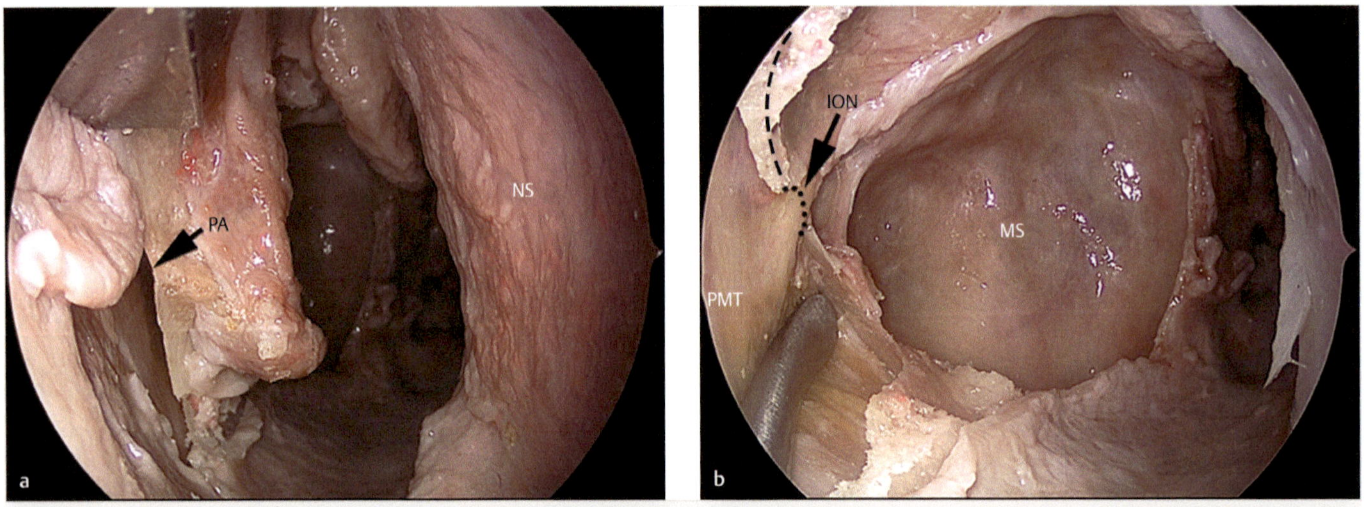

Fig. 5.22 (a, b) Step 9 (part 3). The superior osteotomy (*black dashed line*) is performed along the plane passing through the superior border of the infraorbital foramen (*black dotted line*) and nerve (ION). In this way, complete exposure of the maxillary sinus (MS) is obtained. NS, nasal septum; PA, piriform aperture; PMT, premaxillary tissues.

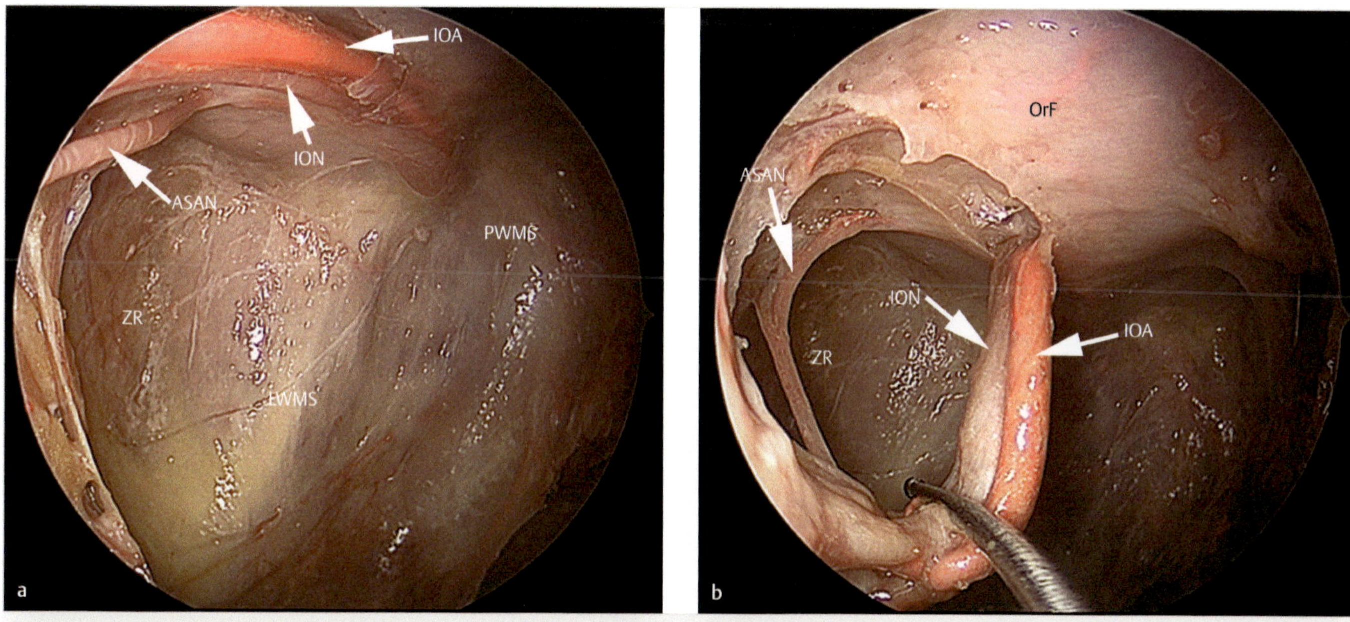

Fig. 5.23 (a, b) Step 10. The infraorbital artery (IOA) and nerve (ION) are completely freed from the surrounding bone that makes up the inferior portion of the infraorbital canal. The anterior superior alveolar nerve (ASAN) is identified where it arises from the lateral surface of the infraorbital nerve (ION). The infraorbital nerve and artery can be transposed inferiorly to reach the cranial portion of the zygomatic recess (ZR) and the lateral portion of the orbital floor (OrF). LWMS, lateral wall of the maxillary sinus; PWMS, posterior wall of the maxillary sinus.

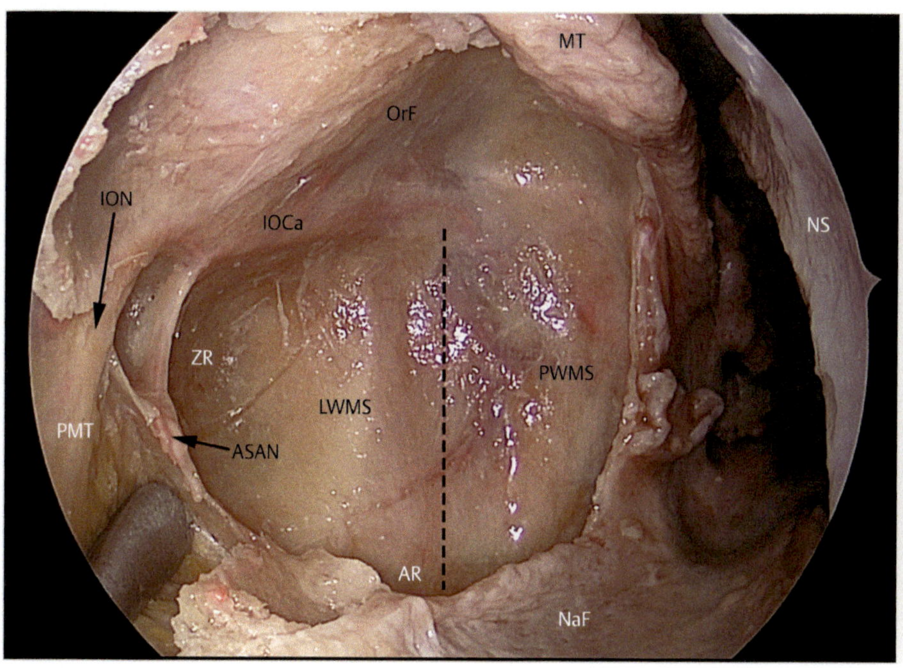

Fig. 5.24 The maxillary sinus. After completing type D endoscopic medial maxillectomy, all the remaining subunits of the maxillary sinus can be identified. The sagittal plane (*black dashed line*) passing through the posterior end of the infraorbital canal (IOCa) can be considered as a landmark for the pterygomaxillary fissure, which is the limit between the pterygopalatine fossa medially and infratemporal fossa laterally. These spaces are covered by the posterior (PWMS) and lateral walls (LWMS) of the maxillary sinus, respectively. The maxillary sinus also shows pneumatization toward the alveolar and zygomatic process of the maxillary bone called the alveolar (AR) and zygomatic recess (ZR), respectively. ASAN, anterior superior alveolar nerve; ION, infraorbital nerve; MT, middle turbinate; NS, nasal septum; NaF, nasal floor; OrF, orbit floor; PMT, premaxillary tissues.

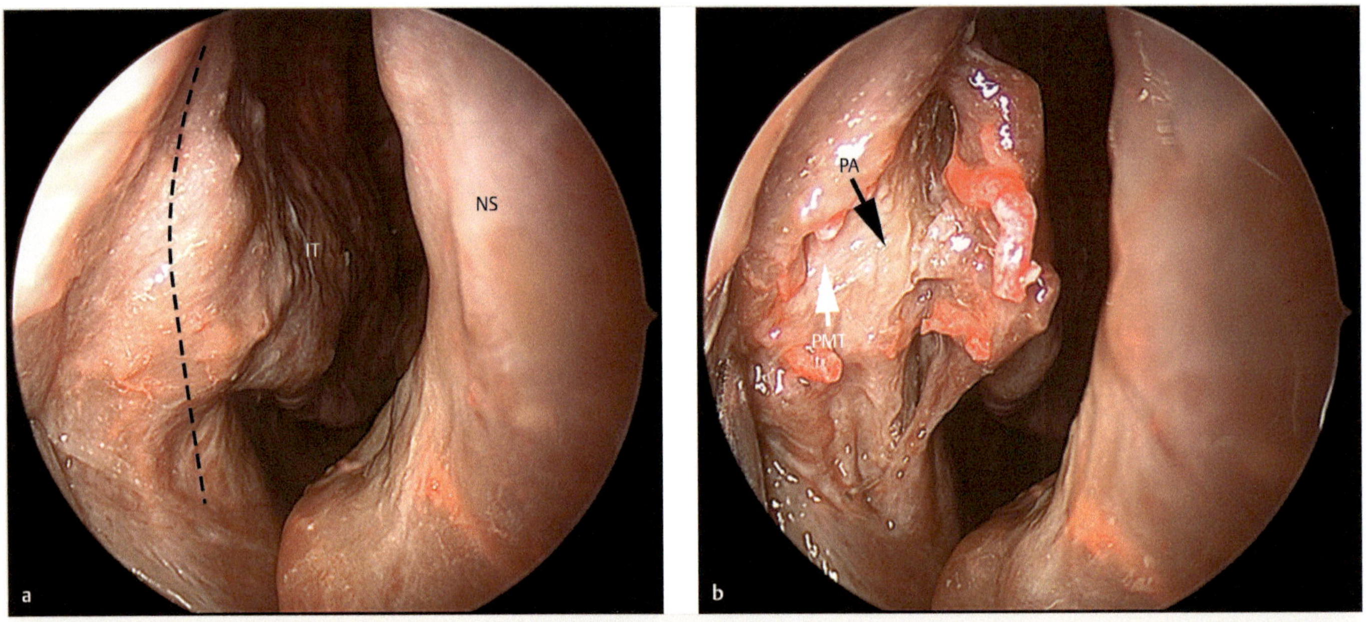

Fig. 5.25 (a, b) Step 11 (part 1). A vertical mucosal incision (*black dashed line*) is made anterior to the head of the inferior turbinate (IT) to expose the piriform aperture (PA) and premaxillary tissues (PMT). NS, nasal septum.

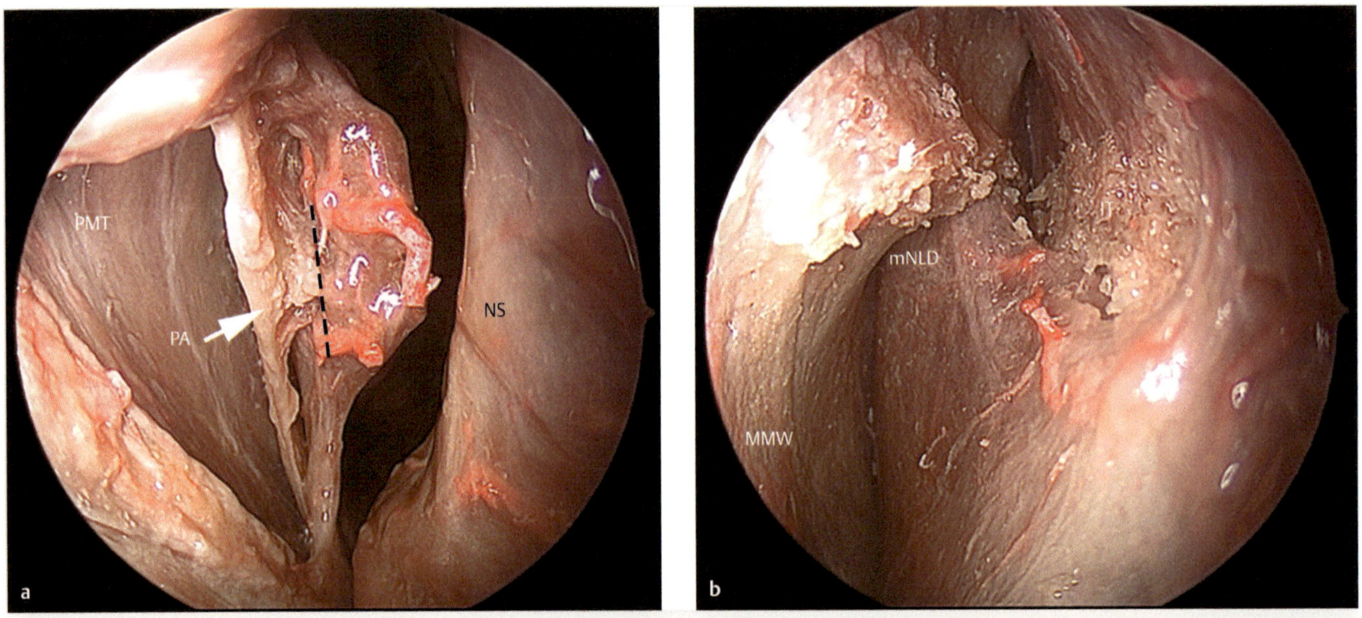

Fig. 5.26 (a, b) Step 11 (part 2). On the lateral side of the incision, subperiosteal dissection is performed laterally to the piriform aperture (PA) to separate premaxillary tissues (PMT) from the anterior maxillary wall. On the medial side of the incision, a cutting instrument is used to detach (*black dashed line*) the inferior turbinate (IT) from the medial maxillary wall (MMW) until reaching the inferior end of the mucosal nasolacrimal duct (mNLD). NS, nasal septum.

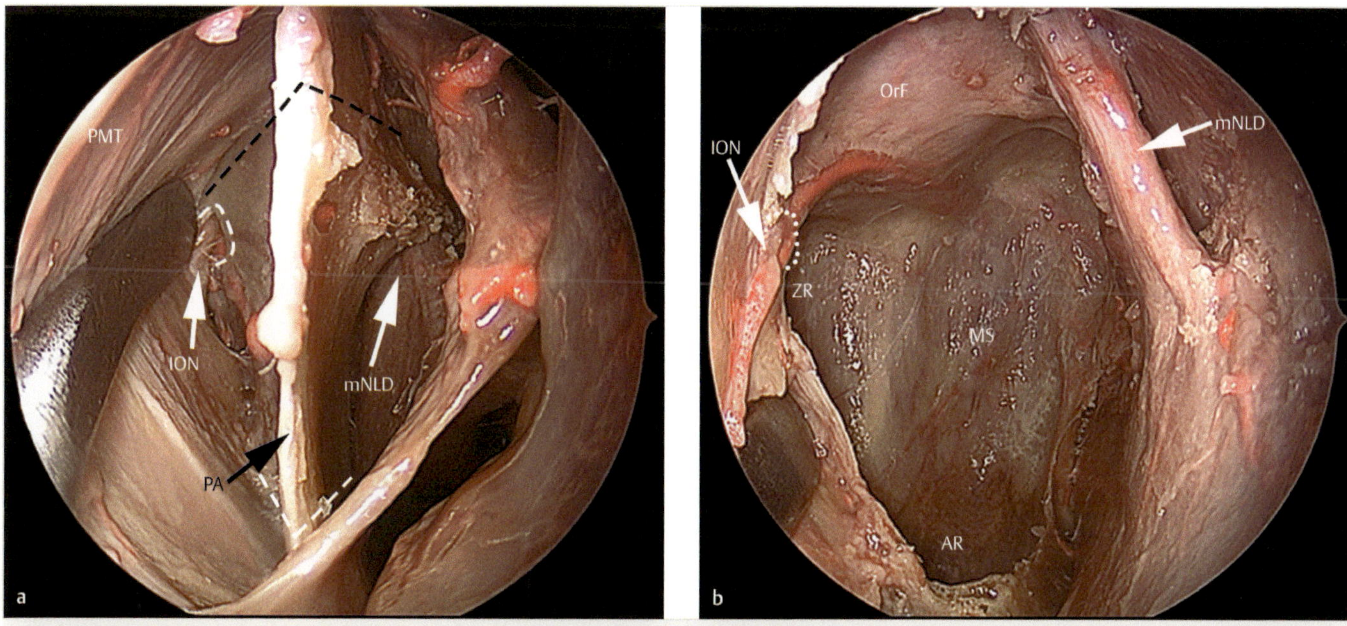

Fig. 5.27 (a, b) Step 11 (part 3). Type D endoscopic medial maxillectomy is completed using the landmarks reported in ▶Fig. 5.21 and ▶Fig. 5.22 and preserving the mucosal nasolacrimal duct (mNLD). The removal of bone can also be limited to the medial maxillary wall as for type C maxillectomy, according to the need for exposure. AR, alveolar recess; ION, infraorbital nerve; OrF, orbital floor; MS, maxillary sinus; PA, piriform aperture; PMT, premaxillary tissues; ZR, zygomatic recess. (*Black dashed line*, superior osteotomy; *white dashed line*, inferior osteotomy; *white dotted line*, infraorbital foramen.

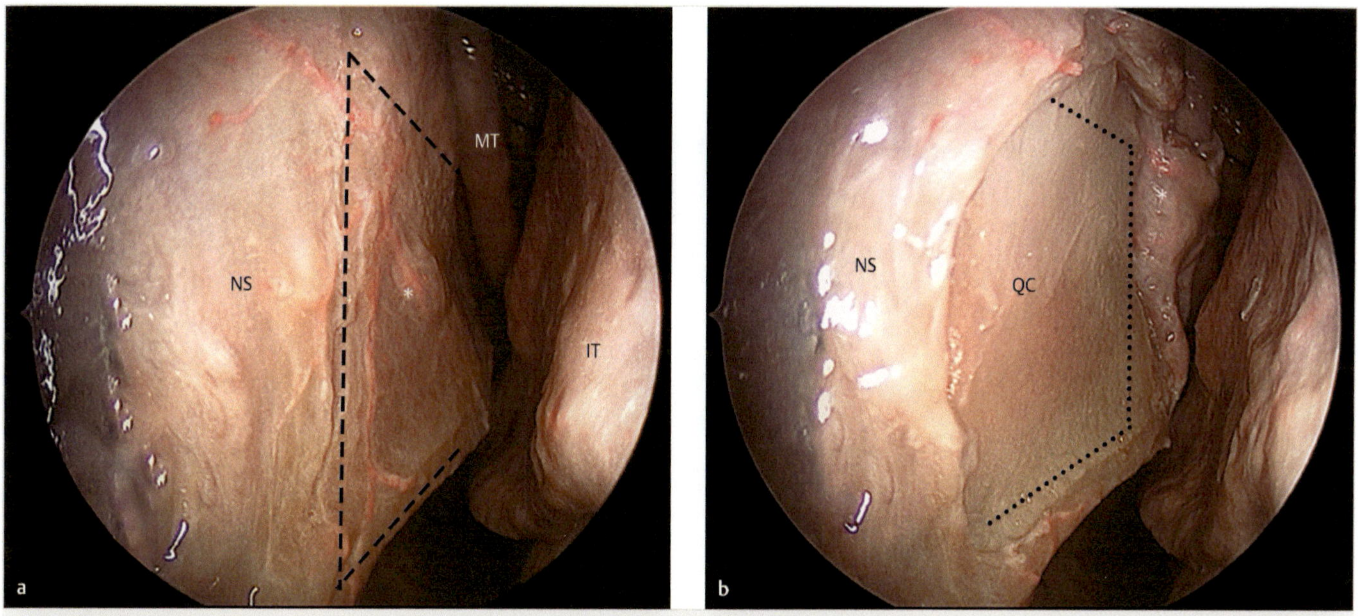

Fig. 5.28 (a, b) Step 12 (part 1). On the contralateral side with respect to the targeted maxillary sinus, a squared incomplete mucosal incision (*black dashed line*) is performed on the nasal septum (NS) to elevate a posterior pedicle mucoperichondrial flap (*white asterisk*), which is stored posteriorly. A squared incomplete incision (*black dotted line*) of the quadrangular cartilage (QC) is performed, leaving the anterior border of the exposed cartilaginous area intact. IT, inferior turbinate; MT, middle turbinate.

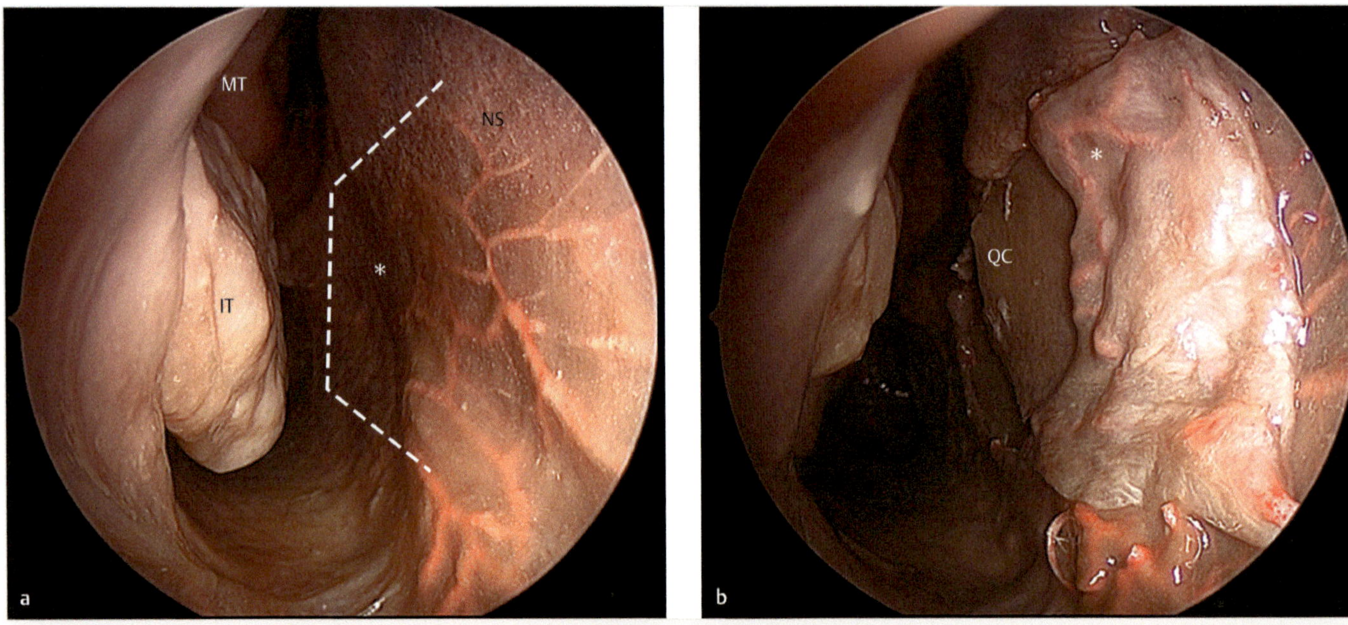

Fig. 5.29 (a, b) Step 12 (part 2). On the ipsilateral side with respect to the targeted maxillary sinus, a squared incomplete mucosal incision (*white dashed line*) is performed on the nasal septum (NS) to elevate an anterior pedicle mucoperichondrial flap (*white asterisk*), which is flipped anteriorly. IT, inferior turbinate; MT, middle turbinate; QC, quadrangular cartilage.

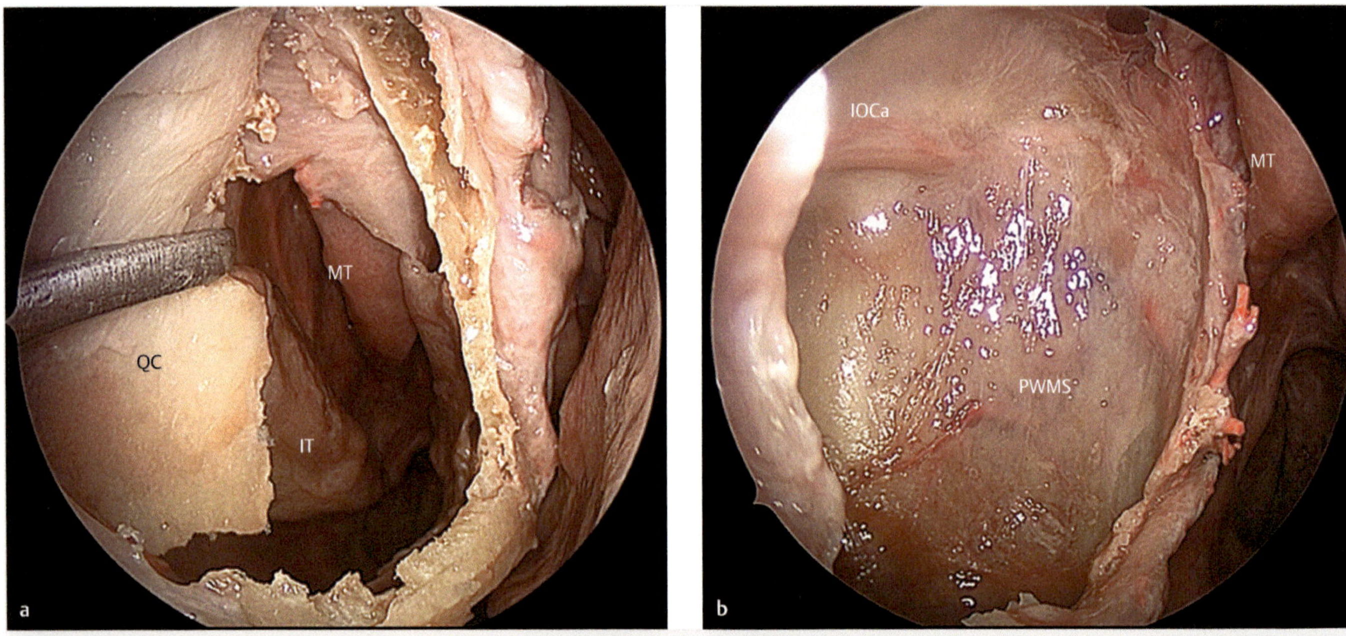

Fig. 5.30 (a, b) Step 12 (part 3). From the contralateral side with respect to the targeted maxillary sinus, a dissector is used to laterally displace the quadrangular cartilage (QC), thus completing the transseptal approach to the maxillary sinus. In this specimen, a type B endoscopic medial maxillectomy was performed. This corridor provides a far-lateral trajectory to the maxillary sinus and adjacent areas without performing more extensive endoscopic medial maxillectomies. IOCa, infraorbital canal; IT, inferior turbinate; MT, middle turbinate; PWMS, posterior wall of the maxillary sinus.

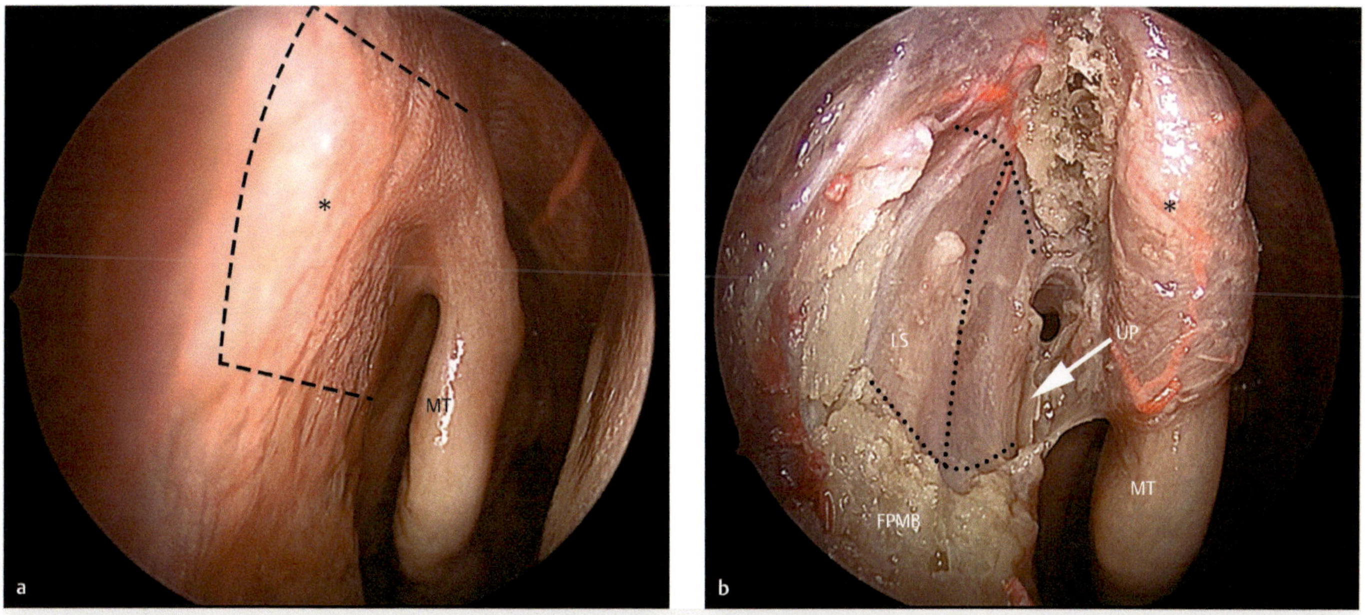

Fig. 5.31 (a, b) Step 13 (part 1). A squared incomplete incision (*black dashed line*) is made anteriorly to the middle turbinate (MT) to elevate the axillary flap (*black asterisk*). The vertical incision is performed from a few millimeters caudal to the axilla of the middle turbinate to a few millimeters above. Horizontal incisions are performed from about 1 cm in front of the axilla of the middle turbinate to the plane passing through the maxillary line. After exposing the frontal process of the maxillary bone (FPMB) and lacrimal bone, they are removed to uncover the lacrimal sac (LS). The uncinate process (UP) can be preserved when it is not inserted far anteriorly onto the medial bony wall of the lacrimal fossa. An H-shaped incision (*black dotted line*) is performed on the lateral mucosal wall of the lacrimal sac.

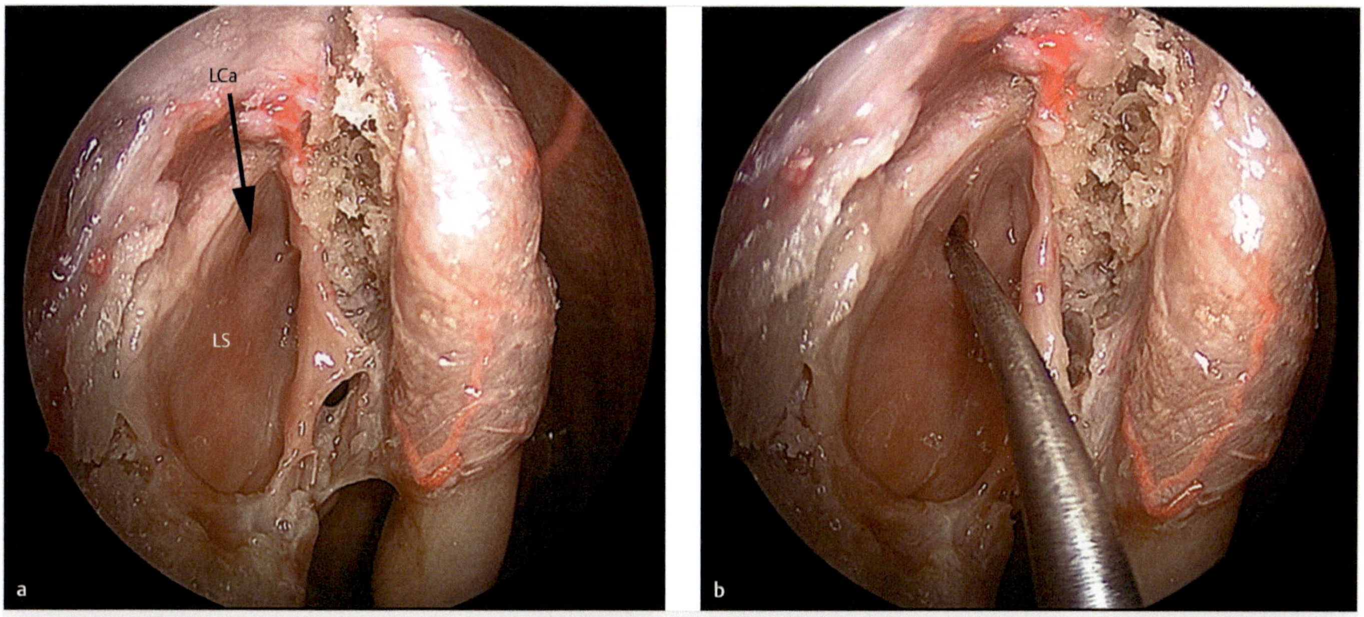

Fig. 5.32 (a, b) Step 13 (part 2). Dacryocystorhinostomy is completed by displacing centrifugally the mucosal flaps of the lacrimal sac (LS). The common lacrimal canaliculus (LCa) is identified on the lateral mucosal surface of the lacrimal sac. This opening marks the midpoint of the craniocaudal height of the sac.

References

[1] Schreiber A, Ferrari M, Rampinelli V, et al. Modular endoscopic medial maxillectomies: quantitative analysis of surgical exposure in a preclinical setting. World Neurosurg 2017;100:44–55

[2] Turri-Zanoni M, Battaglia P, Karligkiotis A, et al. Transnasal endoscopic partial maxillectomy: operative nuances and proposal for a comprehensive classification system based on 1378 cases. Head Neck 2017;39(4):754–766

[3] Canfield R. The submucous resection of the lateral nasal wall in chronic empyema of the antrum, ethmoid and sphenoid. JAMA 1908;51:1136–1141

[4] Denker A. [A new way for the surgery of malignant nasal tumors] Munch Med Wochenschr 1906;53:953–956

[5] Sturmann D. [The intranasal opening of the maxillary sinus] Wien Klin Wochenschr 1907;27:1273–1274

[6] Schreiber A, Mattavelli D, Ferrari M, et al. Anterior superior alveolar nerve injury after extended endoscopic medial maxillectomy: a preclinical study to predict neurological morbidity. Int Forum Allergy Rhinol 2017;7(10):1014–1021

[7] Salzano G, Turri-Zanoni M, Karligkiotis A, et al. Infraorbital nerve transposition to expand the endoscopic transnasal maxillectomy. Int Forum Allergy Rhinol 2017;7(2):149–153

[8] Zhou B, Han DM, Cui SJ, Huang Q, Wang CS. Intranasal endoscopic prelacrimal recess approach to maxillary sinus. Chin Med J (Engl) 2013;126(7):1276–1280

[9] Morrissey DK, Wormald PJ, Psaltis AJ. Prelacrimal approach to the maxillary sinus. Int Forum Allergy Rhinol 2016;6(2):214–218

[10] Suzuki M, Nakamura Y, Yokota M, Ozaki S, Murakami S. Modified transnasal endoscopic medial maxillectomy through prelacrimal duct approach. Laryngoscope 2017;127(10):2205–2209

[11] Guo T, Sun JW, Wang YF, Sun JQ. Endoscopic endonasal surgery for pterygopalatine fossa schwannoma via prelacrimal recess-maxillary sinus. B-ENT 2014;10(1):81–86

[12] He S, Bakst RL, Guo T, Sun J. A combination of modified transnasal endoscopic maxillectomy via transnasal prelacrimal recess approach with or without radiotherapy for selected sinonasal malignancies. Eur Arch Otorhinolaryngol 2015;272(10):2933–2938

[13] Lin YT, Lin CF, Yeh TH. Application of the endoscopic prelacrimal recess approach to the maxillary sinus in unilateral maxillary diseases. Int Forum Allergy Rhinol 2018;8(4):530–536

[14] Harvey RJ, Sheehan PO, Debnath NI, Schlosser RJ. Transseptal approach for extended endoscopic resections of the maxilla and infratemporal fossa. Am J Rhinol Allergy 2009;23(4):426–432

[15] Ramakrishnan VR, Suh JD, Chiu AG, Palmer JN. Septal dislocation for endoscopic access of the anterolateral maxillary sinus and infratemporal fossa. Am J Rhinol Allergy 2011;25(2):128–130

6 Transfrontal Approach

Francesco Belotti, Marco Ravanelli, Marco Angelo Cocchi, Vittorio Rampinelli, Francesco Doglietto

In very selected cases, the frontal sinus can serve as a corridor toward lesions with isolated involvement of the posterior frontal plate,[1-4] which is the most anterior subunit of the midline anterior skull base. They are mostly included in the group of nasofrontal dysembriogenic lesions, which entails dermoid sinuses, dermoid cysts, nasal gliomas, and meningoencephaloceles.[2,5-7] Although based on limited case series, the endoscopic approach provides favorable results with minimal morbidity in adequately selected cases. Given the tendency of these malformations to grow toward the external nose, a combined endoscopic rhinoplasty technique can also be indicated in selected cases.[2] On the other hand, the transfrontal approach can be employed to manage selected benign tumors or tumorlike lesions of the frontal sinus and adjacent skull base (e.g., osteomas, inverted papillomas, glomangiopericytomas, and mucocele) that show no far-lateral extension and no involvement of the anterior frontal plate.[1,3,4,8]

The transfrontal endoscopic corridor, which requires a wide Draf type III frontal sinusotomy, is bounded by the nasal bones anteriorly, nasal septum and cribriform plate posteriorly, and orbital cavity bilaterally. This surgical route is quite challenging due to several reasons: (1) it is oriented in a caudal-to-cranial fashion and shows very narrow anteroposterior and lateral–lateral diameters that hamper surgical maneuvers and facilitate the "sword-fighting" phenomenon during surgery; (2) the boundaries of the corridors must be accurately preserved to avoid injuring the midline anterior skull base, skin of the nose, and anterior orbital content; (3) the reconstruction of the skull base can be made difficult by the three-dimensional geometry of the defect and limited maneuverability of instruments; (4) in cases requiring a transdural resection, attention must be paid to not damage the superior sagittal sinus, bridging veins, and orbitofrontal and frontopolar arteries.

By virtue of its difficulty and rarity of adequate indications, the transfrontal endoscopic approach might arouse limited interest in the reader. However, this approach allows to face an area that is infrequently thoroughly explored with other endoscopic skull base approaches, although its anatomy should be mastered to approach far-anterior lesions of the midline skull base. In fact, secondary involvement of this anterior region from lesions that originate from adjacent skull base areas (i.e., cribriform plate and fovea ethmoidalis/ethmoidal roof) is quite frequent.

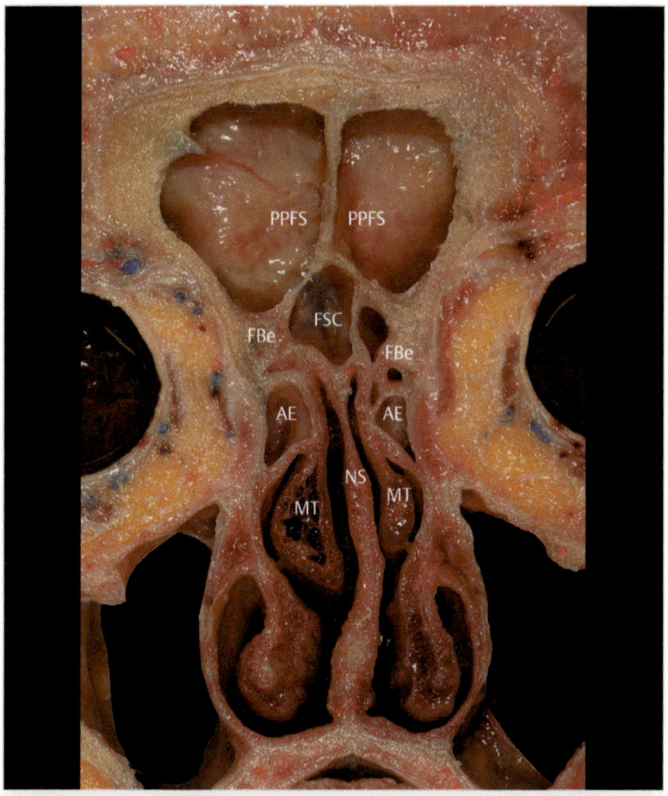

Fig. 6.1 Coronal view of transnasal route toward the posterior plate of the frontal sinus spaces. This coronal cadaver cut shows anatomy of the structures encountered while reaching the posterior plate of the frontal sinus (PPFS) through the nasal cavity and frontal sinuses. AE, anterior ethmoidal compartment; FBe, frontal beak; FSC, frontal septal cell; MT, middle turbinate; NS, nasal septum.

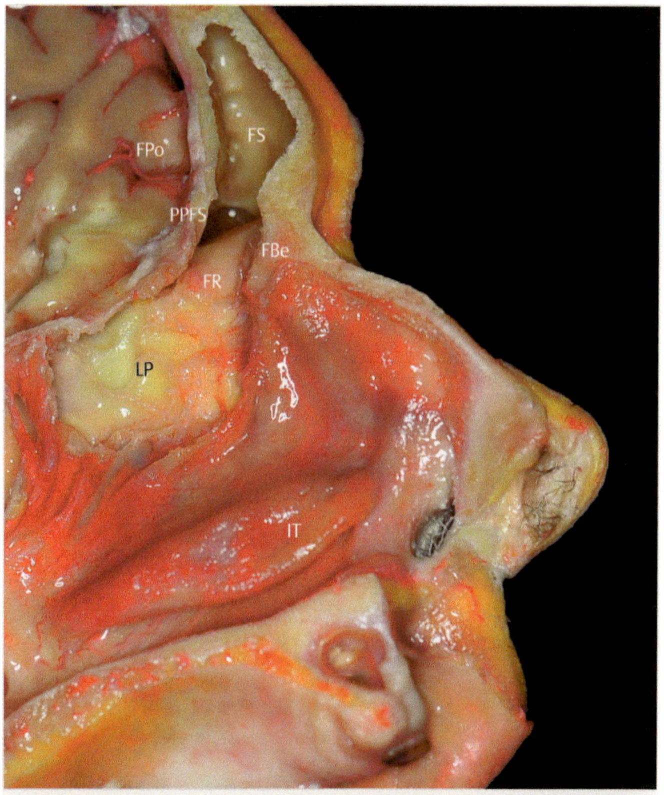

Fig. 6.2 Sagittal view of transnasal route toward the posterior plate of the frontal sinus spaces. This cadaver cut shows anatomy of the route toward the posterior plate of the frontal sinus (PPFS). FBe, frontal beak; FPo, frontal pole; FR, frontal recess; FS, frontal sinus; IT, inferior turbinate; LP, lamina papyracea.

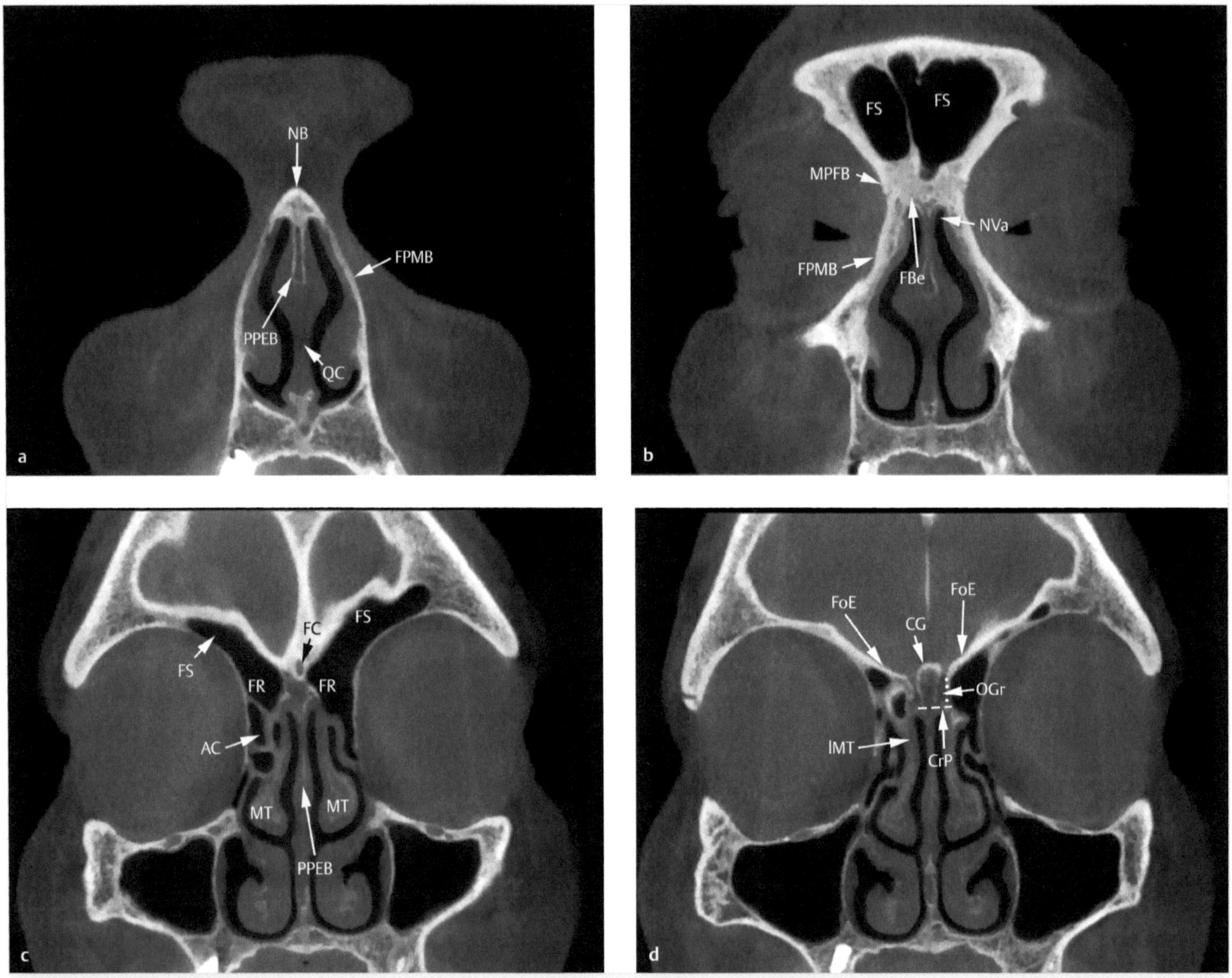

Fig. 6.3 (a–d) Coronal CT of the frontal sinus and adjacent skull base. The panel includes four coronal CT scans, from anterior **(a)** to posterior **(d)**. The transfrontal transnasal corridor lies between the nasal bones (NB) cranially, frontal processes of the maxillary bones (FPMB) laterally, and crista galli (CG) posteriorly. The corridor exploits the space of frontal recesses (FR) and frontal sinuses (FS) to reach the posterior frontal plate, which is exposed removing part of nasal septum and frontal beaks (FBe). AC, agger complex; CrP, cribriform plate; FC, foramen coecum; FoE, fovea ethmoidalis; IMT, laminar portion of the middle turbinate; MPFB, maxillary process of the frontal bone; MT, middle turbinate; NVa, nasal vault; OGr, olfactory groove; PPEB, perpendicular plate of the ethmoid bone; QC, quadrangular cartilage.) (*White dashed line*, horizontal lamella of the cribriform plate; *white dotted line*, vertical lamella of the cribriform plate.

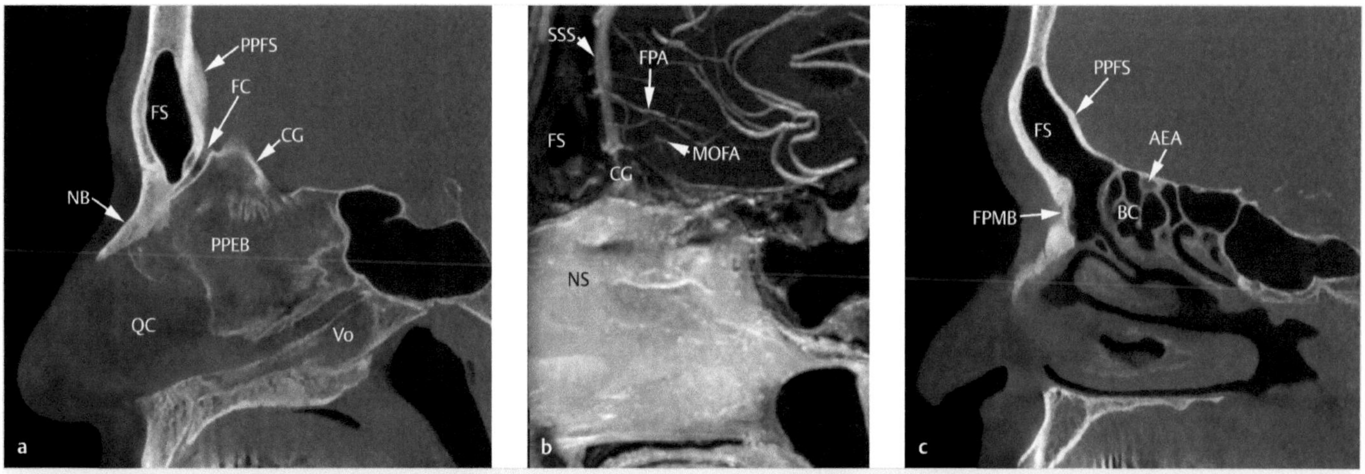

Fig. 6.4 Sagittal CT and MRI anatomy of the posterior plate of the frontal sinus and adjacent structures. The panel is composed by three sagittal images: two CT scans **(a, c)** and one T1-weighted, contrast-enhanced, fat-saturated MRI scan **(b)**. The posterior plate of the frontal sinus (PPFS) lies anterosuperiorly to the foramen coecum (FC) and crista galli (CG). It serves as a barrier between the frontal sinus (FS) and anterior cranial fossa. The medial orbitofrontal (MOFA) and frontopolar arteries (FPA) run toward this plate along the cerebral surface. AEA, anterior ethmoidal artery; BC, bullar complex; FPMB, frontal process of the maxillary bone; NB, nasal bone; NS, nasal septum; PPEB, perpendicular plate of the ethmoid bone; QC, quadrangular cartilage; SSS, superior sagittal sinus; Vo, vomer.

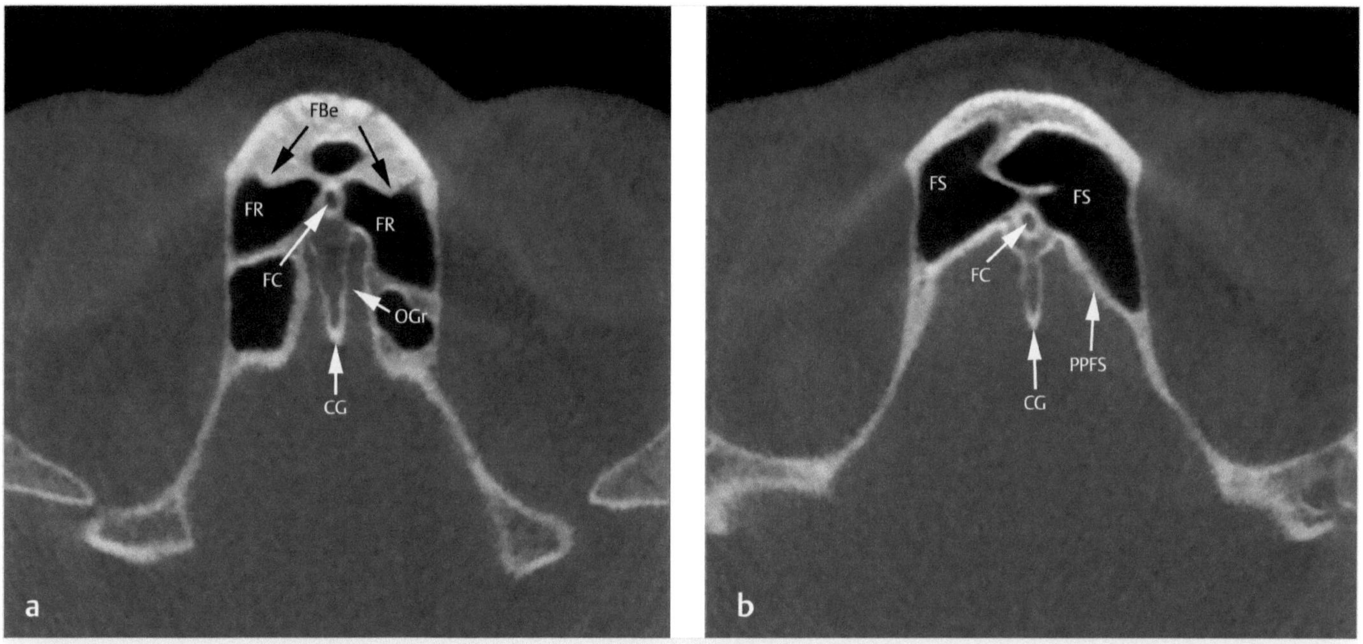

Fig. 6.5 (a, b) Axial CT anatomy of the posterior plate of the frontal sinus and adjacent structures. The frontal recesses (FR) and frontal sinuses (FS) lie anterior to the olfactory grooves (OGr), crista galli (CG), and posterior plate of the frontal sinus (PPFS). FBe, frontal beak; FC, foramen coecum.

Endoscopic Dissection

Skull Base Phase

- Step 1: Anterosuperior septectomy.
- Step 2: Nonmodular Draf III frontal sinusotomy.
- Step 3: Partial removal of nasal bones.
- Step 4: Partial removal of the posterior plate of the frontal sinus.
- Step 5: Removal of crista galli.
- Step 6: Dural incision.
- Step 7: Transection of the falx and removal of the dura of the crista galli.

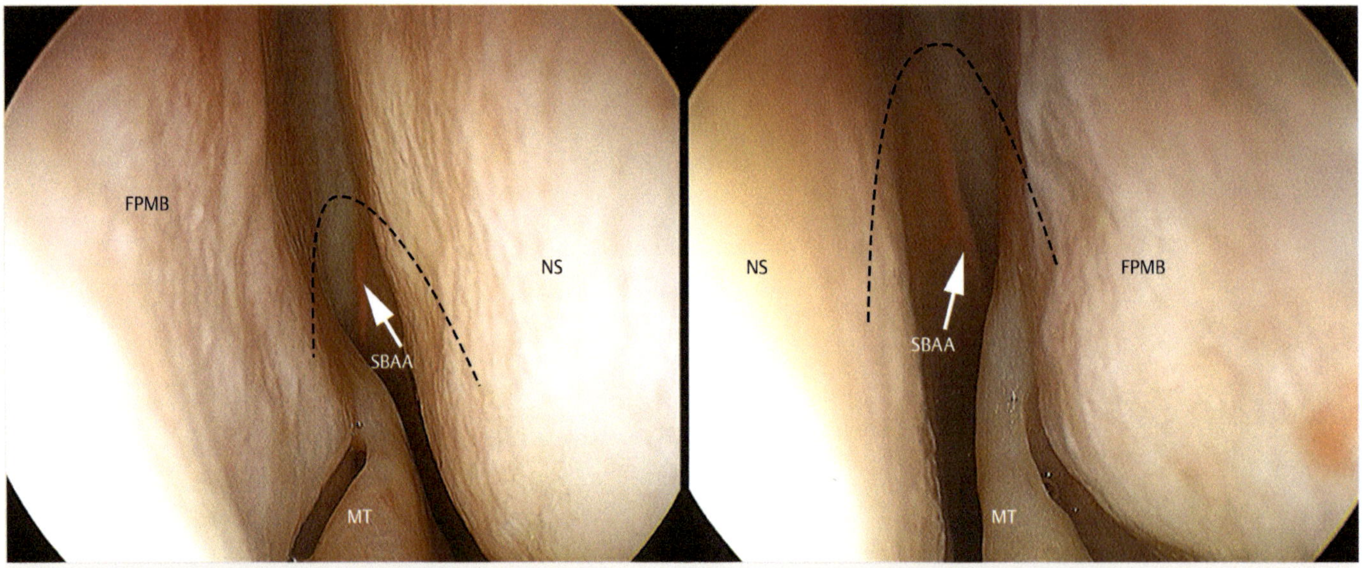

Fig. 6.6 Nasal landmarks. Before performing septectomy, the following landmarks must be identified on each side: the frontal process of the maxillary bone (FPMB) and middle turbinate (MT) laterally and the nasal septum (NS) medially. A curved incision (*black dashed line*) is made from a few millimeters above the axilla of the middle turbinate to the nasal septum, which crosses the trajectory of the septal branch of the anterior ethmoidal artery (SBAA).

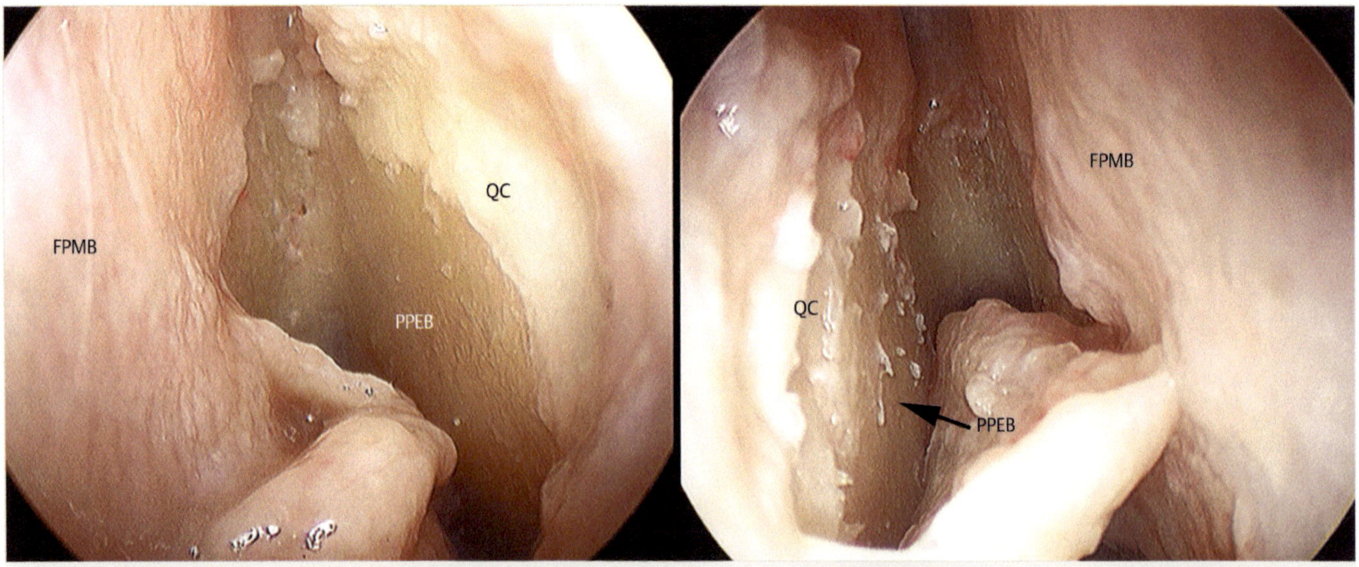

Fig. 6.7 Exposure of the bony cartilaginous septum. Subperichondrial/subperiosteal dissection is performed to expose the quadrangular cartilage (QC) anteriorly and the perpendicular plate of the ethmoid bone (PPEB) posteriorly. FPMB, frontal process of the maxillary bone.

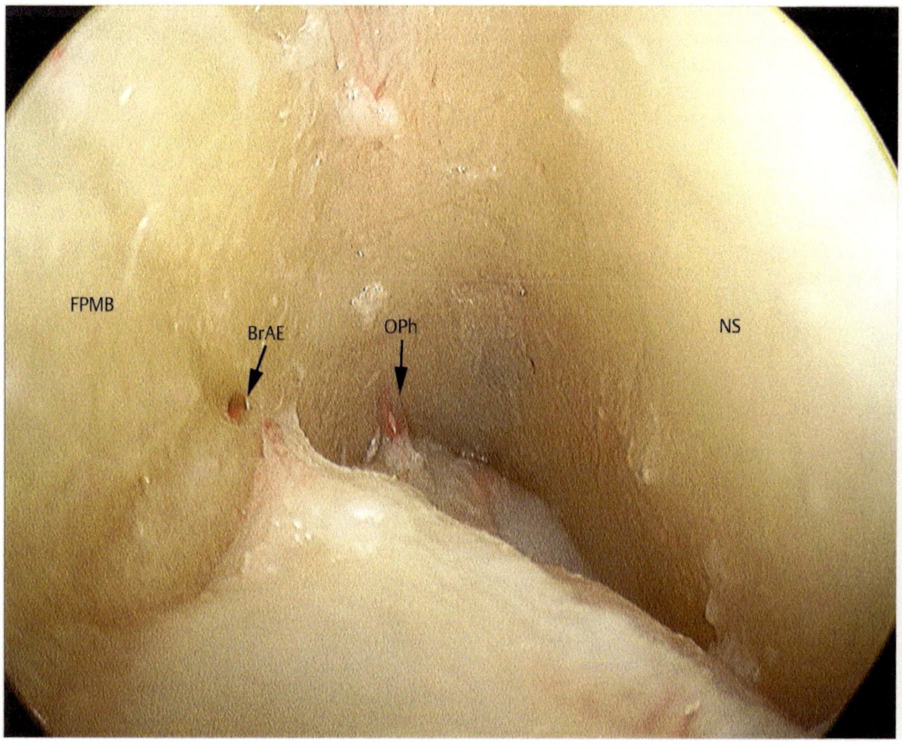

Fig. 6.8 Neurovascular landmarks. The subperiosteal dissection along the top of the frontal process of the maxillary bone (FPMB) reveals some neurovascular structures. The first olfactory phylum (OPh), which marks the anterior limit of the anterior cranial fossa, can be confused with a transosseous branch of the anterior ethmoidal artery (BrAE) that vascularizes the anterior portion of the lateral nasal wall. NS, nasal septum.

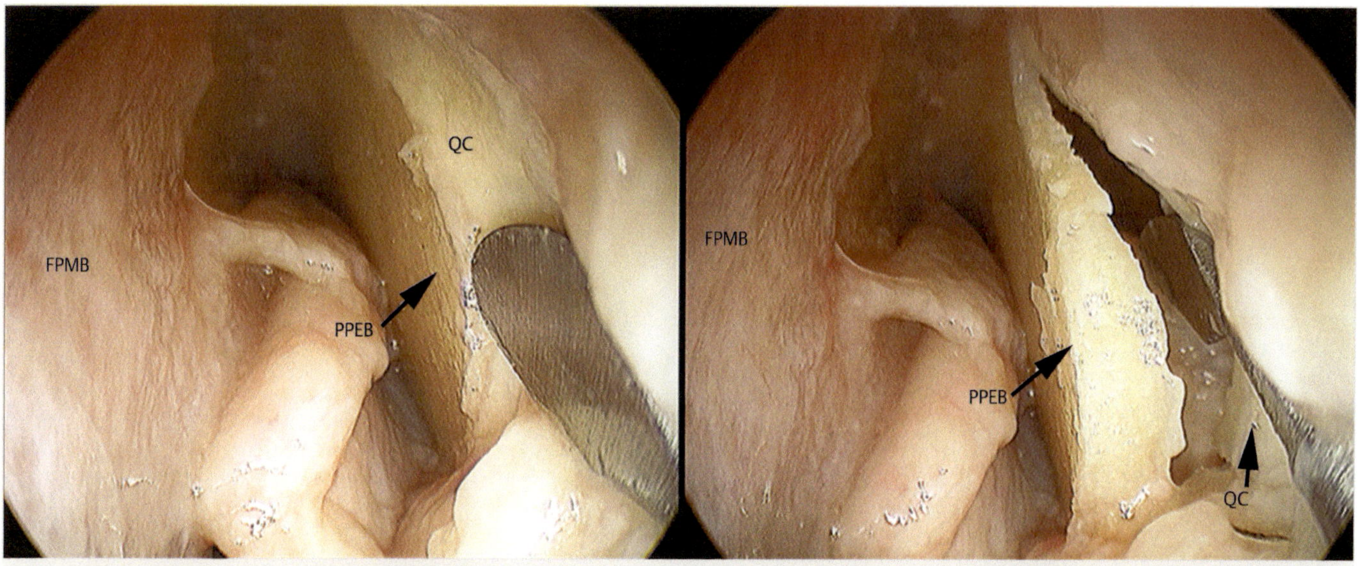

Fig. 6.9 Disarticulation of the septal cartilage from septal bone. The quadrangular cartilage (QC) is disarticulated from the perpendicular plate of the ethmoid bone (PPEB) pushing with a dissector on the bony–cartilaginous junction. FPMB, frontal process of the maxillary bone.

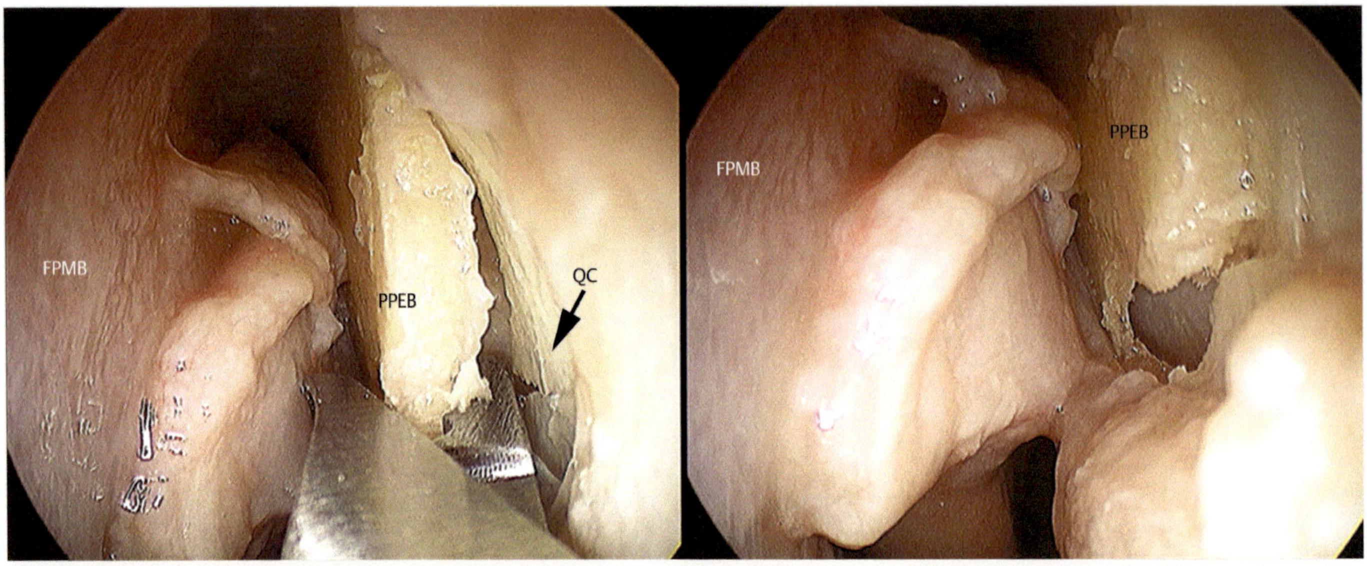

Fig. 6.10 Step 1 (part 1). Cutting forceps are used to perform a small osteotomy in the perpendicular plate of the ethmoid bone (PPEB), roughly at the level of the axilla of the middle turbinate. FPMB, frontal process of the maxillary bone; QC, quadrangular cartilage.

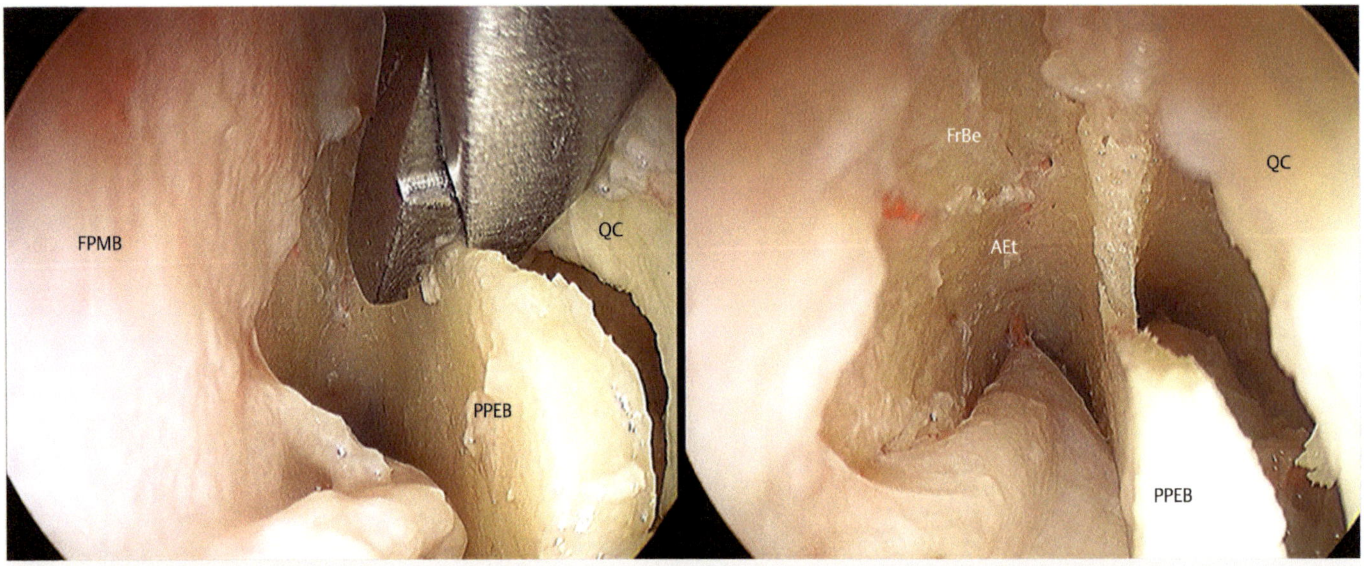

Fig. 6.11 Step 1 (part 2). The perpendicular plate of the ethmoid bone (PPEB) is cut along its attachment to the alae ethmoidalis (AEt). FPMB, frontal process of the maxillary bone; FrBe, frontal beak; QC, quadrangular cartilage.

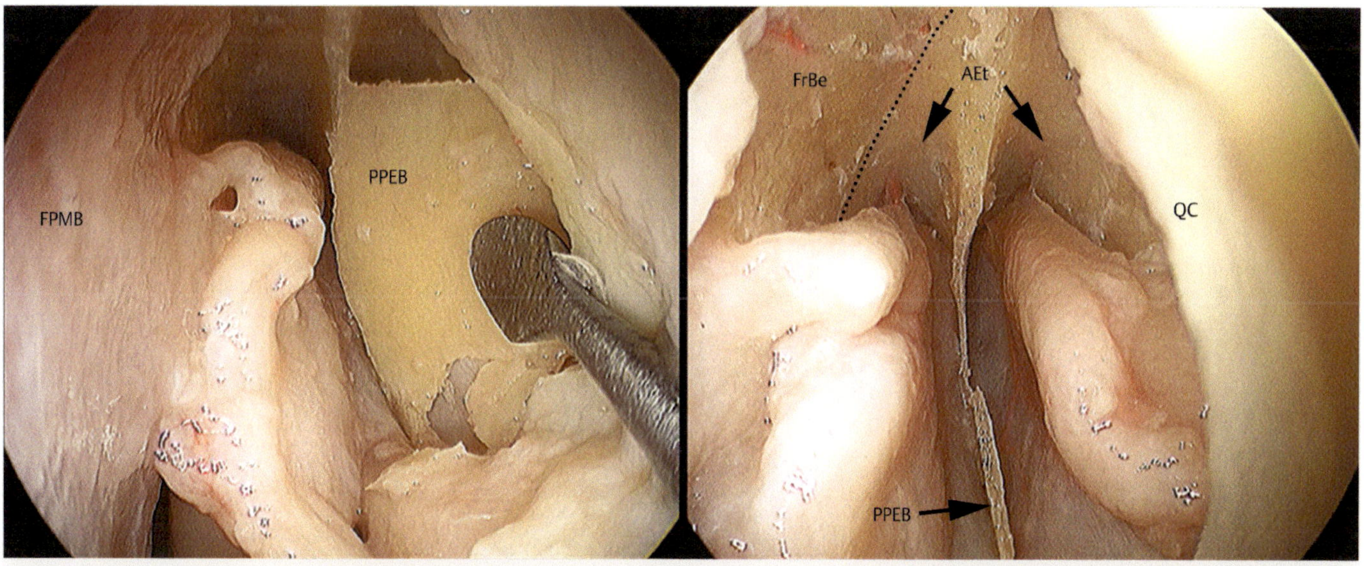

Fig. 6.12 Step 1 (part 3). The anterior septectomy is completed breaking the perpendicular plate of the ethmoid bone (PPEB) in front of the olfactory phyla. In this way, both the alae ethmoidalis (AEt) and frontal beak (FrBe) are exposed. FPMB, frontal process of the maxillary bone; QC, quadrangular cartilage. (*Black dotted line*, ethmoid maxillary suture).

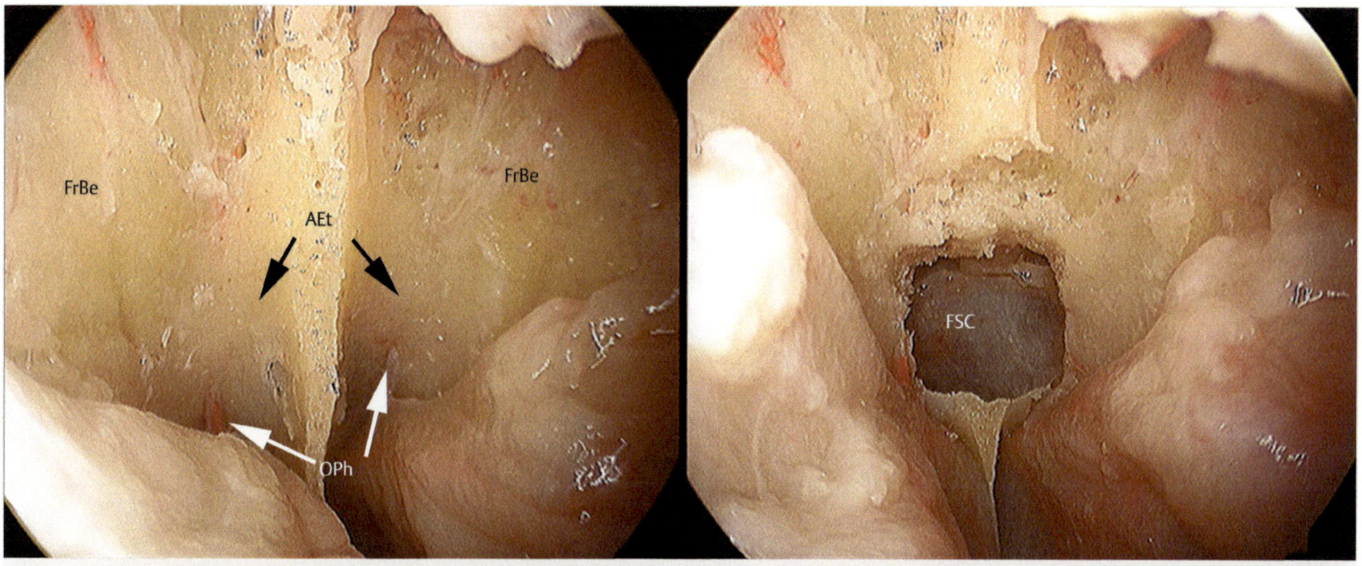

Fig. 6.13 Step 2 (part 1). The bone of the alae ethmoidalis (AEt) is removed between the frontal beak (FrBe) anteriorly and olfactory phyla (OPh) posteriorly. In this specimen, the mucosa of a frontal septal cell (FSC) was identified.

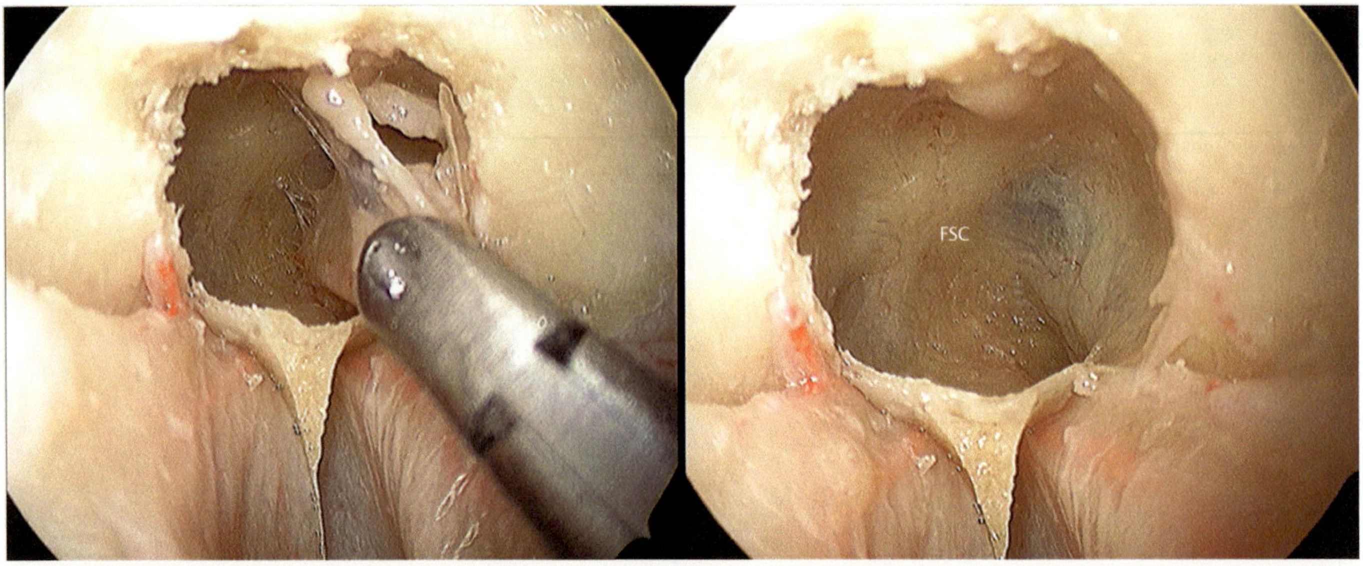

Fig. 6.14 The frontal septal cell. The mucosa of the frontal septal cell (FSC) is removed to identify the bony surface of this air space lying between frontal sinuses.

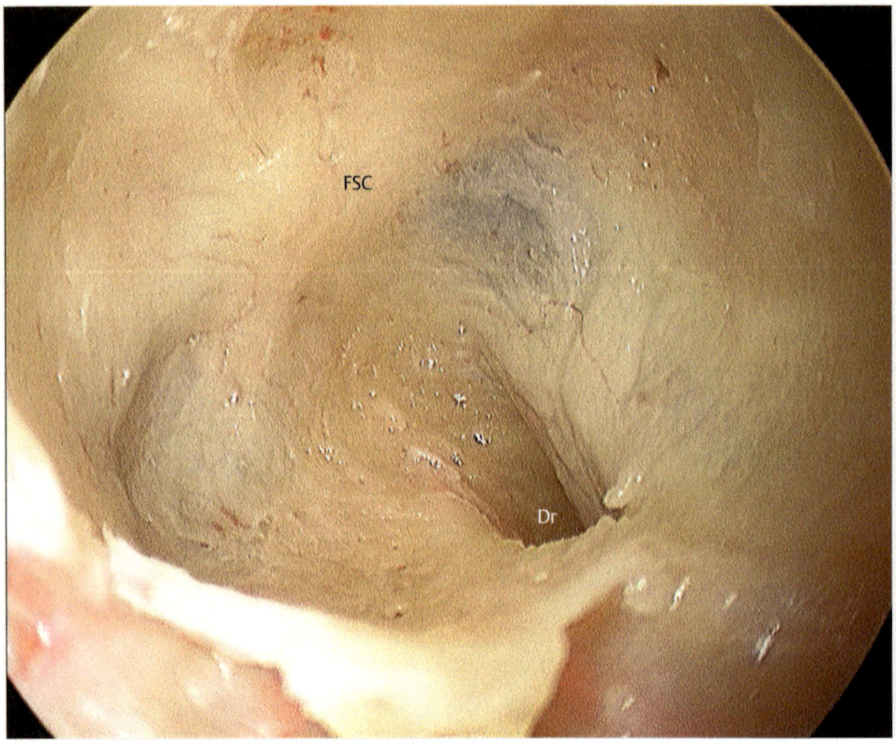

Fig. 6.15 The drainage pathway of the frontal septal cell. Exploring the frontal septal cell (FSC), its drainage pathway (Dr) toward the left frontoethmoidal area is identified.

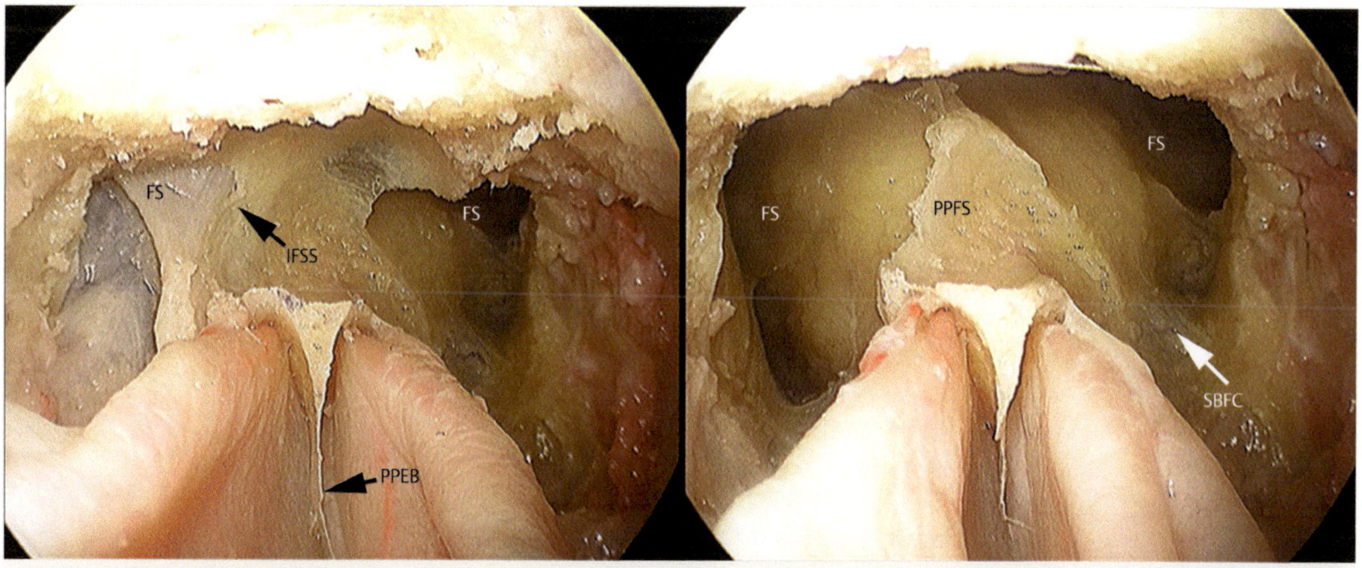

Fig. 6.16 Step 2 (part 2). The frontal beak is removed in a centrifugal fashion starting from the midline and staying in front of the perpendicular plate of the ethmoid bone (PPEB). A Draf type III frontal sinusotomy is completed removing the interfrontal sinus septum (IFSS) and other septa within the inferior portion of the frontal sinuses (FS). Frontal cells, such as the suprabullar frontal cell (SBFC) that was identified in this specimen, can be left intact when they do not extend to the midline portion of the posterior plate of the frontal sinus (PPFS).

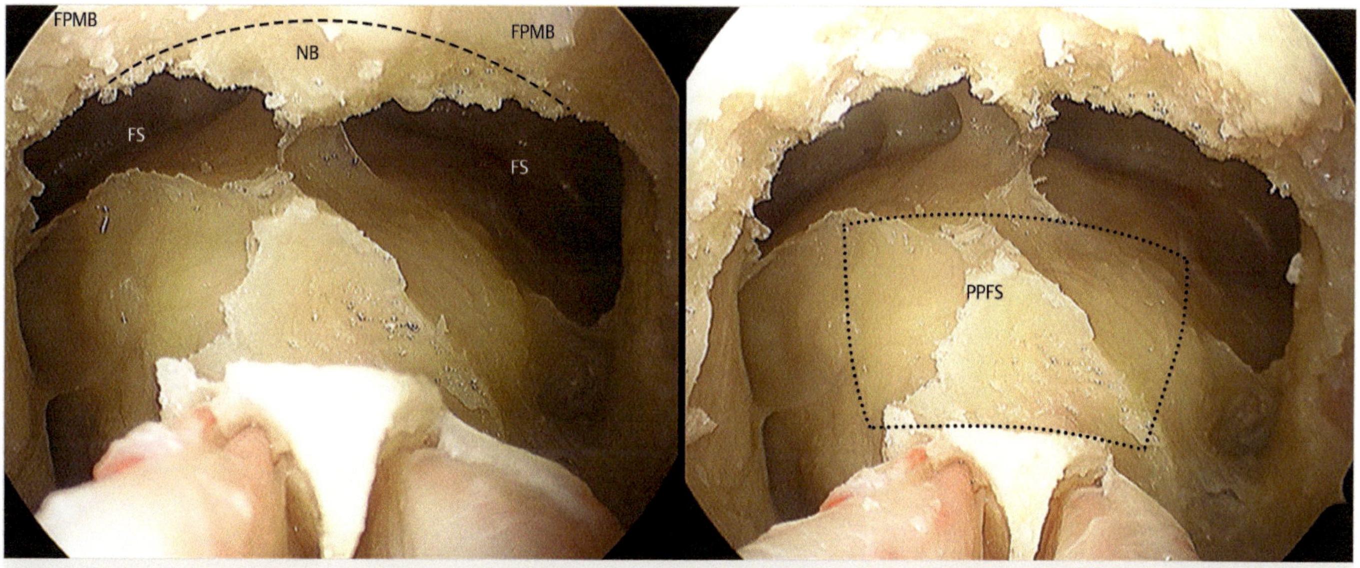

Fig. 6.17 Step 3. The window of the Draf type III sinusotomy is enlarged (*black dashed line*) removing the cranial portion of nasal bones (NB), between the frontal processes of the maxillary bones (FPMB). In this way, frontal sinuses (FS) are completely exposed and the craniectomy (*black dotted line*) can be performed in the inferior and median portions of the posterior plate of the frontal sinus (PPFS).

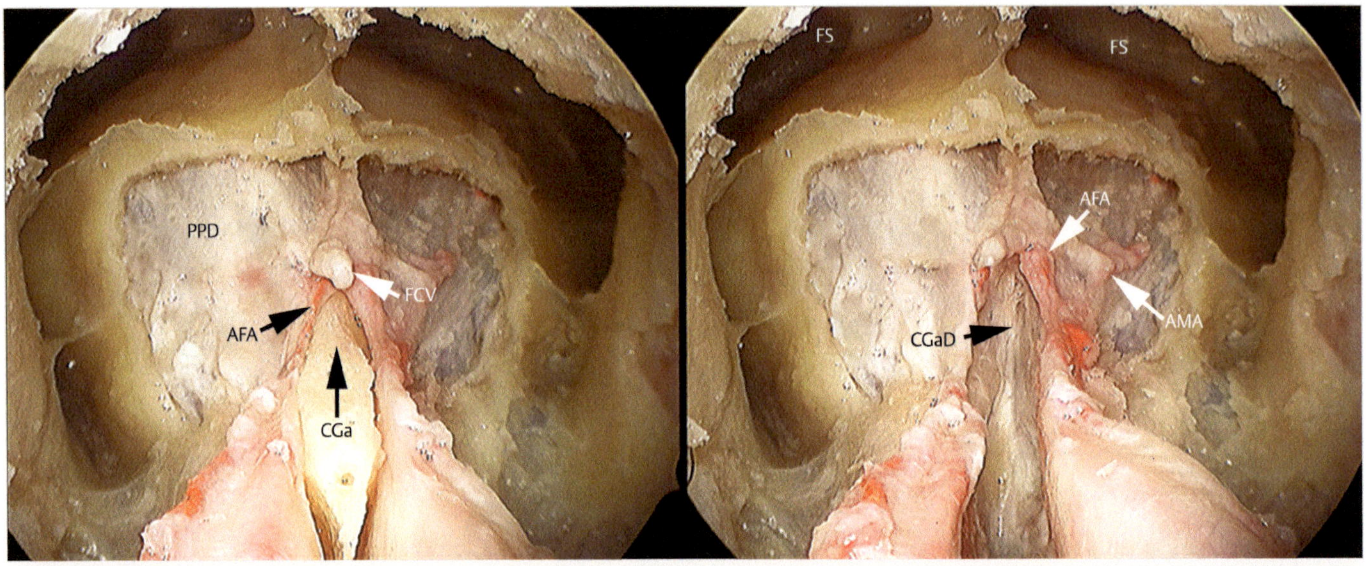

Fig. 6.18 Steps 4 and 5. The inferior and midline portions of the posterior plate of the frontal sinuses are removed preserving the dural lining (PPD). The crista galli (CGa) of the ethmoid bone comes into view in the median portion of the craniectomy. The vein of the foramen caecum (FCV), which is a foramen between the crista galli and the posterior plate of the frontal bone, can be seen above the crista galli. The anterior falcine artery (AFA), one of the terminal branches of the anterior ethmoidal artery, runs beside the crista galli and reaches the falx cerebri. The crista galli is removed to expose its dural envelope (CGaD), which corresponds to the anteroinferior insertion of the falx cerebri. The anterior meningeal artery (AMA), which branches from the anterior ethmoidal artery, can be seen lateral to the anterior falcine artery. FS, frontal sinus.

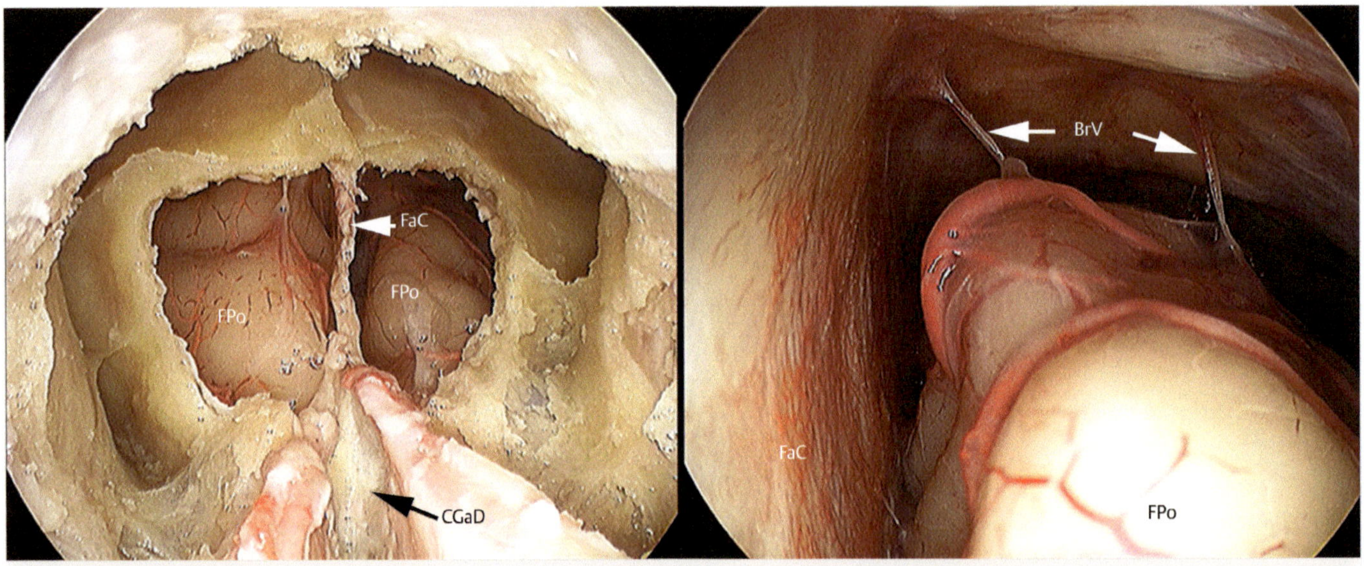

Fig. 6.19 Step 6. The dura is opened and the frontal poles (FPo) become visible beside the falx cerebri (FaC), which is encountered along the median sagittal plane. Moving the scope toward a frontal pole, some bridging veins (BrV) can be identified. These structures extend from the brain cortex to the superior sagittal sinus, which runs along the insertion of the falx cerebri on the cranial vault. CGaD, dura of the crista galli.

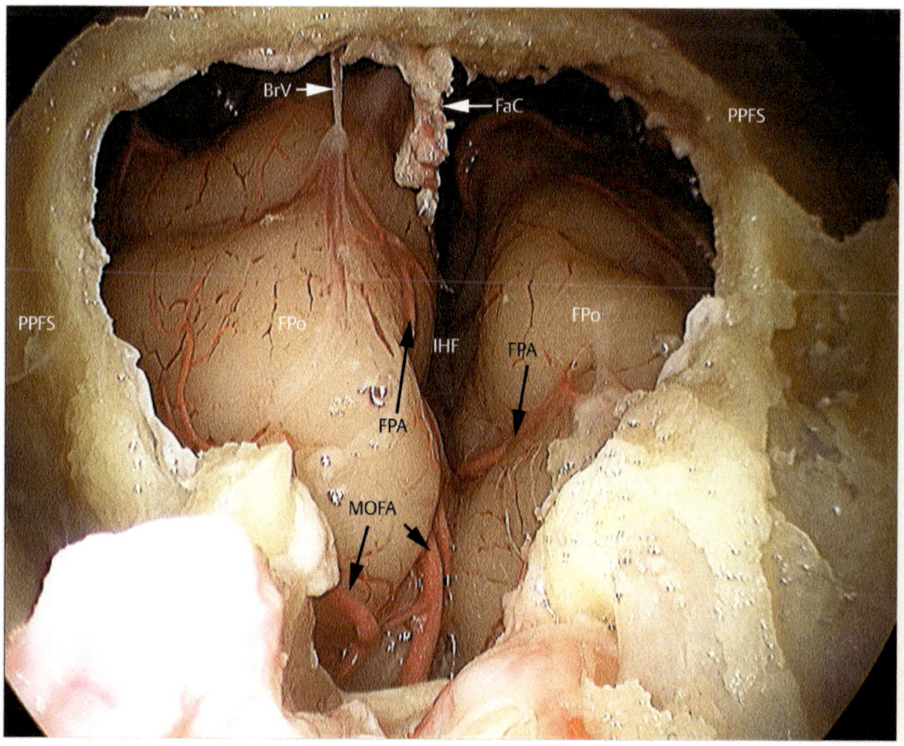

Fig. 6.20 Step 7. The falx cerebri (FaC) is transected and the dura of the crista galli is removed to expose the medial orbitofrontal (MOFA) and frontopolar arteries (FPA). Additionally, the anterior part of the interhemispheric fissure (IHF) becomes accessible. BrV, bridging vein; FPo, frontal pole; PPFS, posterior plate of the frontal sinus.

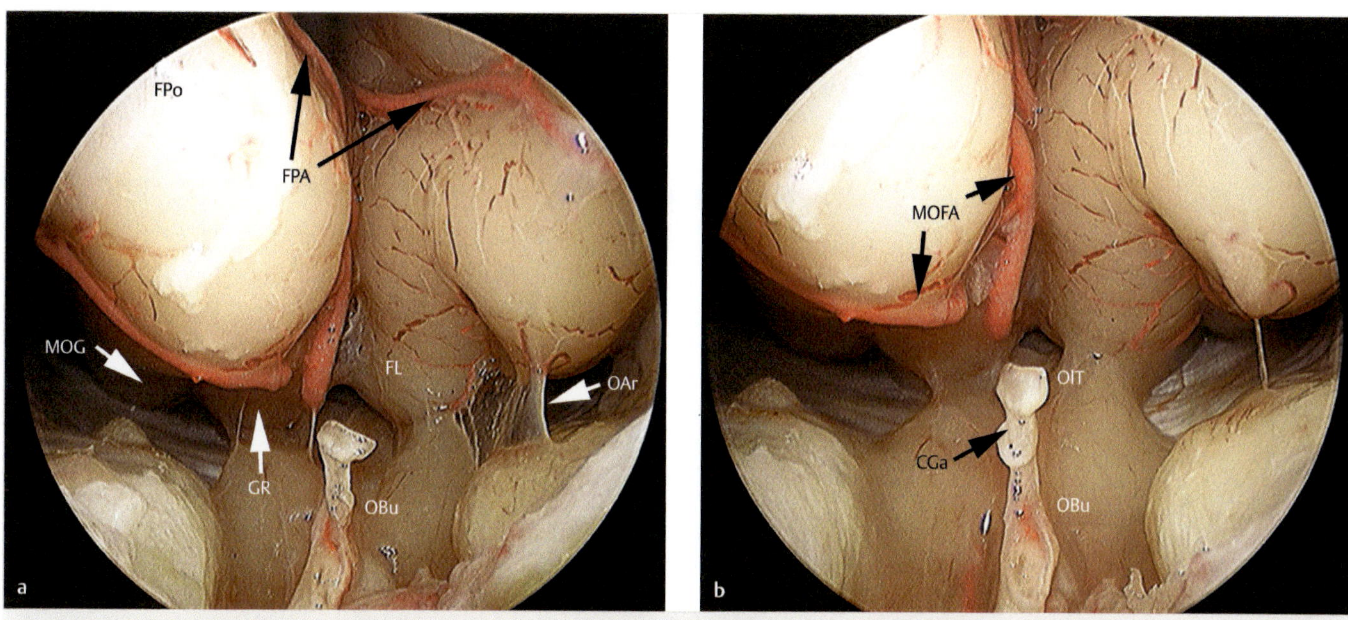

Fig. 6.21 (a, b) Midline anterior cranial fossa. A 70-degree scope turned inferoposteriorly is placed along the dural defect to explore the contents of the anterior cranial fossa. The olfactory bulbs (OBu) can be identified within the olfactory grooves, which are separated by the posterior tail of the crista galli (CGa). After removing the outer arachnoid layer (OAr) connecting the bulbs to the brain, the olfactory tracts (OlT) can be identified behind each bulb while running toward the frontal lobes (FL). The inferior surface of the frontal lobes that faces the midline anterior skull base is composed by the gyrus rectus (GR) medially and the medial orbital gyrus (MOG) laterally. FPA, frontopolar artery; FPo, frontal pole; MOFA, medial orbitofrontal arteries.

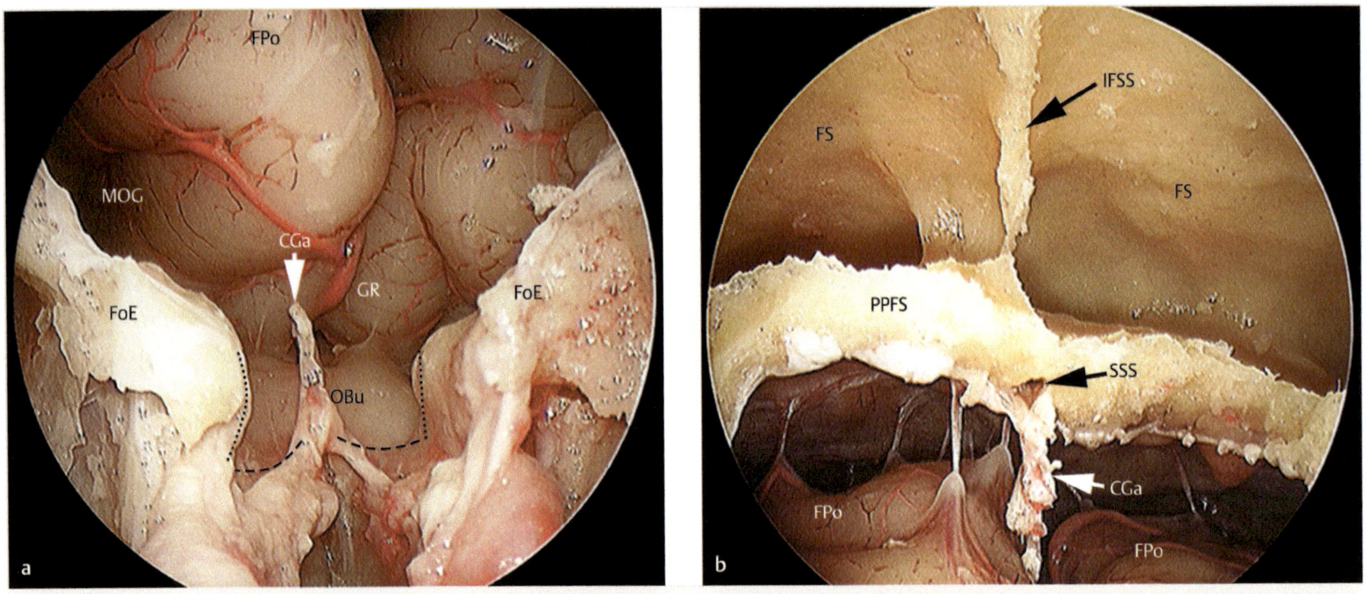

Fig. 6.22 (a, b) Boundaries of the craniectomy. A 70-degree scope turned posteriorly is placed in front of the inferior boundary of the craniectomy to have a coronal perspective of the anterior skull base. The olfactory groove is delimited by the horizontal (*black dashed line*) and vertical (*black dotted line*) portions of the cribriform plate and is located caudally with respect to the foveae ethmoidalis (FoE). Placing the 70-degree scope turned superiorly at the superior boundary of the craniectomy, it is possible to identify the caudal end of the superior sagittal sinus (SSS). CGa, crista galli (residual insertions); FPo, frontal pole; FS, frontal sinus; GR, gyrus rectus; IFSS, interfrontal sinus septum; MOG, medial orbital gyrus; OBu, olfactory bulb; PPFS, posterior plate of the frontal sinus.

References

[1] Cervantes SS, Lal D. Crista galli mucocele: endoscopic marsupialization via frontoethmoid approach. Int Forum Allergy Rhinol 2014;4(7):598–602

[2] Pinheiro-Neto CD, Snyderman CH, Fernandez-Miranda J, Gardner PA. Endoscopic endonasal surgery for nasal dermoids. Otolaryngol Clin North Am 2011;44(4): 981–987, ix

[3] Selleck AM, Desai D, Thorp BD, Ebert CS, Zanation AM. Management of Frontal Sinus Tumors. Otolaryngol Clin North Am 2016;49(4):1051–1065

[4] Shidanshid M, Taghi AS, Kuchai R, Saleh HA. Endoscopic resection of a mucocele of the crista galli. Ear Nose Throat J 2015;94(9):E23–E25

[5] Ma J, Huang Q, Li X, et al. Endoscopic transnasal repair of cerebrospinal fluid leaks with and without an encephalocele in pediatric patients: from infants to children. Childs Nerv Syst 2015;31(9):1493–1498

[6] Nyquist GG, Anand VK, Mehra S, Kacker A, Schwartz TH. Endoscopic endonasal repair of anterior skull base non-traumatic cerebrospinal fluid leaks, meningoceles, and encephaloceles. J Neurosurg 2010;113(5):961–966

[7] Re M, Tarchini P, Macrì G, Pasquini E. Endonasal endoscopic approach for intracranial nasal dermoid sinus cysts in children. Int J Pediatr Otorhinolaryngol 2012;76(8):1217–1222

[8] Thong JF, Chatterjee D, Hwang SY. Endoscopic modified Lothrop approach for the excision of bilateral frontal sinus tumors. Ear Nose Throat J 2014;93(3):116–119

7 Transcribriform Approach

Marco Ferrari, Marco Ravanelli, Davide Lancini, Vittorio Rampinelli, Alberto Schreiber

The transcribriform approach is most frequently employed to resect tumors of the anterior skull base via a transnasal endoscopic route. Formally, the term "transcribriform approach" is anatomically inaccurate as it refers only to the cribriform plate, while almost invariably resection also includes the ethmoidal roof (or fovea ethmoidalis).[1,2] During the last decades, this corridor progressively became the mainstay for the surgical management of a wide array of diseases involving the anterior skull base, including meningiomas,[3-7] schwannomas,[8,9] dysembryogenic lesions,[10] sinonasal malignancies,[11-22] and other tumors or tumorlike lesions.[1] On the other hand, its indications in the management of some tumors of the anterior skull base (i.e., meningiomas of the cribriform plate and/or ethmoidal roof) are controversial and factors like the status of olfaction before surgery and the possibility of its preservation should be considered in the decision-making process.[23,24,25] Moreover, the anatomy of the transcribriform approach should also be mastered when treating cerebrospinal fluid leaks of the cribriform plate or ethmoidal roof, though, in such circumstances, the resection of sinonasal structures is commonly less extensive.[26,27]

The transcribriform route is limited anteriorly by the bony angle joining the posterior frontal plate with midline anterior skull base, posteriorly by the ethmoidal–sphenoidal junction and laterally by the medial orbital walls. To get access to the anterior skull base through the nose, the ethmoidal box must be disassembled according to the needs of resection and exposure. The most extensive variant of this approach, which includes a binostril corridor with a subtotal septectomy, is detailed in the present chapter. Subtotal septectomy is performed for oncologic reasons because most nasal–ethmoidal lesions directly invade the septum and/or with the intent to provide a binostril access to the surgical field with the advantage to work with a four-hand technique. This approach offers to the surgeon a wide and sequential view of the skull base layers that are invaded by tumors arising from nasal–ethmoidal complex,

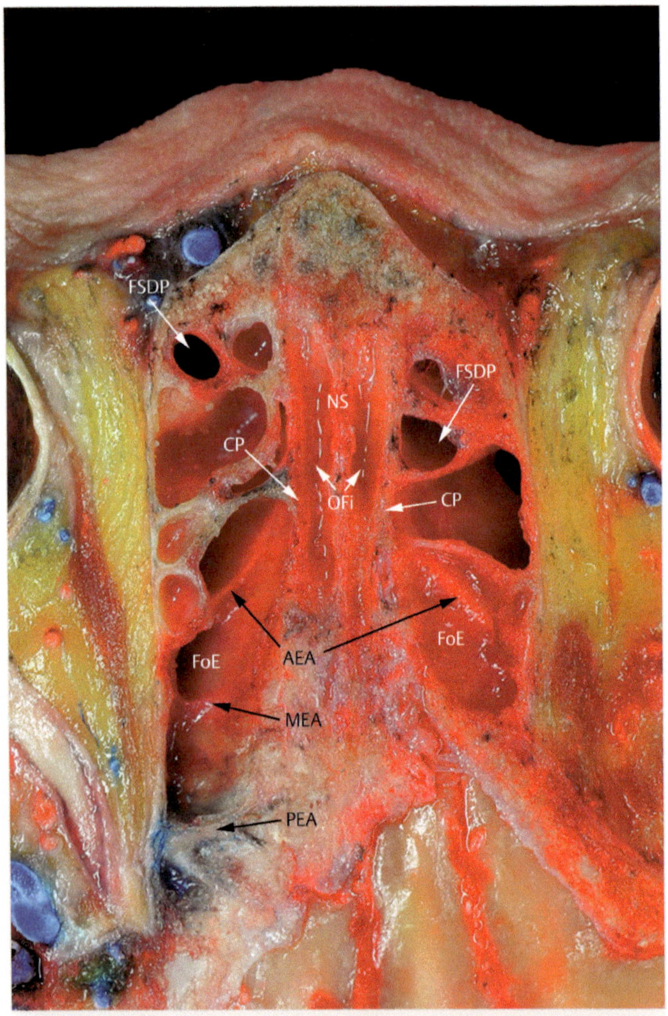

Fig. 7.1 Axial view of the midline anterior skull base as seen from caudal to cranial. This axial cadaver cut shows anatomy of the midline anterior skull base as seen from the sinonasal area. AEA, anterior ethmoidal artery; CP, conchal plate; FoE, fovea ethmoidalis (or ethmoidal roof); FSDP, frontal sinus drainage pathway; MEA, middle ethmoidal artery; NS, nasal septum; OFi, olfactory fissure (or cleft); PEA, posterior ethmoidal artery.

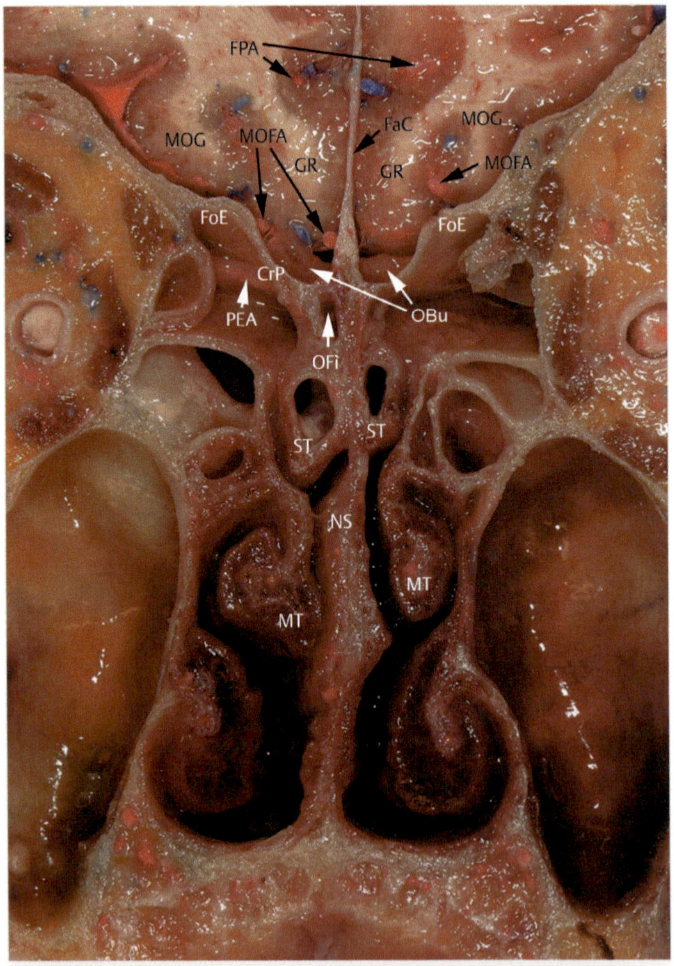

Fig. 7.2 Coronal view of the midline anterior skull base. This coronal cadaver cut shows anatomy of the midline anterior skull base and adjacent structures. CrP, cribriform plate; FaC, falx cerebri; FoE, fovea ethmoidalis (or ethmoidal roof); FPA, frontopolar artery; GR, gyrus rectus; MOFA, medial orbitofrontal artery; MOG, medial orbital gyrus; MT, middle turbinate; NS, nasal septum; OBu, olfactory bulb; OFi, olfactory fissue (or cleft); PEA, posterior ethmoidal artery; ST, superior turbinate.

thus allowing for a tailored and targeted resection. However, it is worth mentioning that a unilateral transcribriform approach gives the patient the possibility to maintain at least partially the sense of smell, as demonstrated by recent studies on the surgical treatment of unilateral tumors without septal extension.[28] With a similar philosophy, spontaneous or post-traumatic/-surgical cerebrospinal fluid leaks and/or meningoencephaloceles are usually managed with conservative variants of the transcribriform approach herein presented, with the aim to minimize postsurgical morbidity. As an additional remark, the transcribriform corridor provides a direct view of the gyrus rectus and medial orbital gyrus, whose minimal invasion can be managed with endoscopic subpial dissection without the need for craniotomy.

The transcribriform approach crosses by its nature the course of ethmoidal arteries, whose variable anatomy must be fully understood to coagulate and cut them safely, minimizing the risk for orbital complications. In addition, when the intradural space is entered, the medial orbitofrontal arteries and veins are encountered; their careful manipulation avoids the risk of intracranial hemorrhage, which might be difficult to manage via a transnasal endoscopic approach.

The bony borders of the craniectomy performed while harvesting the transcribriform pathway are usually thick and well defined. As a consequence, they are particularly suitable for multilayered reconstruction with several grafts and flaps that can be variably positioned with respect to the dura mater and bony edges of the skull base. Despite the unquestionable efficacy of vascularized local flaps,[21,29] they are frequently not available after a transcribriform approach as a consequence of nasal–ethmoidal tumors propensity to invade the nasal septum and turbinates. However, a three-layered reconstruction with fascial grafts (such as the iliotibial tract) demonstrated to be a safe and effective technique that is feasible in almost all cases.[30,31]

The reader is encouraged to pay particular attention to learn the transcribriform approach as it represents one of the most important steps in the tool kit of endoscopic skull base surgeons.

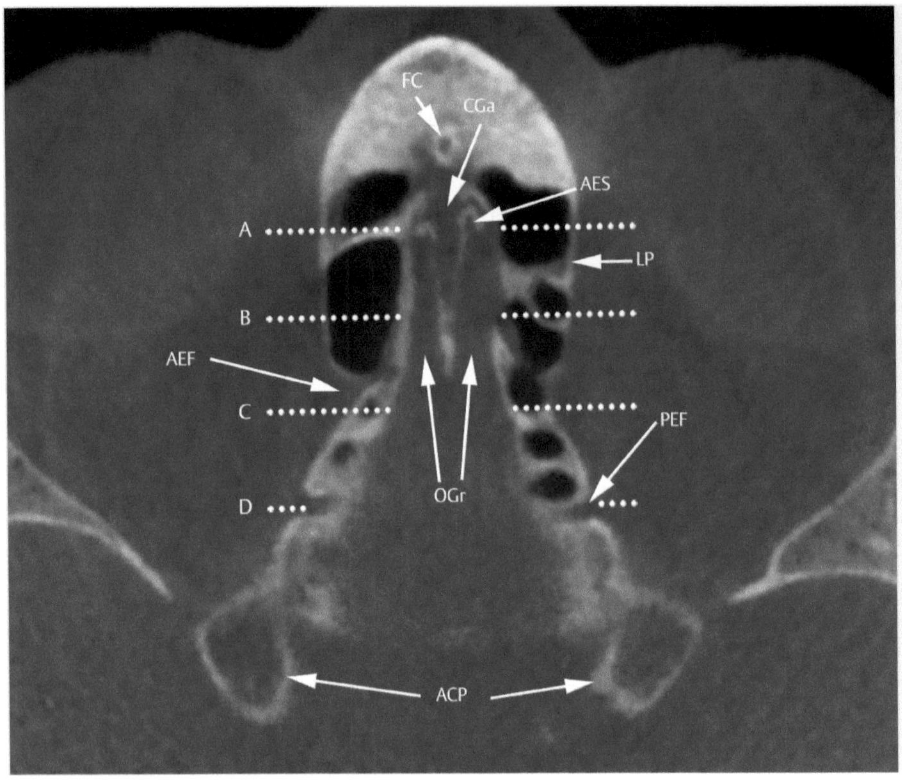

Fig. 7.3 Axial CT of the midline anterior skull base. The midline portion of the anterior skull base lies above the nasal–ethmoidal complex and sphenoid sinus. The crista galli (CGa) serves as anteroinferior insertion of the falx cerebri and separates the olfactory grooves (OGr), which are located cranially to the olfactory fissures. The foramen caecum (FC), which can harbor a small vein, is located anterior to the crista galli. The ethmoidal roof lies above the ethmoidal complex and is crossed by the ethmoidal arteries. The anterior (AEF) and posterior ethmoidal foramina (PEF) can be identified along the lamina papyracea (LP). The anterior (AES) and posterior ethmoidal sulci are small bony douches located in the vertical lamella of the cribriform plate. The position of images composing ▸Fig. 7.4 are shown by *white dotted lines* (A–D). ACP, anterior clinoid process.

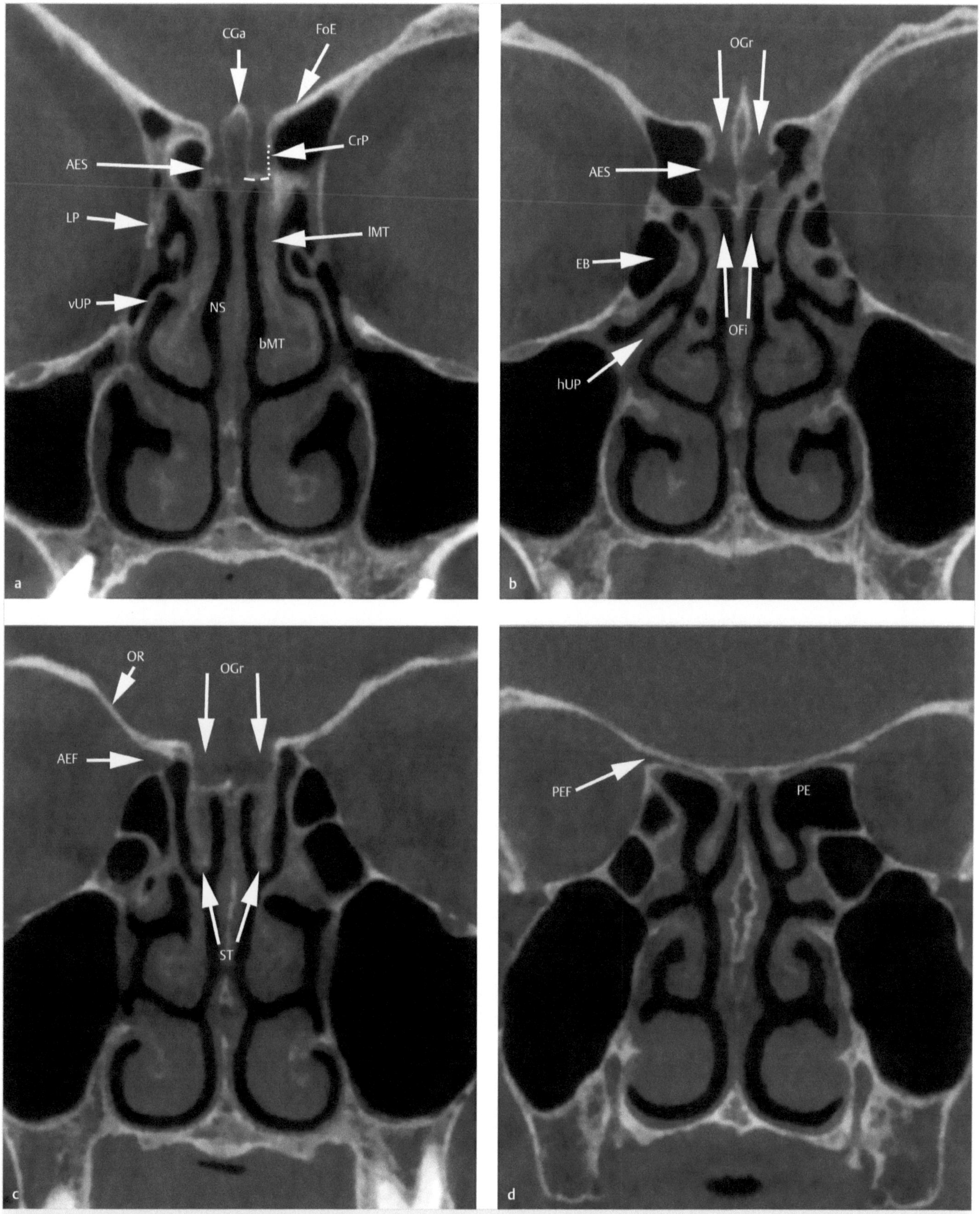

Fig. 7.4 (a–d) Coronal CT anatomy of the midline anterior skull base. The panel includes four coronal CT images, from anterior **(a)** to posterior **(d)**. The midline anterior skull base that lies above the nasal–ethmoidal complex is disposed in three different levels from caudal, medially, to cranial, laterally: the olfactory groove, the ethmoidal roof, and the orbital roof. The inferior boundary of the olfactory groove (OGr) is formed by the horizontal (*white dashed line*) lamella of the cribriform plate (CrP), which joins with the vertical lamella (*white dotted line*) in the area where the laminar portion of the middle (lMT) and superior turbinates (ST) attaches to the skull base. The lateral boundary of the olfactory groove is formed by the vertical lamella of the cribriform plate and by the medial edge of the fovea ethmoidalis (FoE), which is thicker and forms the ethmoidal roof. The orbital roof (OR) lies lateral to the junction between the lamina papyracea (LP) and fovea ethmoidalis and tilts cranially, following the shape of the orbital content. AEF, anterior ethmoidal foramen; AES, anterior ethmoidal sulcus; bMT, bulbous portion of the middle turbinate; CGa, crista galli; EB, ethmoid bulla; hUP, horizontal portion of the uncinate process; NS, nasal septum; OFi, olfactory fissure (or cleft); PE, posterior ethmoidal complex; PEF, posterior ethmoidal foramen; vUP, vertical portion of the uncinate process that inserts on the middle turbinate.

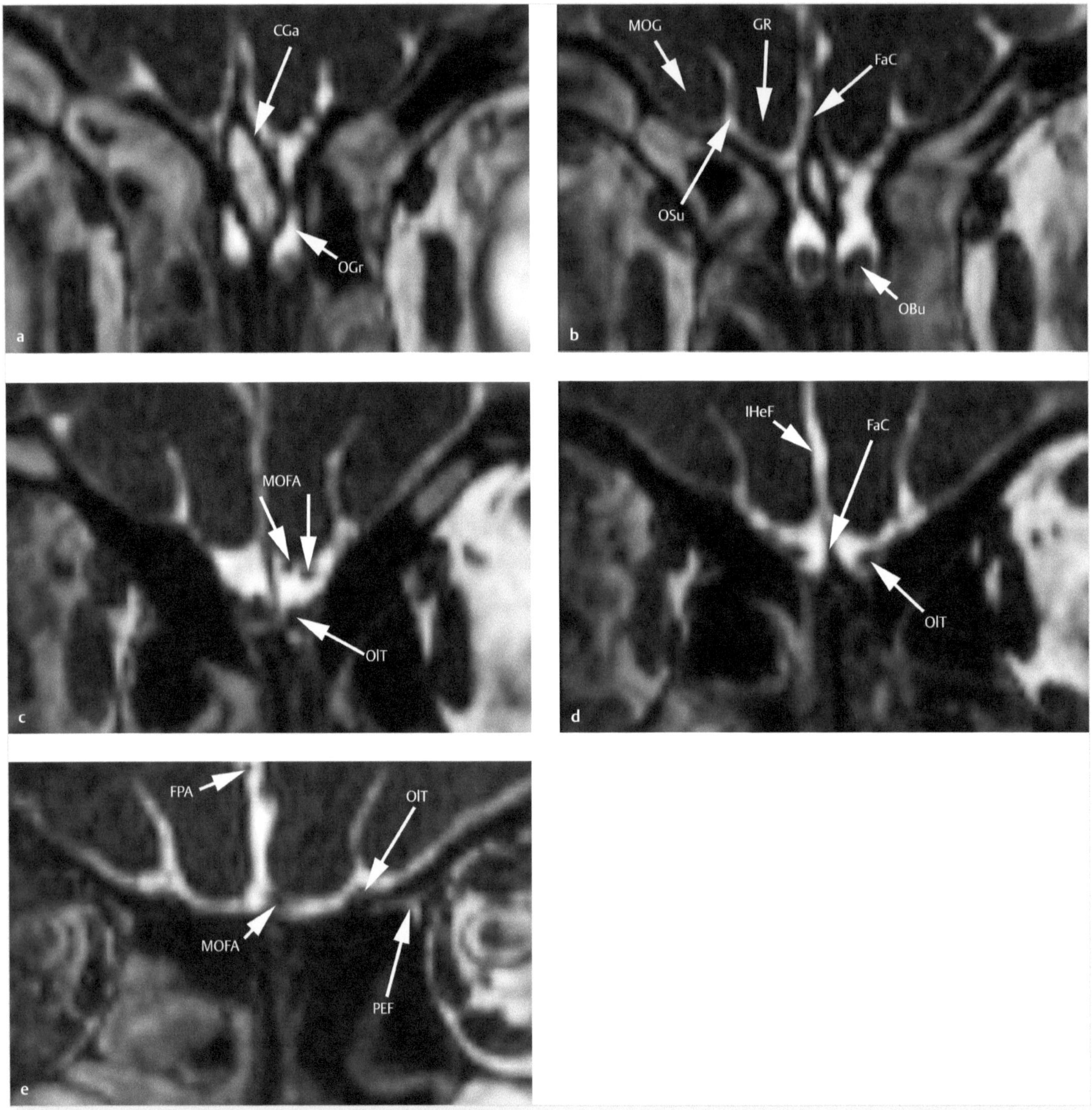

Fig. 7.5 (a–e) Coronal MRI anatomy of the olfactory groove. The panel contains five coronal constructive interference in steady state (CISS) MRI passing through the olfactory groove and adjacent areas, from anterior **(a)** to posterior (lower image) **(e)**. The olfactory grooves (OGr) are separated by the crista galli (CGa) anteriorly and falx cerebri (FaC) posteriorly and house the olfactory bulb (OBu) and the anterior portion of the olfactory tract (OlT). The gyrus rectus (GR) and medial orbital gyrus (MOG) are located above the midline anterior skull base and are divided by the olfactory sulcus (OSu), which harbors the posterior portion of the olfactory tract. The medial orbitofrontal artery (MOFA) is a branch of the anterior cerebral artery and has variable anatomy. Its course can vary from the interhemispheric fissure (IHeF) to the inferior surface of the gyrus rectus, to the olfactory sulcus. Moreover, this artery can be double, as on the left side of the present case. The frontopolar artery (FPA) runs more cranially, passing commonly through the interhemispheric fissure. PEF, posterior ethmoidal foramen.

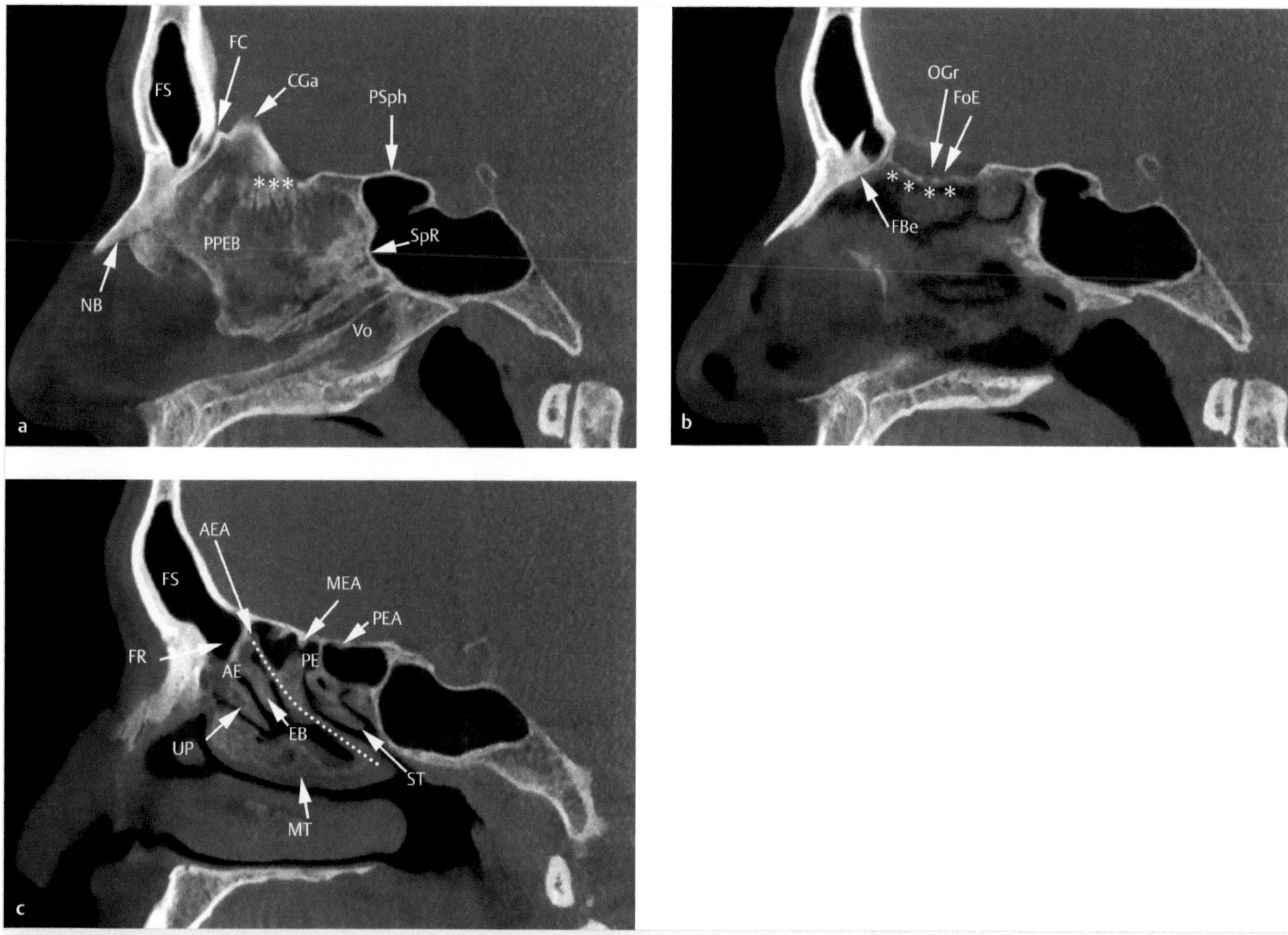

Fig. 7.6 (a–d) Sagittal CT anatomy of the midline anterior skull base. The panel contains three sagittal CT images passing through the midline anterior skull base, from medial **(a)** to lateral **(c)**. The crista galli (CGa) is located posteriorly to the frontal sinus (FS), anteriorly to the planum sphenoidale (PSph), and superiorly to the perpendicular plate of the ethmoid bone (PPEB). The olfactory groove (OGr) lies just lateral to the crista galli and its inferior and lateral walls, which correspond to the cribriform plate, show several defects (*white asterisks*) where the olfactory phyla pass from the olfactory fissure to the olfactory groove. The anterior (AE) and posterior ethmoidal complexes (PE) lie inferior to the fovea ethmoidalis (FoE) and are separated by the basal lamella (*white dotted line*) of the middle turbinate (MT). AEA, anterior ethmoidal artery; EB, ethmoid bulla; FBe, frontal beak; FC, foramen caecum; FR, frontal recess; MEA, middle ethmoidal artery; MT, middle turbinate; NB, nasal bone; PEA, posterior ethmoidal artery; SpR, sphenoid rostrum; ST, superior turbinate; UP, uncinate process; Vo, vomer.

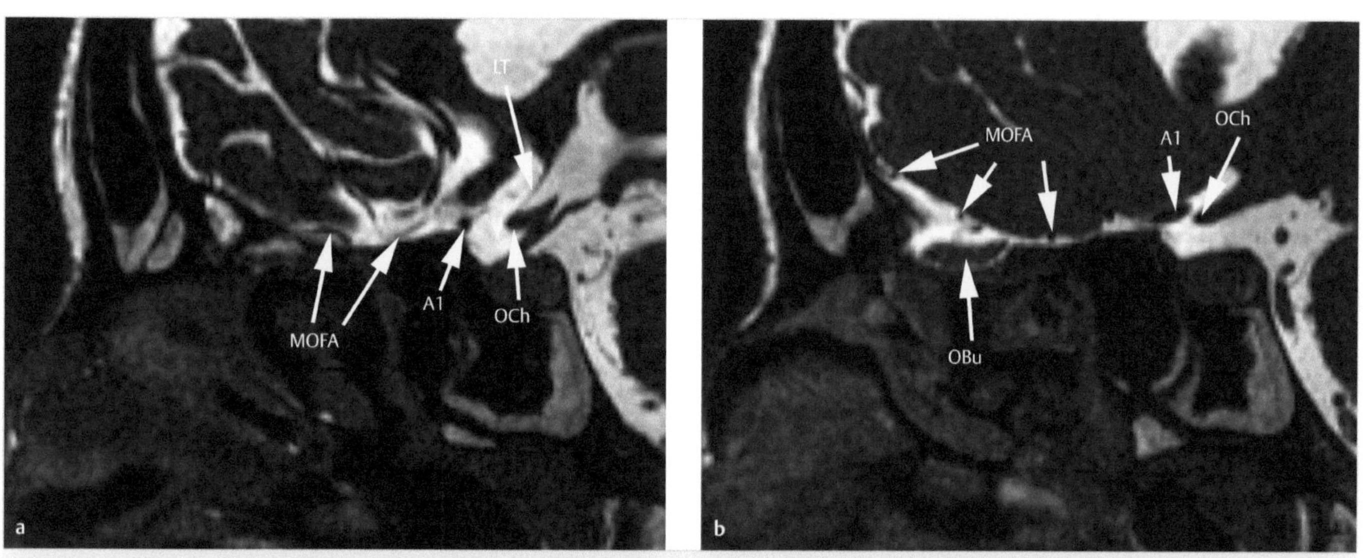

Fig. 7.7 (a, b) Sagittal MRI anatomy of the midline anterior skull base. The panel contains two sagittal constructive interference in steady state (CISS) MRI passing through the midline anterior skull base, from medial **(a)** to lateral **(b)**. The medial orbitofrontal artery (MOFA) runs cranially to the anterior portion of the midline anterior skull base, which houses the olfactory bulb (OBu). The posterior portion of the midline anterior skull base is adjacent to the precommunicating tract of the anterior cerebral artery (A1) and optic chiasm (OCh). LT, lamina terminalis.

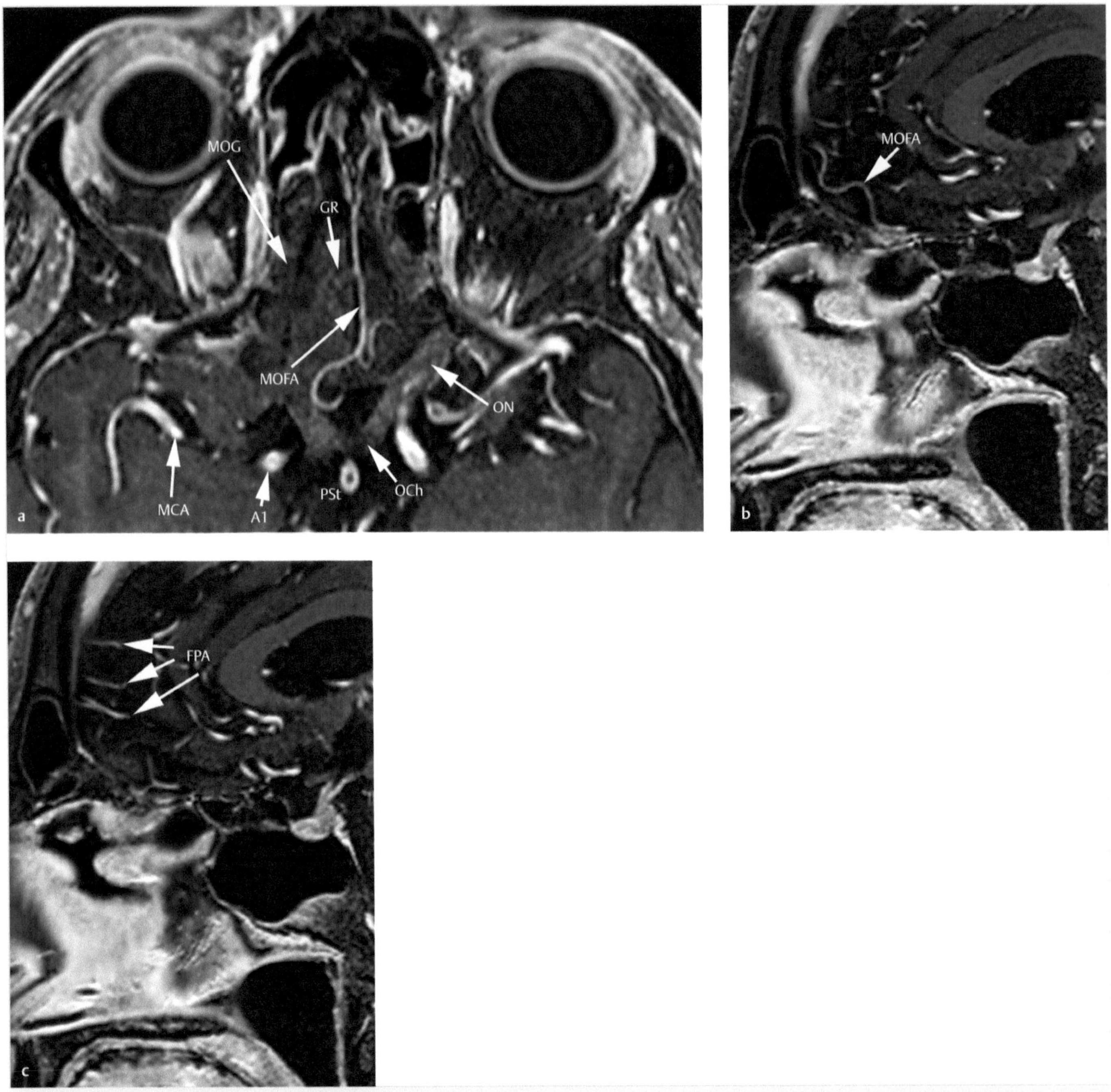

Fig. 7.8 Axial and sagittal MRI anatomy of the midline anterior skull base. The panel contains one axial **(a)** and two sagittal **(b, c)** T1-weighted, fat-saturated MRI passing through the midline anterior skull base. The medial orbitofrontal artery (MOFA) is the first branch of the postcommunicating tract of the anterior cerebral artery and runs along the inferior surface of the frontal lobes or through the caudal portion of the interhemispheric fissure. The frontopolar arteries (FPA) arise from the postcommunicating tract of the anterior cerebral artery in a distal position with respect to the medial orbitofrontal artery and reach the area of the frontal pole. A1, precommunicating tract of the anterior cerebral artery; GR, gyrus rectus; MCA, middle cerebral artery; MOG, medial orbital gyrus; OCh, optic chiasm; ON, optic nerve; PSt, pituitary stalk.

Endoscopic Dissection

Nasal Phase

- Vertical and horizontal uncinectomy.
- Anterior ethmoidectomy.
- Draf I frontal sinusotomy.
- Draf IIa frontal sinusotomy.
- Draf IIb frontal sinusotomy.
- Draf III frontal sinusotomy.
- Paraseptal sphenoidotomy.
- Transrostral sphenoidotomy.
- Expanded transrostral sphenoidotomy.
- Posterior ethmoidectomy.
- Transethmoidal sphenoidotomy.

Skull Base Phase

- Step 1: Subtotal septectomy.
- Step 2: Middle and superior turbinectomies.
- Step 3: Removal of the olfactory mucosa and rostrum sphenoidalis.
- Step 4: Orbital decompression (removal of the medial orbital wall).
- Step 5: Exposure of the anterior, middle, and posterior ethmoidal bundles.
- Step 6: Sectioning of the ethmoidal bundles.
- Step 7: Removal of the fovea ethmoidalis.
- Step 8: Removal of the inferior portion of the posterior frontal plate.
- Step 9: Removal of the cribriform plate and anterior portion of the planum sphenoidalis.
- Step 10: Removal of the crista galli.
- Step 11: Supraorbital epidural dissection.
- Step 12: Lateral dural incisions.
- Step 13: Anterior dural incision.
- Step 14: Falx transection.
- Step 15: Posterior dural sectioning.

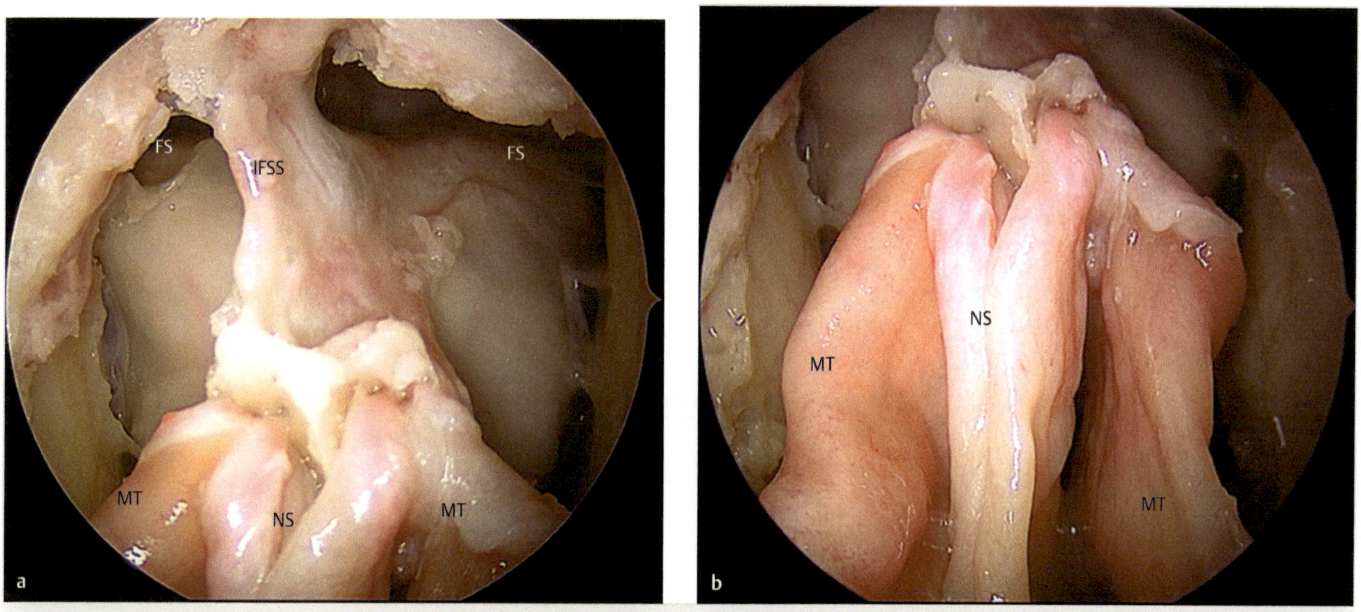

Fig. 7.9 (a, b) Sinonasal landmarks. After completing the nasal phase, both frontal sinuses (FS) are visible through a Draf type III frontal sinusotomy. The interfrontal sinus septum (IFSS) attaches to the posterior frontal plate posteriorly. After performing a complete ethmoidectomy, the middle turbinate (MT) and nasal septum (NS) attachments to the anterior skull base are visible. The nasal septum shows a free edge because of the anterosuperior partial septectomy, which is a step of Draf type III frontal sinusotomy.

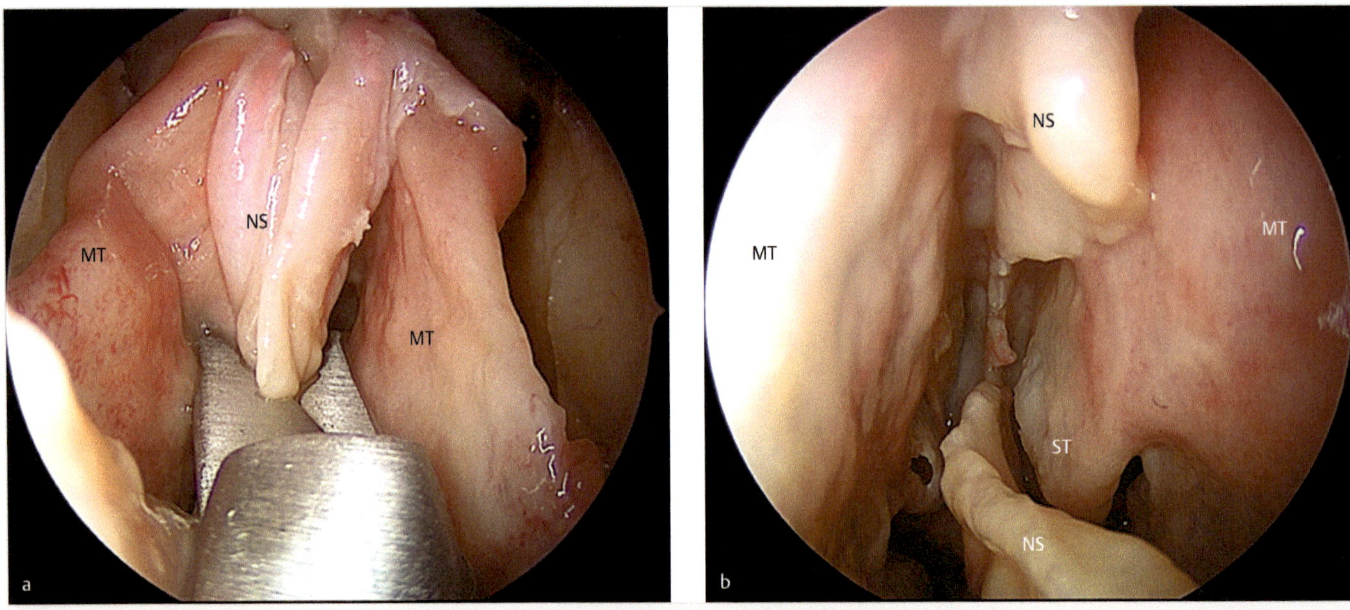

Fig. 7.10 (a, b) Step 1. The nasal septum (NS) is cut through the anterosuperior septal window a few millimeters below its insertion on the anterior skull base. Then, the inferior insertion of the nasal septum on the nasal floor is sectioned. Finally, two vertical incisions are made to complete the septectomy: one in front of the sphenoid rostrum and the other from the posterior edge of the frontal sinusotomy down to the nasal floor. MT, middle turbinate; ST, superior turbinate.

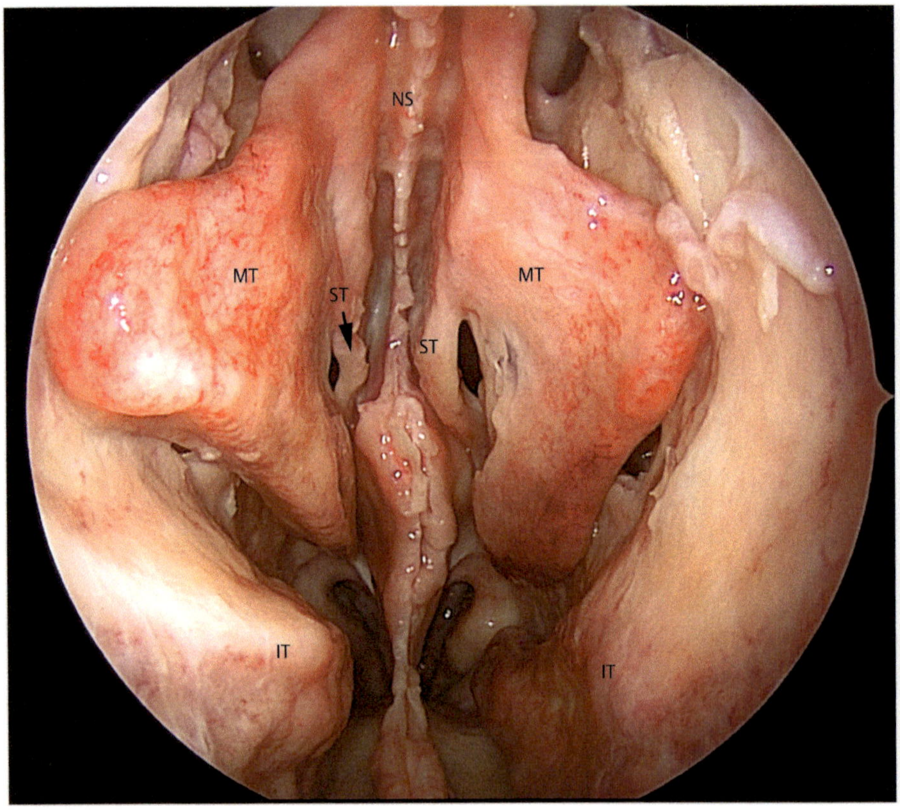

Fig. 7.11 A single sinonasal cavity. After performing septectomy, a single sinonasal cavity is obtained. The olfactory fissures are identified between the common laminae of the middle (MT) and superior turbinates (ST), lateral to the nasal septum (NS). The fovea ethmoidalis is still covered by the middle turbinate on both sides. IT, inferior turbinate.

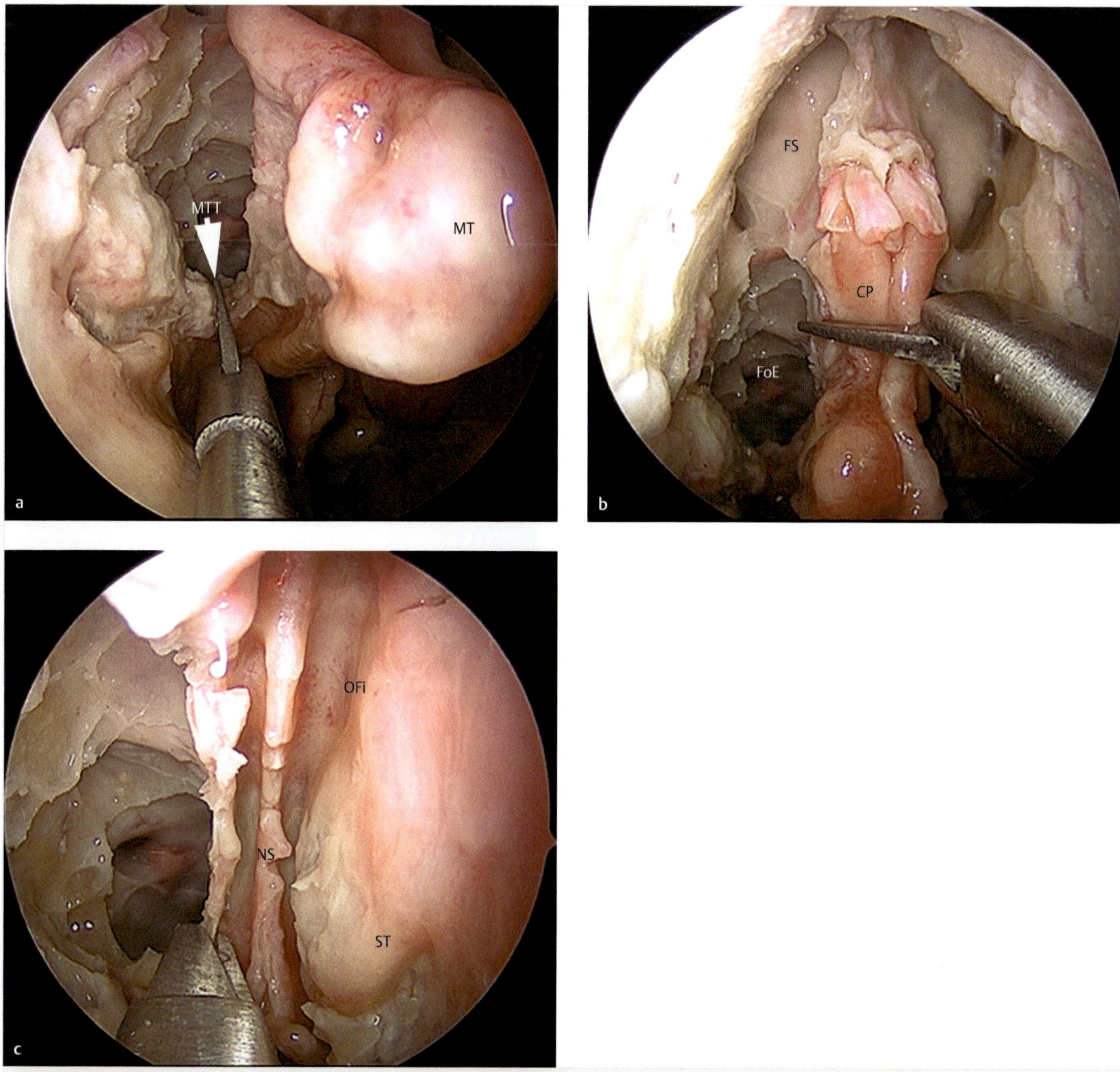

Fig. 7.12 (a–c) Step 2. The horizontal portion of the basal lamella of the middle turbinate is cut along with its tail (MTT) on both sides. Then, the conchal plates (CP), which are the common lamina of the middle (MT) and superior turbinates (ST), are sectioned in an anteroposterior direction until the sphenoid rostrum comes into view. Given the fact that the midline anterior skull base bends toward the nasal cavity from anterior to posterior, this maneuver has to be performed by slightly moving downward the cutting instrument after each cut. FoE, fovea ethmoidalis; FS, frontal sinus; NS, nasal septum; OFi, olfactory fissure.

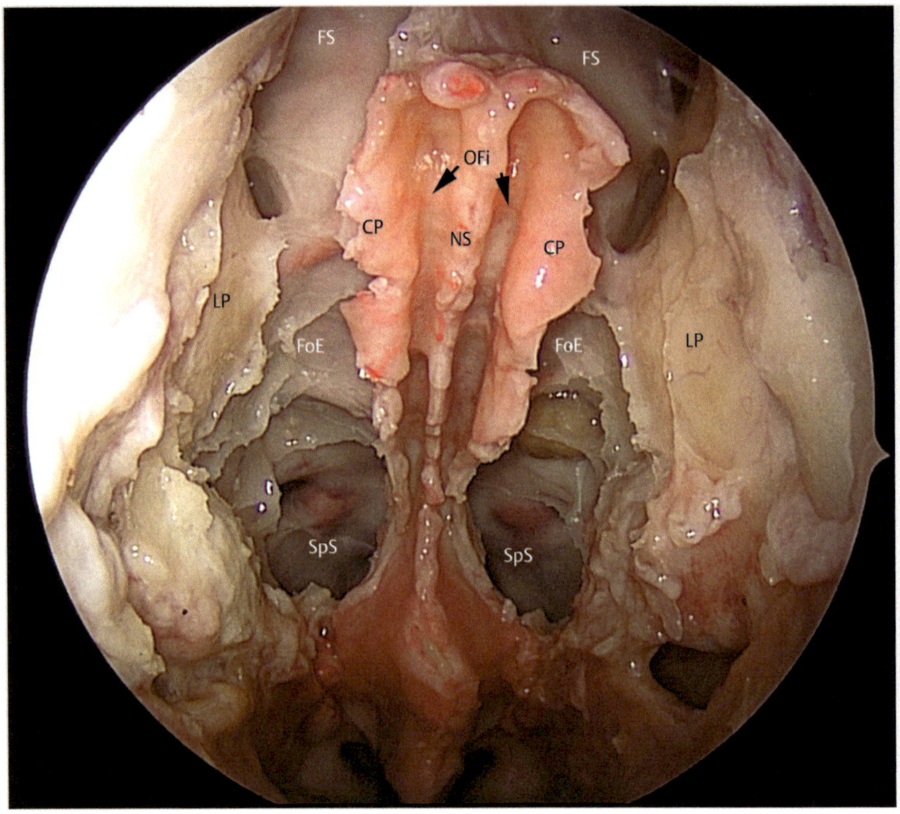

Fig. 7.13 The midline anterior skull base. After removing the nasal septum (NS) and cutting both the conchal plates (CP), the entire midline portion of the anterior skull base comes into view. The two olfactory fissures (OFi) lie medially and are still covered by olfactory mucosa. The foveae ethmoidalis (FoE) lie laterally, close to the laminae papyraceae (LP). From an anteroposterior perspective, the exposure ranges from the frontal (FS) to the sphenoid sinuses (SpS). In this dissection, the planum sphenoidale is still hidden by the sphenoid rostrum.

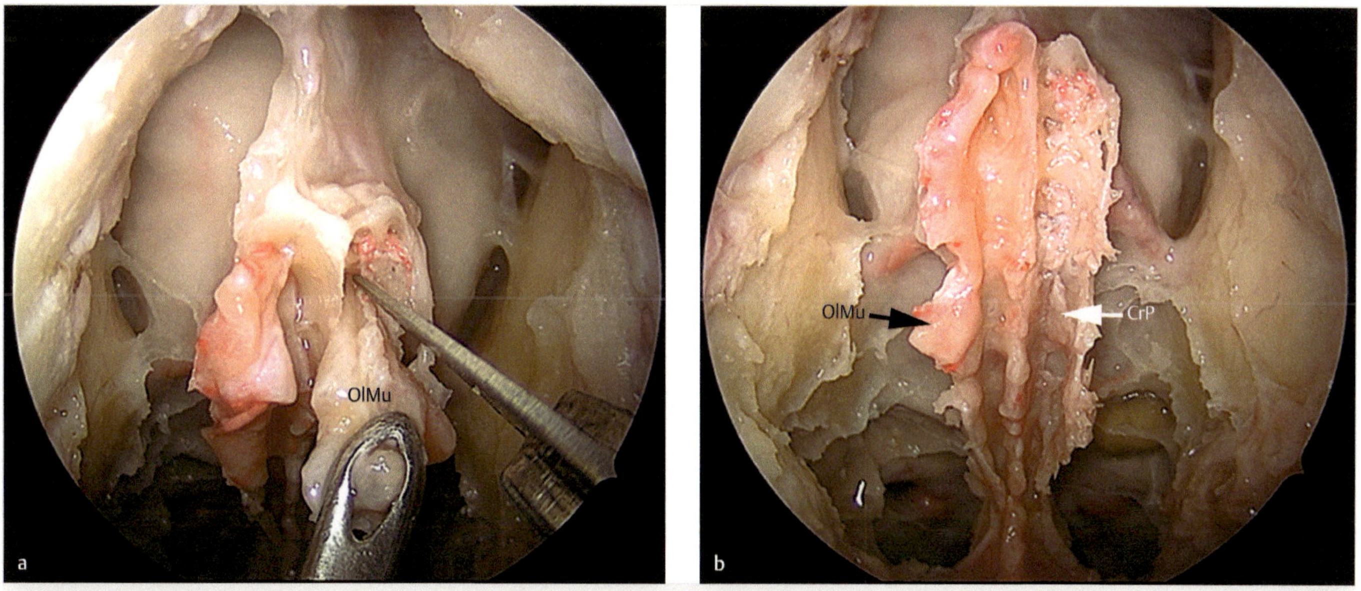

Fig. 7.14 (a, b) Step 3. With a four-hand technique, the anterior portion of the olfactory mucosa (OlMu) is pulled down and a scalpel is used to dissect the mucosal lining from the cribriform plate (CrP).

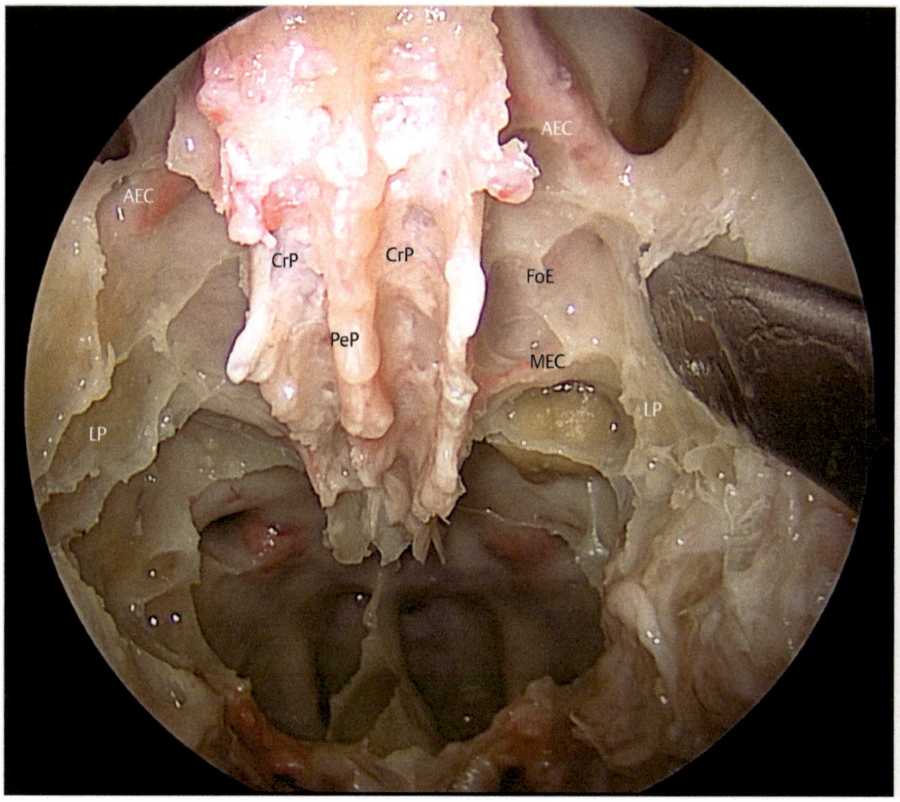

Fig. 7.15 Step 4. A blunt instrument is used to make a small fracture in the lamina papyracea (LP) and dissect the periorbit from the bone. The fovea ethmoidalis (FoE) is then accurately checked to identify the anterior (AEC), middle (MEC), and posterior ethmoidal canal. CrP, cribriform plate; PeP, perpendicular plate of the ethmoid bone.

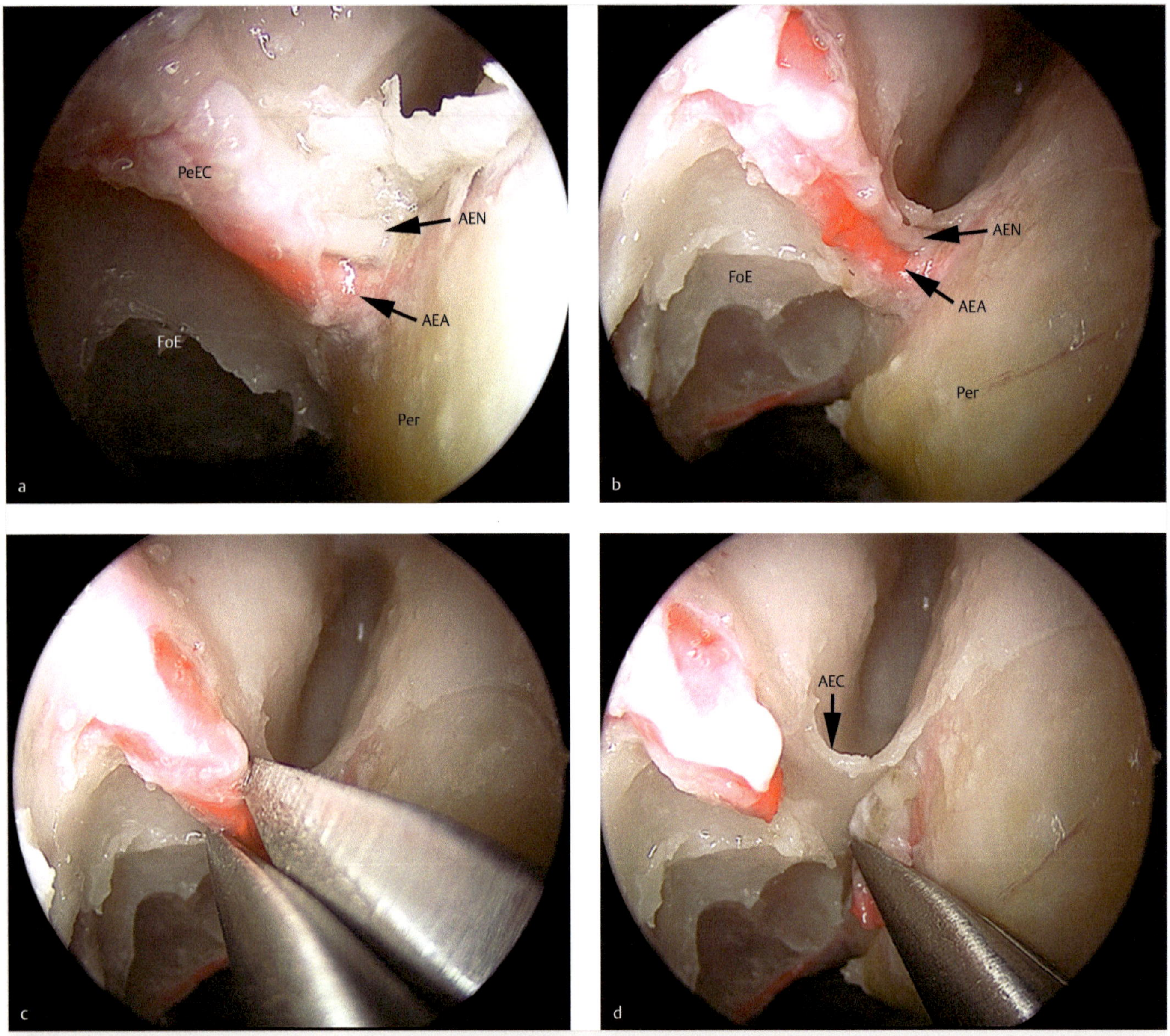

Fig. 7.16 (a–d) Steps 5 and 6 on the anterior ethmoidal canal. The inferior half of the anterior ethmoidal canal (AEC) is removed to expose the periosteum of the ethmoidal canal (PeEC). Incising this thin layer, the anterior ethmoidal artery (AEA) and nerve (AEN) come into view. A small cutting instrument is employed to cut the content of the anterior ethmoidal canal midway between the anterior ethmoidal foramen, where the structures pass from the orbit into the canal, and anterior ethmoidal sulcus, where the structures pass from the canal to the olfactory groove. Finally, the exposure of the superior half of the bony canal is completed by subperiosteal dissection.

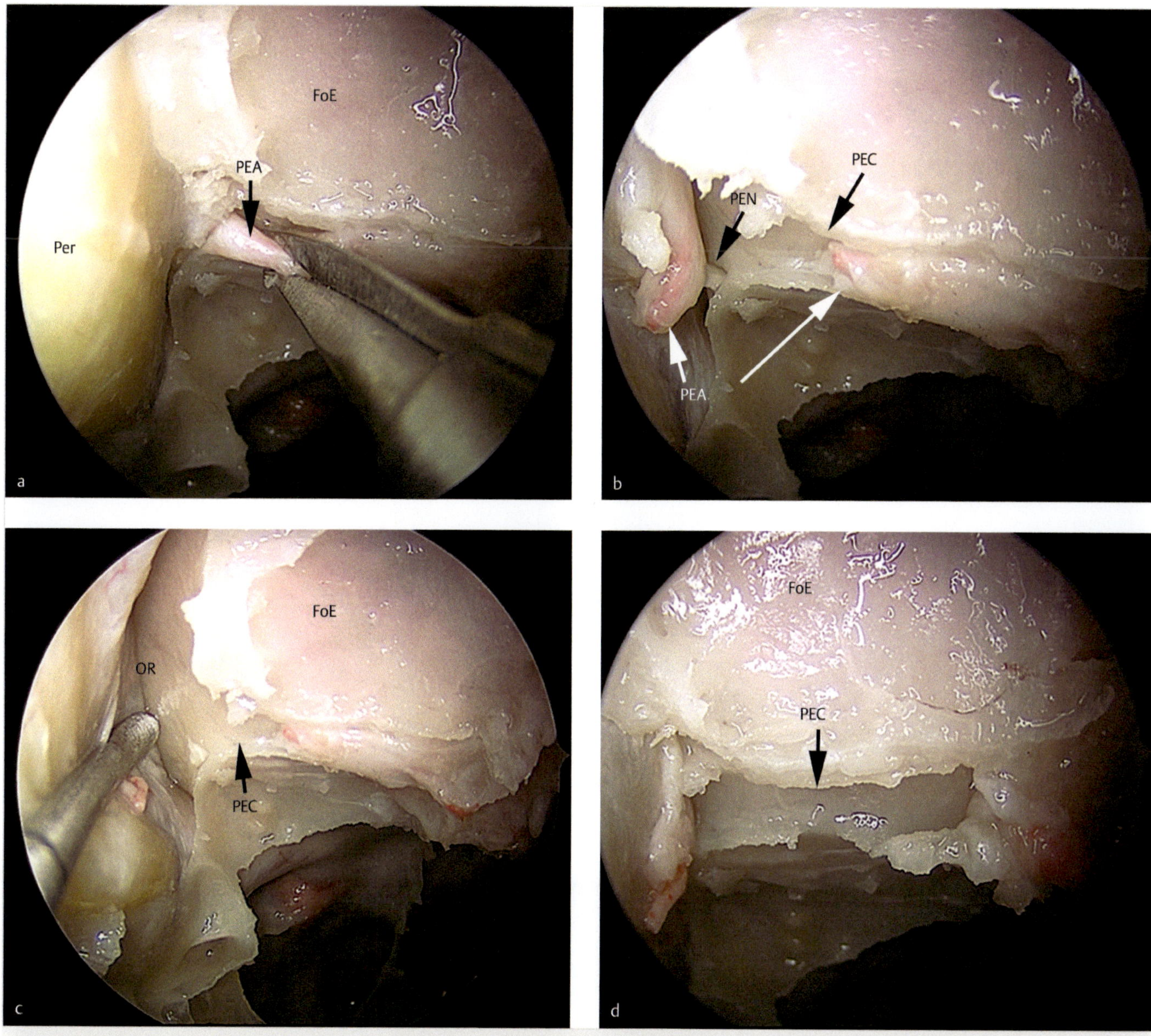

Fig. 7.17 (a–d) Steps 5 and 6 on the posterior ethmoidal canal. The procedure described in ▶Fig. 7.16 is repeated on the posterior ethmoidal canal. Especially for the posterior ethmoidal bundle, the posterior ethmoidal nerve (PEN) is often separated from the posterior ethmoidal artery (PEA) and follows an isolated small bony canal. After cutting both the anterior, middle (when present), and posterior ethmoidal bundles, a subperiorbital dissection allows the exposure of the orbital roof (ORo). FoE, fovea ethmoidalis; PEC, posterior ethmoidal canal; Per, periorbit.

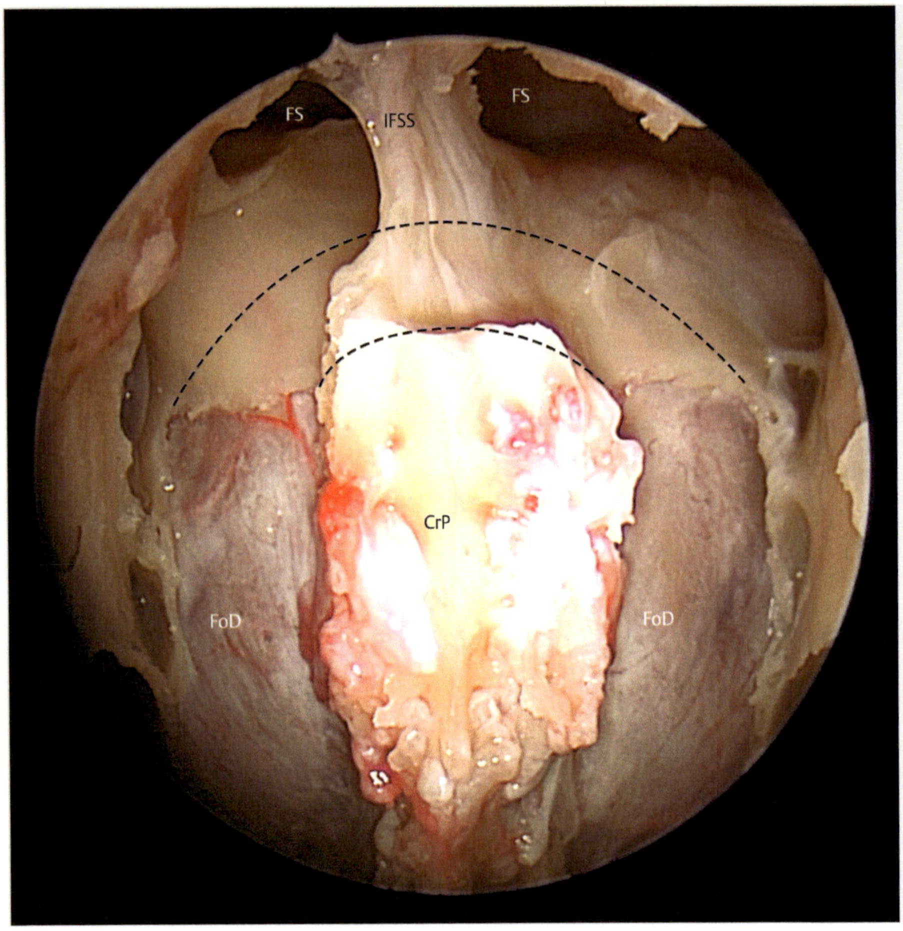

Fig. 7.18 Step 7. The foveae ethmoidalis are removed bilaterally to expose the overlying dura (FoD). Then, the inferior portion of the posterior frontal plate (*black dashed lines*) and the related portion of the interfrontal sinus septum (IFSS) are removed. When the dissection is performed with a two-hand technique, it is advisable to remove this bony area after completing the dissection of the crista galli (▶Fig. 7.22). FS, frontal sinus; CrP, cribriform plates.

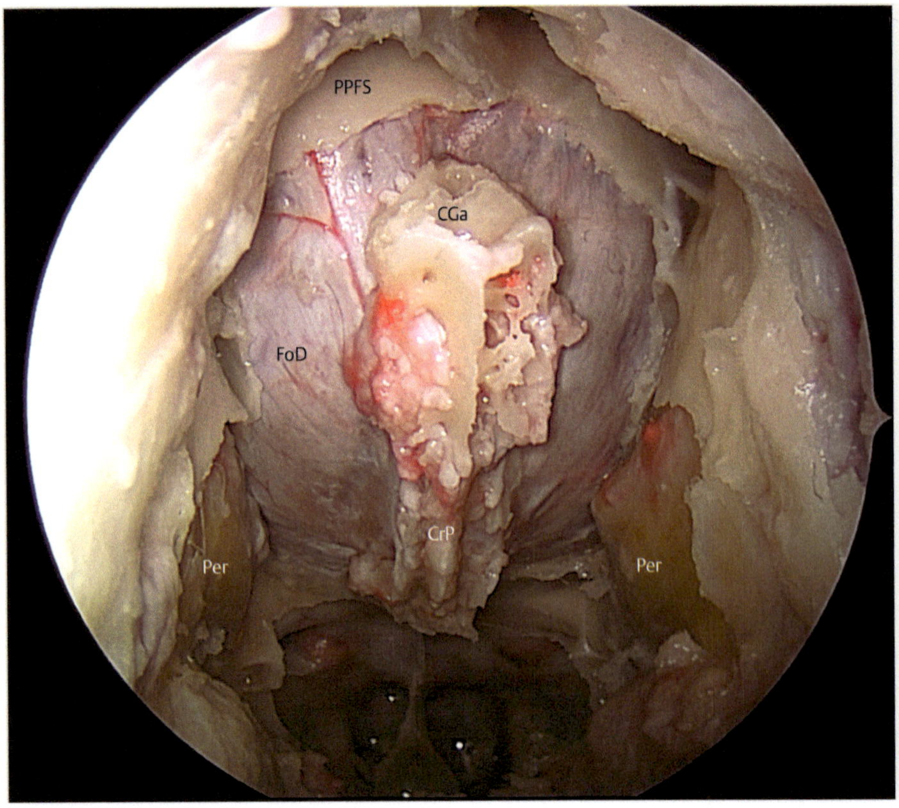

Fig. 7.19 Step 8. The crista galli (CGa) is isolated anteriorly by removing the inferior portion of the posterior plate of the frontal sinus (PPFS). Consequently, this thick bony spur, which is a part of the ethmoid bone, is surrounded by the dura of the posterior frontal plate anteriorly, dura of the fovea ethmoidalis (FoD) laterally, and the cribriform plate (CrP) posteriorly. A small, anterior part of the cribriform plate is very close to the inferior portion of the crista galli. Per, periorbit.

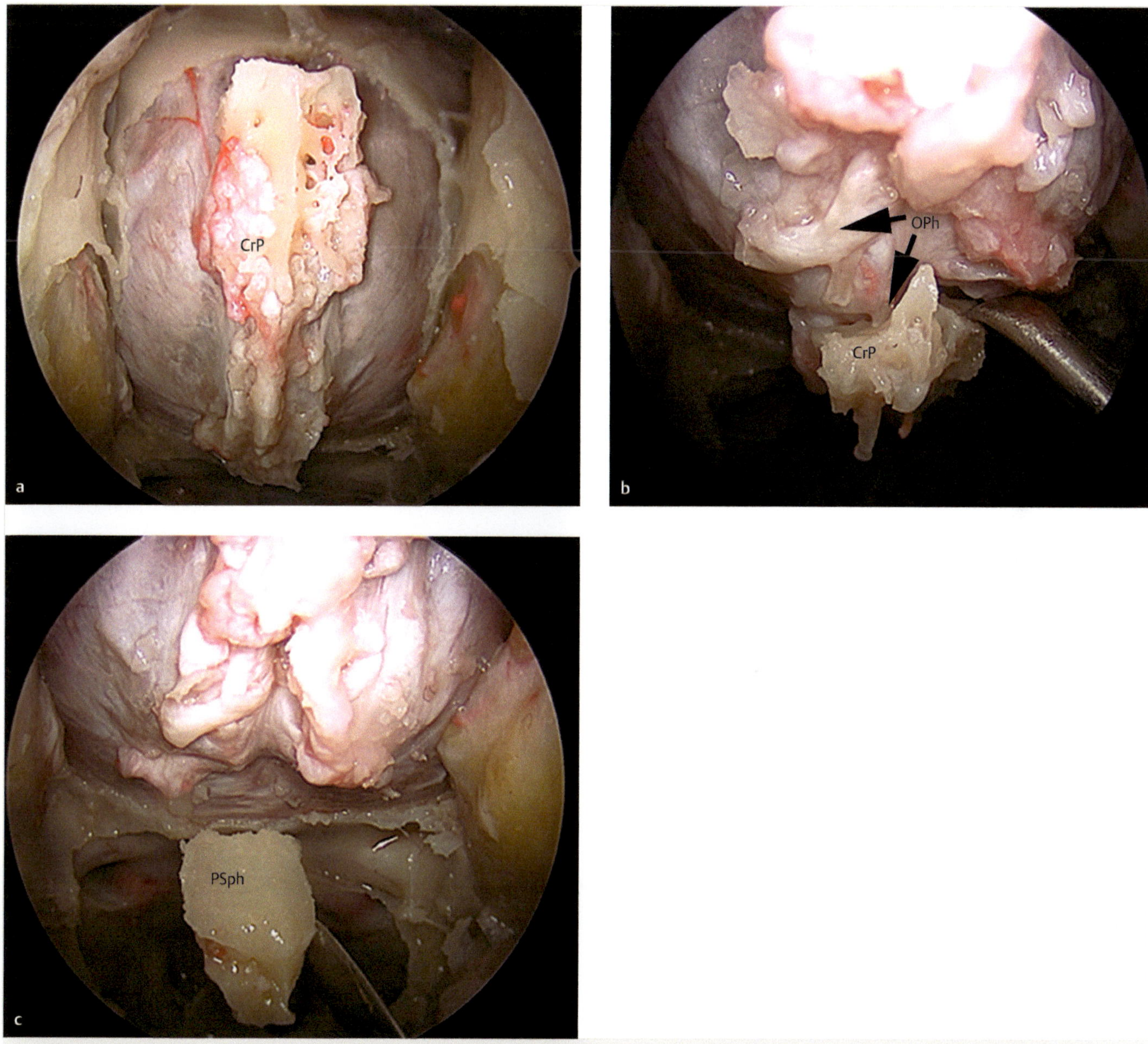

Fig. 7.20 (a–c) Step 9. The cribriform plate (CrP) is fractured posteriorly to the crista galli and gently dissected from the dura of the olfactory groove. While pushing inferiorly the cribriform plate, the olfactory phyla (OPh) are slipped off from it. After completing the removal of the posterior portion of the cribriform plate, the epidural plane is followed posteriorly for a few millimeters over the planum sphenoidale (PSph), which is then fractured almost at the level of posterior ethmoidal canals.

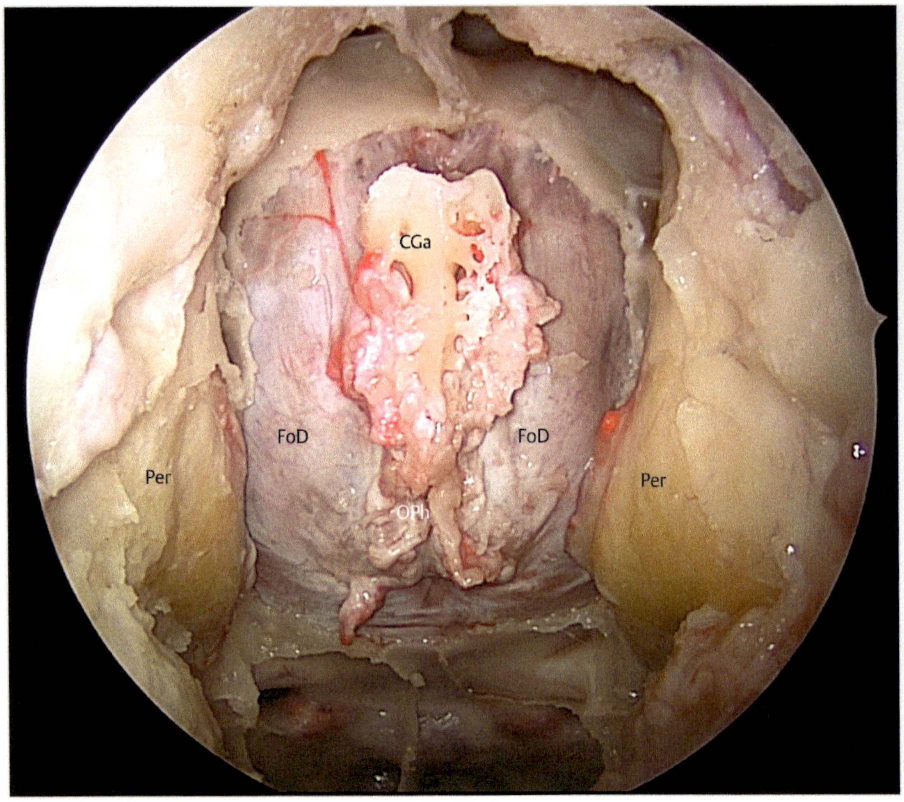

Fig. 7.21 Partial exposure of the olfactory groove. After removing the posterior portion of the cribriform plate, the crista galli (CGa) is completely surrounded by dura. The dura of the fovea ethmoidalis (FoD) lies laterally, the dura of the posterior frontal plate anteriorly, and the dura of the olfactory grooves and olfactory phyla (OPh) posteriorly. At this point, the crista galli has to be removed to complete the exposure of the olfactory groove. Per, periorbit.

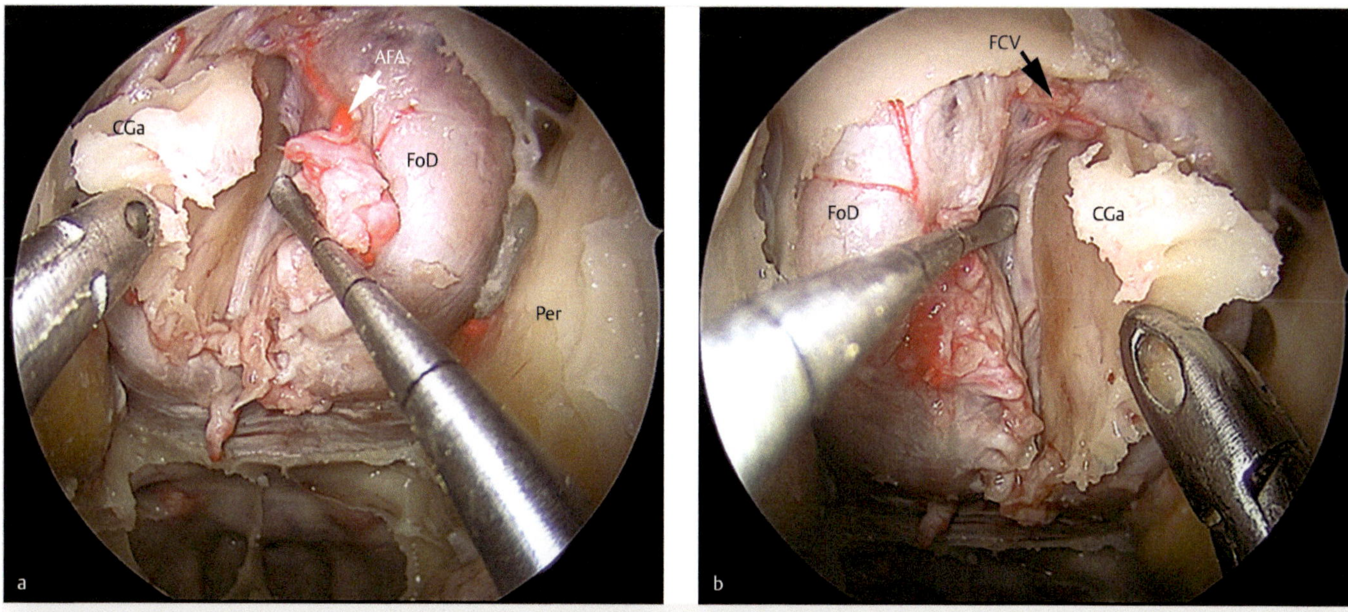

Fig. 7.22 (a, b) Step 10 (part 1). With a four-hand technique, the inferior portion of the crista galli (CGa) is pulled laterally while dissecting the dura on the contralateral side. This dura constitutes the anteroinferior insertion of the falx cerebri. The anterior falcine artery (AFA) is one of the terminal branches of the anterior ethmoidal artery and runs along the anterolateral border of the crista galli. The vein of the foramen caecum (FCV) comes into view while freeing anteriorly the crista galli. FoD, fovea ethmoidalis; Per, periorbit.

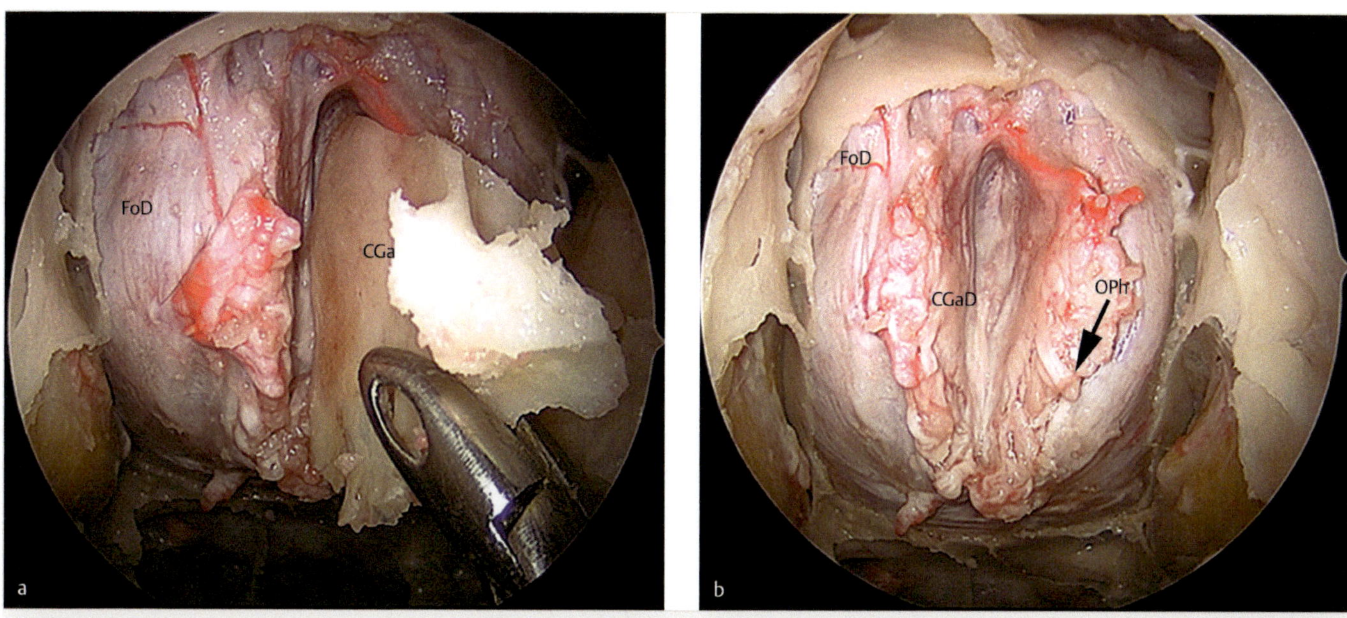

Fig. 7.23 (a, b) Step 10 (part 2). When the crista galli (CGa) is completely freed from the surrounding dura, it is gently taken out to expose the anteroinferior insertion of the falx cerebri, called dura of the crista galli (CGaD). This dura is completely surrounded by the olfactory phyla (OPh) laterally, the vein of the foramen caecum anteriorly, and the dura of the planum sphenoidale posteriorly. FoD, dura mater of the fovea ethmoidalis.

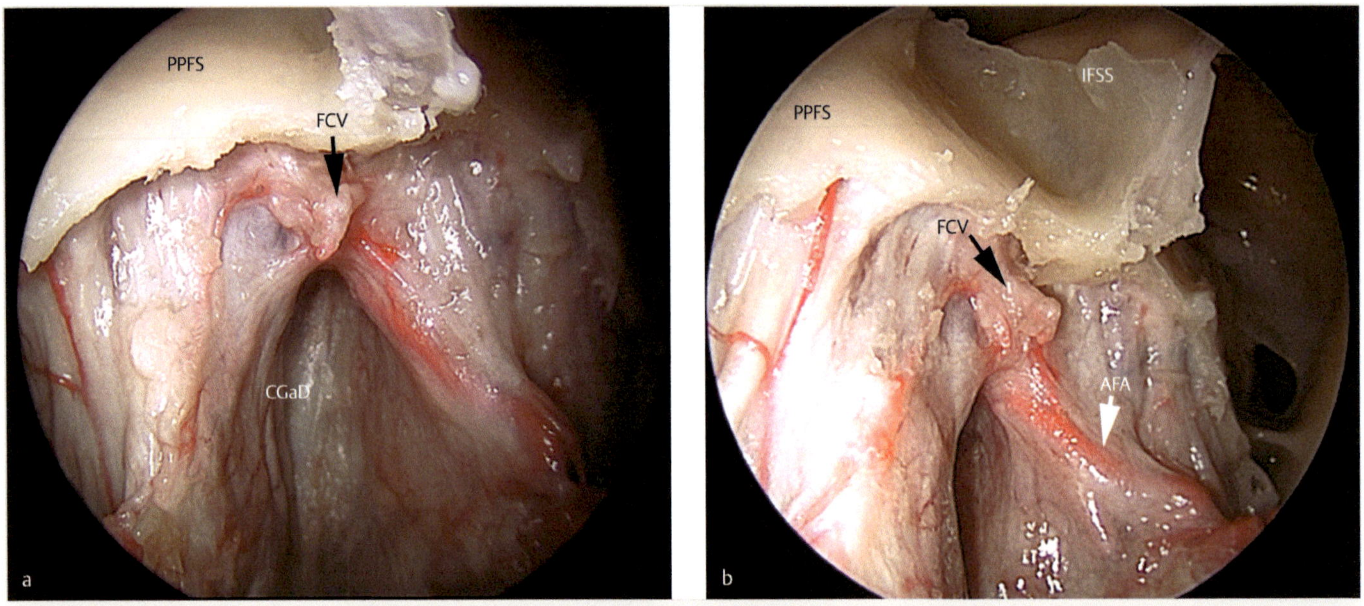

Fig. 7.24 (a, b) The vein of the foramen caecum and anterior falcine artery. The vein of the foramen caecum (FCV) lies in front of the dura of the crista galli (CGaD), at the junction between the posterior plate of the frontal sinus (PPFS) and crista galli. When the interfrontal sinus septum (IFSS) inserts on the midline posteriorly, it could be used as a landmark for the vein. The anterior falcine artery (AFA) runs vertically along the anterior border of the crista galli. Its diameter could be as large as that of the anterior ethmoidal artery (as in **a**). In **b**, both the vein of the foramen caecum and anterior falcine artery are seen with a 70-degree scope turned toward the left side of the specimen.

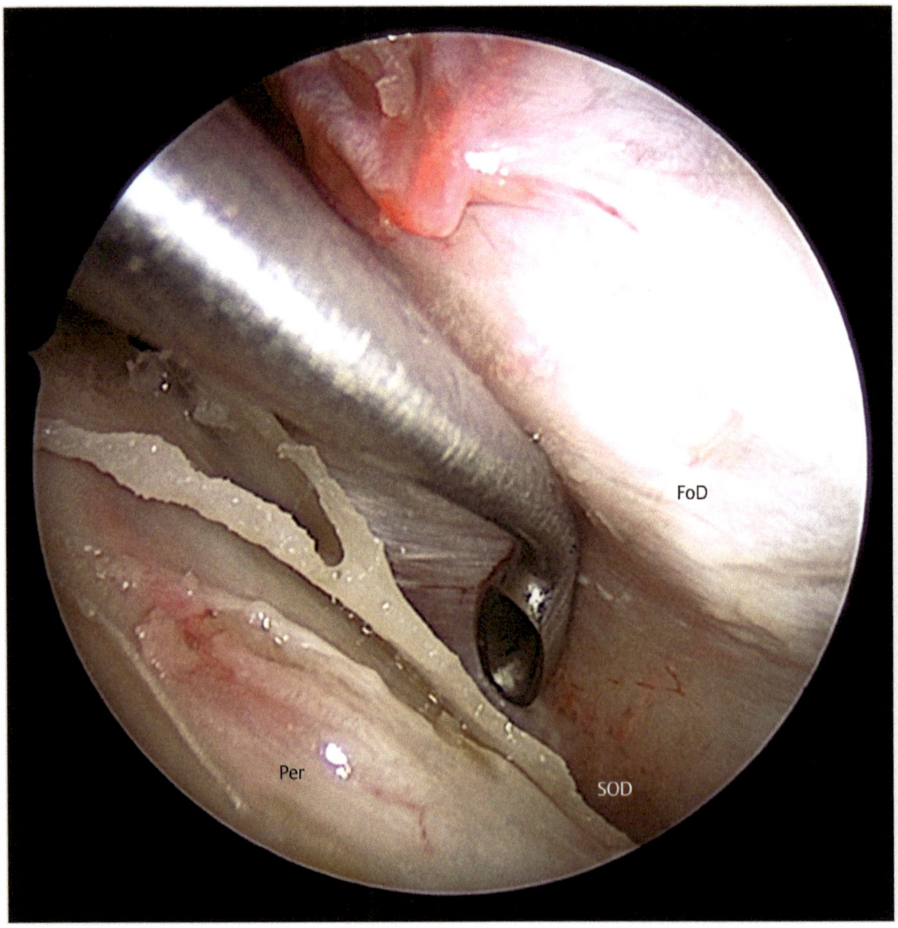

Fig. 7.25 Step 11. A curved curette or dissector is employed under the guidance of a 70-degree scope turned on the right side to perform a supraorbital epidural dissection. The supraorbital dura mater (SOD) is gently dissected from the orbital plate of the frontal bone. FoD, dura mater of the fovea ethmoidalis; Per, periorbit.

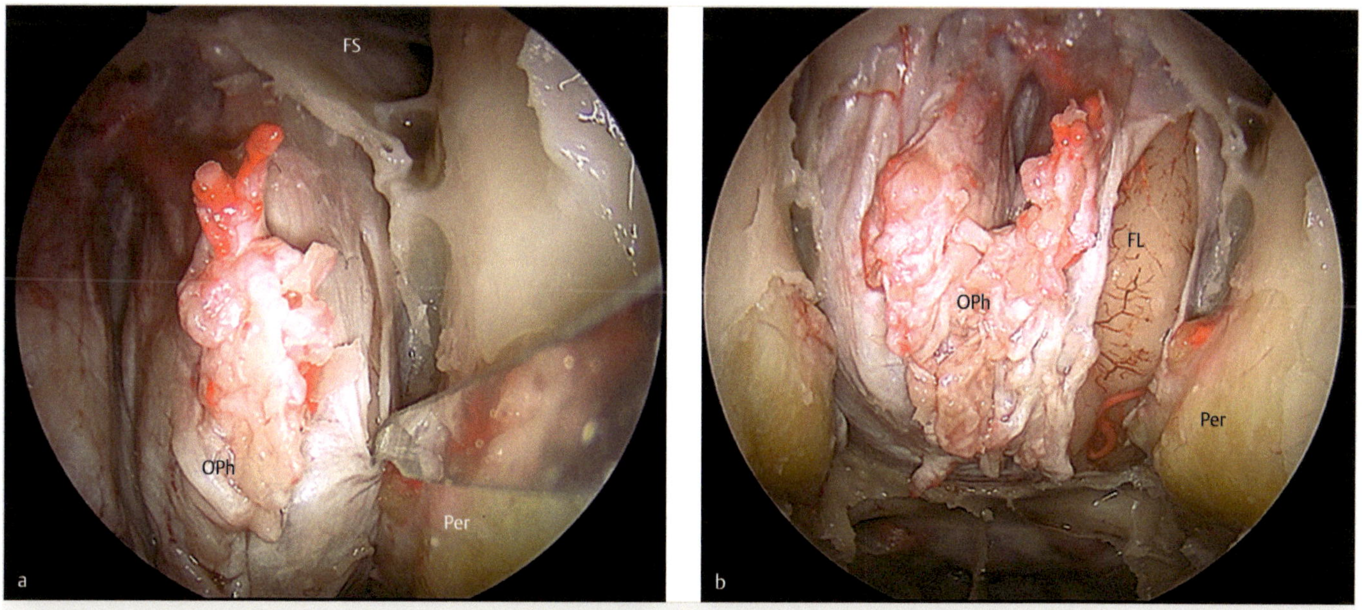

Fig. 7.26 (a, b) Step 12 (part 1). The dura mater of the fovea ethmoidalis is incised following an anteroposterior direction, starting from the posterior bony wall of the frontal sinus (FS) and following the lateral boundary of the craniectomy until the planum sphenoidale is reached. In **(b)** the inferior surface of the frontal lobe (FL) after completing dural incision is shown. OPh, olfactory phyla; Per, periorbit.

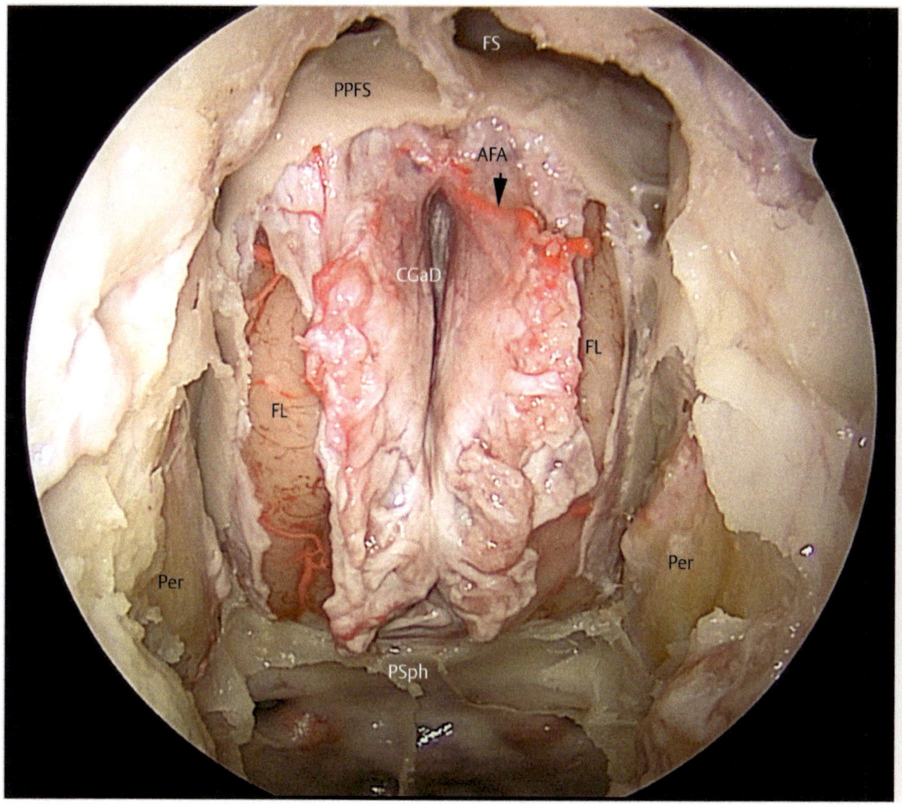

Fig. 7.27 Step 12 (part 2). After performing the contralateral incision, both frontal lobes (FL) come into view. The corridor toward the intracranial structures is surrounded by the two periorbits (Per) laterally, the posterior plate of the frontal sinus (PPFS) anteriorly, and the planum sphenoidale (PSph) posteriorly. The dura mater that surrounds the crista galli (CGaD) lies in the center of the field of view. AFA, anterior falcine artery; FS, frontal sinus.

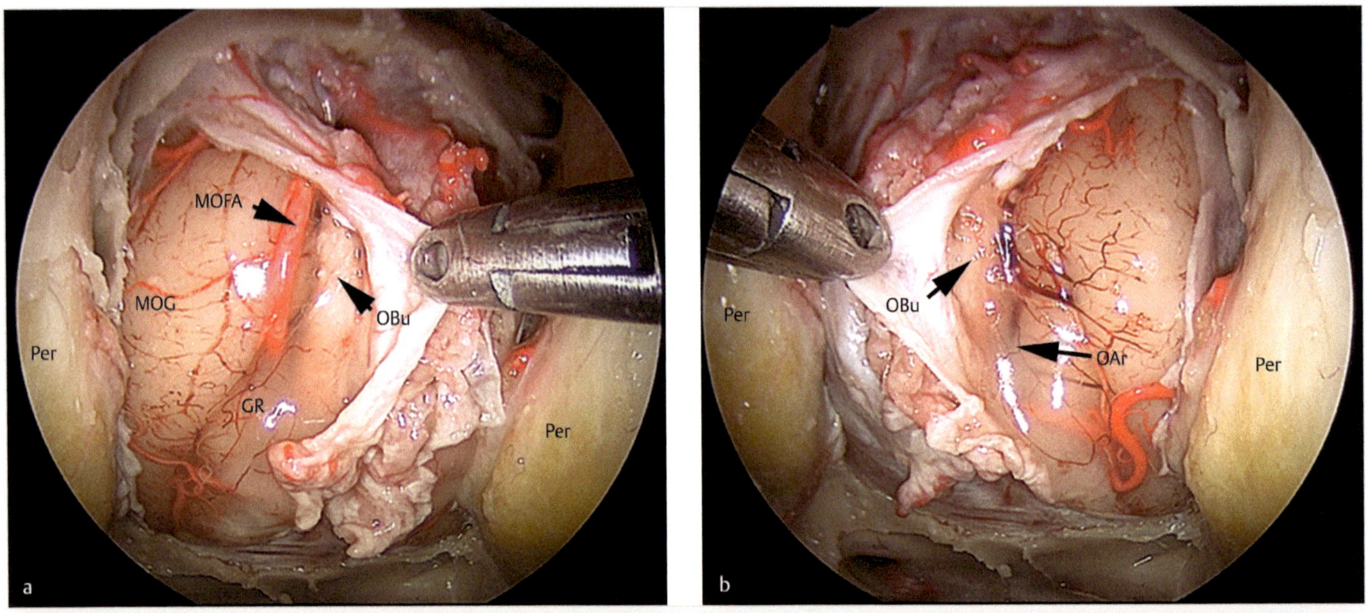

Fig. 7.28 (a, b) Exposure of the olfactory bulbs. The olfactory bulb (OBu), medial orbital gyrus (MOG), and gyrus rectus (GR) can be identified pulling the dural edges toward the midline. In **(a)**, the medial orbitofrontal artery (MOFA) runs within the anterior tract of the olfactory sulcus, which separates the medial orbital gyrus from the gyrus rectus. The olfactory bulb and its phyla are covered by the dura mater of the olfactory groove. The outer arachnoid layer (OAr) connecting the frontal lobe to the olfactory bulb becomes visible by moving medially the dura. Per, periorbit.

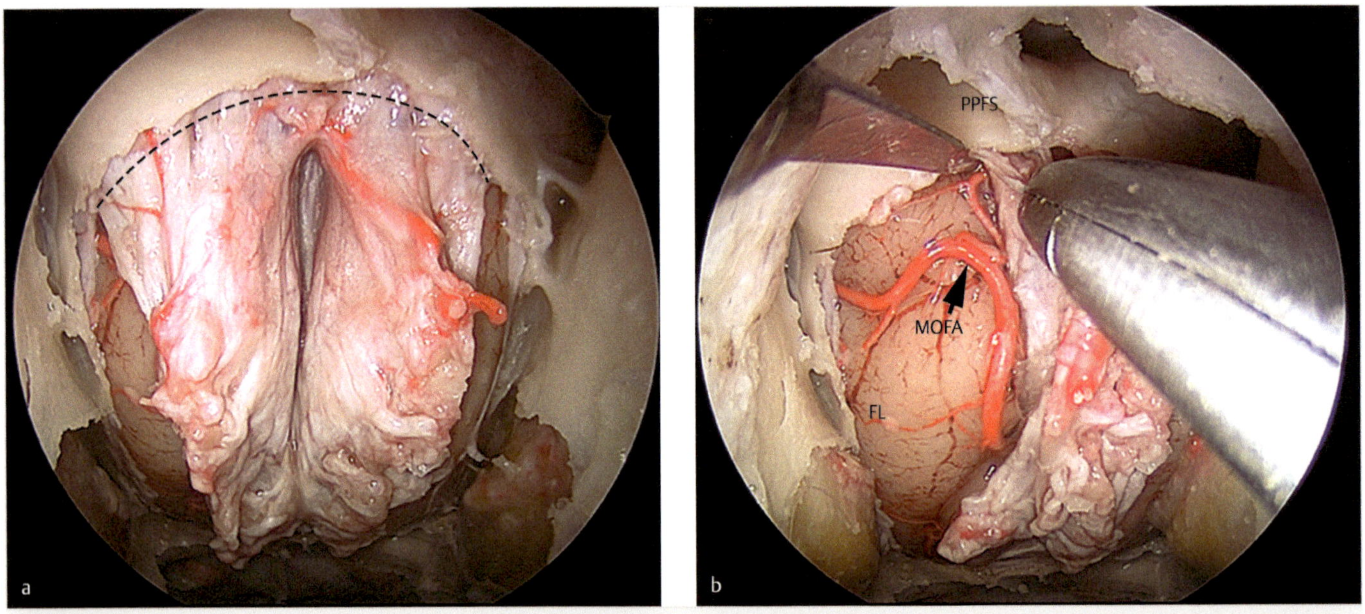

Fig. 7.29 (a, b) Step 13. The anterior dural incision (*black dashed line*) is made anteriorly to the dura of the crista galli along the posterior plate of the frontal sinus (PPFS). On the right, the four-hand dissection is shown. FL, frontal lobe; MOFA, medial orbitofrontal artery.

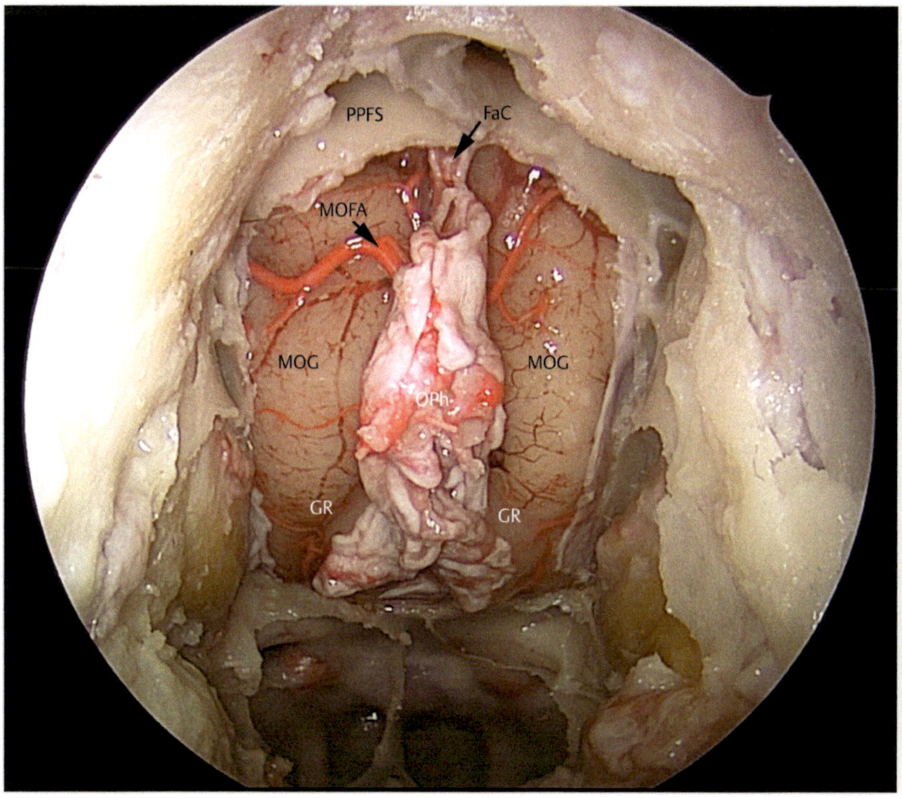

Fig. 7.30 Exposure of the falx cerebri. The anterior dural incision is completed bilaterally to reach the midline. In this way, the anterior insertion of the falx cerebri (FaC) is identified posterior to the posterior plate of the frontal sinus (PPFS). GR, gyrus rectus; MOFA, medial orbitofrontal artery; MOG, medial orbital gyrus; OPh, olfactory phyla.

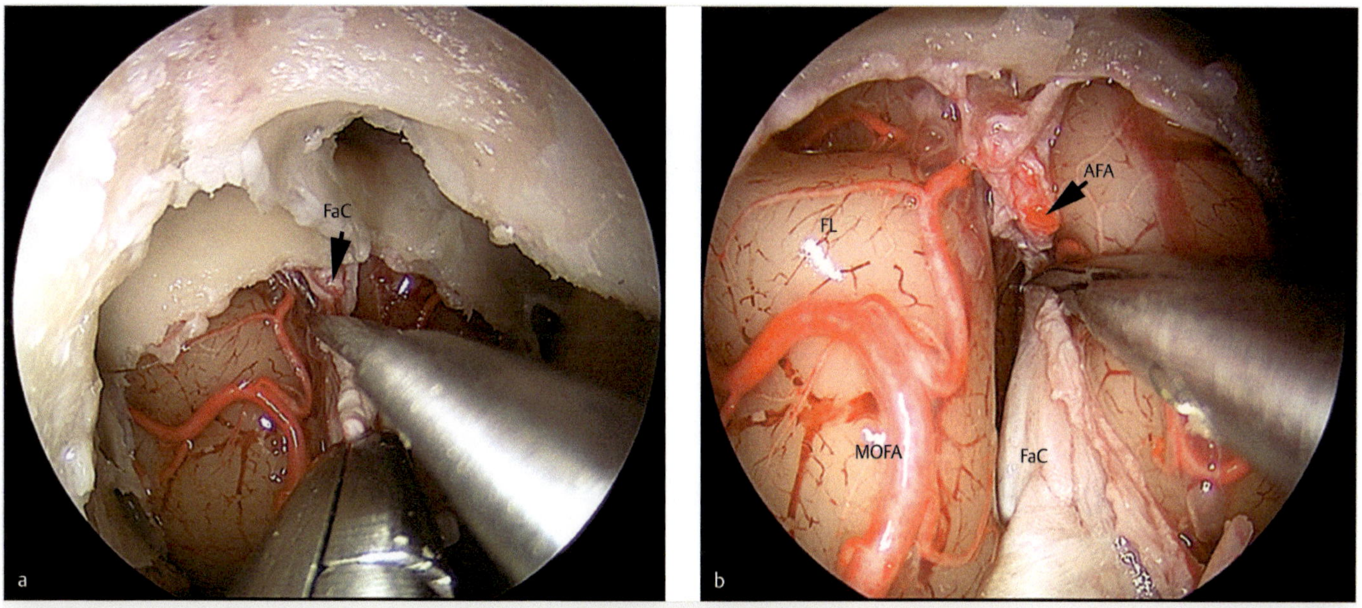

Fig. 7.31 (a, b) Step 14 (part 1). The falx cerebri (FaC) is pulled downward and cut in an anteroposterior direction. In this way, the anterior falcine artery (AFA) is cut as it runs along the anterior insertion of the falx cerebri. FL, frontal lobe; MOFA, medial orbitofrontal artery.

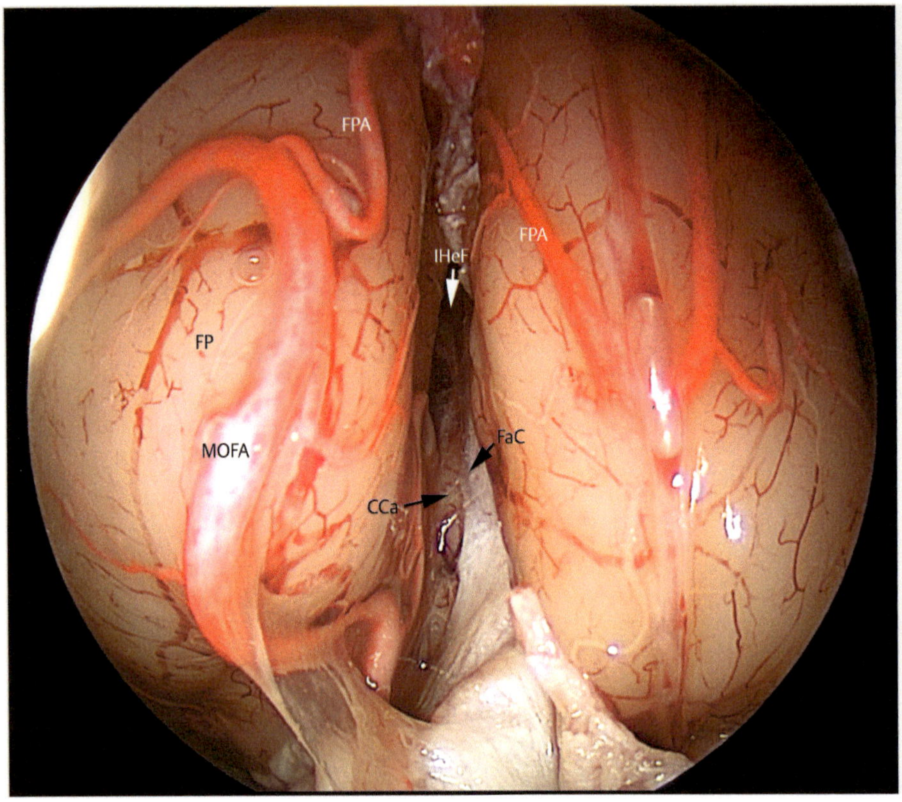

Fig. 7.32 Step 14 (part 2). Falx transection is completed and the interhemispheric fissure (IHeF) is exposed. The posterior border of the falx cerebri (FaC) can be exposed pulling the dura inferiorly, laterally, and anteriorly. The corpus callosum (CCa) is identified behind the free edge of the falx cerebri. Both frontopolar arteries (FPA) reach the frontal pole (FP) from the interhemispheric fissure and form an anastomosis with the medial orbitofrontal artery (MOFA).

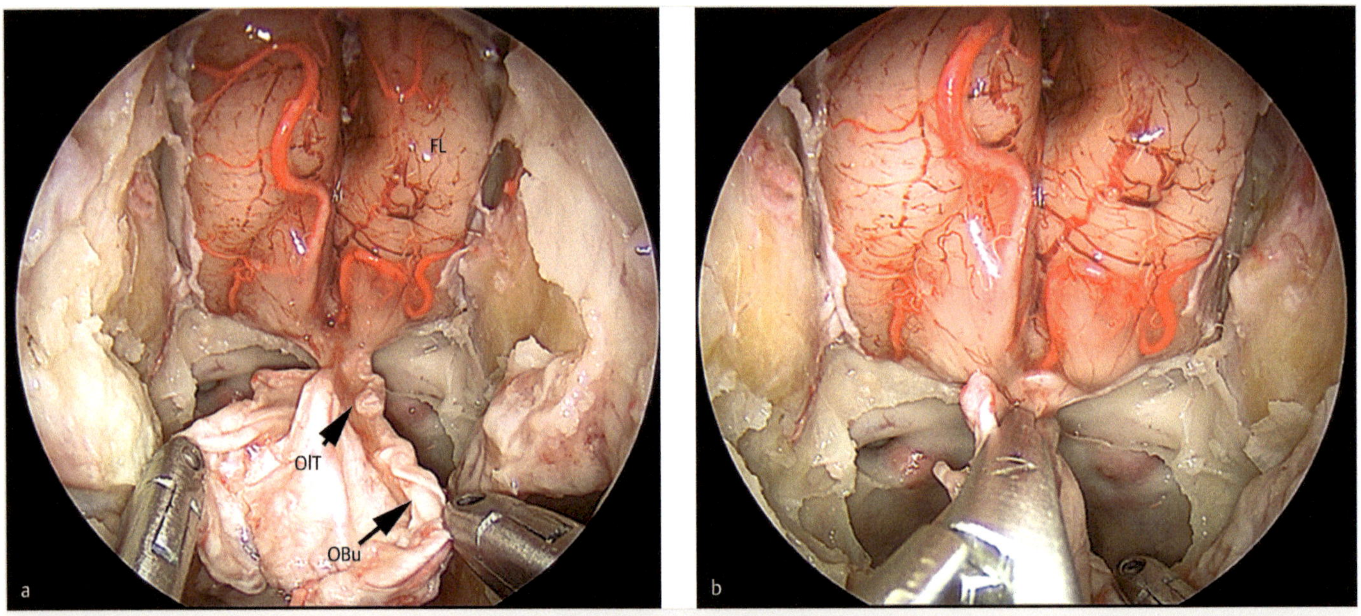

Fig. 7.33 (a, b) Step 15. After completing falx transection, the posterior border remains the only point of attachment of the dural layer to the skull base. The posterior dural incision is performed following the bony edge of the planum sphenoidale. As the olfactory bulb (OBu) is still attached to the olfactory fossa, the olfactory tract (OlT) is pulled together with the dural layer and needs to be cut along with the dura on both sides. FL, frontal lobe.

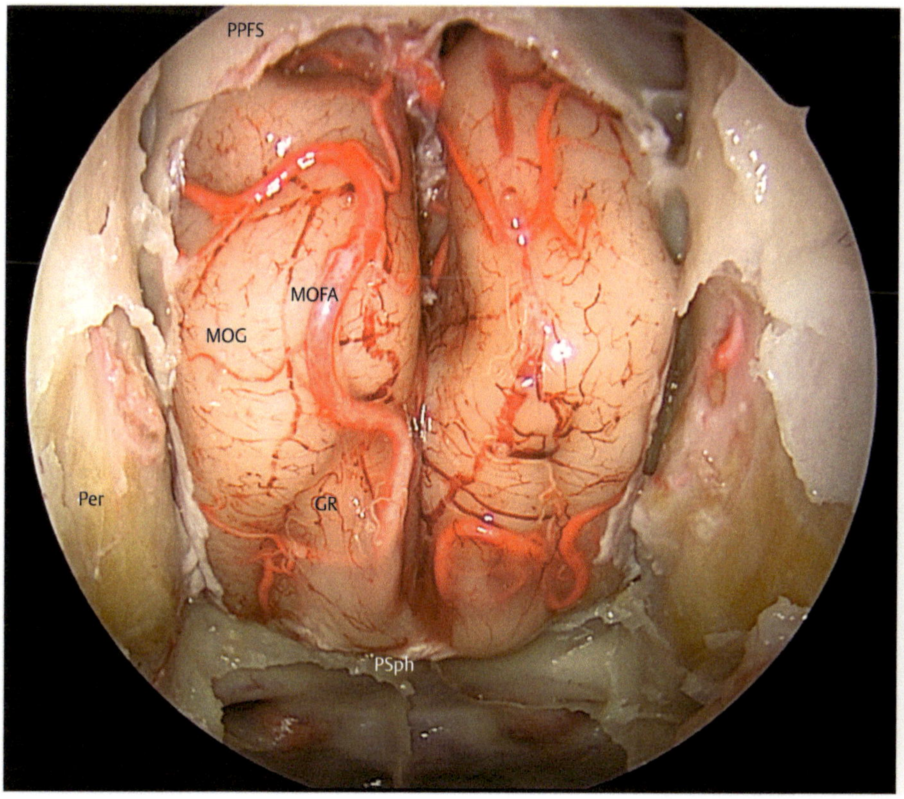

Fig. 7.34 Overview after the dural removal. The limits of the transcribriform defect are the posterior plate of the frontal sinus (PPFS) anteriorly, the anterior limit of the planum sphenoidale (PSph) posteriorly, and the junction between the fovea ethmoidalis and the orbital plate of the frontal sinus bilaterally. GR, gyrus rectus; MOFA, medial orbitofrontal artery; MOG, medial orbital gyrus; Per, periorbit.

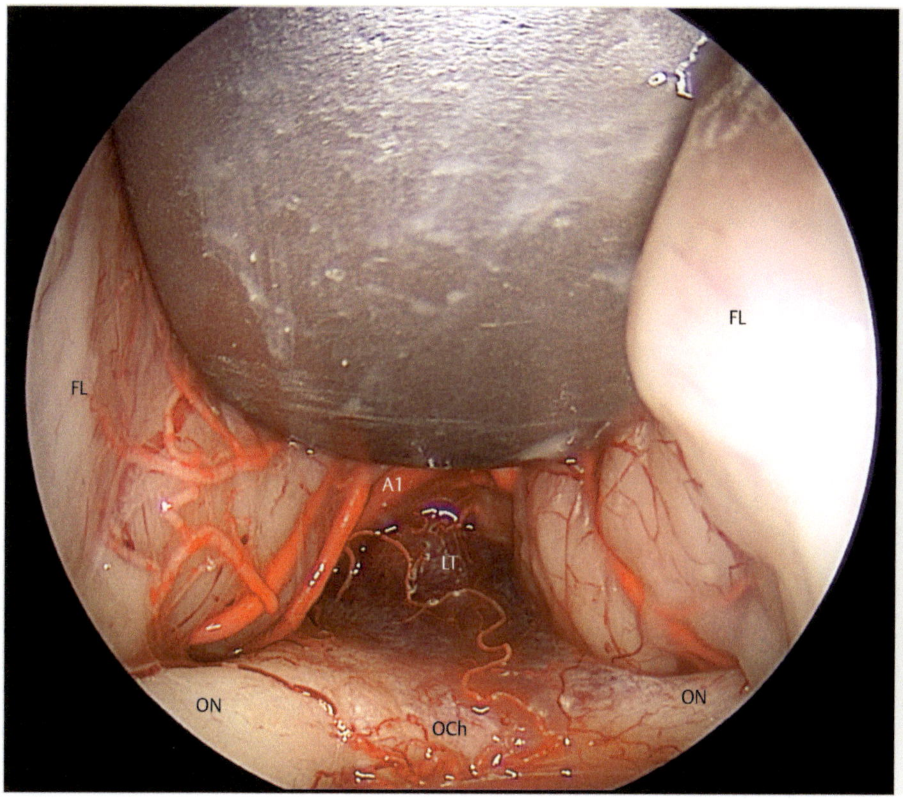

Fig. 7.35 The cistern of the lamina terminalis. The frontal lobes (FL) are gently displaced and a 45-degree scope turned inferiorly and posteriorly is placed in the inferior portion of the interhemispheric fissure until the optic nerves (ON), optic chiasm (OCh), and lamina terminalis (LT) are identified. The precommunicating tract of the anterior cerebral artery (A1) can be seen placing the scope in the interhemispheric fissure.

References

[1] Greenfield JP, Anand VK, Kacker A, et al. Endoscopic endonasal transethmoidal transcribriform transfovea ethmoidalis approach to the anterior cranial fossa and skull base. Neurosurgery 2010;66(5):883–892, discussion 892

[2] Kassam A, Snyderman CH, Mintz A, Gardner P, Carrau RL. Expanded endonasal approach: the rostrocaudal axis. Part I. Crista galli to the sella turcica. Neurosurg Focus 2005;19(1):E3

[3] Verillaud B, Bresson D, Sauvaget E, et al. Transcribriform and transplanum endoscopic approach for skull-base tumors. Eur Ann Otorhinolaryngol Head Neck Dis 2013;130(4):233–236

[4] Koutourousiou M, Fernandez-Miranda JC, Wang EW, Snyderman CH, Gardner PA. Endoscopic endonasal surgery for olfactory groove meningiomas: outcomes and limitations in 50 patients. Neurosurg Focus 2014;37(4):E8

[5] Fernandez-Miranda JC, Gardner PA, Prevedello DM, Kassam AB. Expanded endonasal approach for olfactory groove meningioma. Acta Neurochir (Wien) 2009;151(3):287–288, author reply 289–290

[6] de Divitiis E, Esposito F, Cappabianca P, Cavallo LM, de Divitiis O, Esposito I. Endoscopic transnasal resection of anterior cranial fossa meningiomas. Neurosurg Focus 2008;25(6):E8

[7] Gardner PA, Kassam AB, Thomas A, et al. Endoscopic endonasal resection of anterior cranial base meningiomas. Neurosurgery 2008;63(1):36–52, discussion 52–54

[8] Blake DM, Husain Q, Kanumuri VV, Svider PF, Eloy JA, Liu JK. Endoscopic endonasal resection of sinonasal and anterior skull base schwannomas. J Clin Neurosci 2014;21(8):1419–1423

[9] Liu JK, Eloy JA. Expanded endoscopic endonasal transcribriform approach for resection of anterior skull base olfactory schwannoma. J Neurosurg 2012;32(Suppl):E3

[10] Vaz-Guimaraes F, Koutourousiou M, de Almeida JR, et al. Endoscopic endonasal surgery for epidermoid and dermoid cysts: a 10-year experience. J Neurosurg 2018 (e-pub ahead of print). doi:10.3171/2017.7.JNS162783

[11] Castelnuovo P, Battaglia P, Turri-Zanoni M, et al. Endoscopic endonasal surgery for malignancies of the anterior cranial base. World Neurosurg 2014;82(6, Suppl):S22–S31

[12] Krischek B, Carvalho FG, Godoy BL, Kiehl R, Zadeh G, Gentili F. From craniofacial resection to endonasal endoscopic removal of malignant tumors of the anterior skull base. World Neurosurg 2014;82(6, Suppl):S59–S65

[13] Lund V, Howard DJ, Wei WI. Endoscopic resection of malignant tumors of the nose and sinuses. Am J Rhinol 2007;21(1):89–94

[14] Lund VJ, Stammberger H, Nicolai P, et al; European Rhinologic Society Advisory Board on Endoscopic Techniques in the Management of Nose, Paranasal Sinus and Skull Base Tumours. European position paper on endoscopic management of tumours of the nose, paranasal sinuses and skull base. Rhinol Suppl 2010;22:1–143

[15] Lund VJ, Wei WI. Endoscopic surgery for malignant sinonasal tumours: an eighteen year experience. Rhinology 2015;53(3):204–211

[16] Moya-Plana A, Bresson D, Temam S, Kolb F, Janot F, Herman P. Development of minimally invasive surgery for sinonasal malignancy. Eur Ann Otorhinolaryngol Head Neck Dis 2016;133(6):405–411

[17] Nicolai P, Battaglia P, Bignami M, et al. Endoscopic surgery for malignant tumors of the sinonasal tract and adjacent skull base: a 10-year experience. Am J Rhinol 2008;22(3):308–316

[18] Nicolai P, Castelnuovo P, Bolzoni Villaret A. Endoscopic resection of sinonasal malignancies. Curr Oncol Rep 2011;13(2):138–144

[19] Villaret AB, Yakirevitch A, Bizzoni A, et al. Endoscopic transnasal craniectomy in the management of selected sinonasal malignancies. Am J Rhinol Allergy 2010;24(1):60–65

[20] Snyderman CH, Carrau RL, Kassam AB, et al. Endoscopic skull base surgery: principles of endonasal oncological surgery. J Surg Oncol 2008;97(8):658–664

[21] Hanna E, DeMonte F, Ibrahim S, Roberts D, Levine N, Kupferman M. Endoscopic resection of sinonasal cancers with and without craniotomy: oncologic results. Arch Otolaryngol Head Neck Surg 2009;135(12):1219–1224

[22] Meccariello G, Deganello A, Choussy O, et al. Endoscopic nasal versus open approach for the management of sinonasal adenocarcinoma: a pooled-analysis of 1826 patients. Head Neck 2016;38(Suppl 1):E2267–E2274

[23] Liu JK, Silva NA, Sevak IA, Eloy JA. Transbasal versus endoscopic endonasal versus combined approaches for olfactory groove meningiomas: importance of approach selection. Neurosurg Focus 2018;44(4):E8

[24] Ottenhausen M, Rumalla K, Alalade AF, et al. Decision-making algorithm for minimally invasive approaches to anterior skull base meningiomas. Neurosurg Focus 2018;44(4):E7

[25] Banu MA, Mehta A, Ottenhausen M, et al. Endoscope-assisted endonasal versus supraorbital keyhole resection of olfactory groove meningiomas: comparison and combination of 2 minimally invasive approaches. J Neurosurg 2016;124(3):605–620

[26] Bedrosian JC, Anand VK, Schwartz TH. The endoscopic endonasal approach to repair of iatrogenic and noniatrogenic cerebrospinal fluid leaks and encephaloceles of the anterior cranial fossa. World Neurosurg 2014;82(6, Suppl):S86–S94

[27] Lobo BC, Baumanis MM, Nelson RF. Surgical repair of spontaneous cerebrospinal fluid (CSF) leaks: a systematic review. Laryngoscope Investig Otolaryngol 2017;2(5):215–224

[28] Tajudeen BA, Adappa ND, Kuan EC, et al. Smell preservation following endoscopic unilateral resection of esthesioneuroblastoma: a multi-institutional experience. Int Forum Allergy Rhinol 2016;6(10):1047–1050

[29] Choussy O, Ferron C, Védrine PO, et al; GETTEC Study Group. Adenocarcinoma of Ethmoid: a GETTEC retrospective multicenter study of 418 cases. Laryngoscope 2008;118(3):437–443

[30] Mattavelli D, Schreiber A, Ferrari M, et al. Three-layer reconstruction with iliotibial tract after endoscopic resection of sinonasal tumors. World Neurosurg 2017;101:486–492

[31] Mattavelli D, Schreiber A, Villaret AB, et al. Complications and donor site morbidity of 3-layer reconstruction with iliotibial tract of the anterior skull base: retrospective analysis of 186 patients. Head Neck 2018;40(1):63–69

8 Transplanum–Transtuberculum Approach

Davide Mattavelli, Marco Ravanelli, Davide Lancini, Marco Ferrari, Alberto Schreiber

The transplanum–transtuberculum approach provides direct access to the suprasellar areas through the planum sphenoidale and tuberculum sellae, representing a "frontier" route that can be useful to manage lesions of both the anterior and middle midline skull base. First, this approach has been combined with the transsellar route to resect the cranial portion of suprasellar pituitary adenomas via transnasal endoscopic surgery.[1-4] Subsequently, its employment in the resection of meningiomas of the planum sphenoidale and/or tuberculum sellae led to consider the transplanum–transtuberculum approach an independent corridor that can be combined with other pathways according to the extent of the lesion.[1,5] In view of its natural trajectory toward the optic system, pituitary stalk, hypothalamus, third ventricle, and anterior cerebral arterial system, the indications for the transplanum–transtuberculum approach progressively evolved to include the management of retrochiasmatic/intraventricular craniopharyngiomas,[6-11] hypothalamic gliomas,[12] choroid plexus papillomas[13] and germ cell tumors[14] of the third ventricle, and aneurysms of the anterior cerebral circulation.[15]

The transplanum–transtuberculum craniectomy is bounded by the anterior sellar wall posteriorly, ethmoidal roofs and cribriform plates anteriorly, and optic canals bilaterally. The planum sphenoidale and tuberculum sellae are usually properly exposed through the sphenoid sinus with a transrostral or extended transrostral sphenoidotomy. However, the posterior ethmoid also needs to be dissected when a far-lateral exposure in the area of the optic canal is required. When addressing the skull base, special attention must be paid to the structures corresponding to each side of the craniectomy: at the posterior border, the anterosuperior intercavernous sinus runs usually parallel and in close proximity to the tuberculum sellae, which in fact represent the anterior insertion of the diaphragma sellae; at the anterior border, caution should be paid to not inadvertently injure the posterior portion of the cribriform plate on the midline and posterior ethmoidal artery laterally; at the lateral border, drilling should be carefully performed together with meticulous irrigation to avoid thermal damage of the optic nerve. Within the intracranial compartment, movements should be performed with remarkable attention to avoid damaging the pituitary stalk and optic apparatus, superior hypophyseal arteries, intracranial internal carotid arteries, and anterior cerebral vessels.

After the transplanum–transtuberculum approach, reconstruction must be performed paying attention to the adjacent intracranial structures. A multilayered technique, including fascia and/or fat tissue as inner layer to avoid compression or mechanic damage of the aforementioned intracranial structures, is typically used. The so-called gasket seal technique is based on the embedding of a rigid graft of cartilage or bone to fix the plasty to the edges of craniectomy. Given its indications, which mostly include intracranial lesions, vascularized flaps as the outer layer of the reconstruction are strongly recommended after a transplanum–transtuberculum approach.[16]

After completing the harvesting of the surgical corridor, the reader is suggested to explore both the infrachiasmatic and the suprachiasmatic areas with angled scopes to have a three-dimensional understanding of the anatomy and identify the structures adjacent to this region that will be directly reached with approaches illustrated in other chapters. Furthermore, in specimens with favorable anatomy, an exploration of the third ventricle through the lamina terminalis is also feasible.

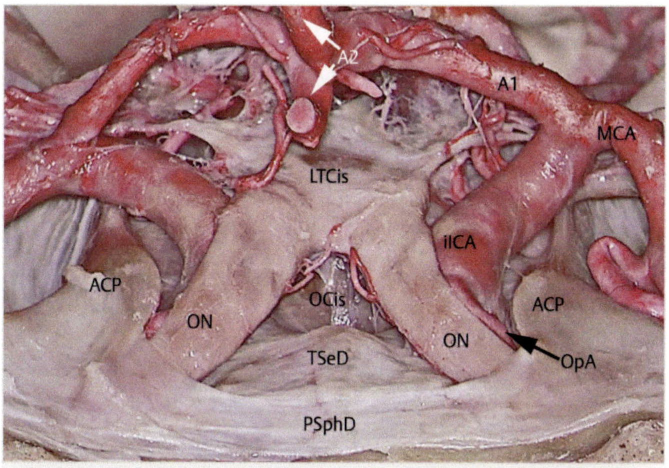

Fig. 8.1 Anterior-to-posterior intracranial view of the suprasellar area. This cadaver picture shows the anatomy of the suprasellar area as seen from an anterior-to-posterior intracranial perspective. A1, precommunicating tract of the anterior cerebral artery; A2, postcommunicating tract of the anterior cerebral artery; ACP, anterior clinoid process; iICA, intracranial tract of the internal carotid artery; LTCis, lamina terminalis cistern; MCA, middle cerebral artery; OCis, optic cistern; ON, optic nerve; OpA, ophthalmic artery; PSphD, dura of the planum sphenoidale; TSeD, dura of the tuberculum sellae.

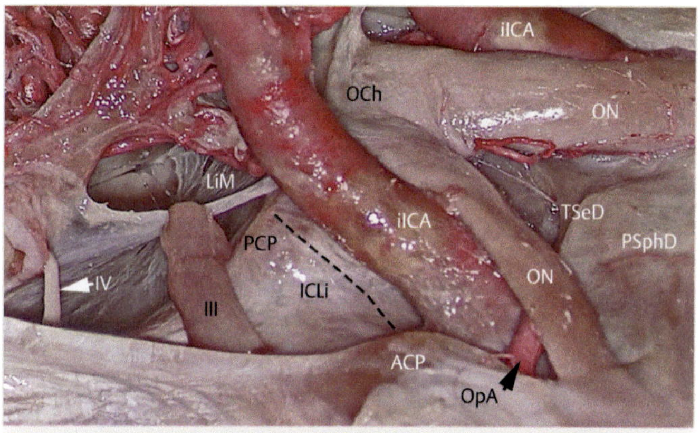

Fig. 8.2 Lateral-to-medial intracranial view of the suprasellar area. This cadaver picture shows the anatomy of the suprasellar area as seen from an lateral-to-medial intracranial perspective. III, oculomotor nerve; IV, trochlear nerve; ACP, anterior clinoid process; ICLi (*black dashed line*), interclinoid ligament; iICA, intracranial tract of the internal carotid artery; LiM, Liliequist's membrane; OCh, optic chiasm; OpA, ophthalmic artery; ON, optic nerve; PCP, posterior clinoid process; PSphD, dura of the planum sphenoidale; TSeD, dura of the tuberculum sellae.

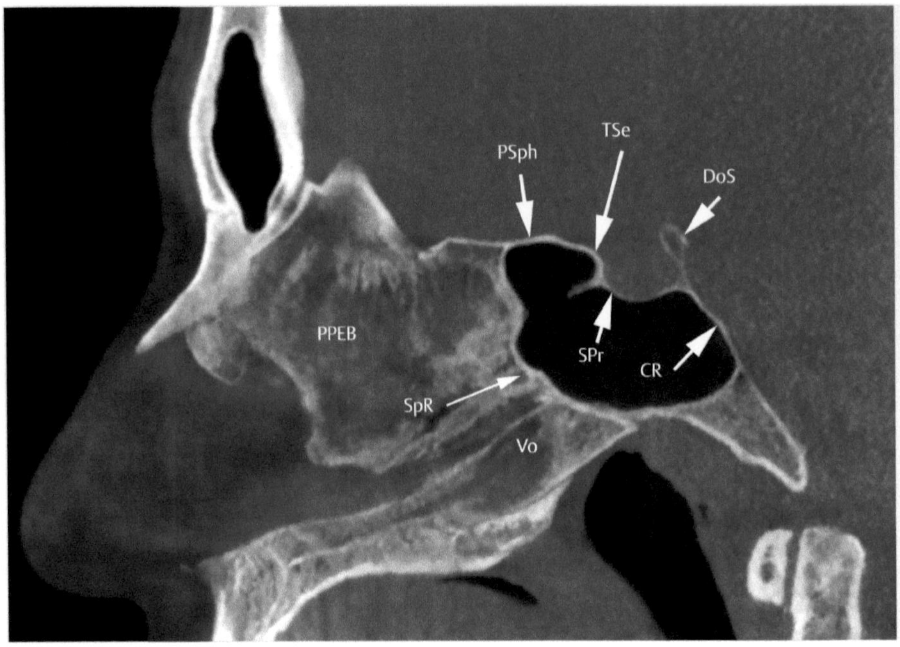

Fig. 8.3 Sagittal CT of the midline anterior skull base. The planum sphenoidale (PSph) is the roof of the sphenoid sinus. The tuberculum sellae (TSe) is a thickening of the bone serving as a junction between planum sphenoidale and sellar prominence (SPr). The trajectory of the transplanum–transtuberculum approach passes through the sphenoid rostrum (SpR). CR, clival recess; DoS, dorsum sellae; PPEB, perpendicular plate of the ethmoid bone; Vo, vomer.

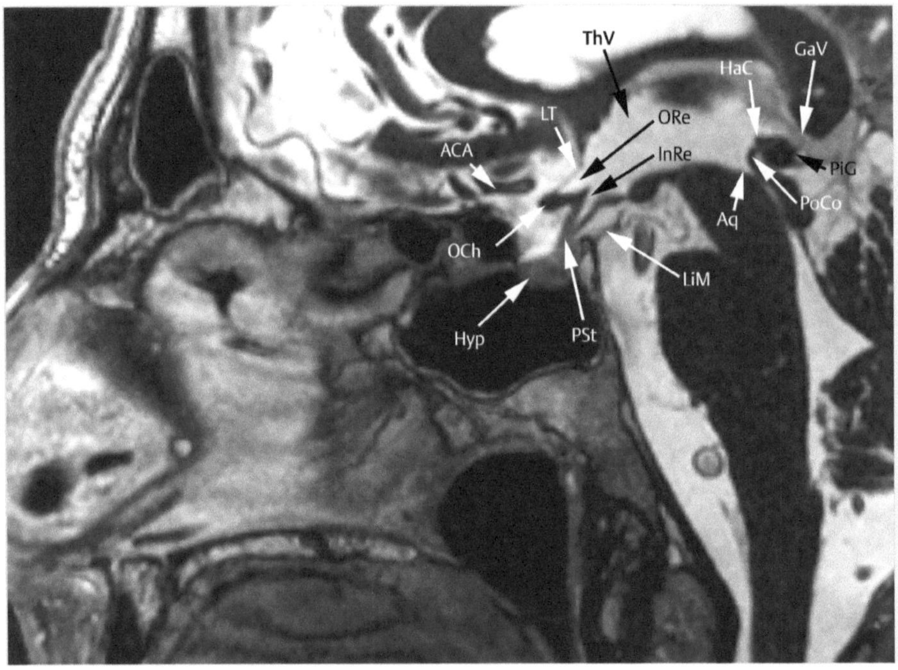

Fig. 8.4 Sagittal MRI anatomy of the suprasellar area. The lamina terminalis cistern and optic cistern are located superiorly and inferiorly to the optic chiasm (OCh), respectively, and form the suprasellar area. The optic cistern is bounded by the optic system anterosuperiorly and Liliequist membrane (LiM) posteroinferiorly and includes the pituitary stalk (PSt) and superior hypophyseal arteries. The lamina terminalis cistern is bounded by the lamina terminalis (LT) posteriorly and continues into the interhemispheric fissure anteriorly. This cisternal space includes the proximal portion of the anterior cerebral arteries (ACA). The lamina terminalis serves as anterior door toward the third ventricle (ThV). Aq, cerebral aqueduct; GaV, vein of Galen; HaC, habenular commissure; Hyp, hypophysis; InRe, infundibular recess; ORe, optic recess; PiG, pineal gland; PoCo, posterior commissure.

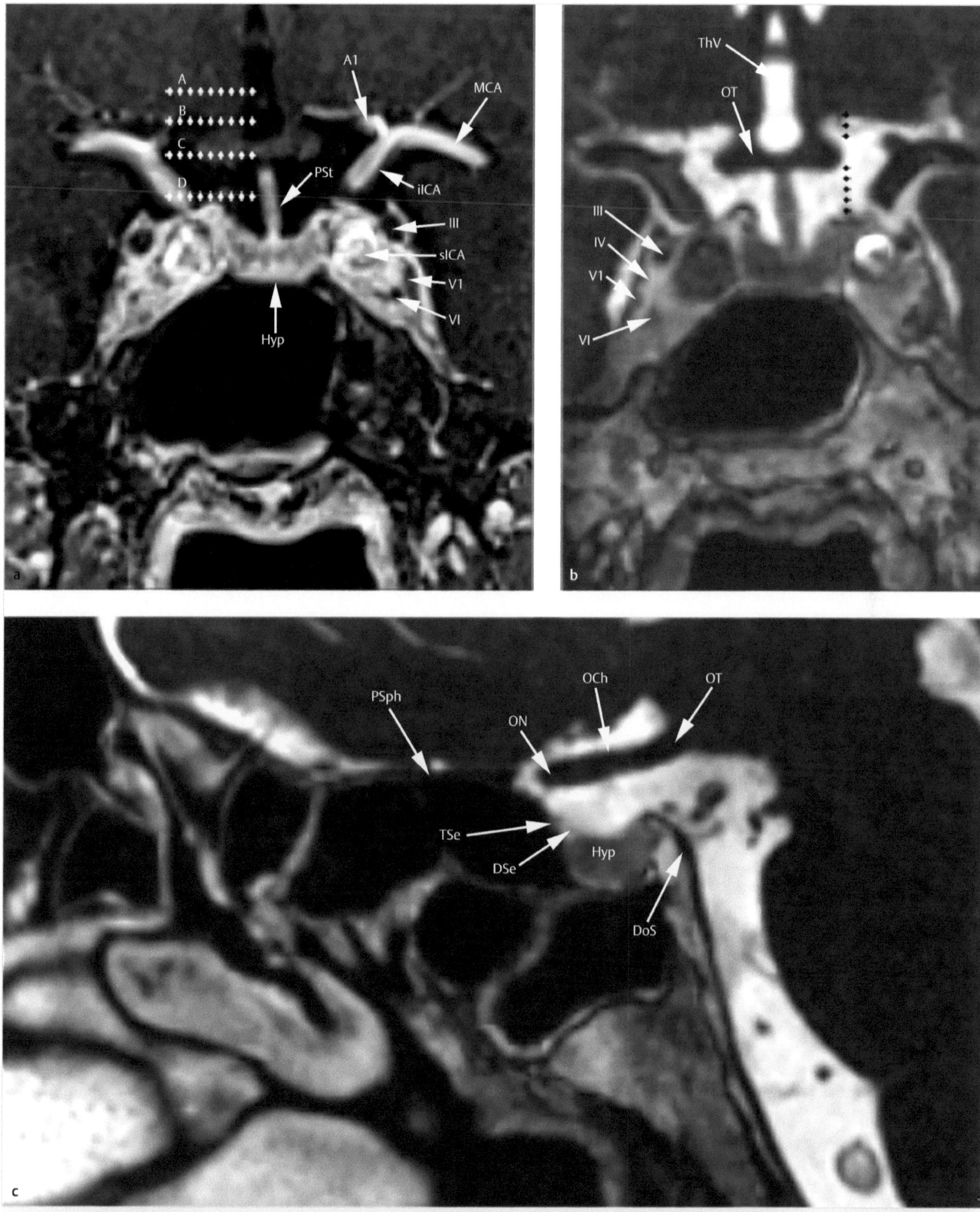

Fig. 8.5 Coronal and sagittal MRI anatomy of the suprasellar area. The panel contains a paracoronal T1-weighted, fat-saturated, contrast-enhanced MRI **(a)** along with a sagittal paramedian and a paracoronal constructive interference in steady state (CISS) MRI **(b, c)** passing through the suprasellar area. The position of the sagittal image is depicted in the upper right image (*black dotted line*). The optic cistern lies cranially to the diaphragma sellae (DSe), which serves as the roof of the sellar region, and below the optic system, which is formed from posterior to anterior by the optic tract (OT), optic chiasm (OCh), and optic nerve (ON). The intracranial tract of the internal carotid artery (iICA) runs at the lateral boundary of the optic cistern and bifurcates into the precommunicating tract of the anterior cerebral artery (A1) and middle cerebral artery (MCA) just cranially to the plane passing through the optic system. *White dotted lines* in the upper left image depict the position of images composing ▶Fig. 8.6. III, oculomotor nerve; V1, ophthalmic nerve; VI, abducens nerve; DoS, dorsum sellae; Hyp, hypophysis; PSph, planum sphenoidale; PSt, pituitary stalk; sICA, parasellar tract of the internal carotid artery; ThV, third ventricle; TSe, tuberculum sellae.

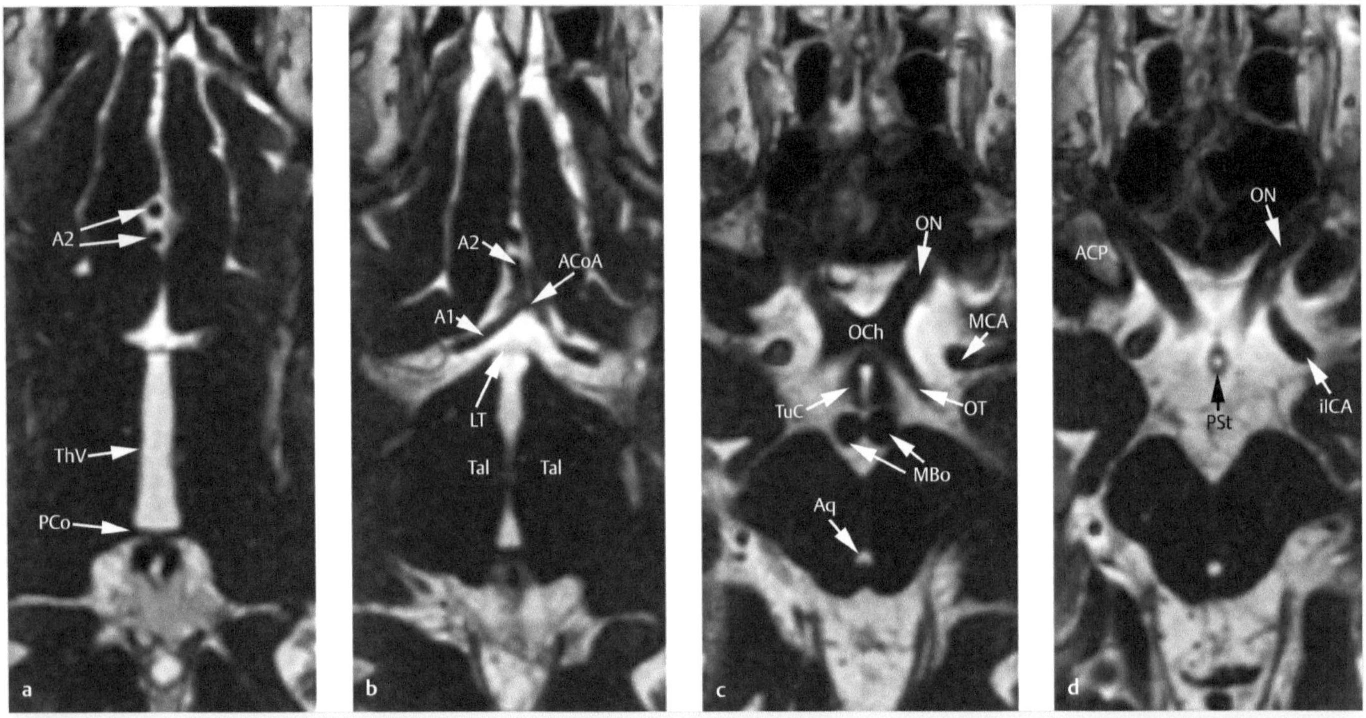

Fig. 8.6 Axial MRI anatomy of the third ventricle, lamina terminalis cistern, and optic cistern. The panel contains four axial constructive interference in steady state (CISS) MRI passing through the suprasellar area and third ventricle, from cranial **(a)** to caudal **(d)**. The third ventricle (ThV) is bounded by the lamina terminalis (LT) anteriorly and by the posterior commissure (PCo) posteriorly. Inferiorly, the floor of the third ventricle is mostly formed by the mammillary bodies (MBo) and tuber cinereum (TuC). The lamina terminalis cistern lies in front of the lamina terminalis and houses the anterior cerebral artery system, which is formed by the pre- (A1) and postcommunicating tract (A2) of the vessel and by the anterior communicating artery (ACoA). The optic cistern lies below the optic system, which is formed by the optic tract (OT), optic chiasm (OCh), and optic nerve (ON), and includes the pituitary stalk (PSt). ACP, anterior clinoid process; Aq, cerebral aqueduct; iICA, intracranial tract of the internal carotid artery; MCA, middle cerebral artery; Tal, thalamus.

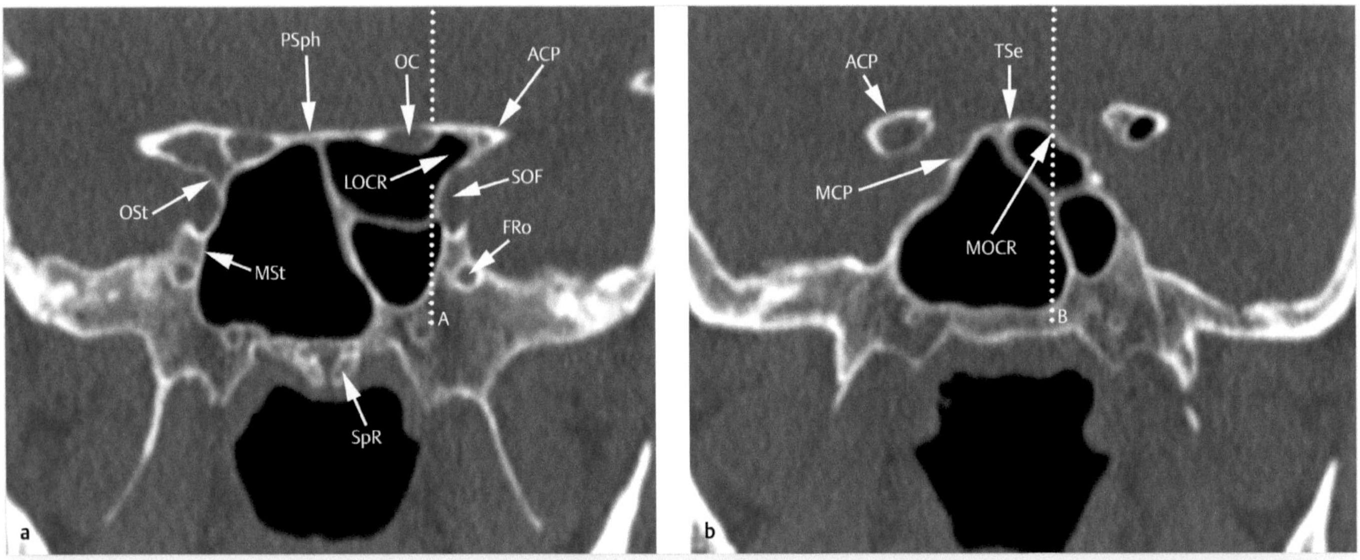

Fig. 8.7 (a, b) Coronal CT anatomy of the planum sphenoidale and tuberculum sellae. The panel contains two coronal CT images passing through the planum sphenoidale (PSph) and tuberculum sellae (TSe). The lateral boundary of the planum sphenoidale is the optic canal (OC), while the lateral limit of the tuberculum sellae is the medial optic-carotid recess (MOCR). The middle clinoid process (MCP) lies inferiorly and medially with respect to the medial optic-carotid recess and can fuse with the apex of the anterior clinoid process (ACP) forming the carotid clinoid bony ring. The lateral optic-carotid recess (LOCR) can considerably extend within the anterior clinoid process through the optic strut (OSt), which separates the optic canal, superior orbital fissure (SOF), and the parasellar and paraclinoid tracts of the internal carotid artery. Similarly, the maxillary strut (MSt) is defined as the upper portion of the foramen rotundum (FRo), which separates the maxillary nerve from the content of the superior orbital fissure. The white dotted lines (A, B) show the position of images composing ▶ Fig. 8.8. SpR, sphenoidal rostrum.

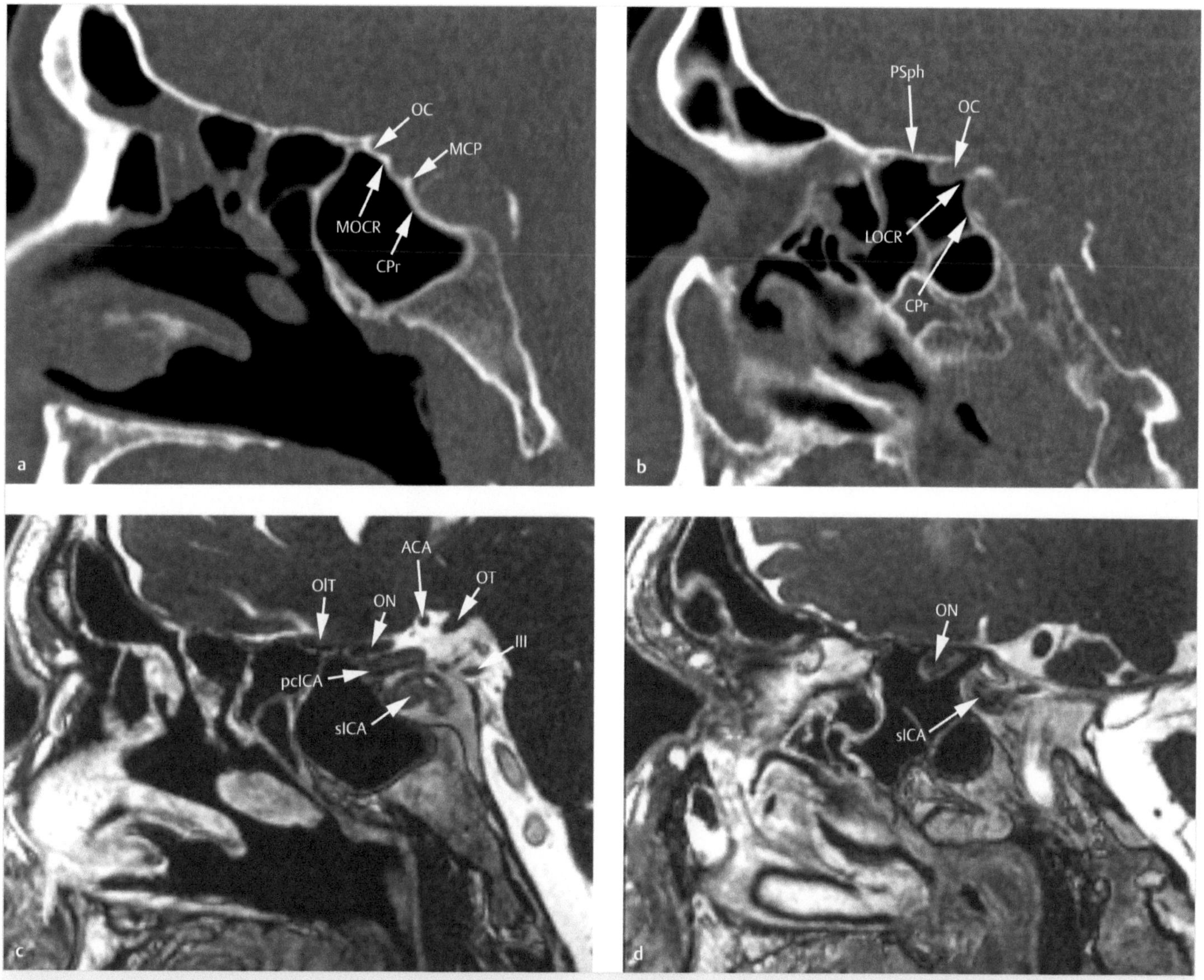

Fig. 8.8 Sagittal CT and MRI anatomy of the lateral boundaries of the transplanum–transtuberculum approach. The panel contains two sagittal CT scans **(a, b)** and two sagittal constructive interference in steady state (CISS) MRI scans **(c, d)**. The position of images on the right and left columns is depicted in ▶ Fig. 8.7 (A and B, respectively). The lateral boundary of the tuberculum sellae is the medial optic-carotid recess (MOCR), which lies between the carotid prominence (CPr) and the optic canal (OC), thus serving as a landmark to identify the interface between the paraclinoid tracts of the internal carotid artery (pcICA) and optic nerve (ON). Similarly, the lateral optic-carotid recess (LOCR) can be used to identify the plane between the parasellar tract of the internal carotid artery (sICA) and optic canal. The olfactory tract (OlT) runs at the posterolateral corner of the planum sphenoidale (PSph). III, oculomotor nerve; ACA, anterior cerebral artery; MCP, middle clinoid process; OT, optic tract.

Endoscopic Dissection

Nasal Phase

- Paraseptal sphenoidotomy.
- Transrostral sphenoidotomy.
- Expanded transrostral sphenoidotomy.
- Vertical uncinectomy.
- Anterior ethmoidectomy.
- Posterior ethmoidectomy.
- Superior turbinectomy.
- Transethmoidal sphenoidotomy.
- Middle turbinectomy.

Skull Base Phase

- Step 1: Removal of the mucosa of the sphenoid sinus.
- Step 2: Removal of the tuberculum sellae and planum sphenoidale.
- Step 3: Incision of the periosteum of the tuberculum sellae and planum sphenoidale.
- Step 4: Removal of the anterior arachnoid of the optic cistern.
- Step 5: Removal of the anterior arachnoid of the lamina terminalis cistern.
- Step 6: Translamina terminalis ventriculostomy.

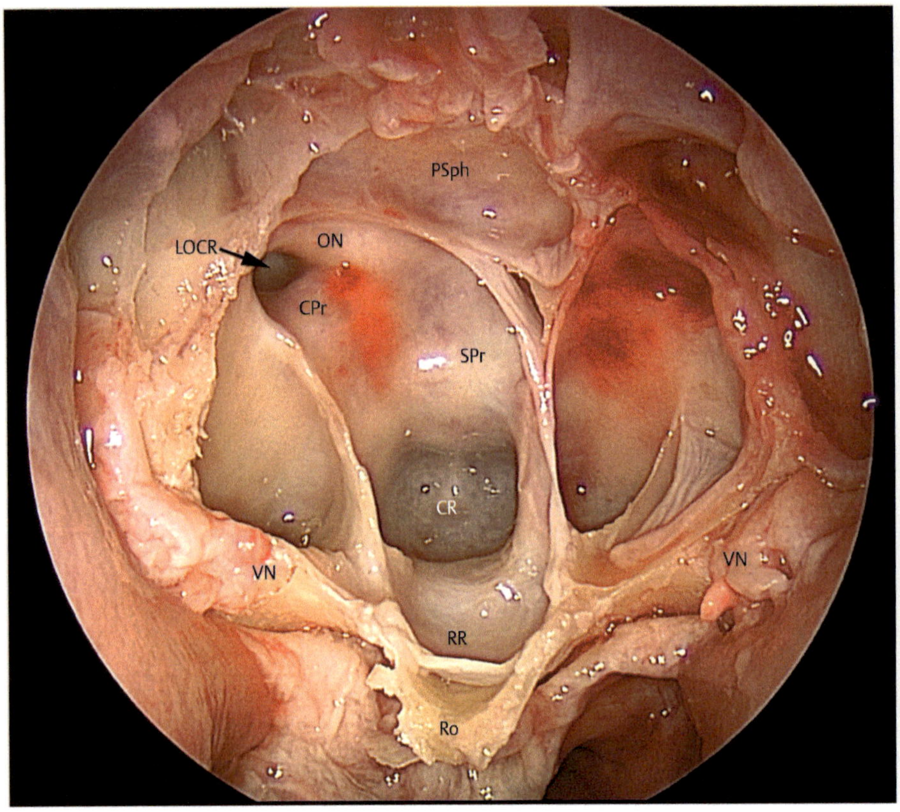

Fig. 8.9 Sphenoid sinus. Through a transethmoidal sphenoidotomy, the sphenoid sinus is widely opened. The roof of the sinus consists of the planum sphenoidale (PSph). The lateral optic-carotid recess lies between the optic nerve (ON) and the carotid prominence (CPr). The posterior wall of the sphenoid sinus is composed by the sellar protuberance (SPr) superiorly and the clival recess (CR) inferiorly; this recess is present only when the sinus is well pneumatized. Ro, rostrum sphenoidale; RR, rostral recess; VN, vidian nerve.

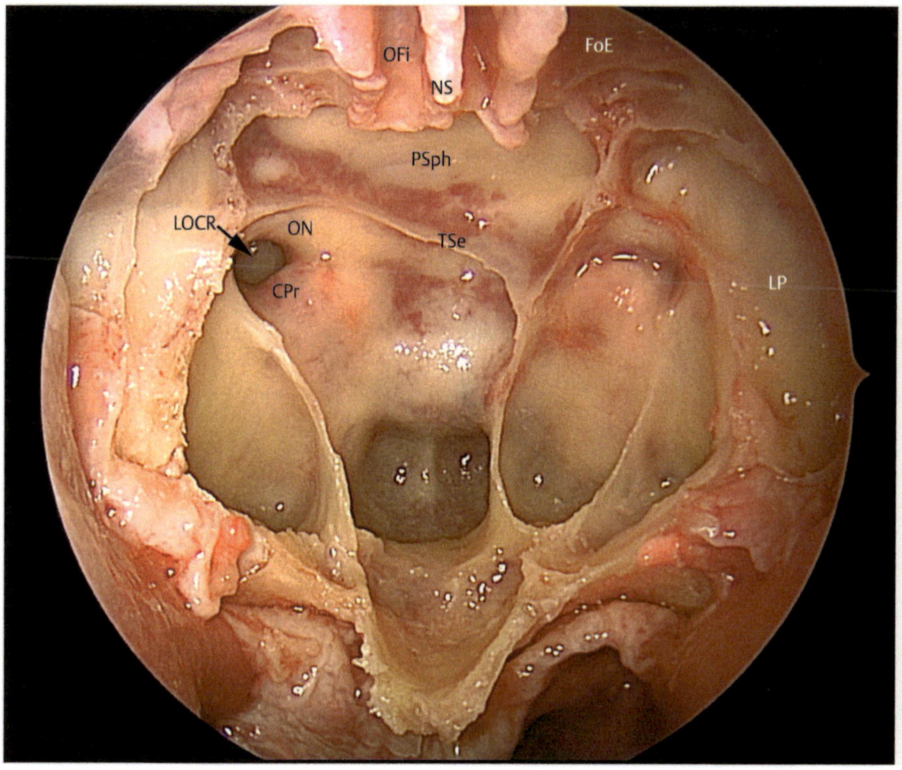

Fig. 8.10 Step 1. The mucosa of the sphenoid sinus is removed to identify the bony landmarks on the sphenoid sinus walls. The tuberculum sellae (TSe) is bounded by the optic nerve (ON) laterally, the planum sphenoidale (PSph) anteriorly, and the sellar prominence inferiorly. CPr, carotid prominence; FoE, fovea ethmoidalis; LOCR, lateral optic-carotid recess; LP, lamina papyracea; NS, nasal septum; OFi, olfactory fissure.

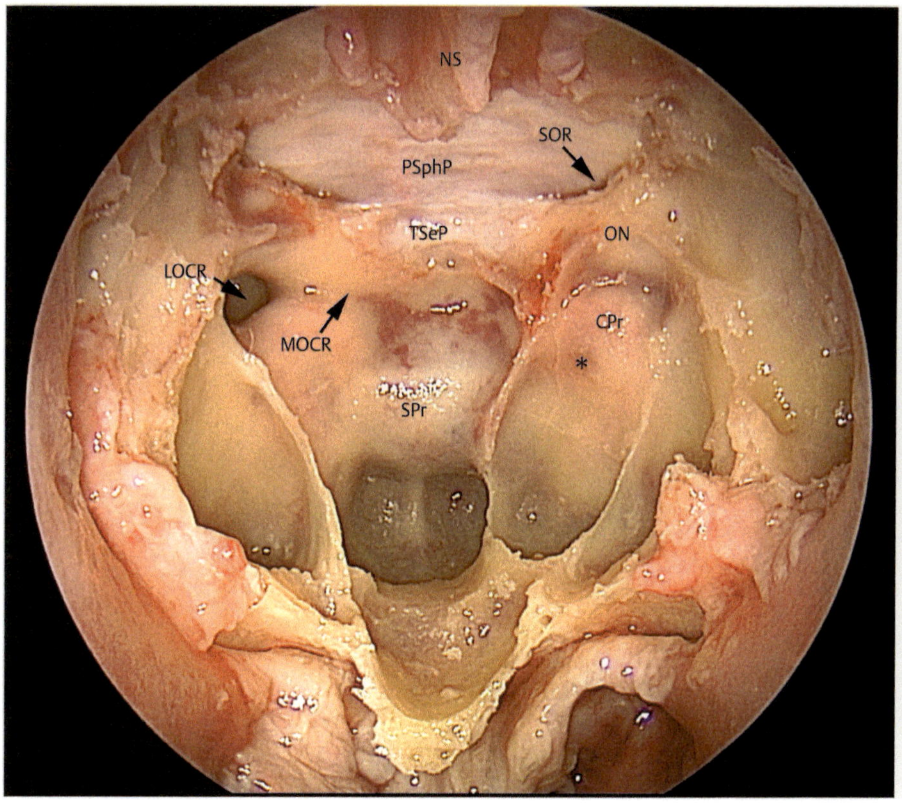

Fig. 8.11 Step 2. The bone corresponding to the planum sphenoidale and tuberculum sellae is removed to expose the underlying periosteum (PSphP and TSeP). Bone removal can be extended to the supraoptic recess (SOR). The tuberculum sellae is removed up to the optic nerve (ON) and medial optic-carotid recess (MOCR). Notably, the position of the middle clinoid process (*black asterisk*) is caudal to the area of the medial optic-carotid recess. CPr, carotid prominence; LOCR, lateral optic-carotid recess; NS, nasal septum; SPr, sellar prominence.

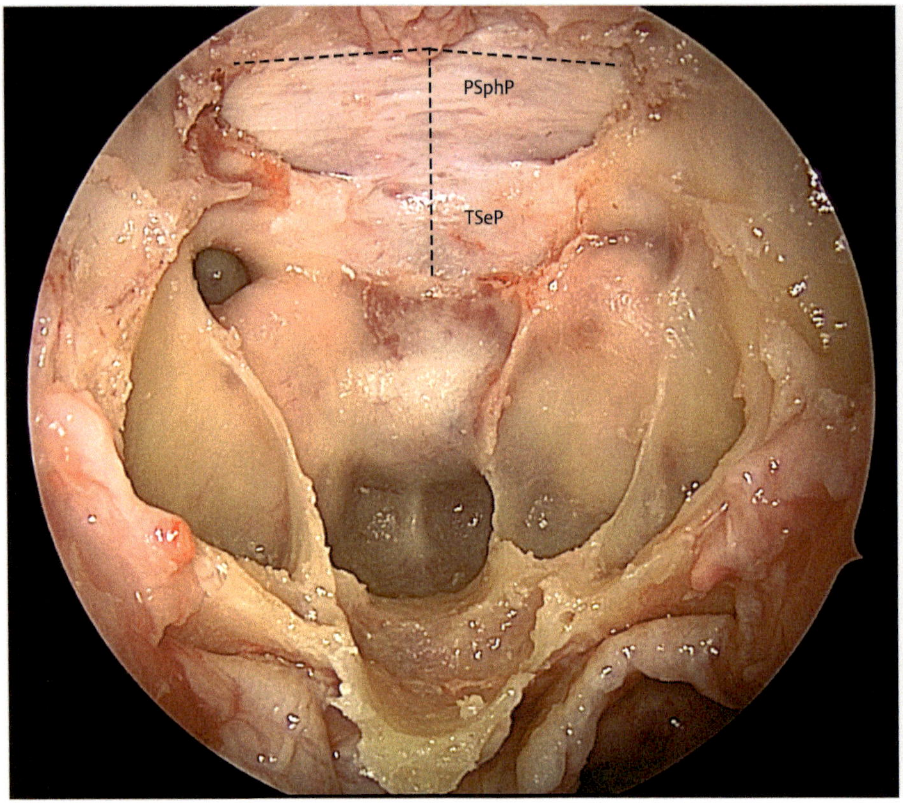

Fig. 8.12 Step 3. (part 1) The periosteum of the planum sphenoidale (PSphP) and tuberculum sellae (TSeP) is incised together with the underlying dura along the midline (*vertical black dashed line*). A horizontal incision is then made along the anterior limit of the planum sphenoidale (*horizontal black dashed line*).

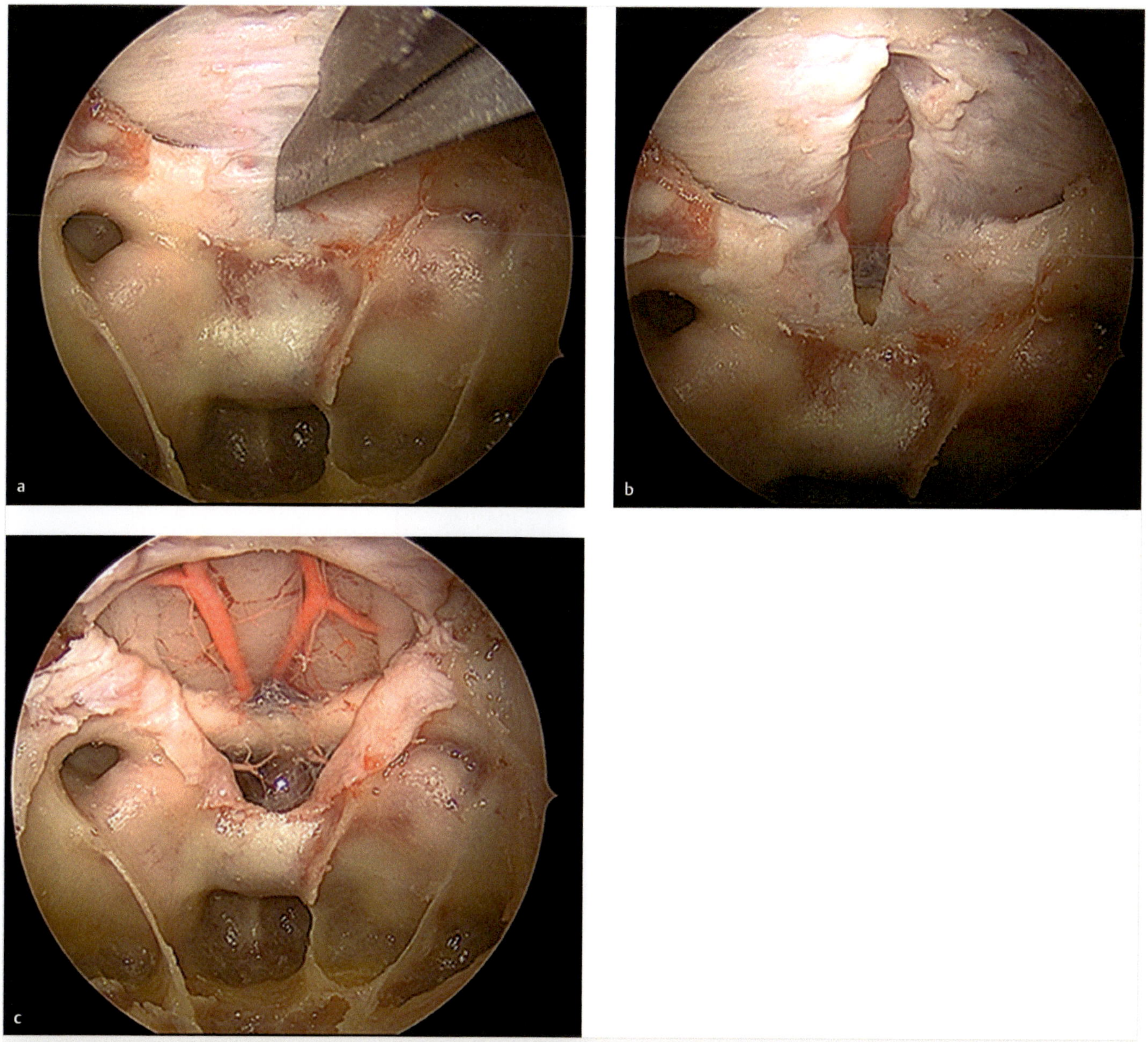

Fig. 8.13 (a–c) Step 3 (part 2). After completing the incisions, the periosteal dural flaps are turned laterally to cover the optic canals and identify the arachnoid layer.

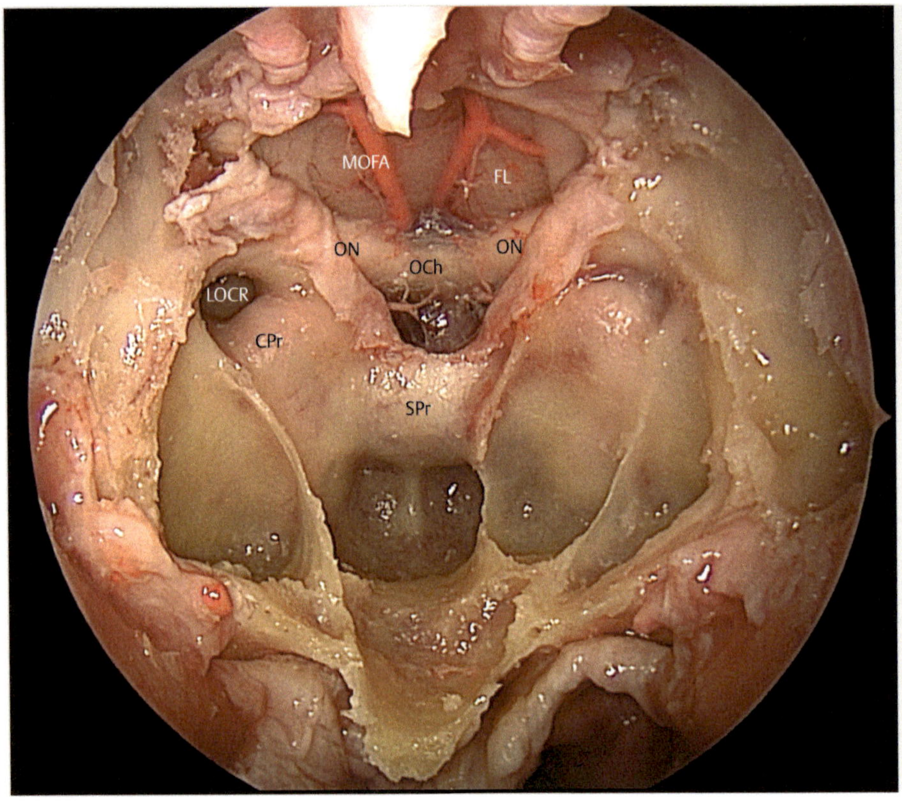

Fig. 8.14 The intradural space. The intracranial structures, which are covered by arachnoid, come into view. The medial orbitofrontal artery (MOFA) runs along the inferior surface of the frontal lobes (FL). The optic nerves (ON) merge to form the optic chiasm (OCh). CPr, carotid prominence; LOCR, lateral optic-carotid recess; SPr, sella prominence.

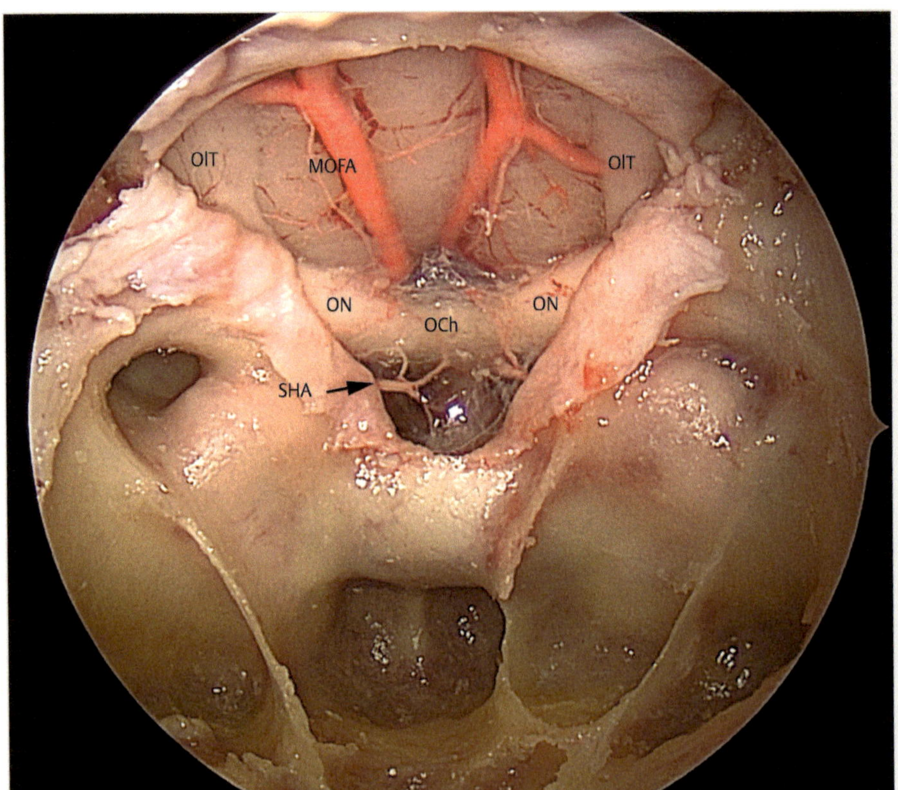

Fig. 8.15 Doors of the supra- and infrachiasmatic corridors. The optic chiasm (OCh) and optic nerves (ON) are located in the middle of the transplanum–transtuberculum window. The superior hypophyseal arteries (SHA) can be identified below the optic chiasm, within the optic cistern. The medial orbitofrontal arteries (MOFA) arise from the anterior cerebral artery in the lamina terminalis cistern and run above the optic system. The olfactory tracts (OlT) can be identified superiorly to the lateral margin of the periosteal opening. The anterior arachnoid of the lamina terminalis and optic cisterns can be considered the doors toward the supra- and infrachiasmatic corridors of the transplanum–transtuberculum approach, respectively.

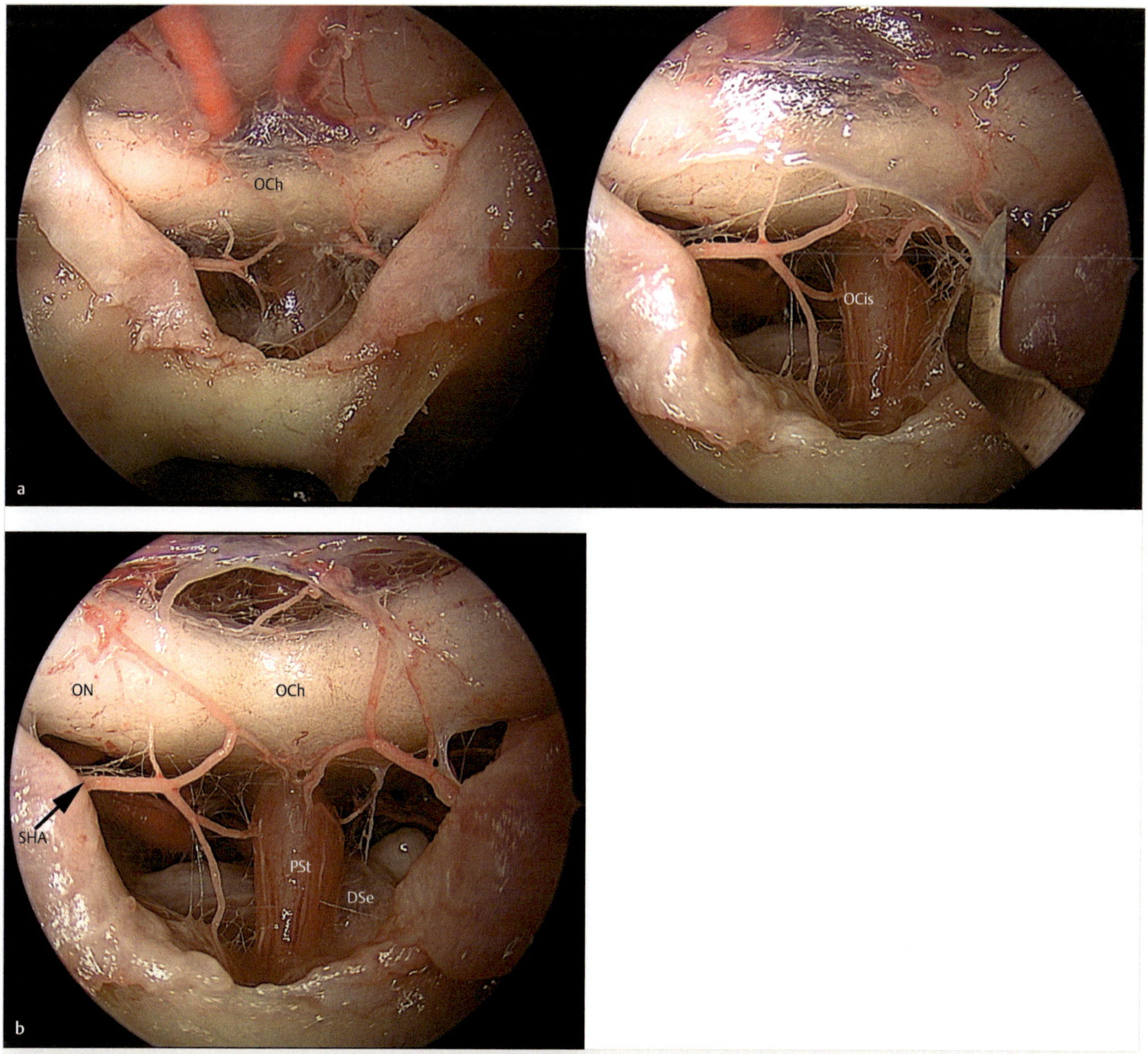

Fig. 8.16 (a, b) Step 4. The anterior arachnoid of the optic cistern (OCis) is removed to get access to the infrachiasmatic corridor. The pituitary stalk (PSt) can be more clearly identified after removing the arachnoid. The superior hypophyseal arteries (SHA) run within the optic cistern and give branches to the optic nerve (ON), optic chiasm (OCh), pituitary stalk, and diaphragma sellae (DSe).

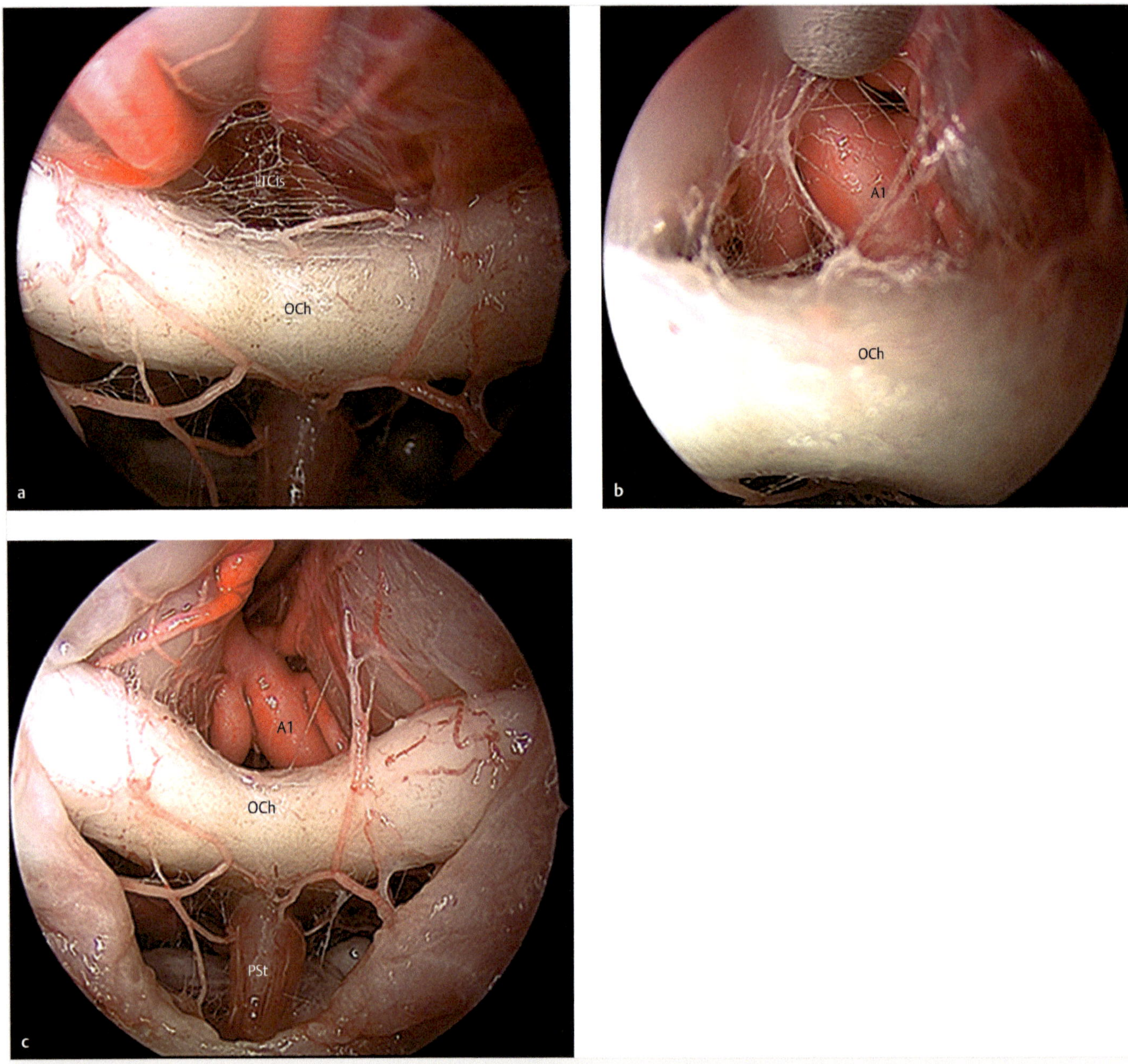

Fig. 8.17 (a–c) Step 5. To get access to the suprachiasmatic corridor, the anterior arachnoid of the lamina terminalis cistern (LTCis) is removed. The lamina terminalis cistern is located above the optic chiasm (OCh). The precommunicating tract of the anterior cerebral artery (A1) is first identified within the cistern. PSt, pituitary stalk.

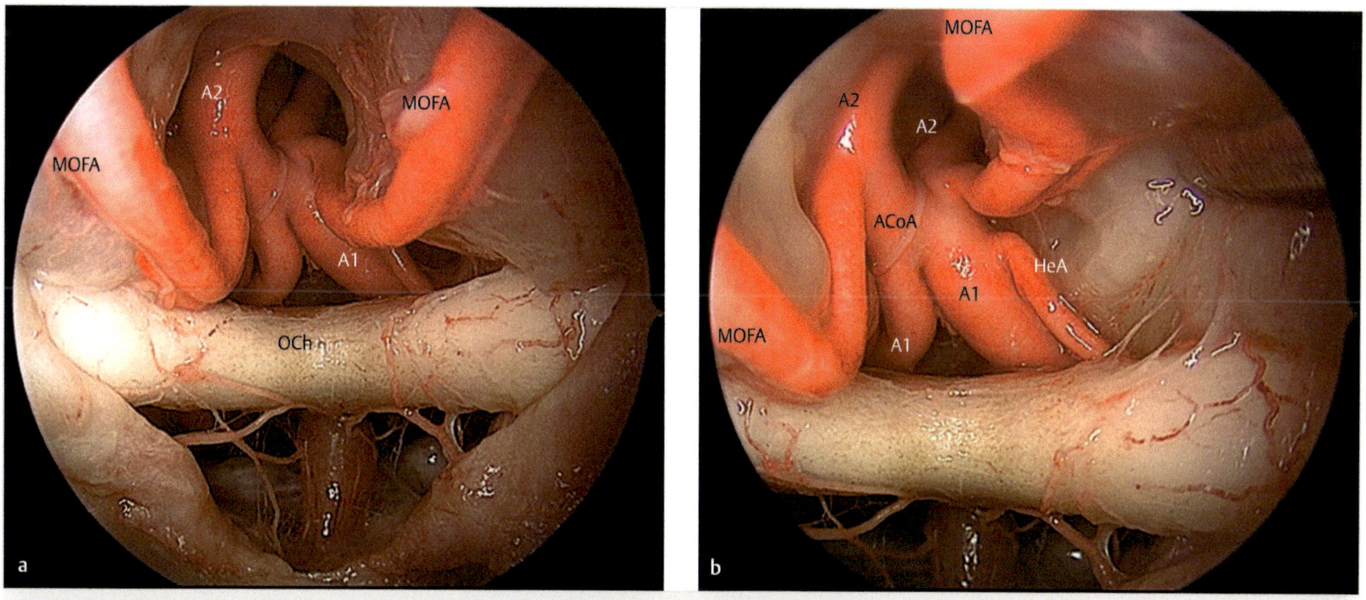

Fig. 8.18 (a, b) The anterior cerebral arteries. The arachnoid is gently removed to identify the system of the anterior cerebral arteries. The anterior cerebral arteries are connected through the anterior communicating artery (ACoA). The precommunicating tract of the anterior cerebral artery (A1) runs from the internal carotid artery to the anterior communicating artery, and the postcommunicating tract of the anterior cerebral artery (A2) lies distally to the anterior communicating artery. The medial orbitofrontal artery (MOFA) is the first branch of the postcommunicating tract of the anterior cerebral artery. The recurrent artery of Heubner (HeA), which reaches the internal capsule and basal nuclei, arises from the lateral surface of the anterior cerebral artery, close to the anterior communicating artery.

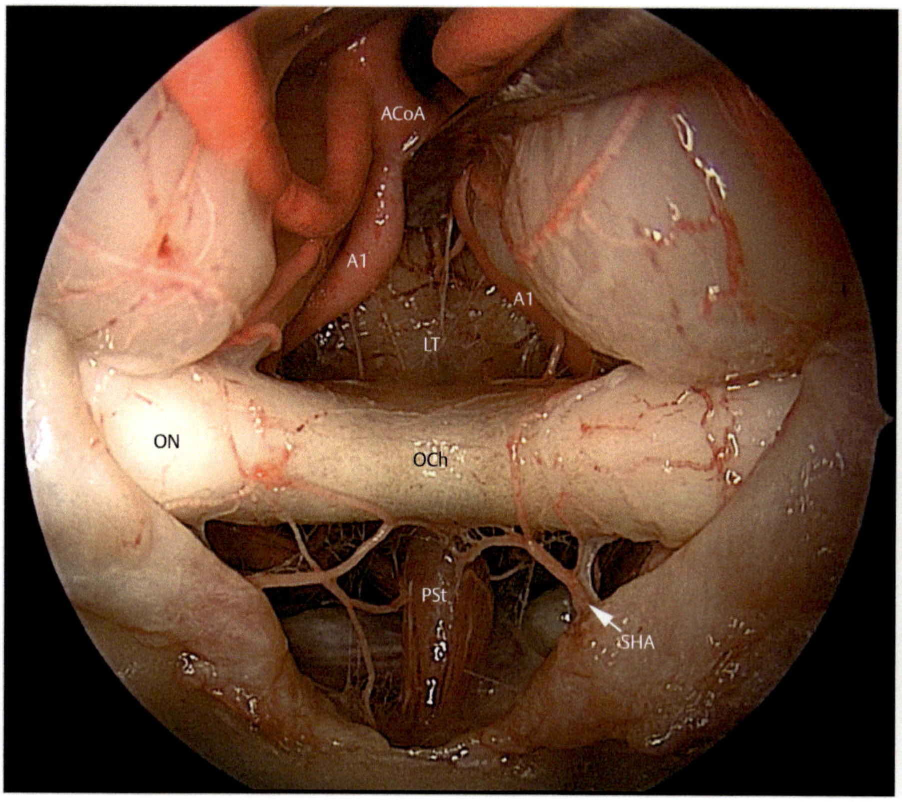

Fig. 8.19 The lamina terminalis. The anterior cerebral artery (A1) and anterior communicating artery (ACoA) are cranially displaced to identify the lamina terminalis (LT), which continues posterosuperiorly from the optic chiasm (OCh). The lamina terminalis is the anterior boundary of the hypothalamus and represents the anterior wall of the third ventricle. ON, optic nerve; PSt, pituitary stalk; SHA, superior hypophyseal artery.

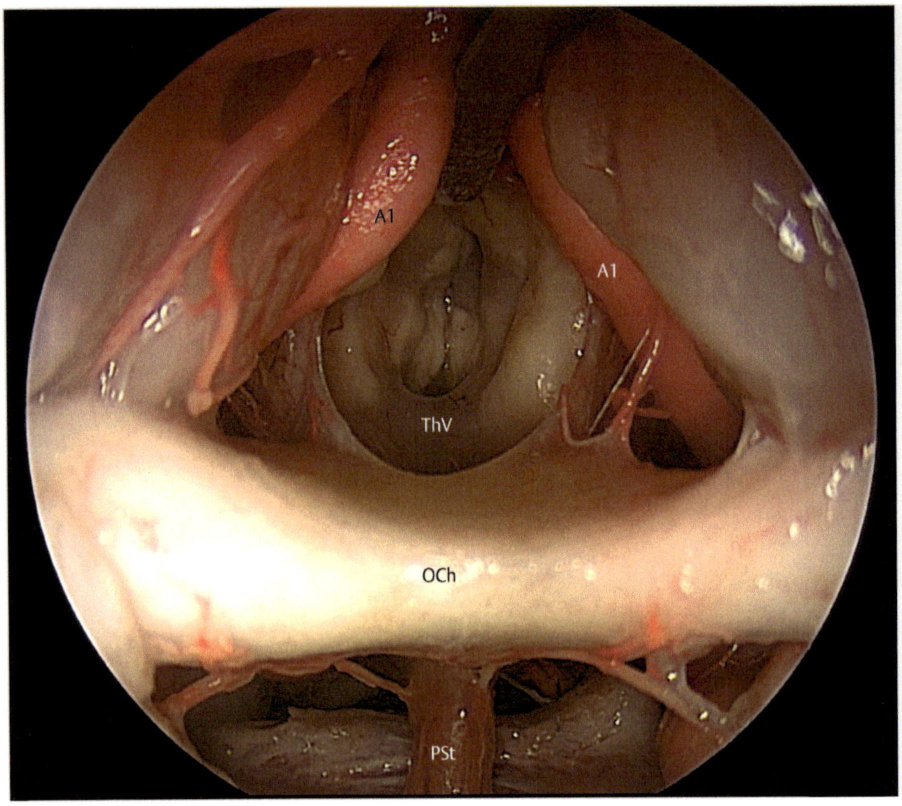

Fig. 8.20 Step 6. The lamina terminalis is opened to expose the third ventricle (ThV). A1, precommunicating tract of the anterior cerebral artery; OCh, optic chiasm; PSt, pituitary stalk.

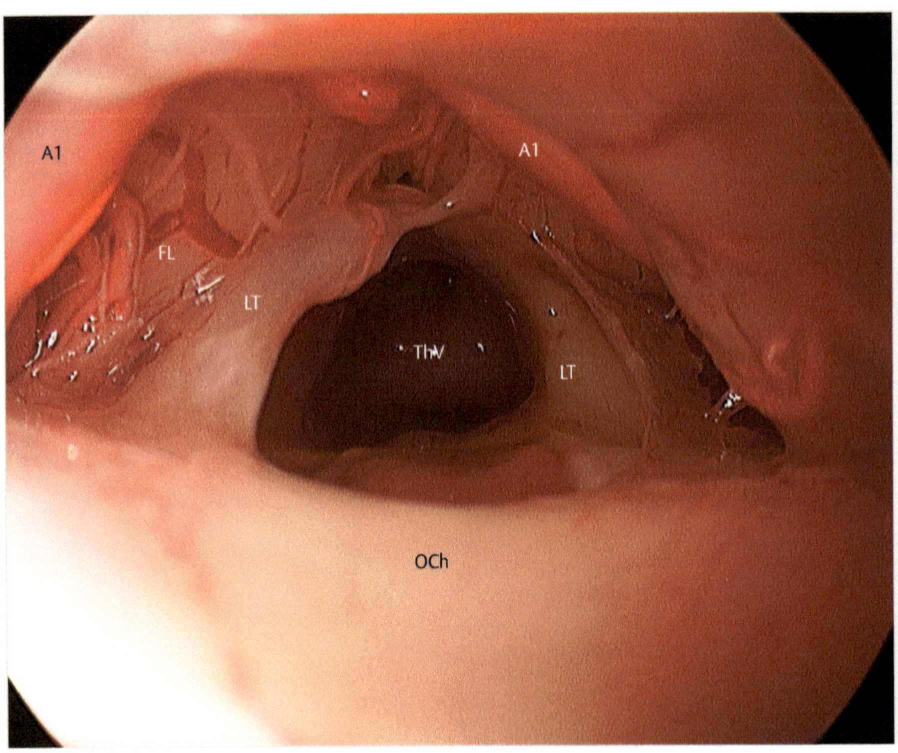

Fig. 8.21 The translamina terminalis window. Once the lamina terminalis (LT) is opened, a straight scope is placed below the precommunicating tract of the anterior cerebral artery (A1) and above the optic chiasm (OCh) to get access to the third ventricle (ThV). FL, frontal lobe.

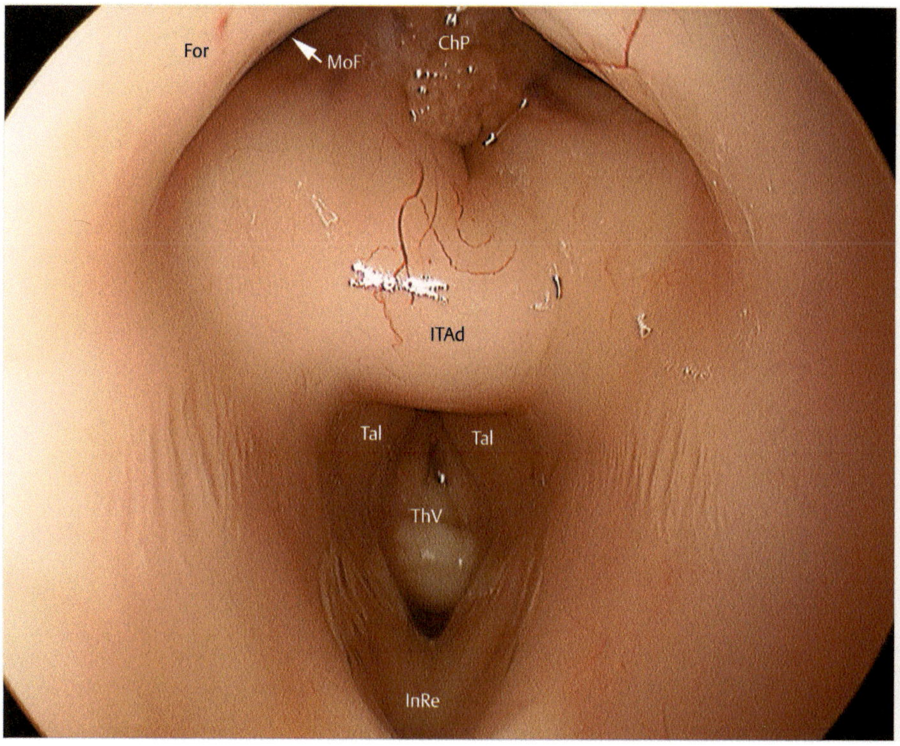

Fig. 8.22 Intraventricular anatomy (part 1). After entering the third ventricle (ThV), the interthalamic adherence (ITAd) appears in the center of the field. This adherence, also called massa intermedia, connects the two thalami (Tal). The choroid plexus (ChP) lies above the interthalamic adherence in the midline, and the columns of the fornix (For) are identified laterally, where they serve as main boundaries of the foramen of Monro (MoF). InRe, infundibular recess of the third ventricle.

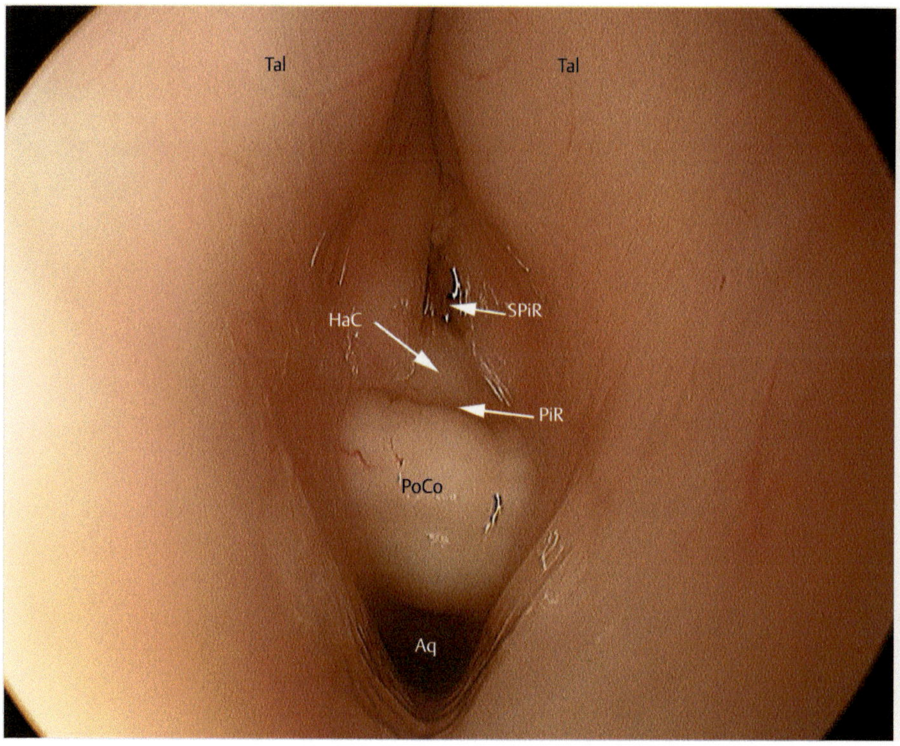

Fig. 8.23 Intraventricular anatomy (part 2). The scope is moved inferiorly and posteriorly to show the posterior region of the third ventricle and the posterior commissure (PoCo). The cerebral aqueduct (Aq) is identified below the posterior commissure. The pineal (PiR) and suprapineal (SPiR) recesses are sequentially identified above the posterior commissure, being located caudally and cranially to the habenular commissure (HaC), respectively. These small pouches are the landmarks for the pineal gland, as its base lies between these recesses. The suprapineal recess can be used as a landmark for the great cerebral vein of Galen. Tal, thalamus.

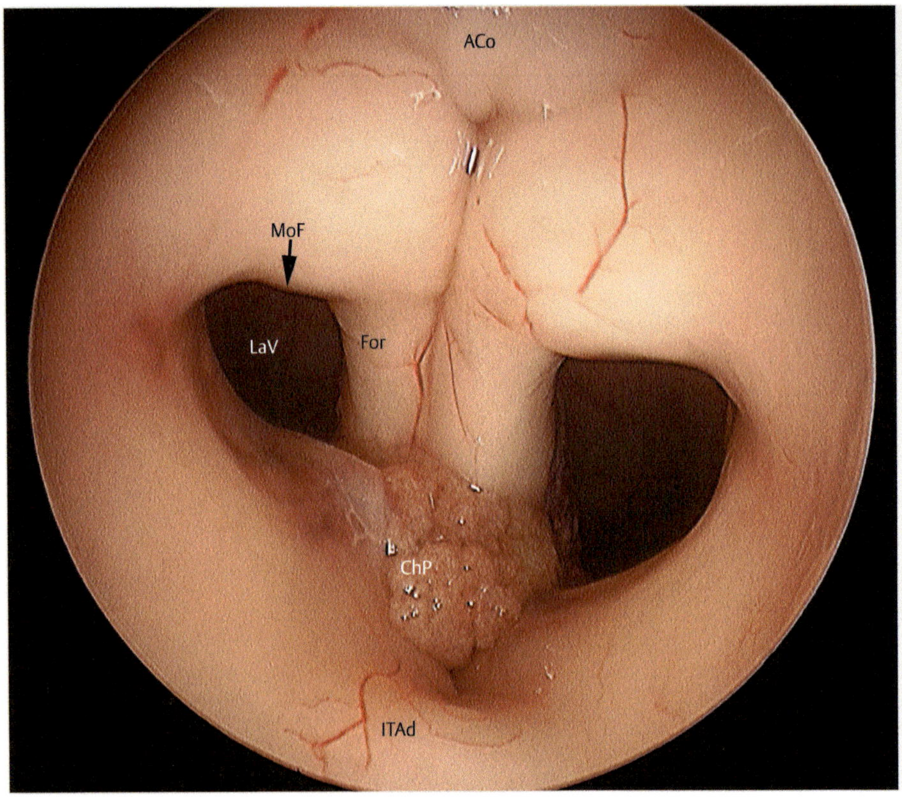

Fig. 8.24 Intraventricular anatomy (part 3). A 70-degree scope is employed, turned cranially, and placed anterior to the interthalamic adherence (ITAd). In this way, the choroid plexus (ChP) and columns of the fornix (For) are identified. Each foramen of Monro (MoF) is surrounded by the column of the fornix and gives access to the lateral ventricle (LaV). At the top of the field of view, the anterior commissure (ACo) is identified.

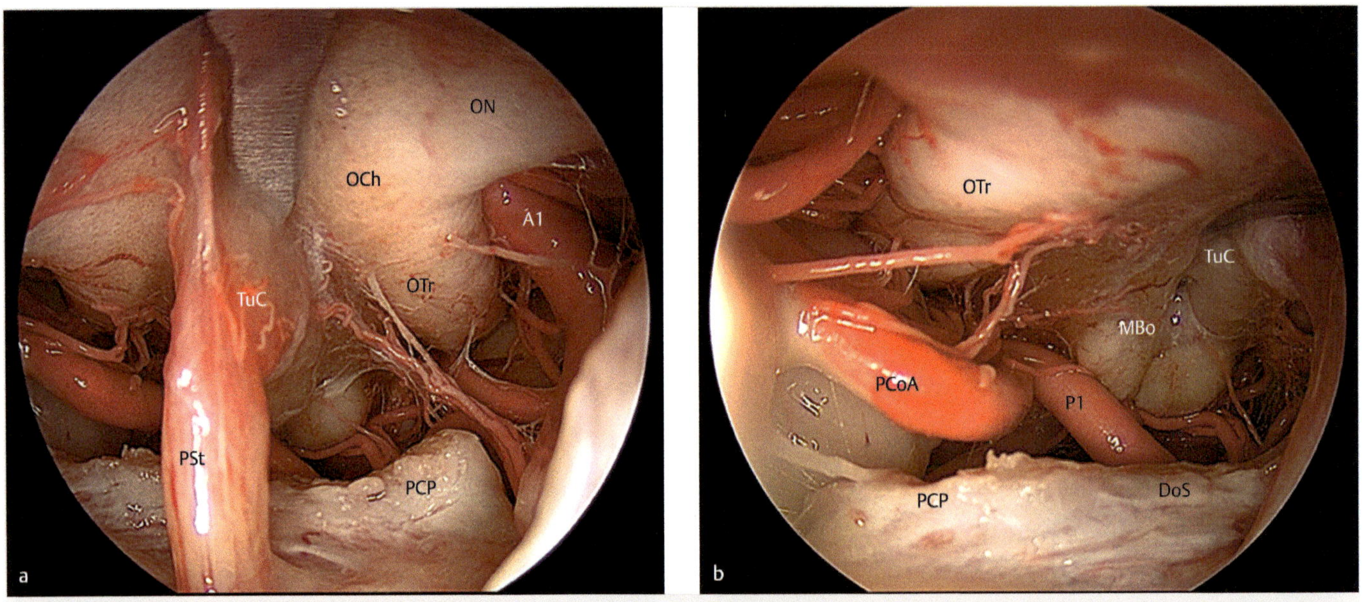

Fig. 8.25 (a, b) The optic cistern. The optic nerve (ON) arises from the optic chiasm (OCh), which is formed by the union of the optic tracts (OTr). The pituitary stalk (PSt) arises from the tuber cinereum (TuC), which lies anteriorly to the mammillary bodies (MBo). The dorsum sellae (DoS) and posterior clinoid processes (PCP) hinder the view of interpeduncular cistern and its contents. The posterior communicating artery (PCoA) can be identified above the posterior clinoid process. A1, precommunicating tract of the anterior cerebral artery; P1, precommunicating tract of the posterior cerebral artery.

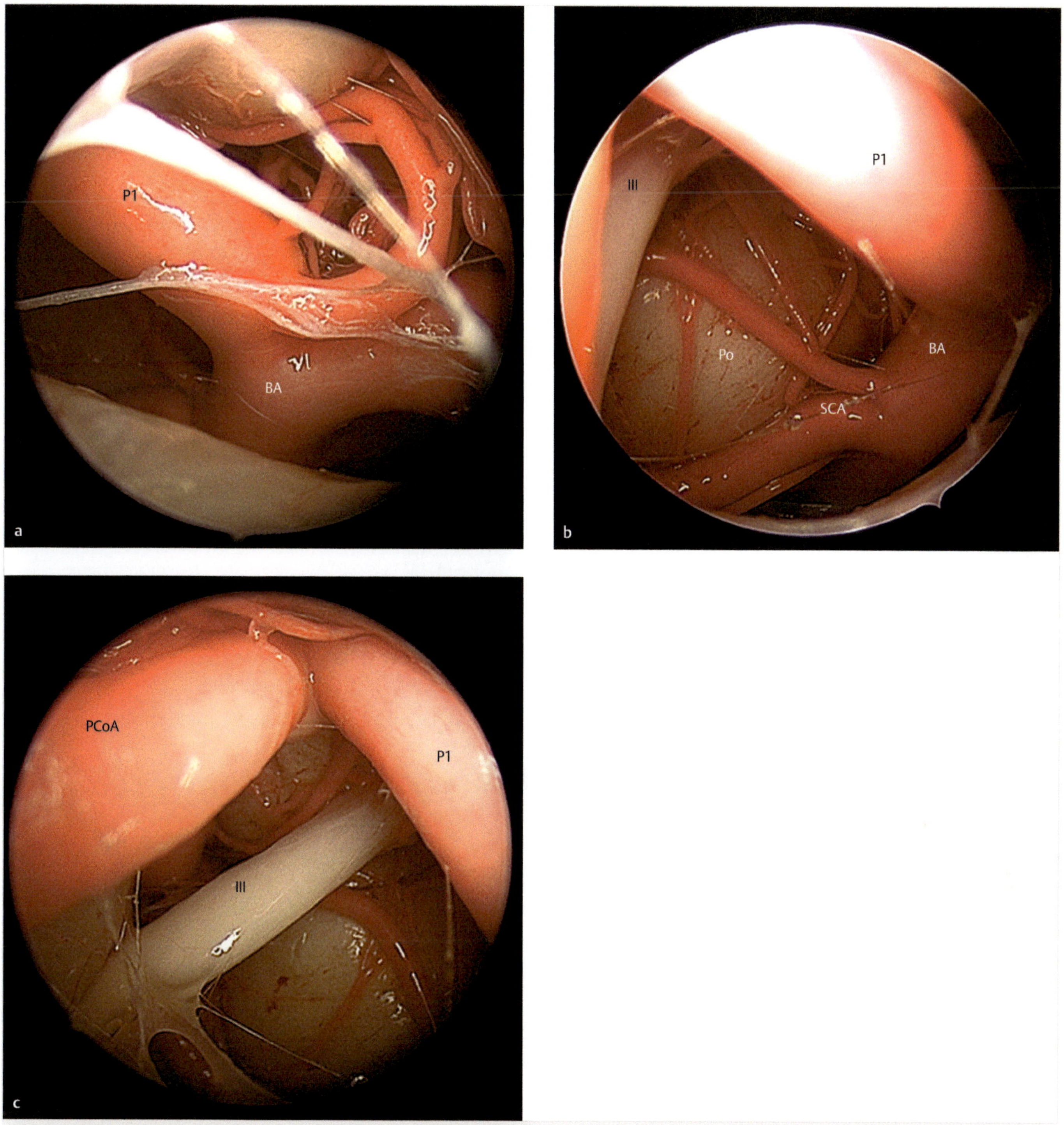

Fig. 8.26 (a–c) The interpeduncular and prepontine cisterns. A 70-degree scope is placed at the edge of the dorsum sellae and progressively turned from inferiorly to inferolaterally (toward the right side in the present figure). In this way, the precommunicating tract of the posterior cerebral artery (P1) comes into view together with the posterior communicating artery (PCoA), which runs parallel to the third cranial nerve (III). The posterior cerebral artery arises from the terminal bifurcation of the basilar artery (BA), which runs on the anterior surface of the pons (Po). The superior cerebellar artery (SCA) arises from the basilar artery, inferior to the posterior cerebral artery; the oculomotor nerve passes between the superior cerebellar artery inferiorly and the posterior cerebral artery superiorly.

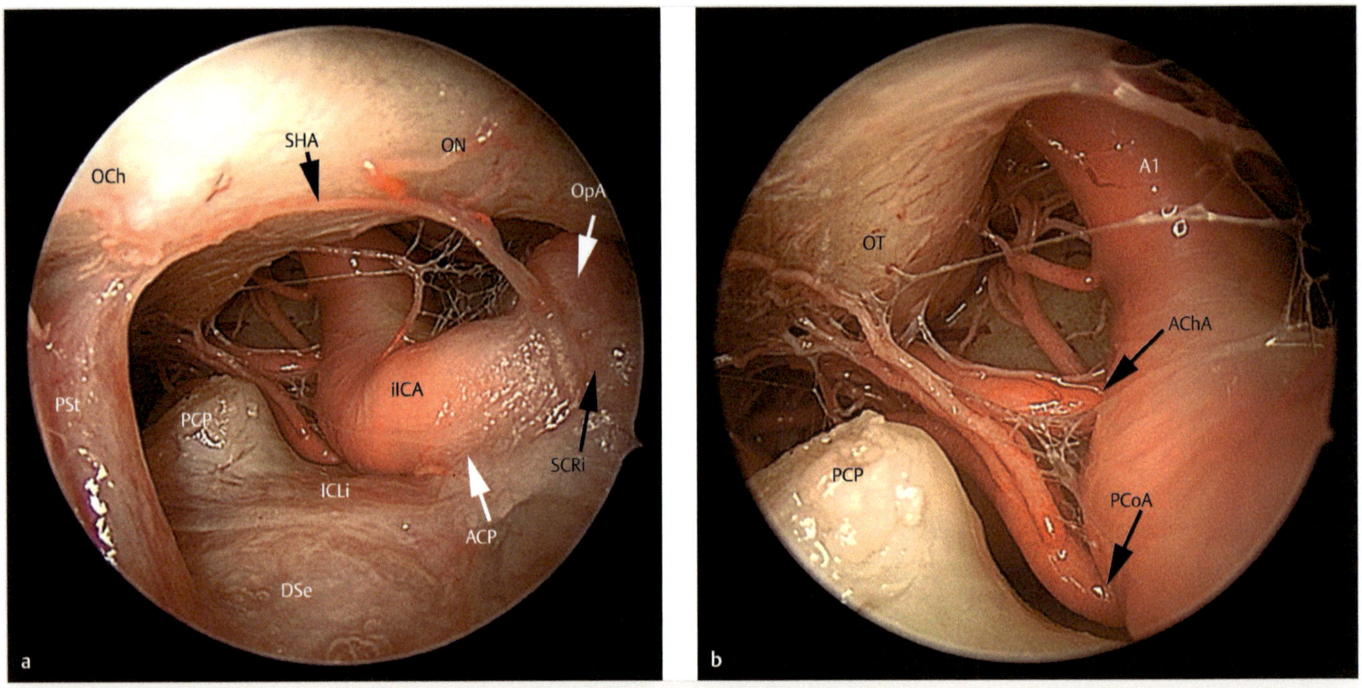

Fig. 8.27 (a, b) The intracranial tract of the internal carotid artery. A 70-degree scope turned laterally (toward the left side in this figure) is placed above the diaphragma sellae (DSe) and beside the pituitary stalk (PSt) to identify the intracranial portion of the internal carotid artery (iICA). This tract begins just distally to the superior (or distal) carotid ring (SCRi), which is attached to the anterior clinoid process (ACP). The ophthalmic artery (OpA) arises just after the internal carotid artery passes through the superior dural ring, usually from the superior surface of the vessel. However, sometimes this artery can arise from other portions of the internal carotid artery, including the parasellar or paraclinoid tracts, as well as from other intracranial vessels. The superior hypophyseal arteries (SHA), which are classified in anterior and posterior with respect to the pituitary stalk, arise from the medial surface of the intracranial tract of the internal carotid artery and run toward the optic nerve (ON), chiasm (OCh), optic tract (OT), and pituitary stalk. Before bifurcating into the anterior (A1) and middle cerebral arteries, the internal carotid artery gives two further branches: the posterior communicating artery (PCoA) proximally and the anterior choroidal artery (AChA) distally. These arteries commonly arise from the medial surface of the internal carotid artery, superolaterally to the posterior clinoid process (PCP) and interclinoid ligament (ICLi), and give some branches to the optic tract. The intracranial tract of the internal carotid artery is further classified in ophthalmic, communicating, and choroidal segments, which are centered on the point of origin of the respective vessel.

References

[1] Laufer I, Anand VK, Schwartz TH. Endoscopic, endonasal extended transsphenoidal, transplanum transtuberculum approach for resection of suprasellar lesions. J Neurosurg 2007;106(3):400–406

[2] Cavallo LM, de Divitiis O, Aydin S, et al. Extended endoscopic endonasal transsphenoidal approach to the suprasellar area: anatomic considerations—part 1. Neurosurgery 2007;61(3, Suppl):24–33, discussion 33–34

[3] Kassam A, Snyderman CH, Mintz A, Gardner P, Carrau RL. Expanded endonasal approach: the rostrocaudal axis. Part I. Crista galli to the sella turcica. Neurosurg Focus 2005;19(1):E3

[4] Barazi SA, Pasquini E, D'Urso PI, et al. Extended endoscopic transplanum-transtuberculum approach for pituitary adenomas. Br J Neurosurg 2013;27(3):374–382

[5] Liu JK, Christiano LD, Patel SK, Tubbs RS, Eloy JA. Surgical nuances for removal of tuberculum sellae meningiomas with optic canal involvement using the endoscopic endonasal extended transsphenoidal transplanum transtuberculum approach. Neurosurg Focus 2011;30(5):E2

[6] Sankhla SK, Jayashankar N, Khan GM. Extended endoscopic endonasal transsphenoidal approach for retrochiasmatic craniopharyngioma: surgical technique and results. J Pediatr Neurosci 2015;10(4):308–316

[7] Liu JK, Christiano LD, Patel SK, Eloy JA. Surgical nuances for removal of retrochiasmatic craniopharyngioma via the endoscopic endonasal extended transsphenoidal transplanum transtuberculum approach. Neurosurg Focus 2011;30(4):E14

[8] Liu JK, Eloy JA. Endoscopic endonasal transplanum transtuberculum approach for resection of retrochiasmatic craniopharyngioma. J Neurosurg 2012;32(Suppl):E2

[9] Cavallo LM, Solari D, Esposito F, Cappabianca P. The endoscopic endonasal approach for the management of craniopharyngiomas involving the third ventricle. Neurosurg Rev 2013;36(1):27–37, discussion 38

[10] Hardesty DA, Montaser AS, Beer-Furlan A, Carrau RL, Prevedello DM. Limits of endoscopic endonasal surgery for III ventricle craniopharyngiomas. J Neurosurg Sci 2018;62(3):310–321

[11] Nishioka H, Fukuhara N, Yamaguchi-Okada M, Yamada S. Endoscopic endonasal surgery for purely intrathird ventricle craniopharyngioma. World Neurosurg 2016;91:266–271

[12] Zoli M, Mazzatenta D, Valluzzi A, et al. Expanding indications for the extended endoscopic endonasal approach to hypothalamic gliomas: preliminary report. Neurosurg Focus 2014;37(4):E11

[13] Kulwin C, Chan D, Ting J, Hattab EM, Cohen-Gadol AA. Endoscopic endonasal transplanum transtuberculum resection of a large solid choroid plexus papilloma of the third ventricle. J Clin Neurosci 2014;21(7):1263–1266

[14] Yoneoka Y, Yoshimura J, Sano M, Okada M, Kakita A, Fujii Y. Third ventricle germ cell tumor originating from the infundibulum with rapidly expansive enlargement. Pediatr Neurosurg 2018;53(1):49–54

[15] Froelich S, Cebula H, Debry C, Boyer P. Anterior communicating artery aneurysm clipped via an endoscopic endonasal approach: technical note. Neurosurgery 2011;68(2, Suppl Operative):310–316, discussion 315–316

[16] Mascarenhas L, Moshel YA, Bayad F, et al. The transplanum transtuberculum approaches for suprasellar and sellar-suprasellar lesions: avoidance of cerebrospinal fluid leak and lessons learned. World Neurosurg 2014;82(1–2):186–195

9 Transsellar Approach

Francesco Doglietto, Marco Ravanelli, Francesco Belotti, Marco Maria Fontanella

The transsellar endoscopic approach to remove pituitary adenomas represented the first application of the endoscopic technique to transnasal skull base surgery.[1–6] Subsequently, the same route was adopted for other rarer sellar tumors and tumorlike lesions.[7–10] This approach takes advantage of the natural corridor formed by the nasal cavities and sphenoid sinuses to approach lesions within the sella turcica through its anterior and inferior bony walls.

Different types of transsphenoidal accesses have been proposed in the literature, with the intent to minimize morbidity by precisely tailoring the sphenoidotomy to the need for cranial–caudal and medial–lateral exposure.[11,12] In line with this principle, submucoperiosteal–submucoperichondrial routes similar to those used for microsurgical resection of sellar lesions were developed to maximize the possibility of sparing nasal structures.[13] In summary, the basic concept is that the aperture of the sphenoid sinus should be tailored case by case, providing adequate exposure to safely and radically remove a sellar lesion.

As in general with endoscopic skull base surgery, the identification of bony landmarks is of utmost importance in transsphenoidal approaches. The transsellar corridor passes through the anterior and inferior sellar walls, whose boundaries are the tuberculum sellae superiorly, carotid prominences laterally, and clival recess inferiorly. Bony landmarks are not well evident in poorly pneumatized and/or multiseptated sphenoid sinuses. In fact, it is not infrequent that sphenoid sinus septa have a diagonal orientation inserting on the carotid prominence or sulcus, thus partially preventing a complete visualization of the sinus. More rarely, the sphenoid sinus can be poorly or nonpneumatized, thus requiring high expertise and possibly dedicated instrumentation (i.e., navigation and Doppler probe) to safely drill the sphenoid body to create an adequate corridor toward the sella.

The removal of the anterior and inferior sellar walls allows the exposure of the sellar periosteum. Within the sella, three planes of dissection in relation to the pituitary gland can be identified: the suprahypophyseal plane is enclosed between the pituitary gland and diaphragma sellae (this corridor can be considerably narrowed by arachnoid prolapse toward the sellar region or tumor expansion in the cranial direction); the infrahypophyseal plane guides toward the dorsum sellae and can be fully marsupialized toward the sphenoid sinuses by removing the sellar inferior wall; and the parahypophyseal plane lies between the gland and the medial wall of the cavernous sinus and is crossed in the inferior portion by the inferior hypophyseal artery. At surgery, these corridors of dissections within the sellar area are rarely required; however, their analysis in the anatomic laboratory can be helpful to fully understand the relationships of the sellar content with neighboring anatomical regions.

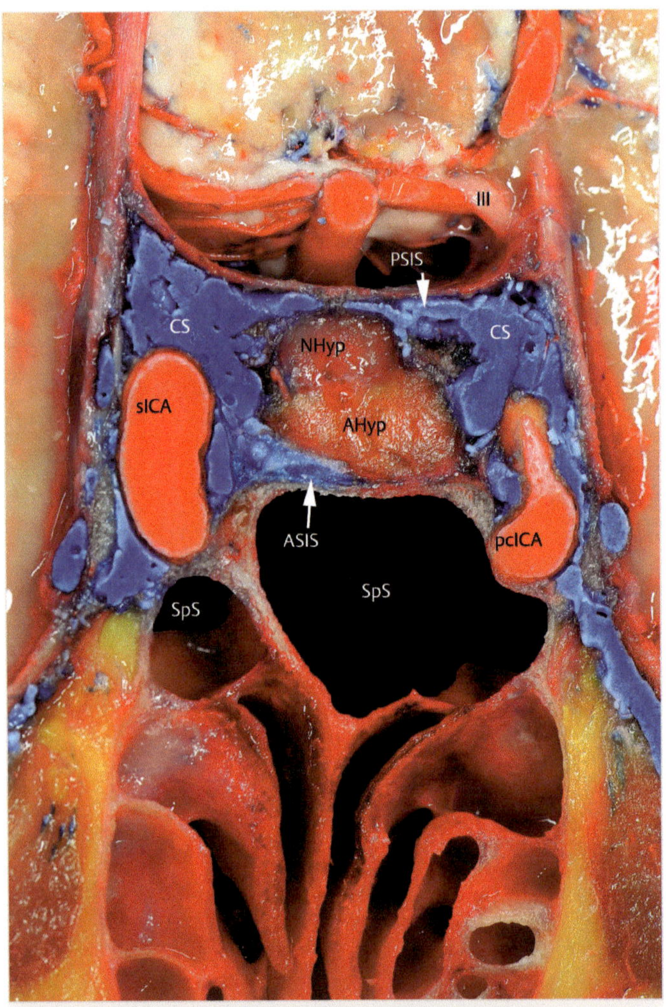

Fig. 9.1 Axial view of the sellar area. This cadaver axial cut shows the anatomy of the sellar area. III, oculomotor nerve; AHyp, adenohypophysis; ASIS, anterosuperior cavernous sinus; CS, cavernous sinus; NHyp, neurohypophysis; PSIS, posterosuperior intercavernous sinus; sICA, parasellar tract of the internal carotid artery; SpS, sphenoid sinus.

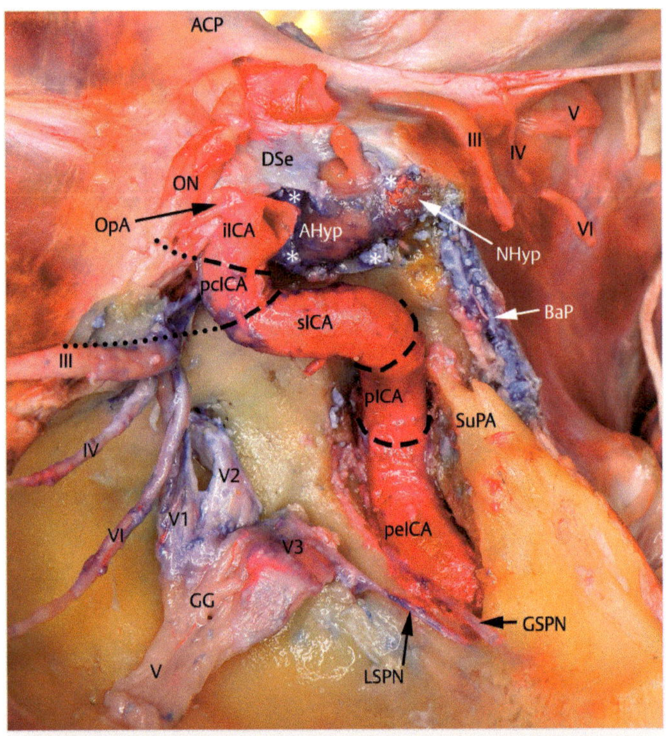

Fig. 9.2 Intracranial view of the sellar area. This cadaver picture shows the anatomy of the sellar area as seen from superolateral to inferomedial. Cranial nerves on the left side have been displaced anteriorly to show the underlying skull base. III, oculomotor nerve; IV, trochlear nerve; V, trigeminal stem; V1, ophthalmic nerve; V2, maxillary nerve; V3, mandibular nerve; VI, abducens nerve; ACP, anterior clinoid process; AHyp, adenohypophysis; DSe, diaphragma sellae; GG, gasserian ganglion; GSPN, greater superficial petrosal nerve; iICA, intracranial tract of the internal carotid artery; LSPN, lesser superficial petrosal nerve; NHyp, neurohypophysis; ON, optic nerve; OpA, ophthalmic artery; pcICA, paraclinoid tract of the internal carotid artery; peICA, petrous tract of the internal carotid artery; pICA, paraclival tract of the internal carotid artery; sICA, parasellar tract of the internal carotid artery; SuPA, superior portion of the petrous apex. (*Black dashed lines*, boundaries between different tracts of the internal carotid artery; *black dotted lines*, profile of the left anterior clinoid process [removed]; *white asterisks*, intercavernous sinuses).

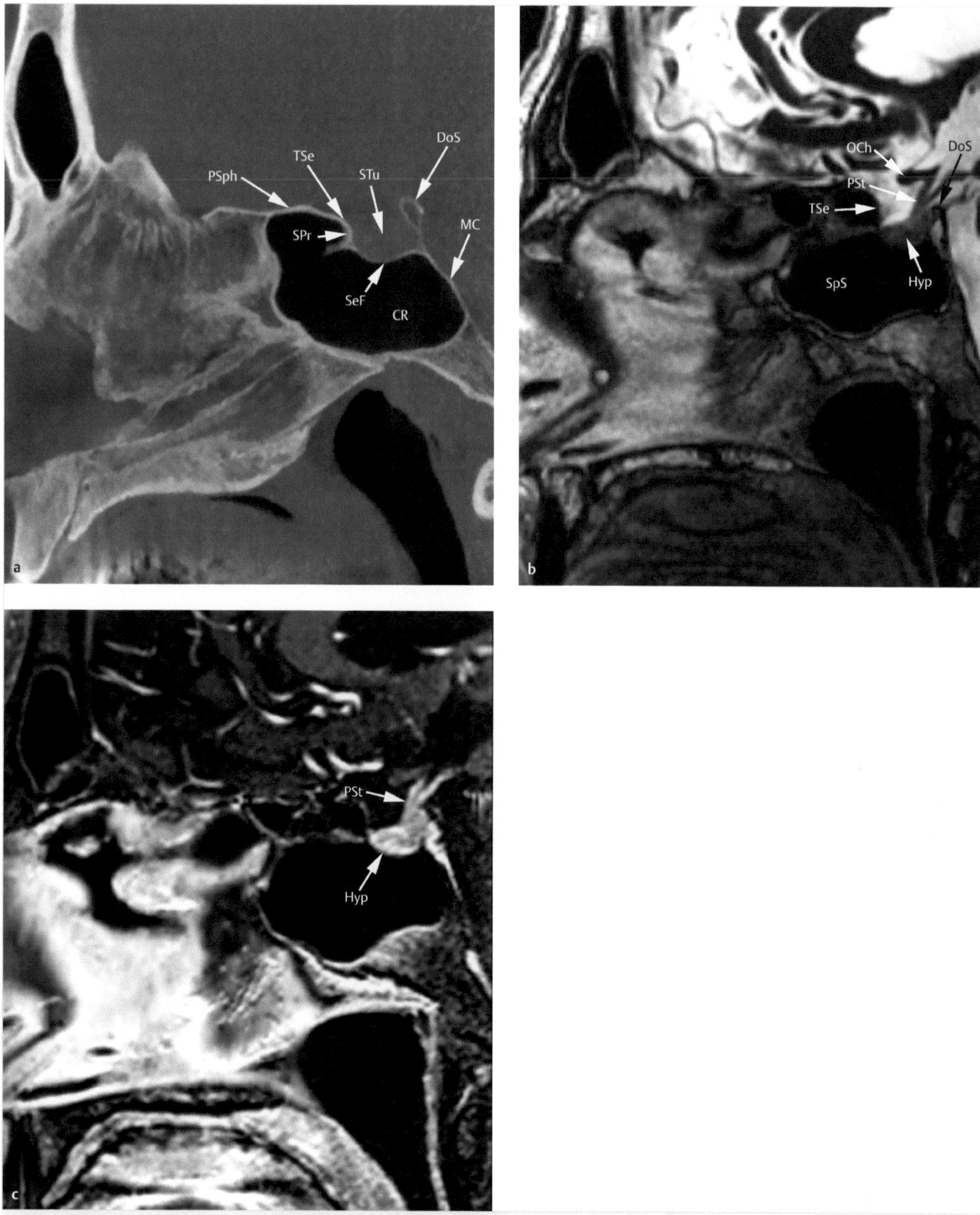

Fig. 9.3 Sagittal CT and MRI anatomy of the sellar region. The panel includes a midline sagittal CT **(a)**, constructive interference in steady state (CISS) MRI **(b)**, and T1-weighted contrast-enhanced fat-saturated MRI scan **(c)** passing through the sellar region. The sella turcica (STu) is bounded by the tuberculum sellae (TSe) and sellar prominence (SPr) anteriorly, sellar floor (SeF) inferiorly, and dorsum sellae (DoS) posteriorly. This space houses the hypophysis (Hyp), also called the pituitary gland. CR, clival recess; MC, midclivus; OCh, optic chiasm; PSph, planum sphenoidale; PSt, pituitary stalk; SpS, sphenoid sinus.

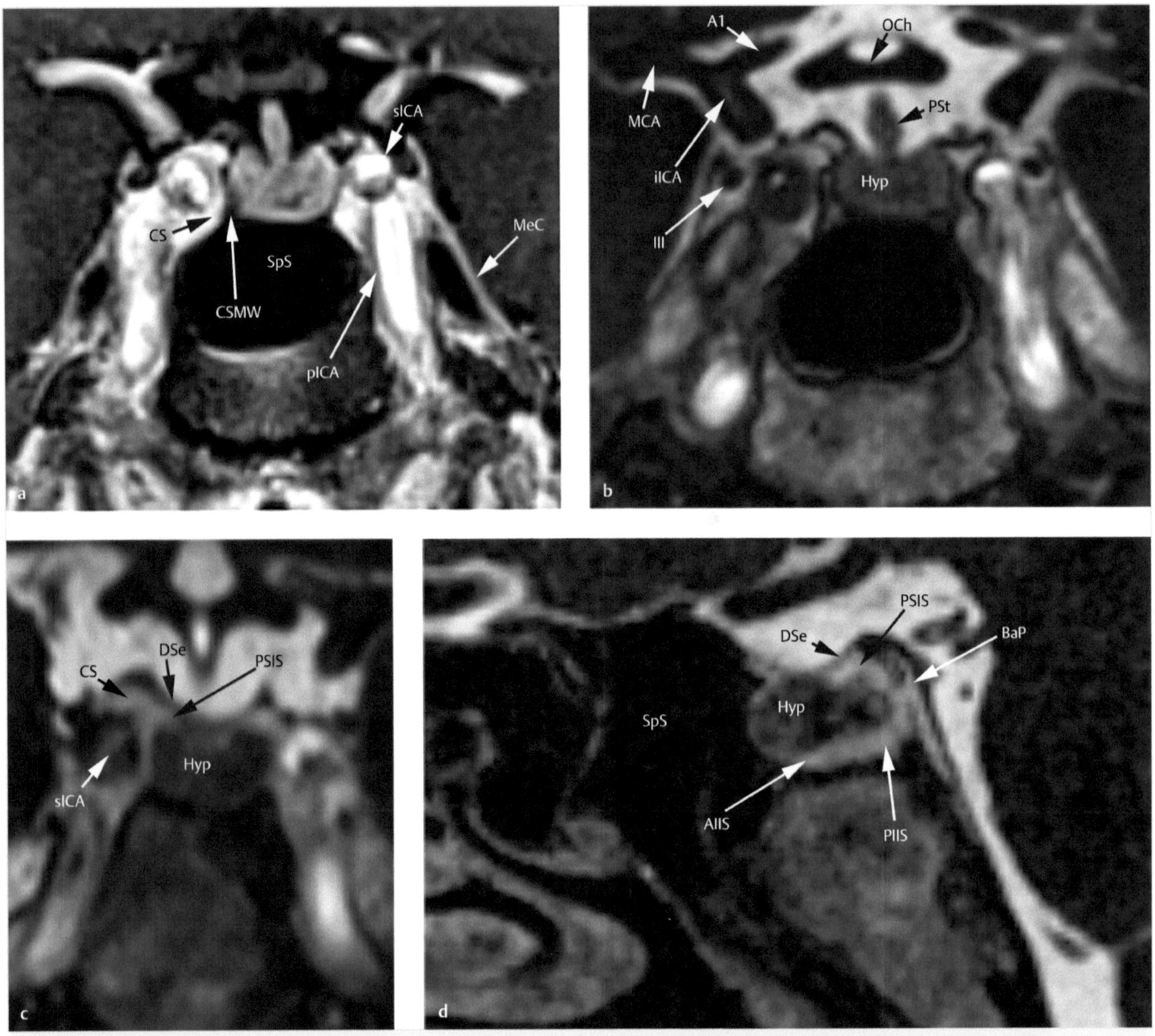

Fig. 9.4 Coronal and sagittal MRI anatomy of the sellar region. The panel includes a coronal T1-weighted contrast-enhanced fat-saturated **(a)**, two coronal **(b, c)**, and a sagittal constructive interference in steady state (CISS) MRI scans (lower right image) passing through the sellar region **(d)**. The hypophysis (Hyp) is bounded by the cavernous sinuses (CS) and para sellar tract of the internal carotid artery (sICA) bilaterally. A thin layer of connective tissue called medial wall of the cavernous sinus (CSMW) separates the sellar region from the cavernous sinus. The two cavernous sinuses are connected via the anterosuperior, anteroinferior (AIIS), posteroinferior (PIIS), and posterosuperior (PSIS) intercavernous sinuses. Cranially, the diaphragma sellae (DSe) separates the sellar region from the suprasellar cisterns. III, oculomotor nerve; A1, precommunicating tract of the anterior cerebral artery; BaP, basilar plexus; iICA, intracranial tract of the internal carotid artery; MCA, middle cerebral artery; MeC, Meckel's cave; OCh, optic chiasm; pICA, paraclival tract of the internal carotid artery; PSt, pituitary stalk; SpS, sphenoid sinus.

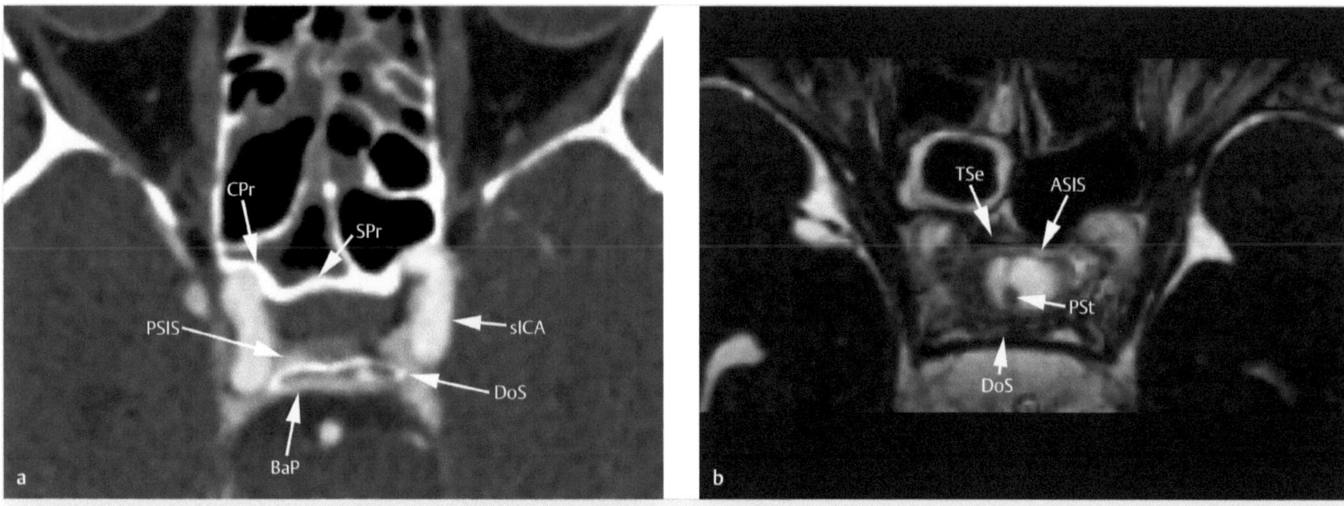

Fig. 9.5 Axial CT and MRI anatomy of the sellar region. The panel contains an axial CT **(a)** and an axial constructive interference in steady state (CISS) MRI scans **(b)**. The sellar region is bounded by the sellar prominence (SPr) anteriorly, which lies between the carotid prominences (CPr). The anterosuperior intercavernous sinus (ASIS) is located posterior to the tuberculum sellae (TSe). The posterosuperior intercavernous sinus (PSIS) and basilar plexus (BaP) lie anterior and posterior to the dorsum sellae (DoS), respectively. PSt, pituitary stalk; sICA, para sellar tract of the internal carotid artery.

Endoscopic Dissection

Nasal Phase

- Paraseptal sphenoidotomy.
- Transrostral sphenoidotomy.
- Facultative: extended transrostral sphenoidotomy.

Skull Base Phase

- Step 1: Removal of the sellar prominence.
- Step 2: Incision of the sellar periosteum.
- Step 3: Suprahypophyseal dissection.
- Step 4: Parahypophyseal dissection.
- Step 5: Infrahypophyseal dissection.

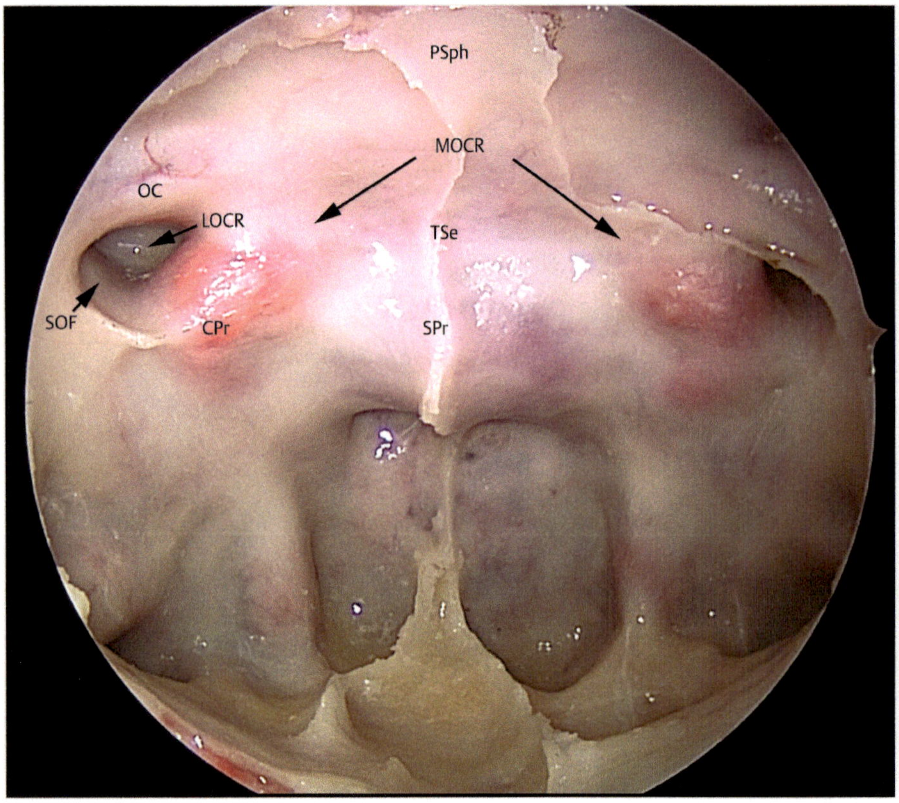

Fig. 9.6 Bony landmarks. After completing a transrostral sphenoidotomy and removal of sphenoid sinus septa, the anatomical landmarks of the posterior wall are visible. The sellar prominence (SPr) is located on the midline, between the carotid prominences (CPr). The tuberculum sellae (TSe) is visible between the medial optic-carotid recesses (MOCR), above the sellar prominence. The optic canal (OC) can have a variable appearance according to the lateral optic-carotid recess (LOCR) pneumatization. PSph, planum sphenoidale; SOF, superior orbital fissure.

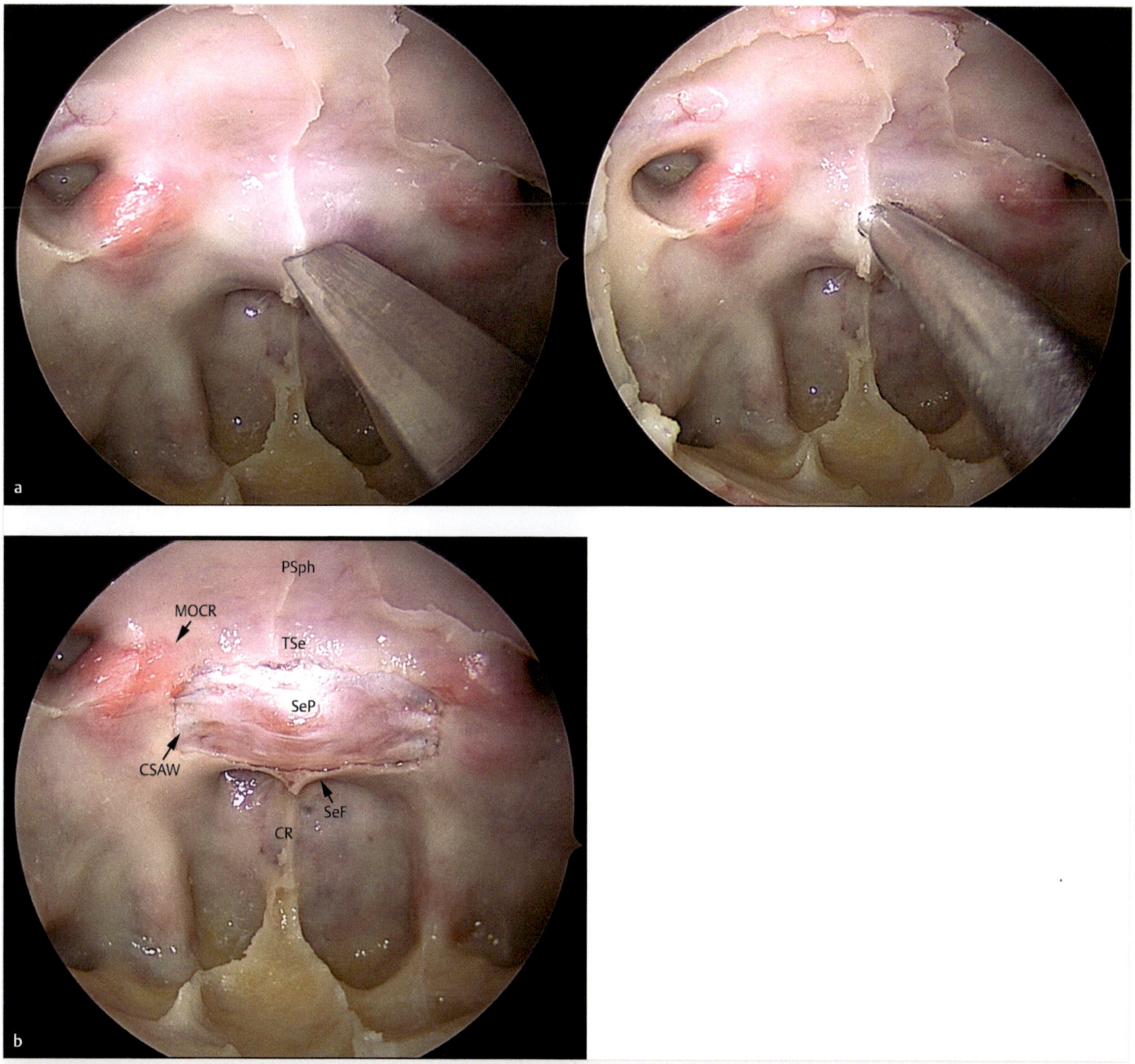

Fig. 9.7 (a, b) Step 1. The sellar prominence is fractured and removed to create a window from the tuberculum sellae (TSe) superiorly to the sellar floor (SeF) inferiorly and cavernous sinus anterior wall (CSAW) bilaterally. The sellar periosteum (SeP) is exposed. CR, clival recess; MOCR, medial optic-carotid recess; PSph, planum sphenoidale.

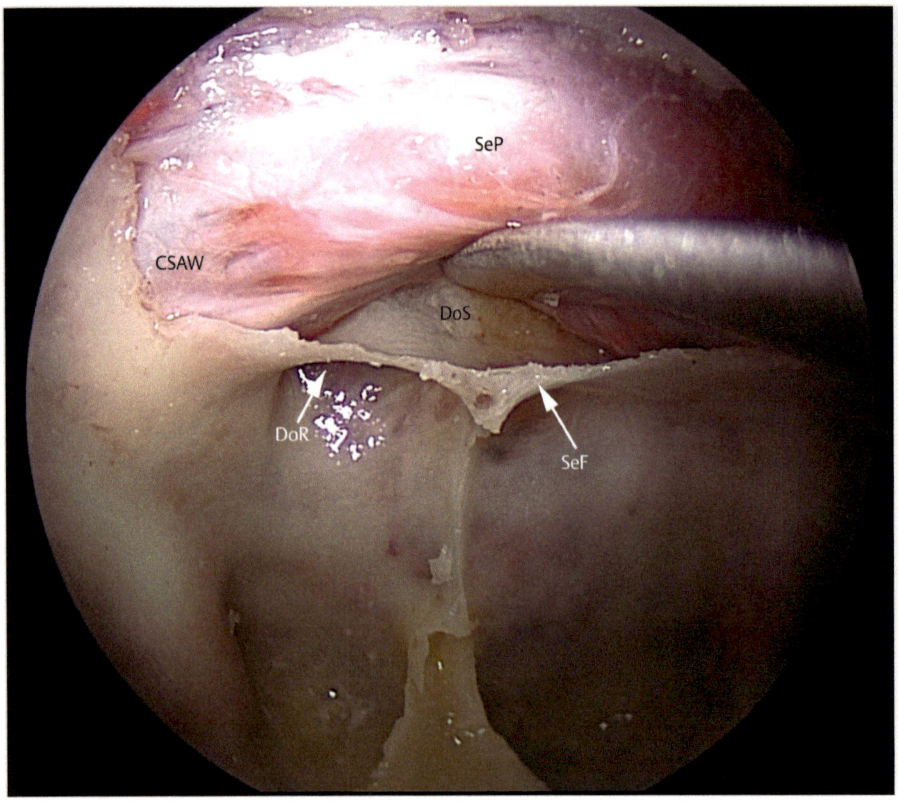

Fig. 9.8 Subsellar dissection. The dissection between the sellar periosteum (SeP) and sellar floor (SeF) exposes the inferior portion of the dorsum sellae (DoS). In this specimen, the dorsum sellae was pneumatized by a dorsal recess (DoR). CSAW, cavernous sinus anterior wall.

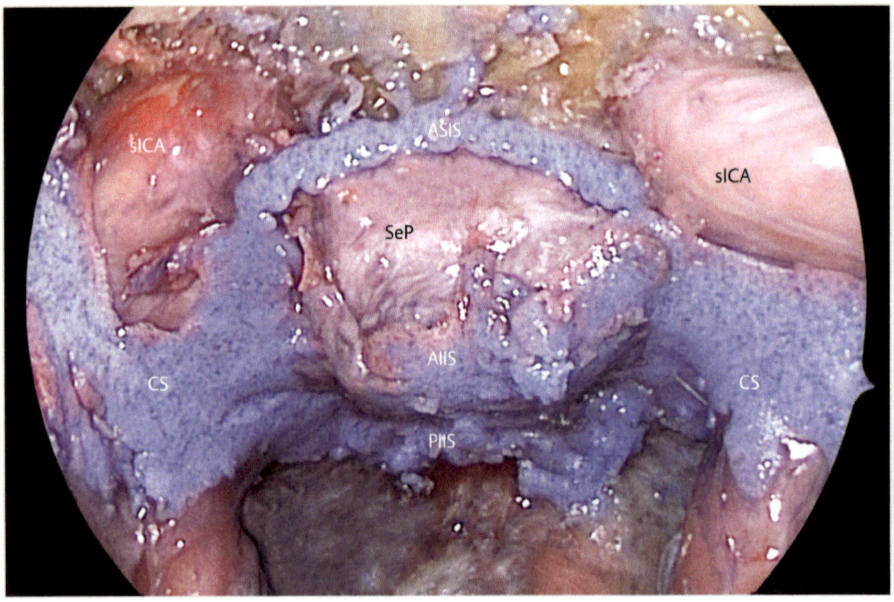

Fig. 9.9 Venous sinuses surrounding the pituitary gland. Four venous sinuses constitute the vascular boundaries of the anterior aspect of the pituitary gland. The superior border is represented by the anterosuperior intercavernous sinus (ASIS); the lateral borders are constituted by the cavernous sinuses (CS); the inferior border is the inferior intercavernous sinus, which is formed by the anteroinferior intercavernous sinus (AIIS) and posteroinferior intercavernous sinus (PIIS). SeP, sellar periosteum; sICA, para sellar portion of the internal carotid artery.

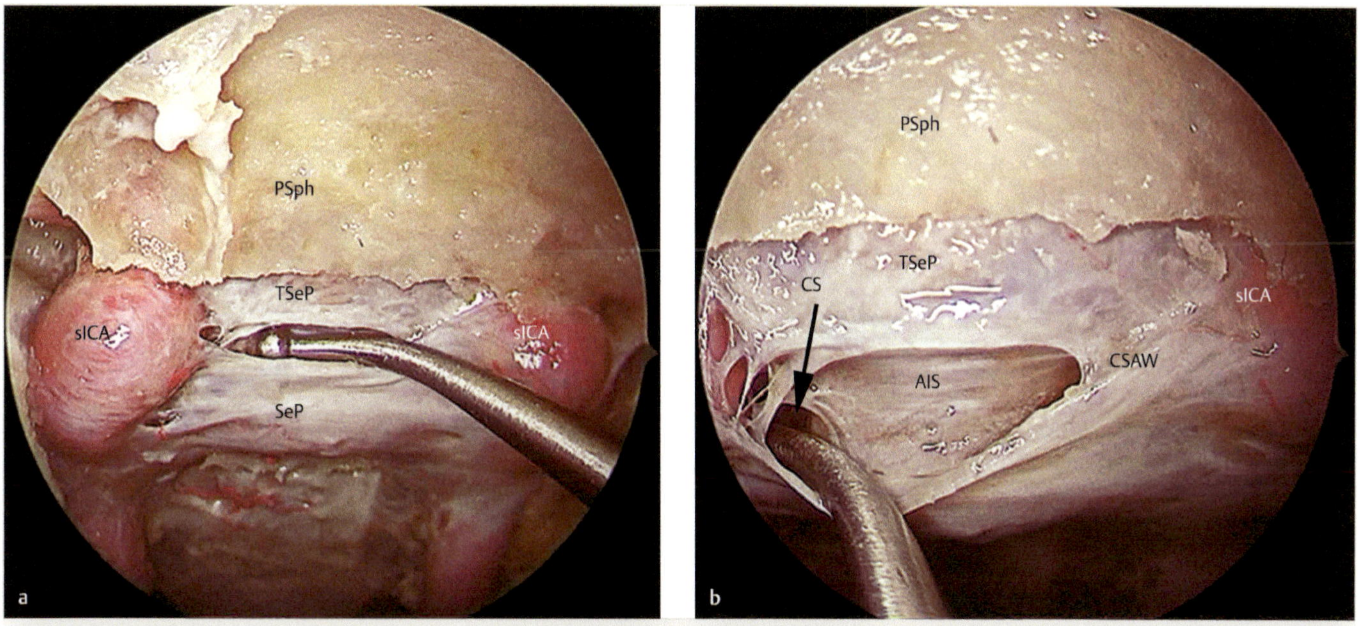

Fig. 9.10 (a, b) The anterosuperior intercavernous sinus. After opening the anterior wall of the anterosuperior intercavernous sinus (ASIS), a ball probe is inserted into the sinus to demonstrate the continuity with the cavernous sinus (CS). CSAW, cavernous sinus anterior wall; PSph, planum sphenoidale; SeP, sellar periosteum; sICA, para sellar portion of the internal carotid artery; TSeP, tuberculum sellae periosteum.

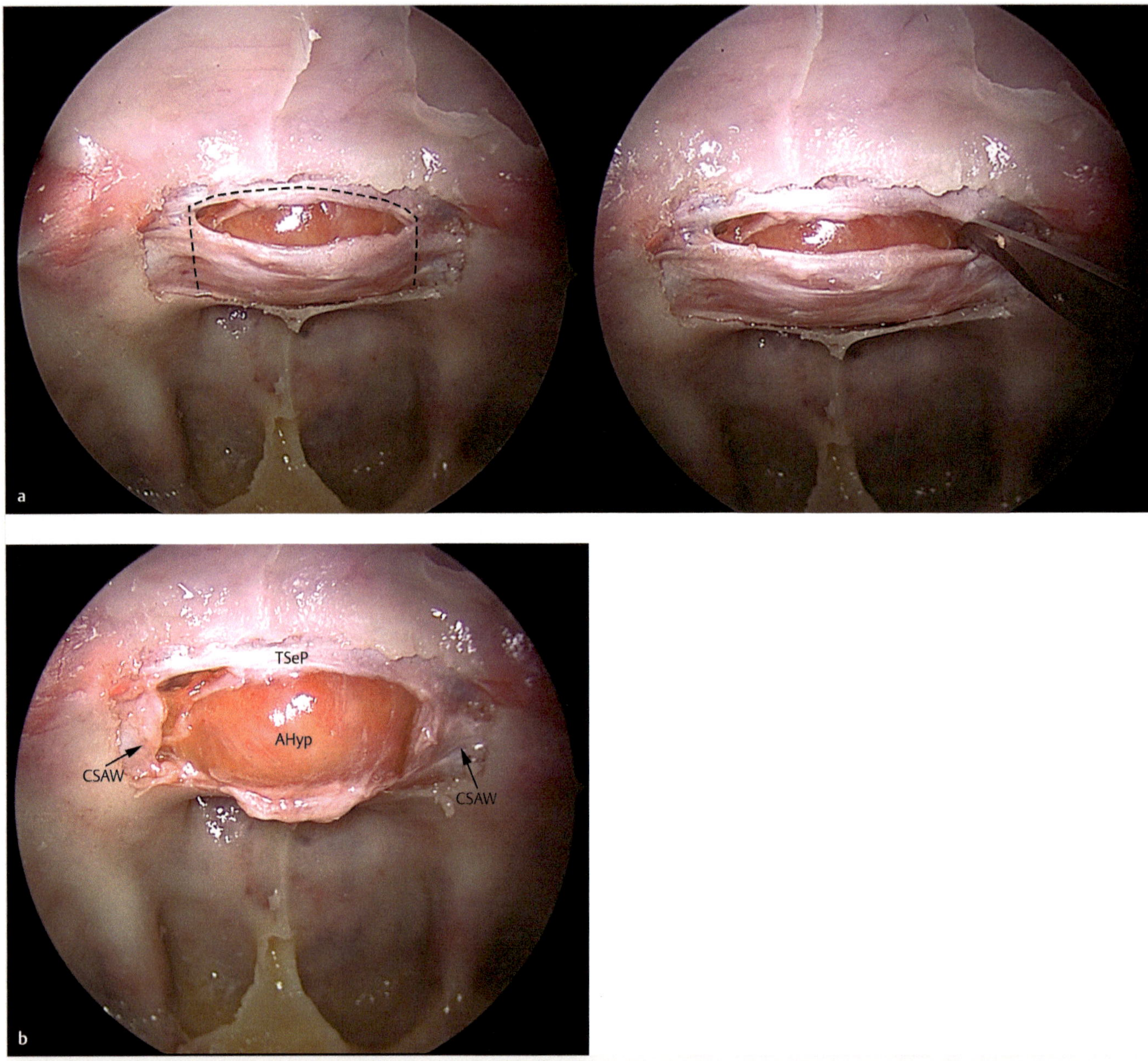

Fig. 9.11 (a, b) Step 2. A rectangular periosteal incision (*black dashed line*) is made on the sellar periosteum. The adenohypophysis (AHyp) is exposed medially to the cavernous sinus anterior walls (CSAW). TSeP, tuberculum sellae periosteum.

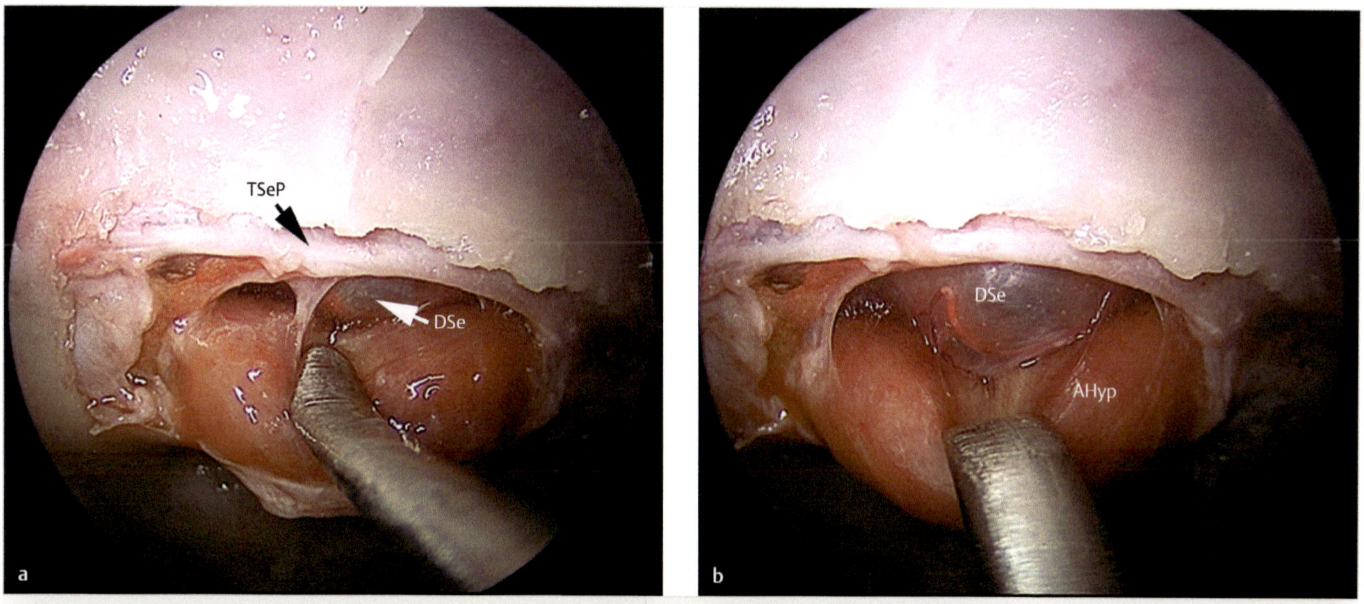

Fig. 9.12 (a, b) Step 3 (part 1). The adenohypophysis (AHyp) is pushed downward to create enough space between the gland and the tuberculum sellae periosteum (TSeP). Subsequently, the diaphragma sellae (DSe) comes into view above the adenohypophysis. The diaphragma sellae can variably bulge downward and adhere to the adenohypophysis, reducing the space granted by this plane of dissection. If the central opening of the diaphragma sellae is relatively wide, the suprasellar arachnoid can be visualized, as in this case.

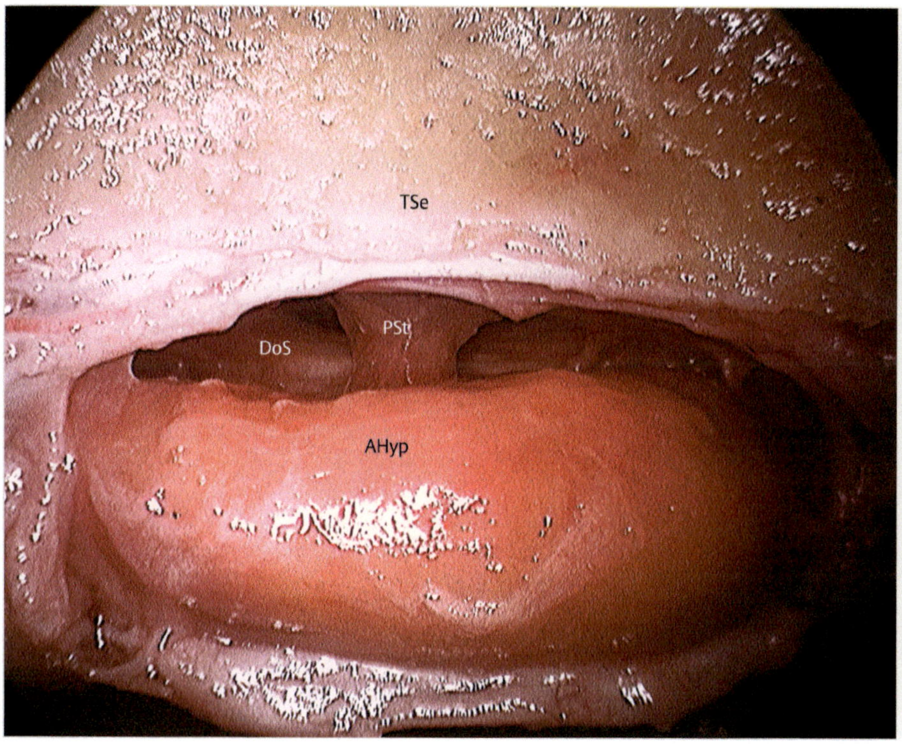

Fig. 9.13 Step 3 (part 2). The suprahypophyseal dissection provides exposure of the dorsum sellae (DoS) between the adenohypophysis (AHyp) and the tuberculum sellae (TSe). The pituitary stalk (PSt) is visible in the midline, above the pituitary gland.

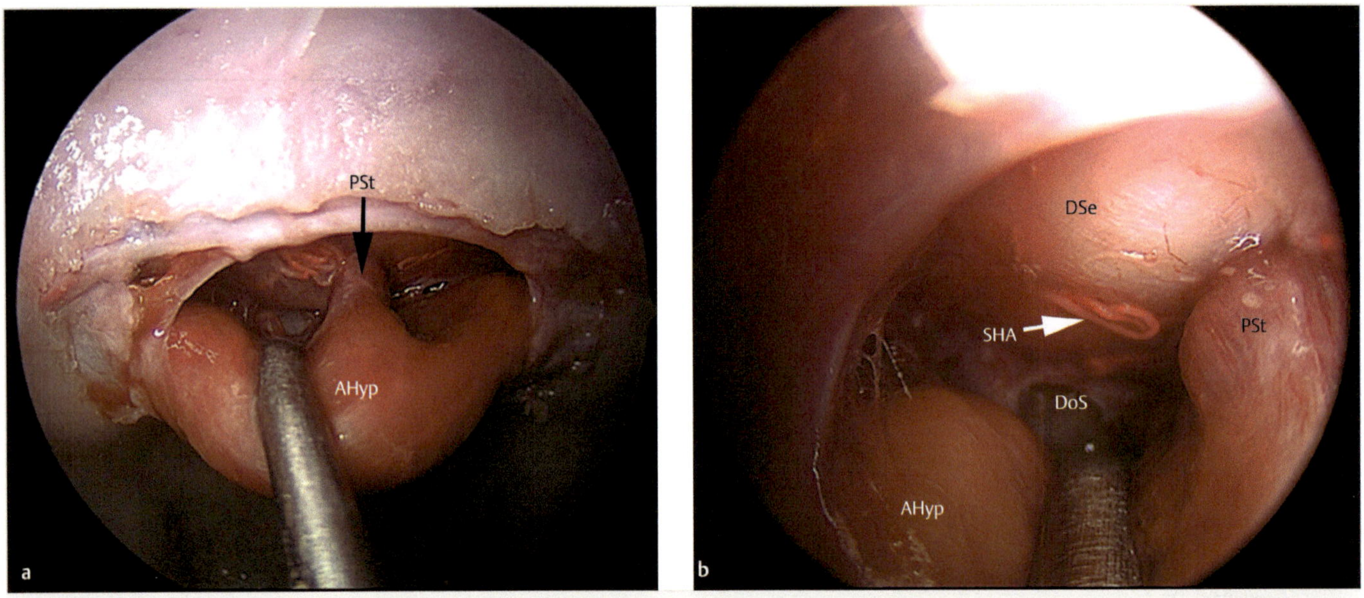

Fig. 9.14 (a, b) Step 3 (part 3). The hypophysis (or pituitary gland) is pushed downward to reach the dorsum sellae (DoS). The diaphragma sellae (DSe), which is thinned and dehiscent in this specimen, and the superior hypophyseal artery (SHA) are visible. AHyp, adenohypophysis; PSt, pituitary stalk.

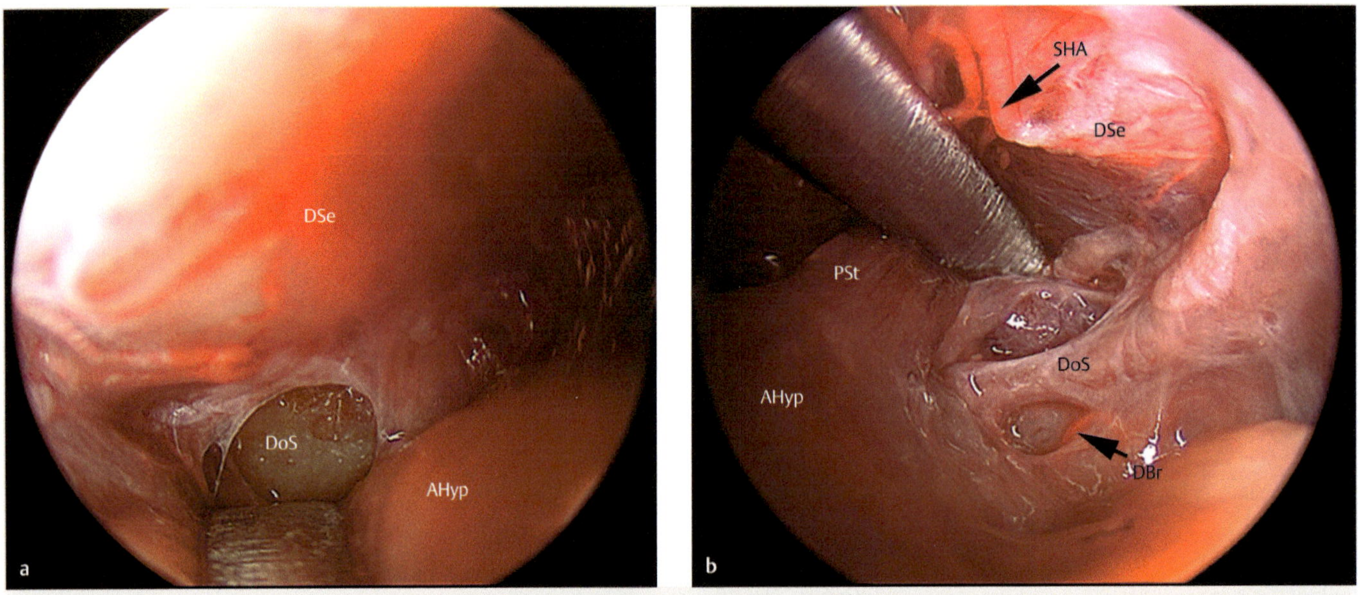

Fig. 9.15 (a, b) The superior portion of the dorsum sellae. The endoscope is placed above the hypophysis. The superior portion of the dorsum sellae (DoS), the superior hypophyseal artery (SHA), and the dorsal branch (DBr) of the meningohypophyseal artery are identified. AHyp, adenohypophysis; DSe, diaphragma sellae; PSt, pituitary stalk.

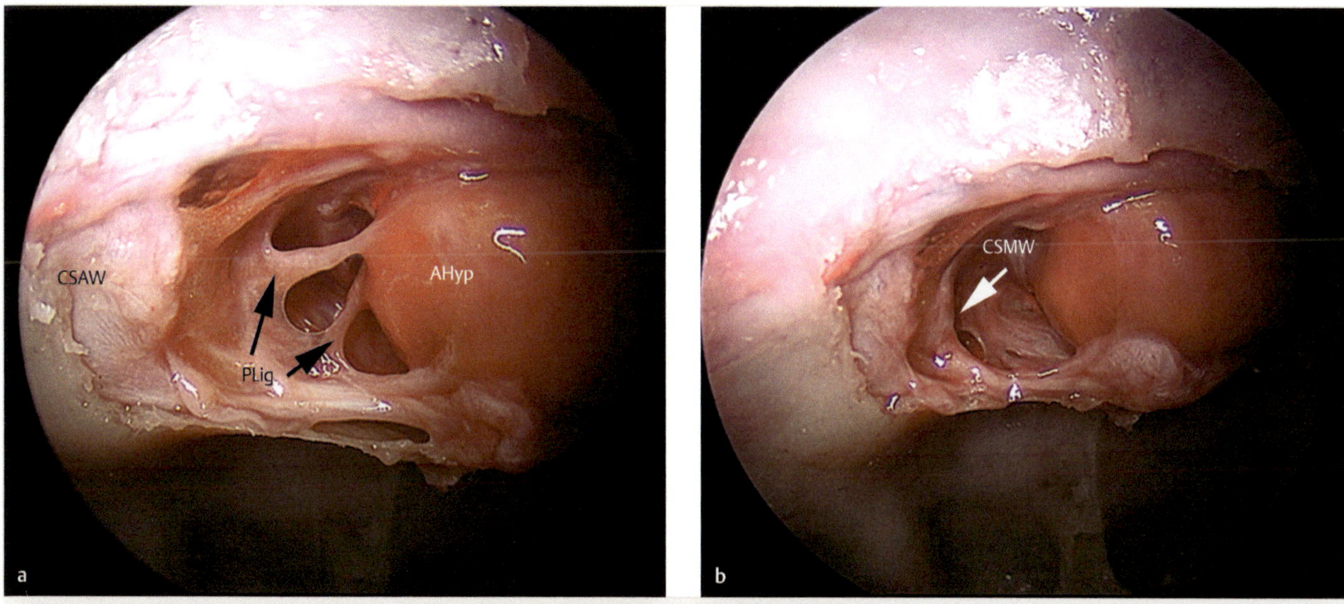

Fig. 9.16 (a, b) Step 4. The space between the cavernous sinus and the adenohypophysis (AHyp) is gently dissected to visualize the pituitary ligaments (PLig), which are cut to separate the cavernous sinus medial wall (CSMW) from the pituitary gland. In this specimen, the pituitary ligaments were multiple and thin, differently from those in the next figure. CSAW, cavernous sinus anterior wall.

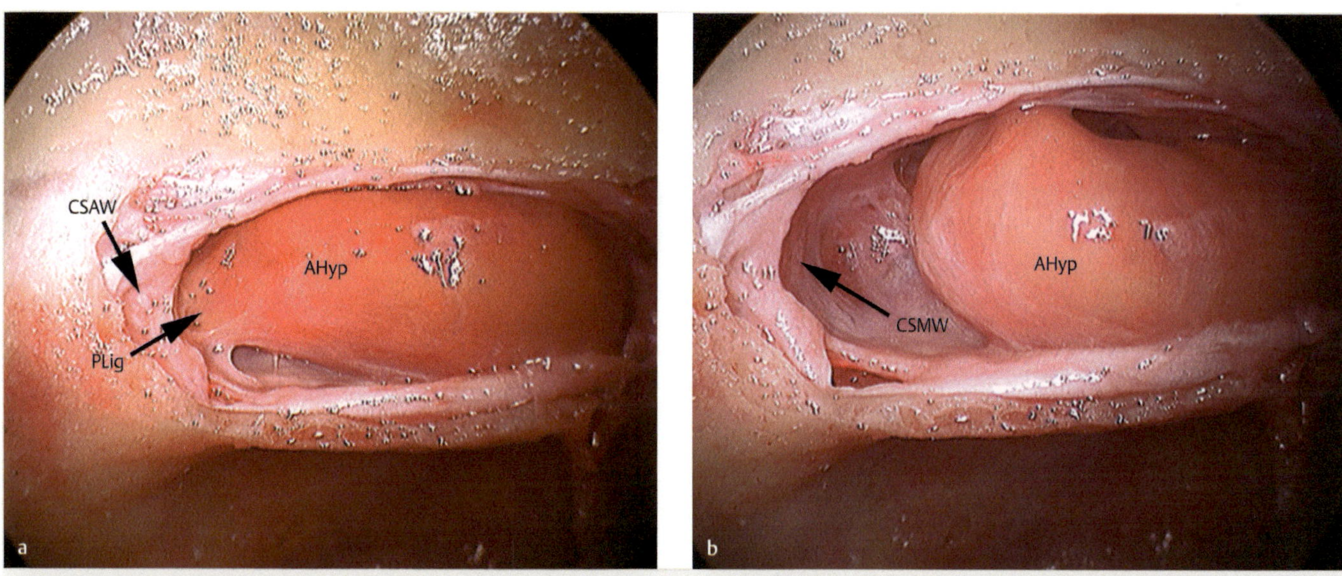

Fig. 9.17 (a, b) Variability of pituitary ligaments. Contrary to the previous figure, this specimen showed a single and thick pituitary ligament (PLig), which anchors the medial wall of the cavernous sinus to the adenohypophysis (AHyp). CSAW, cavernous sinus anterior wall.

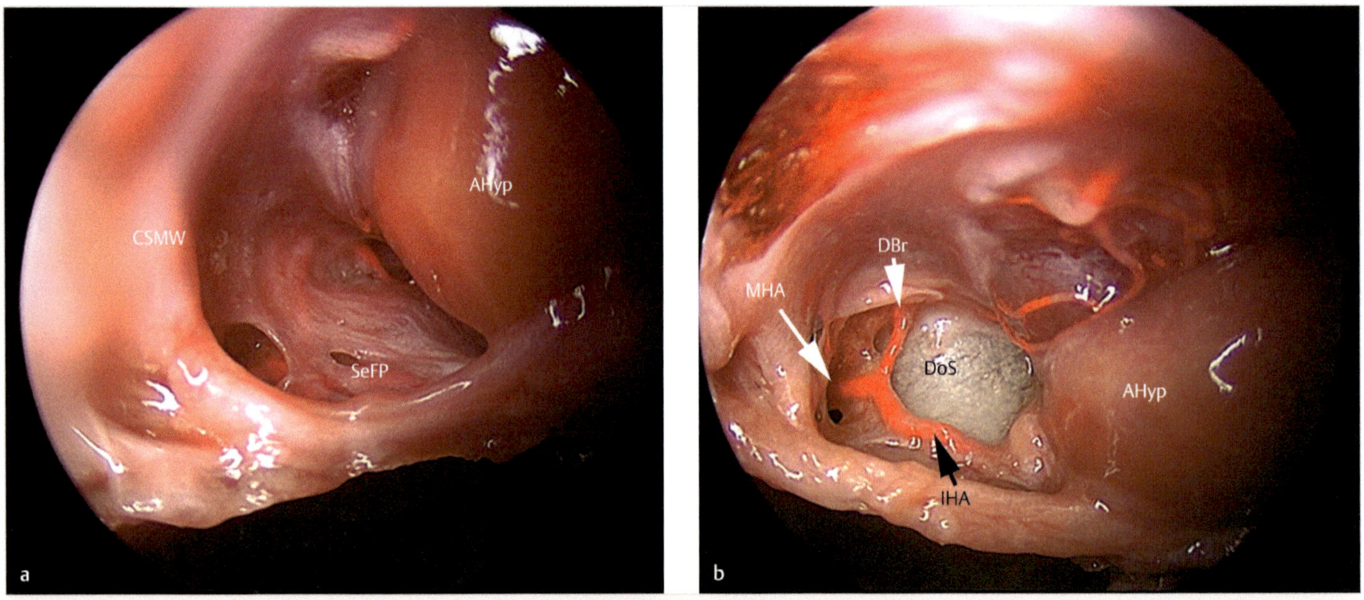

Fig. 9.18 (a, b) The inferolateral portion of the dorsum sellae. A 0-degree scope is inserted along the parahypophyseal plane of dissection to identify the dorsum sellae (DoS), medial wall of the cavernous sinus (CSMW), adenohypophysis (AHyp), and periosteum of the sellar floor (SeFP). The entire course of the inferior hypophyseal artery (IHA) can be seen, from the meningohypophyseal artery (MHA) to the pituitary gland. DBr, dorsal branch of the meningohypophyseal artery.

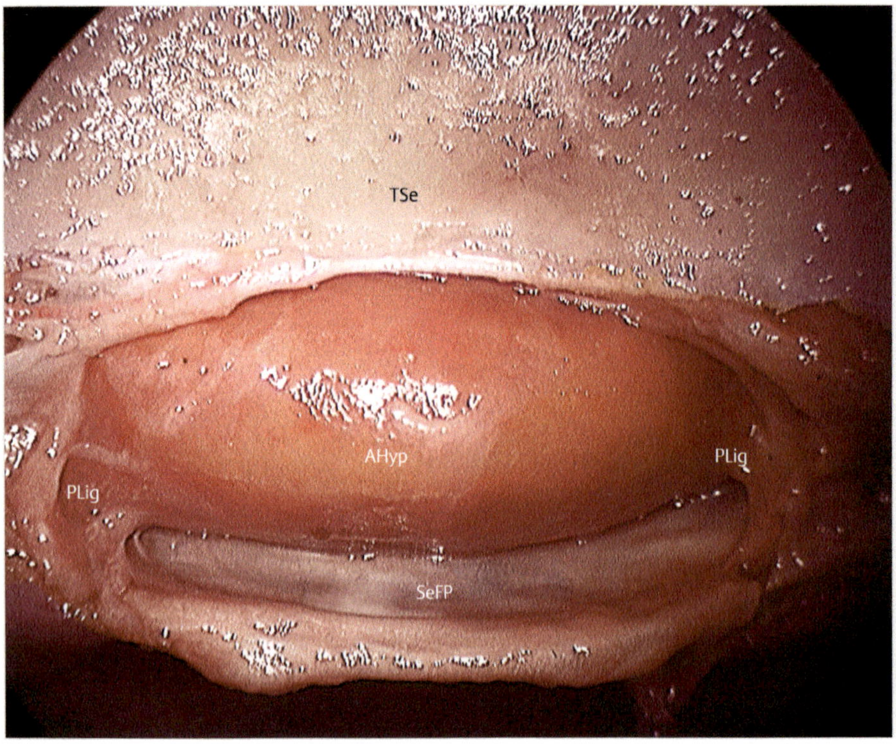

Fig. 9.19 Step 5. The hypophysis is gently separated from the periosteum of the sellar floor periosteum (SeFP). The preservation of the tuberculum sellae (TSe) prevents further elevation of the pituitary gland. AHyp, adenohypophysis; PLig, pituitary ligament.

References

[1] Doglietto F, Prevedello DM, Jane JA Jr, Han J, Laws ER Jr. Brief history of endoscopic transsphenoidal surgery—from Philipp Bozzini to the First World Congress of Endoscopic Skull Base Surgery. Neurosurg Focus 2005;19(6):E3

[2] Prevedello DM, Doglietto F, Jane JA Jr, Jagannathan J, Han J, Laws ER Jr. History of endoscopic skull base surgery: its evolution and current reality. J Neurosurg 2007;107(1):206–213

[3] Li A, Liu W, Cao P, Zheng Y, Bu Z, Zhou T. Endoscopic versus microscopic transsphenoidal surgery in the treatment of pituitary adenoma: a systematic review and meta-analysis. World Neurosurg 2017;101:236–246

[4] Dehdashti AR, Ganna A, Karabatsou K, Gentili F. Pure endoscopic endonasal approach for pituitary adenomas: early surgical results in 200 patients and comparison with previous microsurgical series. Neurosurgery 2008;62(5):1006–1015, discussion 1015–1017

[5] Jho HD. Endoscopic pituitary surgery. Pituitary 1999;2(2):139–154

[6] Jho HD, Carrau RL. Endoscopic endonasal transsphenoidal surgery: experience with 50 patients. J Neurosurg 1997;87(1):44–51

[7] de Divitiis E, Cappabianca P, Cavallo LM. Endoscopic transsphenoidal approach: adaptability of the procedure to different sellar lesions. Neurosurgery 2002;51(3):699–705, discussion 705–707

[8] Somma T, Solari D, Beer-Furlan A, et al. Endoscopic endonasal management of rare sellar lesions: clinical and surgical experience of 78 cases and review of the literature. World Neurosurg 2017;100:369–380

[9] Zoli M, Milanese L, Faustini-Fustini M, et al. Endoscopic endonasal surgery for pituitary apoplexy: evidence on a 75-case series from a tertiary care center. World Neurosurg 2017;106:331–338

[10] Bresson D, Herman P, Polivka M, Froelich S. Sellar lesions/pathology. Otolaryngol Clin North Am 2016;49(1):63–93

[11] Belotti F, Doglietto F, Schreiber A, et al. Modular classification of endoscopic endonasal transsphenoidal approaches to sellar region: anatomic quantitative study. World Neurosurg 2018;109:e281–e291

[12] Schreiber A, Bertazzoni G, Ferrari M, et al. Nasal morbidity and quality of life after endoscopic trans-sphenoidal surgery: a single-center, prospective study. World Neurosurg 2019;123:e557–e565

[13] Hong SD, Nam DH, Kong DS, Kim HY, Chung SK, Dhong HJ. Endoscopic modified transseptal transsphenoidal approach for maximal preservation of sinonasal quality of life and olfaction. World Neurosurg 2016;87:162–169

10 Transsellar Transdorsal Approach

Marco Ferrari, Marco Ravanelli, Francesco Belotti, Francesco Doglietto

The transdorsal approach constitutes the transnasal pathway through the upper third of the clivus and interpeduncular fossa. This surgical route requires a pituitary transposition (or hypophysiopexy) to create a straight transsphenoidal trajectory toward the dorsum sellae.[1,2] It has been adopted by expert teams to manage selected cases of chordomas, craniopharyngiomas, or meningiomas invading the dorsum sellae, interpeduncular fossa, and/or third ventricle.[1–5] Pioneering reports on the employment of transdorsal approaches to manage intracranial aneurysms have also been published.[6]

Three types of hypophysiopexy with increasing difficulty and risk for postoperative hypopituitarism have been described.[1,3] Extradural hypophysiopexy consists of a dislocation of the sellar content still protected by its periosteal envelope; this procedure (which is described in Chapter 11) represents an extension of the approach to the midclivus rather than a true transsellar transdorsal approach.[1,3] The interdural hypophysiopexy takes advantage of the corridor between the pituitary gland and sellar tract of the internal carotid artery, requiring the sacrifice of the ipsilateral inferior hypophyseal artery.[2,5] This anatomical route leads to the junction between the posterior wall of the cavernous sinus and the oculomotor triangle (i.e., the posterior half of the roof of the cavernous sinus) and can be exploited to reach the medial portion of the sylvian fissure.[7–9] Theoretically, this corridor can be harvested preserving the medial wall of the cavernous sinus, along either its medial (transsellar) or lateral (transcavernous) side. However, the medial wall of the cavernous sinus is frequently dehiscent and exceedingly delicate, thus being prone to laceration. Consequently, the variant of this approach, including the removal of the medial wall of the cavernous sinus, is described in the present chapter. Intradural hypophysiopexy consists of sectioning the diaphragma sellae on the midline, together with both inferior hypophyseal arteries, and transposing the pituitary gland in a cranial direction. This approach provides the widest upper transclival exposure among transnasal routes.[10] A partial transplanum–transtuberculum approach can be useful to control the most cranial portion of the surgical field. It is worth mentioning that most of the vascular supply of the pituitary gland comes from the inferior hypophyseal arteries. As a consequence, intradural hypophysiopexy is a procedure with a high risk for postoperative hypopituitarism.

Regardless of the specific type of hypophysiopexy, transdorsal approaches provide exposure of the interpeduncular fossa and related meningeal, vascular, and neural structures, creating the

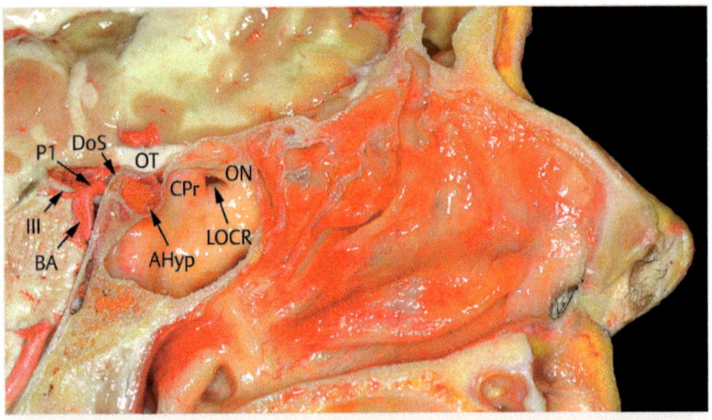

Fig. 10.1 Sagittal view of the route toward the dorsum sellae and interpeduncular area. This sagittal cadaver cut shows the trajectory from the nasal cavity to the sellar region and dorsum sellae. III, oculomotor nerve; AHyp, adenohypophysis; BA, basilar artery; CPr, carotid prominence; DoS, dorsum sellae; LOCR, lateral optic carotid recess; ON, optic nerve; OT, optic tract; P1, precommunicating tract of the posterior cerebral artery

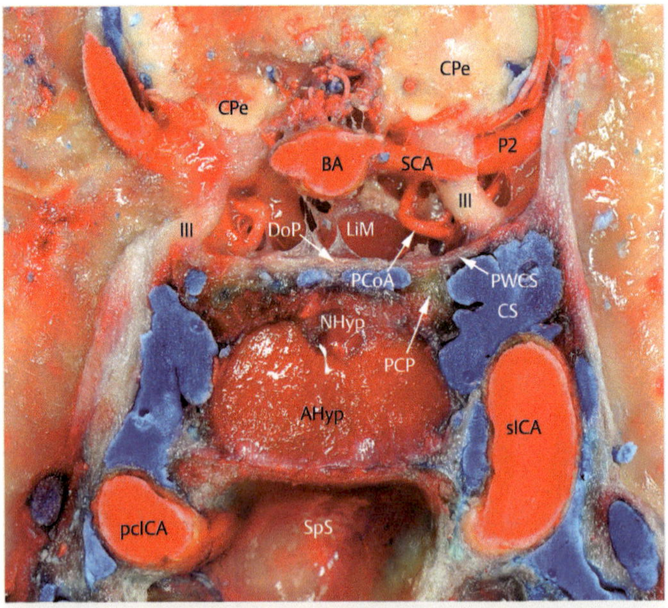

Fig. 10.2 Axial view of the dorsum sellae and adjacent structures. This axial cadaver cut shows the dorsum sellae and neighboring structures. III, oculomotor nerve; AHyp, adenohypophysis; BA, basilar artery; CPe, cerebral peduncle; CS, cavernous sinus; DoP, periosteum of the dorsum sellae; LiM, Liliequist's membrane; NHyp, neurohypophysis; P2, postcommunicating tract of the posterior cerebral artery; pcICA, paraclinoid tract of the internal carotid artery; PCoA, posterior communicating artery; PCP, posterior clinoid process; PWCS, posterior wall of the cavernous sinus; SCA, superior cerebellar artery; sICA, parasellar tract of the internal carotid artery; SpS, sphenoid sinus

route between parasellar carotid arteries bilaterally, sellar floor inferiorly, and transposed pituitary gland superiorly (or medially for the interdural hypophysiopexy).

After transgressing the dural layer, the arachnoid system of the posterior cranial fossa comes into view. The architecture and nomenclature of arachnoid membranes in this region are exceedingly complex and not universally accepted. Briefly, three groups of arachnoid membranes can be identified around the brainstem and cerebellum: (1) the tentorial group (which includes the posterior cerebral, lateral mesencephalic, superior cerebellar, and trigeminal membranes) is located adjacently to the tentorium and nearby the lateral surfaces of the mesencephalon and upper pons; (2) the clival group (which includes the Liliequist and anterior pontine membranes) lies between the clivus and the ventral surface of the mesencephalon and pons; (3) the perimedullary group (which includes the rhomboid membrane and denticulate ligaments) is formed by the arachnoid membranes surrounding the medulla oblongata and upper spinal cord.[11] The key arachnoid structure in this area is the Liliequist membrane, which compartmentalizes the cisterns in front of the brainstem and surrounds cranial nerves and vessels of this area. In the anatomy laboratory, meticulous removal of arachnoid is of paramount importance to completely expose the neurovascular structures of the cisterns.

As an additional anatomical exercise, the reader is suggested to perform an inferior third ventriculostomy to analyze one of the possible pathways followed by chordomas and craniopharyngiomas to reach the third ventricle.

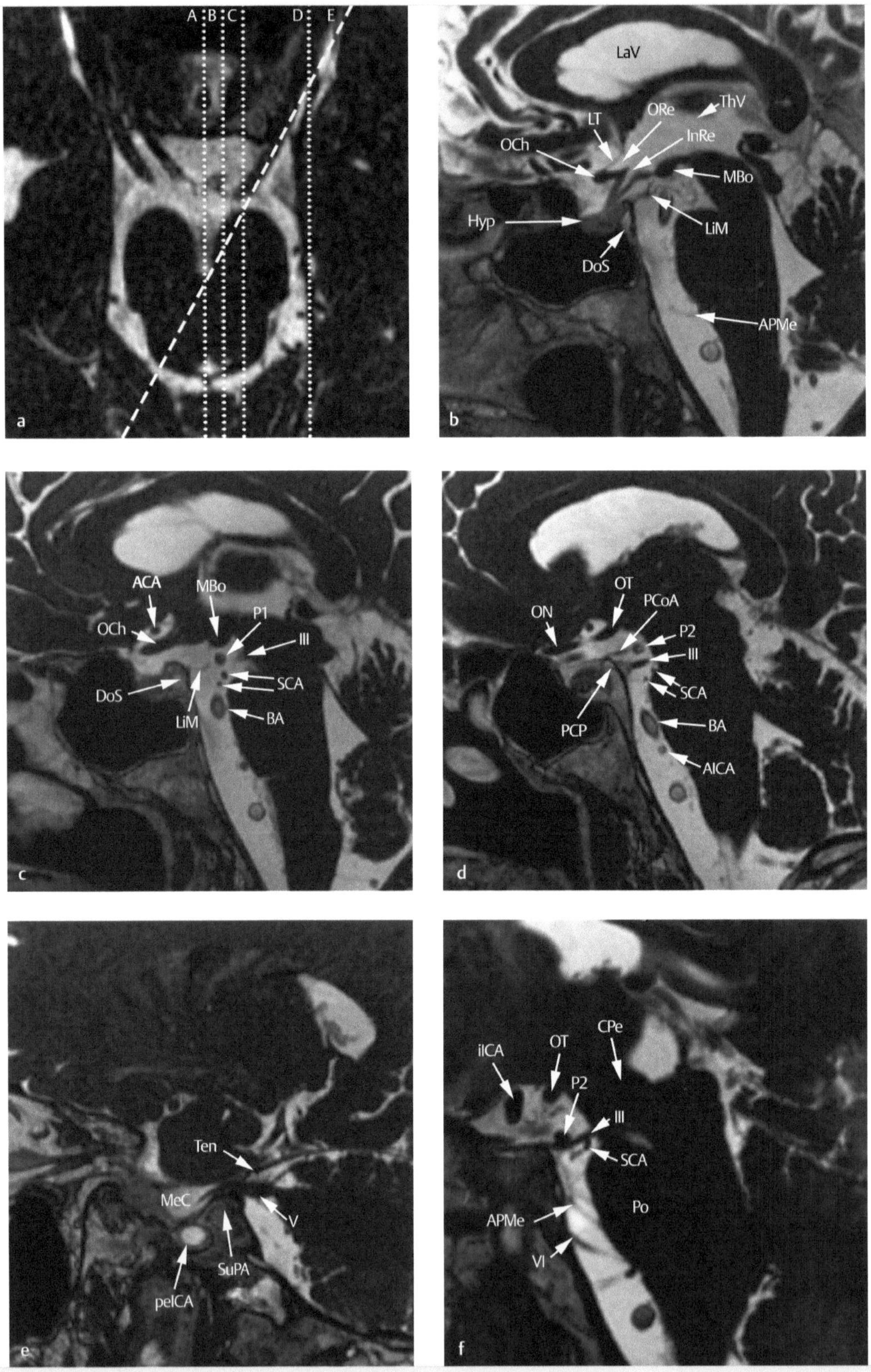

Fig. 10.3 Sagittal and parasagittal MRI anatomy of the lamina terminalis, optic, interpeduncular, and prepontine cisterns. (a) The upper left axial image summarizes the position of the following five sagittal (*white dotted lines*) and parasagittal (*white dashed line*) constructive interference in steady state (CISS) MRI **(b–f)**. The lamina terminalis cistern lies in front of the lamina terminalis (LT) and above the optic tract (OT) and chiasm (OCh). The optic cistern is enclosed between the optic chiasm and nerve (ON) superiorly and Liliequist's membrane (LiM) posteroinferiorly. The interpeduncular cistern is delimited by the cerebral pedicles (CPe) bilaterally and Liliequist's membrane anteriorly. Finally, the prepontine cistern is bounded by the anterior pontine membrane (APMe) anteriorly and pons (Po) posteriorly. The third ventricle (ThV) lies cranial to the interpeduncular cistern and shows an optic (ORe) and infundibular recess (InRe) toward the optic nerve and pituitary stalk, respectively. The oculomotor nerve (III) arises in the interpeduncular cistern and runs toward the cavernous sinus passing between the posterior cerebral artery and superior cerebellar artery (SCA), which can be double as in the present case. The posterior communicating artery (PCoA) runs parallel to the oculomotor nerve and above the posterior clinoid process (PCP), connecting the intracranial tract of the internal carotid artery (iICA) with the posterior cerebral artery. V, trigeminal stem; VI, abducens nerve; ACA, anterior communicating artery; AICA, anterior inferior cerebellar artery; BA, basilar artery; DoS, dorsum sellae; Hyp, hypophysis (pituitary gland); LaV, lateral ventricle; MBo, mammillary bodies; MeC, Meckel's cave; P1, precommunicating tract of the posterior cerebral artery; P2, postcommunicating tract of the posterior cerebral artery; peICA, petrous tract of the internal carotid artery; SuPA, superior portion of the petrous apex; Ten, tentorium.

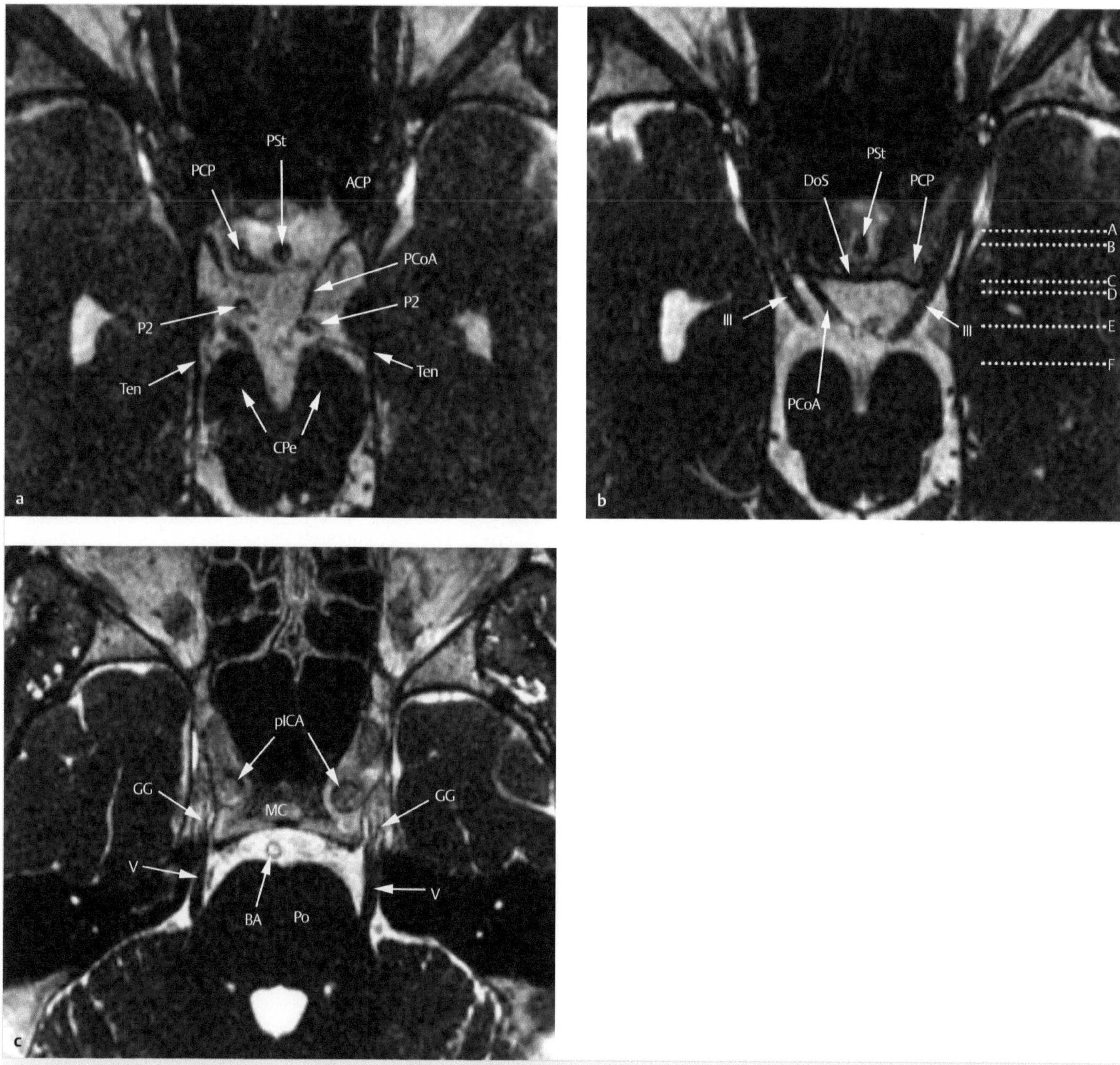

Fig. 10.4 Axial MRI anatomy of the interpeduncular and prepontine cisterns. The panel includes three axial constructive interference in steady state (CISS) MRI, from cranial **(a)** to caudal (lower image) **(c)**. The *white dotted lines* represent the position of the coronal images making up ▶Fig. 10.5. The posterior communicating artery (PCoA) arises from the posterior cerebral artery and reaches the intracranial tract of the internal carotid artery passing above the posterior clinoid process (PCP). This artery can maintain a remarkable caliber as a result of noninvolution of the fetal internal carotid artery. In particular, it is defined as "fetal posterior communicating artery" when it is larger than the precommunicating tract of the posterior cerebral artery. The oculomotor nerve (III) runs in the interpeduncular cistern, immediately below the posterior communicating artery, whereas the trigeminal stem (V) is located at the lateral boundary of the prepontine cistern. ACP, anterior clinoid process; BA, basilar artery; CPe, cerebral pedicle; DoS, dorsum sellae; GG, gasserian ganglion; MC, midclivus; P2, postcommunicating tract of the posterior cerebral artery; pICA, paraclival tract of the internal carotid artery; Po, pons; PSt, pituitary stalk; Ten, tentorium.

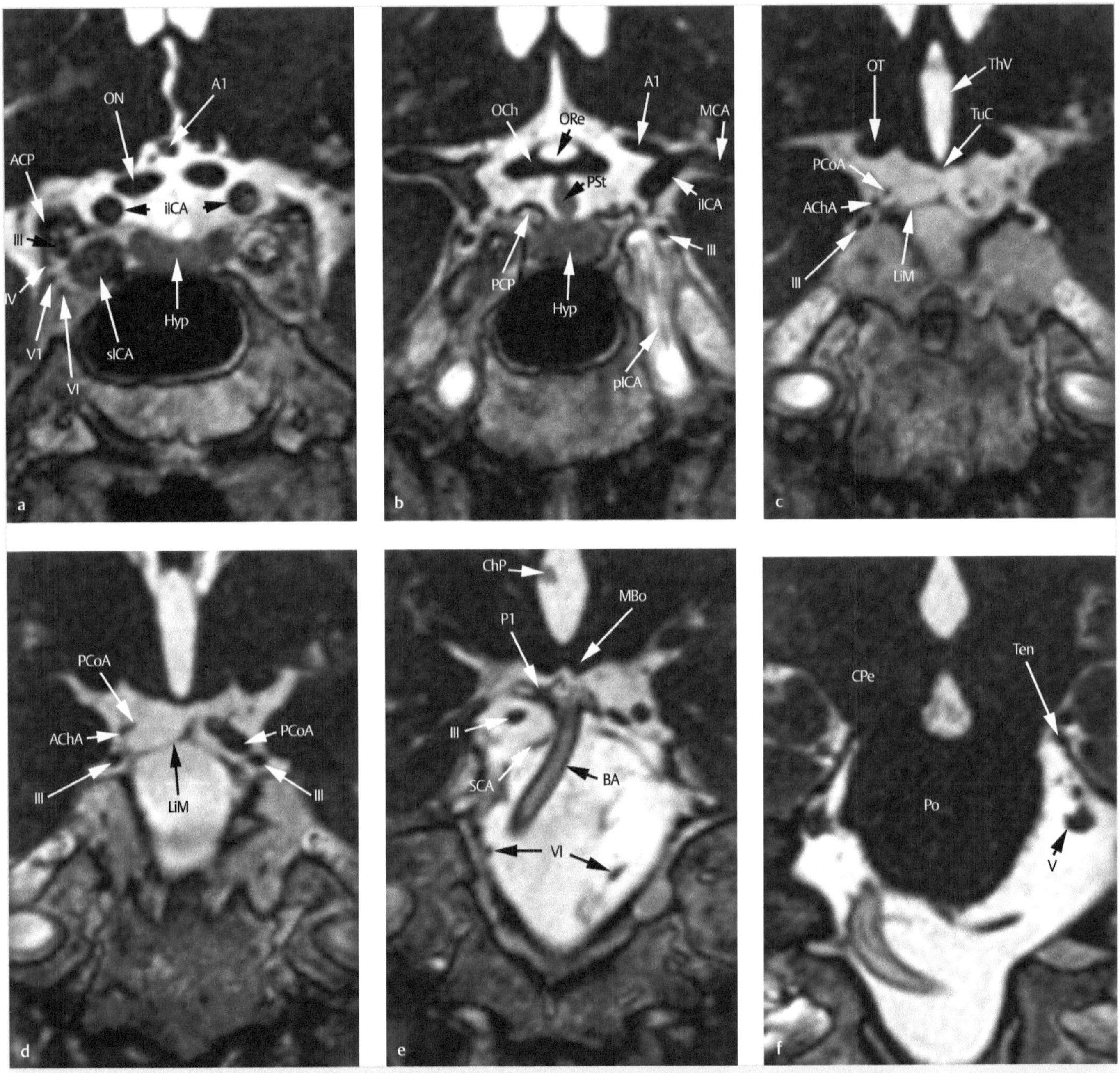

Fig. 10.5 (a–f) Coronal MRI anatomy of the interpeduncular and prepontine cisterns. The panel contains six coronal constructive interference in steady state (CISS) MRI passing through the interpeduncular and prepontine cisterns, from anterior **(a)** (upper left image) to posterior (lower right image) **(f)**. Liliequist's membrane (LiM) inserts anteriorly on the dorsum sellae and posterior clinoid processes (PCP) and reaches laterally the oculomotor nerve (III). This nerve enters the posterior half of the roof of the cavernous sinus and is surrounded by a narrow cistern. The anterior choroidal artery (AChA) and posterior communicating artery (PCoA) arise from the intracranial tract of the internal carotid artery (iICA) and run above the oculomotor nerve. IV, trochlear nerve; V, trigeminal stem; V1, ophthalmic nerve; VI, abducens nerve; A1, precommunicating tract of the anterior cerebral artery; ACP, anterior clinoid process; BA, basilar artery; ChP, choroidal plexus; CPe, cerebral peduncle; Hyp, hypophysis (pituitary gland); MBo, mammillary bodies; MCA, middle cerebral artery; OCh, optic chiasm; ON, optic nerve; ORe, optic recess; OT, optic tract; Po, pons; P1, precommunicating tract of the posterior cerebral artery; pICA, paraclival tract of the internal carotid artery; PSt, pituitary stalk; SCA, superior cerebellar artery; sICA, parasellar tract of the internal carotid artery; Ten, tentorium; ThV, third ventricle; TuC, tuber cinereum.

Endoscopic Dissection

Nasal Phase

- Paraseptal sphenoidotomy.
- Transrostral sphenoidotomy.
- Expanded transrostral sphenoidotomy.
- Facultative: anterior ethmoidectomy.
- Facultative: posterior ethmoidectomy.
- Facultative: transethmoidal sphenoidotomy.

Skull Base Phase

Intradural Hypophysiopexy

- Transsellar approach.
- Transplanum–transtuberculum approach.
- Step 1: Opening of the optic cistern, incision, and removal of the diaphragma sellae.
- Step 2: Opening of the lamina terminalis cisterns.
- Step 3: Infrahypophyseal dissection and sectioning of the inferior hypophyseal artery.
- Step 4: Intradural hypophysiopexy.
- Step 5: Removal of the posterior sellar periosteum.
- Step 6: Removal of the dorsum sellae and posterior clinoid processes.
- Step 7: Incision of the dorsal periosteum and dura mater.
- Step 8: Incision of the anterior pontine membrane.
- Step 9: Incision of the sellar and mesencephalic portions of the Liliequist membrane.
- Step 10: Removal of the diencephalic portion of the Liliequist membrane and other arachnoid membranes.
- Step 11: Ventriculostomy between the mammillary bodies and tuber cinereum.

Interdural Hypophysiopexy

- Transsellar approach (until exposing the sellar periosteum).
- Step 1: Incision of the sellar periosteum.
- Step 2: Parahypophyseal dissection.
- Step 3: Section of the inferior hypophyseal artery.
- Step 4: Posterior clinoidectomy.
- Step 5: Incision of the dorsal periosteum and dura mater.
- Step 6: Removal of the Liliequist membrane.
- Step 7: Removal of the anterior pontine membrane.

Intradural Hypophysiopexy

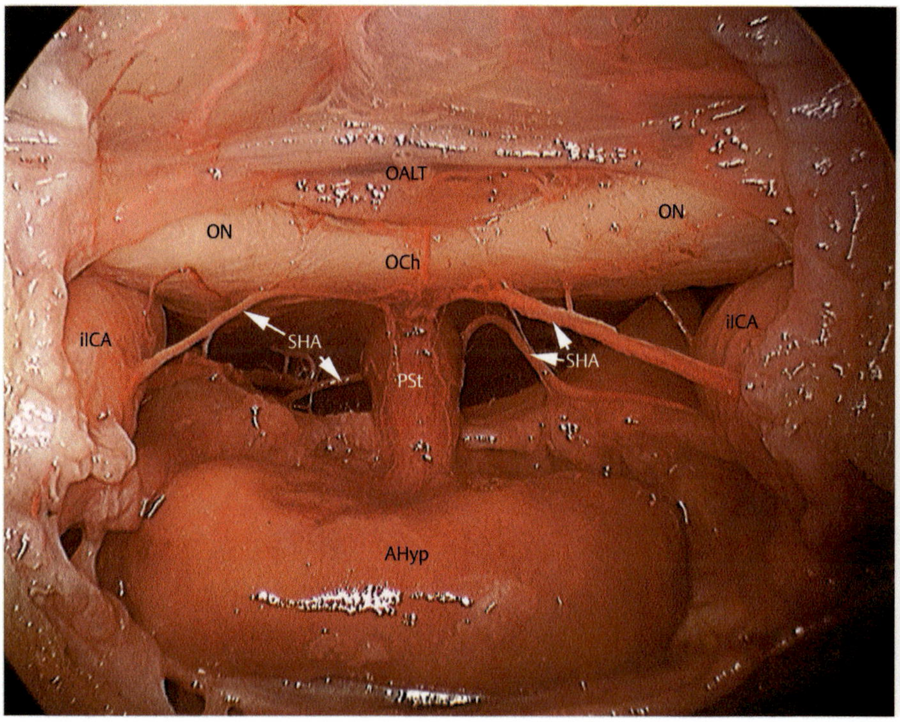

Fig. 10.6 Step 1 (part 1). After performing the transsellar and transplanum–transtuberculum approaches, the optic cistern is opened and the diaphragm sellae is incised along the midline and removed after isolating the pituitary stalk (PSt). The superior hypophyseal arteries (SHA) are cleaned from the arachnoid and their origin from the intracranial tracts of the internal carotid arteries (iICA) is demonstrated. Optic nerves and outer arachnoid of the lamina terminalis cistern (OALT) are identified in the cranial portion of the endoscopic field. AHyp, adenohypophysis; OCh, optic chiasm; ON, optic nerve.

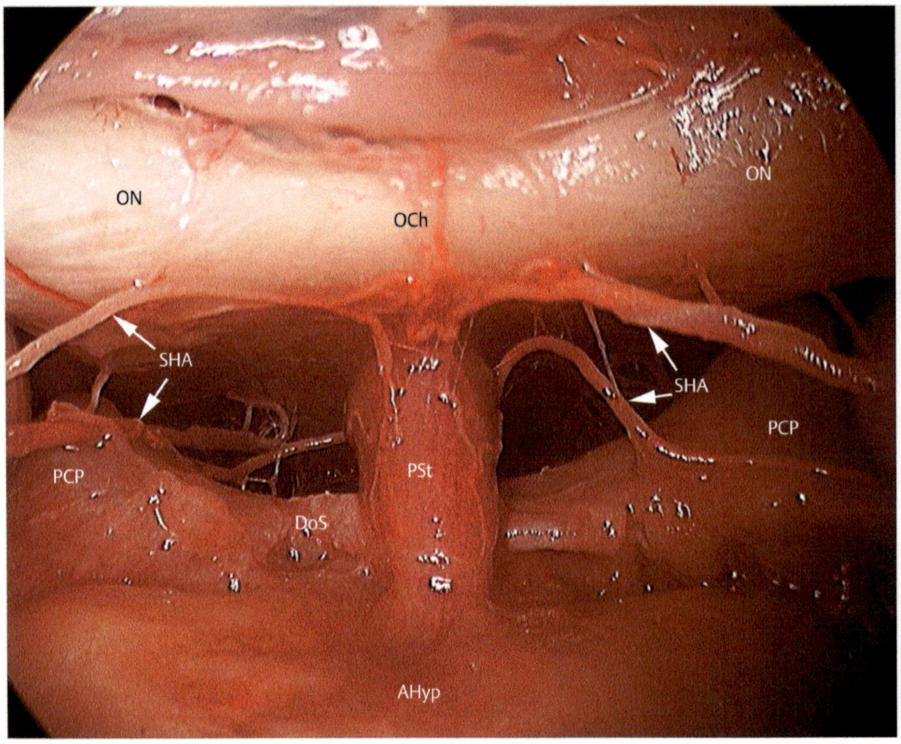

Fig. 10.7 Step 1 (part 2). The three main branches of the superior hypophyseal artery (SHA) can be identified within the optic cistern: one branch reaches the optic nerve (ON), one the optic chiasm (OCh) and pituitary stalk (PSt), and one the optic tract. Frequently, the superior hypophyseal artery is double, with the anterior superior hypophyseal artery arising close to the superior carotid ring and the posterior superior hypophyseal artery originating nearby the posterior clinoid process (PCP). AHyp, adenohypophysis; DoS, dorsum sellae.

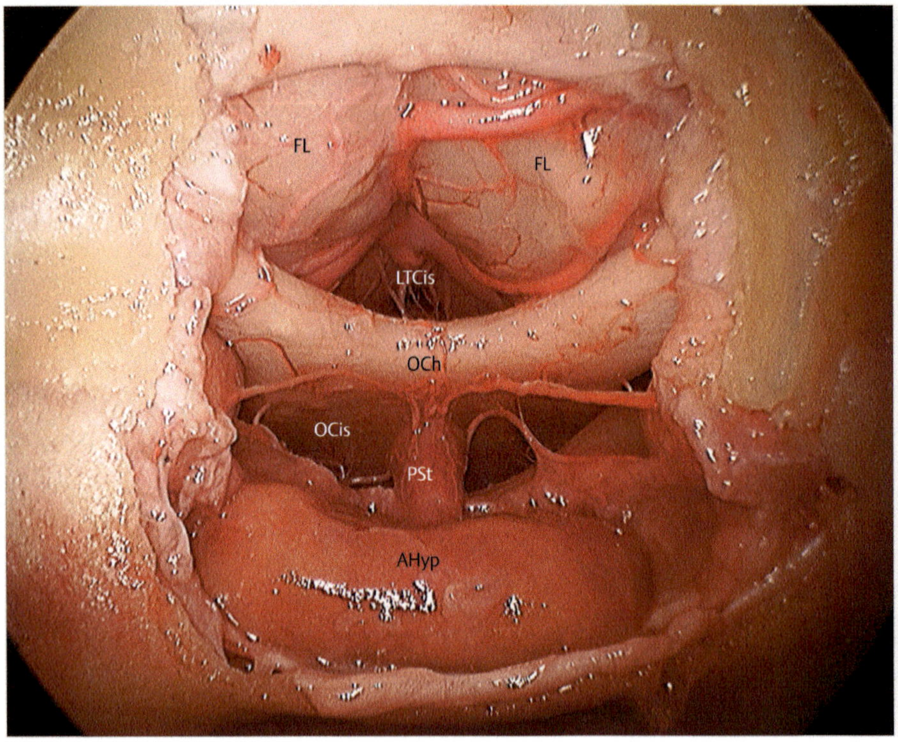

Fig. 10.8 Step 2. The lamina terminalis cistern (LTCis) is opened and the frontal lobes (FL) are exposed above the cistern, which is bounded inferiorly by the optic chiasm (OCh). AHyp, adenohypophysis; OCis, optic cistern; PSt, pituitary stalk.

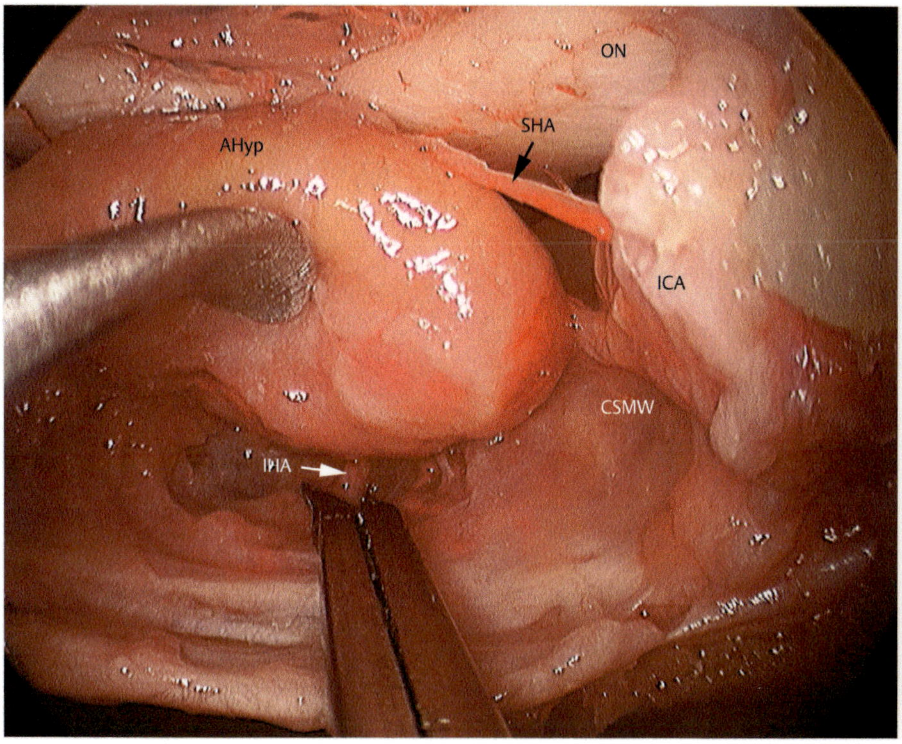

Fig. 10.9 Step 3. After performing a parahypophyseal dissection along the medial wall of the cavernous sinus (CSMW), the hypophyseal gland is gently dissected off the inferior sellar periosteum, isolating the inferior hypophyseal arteries (IHA), which are then sectioned. The superior hypophyseal arteries (SHA) are preserved during this maneuver. AHyp, adenohypophysis; ICA, internal carotid artery; ON, optic nerve.

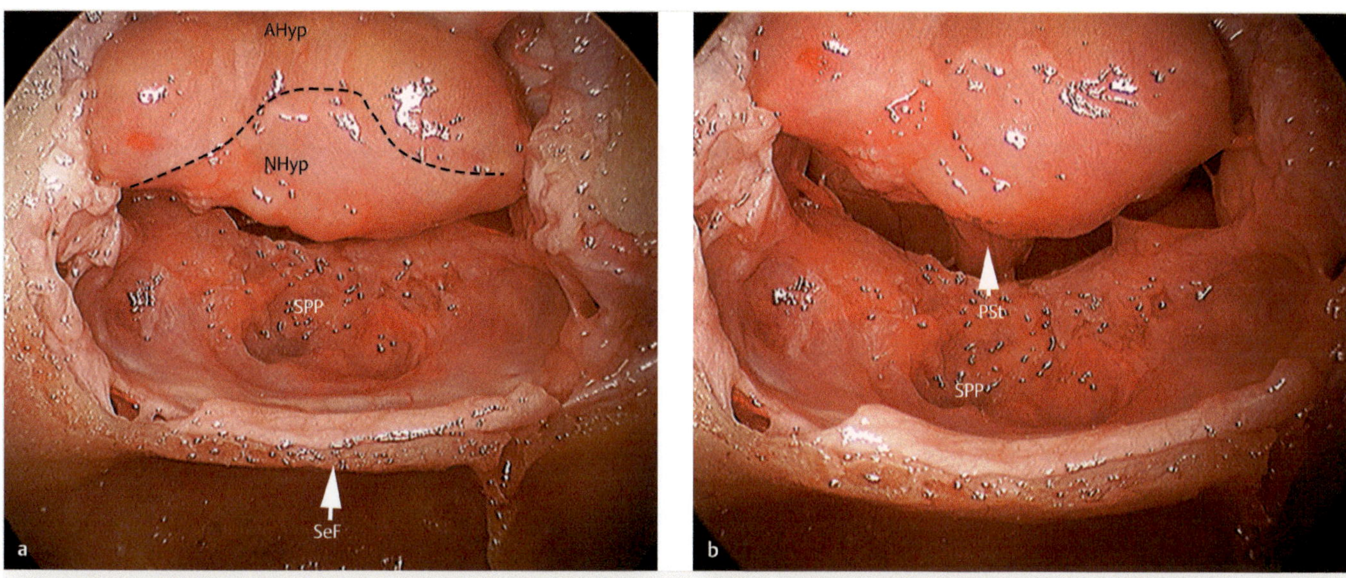

Fig. 10.10 (a, b) Step 4. The pituitary gland is elevated in front of the optic chiasm. The limit (*black dashed line*) between adenohypophysis (AHyp) and neurohypophysis (NHyp) can be better identified from this perspective. The sellar posterior periosteum (SPP) and inferior periosteum, which cover the dorsum sellae and sellar floor (SeF), respectively, are completely exposed. PSt, pituitary stalk.

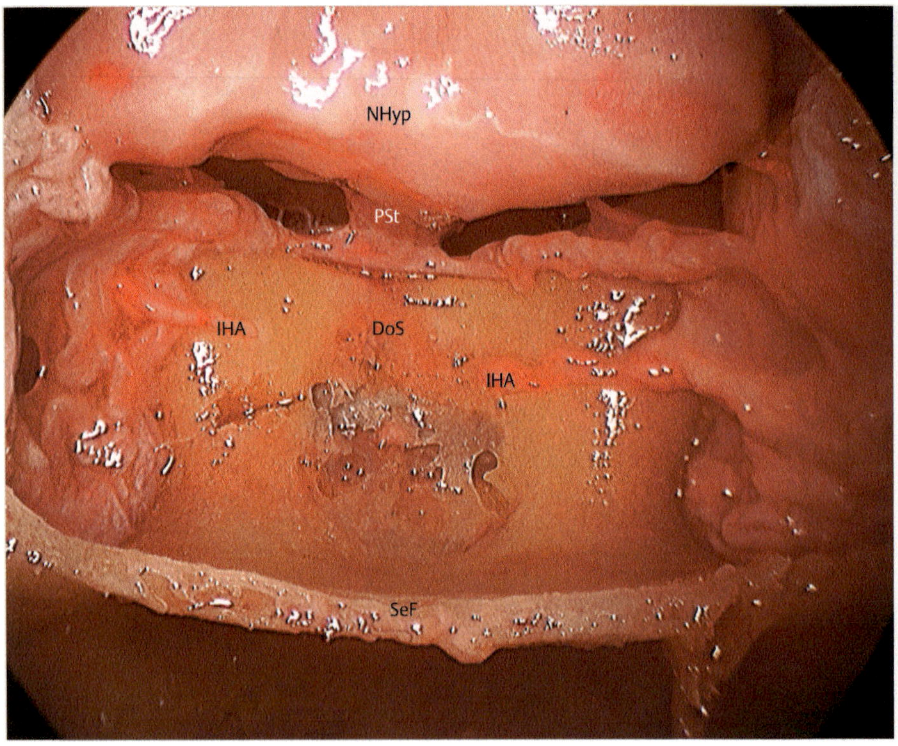

Fig. 10.11 Step 5. The sellar posterior periosteum is removed to expose the bone of the dorsum sellae (DoS), which corresponds to the upper third of the clivus. IHA, inferior hypophyseal artery (sectioned); NHyp, neurohypophysis; PSt, pituitary stalk; SeF, sellar floor.

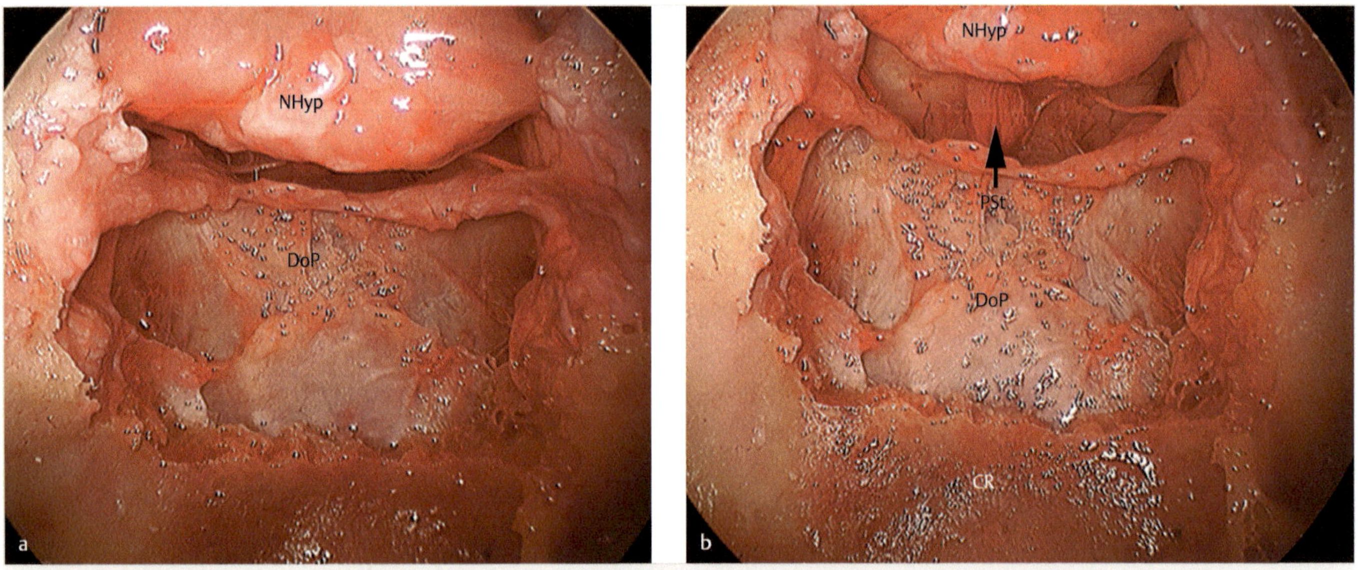

Fig. 10.12 (a, b) Step 6. The bone of the dorsum sellae is removed together with the posterior clinoid processes laterally and bony sellar floor inferiorly. The dorsal periosteum (DoP) is subsequently exposed. CR, clival recess; NHyp, neurohypophysis; PSt, pituitary stalk.

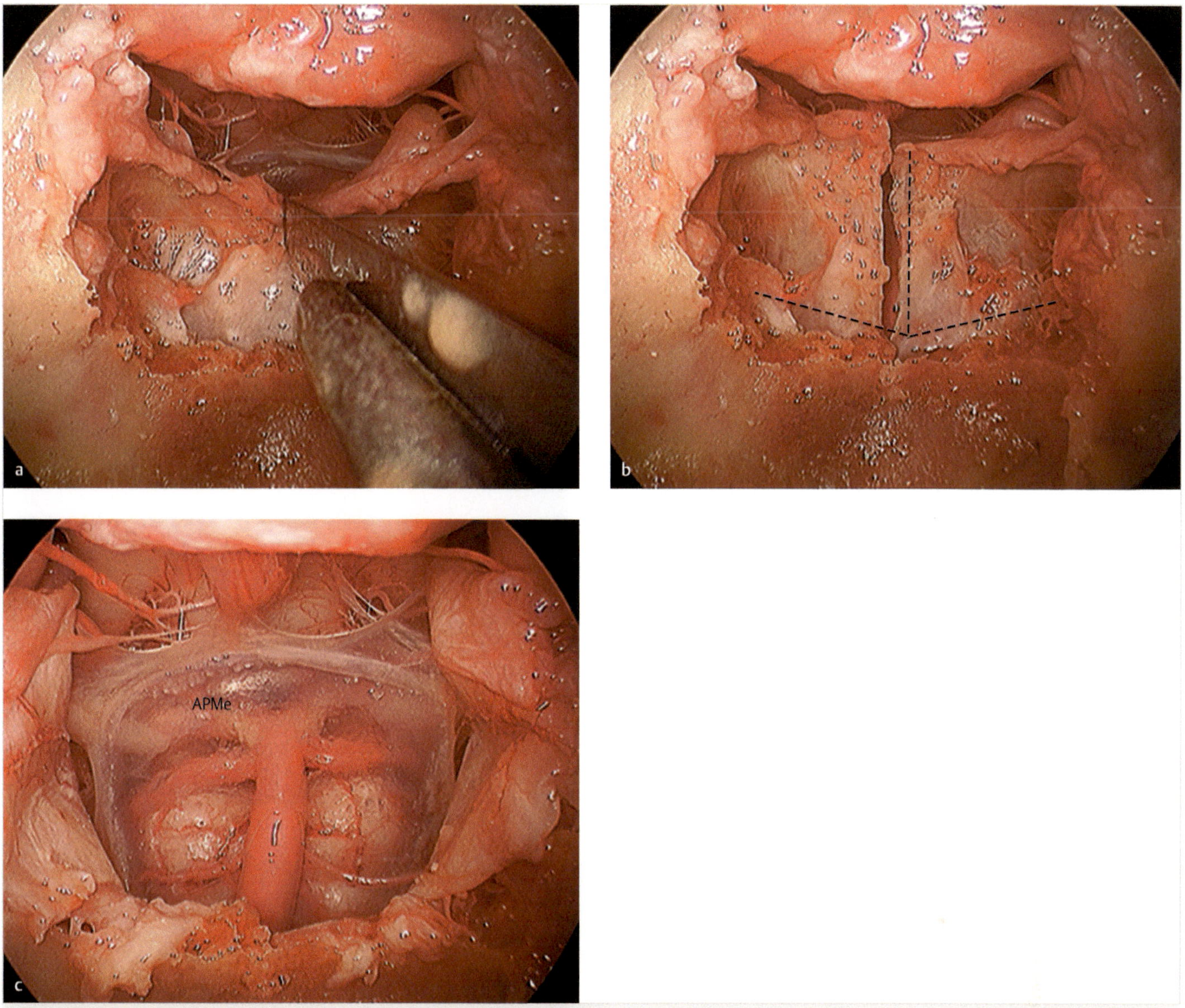

Fig. 10.13 (a–c) Step 7. A midline incision (*vertical black dashed line*) of the dorsal periosteum from the superior free edge down to the upper border of the clival recess is performed. Then, a horizontal incision is made along the inferior border of the bony window (*horizontal black dashed line*). The periosteal dural flaps are turned anterolaterally to cover the medial wall of the cavernous sinus. The anterior pontine membrane (APMe) comes into view.

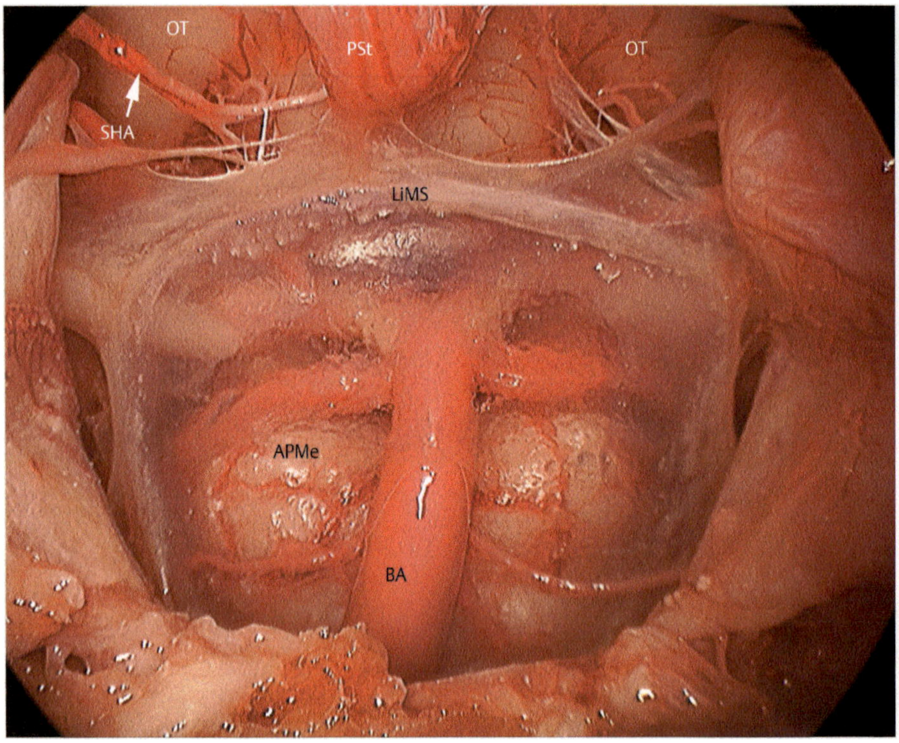

Fig. 10.14 The anterior pontine membrane. The anterior pontine membrane (APMe) is the anterior boundary of the prepontine cistern, which contains the basilar artery (BA). Superiorly, it continues into the sellar portion of the Liliequist membrane (LiMS), which inserts on the dorsum sellae and pituitary stalk (PSt). Laterally, the anterior pontine membrane turns in a posterior direction, following the contour of the brainstem. OT, optic tract; SHA, superior hypophyseal artery.

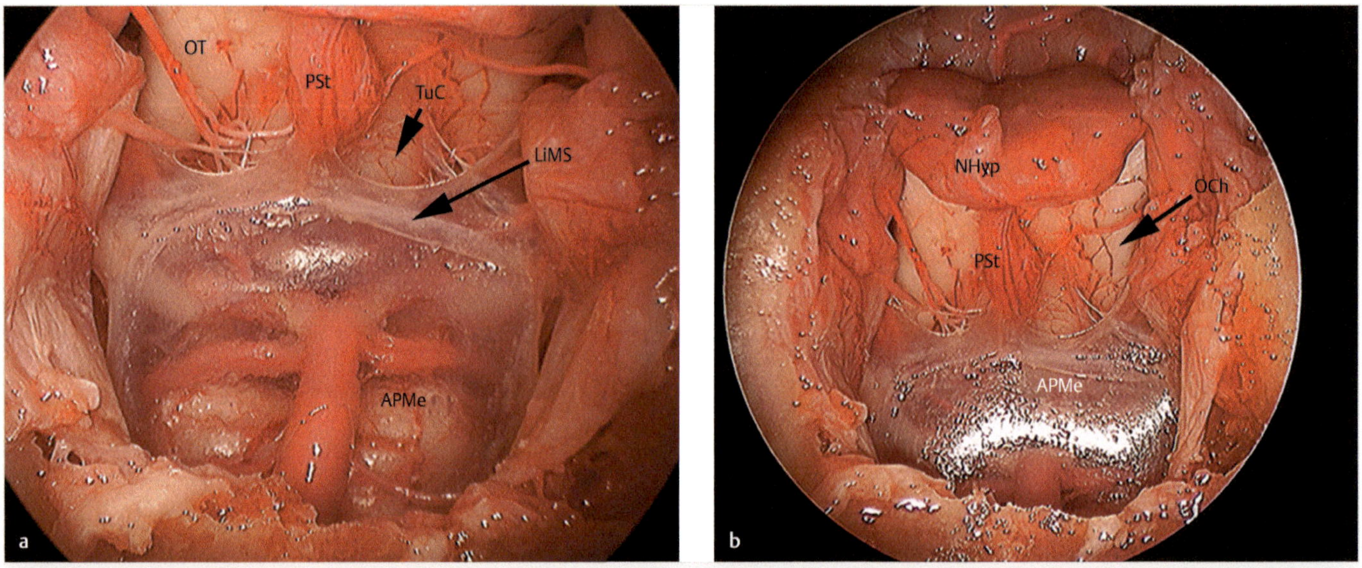

Fig. 10.15 (a, b) The optic cistern. Following superiorly the anterior pontine membrane (APMe), the anterior insertion of the sellar portion of the Liliequist membrane (LiMS) on the dorsum sellae is identified. As the dorsum sellae was removed to harvest the transdorsal corridor, this insertion appears as a free arachnoid edge partially attached to the dorsal surface of the pituitary stalk (PSt). The optic cistern is located above this insertion and below the optic chiasm (OCh). Using a 0-degree scope, the tuber cinereum (TuC) can be identified posteriorly to the pituitary stalk and medially to the optic tracts (OT). With a 70-degree endoscope turned superiorly, an overview of the transposed pituitary gland is obtained. NHyp, neurohypophysis.

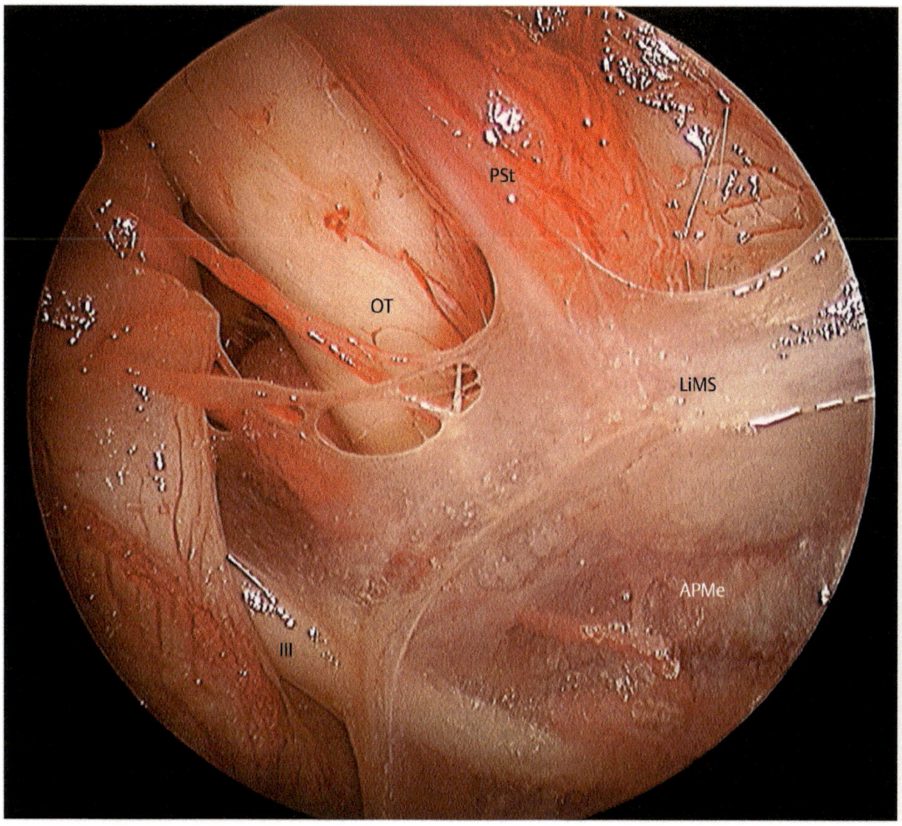

Fig. 10.16 The oculomotor cistern. With a 70-degree scope turned superolaterally (on the right side of the specimen in this figure), it is possible to see how the sellar portion of the Liliequist membrane (LiMS) continues laterally to envelop the oculomotor nerve (III) before it enters the cavernous sinus, forming the oculomotor cistern. APMe, anterior pontine membrane; OT, optic tract; PSt, pituitary stalk.

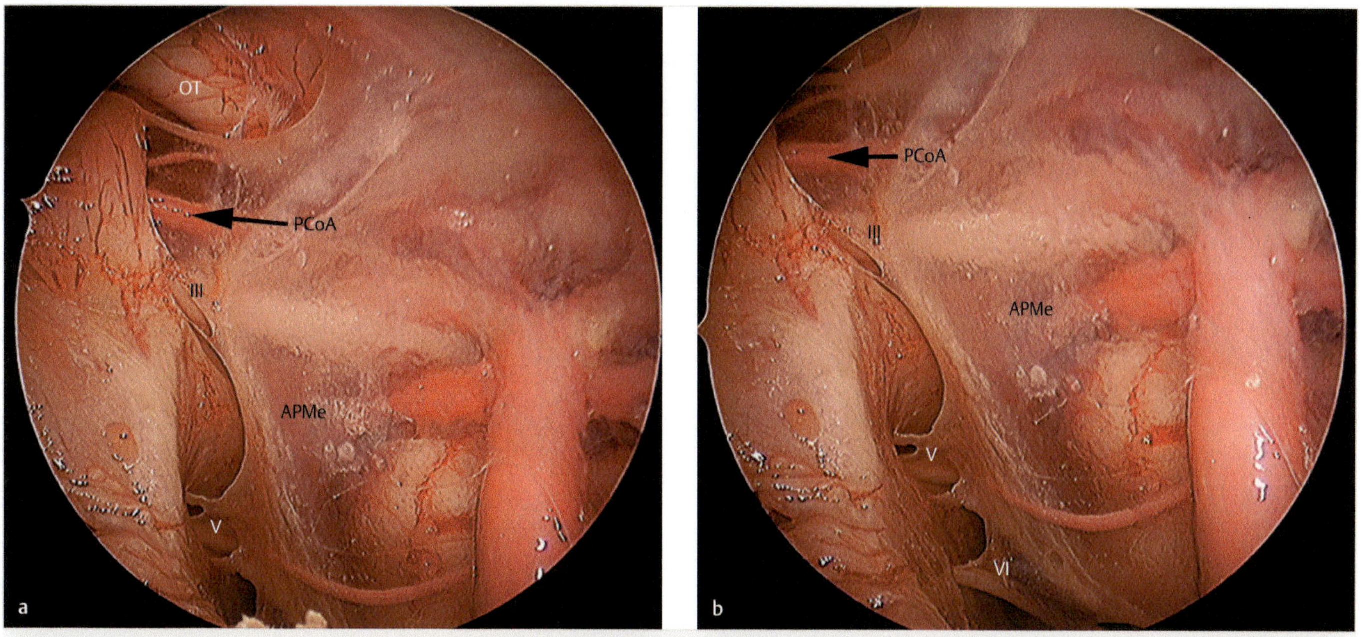

Fig. 10.17 (a, b) The lateral portion of the anterior pontine membrane. Turning laterally the 70-degree scope, it comes into view how the anterior pontine membrane (APMe) envelops the trigeminal stem (V) and abducens nerve (VI) before they enter the Meckel cave and basilar plexus, respectively. III, oculomotor nerve; OT, optic tract; PCoA, posterior communicating artery.

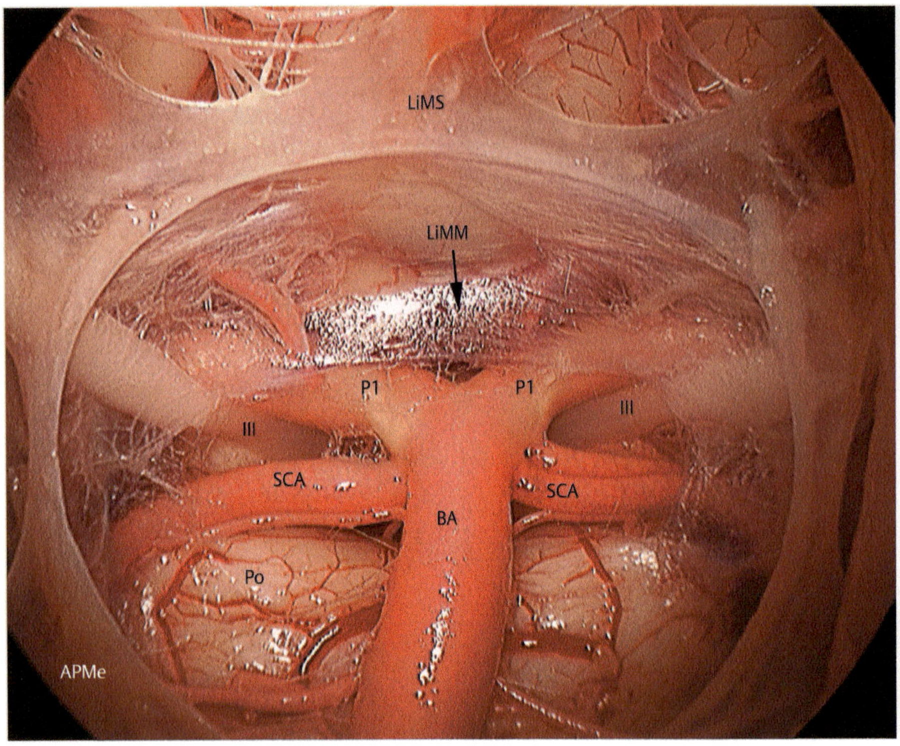

Fig. 10.18 Step 8. The anterior pontine membrane (APMe) is incised along the midline, below the anterior insertion of the sellar portion of the Liliequist membrane (LiMS). In this way, the prepontine cistern is opened and its content becomes visible: the basilar artery (BA) passes through the mesencephalic portion of the Liliequist membrane (LiMM), bifurcating in the precommunicating tracts of the posterior cerebral arteries (P1). The mesencephalic portion of the Liliequist membrane represents the roof of the prepontine cistern and the floor of the interpeduncular cistern. The oculomotor nerve (III) runs between the posterior cerebral artery and the superior cerebellar artery (SCA), which is often double (as on the left side of this specimen). Po, pons.

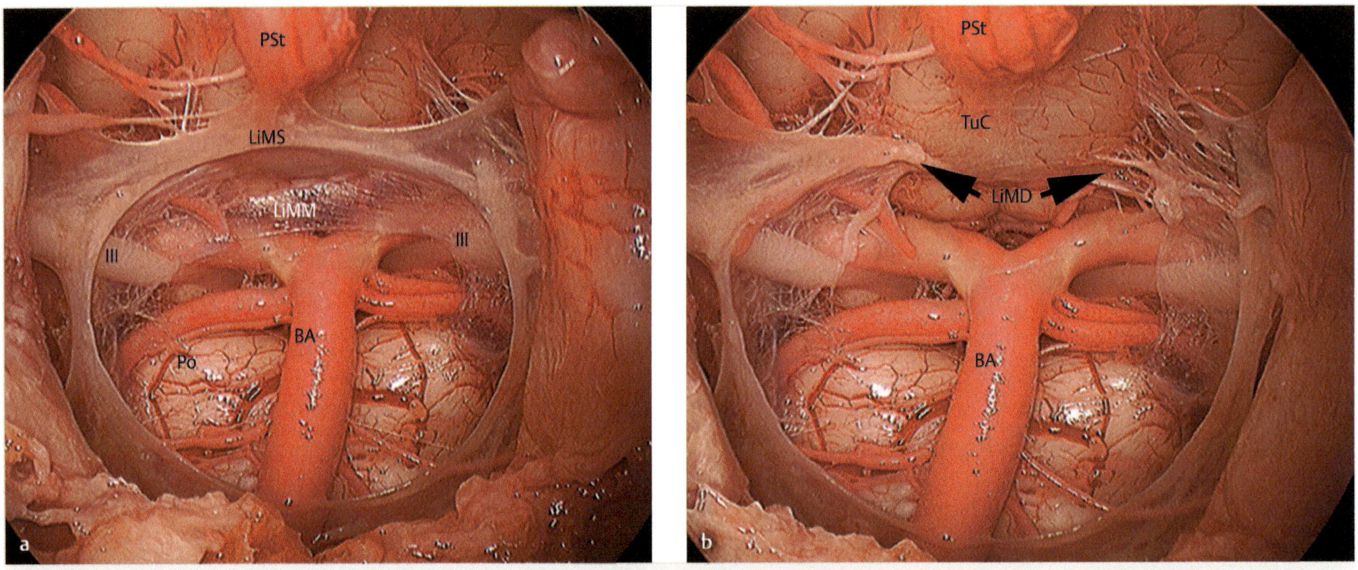

Fig. 10.19 (a, b) Step 9. The sellar (LiMS) and mesencephalic (LiMM) portions of the Liliequist membrane are incised on the midline, from the basilar tip to the pituitary stalk (PSt). In this way, the lateral parts of the diencephalic portion of the Liliequist membrane (LiMD) are preserved. This maneuver joins the prepontine and interpeduncular cisterns, showing the entire tuber cinereum (TuC) behind the pituitary stalk. III, oculomotor nerve; BA, basilar artery; Po, pons.

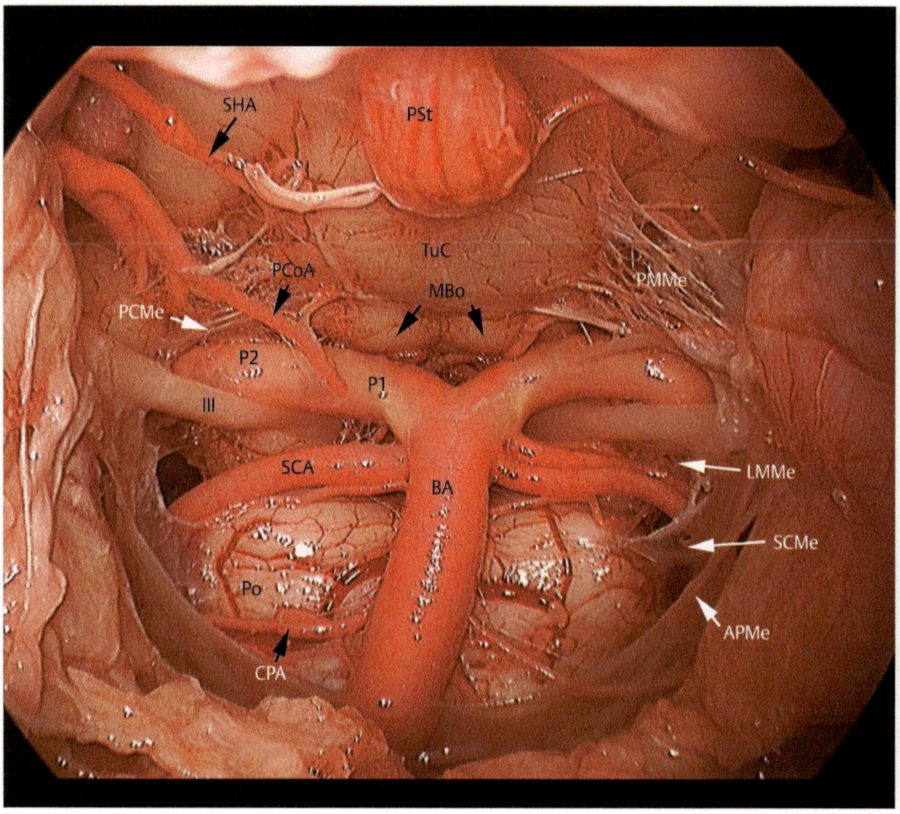

Fig. 10.20 Step 10. The diencephalic portion of the Liliequist membrane is removed to expose the posterior mesencephalic membrane (PMMe), which inserts on the tuber cinereum (TuC) and is the lateral border of the optic cistern. The arachnoid enveloping the oculomotor nerve (III) continues with the posterior mesencephalic membrane superiorly and lateral mesencephalic membrane (LMMe) inferiorly. The postcommunicating tract of the posterior cerebral artery (P2) passes between the oculomotor nerve and the posterior mesencephalic membrane, while the superior cerebellar artery (SCA) passes between the lateral mesencephalic membrane and the area where the anterior pontine membrane (APMe) fuses with the superior cerebellar membrane (SCMe). After removing the posterior mesencephalic membrane (as performed on the right side of the specimen), the posterior cerebral membrane (PCMe) comes into view just superior to the posterior communicating artery (PCoA). BA, basilar artery; CPA, circumferential pontine artery; MBo, mammillary bodies; P1, precommunicating tract of the posterior cerebral artery; Po, pons; PSt, pituitary stalk; SHA, superior hypophyseal artery; TuC, tuber cinereum.

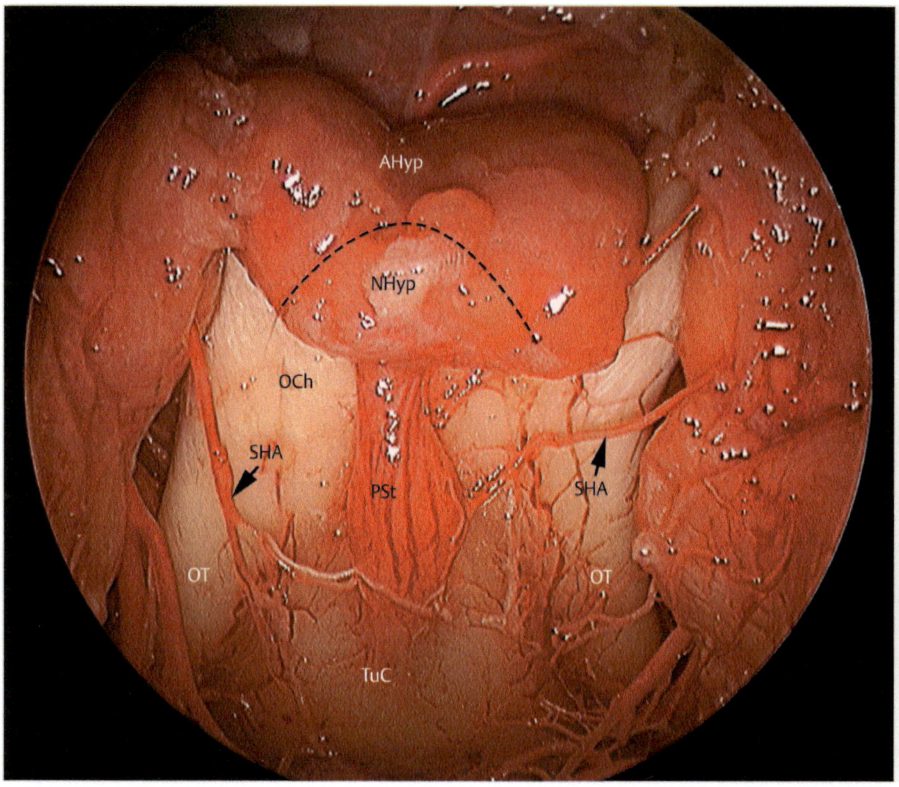

Fig. 10.21 Overview of the optic system and pituitary gland. With a 70-degree scope turned superiorly, an overview of the pituitary gland, which is divided (*black dashed line*) in adeno- (AHyp) and neurohypophysis (NHyp), pituitary stalk (PSt), and tuber cinereum (TuC), is obtained. Laterally and superiorly to these structures, the optic tracts (OT), optic chiasm (OCh), optic nerves, and superior hypophyseal arteries (SHA) can also be identified.

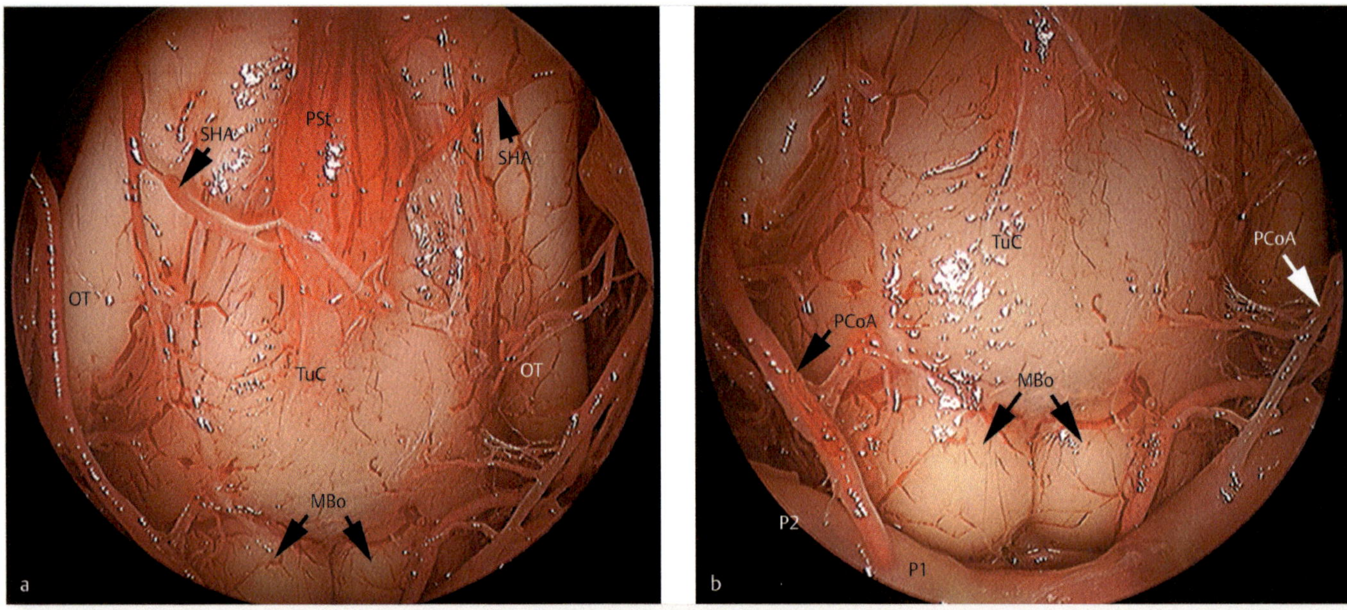

Fig. 10.22 (a, b) The tuber cinereum and mammillary bodies. Moving the 70-degree scope in a posterior direction, the pituitary stalk (PSt), tuber cinereum (TuC), mammillary bodies (MBo), and basilar tip are sequentially identified along the midline. The optic tracts arise from the diencephalon beside the tuber cinereum (TuC). The mammillary bodies lie above the basilar tip and precommunicating tract of the posterior cerebral artery (P1). From this perspective, it becomes evident that the posterior communicating arteries (PCoA) and optic tracts (OT) have a divergent and convergent direction, respectively. P2, postcommunicating tract of the posterior cerebral artery; SHA, superior hypophyseal artery.

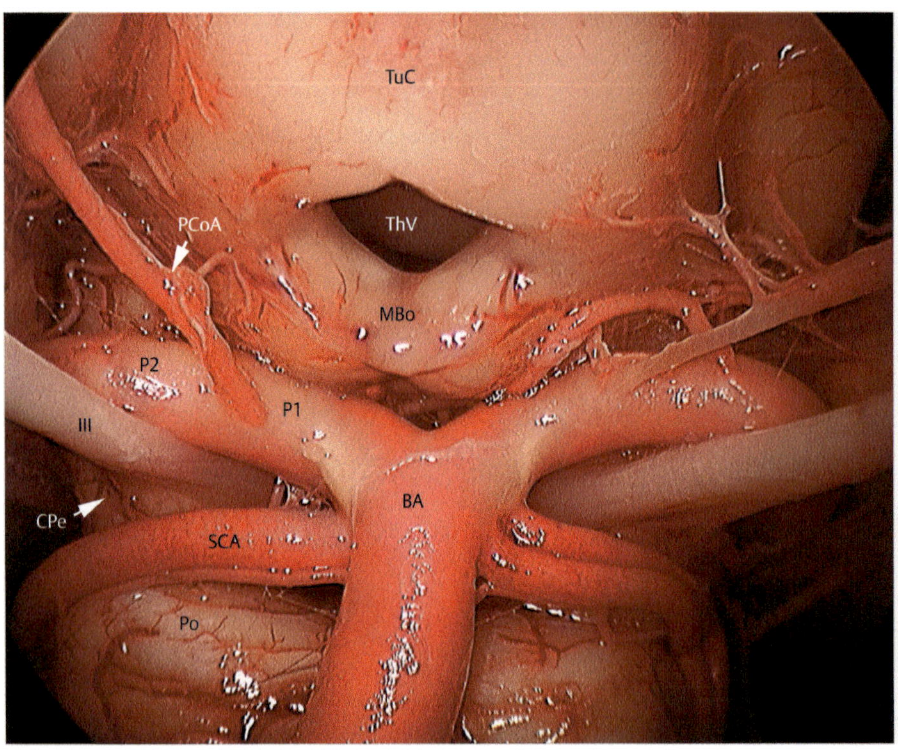

Fig. 10.23 Step 11 (part 1). After completing the removal of the arachnoid membranes, the cerebral peduncle (CPe) is identified behind the pre (P1) and postcommunicating (P2) tracts of the posterior cerebral artery, oculomotor nerve (III), and superior cerebellar artery (SCA). A small horizontal incision of the diencephalon is made between the mammillary bodies (MBo) and tuber cinereum (TuC) to expose the third ventricle (ThV). PCoA, posterior communicating artery; Po, pons.

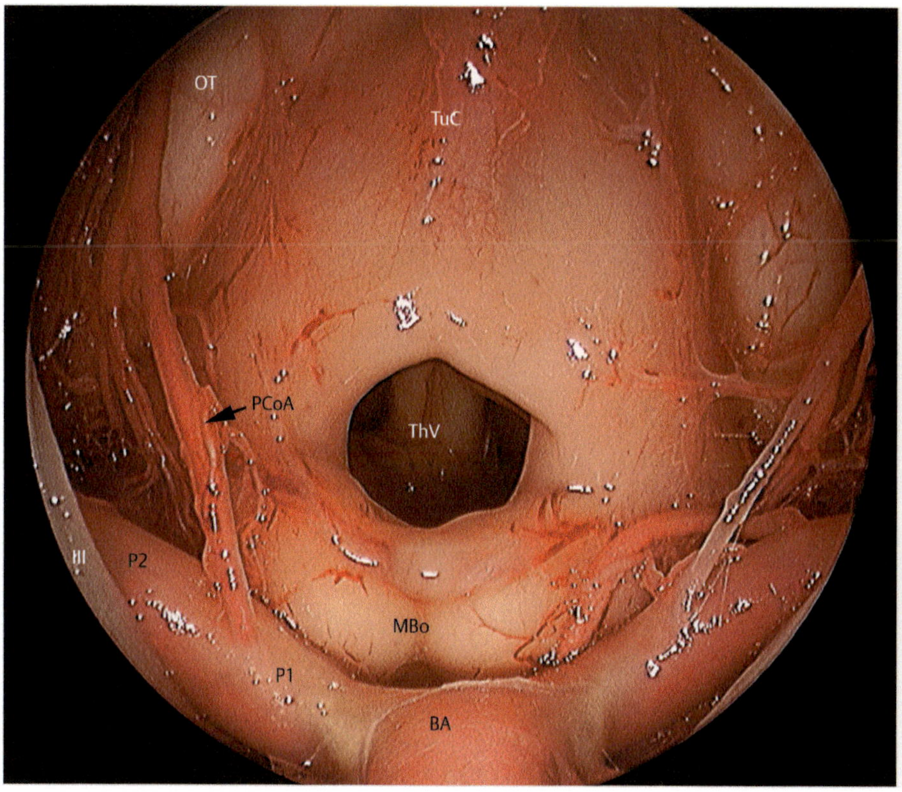

Fig. 10.24 Step 11 (part 2). A 70-degree scope turned superiorly allows a direct view of the third ventricle (ThV) through the defect within its floor, which lies between the mammillary bodies (MBo) and tuber cinereum (TuC). III, oculomotor nerve; BA, basilar artery; OT, optic tract; P1, precommunicating tract of the posterior cerebral artery; P2, postcommunicating tract of the posterior cerebral artery; PCoA, posterior communicating artery.

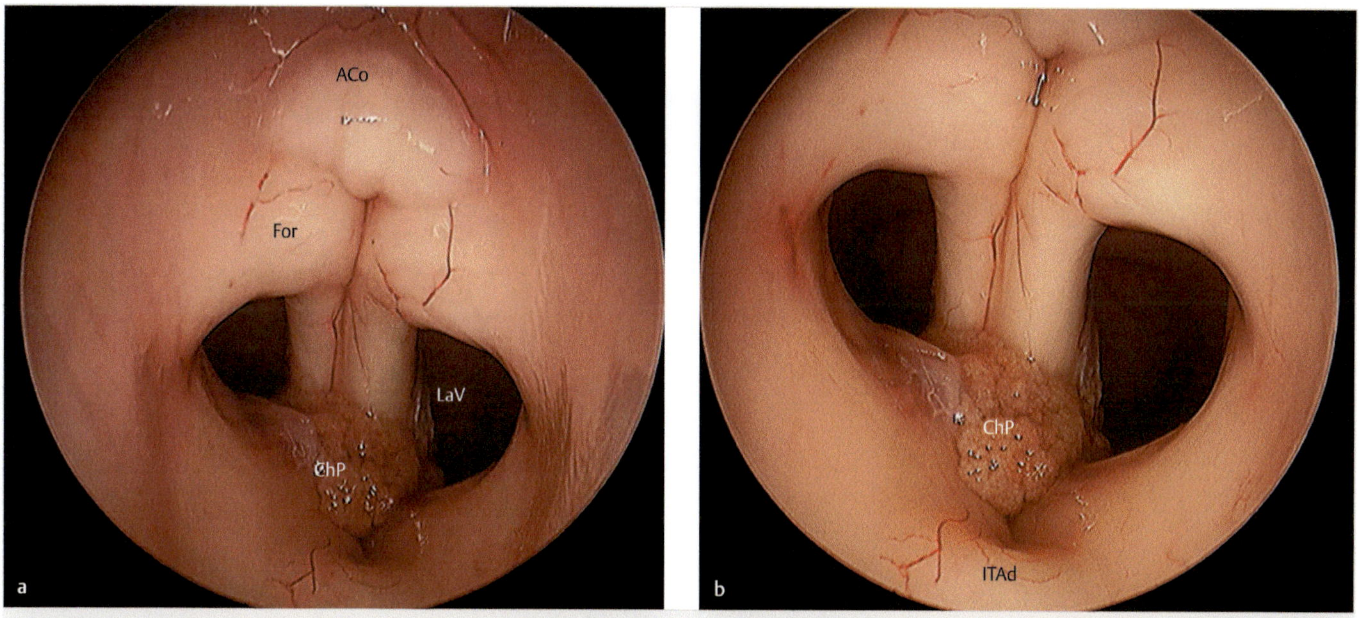

Fig. 10.25 (a, b) The third ventricle. Moving the 70-degree scope within the third ventricle, it is possible to identify the most anterior structures of this space. The anterior commissure (ACo) lies in front of the fornices (For), which surround the passages toward the lateral ventricles (LaV); these passages are called Monroe's foramina. The choroid plexus (ChP) comes from the lateral ventricle and lies anterosuperiorly to the interthalamic adherence (ITAd).

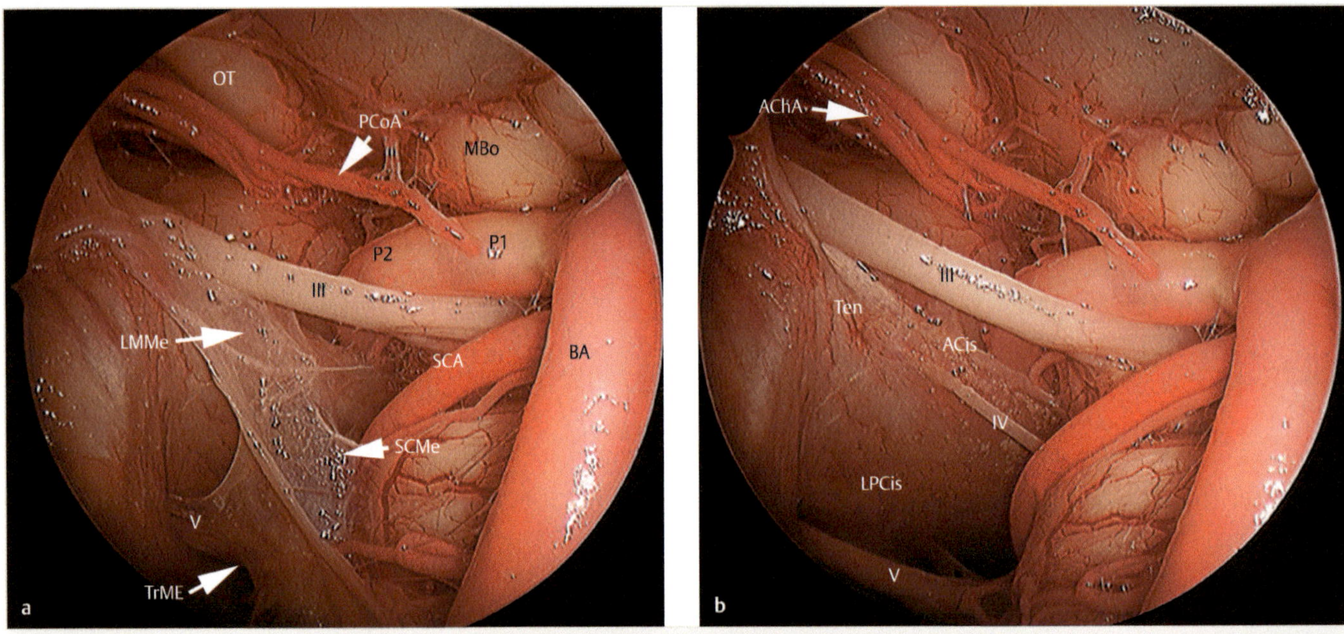

Fig. 10.26 (a, b) Lateral arachnoid membranes. A 70-degree scope is positioned in front of the basilar artery (BA) and turned laterally to the right side. This perspective provides an overview of the cisternal tract of the oculomotor nerve (III), which passes between the posterior cerebral artery and superior cerebellar artery (SCA), running parallel to the posterior communicating artery (PCoA). The anterior choroidal artery (AChA) runs laterally to the posterior communicating artery. The superior cerebellar membrane (SCMe) lies just below the superior cerebellar artery and fuses with the anterior pontine membrane medially, trigeminal membrane (TrME) inferiorly, and lateral mesencephalic membrane (LMMe) superiorly. After removing these arachnoid layers, the trigeminal stem (V) comes into view within the lateral pontine cistern (LPCis), while the trochlear nerve (IV) is identified in ambient cistern (ACis) before it enters the tentorium (Ten). MBo, mammillary bodies; OT, optic tract; P1, precommunicating tract of the posterior cerebral artery; P2, postcommunicating tract of the posterior cerebral artery.

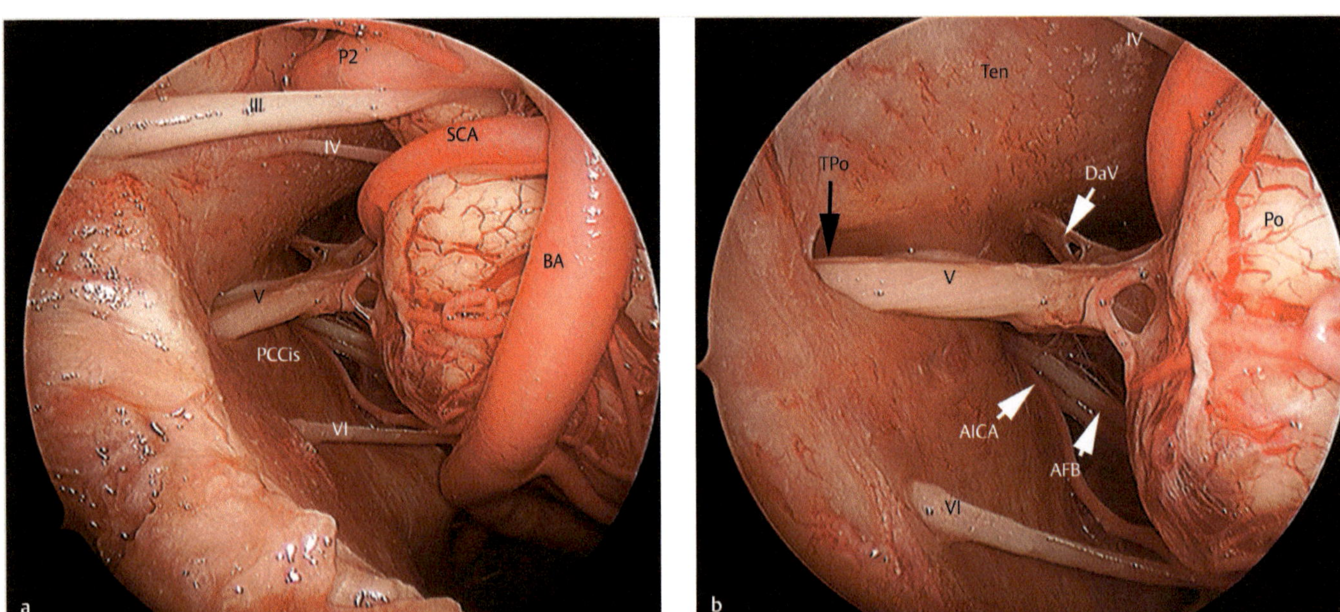

Fig. 10.27 (a, b) The pontocerebellar cistern. Turning inferiorly the 70-degree scope, it is possible to identify, from cranial to caudal, the oculomotor nerve (III), the trochlear nerve (IV) entering the tentorium (Ten), the trigeminal stem (V) entering the trigeminal porus (TPo) medially to Dandy's vein (DaV), the abducens nerve (VI) entering the basilar plexus medial to the trigeminal stem, and the acoustic-facial bundle (AFB) together with the anterior inferior cerebellar artery (AICA) running within the pontocerebellar cistern (PCCis). Po, pons; SCA, superior cerebellar artery.

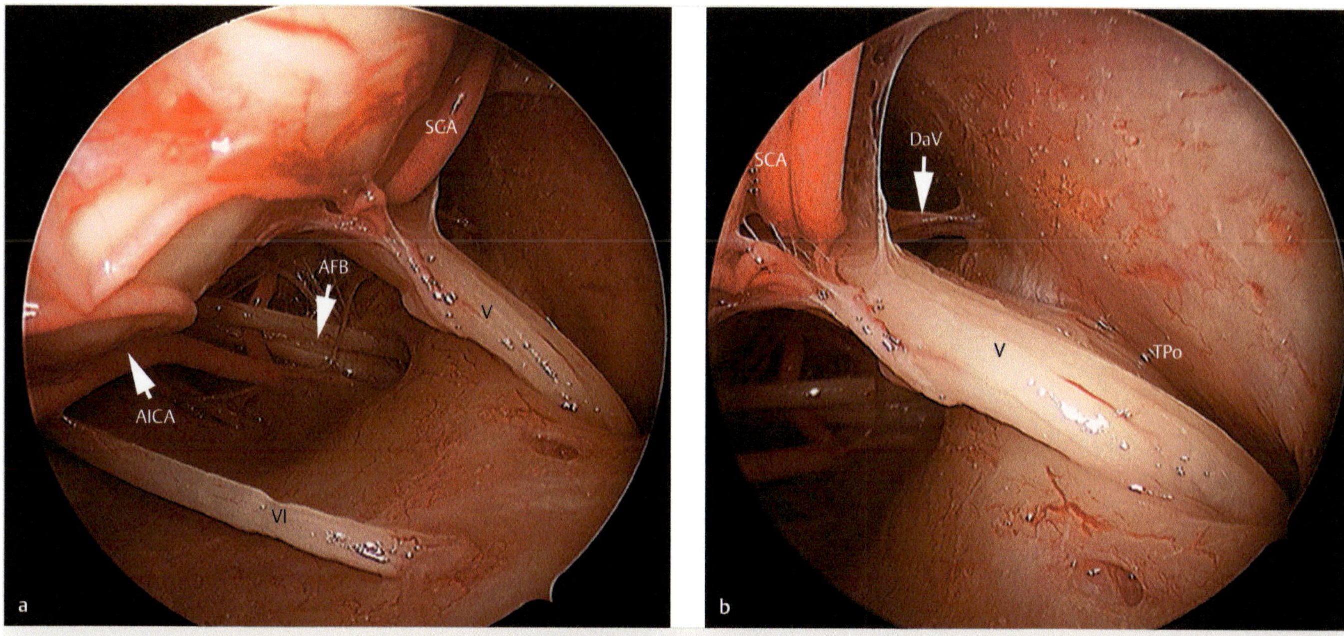

Fig. 10.28 (a, b) Cerebellar arteries, trigeminal stem, and abducens nerve. Moving the 70-degree scope optic laterally, the relationship between cerebellar arteries and cranial nerves can be better analyzed. The anterior inferior cerebellar artery (AICA) commonly runs above the abducens nerve (VI), below the trigeminal stem (V) and between the facial and vestibulocochlear nerve. The superior cerebellar artery (SCA) lies above the trigeminal stem and Dandy's vein (DaV). AFB, acoustic-facial bundle; TPo, trigeminal porus.

Interdural Hypophysiopexy

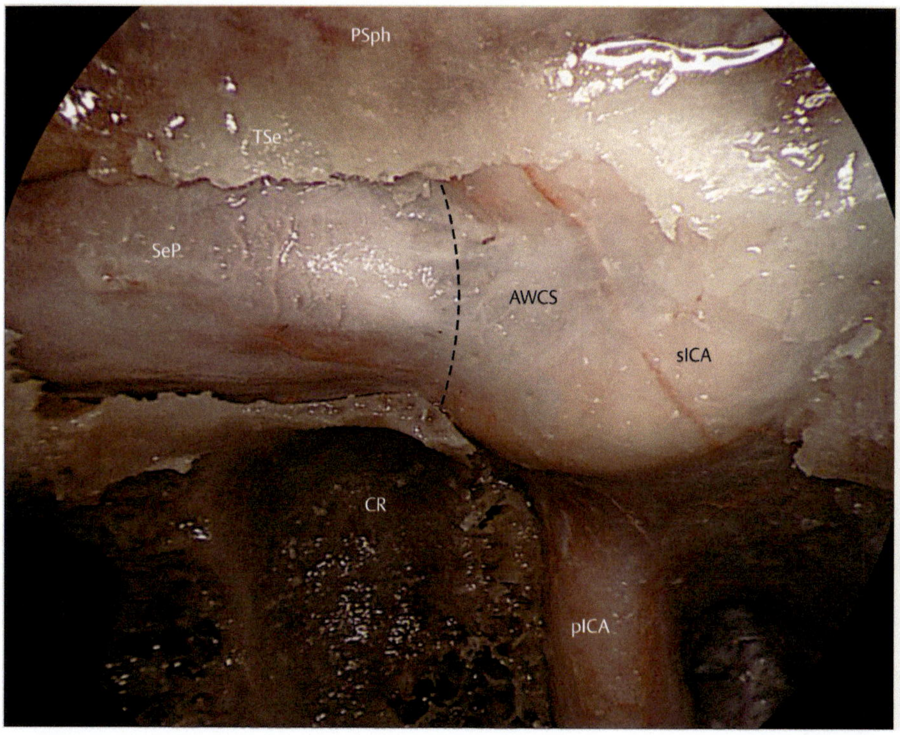

Fig. 10.29 Step 1. A vertical periosteal incision (*black dashed line*) is made between the sellar periosteum (SeP) and the anterior wall of the cavernous sinus (AWCS). CR, clival recess; pICA, paraclival tract of the internal carotid artery; PSph, planum sphenoidale; sICA, parasellar tract of the internal carotid artery; TSe, tuberculum sellae.

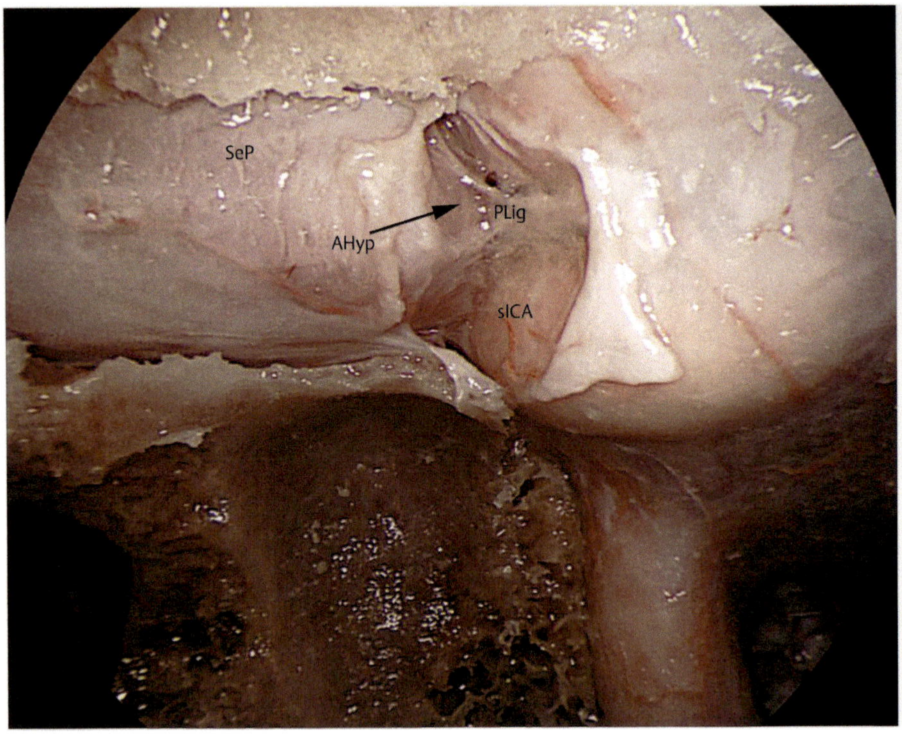

Fig. 10.30 Step 2 (part 1). The pituitary ligament (PLig) is incised to create a plane of dissection between the adenohypophysis (AHyp) and the parasellar tract of the internal carotid artery (sICA). SeP, sellar periosteum.

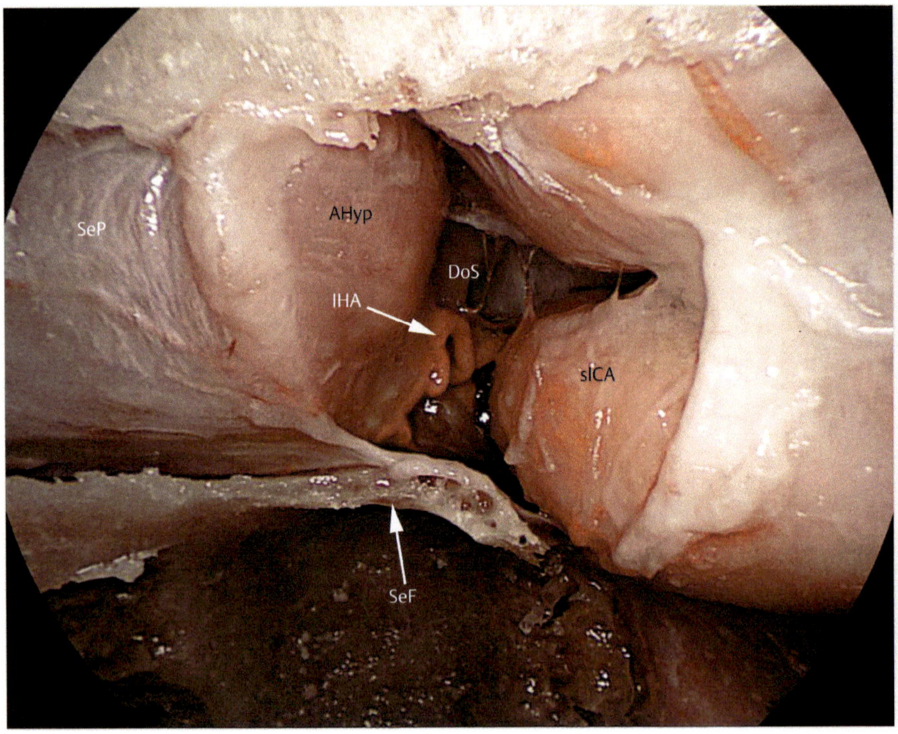

Fig. 10.31 Step 2 (part 2). The parahypophyseal dissection is performed to expose the inferior hypophyseal artery (IHA) and dorsum sellae (DoS). The medial wall of the cavernous sinus can be removed to optimize the width of the corridor. AHyp, adenohypophysis; SeF, sellar floor; SeP, sellar periosteum; sICA, parasellar tract of the internal carotid artery.

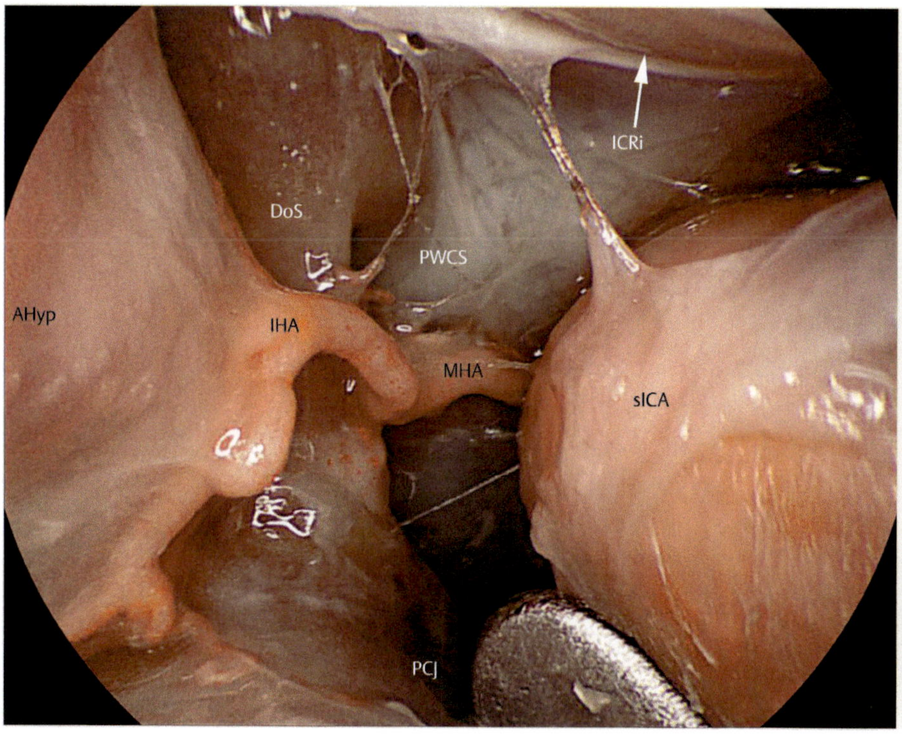

Fig. 10.32 The inferior hypophyseal artery. The parasellar tract of the internal carotid artery (sICA) is gently displaced laterally to expose the inferior hypophyseal artery (IHA), which arises from the meningohypophyseal trunk (MHA). AHyp, adenohypophysis; DoS, dorsum sellae; ICRi, inferior carotid ring; PCJ, petroclival junction; PWCS, posterior wall of the cavernous sinus.

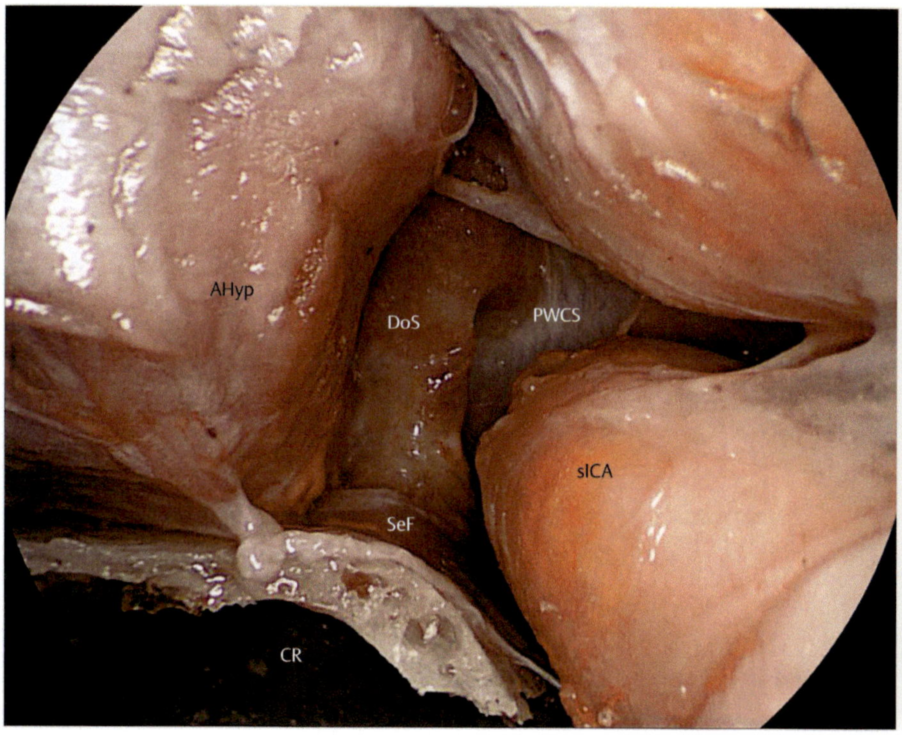

Fig. 10.33 Step 3. After sectioning the inferior hypophyseal artery, a full view of the dorsum sellae (DoS) and posterior wall of the cavernous sinus (PWCS) is obtained. AHyp, adenohypophysis; CR, clival recess; SeF, sellar floor; sICA, parasellar tract of the internal carotid artery.

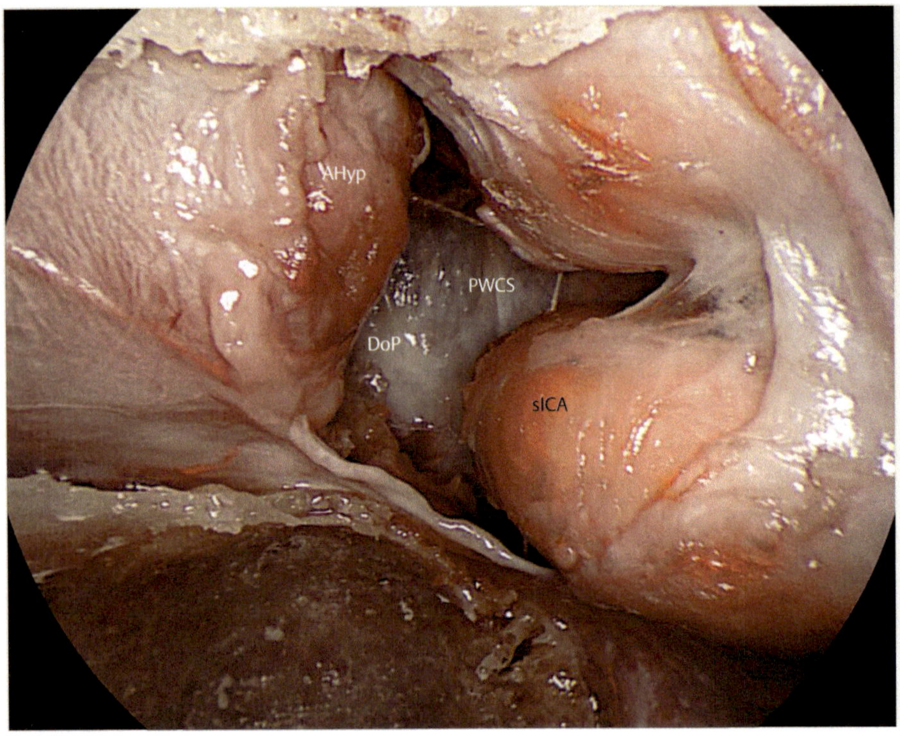

Fig. 10.34 Step 4. The posterior clinoid process, which is the lateral portion of the dorsum sellae, is removed to expose the ipsilateral half of the dorsal periosteum (DoP). The sellar floor can be removed to increase the maneuverability of instruments. AHyp, adenohypophysis; PWCS, posterior wall of the cavernous sinus; sICA, parasellar tract of the internal carotid artery.

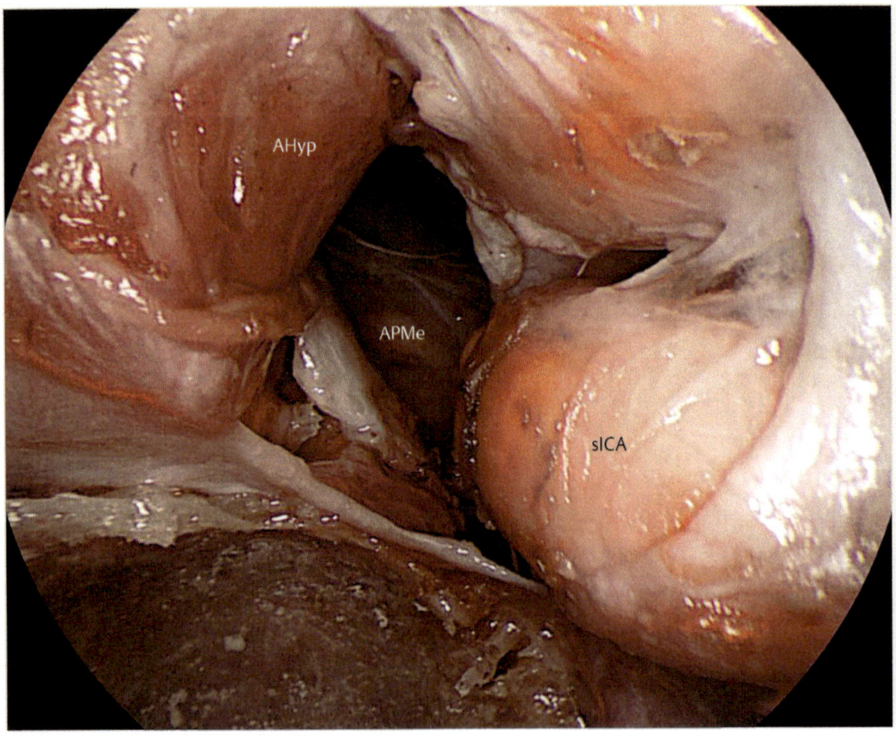

Fig. 10.35 Step 5. A vertical incision between the dorsal periosteum and the posterior wall of the cavernous sinus is performed. The anterior pontine membrane (APMe) comes into view displacing the dural flaps. AHyp, adenohypophysis; sICA, parasellar tract of the internal carotid artery.

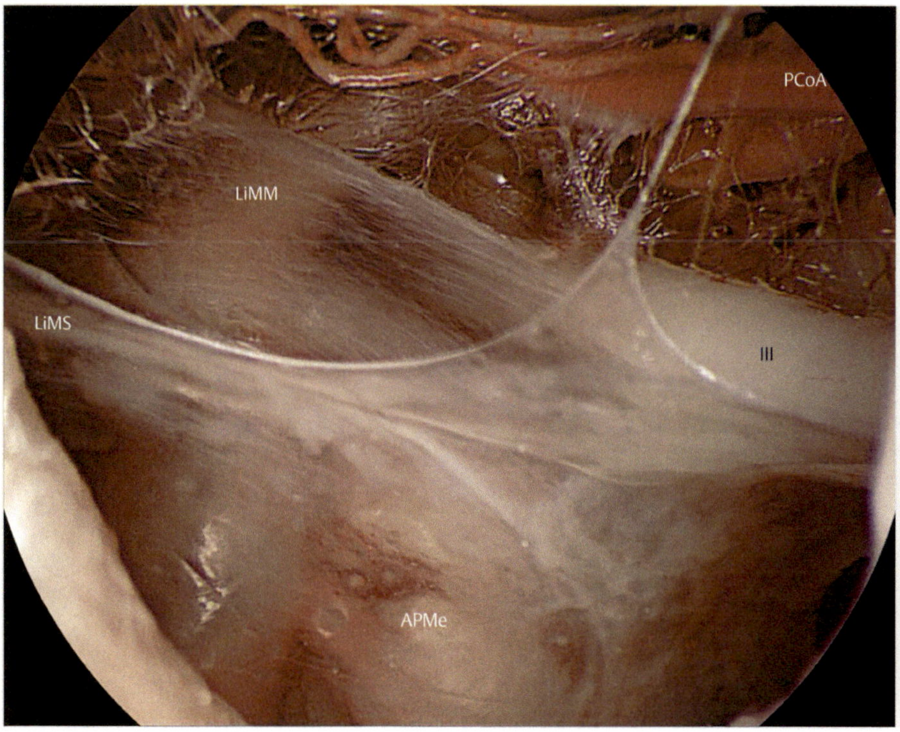

Fig. 10.36 Arachnoid membranes. A 0-degree scope is placed through the dural defect to identify the sellar (LiMS) and mesencephalic (LiMM) portions of the Liliequist membrane and the anterior pontine membrane (APMe). With this paramedian trajectory, the oculomotor (III) nerve is directly faced. PCoA, posterior communicating artery.

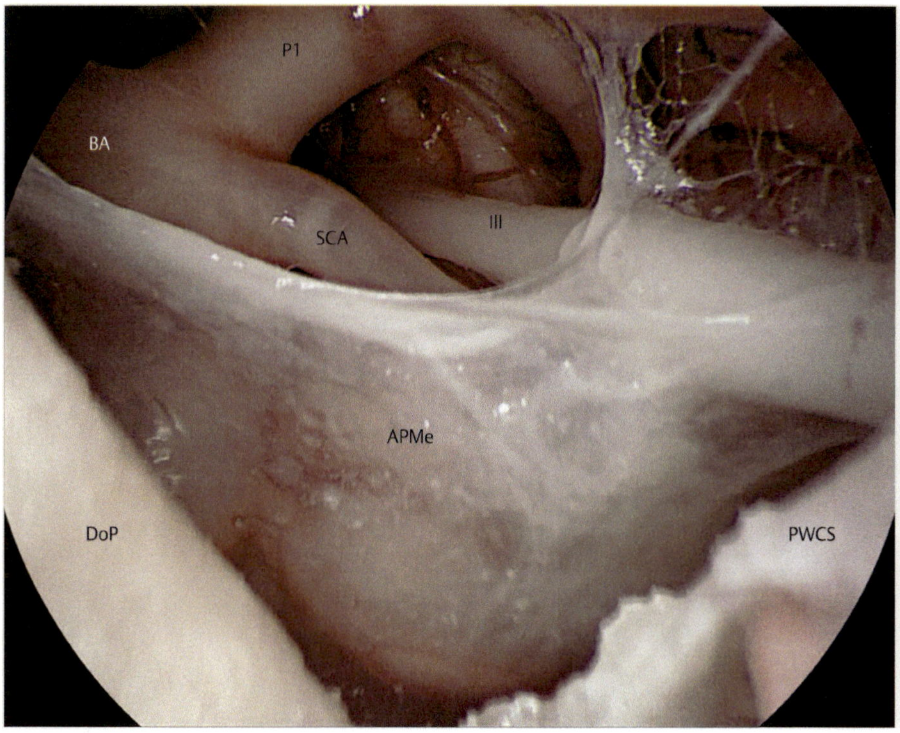

Fig. 10.37 Step 6. The Liliequist membrane is removed to expose the basilar artery (BA) and its branches. The oculomotor nerve (III) arises from the interpeduncular area and passes between the precommunicating tract of the posterior cerebral artery (P1) and the superior cerebellar artery (SCA). APMe, anterior pontine membrane; DoP, dorsal periosteum; PWCS, posterior wall of the cavernous sinus.

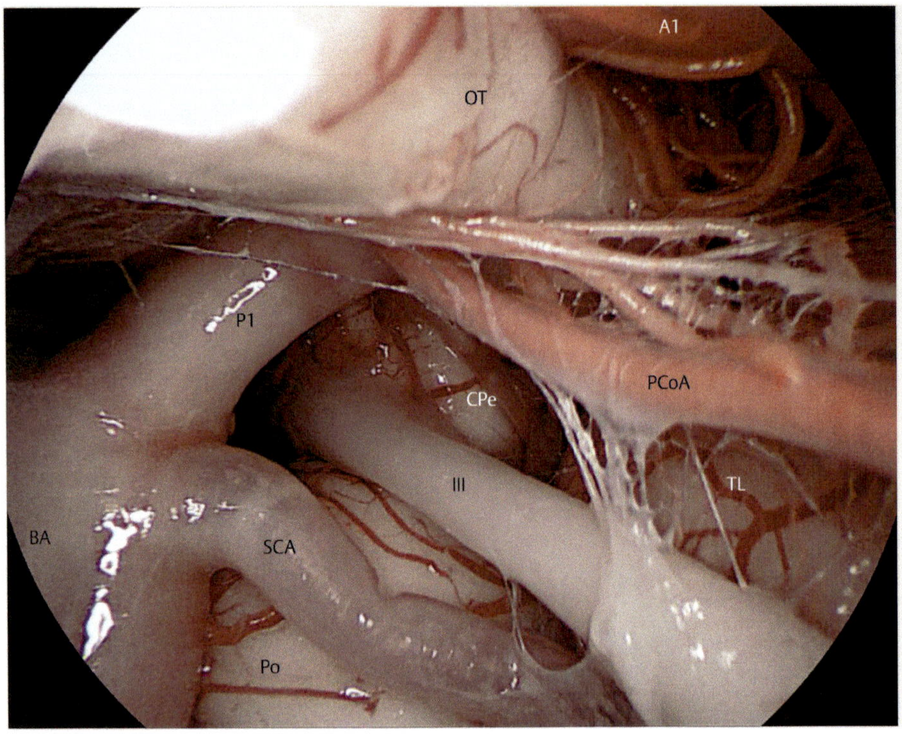

Fig. 10.38 The ambient cistern. By removing the arachnoid membranes of this area, it is possible to expose the interface between the cerebral pedicle (CPe) and temporal lobe (TL). This space is called ambient cistern. III, oculomotor nerve; A1, precommunicating tract of the anterior cerebral artery; BA, basilar artery; OT, optic tract; P1, precommunicating tract of the posterior cerebral artery; PCoA, posterior communicating artery; Po, pons; SCA, superior cerebellar artery.

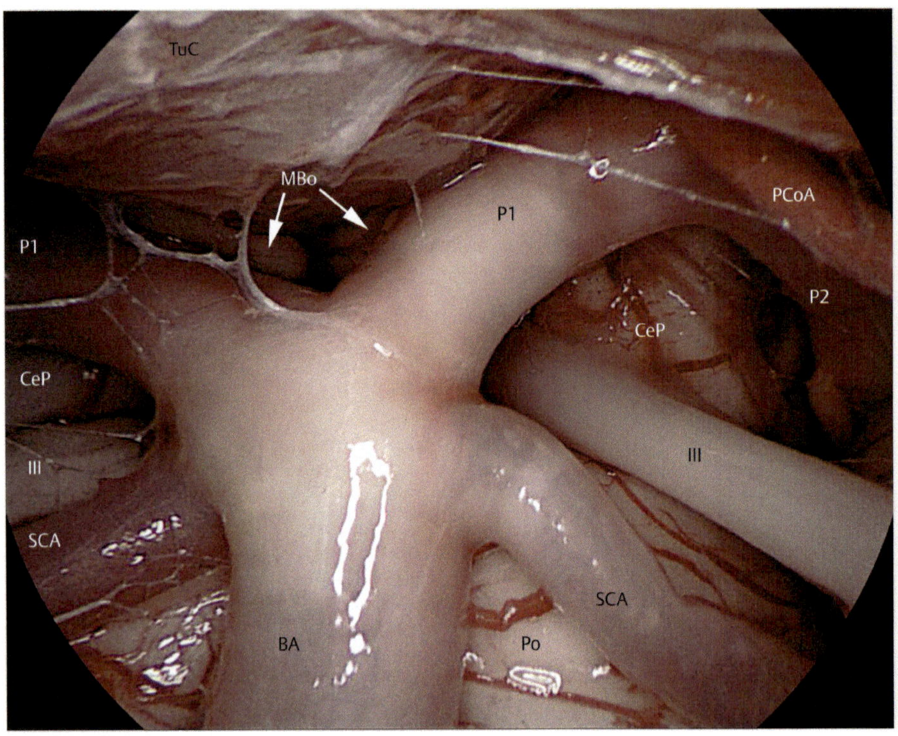

Fig. 10.39 The interpeduncular cistern. The interpeduncular cistern and its content can be seen moving medially the scope. The trajectory toward this area is inevitably paramedian when performing the interdural hypophysiopexy. III, oculomotor nerve; BA, basilar artery; CeP, cerebral pedicle; MBo, mammillary bodies; P1, precommunicating tract of the posterior cerebral artery; P2, postcommunicating tract of the posterior cerebral artery; PCoA, posterior communicating artery; Po, pons; SCA, superior cerebellar artery; TuC, tuber cinereum.

References

[1] Kassam AB, Prevedello DM, Thomas A, et al. Endoscopic endonasal pituitary transposition for a transdorsum sellae approach to the interpeduncular cistern. Neurosurgery 2008;62(3, Suppl 1):57–72, discussion 72–74

[2] Fernandez-Miranda JC, Gardner PA, Rastelli MM Jr, et al. Endoscopic endonasal transcavernous posterior clinoidectomy with interdural pituitary transposition. J Neurosurg 2014;121(1):91–99

[3] Fernandez-Miranda JC, Gardner PA, Snyderman CH, et al. Clival chordomas: a pathological, surgical, and radiotherapeutic review. Head Neck 2014;36(6):892–906

[4] Fernandez-Miranda JC, Gardner PA, Snyderman CH, et al. Craniopharyngioma: a pathologic, clinical, and surgical review. Head Neck 2012;34(7):1036–1044

[5] Montaser AS, Revuelta Barbero JM, Todeschini A, et al. Endoscopic endonasal pituitary gland hemi-transposition for resection of a dorsum sellae meningioma. Neurosurg Focus 2017;43(VideoSuppl2):V7

[6] Gardner PA, Vaz-Guimaraes F, Jankowitz B, et al. Endoscopic endonasal clipping of intracranial aneurysms: surgical technique and results. World Neurosurg 2015;84(5):1380–1393

[7] Ferrareze Nunes C, Lieber S, Truong HQ, et al. Endoscopic endonasal transoculomotor triangle approach for adenomas invading the parapeduncular space: surgical anatomy, technical nuances, and case series. J Neurosurg 2018:1–11.

[8] Theodosopoulos PV, Cebula H, Kurbanov A, et al. The medial extra-sellar corridor to the cavernous sinus: anatomic description and clinical correlation. World Neurosurg 2016;96:417–422

[9] Zenonos GA, Wang EW, Fernandez-Miranda JC. Endoscopic endonasal transoculomotor triangle approach for the resection of a pituitary adenoma with ambient cistern extension. J Neurol Surg B Skull Base 2018;79(Suppl 3):S283

[10] Doglietto F, Ferrari M, Mattavelli D, et al. Transnasal endoscopic and lateral approaches to the clivus: a quantitative anatomic study. World Neurosurg 2018;113:e659–e671

[11] Kurucz P, Baksa G, Patonay L, et al. Endoscopic anatomical study of the arachnoid architecture on the base of the skull. Part II: level of the tentorium, posterior fossa and the craniovertebral junction. Innovative Neurosurg 2013; 1:91–108

11 Transclival (Midclivus) Approach

Vittorio Rampinelli, Davide Mattavelli, Marco Ravanelli, Davide Lancini, Alberto Schreiber

The transclival route can be classified into upper, middle, and lower approaches according to two landmarks: the sellar floor and the sphenoidal floor (or alternatively the axial plane passing through the vidian nerves in poorly pneumatized sphenoid sinuses). Approaches through the upper (corresponding to the dorsum sellae) and lower portions of the clivus are described in Chapters 10 and 12, respectively. The approach through the middle portion of the clivus (also called the midclivus) takes advantage of the space between the paraclival internal carotid arteries laterally, sphenoidal floor inferiorly, and sellar floor superiorly to access the prepontine cistern and related structures. In view of the optimal exposure and adequate working volume provided,[1] during the last decades the transclival approach has been employed to manage lesions of the posterior cranial fossa with increasing grades of complexity,[2–5] ranging from spontaneous cerebrospinal fluid leak (e.g., ecchordosis physaliphora)[6] to skull-arising tumors (e.g., chordomas,[7–10] chondrosarcomas),[11] meningiomas,[12–14] aneurysms of the posterior circulation,[15–19] and cisternal (e.g., meningiomas without dural attachment,[20,21] neuroenteric,[22,23] endodermal,[24] epidermoid cysts),[25] and brainstem lesions (e.g., cavernous malformations,[26–32] ependymomas,[33] gliomas).[34]

When harvesting the transsphenoidal transclival corridor, several anatomical structures must be identified to maintain the orientation and to avoid neurovascular injuries. The vidian nerves and the axial plane passing through them serve as landmarks of the lateral and inferior boundaries of the transsphenoidal corridor. The convex vertical shape of the carotid sulcus as seen from the sphenoid sinus (when sufficiently pneumatized) can be used to trace the course of the paraclival tract of the internal carotid artery. The junction between the carotid sulcus and vidian nerve corresponds to the area of the foramen lacerum, which is filled by the fibrocartilago basalis and serves as a bed for the anterior carotid genu (between the horizontal petrous and paraclival tracts). Of note, variability in terms of pneumatization of the sphenoid sinus and course of the internal carotid artery can remarkably affect the shape and size of the window through the midclivus.[35,36] When dissecting the deep lateral boundary of the corridor through the middle third of the clivus, particular attention should be paid to the abducens nerve. This nerve runs into the basilar plexus with an ascending trajectory, superior, posterior, and lateral to the petrous process of the sphenoid bone, which is a lateral prolongation of the sphenoid body and has variable anatomy.[37] The petrous process of the sphenoid bone lies posterior to the anterior carotid genu and must be removed carefully to prevent injury to the abducens nerve. Notably, the cisternal tract of the abducens nerve can be better exposed with a lower transclival approach rather than through the midclivus.

It is worth mentioning that the transclival corridor encroaches the basilar plexus, which is a venous dural plexus enclosed between the clival periosteum and the dura. The basilar plexus is the crossroad of a number of dural sinuses, thus causing

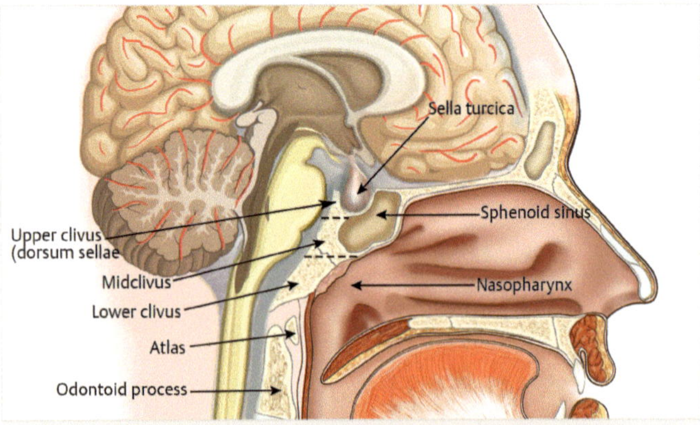

Fig. 11.1 Structure of the clivus and relationship with respect to sella turcica, sphenoid sinus, and nasopharynx. This illustration shows the architecture of the clivus, which is subdivided in upper, middle, and lower segment, as shown by the *black dashed lines*. From an anterior-to-posterior perspective, the upper, middle, and lower portions are related to the sella turcica, sphenoid sinus, and nasopharynx, respectively.

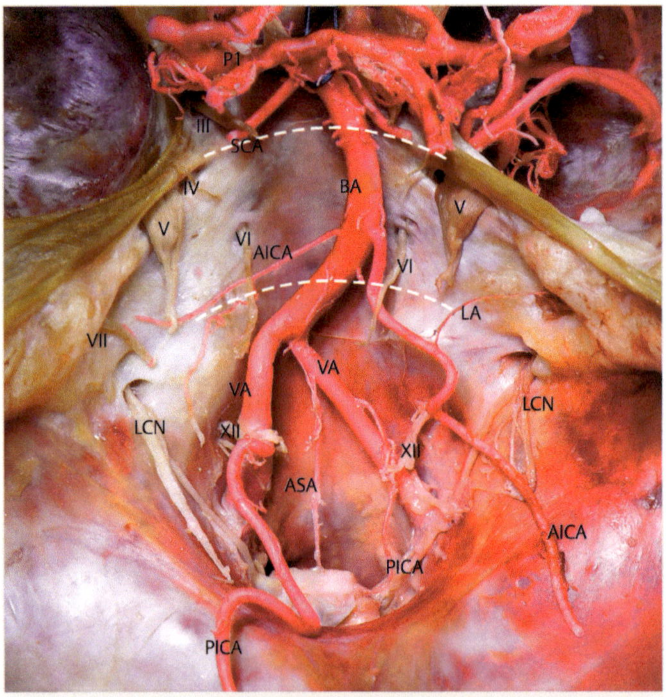

Fig. 11.2 Intracranial neurovascular structures with respect to clival segments. Intracranial view of the neurovascular structures in relation to the upper, middle, and lower clival segments, which are delineated by the *white dashed lines*. III, oculomotor nerve; IV, trochlear nerve; V, trigeminal stem; VI, abducens nerve; VII, facial nerve; XII, hypoglossal nerve; AICA, anterior inferior cerebellar artery; ASA, anterior spinal artery; BA, basilar artery; LA, labyrinthine artery; LCN, lower cranial nerves; P1, precommunicating tract of the posterior cerebral artery; PICA, posterior inferior cerebellar artery; SCA, superior cerebellar artery; VA, vertebral artery.

high-flow bleeding when opened intraoperatively. Moreover, some small veins connected with the basilar plexus can be found within the midclivus, especially in the inferior portion, where the spheno-occipital synchondrosis is located.[38] Injection of cadaver veins for laboratory training provides the reader with a direct perception of the position and density of such plexus. At the same time, vein injection may contribute to obscure other anatomical details of the area. Ideally, multiple sessions with differently injected specimens are recommended.

Within the intradural space, an in-depth analysis of the basilar artery (whose course varies from straight and median to exceedingly tortuous) and its collateral and terminal branches is of utmost importance. For this purpose, delicate and complete dissection of the anterior pontine arachnoid membrane is required to identify the neurovascular structures of the prepontine area.

As a final exercise after harvesting the approach through the midclivus, the reader is asked to accomplish an extradural hypophysiopexy by removing the sellar floor and dorsum sellae without opening the sellar periosteum. Though less extended compared with the interdural and intradural variants (described in Chapter 10), this corridor provides substantial exposure of the interpeduncular fossa and related structures with minimal manipulation of the pituitary gland.

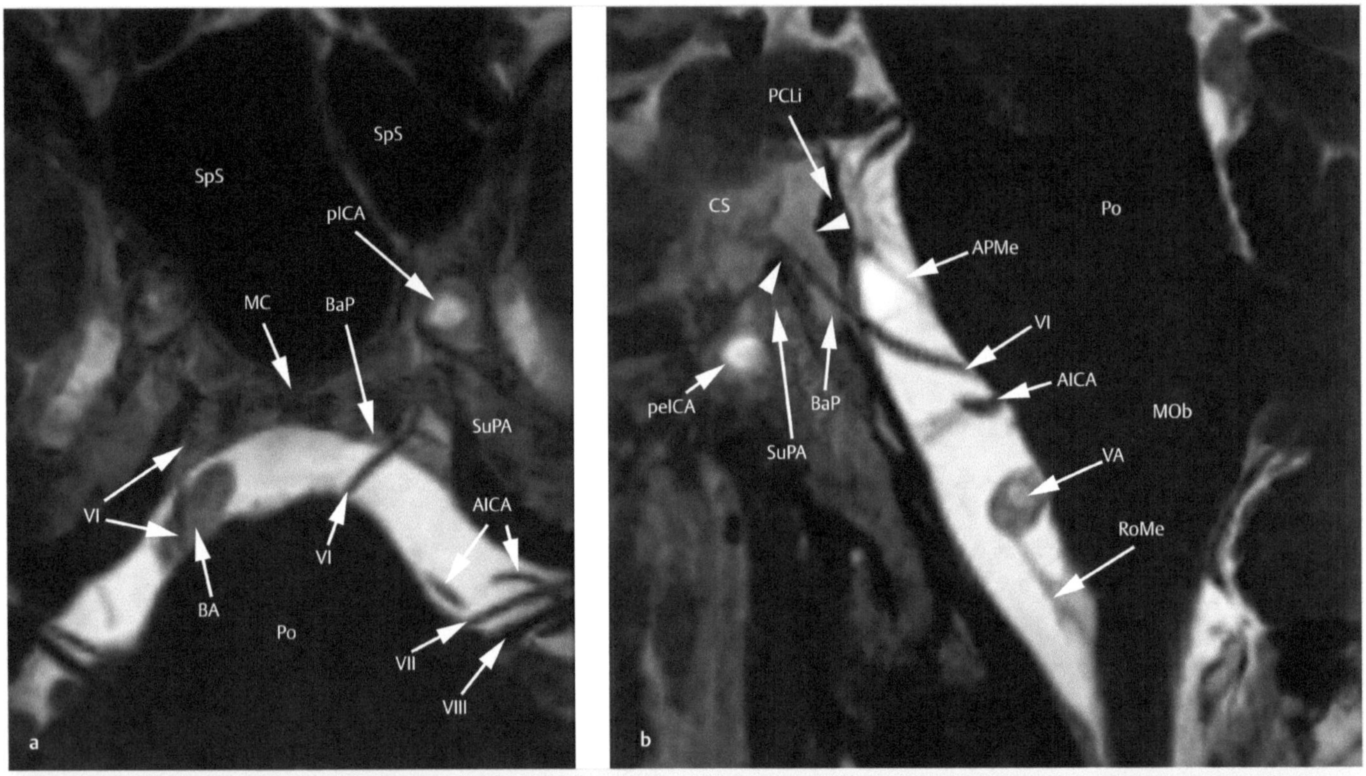

Fig. 11.3 Axial and parasagittal MRI anatomy of the abducens nerve. Panel including a para-axial **(a)** and a parasagittal **(b)** constructive interference in steady state (CISS) MRI scans following the orientation of the left abducens nerve. The abducens nerve (VI) arises from the passage between the medulla oblongata (MOb) and the pons (Po) and runs with an ascending trajectory toward the basilar plexus (BaP). Following a course from inferoposterior to superoanterior, the abducens nerve passes through the Dorello canal (between *arrowheads*), which lies between the superior petrous apex (SuPA), inferiorly, and petroclinoid (or Gruber's) ligament (PCLi), and reaches the cavernous sinus (CS). The abducens nerve crosses the basilar artery (BA) and anterior inferior cerebellar artery (AICA). VII, facial nerve; VIII, vestibulocochlear nerve; APMe, anterior pontine membrane; MC, midclivus; peICA, petrous tract of the internal carotid artery; pICA, paraclinoid tract of the internal carotid artery; RoMe, rhomboid membrane; SpS, sphenoid sinus; SuPA, superior petrous apex; VA, vertebral artery.

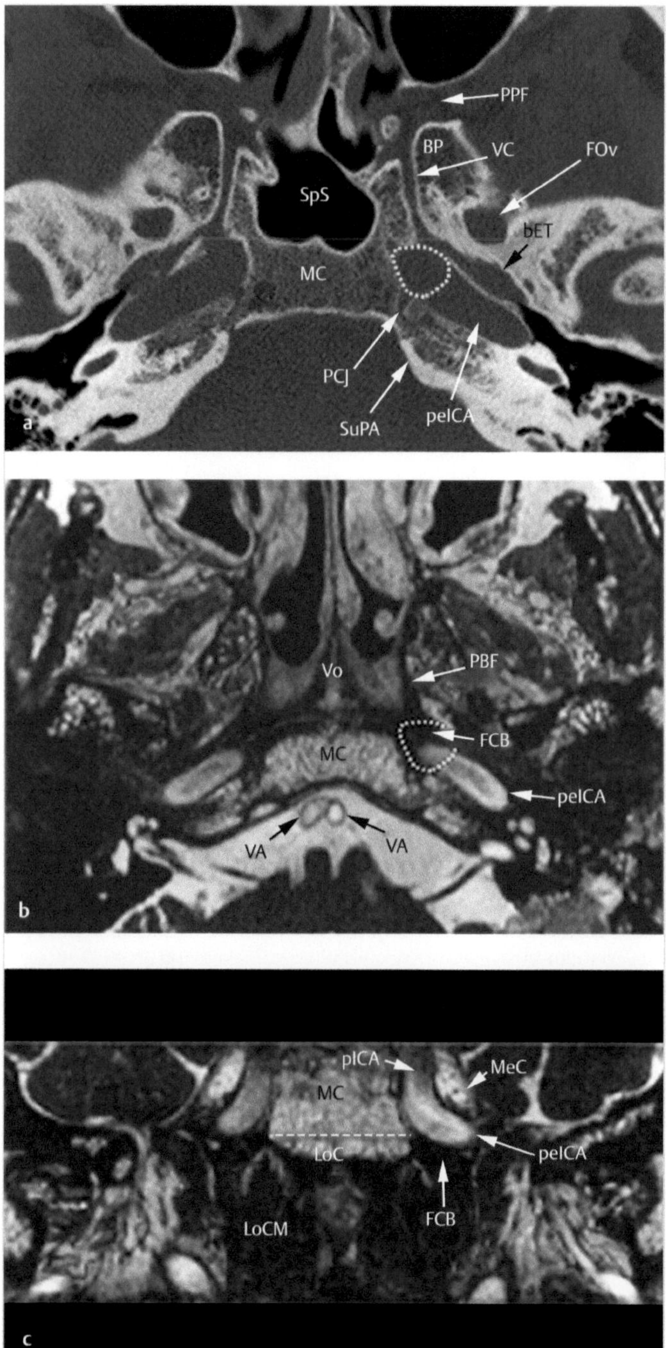

Fig. 11.4 Axial and coronal CT and MRI anatomy of the midclivus. The panel includes one axial CT **(a)** and an axial **(b)** and coronal constructive interference in steady state (CISS) MRI scan **(c)** passing through the midclivus (MC). The midclivus separates the sphenoid sinuses (SpS) from the posterior cranial fossa. It lies medial to the petroclival junction (PCJ), superior petrous apex (SuPA), and foramen lacerum (*white dotted line*), which houses the anterior genu between the petrous tract of the internal carotid artery (peICA) and the paraclival tract of the internal carotid artery (pICA) along with the fibrocartilago basalis (FCB). *White dashed line*, plane passing through the vidian canals. bET, bony portion of the eustachian tube; BP, base of the pterygoid process; FOv, foramen ovale; LoC, lower clivus; LoCM, longus capitis muscle; MeC, Meckel's cave; PBF, pharyngobasilar fascia; PPF, pterygopalatine fossa; VA, vertebral artery; VC, vidian canal; Vo, vomer.

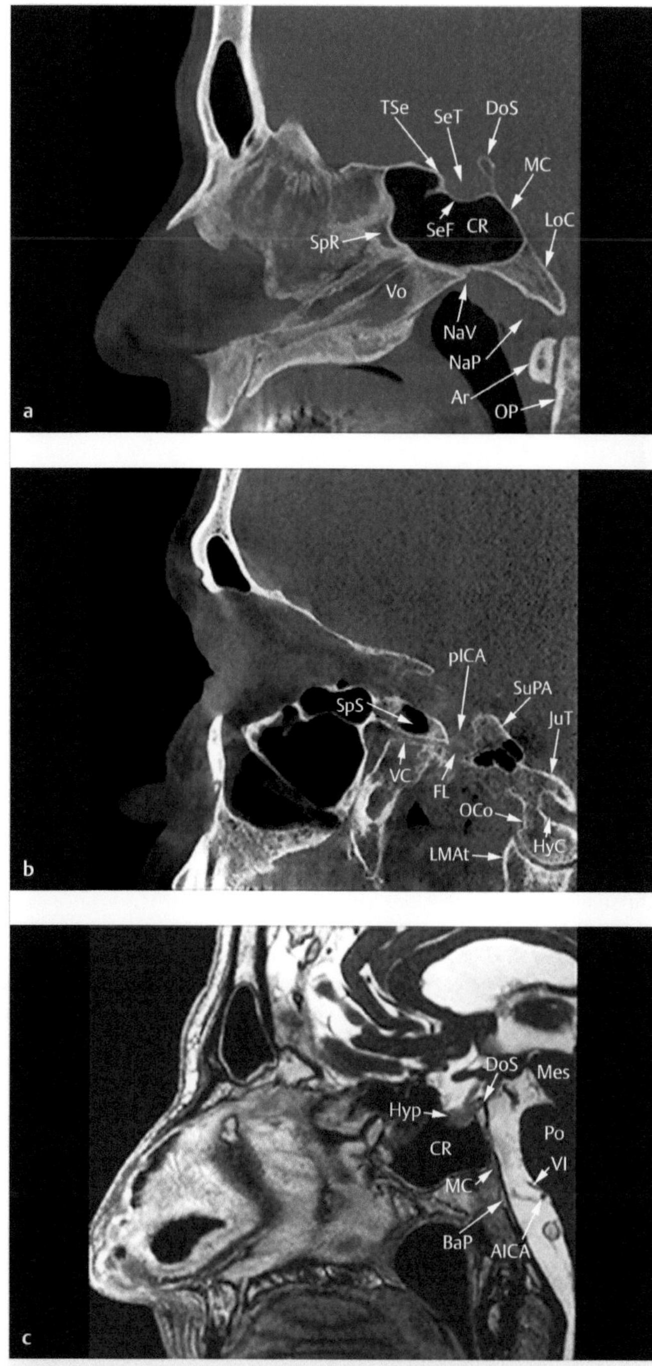

Fig. 11.5 Sagittal CT and MRI anatomy of the midclivus. The panel contains a median **(a)** and paramedian **(b)** CT and one sagittal constructive interference in steady state (CISS) MRI scans **(c)** passing through the midclivus (MC) and adjacent areas. The midclivus lies posterior to the clival recess (CR) of the sphenoid sinus, which can be variably pneumatized. The planes separating the midclivus from the dorsum sellae (DoS) and lower clivus (LoC) pass through sellar floor (SeF) and nasopharyngeal vault (NaV), respectively. As a consequence, the upper, middle, and lower thirds of the clivus lie behind the sella turcica (SeT), clival recess of the sphenoid sinus, and nasopharyngeal posterior wall (NaP), respectively. The lateral boundary of the midclivus can be considered the sagittal plane passing through the vidian canal (VC), foramen lacerum (FL), paraclival tract of the internal carotid artery (pICA), and superior petrous apex (SuPA). The posterior surface of the midclivus is lined by the basilar venous plexus (BaP). The most important intradural structures behind the midclivus are the pons (Po), abducens nerve (VI), basilar artery, and anterior inferior artery (AICA), which are wrapped within the anterior pontine membrane. Ar, anterior arch of the atlas; HyC, hypoglossal canal; Hyp, hypophysis; JuT, jugular tuberculum; LMAt, lateral mass of the atlas; Mes, mesencephalon; OCo, occipital condyle; OP, odontoid process; SpR, sphenoid rostrum; TSe, tuberculum sellae; Vo, vomer.

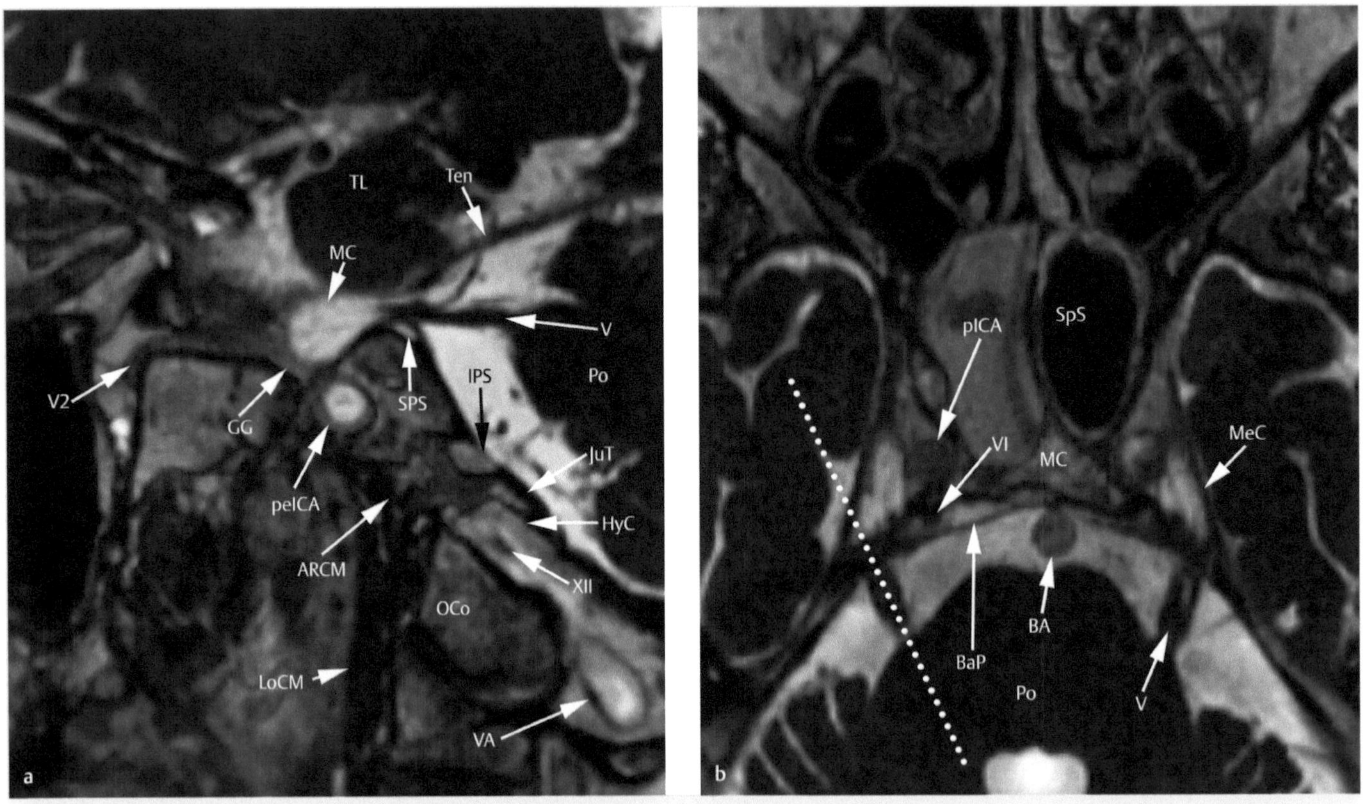

Fig. 11.6 Sagittal and axial MRI anatomy of the structures adjacent to the midclivus. The panel contains a paramedian sagittal **(a)** and an axial constructive interference in steady state (CISS) MRI scans **(b)** depicting the structures lateral to the midclivus. The white dotted line depicts the orientation of the parasagittal CISS MRI. The corridor passing through the midclivus lies immediately medial to several structures, which are, from anterior to posterior, the maxillary nerve (V2), Gasserian ganglion (GG) within the Meckel cave (MeC), petrous tract of the internal carotid artery (peICA), superior petrous apex, superior petrosal sinus (SPS), inferior petrosal sinus (IPS), and trigeminal stem (V). The abducens nerve (VI) runs with a superior–lateral–anterior trajectory from the bulbopontine sulcus toward the cavernous sinus. Therefore, while passing through the prepontine cistern and basilar plexus (BaP), it progressively moves away from the midline to reach the lateral surface of the internal carotid artery. XII, hypoglossal nerve; ARCM, anterior rectus capitis muscle; BA, basilar artery; HyC, hypoglossal canal; JuT, jugular tuberculum; LoCM, longus capitis muscle; OCo, occipital condyle; SpS, sphenoid sinus; Ten, tentorium cerebri; TL, temporal lobe of the brain; VA, vertebral artery.

Endoscopic Dissection

Nasal Phase

- Paraseptal sphenoidotomy.
- Transrostral sphenoidotomy.
- Expanded transrostral approach.
- Vertical uncinectomy.
- Anterior ethmoidectomy.
- Posterior ethmoidectomy.
- Transethmoidal sphenoidotomy.

Skull Base Phase

- Step 1: Removal of the floor of the sphenoid sinus.
- Step 2: Removal of the midclivus and medial portion of the carotid sulcus.
- Step 3: Removal of the petrous process of the sphenoid bone.
- Step 4: Incision of the clival periosteum.
- Step 5: Incision of the clival dura mater.
- Step 6: Removal of the sellar prominence, sellar floor, and dorsum sellae.
- Step 7: Removal of the periosteum and dura mater of the dorsum sellae.

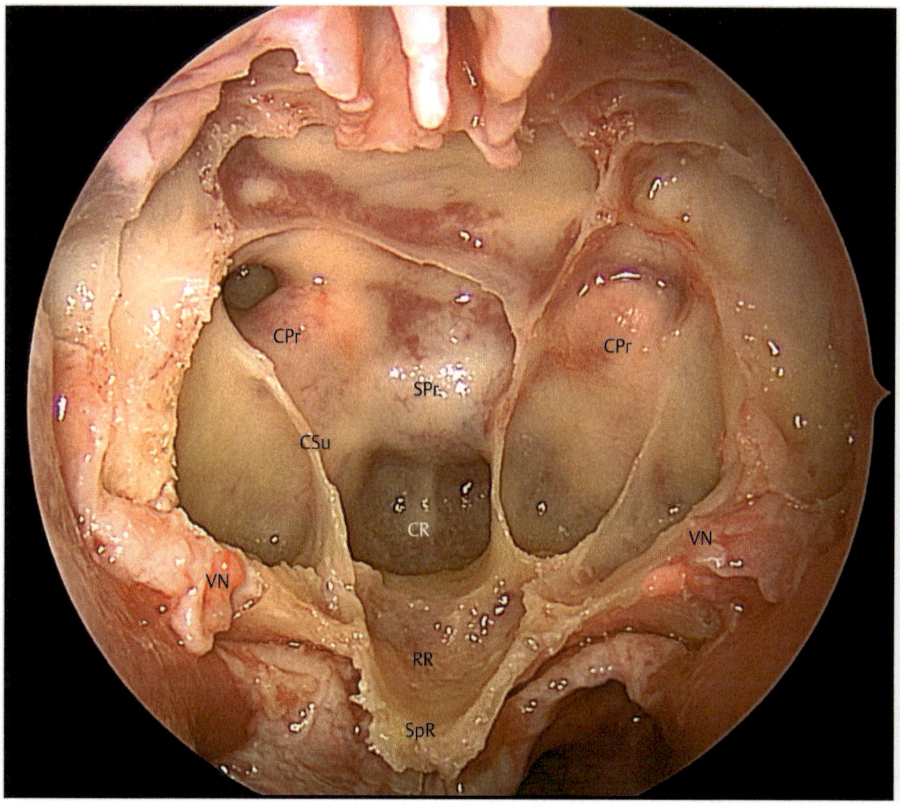

Fig. 11.7 Overview of the sphenoid sinus after an expanded transrostral sphenoidotomy. In a well-pneumatized sphenoid sinus, the clival recess (CR) is clearly visible below the sellar prominence (SPr) and medial to the carotid sulci (CSu). In a medial-to-lateral axis, the vidian nerve serves as a limit between the floor of the sphenoid sinus, which is pneumatized by a rostral recess (RR) in this specimen, and the lateral recess. In a cranial-to-caudal axis, the vidian canal marks the passage from the midclivus to the lower clivus. CPr, carotid prominence; SpR, sphenoidal rostrum.

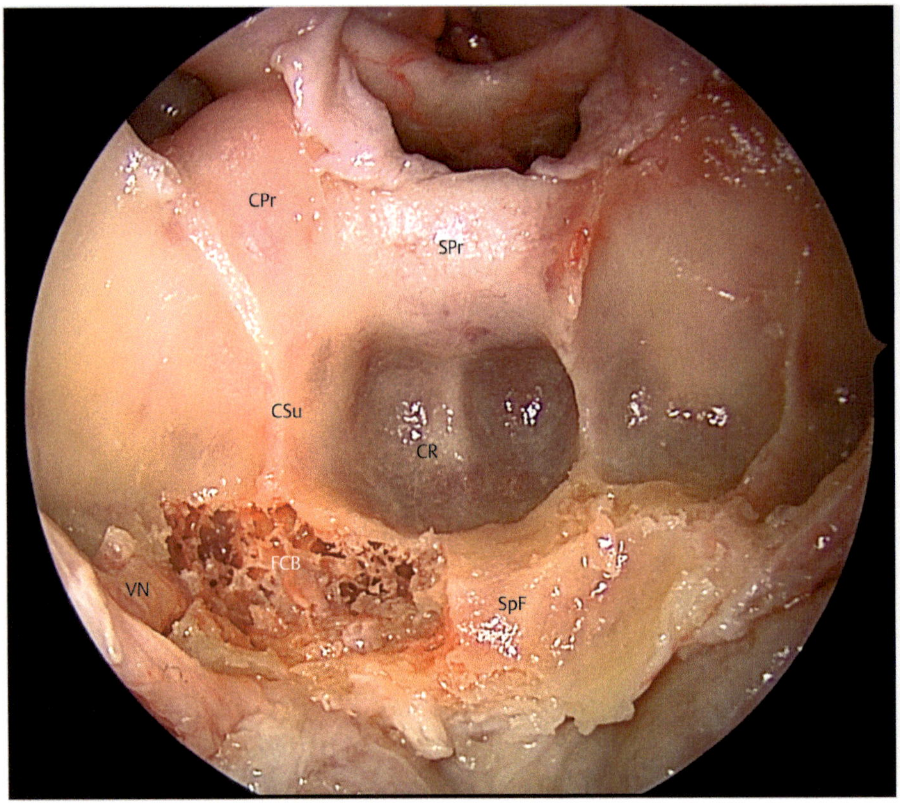

Fig. 11.8 Step 1. The sphenoidal rostrum and floor of the sphenoid sinus (SpF) are removed medially to the vidian nerve (VN), until the fibrocartilago basalis (FCB) is reached. This fibrocartilaginous tissue fills the foramen lacerum whose limits are the sphenoid body bone anteriorly, the anteroinferior petrous apex posterolaterally, and the clival portion of the occipital bone and petrous process of the sphenoid bone posteromedially. When the sphenoid sinus is sufficiently pneumatized, the carotid sulcus (CSu) can be identified and used as a landmark for the foramen lacerum and the paraclival tract of the internal carotid artery. CPr, carotid prominence; CR, clival recess; SPr, sellar prominence.

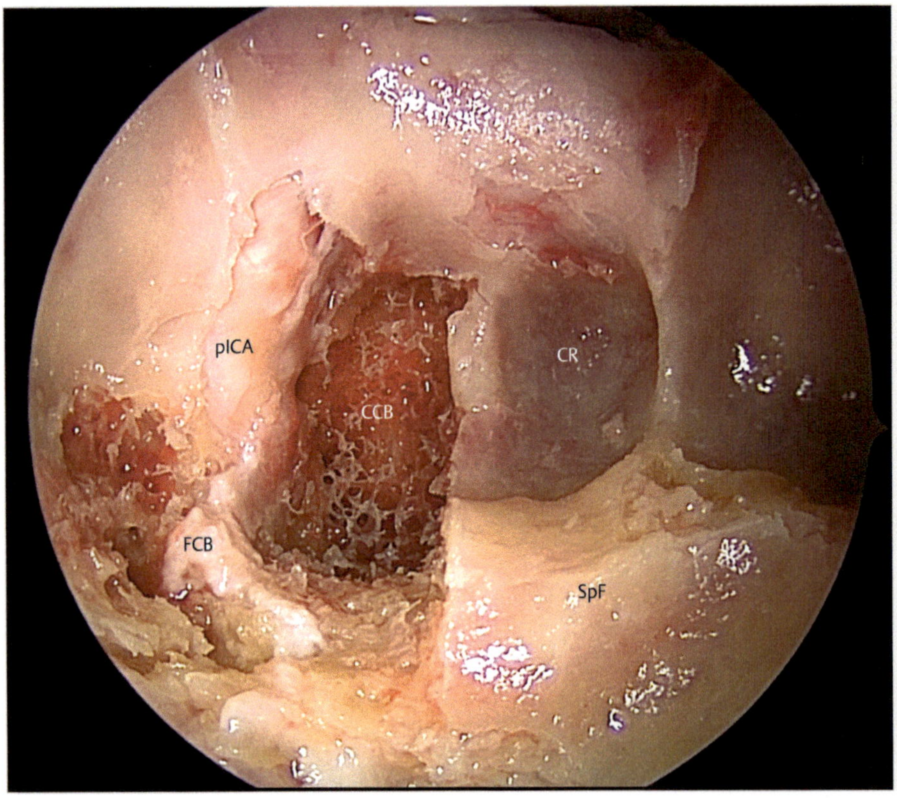

Fig. 11.9 Step 2. Starting from the floor of the sphenoid sinus (SpF), the anterior cortical and medullary bones of the midclivus are removed sparing the sellar floor and sellar prominence. In this way, the posterior clival cortical bone (CCB) is reached. Then, the medial portion of the carotid sulcus is removed to expose the paraclival tract of the internal carotid artery (pICA). FCB, fibrocartilago basalis; CR, clival recess.

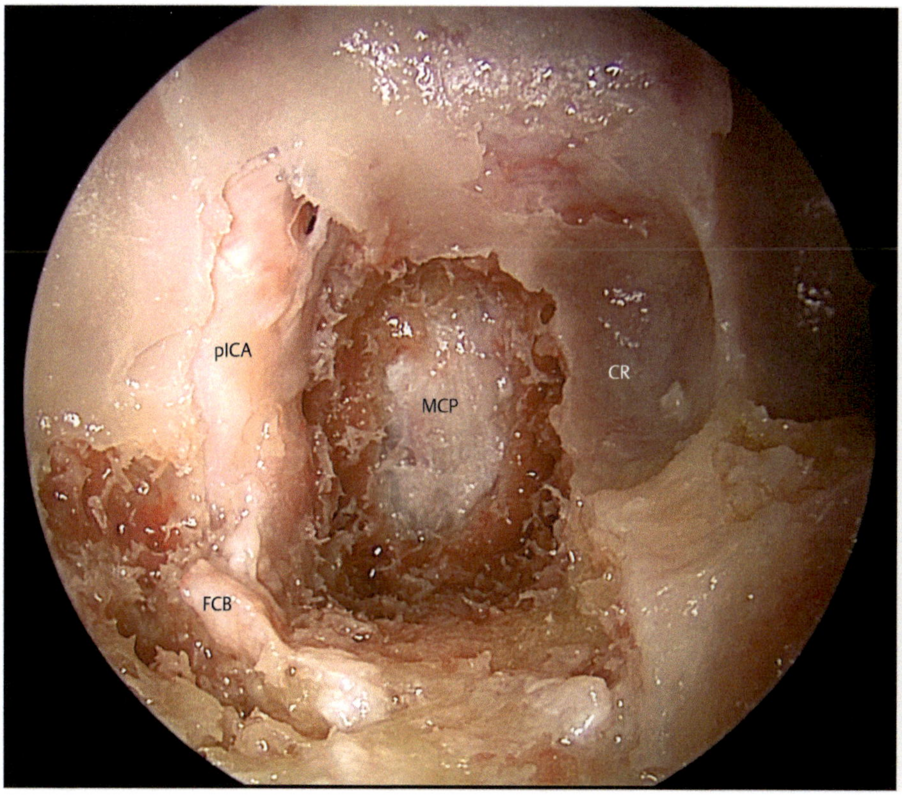

Fig. 11.10 The periosteum of the midclivus. The posterior cortical bone of the midclivus is removed to expose its periosteum (MCP). CR, clival recess; FCB, fibrocartilago basalis; pICA, paraclival tract of the internal carotid artery.

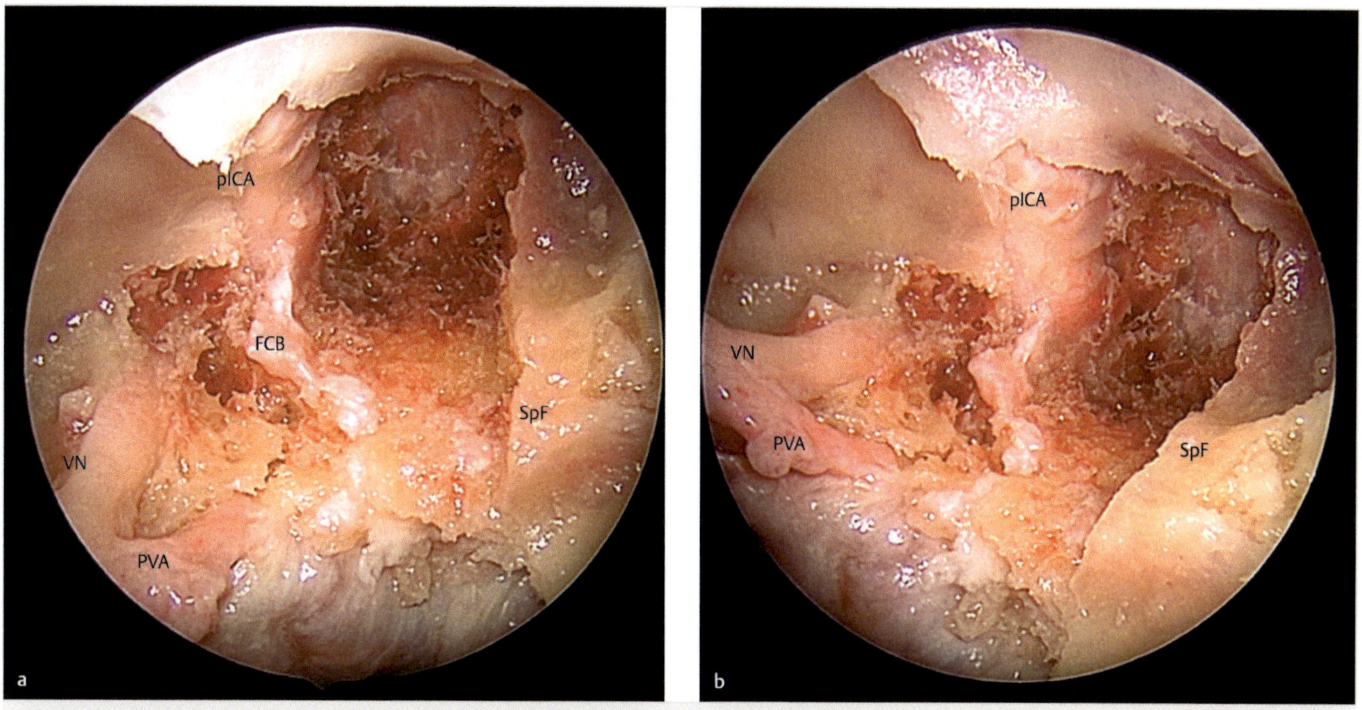

Fig. 11.11 The vidian nerve, fibrocartilago basalis, and internal carotid artery. A 45-degree scope is employed and turned inferiorly **(a)** and inferolaterally **(b)**. The vidian nerve (VN) follows the plane of the sphenoidal floor within a bony canal that begins just in front of the foramen lacerum. The fibrocartilago basalis serves as a bed for the anterior carotid genu, which is defined as the area where the petrous portion of the internal carotid artery turns into the paraclival tract (pICA). The palatovaginal artery (PVA), a branch of the sphenopalatine artery, passes through the palatovaginal canal, which is a bony tunnel formed by the upper edge of the sphenoid process of the palatine bone and the anteroinferior wall of the sphenoid body. This artery runs below the floor of the sphenoid sinus (SpF). Notably, the medial portion of the anterior carotid genu lies slightly medially to the trajectory of the vidian canal. Consequently, drilling medial to the vidian nerve can be considered safe only anterior to the area of the fibrocartilago basalis.

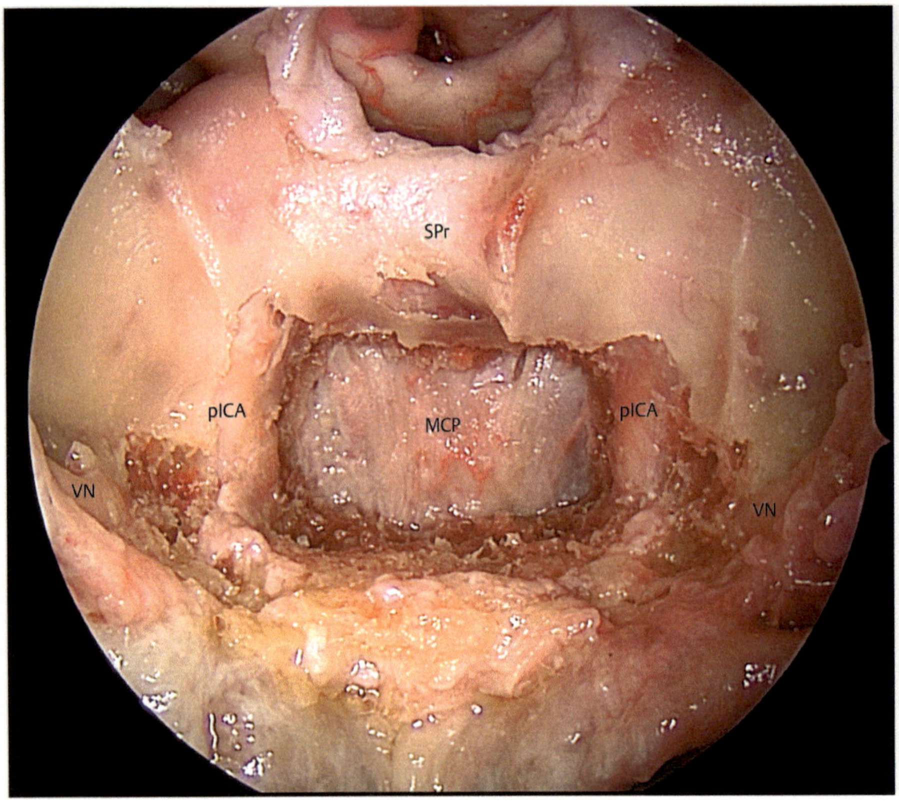

Fig. 11.12 Bilateral window through the midclivus. The periosteum of the midclivus (MCP) is completely exposed between the paraclival tracts of the internal carotid arteries (pICA). SPr, sellar prominence; VN, vidian nerve.

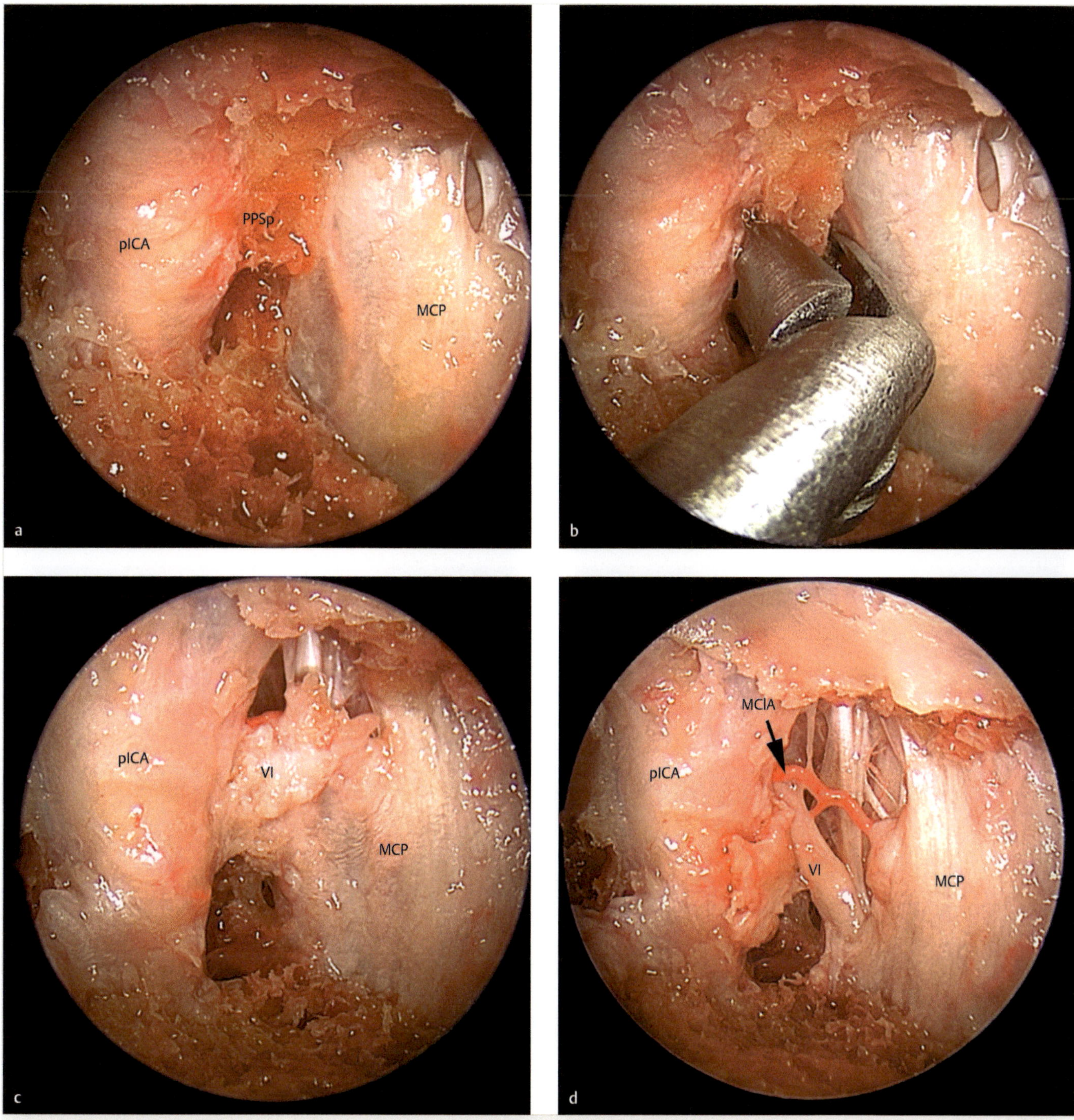

Fig. 11.13 (a–d) Step 3. The petrous process of the sphenoid bone (PPSp) lies between the periosteum of the midclivus (MCP) and the posterior surface of the paraclival tract of the internal carotid artery (pICA). This process of the sphenoidal portion of the clivus reaches the petrous apex, forming the petroclival junction. After removing the petrous process of the sphenoid bone, a periosteal fold directed toward the internal carotid artery is identified and opened to expose the abducens nerve (VI) within the basilar plexus. This tract of the abducens nerve runs in a vertical fashion and is often close to the medial clival artery (MClA).

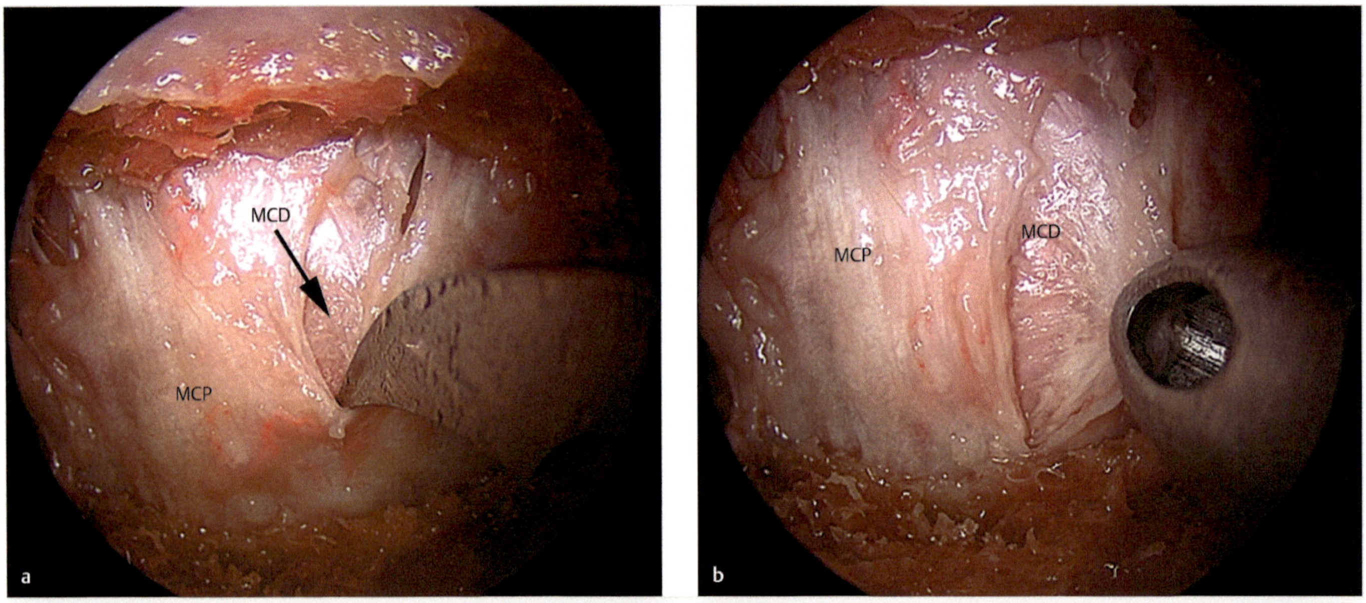

Fig. 11.14 (a, b) Step 4. A vertical incision of the periosteum of the midclivus (MCP) is made on the midline. Then, the periosteal flap is pulled laterally to identify the dura mater of the midclivus (MCD).

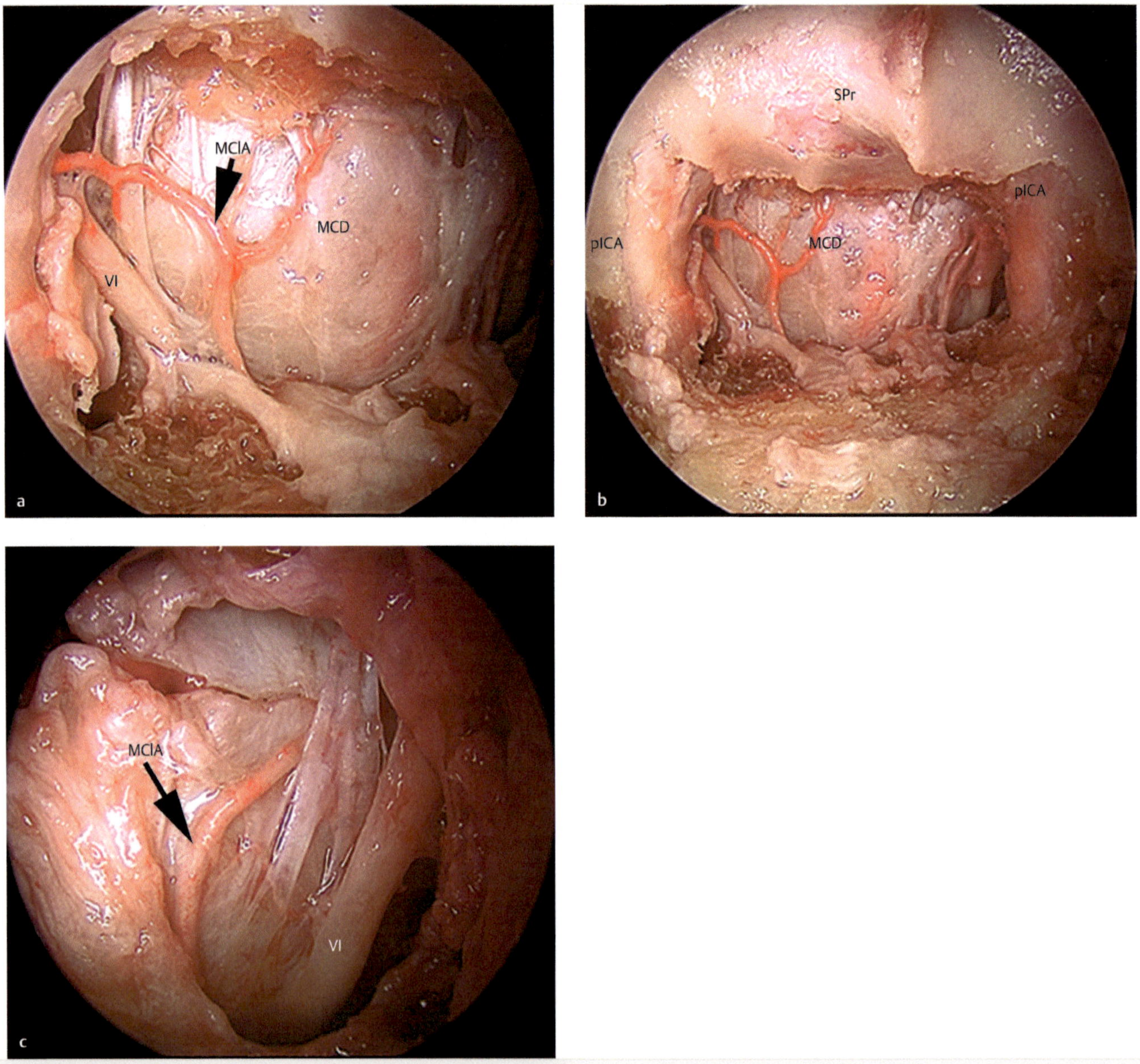

Fig. 11.15 (a–c) The dura mater of the midclivus. The dura mater of the midclivus (MCD) is separated completely from the adjacent periosteum. VI, abducens nerve; MClA, medial clival artery; pICA, paraclival tract of the internal carotid artery; SPr, sellar prominence.

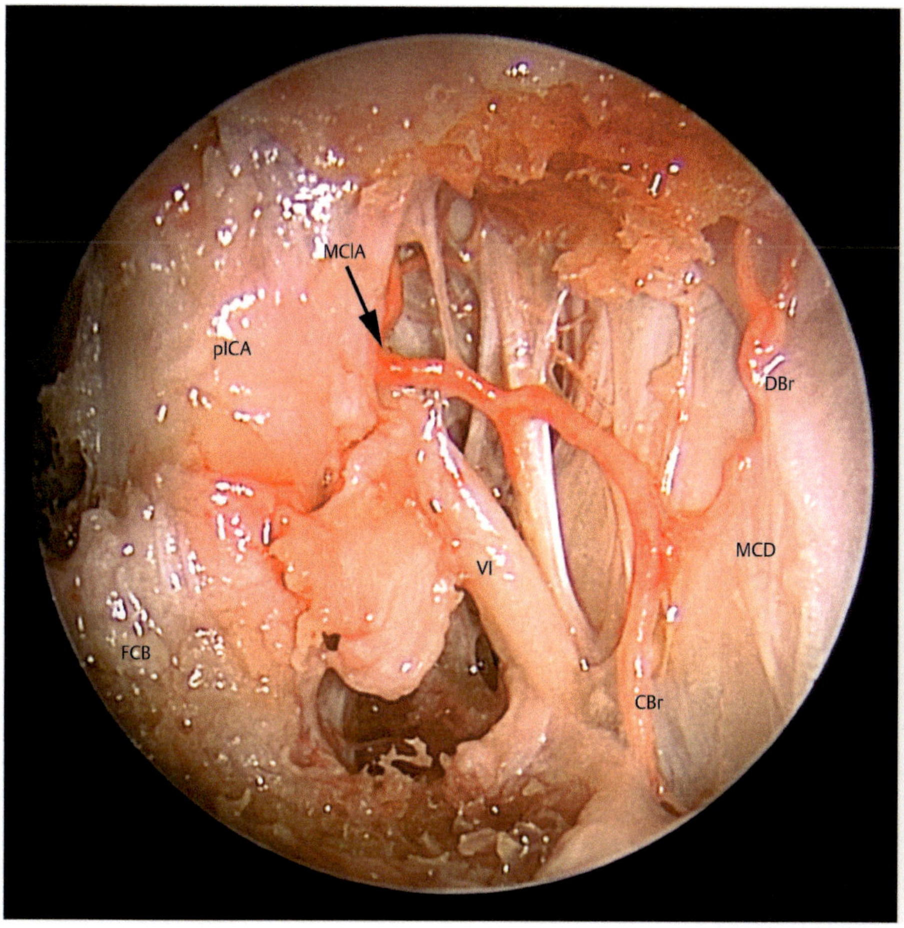

Fig. 11.16 The medial clival artery. The medial clival artery (MClA) arises from the meningohypophyseal artery, runs toward the midclivus, and bifurcates into the dorsal branch (DBr), which ascends to the dorsum sellae, and the clival branch (CBr), which descends to the midclivus and lower third of the clivus. Both the abducens nerve (VI) and medial clival artery run within the basilar plexus between the dura mater posteriorly and periosteum anteriorly.

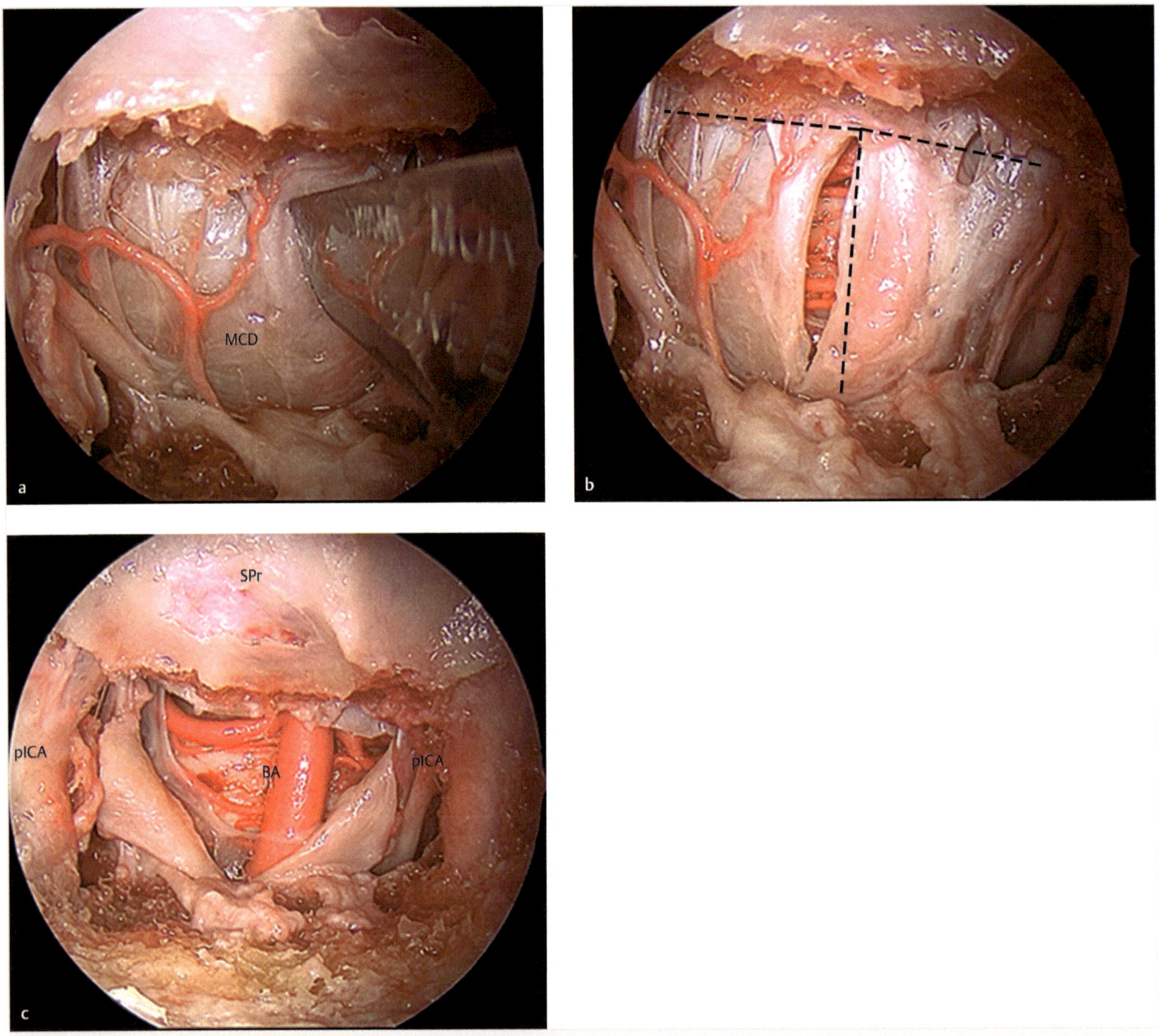

Fig. 11.17 (a–c) Step 5. Using a knife, a T-shaped incision (*black dashed line*) is made on the dura mater of the midclivus (MCD). The resulting dural flaps are pulled laterally to show intradural structures. BA, basilar artery; pICA, paraclival tract of the internal carotid artery; SPr, sellar prominence.

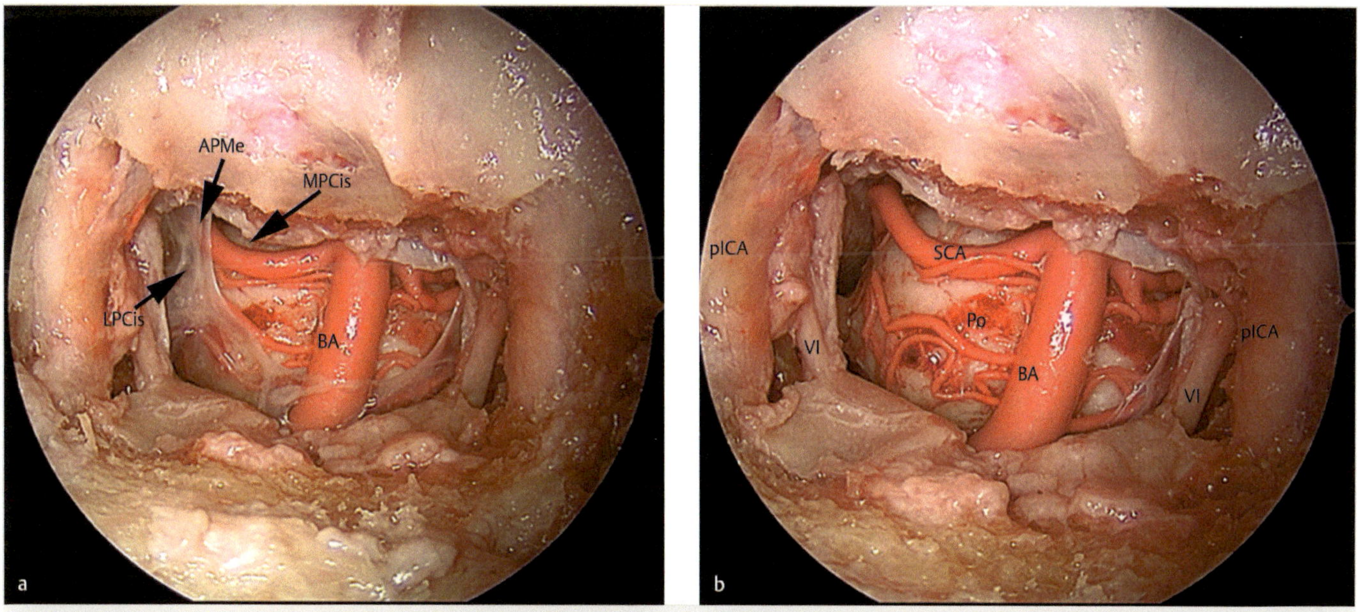

Fig. 11.18 (a, b) The anterior pontine membrane. A dural incision parallel to the abducens nerve is made on both sides. The anterior pontine membrane (APMe) continues from the mesencephalic portion of the Liliequist membrane and forms the anterior and lateral walls of the prepontine cistern. It lies between the clival dura mater and neurovascular structures of the brainstem and divides the medial pontine (or prepontine) cistern (MPCis) from the lateral pontine cistern (LPCis). The superior cerebellar artery (SCA) arises from the lateral surface of the basilar artery (BA) and runs toward the cerebellum. The pons (Po) is identified beneath these structures. The abducens nerves (VI) and paraclival tract of the internal carotid artery (pICA) bound laterally the transclival window.

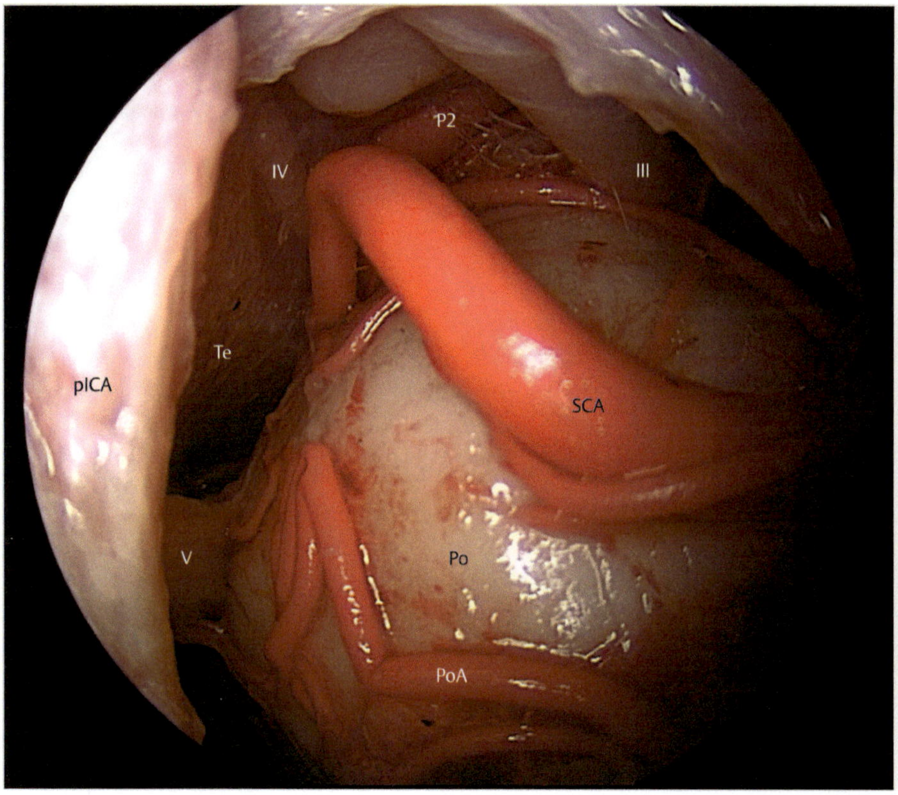

Fig. 11.19 The lateral pontine cistern. The endoscope is placed next to the paraclival tract of the internal carotid artery (pICA) to explore the lateral pontine cistern. The superior cerebellar artery (SCA) and the pontine arteries (PoA) arise from the basilar artery and run horizontally in front of the pons (Po). The oculomotor nerve (III) runs above the superior cerebellar artery. The trochlear nerve (IV) runs toward the tentorium cerebri (Te) and enters its free edge. In the space between the trochlear and oculomotor nerves, the postcommunicating tract of the posterior cerebral artery (P2) can be identified. The trigeminal stem arises from the lateral portion of the pons and runs laterally to the paraclival tract of the internal carotid artery. V, trigeminal stem

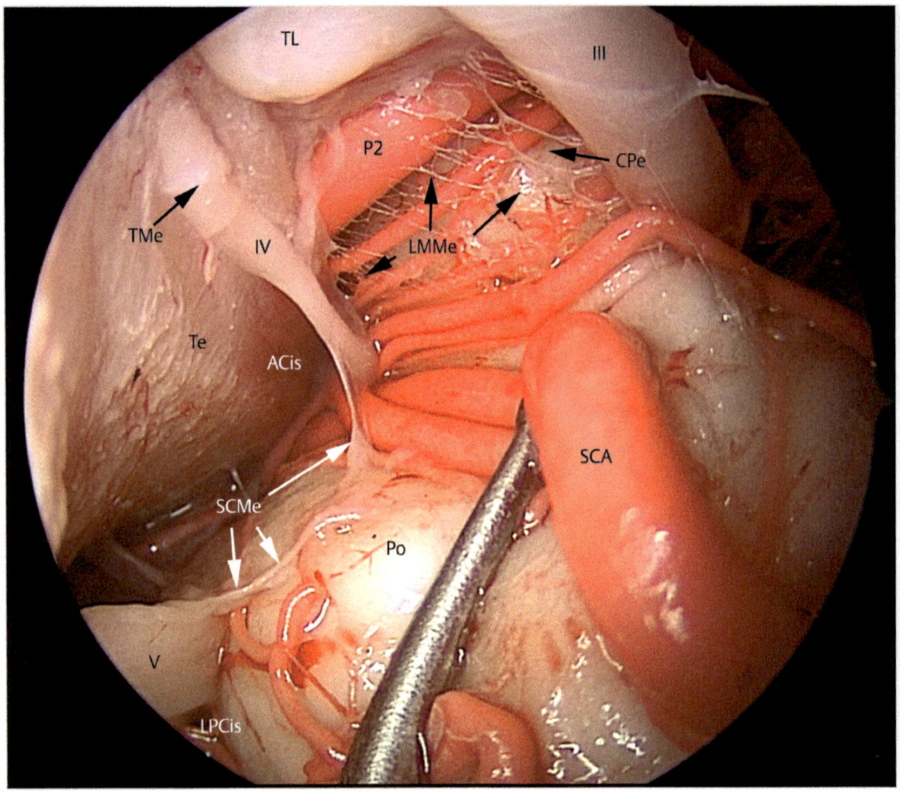

Fig. 11.20 The tentorium cerebri and related arachnoid membranes. The superior cerebellar membrane (SCMe) follows the superior cerebellar artery (SCA) and attaches to the trigeminal stem (V) and the trochlear nerve (IV). The lateral mesencephalic membrane (LMMe) lies between the tentorium cerebri (Te) and the oculomotor nerve (III), inferolaterally to the postcommunicating tract of the posterior cerebral artery (P2) and cerebral peduncle (CPe). The tentorium cerebri serves as lateral limit of this portion of the basal cisterns. ACis, ambient cistern; LPCis, lateral pontine cistern; Po, pons; TL, temporal lobe; TMe, trochlear membrane.

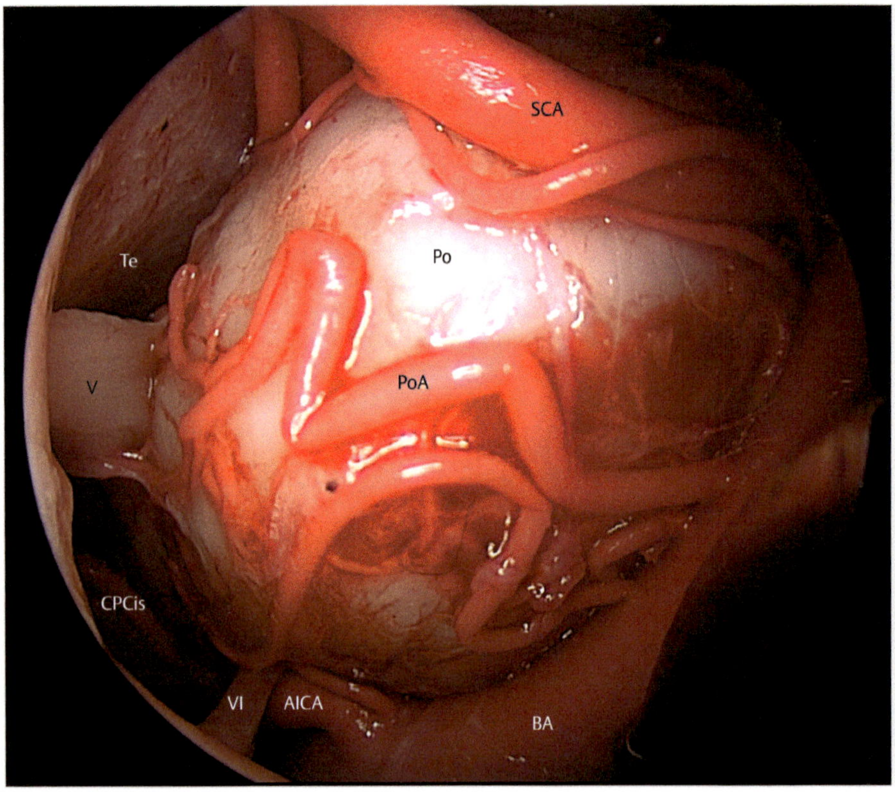

Fig. 11.21 The cisternal tract of the abducens nerve. By moving the 0-degree scope inferiorly, the abducens nerve (VI), is identified. It arises from the bulbopontine junction, runs upward, and crosses the anterior inferior cerebellar artery (AICA), which originates from the basilar artery (BA). The cerebellopontine angle cistern (CPCis) lies between the pons (Po), the medulla oblongata, the cerebellum, and the petrous bone and corresponds to the inferior prolongation of the lateral pontine cistern. V, trigeminal stem; PoA, pontine arteries; SCA, superior cerebellar artery; Te, tentorium cerebri.

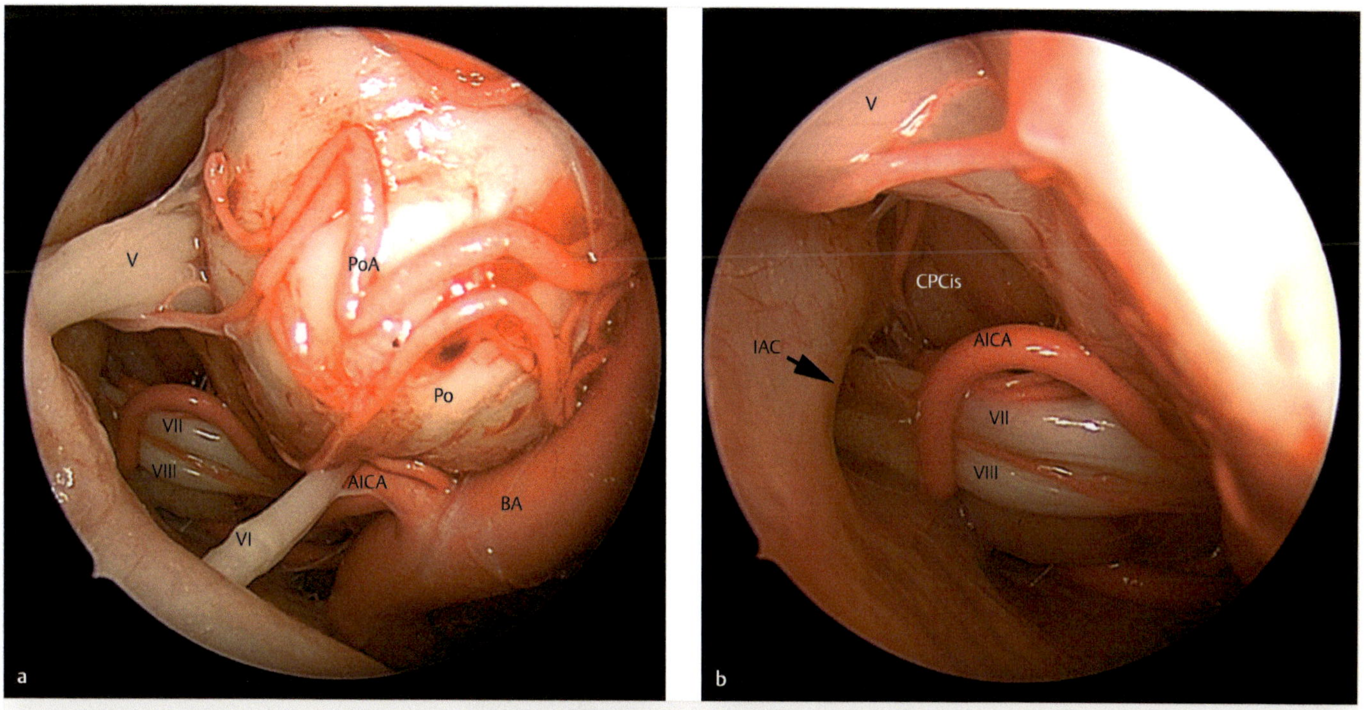

Fig. 11.22 (a, b) The acoustic-facial bundle. A 70-degree scope is inserted and turned inferolaterally. The acoustic-facial bundle includes the facial (VII) and vestibulocochlear (VIII) nerves and enters the internal auditory canal (IAC) after crossing the cerebellopontine angle cistern (CPCis). The anterior inferior cerebellar artery (AICA) crosses this structure, giving origin to the labyrinthine artery. V, trigeminal stem; VI, abducens nerve; BA, basilar artery; Po, pons; PoA, pontine artery.

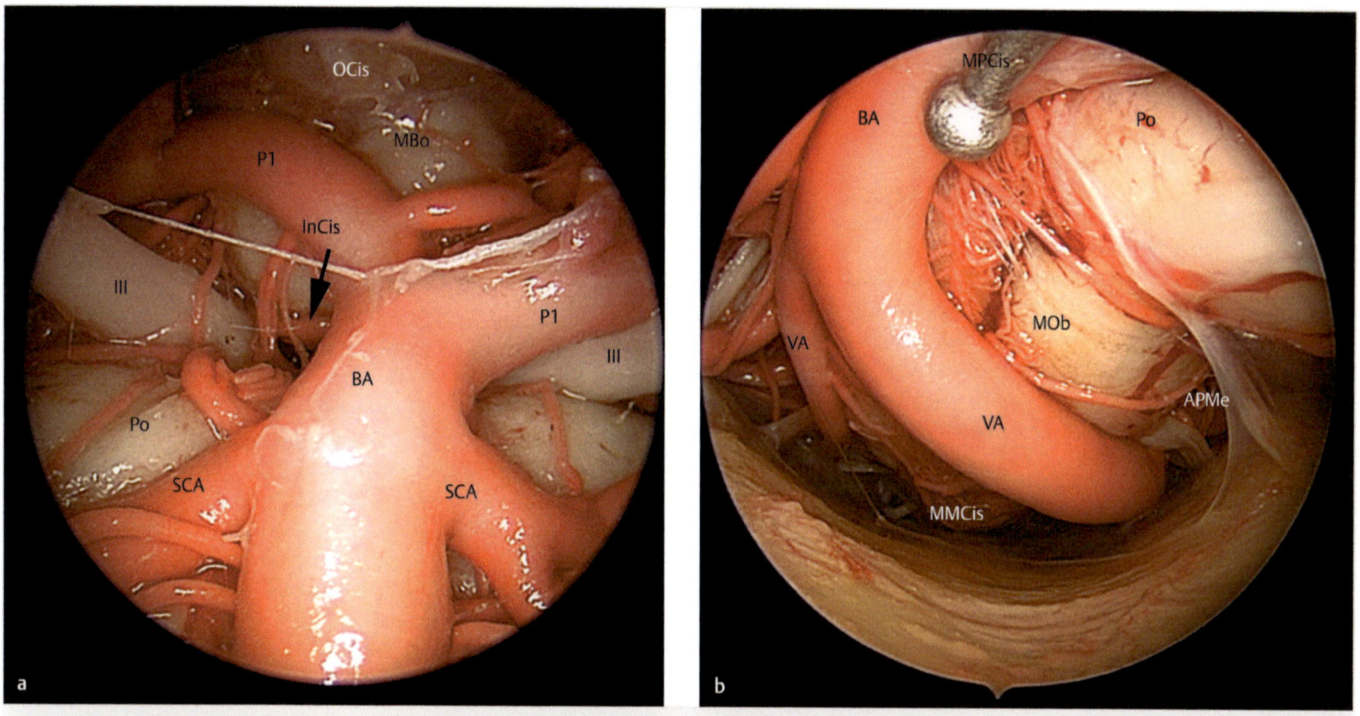

Fig. 11.23 The basilar tip and the vertebrobasilar junction. View with a 70-degree scope turned superiorly **(a)**: the basilar artery (BA) bifurcates into the precommunicating tracts of the posterior cerebral arteries (P1), just below the mammillary bodies (MBo). The interpeduncular (InCis) and optic (OCis) cisterns lie superoposteriorly and superoanteriorly to this area, respectively. The oculomotor nerves (III) run between the ipsilateral posterior cerebral artery and the superior cerebellar artery (SCA). The scope is then turned inferiorly **(b)**: the basilar artery arises from the two vertebral arteries (VA), which are generally asymmetric. The vertebral arteries run in front of the medulla oblongata (MOb), within the medial medullary cistern, which is covered anteriorly by the rhomboid membrane. APMe, anterior pontine membrane (sectioned); MPCis, median pontine cistern; Po, pons.

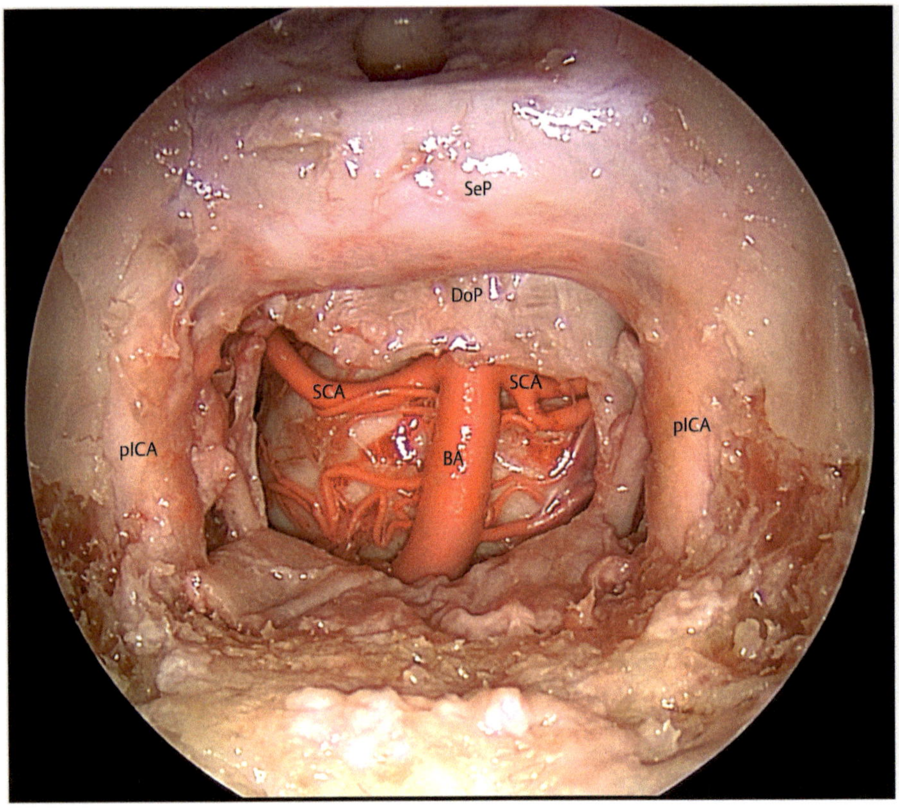

Fig. 11.24 Step 6. To perform the subsellar expansion of the transclival (midclivus) approach, the sellar prominence, sellar floor, and dorsum sellae are removed to expose the sellar (SeP) and dorsal periosteal linings (DoP). BA, basilar artery; pICA, paraclival tract of the internal carotid artery; SCA, superior cerebellar artery.

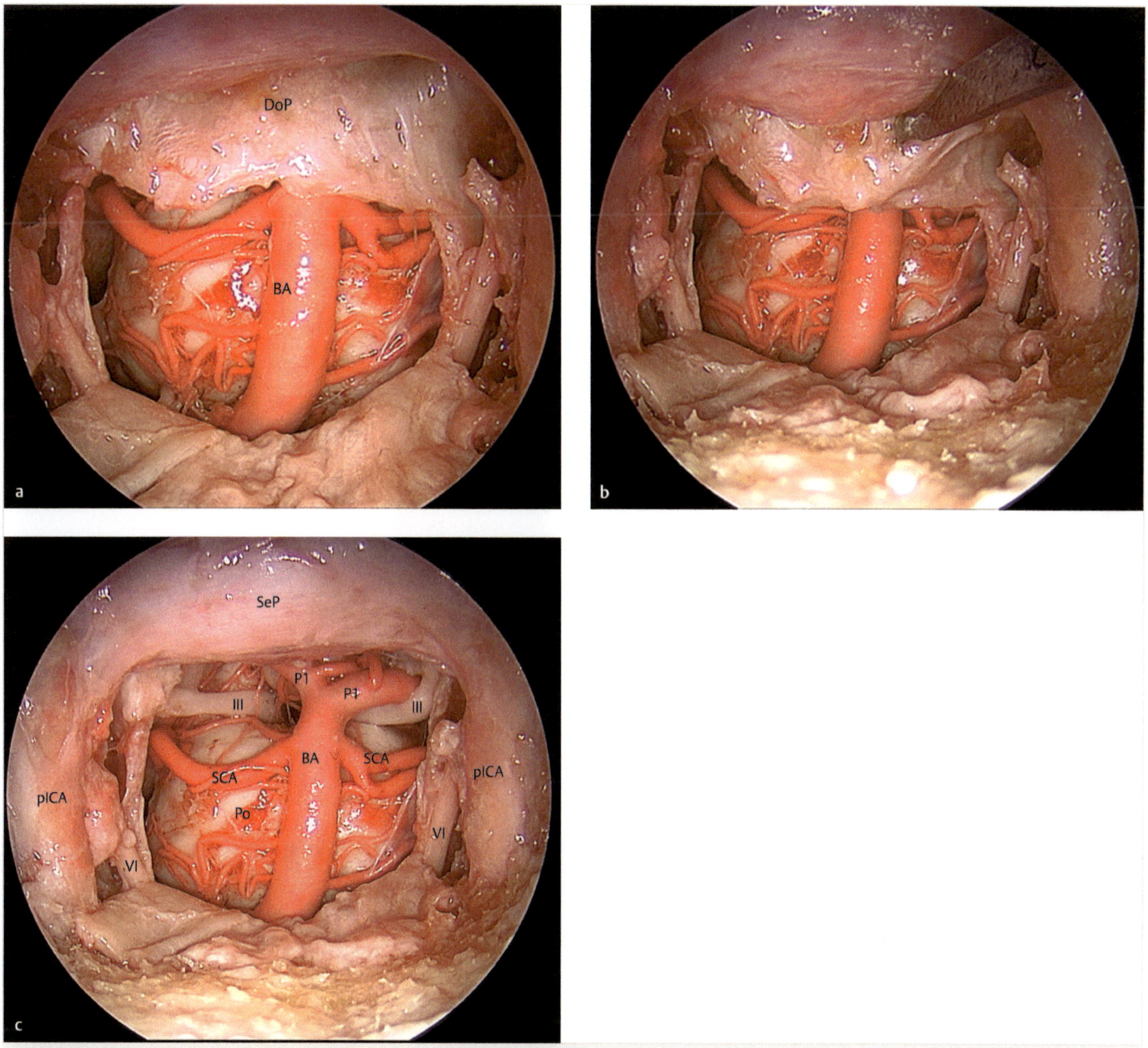

Fig. 11.25 (a–c) Step 7. The periosteum of the dorsum sellae (DoP) is removed preserving the periosteum of the sella turcica (SeP). This step represents the subsellar transdorsal extension of the transclival (midclivus) approach (also defined as extradural hypophysiopexy) and allows us to directly reach the tip of the basilar artery (BA), precommunicating tract of the posterior cerebral artery (P1), oculomotor nerves (III), and superior cerebellar arteries (SCA) with a 0-degree scope and instruments. The lateral boundaries of the approach are the abducens nerves (VI) and the paraclival tracts of the internal carotid arteries (pICA). Po, pons.

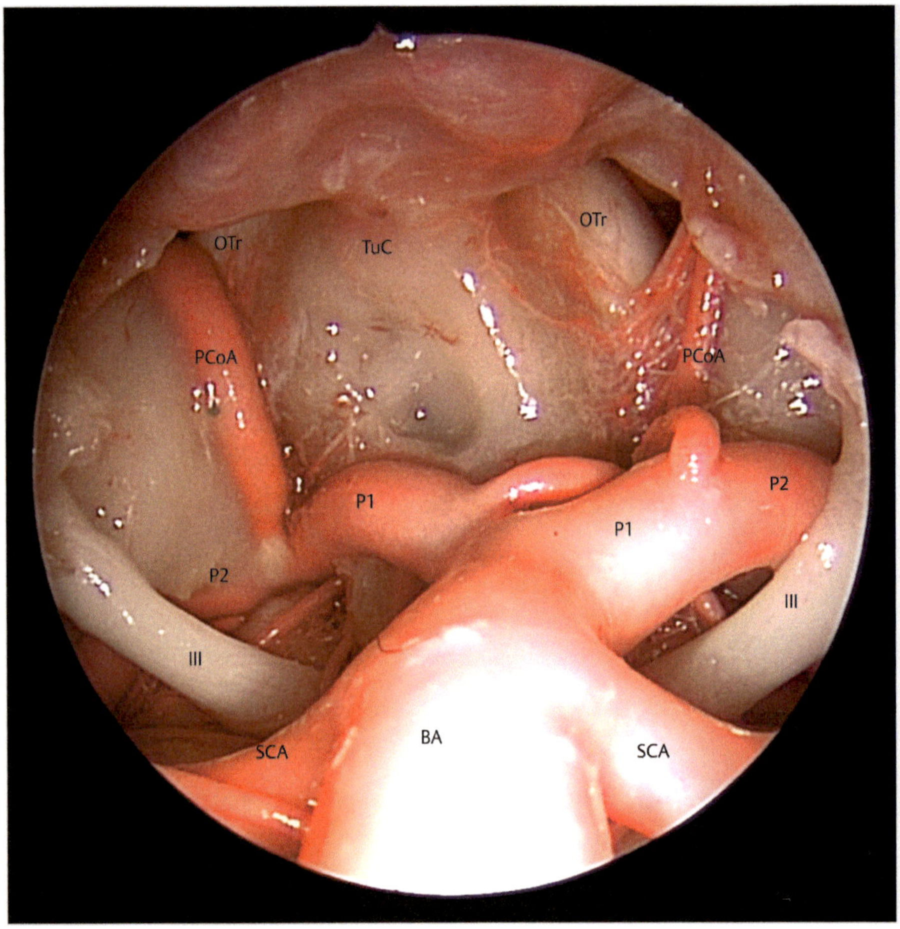

Fig. 11.26 The optic cistern. View with a 70-degree scope turned superiorly, and placed in front of the basilar artery (BA). In this way, the optic cistern can be identified posteriorly to the tuber cinereum (TuC) and inferiorly to the optic tracts (OTr). The posterior communicating artery (PCoA) marks the passage from the precommunicating tract (P1) to the postcommunicating tract (P2) of the posterior cerebral artery. The oculomotor nerves (III) pass below the posterior cerebral arteries, running parallel to the posterior communicating artery. SCA, superior cerebellar artery.

References

[1] Doglietto F, Ferrari M, Mattavelli D, et al. Transnasal endoscopic and lateral approaches to the clivus: a quantitative anatomic study. World Neurosurg 2018;113:e659–e671

[2] Shkarubo AN, Koval KV, Chernov IV, et al. Endoscopic endonasal transclival approach to tumors of the clivus and anterior region of the posterior cranial fossa (results of surgical treatment of 136 patients). World Neurosurg 2018

[3] Vellutini EdeA, Balsalobre L, Hermann DR, Stamm AC. The endoscopic endonasal approach for extradural and intradural clivus lesions. World Neurosurg 2014;82(6, Suppl):S106–S115

[4] Kim YH, Jeon C, Se YB, et al. Clinical outcomes of an endoscopic transclival and transpetrosal approach for primary skull base malignancies involving the clivus. J Neurosurg 2018;128(5):1454–1462

[5] Little RE, Taylor RJ, Miller JD, et al. Endoscopic endonasal transclival approaches: case series and outcomes for different clival regions. J Neurol Surg B Skull Base 2014;75(4):247–254

[6] Dias LA, Nakanishi M, Mangussi-Gomes J, Canuto M, Takano G, Oliveira CA. Successful endoscopic endonasal management of a transclival cerebrospinal fluid fistula secondary to ecchordosis physaliphora: an ectopic remnant of primitive notochord tissue in the clivus. Clin Neurol Neurosurg 2014;117:116–119

[7] Fernandez-Miranda JC, Gardner PA, Snyderman CH, et al. Clival chordomas: a pathological, surgical, and radiotherapeutic review. Head Neck 2014;36(6):892–906

[8] Fraser JF, Nyquist GG, Moore N, Anand VK, Schwartz TH. Endoscopic endonasal transclival resection of chordomas: operative technique, clinical outcome, and review of the literature. J Neurosurg 2010;112(5):1061–1069

[9] Komotar RJ, Starke RM, Raper DM, Anand VK, Schwartz TH. The endoscope-assisted ventral approach compared with open microscope-assisted surgery for clival chordomas. World Neurosurg 2011;76(3–4):318–327, discussion 259–262

[10] Mangussi-Gomes J, Beer-Furlan A, Balsalobre L, Vellutini EA, Stamm AC. Endoscopic endonasal management of skull base chordomas: surgical technique, nuances, and pitfalls. Otolaryngol Clin North Am 2016;49(1):167–182

[11] Ditzel Filho LF, Prevedello DM, Dolci RL, et al. The endoscopic endonasal approach for removal of petroclival chondrosarcomas. Neurosurg Clin N Am 2015;26(3):453–462

[12] Beer-Furlan A, Abi-Hachem R, Jamshidi AO, Carrau RL, Prevedello DM. Endoscopic trans-sphenoidal surgery for petroclival and clival meningiomas. J Neurosurg Sci 2016;60(4):495–502

[13] Koutourousiou M, Fernandez-Miranda JC, Vaz-Guimaraes Filho F, et al. Outcomes of endonasal and lateral approaches to petroclival meningiomas. World Neurosurg 2017;99:500–517

[14] Prosser JD, Vender JR, Alleyne CH, Solares CA. Expanded endoscopic endonasal approaches to skull base meningiomas. J Neurol Surg B Skull Base 2012;73(3):147–156

[15] Gardner PA, Vaz-Guimaraes F, Jankowitz B, et al. Endoscopic endonasal clipping of intracranial aneurysms: surgical technique and results. World Neurosurg 2015;84(5):1380–1393

[16] Kourtopoulos H, Shamsgovara P, Dahlkvist A, Jonasson P. Transclival decompression of brainstem from a compressing coiled aneurysm of the midbasilar artery. Acta Neurochir (Wien) 2005;147(12):1291–1295, discussion 1295–1296

[17] Labib M, Dehdashti AR. Extended endoscopic endonasal transclival clipping of posterior circulation aneurysms: an alternative to the transcranial approach. Acta Neurochir (Wien) 2015;157(12):2087–2088

[18] Lemos-Rodríguez AM, Sreenath S, Unnithan A, et al. A new window for the treatment of posterior cerebral artery, superior cerebellar artery, and basilar apex aneurysm: the expanded endoscopic endonasal approach. J Neurol Surg B Skull Base 2016;77(4):308–313

[19] Sanmillan JL, Lawton MT, Rincon-Torroella J, et al. Assessment of the endoscopic endonasal transclival approach for surgical clipping of anterior pontine anterior-inferior cerebellar artery aneurysms. World Neurosurg 2016; 89:368–375

[20] Gonzalez-Quarante LH, Ruiz-Juretschke F, Iza-Vallejo B, Scola-Pliego E, Poletti D, Sola Vendrell E. Expanded endoscopic transclival approach for resection of a chordoid meningioma without dural attachment (MWODA) located in the prepontine cistern. World Neurosurg 2016;91:675.e5–675.e10

[21] Simal Julian JA, Sanromán Álvarez P, Miranda Lloret P, Plaza Ramirez E, Pérez Borreda P, Botella Asunción C. Full endoscopic endonasal transclival approach: meningioma attached to the ventral surface of the brainstem. Neurocirugia (Astur) 2014;25(3):140–144

[22] Prevedello DM, Fernandez-Miranda JC, Gardner P, et al. The transclival endoscopic endonasal approach (EEA) for prepontine neuroenteric cysts: report of two cases. Acta Neurochir (Wien) 2010;152(7):1223–1229

[23] Cobb WS, Makosch G, Anand VK, Schwartz TH. Endoscopic transsphenoidal, transclival resection of an enterogenous cyst located ventral to the brainstem: case report. Neurosurgery 2010;67(2, Suppl Operative):522–526

[24] Fomichev D, Kalinin P, Gavrushin A. Endoscopic transnasal transclival resection of endodermal cyst on ventral surface of brainstem. World Neurosurg 2017;97:756.e7–756.e11

[25] Esposito F, Becker DP, Villablanca JP, Kelly DF. Endonasal transsphenoidal transclival removal of prepontine epidermoid tumors: technical note. Neurosurgery 2005;56(2, Suppl):E443–, discussion E443

[26] Dallan I, Battaglia P, de Notaris M, Caniglia M, Turri-Zanoni M. Endoscopic endonasal transclival approach to a pontine cavernous malformation: case report. Int J Pediatr Otorhinolaryngol 2015;79(9):1584–1588

[27] Erickson N, Siu A, Sherman JH, Gragnaniello C, Singh A, Litvack Z. Endoscopic transnasal transclival approach to a pontine cavernoma with associated developmental venous anomaly. World Neurosurg 2018;118:212–218

[28] Gómez-Amador JL, Ortega-Porcayo LA, Palacios-Ortíz IJ, Perdomo-Pantoja A, Nares-López FE, Vega-Alarcón A. Endoscopic endonasal transclival resection of a ventral pontine cavernous malformation: technical case report. J Neurosurg 2017;127(3):553–558

[29] He SM, Wang Y, Zhao TZ, et al. Endoscopic endonasal approach to mesencephalic cavernous malformations. World Neurosurg 2016;90:701.e7–701.e10

[30] Linsler S, Oertel J. Endoscopic endonasal transclival resection of a brainstem cavernoma: a detailed account of our technique and comparison with the literature. World Neurosurg 2015;84(6):2064–2071

[31] Nayak NR, Thawani JP, Sanborn MR, Storm PB, Lee JY. Endoscopic approaches to brainstem cavernous malformations: case series and review of the literature. Surg Neurol Int 2015;6:68

[32] Sanborn MR, Kramarz MJ, Storm PB, Adappa ND, Palmer JN, Lee JY. Endoscopic, endonasal, transclival resection of a pontine cavernoma: case report. Neurosurgery 2012;71(1, Suppl Operative):198–203

[33] Rajappa P, Margetis K, Sigounas D, Anand V, Schwartz TH, Greenfield JP. Endoscopic endonasal transclival approach to a ventral pontine pediatric ependymoma. J Neurosurg Pediatr 2013;12(5):465–468

[34] Fernandes Cabral DT, Zenonos GA, Nuñez M, et al. Endoscopic endonasal transclival approach for resection of a pontine glioma: surgical planning, surgical anatomy, and technique. Oper Neurosurg (Hagerstown) 2018;15(5):589–599

[35] Wang J, Bidari S, Inoue K, Yang H, Rhoton A Jr. Extensions of the sphenoid sinus: a new classification. Neurosurgery 2010;66(4):797–816

[36] Cebula H, Kurbanov A, Zimmer LA, et al. Endoscopic, endonasal variability in the anatomy of the internal carotid artery. World Neurosurg 2014;82(6): e759–e764

[37] Pérez de San Román-Mena L, Simal-Julián JA, Miranda-Lloret P, Sanromán-Álvarez P, Botella-Asunción C. Radiological study of the carotid-clival window and its application in endoscopic endonasal expanded approaches. World Neurosurg 2017;104:356–360

[38] Altafulla JJ, Rai R, Shrager S, et al. Transclival venous circulation: anatomic study. World Neurosurg 2019;121:e136–e139

12 Transclival (Lower Clivus) Approach

Marco Ferrari, Marco Ravanelli, Davide Mattavelli, Alberto Schreiber, Francesco Doglietto

As seen from the transnasal perspective, the lower third of the clivus almost corresponds to the sphenoidal floor and the most superior portion of the posterior nasopharyngeal vault.[1] The resection of the lower third of the clivus is most frequently combined with other corridors through the midclivus or craniocervical junction (illustrated in Chapters 11 and 13, respectively). However, for the purpose of providing the reader with a modular understanding of transclival approaches,[2] this chapter specifically focuses on the surgical route through the lower third of the clivus. This corridor has been adopted alone or in combination with other transnasal endoscopic approaches for treating chordomas,[3-6] meningiomas,[7] chondrosarcomas,[4,8] nasopharyngeal carcinomas,[9] cholesterol granulomas,[10] craniopharyngiomas,[10] aneurysms,[11-13] and other rare lesions of the lower clivus and adjacent areas.[10,14-17]

The lower transclival corridor is bounded by the occipital condyle, the hypoglossal canal, and the jugular tubercle bilaterally, the midclivus superiorly, and the craniocervical junction inferiorly. Differently from other transclival approaches, the lateral boundary does not include the internal carotid artery, since the petrous and parapharyngeal tracts run more laterally compared with the paraclival and parasellar portions.

Even though it is theoretically possible to reach the inferior third of the clivus without opening the sphenoid sinus, an extended transrostral sphenoidotomy is recommended to get oriented with the bony landmarks of the sphenoid sinus. The most important bony landmarks of this route are located in a vertical fashion along the lateral boundary of the transclival corridor. From cranial to caudal, the jugular tubercle, the hypoglossal canal, and the occipital condyle can be easily recognized based on the type of bone: the jugular tubercle and the occipital condyle are mostly made of the medullary bone, while the hypoglossal canal is formed by thick cortical bone. The posterior projection of the tail of the inferior turbinate can be adopted as a landmark to identify in advance the position of the hypoglossal canal.

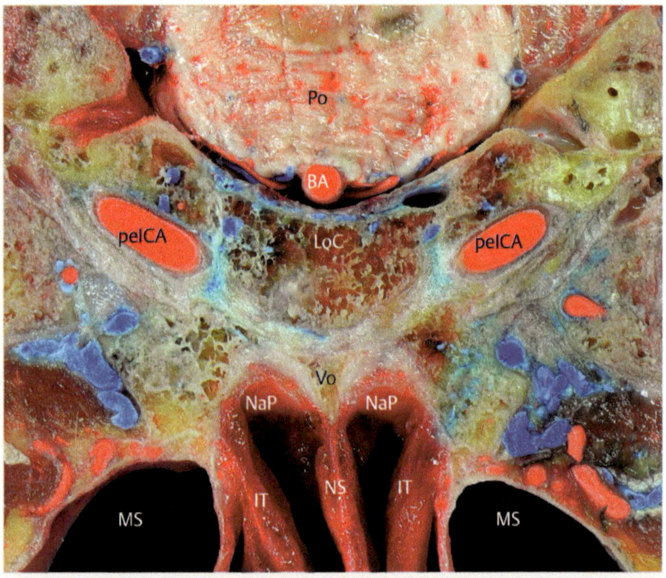

Fig. 12.2 Axial view of the lower clivus. This axial cadaver cut passes through the sphenoidal floor and shows the anatomy of the lower third of the clivus. BA, basilar artery; IT, inferior turbinate; LoC, lower clivus; MS, maxillary sinus; NaP, nasopharyngeal posterior wall; NS, nasal septum; peICA, petrous tract of the internal carotid artery; Po, pons; Vo, vomer.

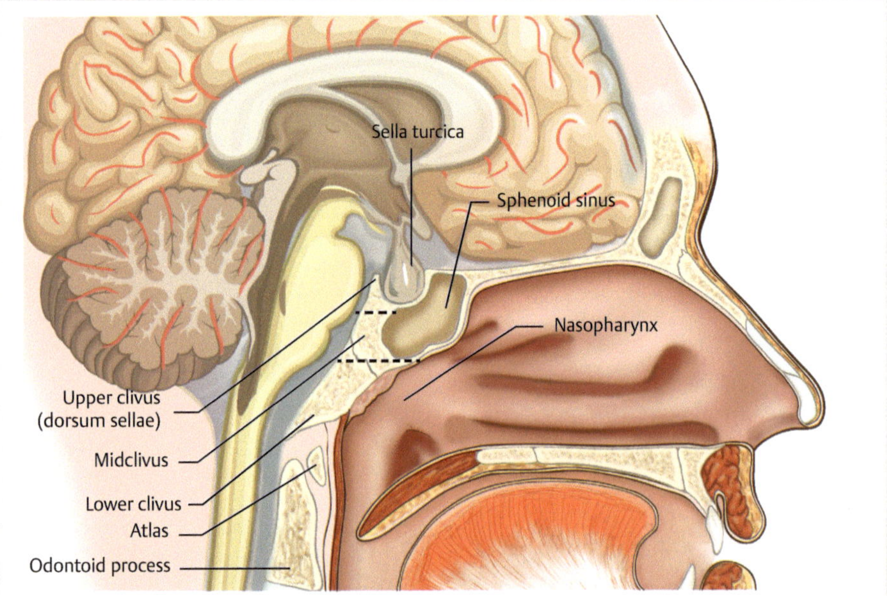

Fig. 12.1 Structure of the clivus and relationship with respect to nasopharynx, palate, and prevertebral muscles. This illustration shows the architecture of the clivus, which is subdivided in upper, middle, and lower segment, as shown by the *black dashed lines.* From an anterior-to-posterior perspective, the lower portion of the clivus is contiguous to the nasopharynx.

After incising the clival dura, meticulous dissection of the rhomboid arachnoid membrane allows us to expose the medulla oblongata, the cranial portion of the spinal cord, and related neurovascular structures.[18] In particular, the vertebral arteries and their branches can be analyzed from the entrance into the cisternal space through the suboccipital cavernous sinus to the vertebrobasilar junction.[19,20]

Transnasal transclival approaches provide unparalleled exposure of the median posterior cranial fossa, ventral surface of the brainstem, and neighboring neurovascular structures, which prompted pioneering groups to employ these routes to manage several challenging lesions of the skull base and adjacent areas. However, two major drawbacks have emerged: (1) the transnasal trajectory is unfavorable to cross the cranial nerves and (2) reconstruction is challenging as a consequence of high cerebrospinal fluid pressure and several geometrical-anatomical features of the defect (i.e., size, inclination, presence of cranial nerves and major vessels close to the bony edges of the craniectomy). In fact, although multilayered reconstruction with vascularized local or regional flaps is the recommended strategy, a non-negligible rate of postoperative cerebrospinal fluid leak has been reported.

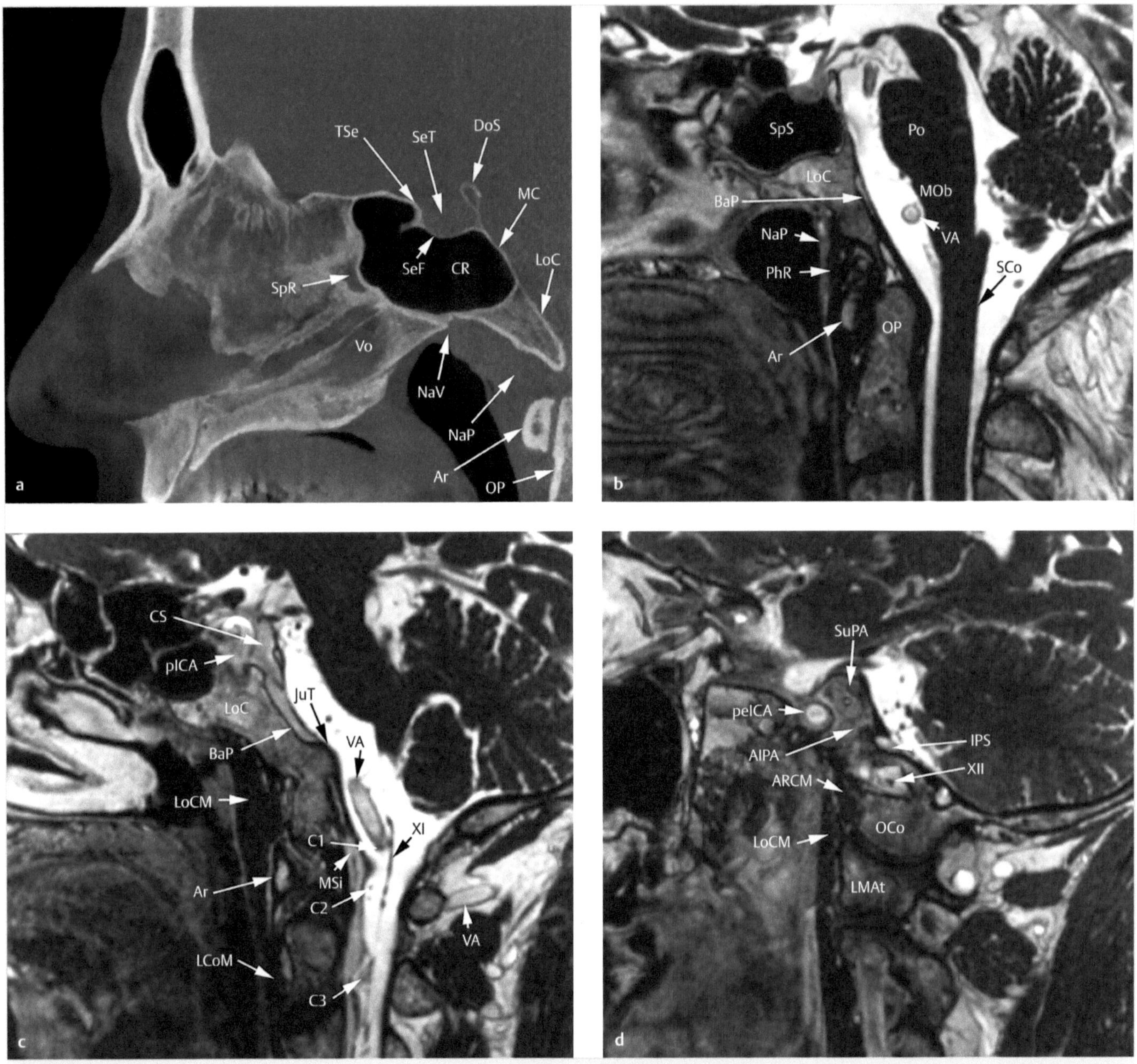

Fig. 12.3 Sagittal CT and MRI anatomy of the lower clivus and adjacent areas. The panel includes four sagittal images: a median CT and constructive interference in steady state (CISS) MRI **(a, b)** and two paramedian CISS MRI **(c, d)**. The lower clivus (LoC) lies posterior to the nasopharyngeal posterior (NaP) wall and the nasopharyngeal vault (NaV). Therefore, when the clival recess (CR) is well pneumatized, the plane parallel to the sphenoidal floor can be used as landmark to define the limit between the midclivus (MC) and the lower clivus. The lower clivus is located above the odontoid process (OP), anterior arch of the atlas (Ar), and other structures of the craniocervical junction. Posteriorly, the inner cortex of the lower clivus is covered by the basilar plexus (BaP), which is adjacent to the vertebral arteries (VA), medulla oblongata (MOb), and upper spinal cord (SCo). Laterally and inferiorly, the lower clivus continues into the jugular tubercle and occipital condyle (OCo). XI, spinal accessory nerve; XII, hypoglossal nerve; AIPA, anteroinferior petrous apex; ARCM, anterior rectus capitis muscle; C1, first cervical nerve; C2, second cervical nerve; C3, third cervical nerve; CS, cavernous sinus; DoS, dorsum sellae; IPS, inferior petrosal sinus; LMAt, lateral mass of the atlas; LCoM, longus colli muscle; LoCM, longus capitis muscle; MSi, marginal sinus; PhR, pharyngeal raphe; pICA, paraclival tract of the internal carotid artery; peICA, petrous tract of the internal carotid artery; Po, pons; SeF, sellar floor; SeT, sella turcica; SpR, sphenoidal rostrum; SpS, sphenoid sinus; SuPA, superior petrous apex; TSe, tuberculum sellae; Vo, vomer.

212

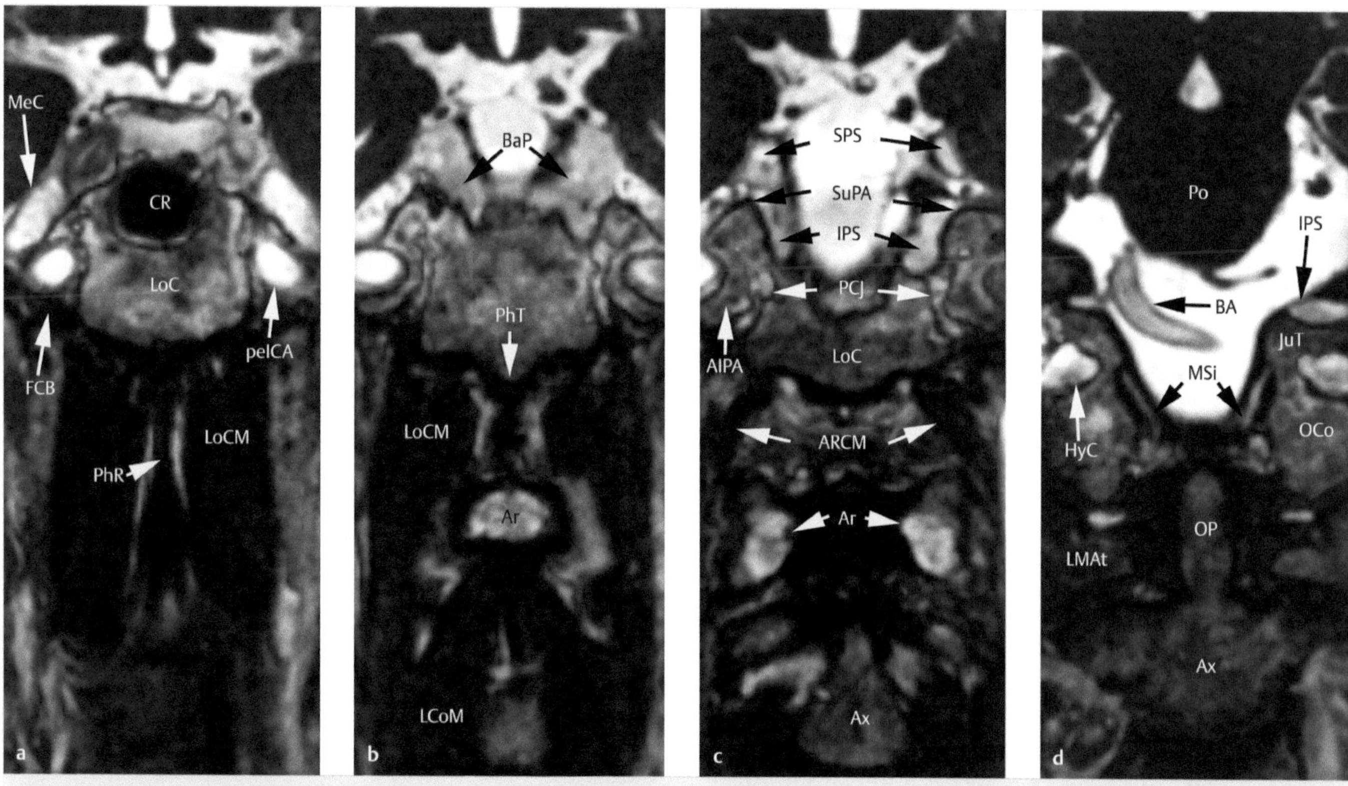

Fig. 12.4 (a–d) Coronal MRI anatomy of the lower clivus and the craniocervical junction. The panel includes four coronal constructive interference in steady state (CISS) MRI scans, from anterior **(a)** to posterior **(d)**. The lower clivus (LoC) has an inferior, median protuberance called pharyngeal tubercle (PhT), where the pharyngeal raphe (PhR) is attached. The longus capitis muscle (LoCM) and anterior rectus capitis muscle (ARCM) are inserted on the lateroinferior surface of the lower clivus. Laterally, the lower clivus continues, from cranial to caudal with the anteroinferior petrous apex (AIPA), jugular tubercle (JuT), and occipital condyle (OCo). The intracranial face of these bony structures is covered by the inferior petrosal (IPS) and marginal sinuses (MSi), which are connected to the basilar plexus (BaP). Ar, anterior arch of the atlas; Ax, axis; BA, basilar artery; CR, clival recess; FCB, fibrocartilago basalis; HyC, hypoglossal canal; LCoM, longus colli muscle; LMAt, lateral mass of the atlas; MeC, Meckel's cave; OP, odontoid process; PCJ, petroclival junction; peICA, petrous tract of the internal carotid artery; Po, pons; SPS, superior petrosal sinus; SuPA, superior petrous apex.

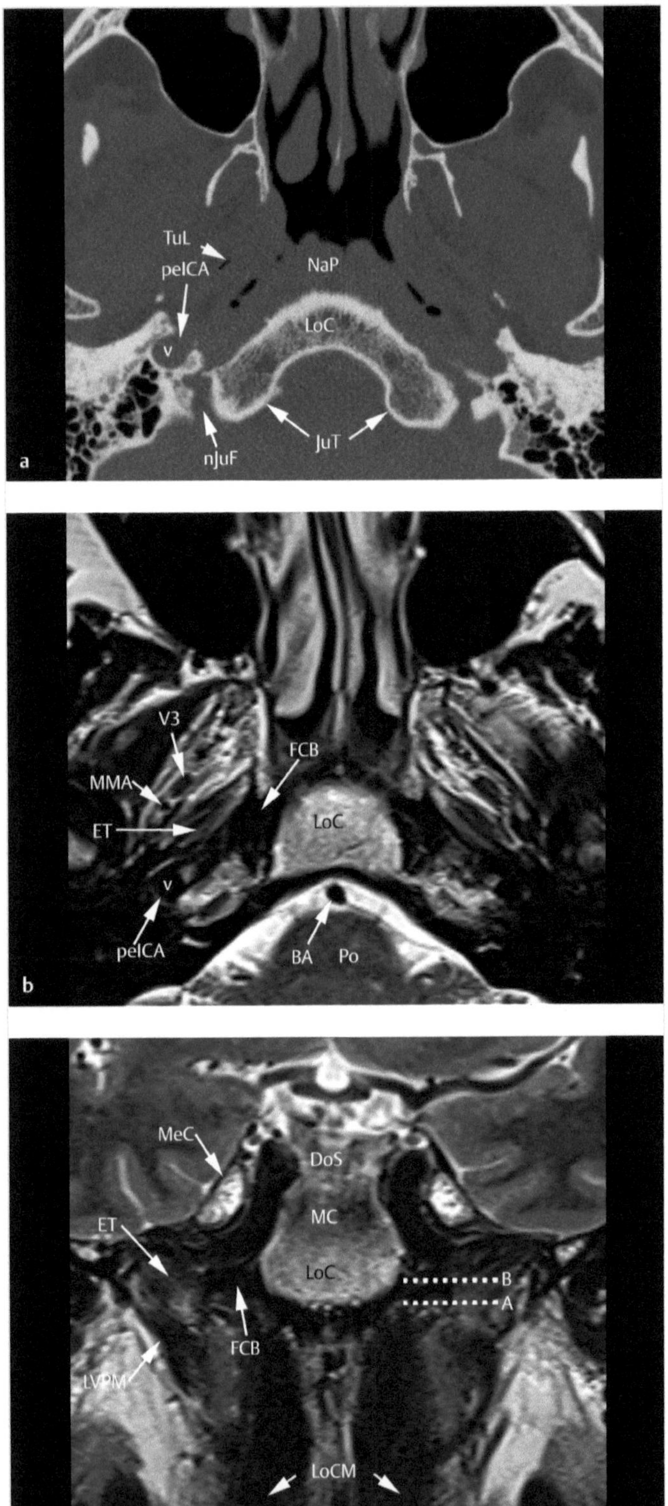

Fig. 12.5 Axial CT and MRI anatomy of the lower clivus. The panel shows an axial CT **(a)**, an axial MRI **(b)**, and a coronal MRI scan **(c)** passing through the lower clivus. The *white dotted lines* in **c** depict the position of **a** and **b** cuts. The lower clivus (LoC) is located posterior to the nasopharyngeal posterior wall (NaP). It extends laterally into the jugular tubercles (JuT) and occipital condyles. Laterally, the jugular tubercle is adjacent to the nervous compartment of the jugular foramen (nJuF). Both the midclivus (MC) and lower clivus are closely contiguous to the fibrocartilago basalis (FCB) that fills the foramen lacerum. V3, mandibular nerve; BA, basilar artery; DoS, dorsum sellae; ET, eustachian tube; LoCM, longus capitis muscle; LVPM, levator veli palatini muscle; MeC, Meckel's cave; MMA, middle meningeal artery; peICA, petrous tract of the internal carotid artery; Po, pons; TuL, tubal lumen; v, vertical portion of the petrous tract of the internal carotid artery.

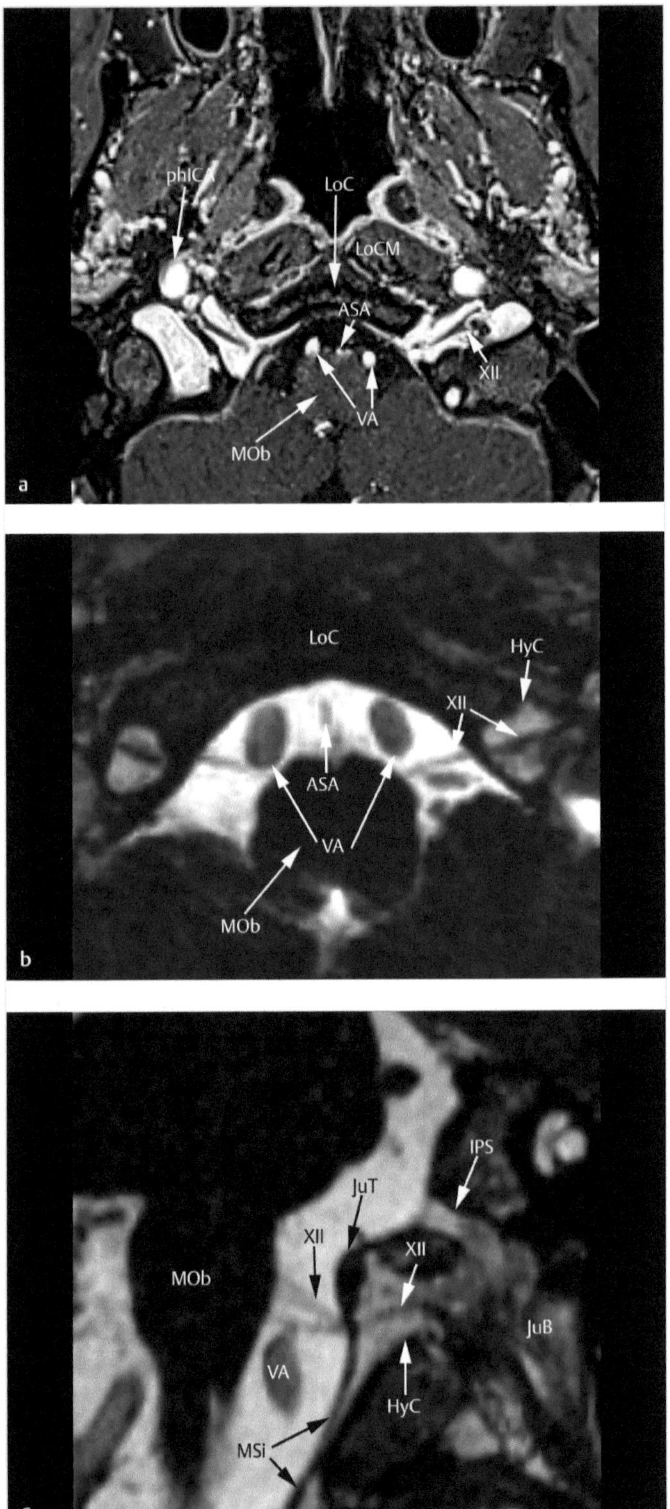

Fig. 12.6 Axial and paracoronal MRI anatomy of the hypoglossal nerve. The panel contains an axial T1-weighted, contrast-enhanced, fat-saturated MRI **(a)**, an axial constructive interference in steady state (CISS) MRI **(b)**, and a paracoronal CISS MRI passing through the hypoglossal nerve **(c)**. The hypoglossal nerve (XII) arises from the medulla oblongata (MOb) and runs in the cisternal space passing behind the ipsilateral vertebral artery (VA) with a posterior and lateral course with respect to the lower clivus (LoC). Then, the nerve enters the hypoglossal canal (XII), also called the anterior condylar canal, which contains a venous plexus and a small arterial branch coming from the ascending pharyngeal artery. Together with the venous plexus of the hypoglossal canal, the inferior petrosal sinus (IPS) and marginal sinus (MSi) drain into the system of the jugular bulb (JuB) and internal jugular vein. ASA, anterior spinal artery; LoCM, longus capitis muscle; phICA, parapharyngeal tract of the internal carotid artery.

Endoscopic Dissection

Nasal Phase

- Inferior turbinectomy.
- Posterior septectomy.
- Paraseptal sphenoidotomy.
- Transrostral sphenoidotomy.
- Expanded transrostral sphenoidotomy.
- Facultative: Vertical and horizontal uncinectomy.
- Facultative: Type A endoscopic medial maxillectomy.
- Facultative: Anterior ethmoidectomy.
- Facultative: Posterior ethmoidectomy.
- Facultative: Transethmoidal sphenoidotomy.

Skull Base Phase

- Step 1: Incision of the posterior wall of the nasopharynx.
- Step 2: Incision of the longus capitis muscle and the pharyngeal raphe.
- Step 3: Removal of the sphenoidal floor and anterior cortical bone of the lower third of the clivus.
- Step 4: Removal of the posterior cortical bone of the clivus.
- Step 5: Incision of the periosteum and dura of the lower third of the clivus.
- Step 6: Removal of the anterior pontine membrane and the rhomboid membrane.
- Step 7: Medialization of the vertebral artery.

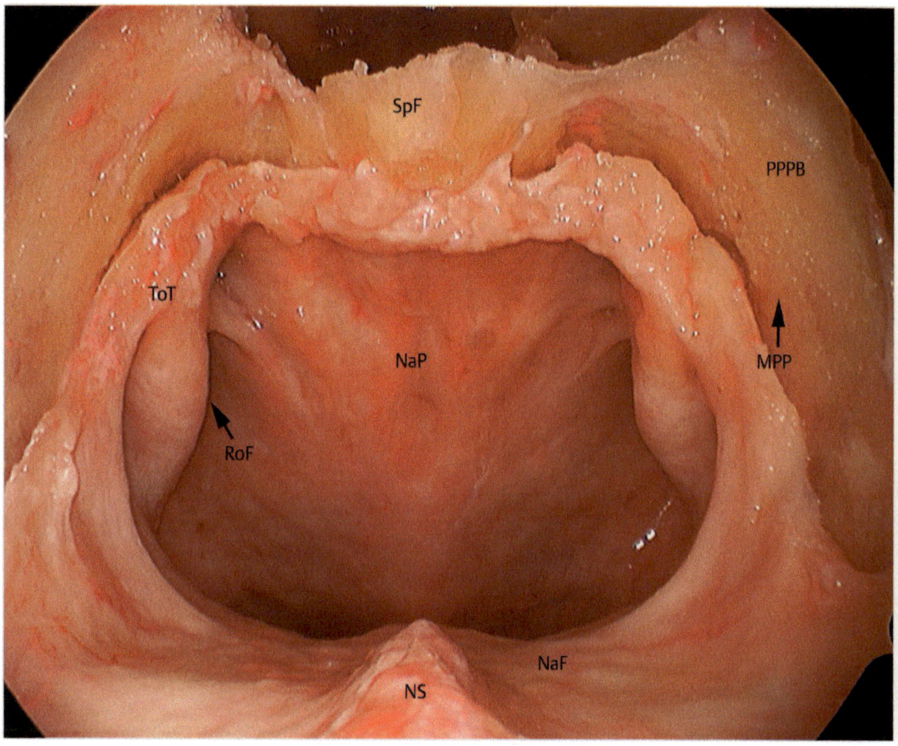

Fig. 12.7 The nasopharynx. The craniocervical junction lies behind the posterior wall of the nasopharynx (NaP). The lateral walls of the nasopharynx show a prominence, called the torus tubarius (ToT), which represents the inferomedial end of the eustachian tube. The fossa of Rosenmüller (RoF) is located superior and posterior to the torus tubarius and separates it from the posterior nasopharyngeal wall. Superiorly, the posterior wall continues into the nasopharyngeal vault, which corresponds to the sphenoidal floor (SpF). PPPB, perpendicular process of the palatine bone; MPP, medial pterygoid plate; NaF, floor of the nasal cavity; NS, nasal septum.

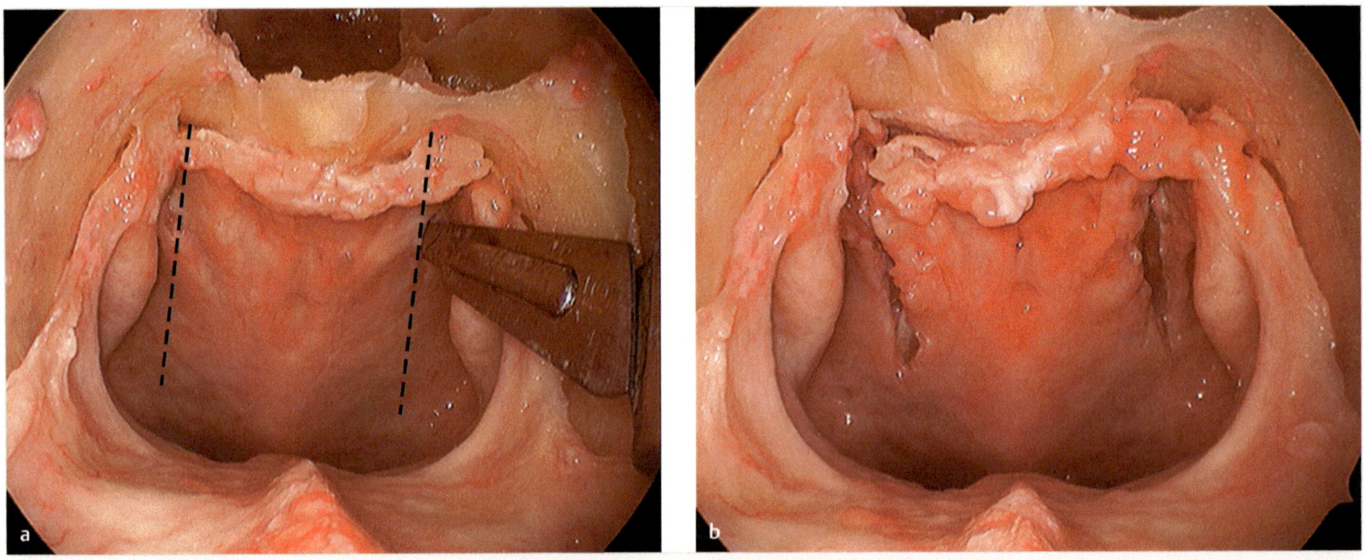

Fig. 12.8 (a, b) Step 1. Two vertical incisions (*black dashed lines*) are made at the junction between the posterior wall of the nasopharynx and the fossae of Rosenmüller.

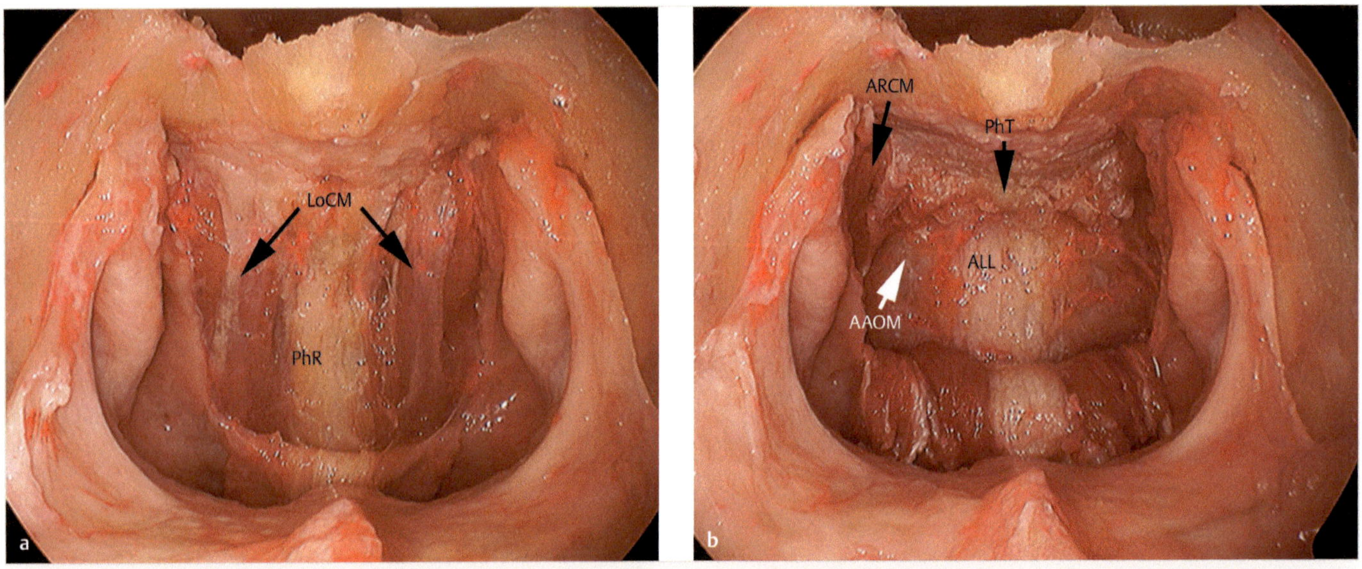

Fig. 12.9 (a, b) Step 2. The mucosal flap is moved inferiorly; the longus capitis muscles (LoCM) come into view together with the pharyngeal raphe (PhR) on the midline. A horizontal incision is made along the posterior border of the sphenoidal floor. The pharyngeal raphe and longus capitis muscles are then detached from the median pharyngeal tubercle (PhT) and sphenoidal floor to expose the anterior rectus capitis muscles (ARCM). Posteriorly, the anterior longitudinal ligament (ALL) and the anterior atlanto-occipital membrane (AAOM) are exposed.

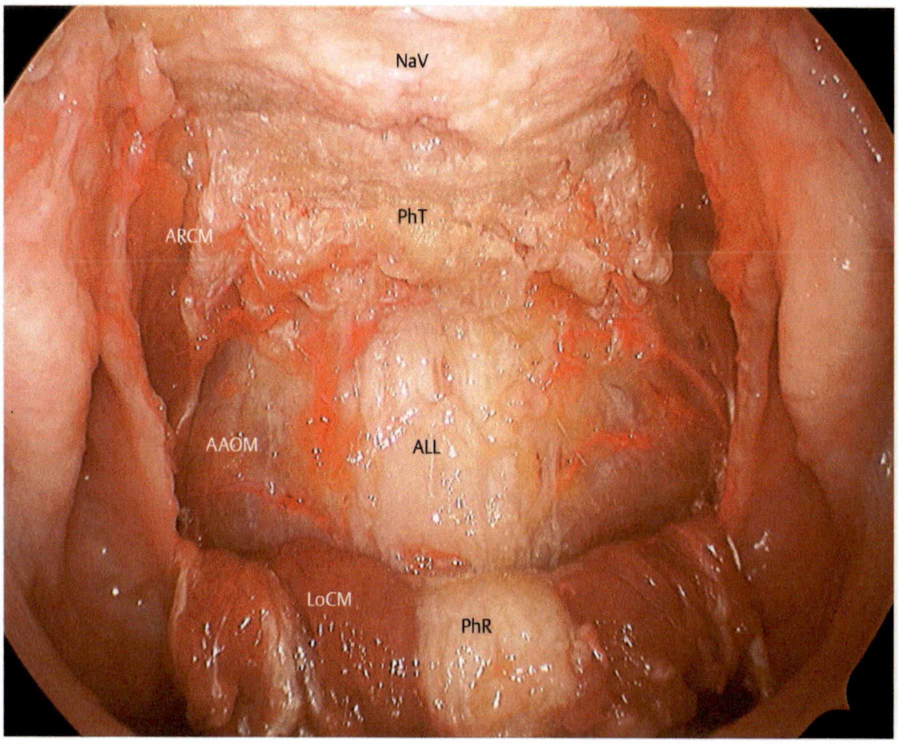

Fig. 12.10 The anterior atlanto-occipital membrane. The anterior atlanto-occipital membrane joins the upper border of the anterior arch of the atlas to the outer margin of the foramen magnum. The anterior longitudinal ligament (ALL) arises from the basion, which is the most anterior midline point of the foramen magnum, and travels down to the sacrum, in front of the vertebral bodies and intervertebral disks. On the lower surface of the basilar part of occipital bone, the pharyngeal tubercle (PhT) gives attachment to the pharyngeal raphe (PhR). The anterior rectus capitis muscle (ARCM) lies beside this tubercle and connects the lower third of the clivus to the lateral mass of the atlas. LoCM, longus capitis muscle; NaV, nasopharyngeal vault.

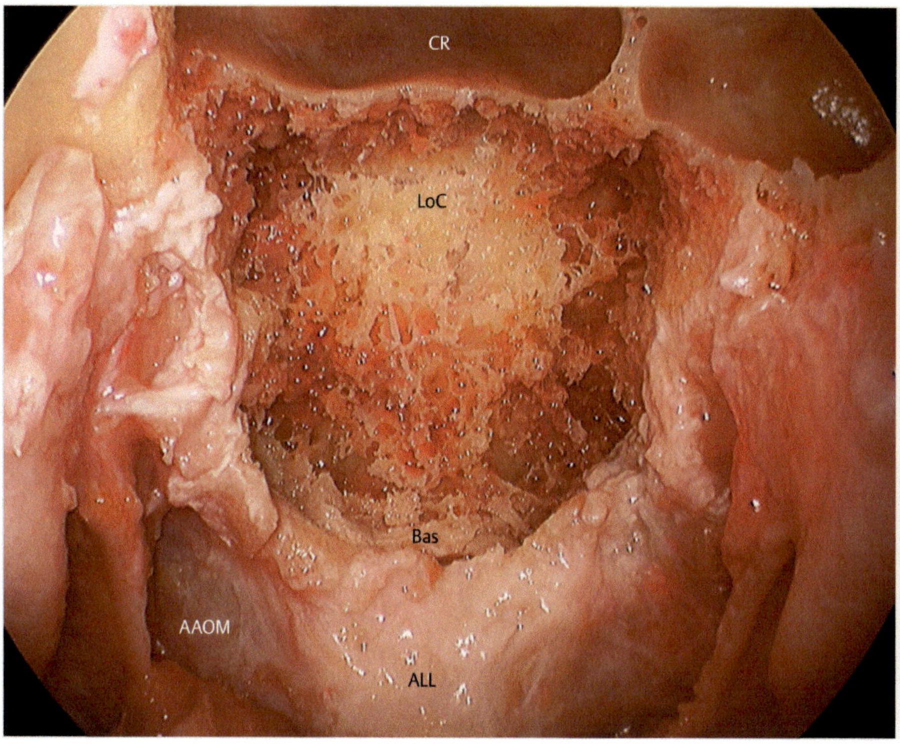

Fig. 12.11 Step 3. The sphenoidal floor and the anterior cortical bone of the lower third of the clivus (LoC) are removed from the clival recess (CR) down to the basion (Bas). ALL, anterior longitudinal ligament; AAOM, anterior atlanto-occipital membrane.

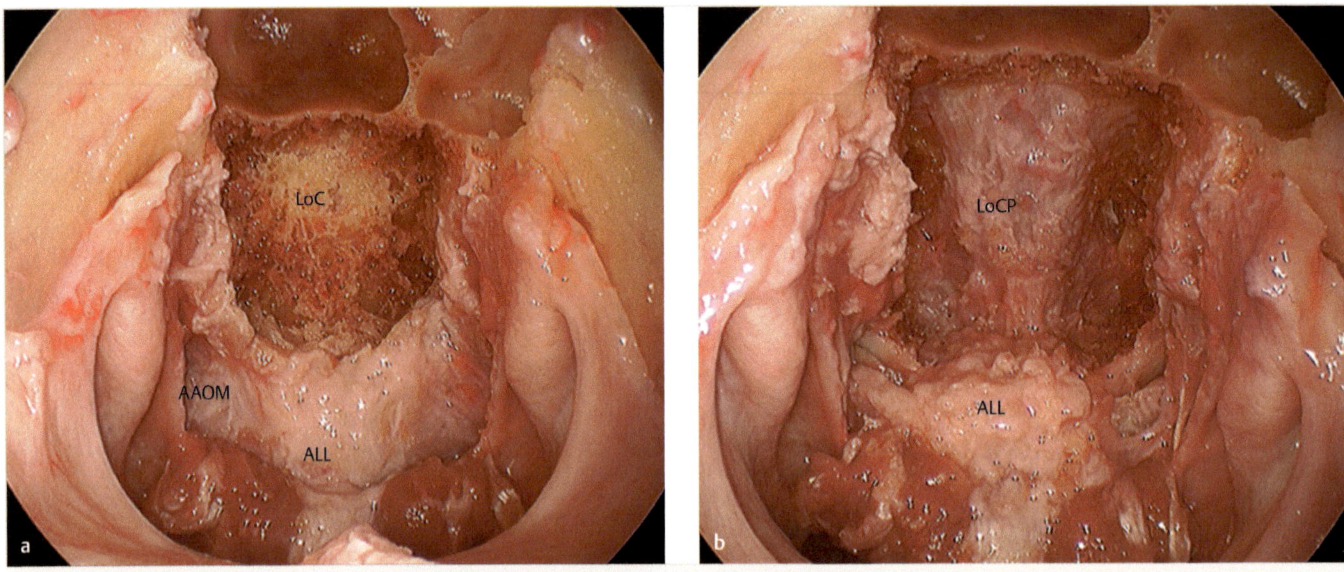

Fig. 12.12 (a, b) Step 4. The posterior cortical bone of the clivus (LoC) is removed to expose the periosteum of the lower third of the clivus (LoCP). AAOM, anterior atlanto-occipital membrane; ALL, anterior longitudinal ligament.

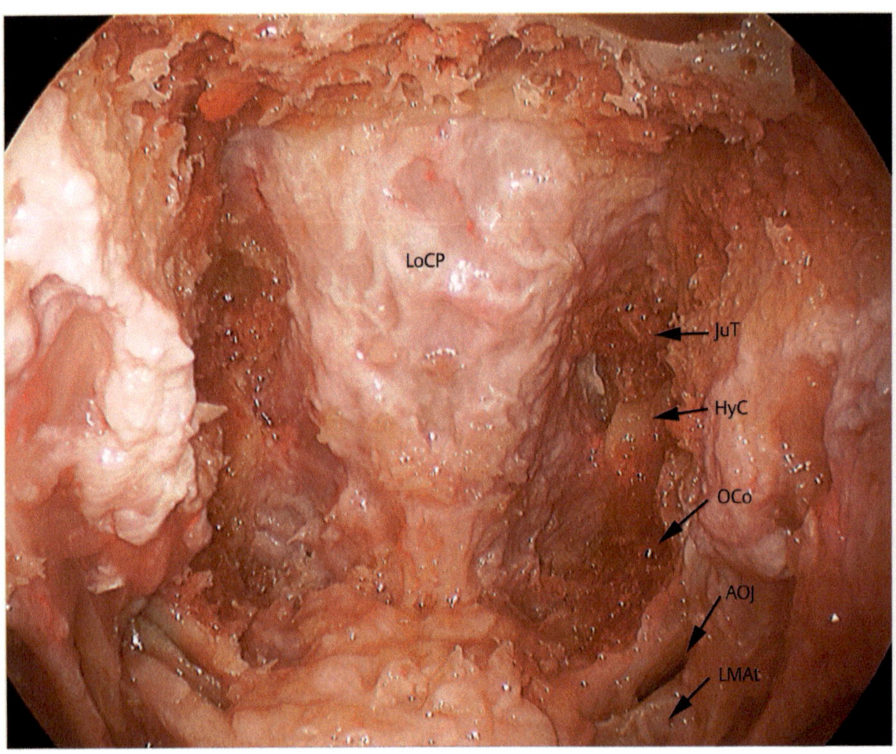

Fig. 12.13 The hypoglossal canal. The hypoglossal canal (HyC) runs within the occipital condyle (OCo), just below the jugular tubercle (JuT). The lateral mass of the atlas (LMAt) forms the atlanto-occipital joint (AOJ) with the occipital condyle. LoCP, periosteum of the lower third of the clivus.

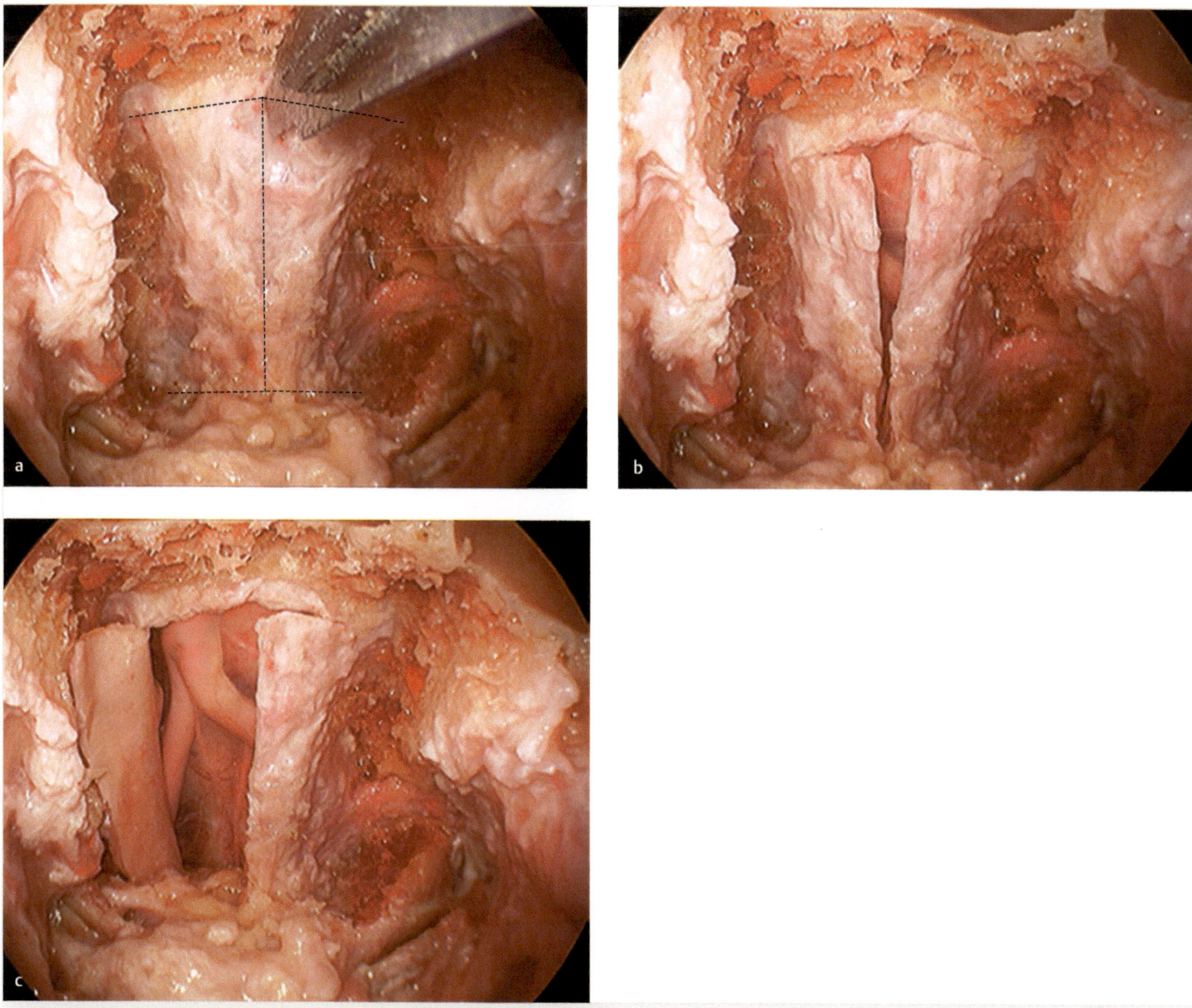

Fig. 12.14 (a–c) Step 5. The periosteum of the lower third of the clivus is incised horizontally along the superior and inferior border of the craniectomy (*horizontal black dashed lines*). Then, a vertical craniocaudal incision is made on the midline (*vertical black dashed line*).

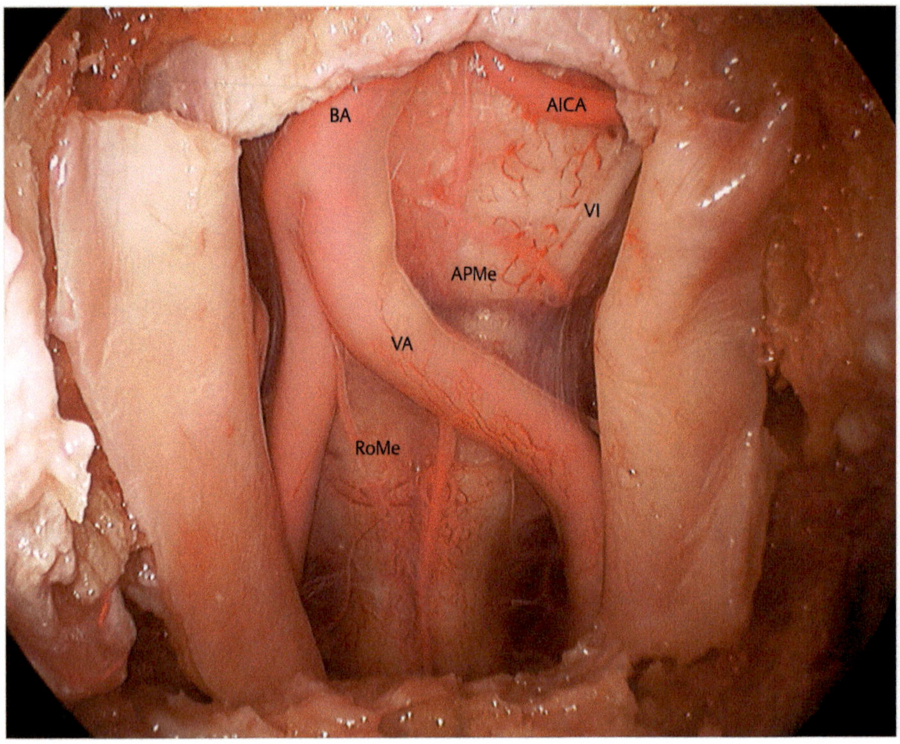

Fig. 12.15 The anterior pontine membrane. The anterior pontine membrane (APMe) is the arachnoid membrane forming the prepontine cistern. The two vertebral arteries (VA) merge to form the basilar artery (BA). The anterior inferior cerebellar artery (AICA) arises from the basilar artery and supplies the brainstem and cerebellum. The rhomboid membrane (RoMe) lies in front of the medulla oblongata and is attached to the intradural tract of the vertebral arteries. VI, abducens nerve.

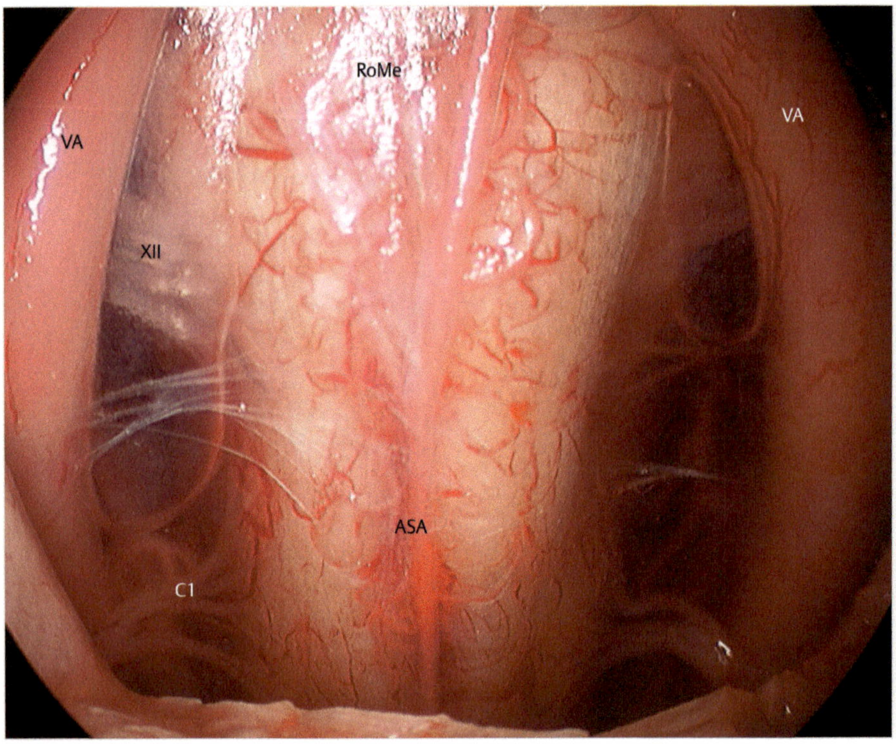

Fig. 12.16 The rhomboid membrane. The hypoglossal nerve (XII) and first cervical nerve (C1) nerves lie behind the rhomboid membrane (RoMe). This membrane attaches bilaterally to the medial surface of the vertebral arteries (VA). The hypoglossal nerve and the rootlets of first cervical nerve arise from the ventromedial part of the medulla oblongata and the spinal cord, respectively. These structures run posterior and anterior to the vertebral artery, respectively. ASA, anterior spinal artery.

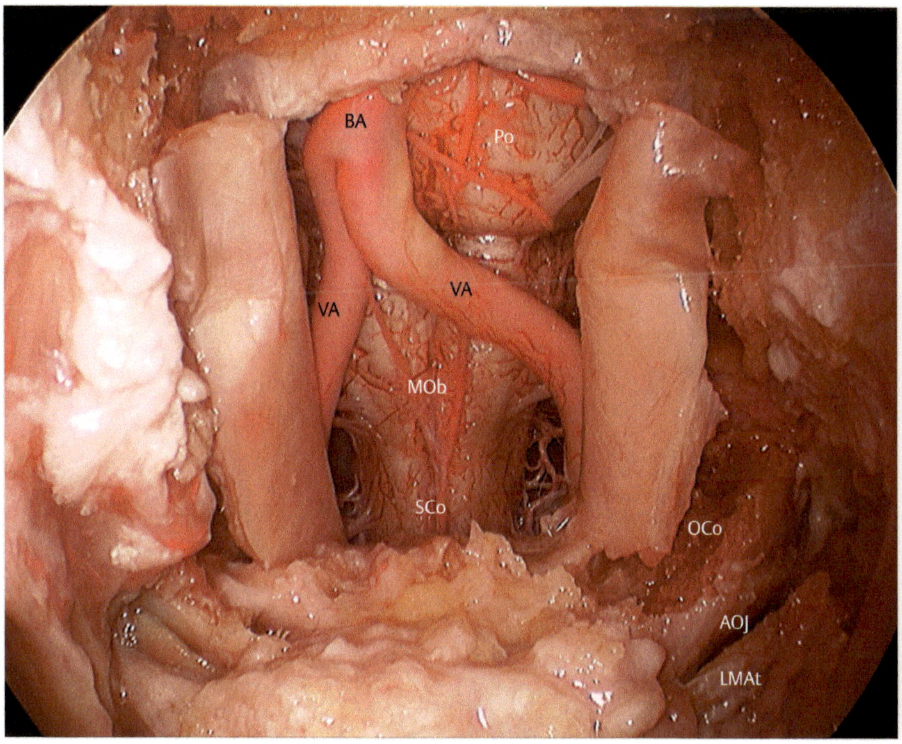

Fig. 12.17 Step 6. The anterior pontine and rhomboid membranes are removed to get access to the subarachnoid space. AOJ, atlanto-occipital joint; BA, basilar artery; LMAt, lateral mass of the atlas; MOb, medulla oblongata; OCo, occipital condyle; Po, pons; SCo, spinal cord; VA, vertebral artery.

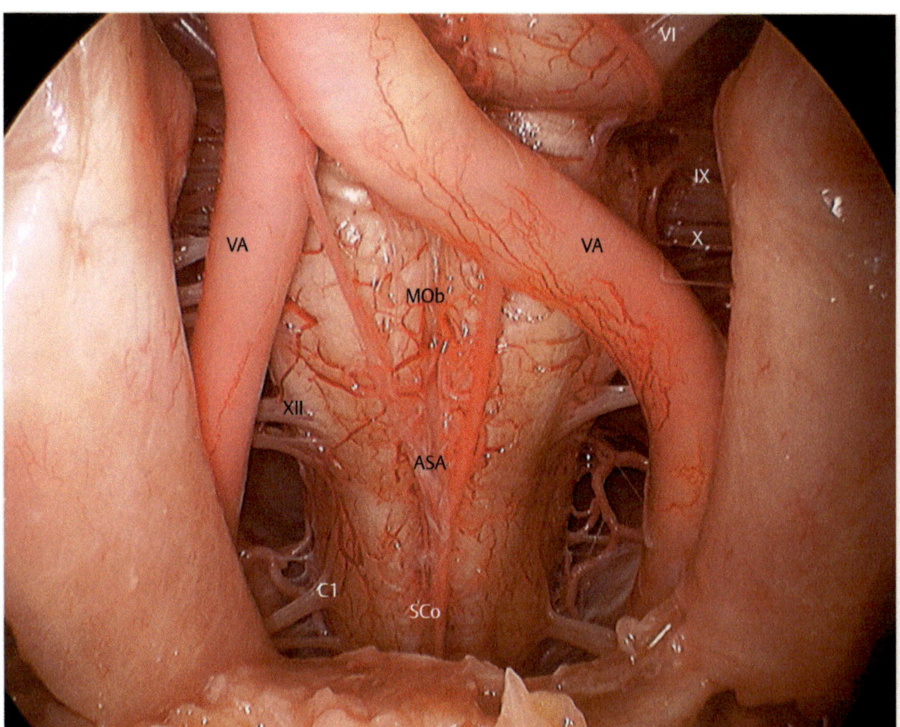

Fig. 12.18 The inferior portion of the transclival window. The anterior spinal artery (ASA) arises from the junction of two branches of vertebral arteries (VA) and runs along the anterior surface of the spinal cord (SCo). The abducens nerve (VI) arises from the brainstem at the junction between the pons and the medulla oblongata (MOb); the glossopharyngeal nerve (IX) arises from the anterolateral surface of the medulla oblongata, superiorly to the vagus nerve (X) and cranial accessory nerve. The hypoglossal nerve (XII) arises from the medulla oblongata and runs anterolaterally passing behind the vertebral artery. C1, first cervical nerve; SCo, spinal cord.

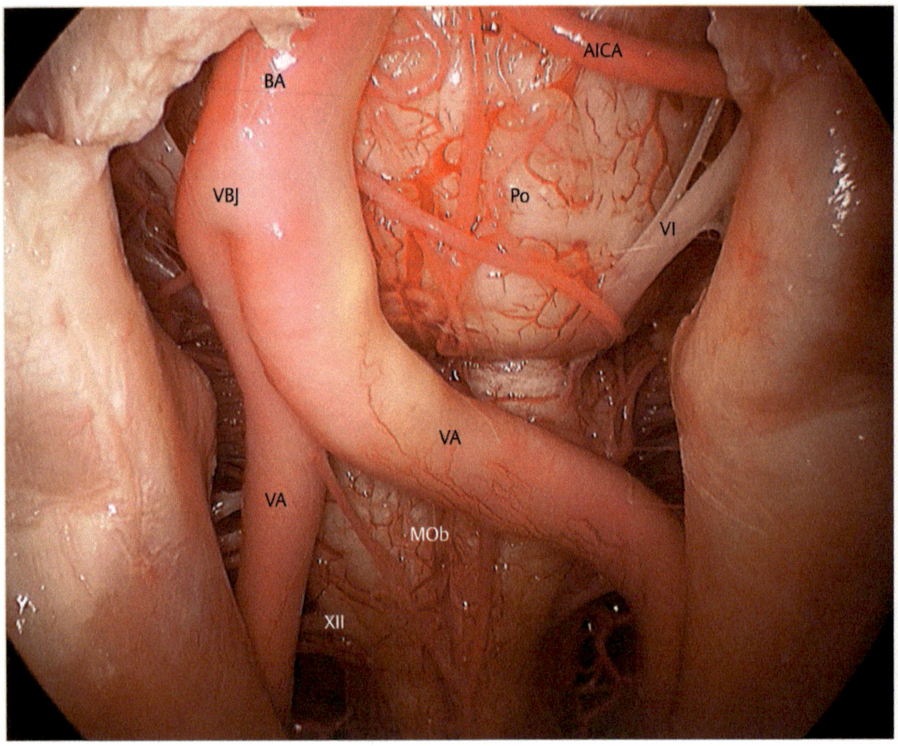

Fig. 12.19 The superior part of the transclival window. The basilar artery (BA) arises from the confluence of the two vertebral arteries (VA), which is called vertebrobasilar junction (VBJ). In this specimen, the left abducens nerve (VI) is split by the anterior inferior cerebellar artery (AICA). This splitting is found most frequently on the left side. Po, pons; MOb, medulla oblongata; XII, hypoglossal nerve.

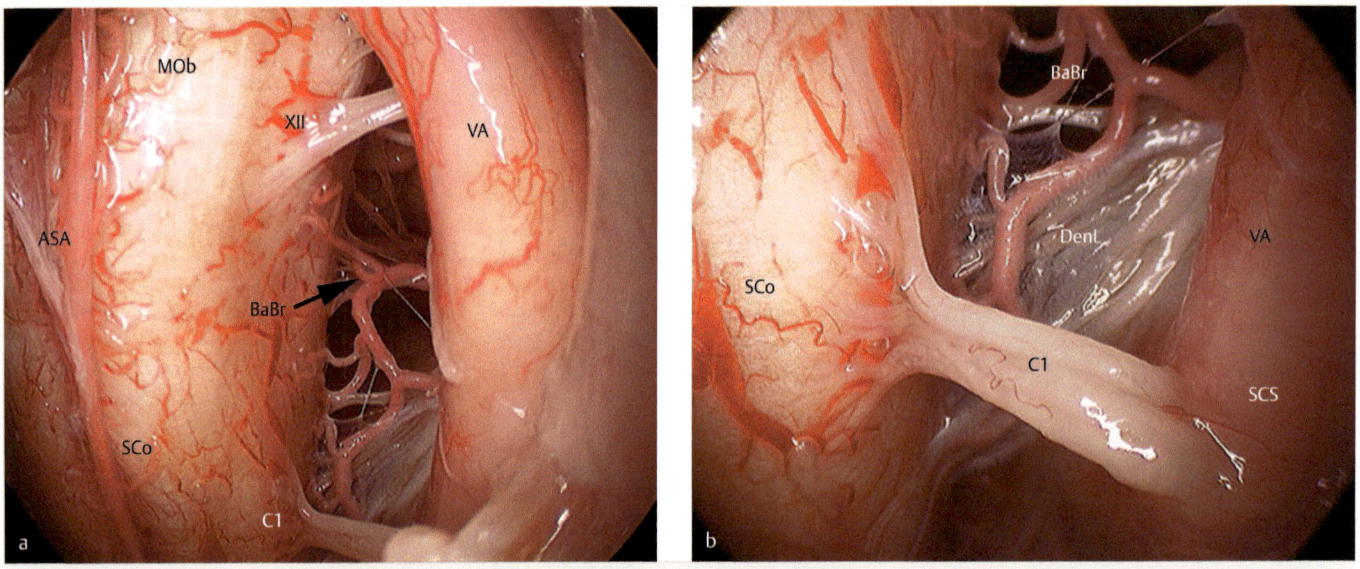

Fig. 12.20 (a, b) The inferior portion of the vertebral artery. The hypoglossal nerve (XII), after arising from the medulla oblongata (MOb), runs posterolaterally to the vertebral artery (VA), while the first cervical nerve (C1), after arising from the spinal cord (SCo), passes anteriorly to the same artery. The basilar branch (BaBr) of the posterior inferior cerebellar artery is found in the window between the hypoglossal nerve and the first cervical nerve. The denticulate ligament (DenL), which connects the spinal cord with the medullary canal posteriorly to the vertebral artery (VA), is visible behind the first cervical nerve. The vertebral artery enters the intradural space after passing through the suboccipital cavernous sinus (SCS). ASA, anterior spinal artery.

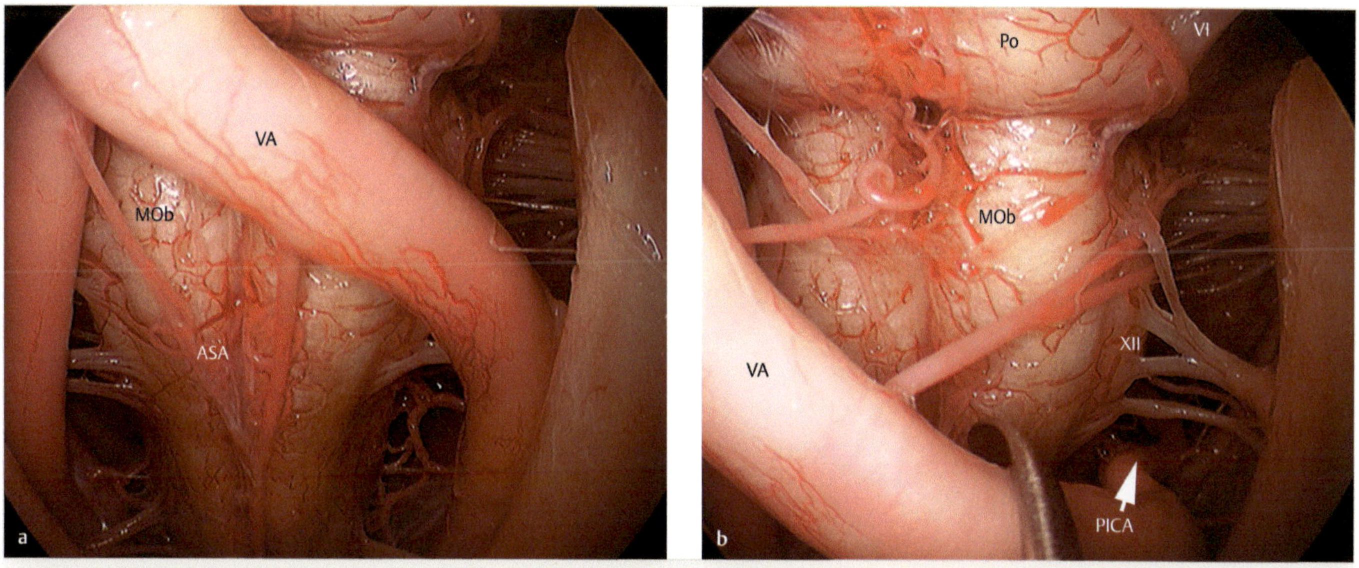

Fig. 12.21 (a, b) Step 7 (part 1). Medialization of the vertebral artery (VA) allows identification of the posterior inferior cerebellar artery (PICA) and the hypoglossal nerve (XII). VI, abducens nerve; ASA, anterior spinal artery; MOb, medulla oblongata; Po, pons.

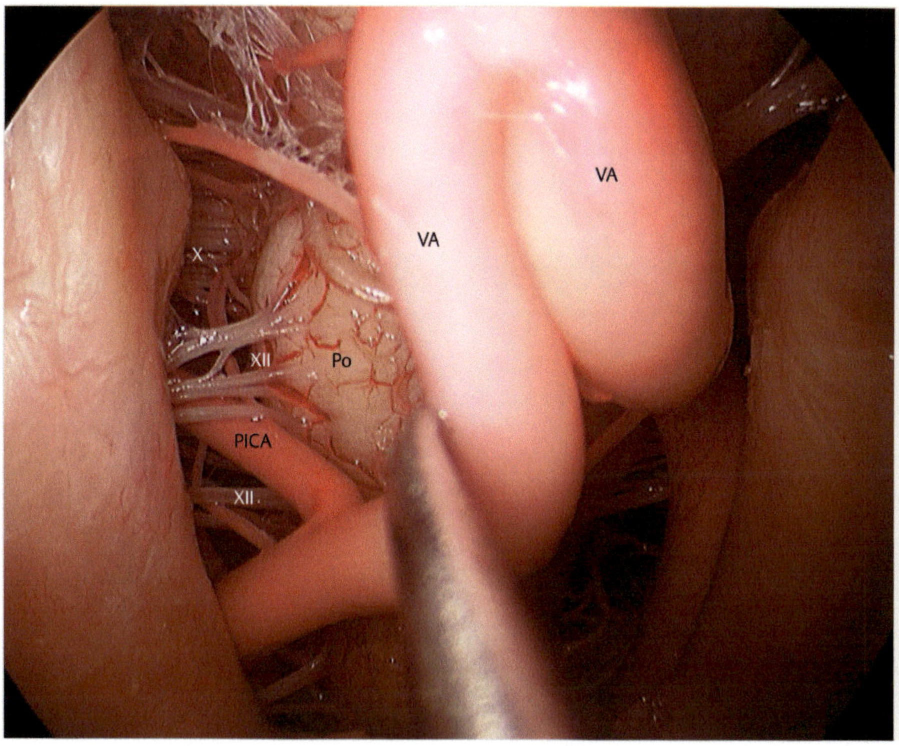

Fig. 12.22 Step 7 (part 2). Medialization of the right vertebral artery (VA) demonstrates how multiple posterior inferior cerebellar arteries (PICA) can be found. All these vessels cross the rootlets of the hypoglossal nerve (XII). X, vagus nerve; Po, pons.

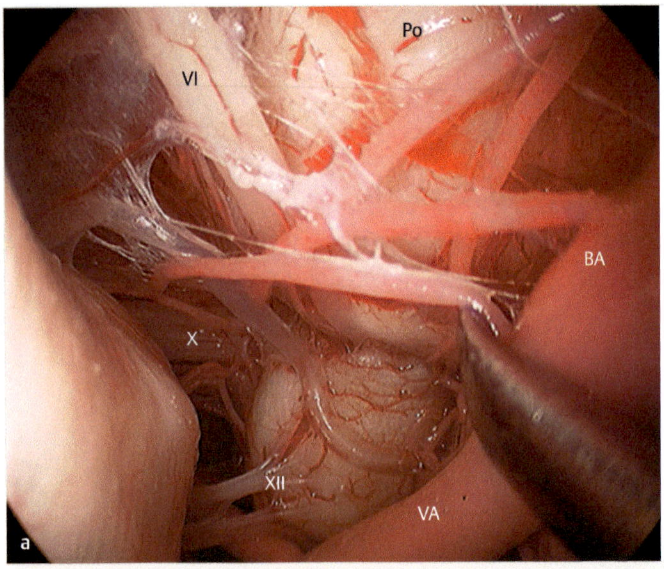

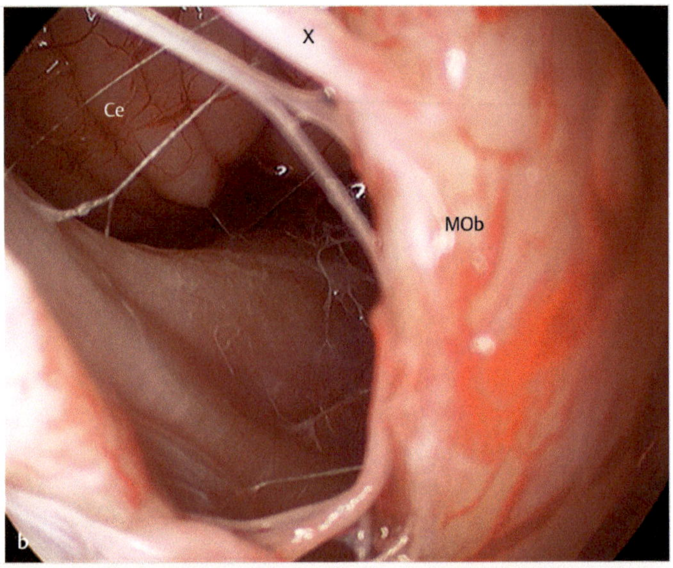

Fig. 12.23 (a, b) The window between the hypoglossal nerve and the lower cranial nerves. After medializing the vertebral artery (VA), a 0-degree scope placed between the hypoglossal nerve (XII) and the vagus nerve (X), beside the medulla oblongata (MOb), allows the visualization of the cerebellum (Ce). VI, abducens nerve; BA, basilar artery; Po, pons.

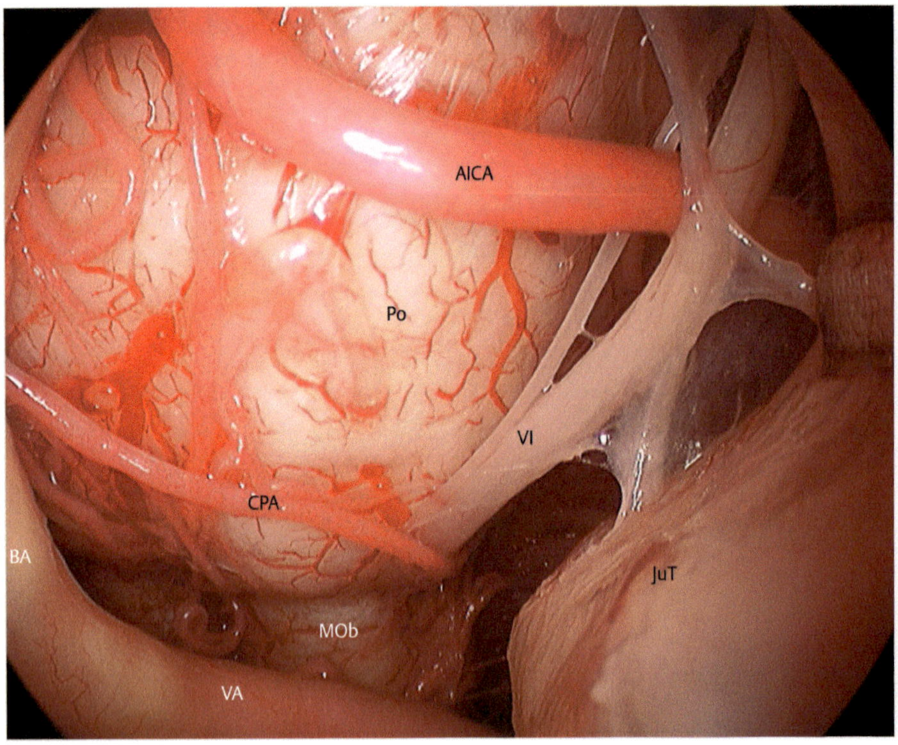

Fig. 12.24 The splitting of the abducens nerve. The anterior inferior cerebellar artery (AICA) runs cranially to the abducens nerve (VI) in most of the cases. Less frequently, this artery splits the abducens nerve in two parts. The circumferential pontine artery (CPA) runs frequently close to the abducens nerve. BA, basilar artery; JuT, jugular tubercle; MOb, medulla oblongata; Po, pons; VA, vertebral artery.

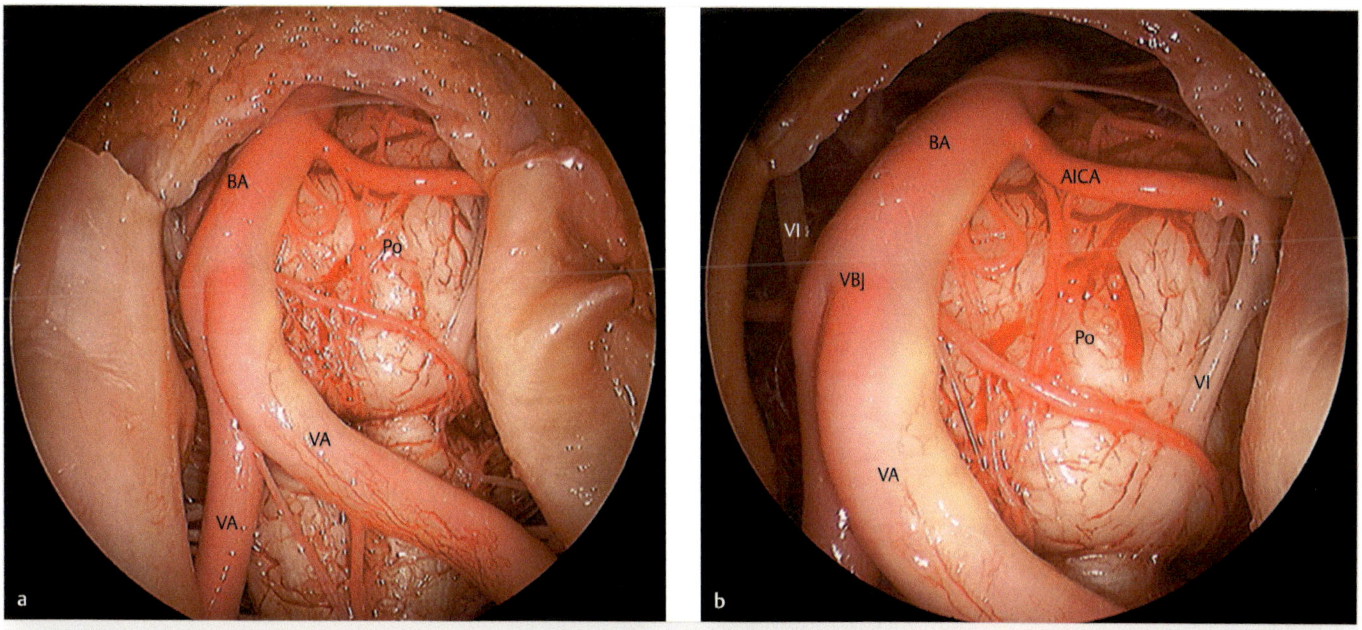

Fig. 12.25 (a, b) The upper portion of the prepontine cistern. A 0-degree scope **(a)** allows the view of the two vertebral arteries (VA) forming the basilar artery (BA) through the vertebrobasilar junction (VBJ). A 70-degree scope turned cranially better identifies the abducens nerves (VI) and anterior inferior cerebellar artery (AICA). Po, pons.

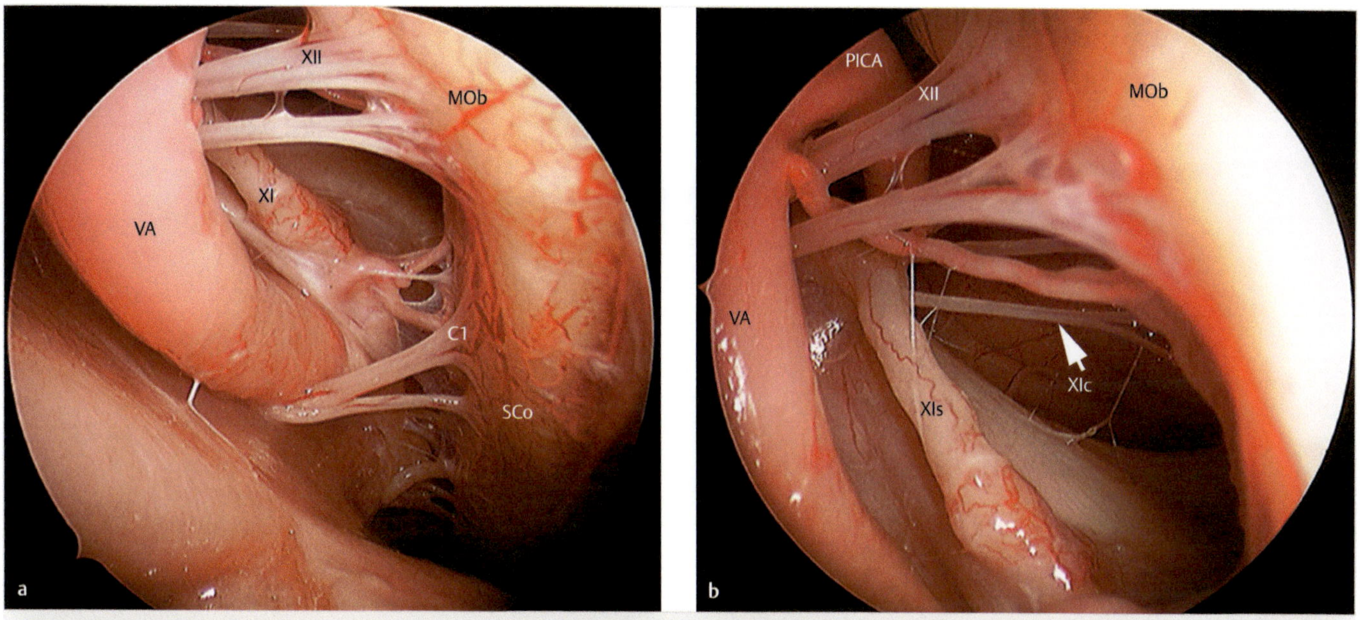

Fig. 12.26 The spinal accessory nerve. With a 70-degree scope turned inferolaterally **(a)** and laterally **(b)**, the three-dimensional relationships among vertebral artery (VA), first cervical nerve (C1), accessory nerve (XI), and hypoglossal nerve (XII) can be better depicted. The first cervical nerve passes anterior to the vertebral artery and the denticulate ligament (DenL) is located behind the vertebral artery and anterior to the spinal accessory nerve (XIs), whereas the hypoglossal nerve passes behind the vertebral artery and anterior to the spinal and cranial accessory nerve (XIc). MOb, medulla oblongata; SCo, spinal cord.

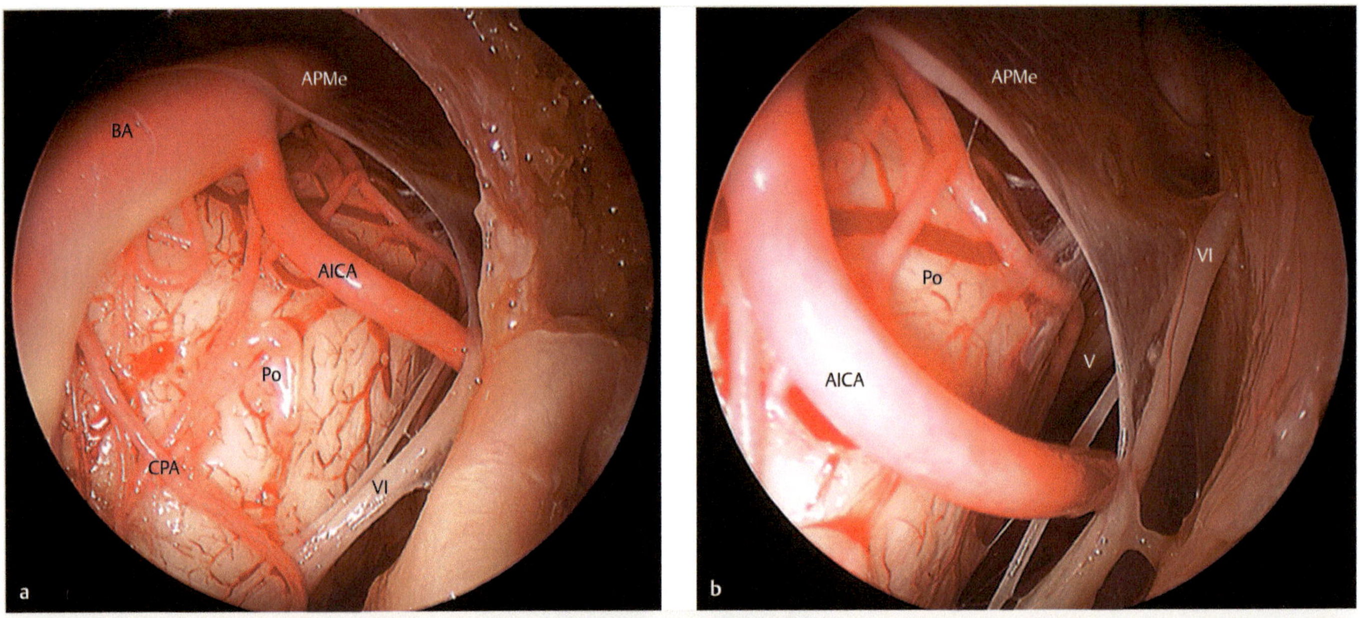

Fig. 12.27 (a, b) The abducens nerve. A 70-degree scope turned superolaterally towards the left side of this specimen allows us to identify the cisternal tract of the abducens nerve (VI). This tract runs in front of the pons (Po) and enters the basilar plexus. The cisternal tract of the abducens nerve is surrounded by the anterior pontine membrane (APMe). V, trigeminal stem; AICA, anterior inferior cerebral artery; BA, basilar artery; CPA, circumferential pontine artery.

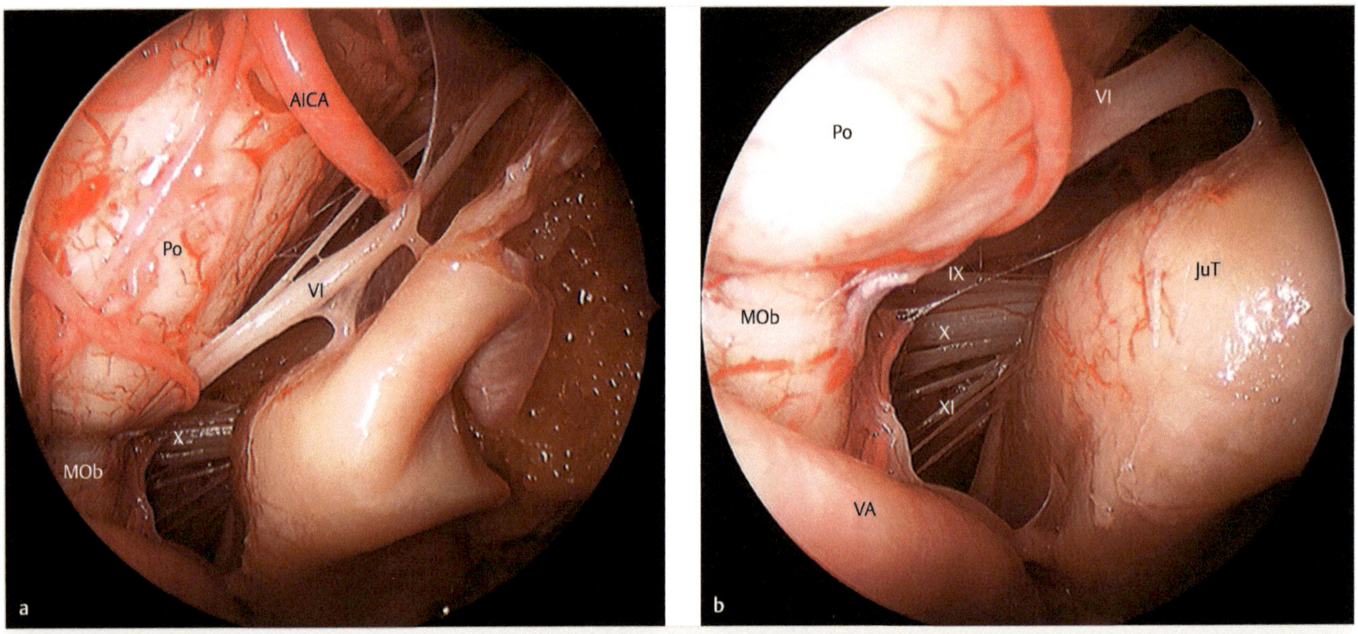

Fig. 12.28 (a, b) The lower cranial nerves. A 70-degree scope turned laterally towards the left side of this specimen and placed at the lower border of the craniectomy allows the identification of the glossopharyngeal (IX), vagus (X), and the accessory (XI) nerves, which are located posterolaterally to the jugular tubercle (JuT). VI, abducens nerve; AICA, anterior inferior cerebellar artery; MOb, medulla oblongata; Po, pons; VA, vertebral artery.

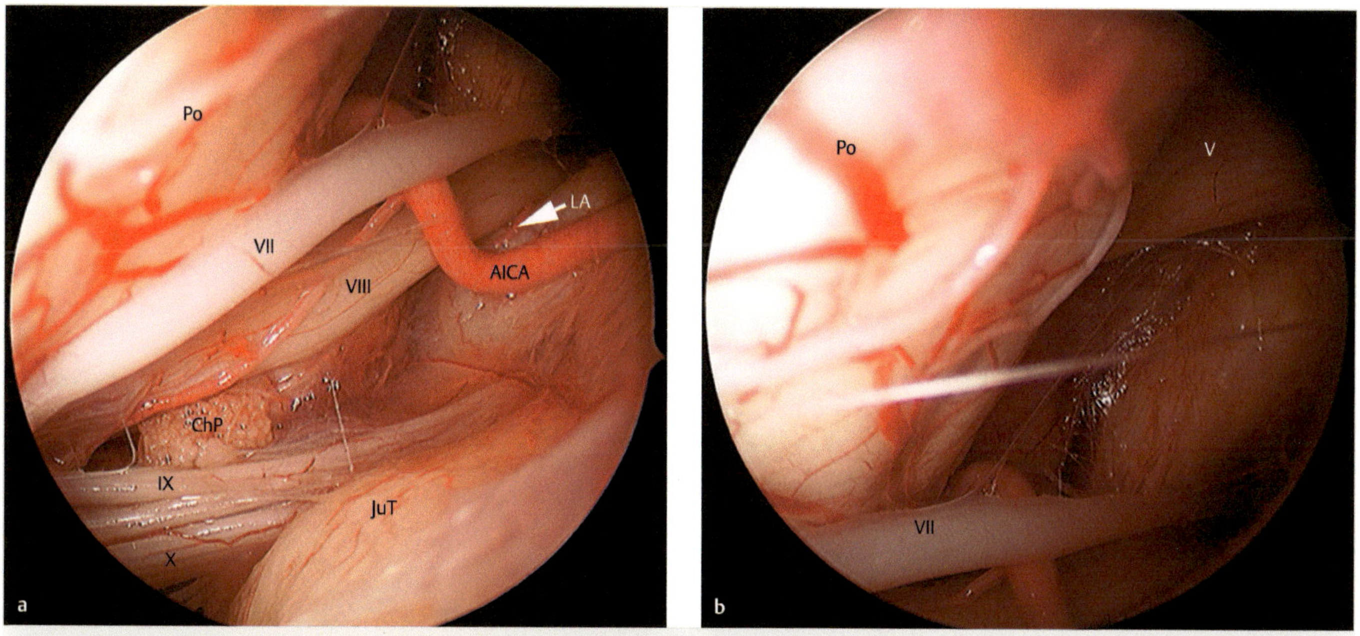

Fig. 12.29 (a, b) The acoustic-facial bundle. The facial (VII) and vestibulocochlear (VIII) nerves form the acoustic-facial bundle. The anterior inferior cerebellar artery (AICA) crosses this bundle and gives the labyrinthine artery (LA), which runs toward the internal auditory canal. The choroid plexus (ChP), which originates from the fourth ventricle and protrudes through Luschka's foramen, separates the lower cranial nerves, namely, the glossopharyngeal (IX), vagus (X), and spinal accessory (XI) nerves, from the acoustic-facial bundle. V, trigeminal stem; JuT, jugular tubercle; Po, pons.

References

[1] Cavallo LM, Cappabianca P, Messina A, et al. The extended endoscopic endonasal approach to the clivus and cranio-vertebral junction: anatomical study. Childs Nerv Syst 2007;23(6):665–671

[2] Doglietto F, Ferrari M, Mattavelli D, et al. Transnasal endoscopic and lateral approaches to the clivus: a quantitative anatomic study. World Neurosurg 2018;113:e659–e671

[3] Fernandez-Miranda JC, Gardner PA, Snyderman CH, et al. Clival chordomas: a pathological, surgical, and radiotherapeutic review. Head Neck 2014;36(6):892–906

[4] Kim YH, Jeon C, Se YB, et al. Clinical outcomes of an endoscopic transclival and transpetrosal approach for primary skull base malignancies involving the clivus. J Neurosurg 2018;128(5):1454–1462

[5] Koutourousiou M, Gardner PA, Tormenti MJ, et al. Endoscopic endonasal approach for resection of cranial base chordomas: outcomes and learning curve. Neurosurgery 2012;71(3):614–624, discussion 624–625

[6] Labidi M, Watanabe K, Bouazza S, et al. Clivus chordomas: a systematic review and meta-analysis of contemporary surgical management. J Neurosurg Sci 2016;60(4):476–484

[7] Beer-Furlan A, Abi-Hachem R, Jamshidi AO, Carrau RL, Prevedello DM. Endoscopic trans-sphenoidal surgery for petroclival and clival meningiomas. J Neurosurg Sci 2016;60(4):495–502

[8] Vaz-Guimaraes F, Fernandez-Miranda JC, Koutourousiou M, et al. Endoscopic endonasal surgery for cranial base chondrosarcomas. Oper Neurosurg (Hagerstown) 2017;13(4):421–434

[9] Castelnuovo P, Nicolai P, Turri-Zanoni M, et al. Endoscopic endonasal nasopharyngectomy in selected cancers. Otolaryngol Head Neck Surg 2013;149(3):424–430

[10] Kooshkabadi A, Choi PA, Koutourousiou M, et al. Atlanto-occipital instability following endoscopic endonasal approach for lower clival lesions: experience with 212 cases. Neurosurgery 2015;77(6):888–897, discussion 897

[11] Gardner PA, Vaz-Guimaraes F, Jankowitz B, et al. Endoscopic endonasal clipping of intracranial aneurysms: surgical technique and results. World Neurosurg 2015;84(5):1380–1393

[12] Kassam AB, Mintz AH, Gardner PA, Horowitz MB, Carrau RL, Snyderman CH. The expanded endonasal approach for an endoscopic transnasal clipping and aneurysmorrhaphy of a large vertebral artery aneurysm: technical case report. Neurosurgery 2006;59(1, Suppl 1):E162–E165, discussion E162–E165

[13] Enseñat J, Alobid I, de Notaris M, et al. Endoscopic endonasal clipping of a ruptured vertebral-posterior inferior cerebellar artery aneurysm: technical case report. Neurosurgery 2011;69(1, Suppl Operative):E121–E127, discussion E127–E128

[14] Marchioni D, Musumeci A, Fabbris C, De Rossi S, Soloperto D. Endoscopic transnasal surgery of clival lesions: our experience. Eur Arch Otorhinolaryngol 2018;275(5):1149–1156

[15] Mathkour M, Garces J, Beard B, Bartholomew A, Sulaiman OA, Ware ML. Primary high-grade osteosarcoma of the clivus: a case report and literature review. World Neurosurg 2016;89:730.e9–730.e13

[16] Beer-Furlan A, Balsalobre L, Vellutini EA, Stamm AC. Endoscopic endonasal approach in invasive aspergillosis of the clivus in an immunocompetent patient. Acta Neurochir (Wien) 2015;157(12):2221–2222

[17] Vellutini EdeA, Balsalobre L, Hermann DR, Stamm AC. The endoscopic endonasal approach for extradural and intradural clivus lesions. World Neurosurg 2014;82(6, Suppl):S106–S115

[18] Kurucz P, Baksa G, Patonay L, et al. Endoscopic anatomical study of the arachnoid architecture on the base of the skull. Part II: level of the tentorium, posterior fossa and the craniovertebral junction. Innovative Neurosurg 2013;1:91–108

[19] Arnautović KI, al-Mefty O, Pait TG, Krisht AF, Husain MM. The suboccipital cavernous sinus. J Neurosurg 1997;86(2):252–262

[20] Parkinson D. The suboccipital cavernous sinus. J Neurosurg 1997;86(2):315–316

13 Transodontoid Approach

Francesco Doglietto, Francesco Belotti, Andrea Bolzoni Villaret, Marco Ravanelli

Being parallel to Kassam's line,[1] which is considered the inferior anatomical boundary of transnasal endoscopic surgery, the transodontoid route is the most caudal corridor among sagittal approaches. This route exploits the nasal cavities and nasopharynx to expose the anterior portion of the craniocervical junction.[2,3] The most relevant indications for the transodontoid approach include bulbomedullary compression caused by basilar invagination, os odontoideum, tumors (especially chordomas), irreducible atlantoaxial subluxation, rheumatoid arthritis pannus (especially if severe and/or unresolved by posterior fixation), or other rarer conditions.[3–8]

The first phases of the dissection consist of progressively detaching the prevertebral muscles, ligaments, and fasciae to expose the craniocervical junction. The main bony landmarks to get oriented within this area are the lower clival border and the anterior arch of the atlas. Two variants of the transodontoid approach are illustrated in this chapter.[9,10] The first variant is performed by removing the cranial portion of the anterior arch of the atlas and the caudal portion of the lower clivus, thus enabling us to reach and resect the apex of the odontoid process. The second variant includes complete removal of both the anterior arch of the atlas and the odontoid process. The former variant allows the reader to understand the boundary between the transclival approach through the lower clivus and the transodontoid approach. As demonstrated by large clinical series, this concept is particularly important in view of the frequent need to adapt the approach according to the extent of clival or craniocervical lesions.[11] Notably, the removal of bony and ligamentous components of the craniocervical junction causes variable grades of joint instability, which can require craniocervical fixation.[11,12]

The anatomy of ligaments and membranes of the craniocervical junction is exceedingly complex. The laboratory setting enables the analysis of each ligament by taking advantage of high magnification and absence of bleeding. Being frequently aimed to decompress the spinal cord and/or medulla oblongata, the transodontoid approach usually does not include a transdural extension. Nevertheless, dural resection is required when tumors of the craniocervical area invade or arise from the dura.[4] The transdural view through the transodontoid corridor faces the caudal portion of the medulla oblongata and the first, second, and cranial portion of the third neuromeres of the spinal cord with related nerves and vessels, which can be exposed after accurately removing the rhomboid arachnoid membrane.

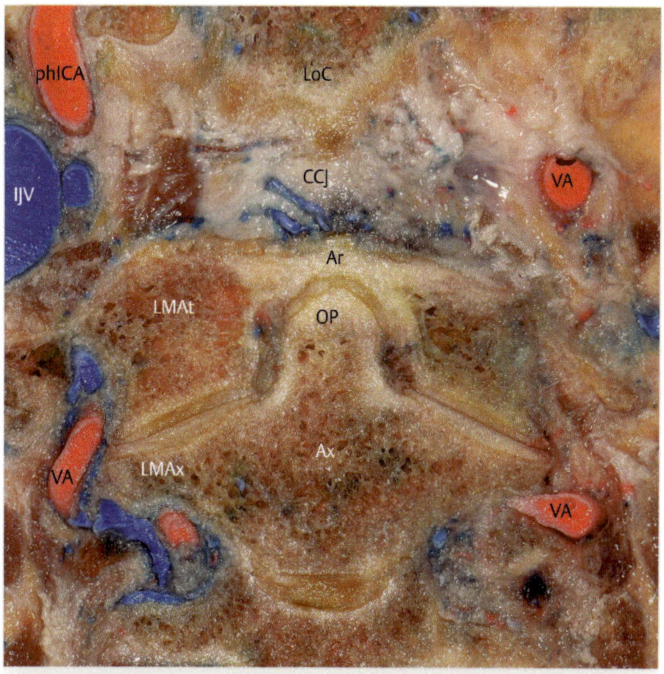

Fig. 13.2 Coronal view of the craniocervical junction. This coronal cadaver cut passes through the craniocervical junction and shows the basic anatomy of its bony boundaries and adjacent structures.
Ar, anterior arch of the atlas; Ax, axis (body); CCJ, craniocervical junction (soft tissues); IJV, internal jugular vein; LMAt, lateral mass of the atlas; LMAx, lateral mass of the axis; LoC, lower clivus; OP, odontoid process; phICA, parapharyngeal tract of the internal carotid artery; VA, vertebral artery.

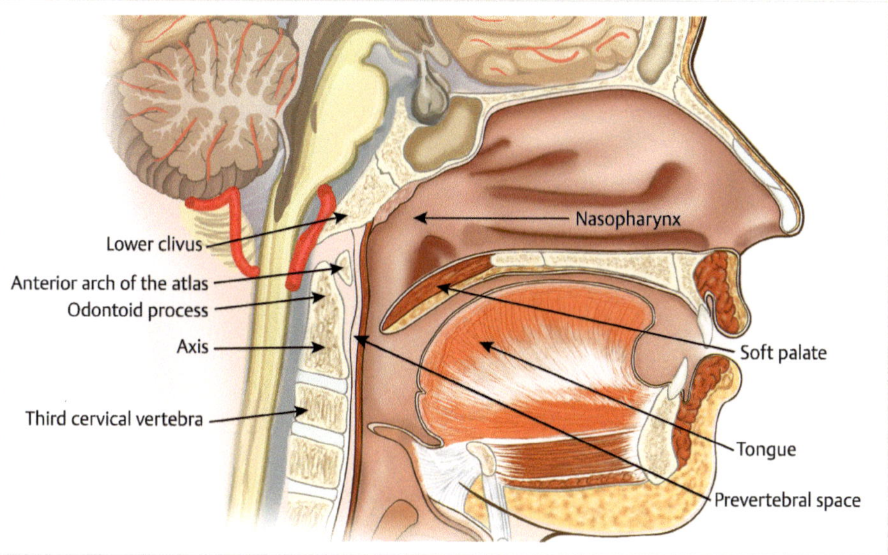

Fig. 13.1 Sagittal view of the transnasal route toward the craniocervical junction. This illustration shows the route toward the craniocervical junction via the nasal cavity.

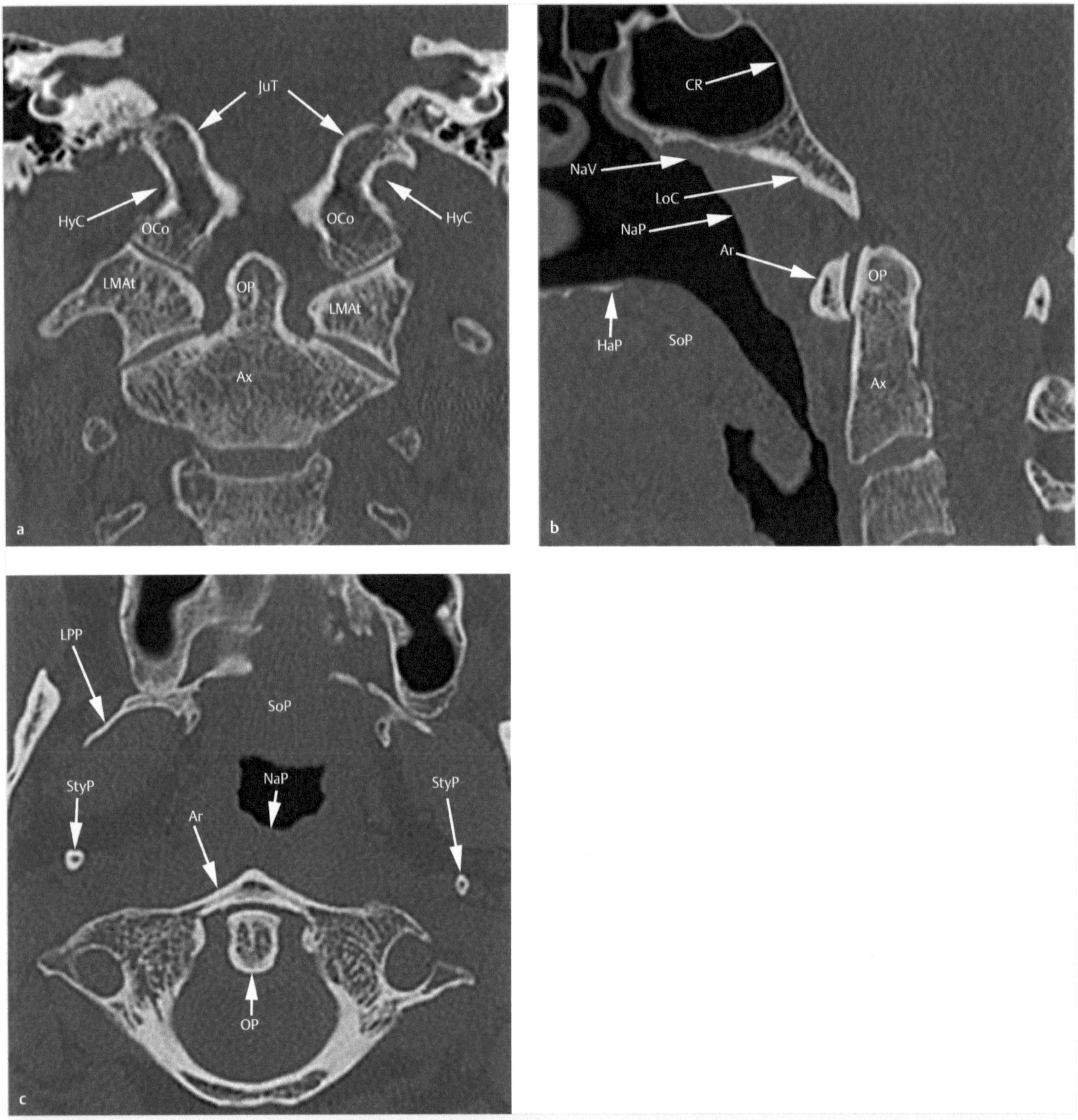

Fig. 13.3 Multiplanar CT of the craniocervical junction. The panel includes a coronal **(a)**, sagittal **(b)**, and axial CT image **(c)** passing through the craniocervical junction. The bony component of the craniocervical junction is made up by occipital condyles (OCo), anterior (Ar) and posterior arches of the atlas, lateral masses of the atlas (LMAt), the axis (Ax), and its odontoid process (OP). All these bony structures lie posterior to the passage from the nasopharynx to the oropharynx. CR, clival recess; HaP, hard palate; HyC, hypoglossal canal; JuT, jugular tubercle; LoC, lower clivus; LPP, lateral pterygoid process; NaP, nasopharyngeal posterior wall; NaV, nasopharyngeal vault; SoP, soft palate; StyP, styloid process.

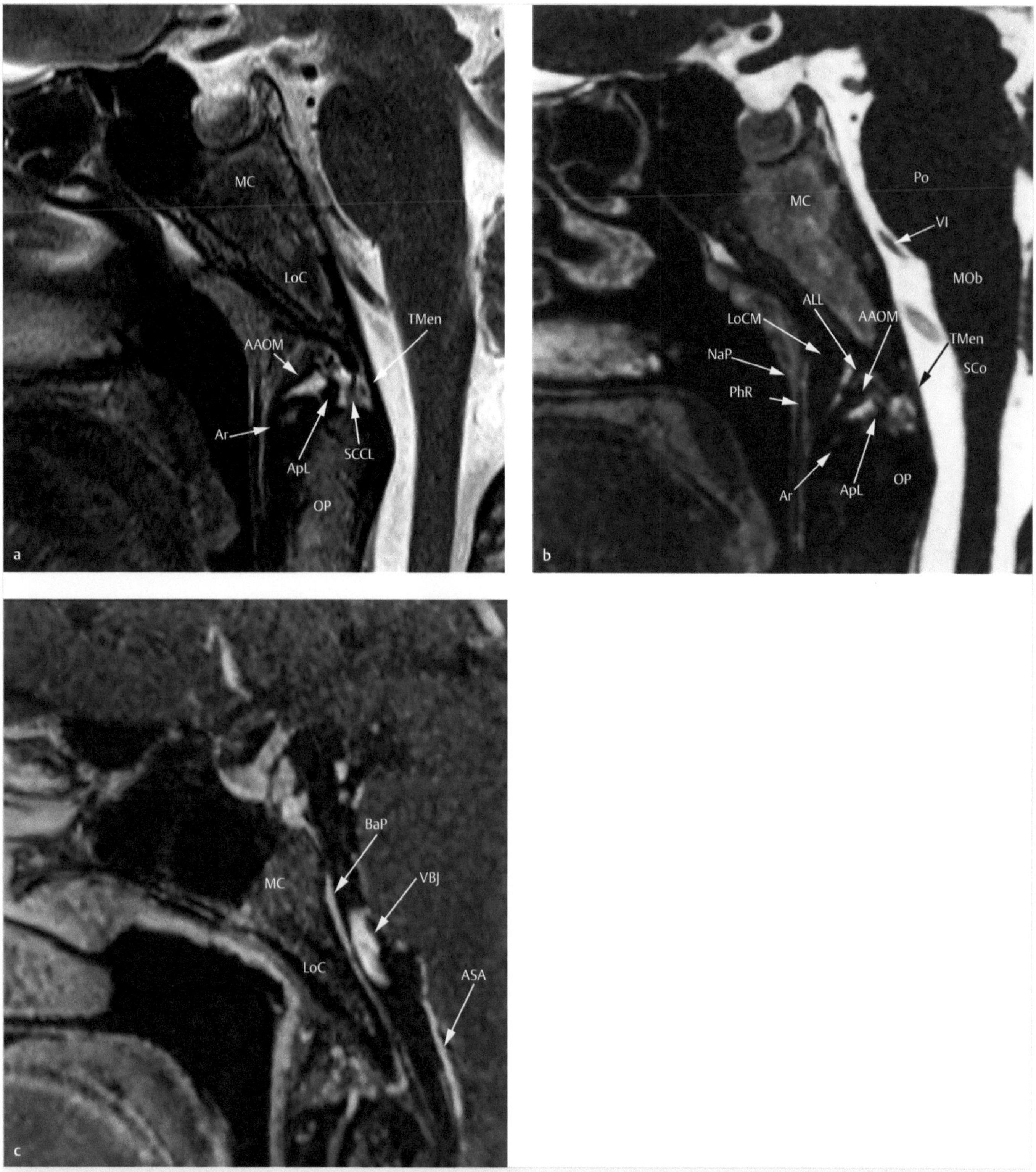

Fig. 13.4 Sagittal MRI anatomy of the craniocervical junction. The panel is formed by sagittal T2-weighted **(a)**, CISS (constructive interference in steady state) **(b)**, and contrast-enhanced T1-weighted fat-saturated images **(c)** passing through the craniocervical junction. The soft-tissue component of the craniocervical junction includes, from anterior to posterior, the pharyngeal raphe (PhR), anterior longitudinal ligament (ALL), anterior atlanto-occipital membrane (AAOM), apical ligament (ApL), superior crus of the cruciform ligament (SCCL), and tectorial membrane (TMen). This complex system of ligaments and membranes anchors the lower clivus (LoC) and occipital condyles to the atlas and axis. VI, abducens nerve; Ar, anterior arch of the atlas; ASA, anterior spinal artery; BaP, basilar plexus; MC, midclivus; MOb, medulla oblongata; NaP, nasopharyngeal posterior wall; OP, odontoid process; Po, pons; SCo, spinal cord; VBJ, vertebrobasilar junction.

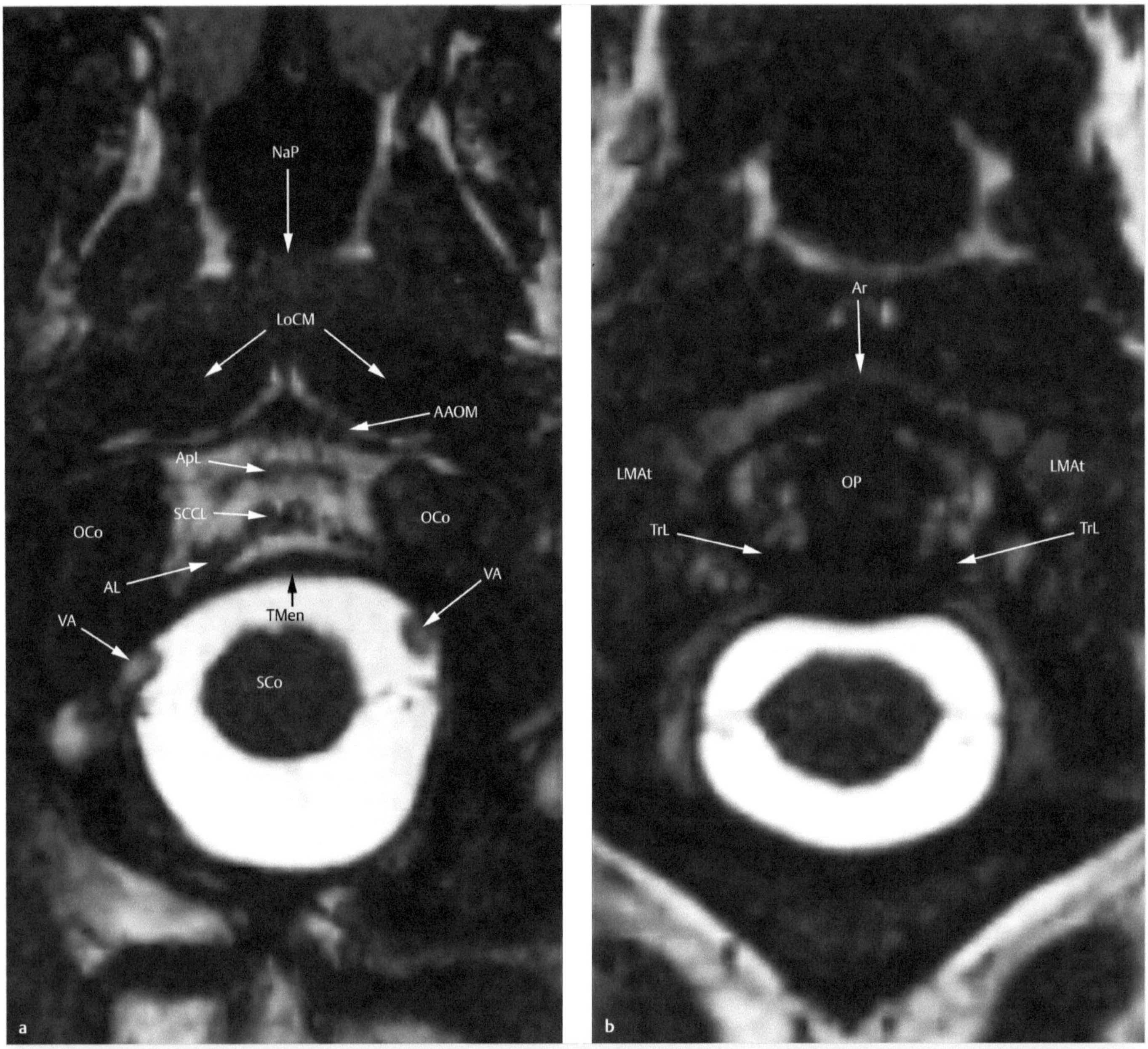

Fig. 13.5 Coronal MRI anatomy of the craniocervical junction. The panel includes two CISS (constructive interference in steady state) MRI axial images passing through the lower portion of occipital condyles **(a)** and through the atlas and odontoid process **(b)**. The connective space between the odontoid process (OP), occipital condyles (OCo), and lower clivus is filled by fat tissue, ligaments, and a venous plexus. From anterior to posterior, the systems of ligaments and membrane is formed by the anterior atlanto-occipital membrane (AAOM), apical ligament (ApL), superior crus of the cruciform ligament (SCCL), alar ligament (AL), and tectorial membrane (TMen). More inferiorly, the transverse ligaments (TrL) serve as the horizontal portion of the cruciform ligament, extending from the odontoid process to the lateral masses of the atlas (LMAt). LoCM, longus capitis muscle; SCo, spinal cord; VA, vertebral artery.

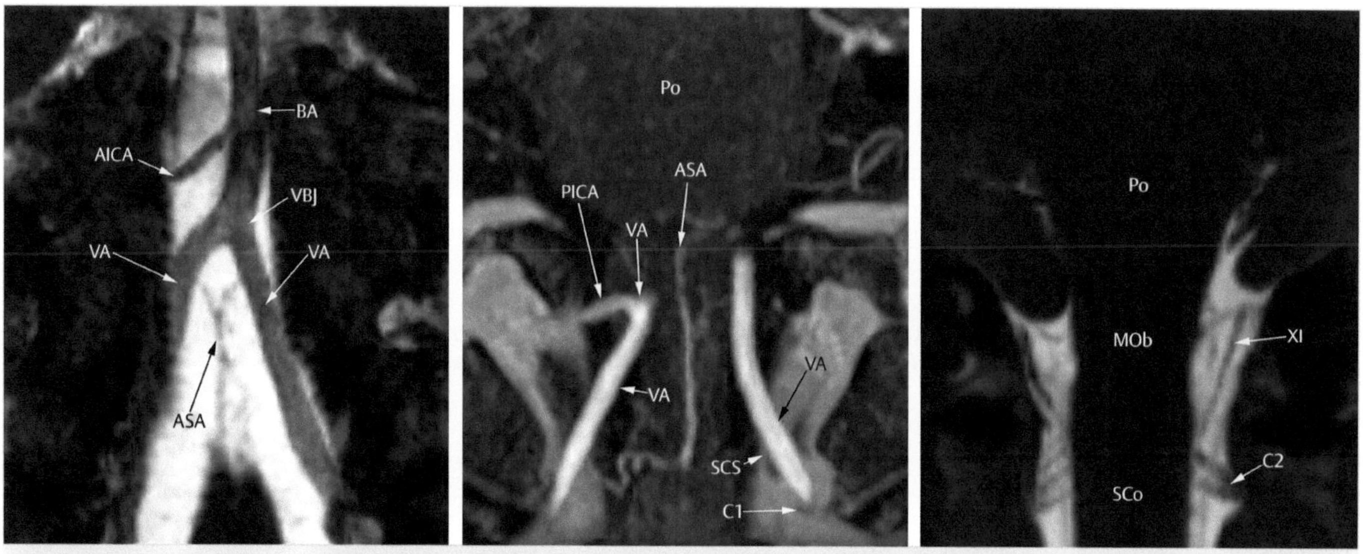

Fig. 13.6 Coronal MRI anatomy of the craniocervical junction. The panel includes three MRI coronal images (two CISS [constructive interference in steady state] MRI scan, top and bottom images, and one T1-weighted contrast-enhanced fat-saturated scan, middle image). The vertebral artery (VA) enters the intradural space through a venous plexus that is defined suboccipital cavernous sinus (SCS), almost at the level of the first cervical nerve (C1). Both the vertebral arteries merge in the vertebrobasilar junction (VBJ), which lies in front of the passage between the pons (Po) and the medulla oblongata (MOb). The anterior spinal artery (ASA) arises from small branches coming from the vertebral arteries. The anterior inferior cerebellar artery (AICA) and the posterior inferior cerebellar artery (PICA) arise from the basilar artery (BA) and the VA, respectively. XI, spinal accessory nerve; C2, second cervical nerve.

Endoscopic Dissection

Nasal Phase

- Paraseptal sphenoidotomy.
- Transrostral sphenoidotomy.
- Facultative: Expanded transrostral sphenoidotomy.
- Posterior septectomy.

Skull Base Phase

Transclival-transodontoid approach

- Step 1: Incision of the posterior wall of the nasopharynx.
- Step 2: Removal of the prevertebral fascia.
- Step 3: Partial removal of the longus capitis muscle and removal of the pharyngeal raphe.
- Step 4: Removal of the anterior longitudinal ligament.
- Step 5: Removal of the anterior atlanto-occipital membrane.
- Step 6: Removal of the apical ligament.
- Step 7: Partial removal of the anterior arch of the atlas.
- Step 8: Partial removal of the lower third of the clivus and removal of the superior crus of the cruciform ligament.
- Step 9: Incision of the tectorial membrane.
- Step 10: Superior odontoidectomy.

Complete transodontoid approach

- Step 11: Total removal of the anterior arch of the atlas.
- Step 12: Total odontoidectomy.
- Step 13: Removal of the tectorial membrane.
- Step 14: Removal of the dura of the craniocervical junction.
- Step 15: Removal of the rhomboid membrane.

Transclival-Transodontoid Approach

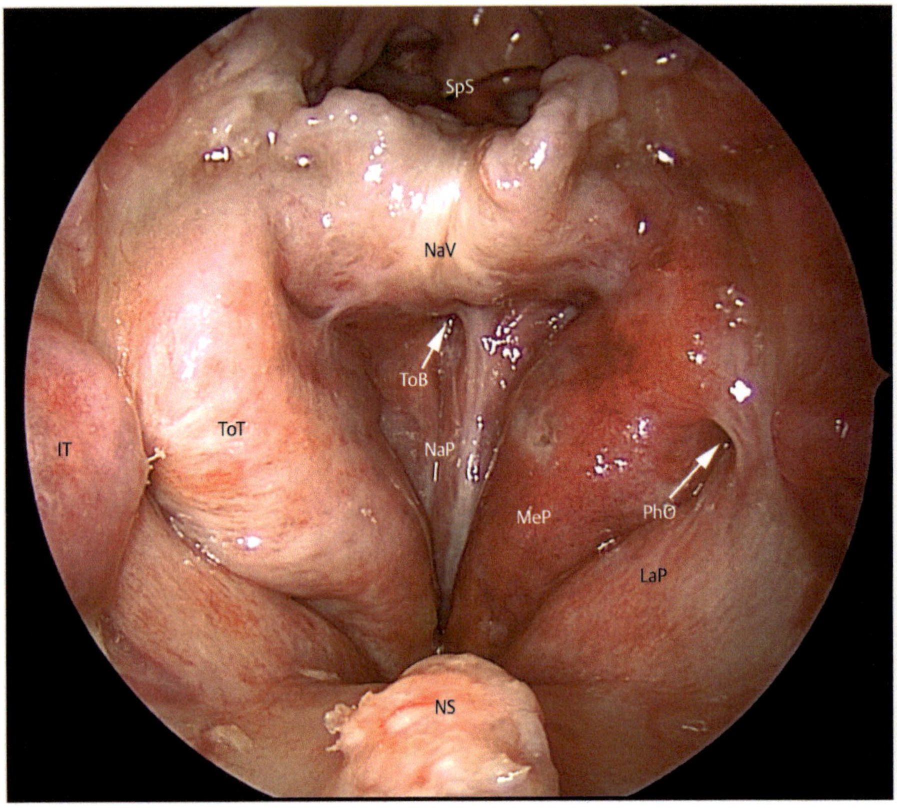

Fig. 13.7 Nasopharyngeal landmarks. The craniocervical junction lies behind the posterior wall of the nasopharynx (NaP). In this specimen, the medial plate (MeP) of torus tubarius (ToT) is remarkably bulky, thus requiring its partial removal to harvest the transodontoid corridor. Thornwaldt's bursa (ToB) is a mucosal recess that lies at the junction between the posterior wall and the vault of the nasopharynx (NaV). IT, inferior turbinate; LaP, lateral plate of the torus tubarius; NS, nasal septum (partially removed); PhO, pharyngeal ostium of the eustachian tube; SpS, sphenoid sinus (previously opened).

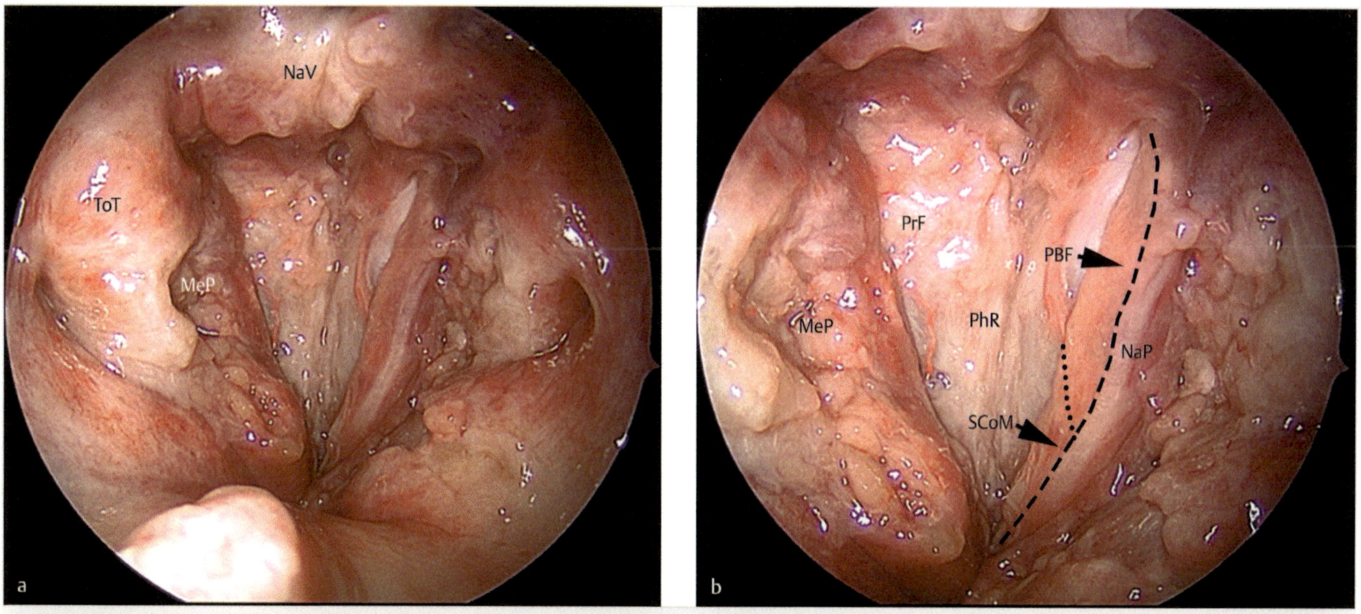

Fig. 13.8 (a, b) Step 1. A vertical incision (*black dashed line*) is made along the posterior wall of the nasopharynx (NaP). The superior constrictor muscle (SCoM) reaches the pharyngeal raphe (PhR) on the midline. Cranially, this muscle has a free edge (*black dotted line*) that continues with the pharyngobasilar fascia (PBF) up to the skull base. As previously mentioned, the partial removal of the medial plate (MeP) of the torus tubarius (ToT) might be necessary. At the end of this step, the prevertebral fascia (PrF) is exposed. NaV, nasopharyngeal vault.

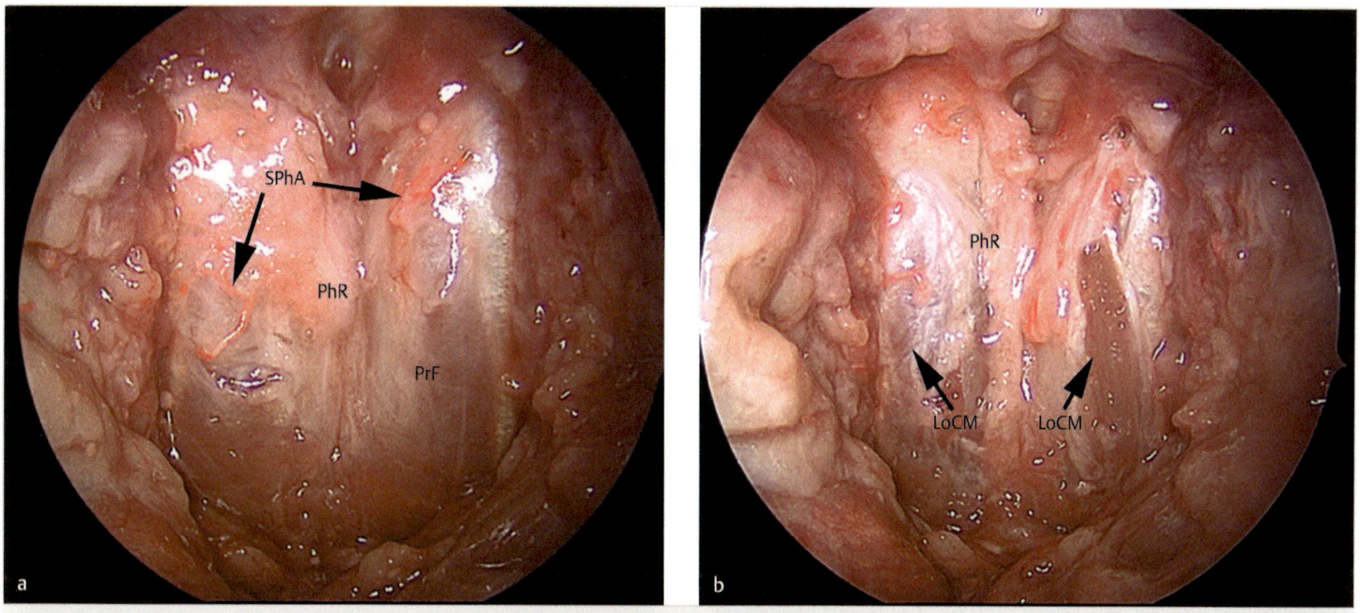

Fig. 13.9 (a, b) Step 2. The prevertebral fascia (PrF) is removed bilaterally preserving the pharyngeal raphe (PhR) to expose the longus capitis muscle (LoCM). The superior pharyngeal arteries (SPhA) are branches of the ascending pharyngeal artery that supply the nasopharynx.

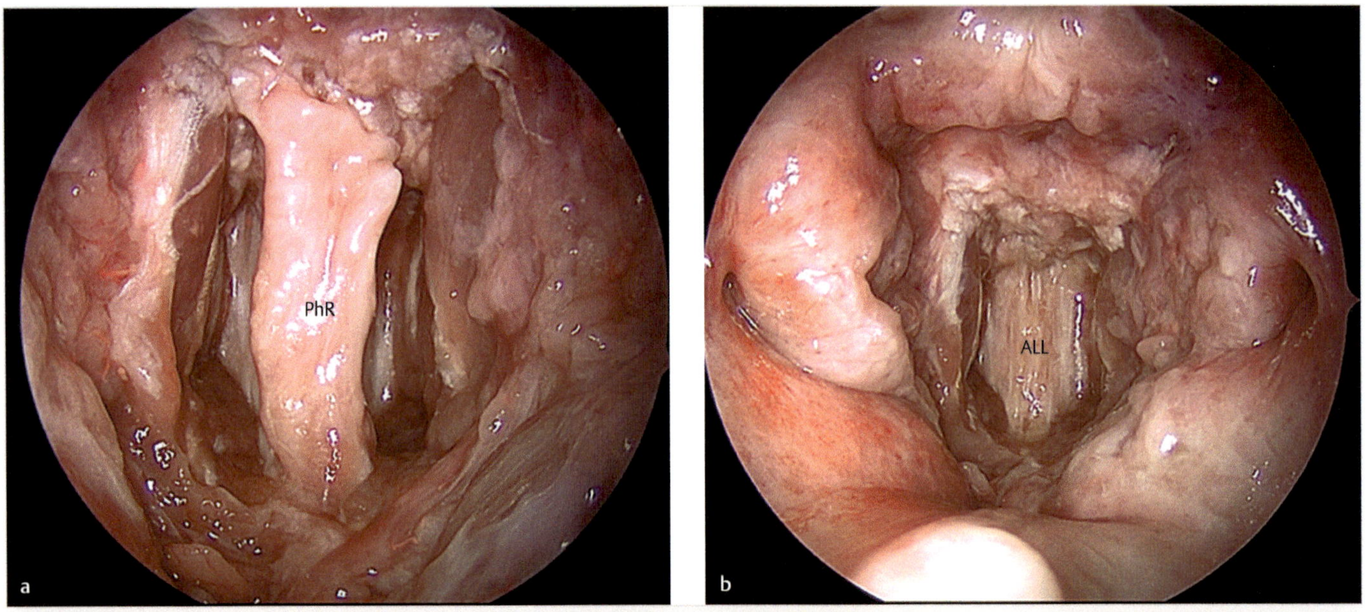

Fig. 13.10 (a, b) Step 3. The most medial portion of the longus capitis muscles is removed to identify the anterior longitudinal ligament (ALL). The pharyngeal raphe (PhR) is therefore isolated on the midline and subsequently removed to complete the exposure of the anterior longitudinal ligament.

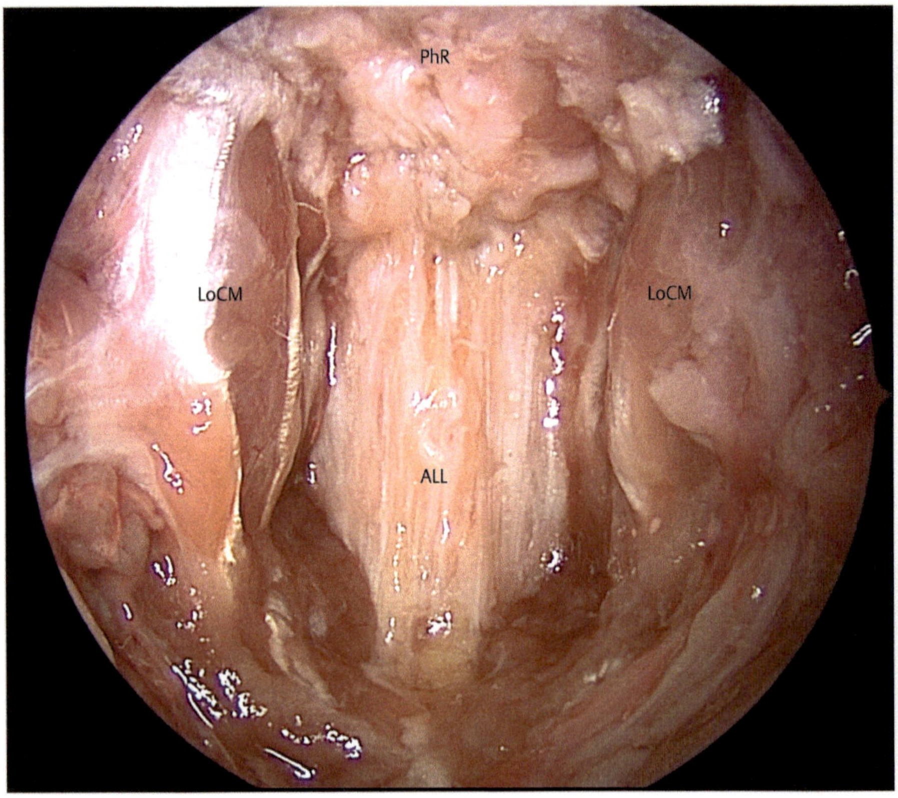

Fig. 13.11 The anterior longitudinal ligament. The anterior longitudinal ligament (ALL) is recognized due to the craniocaudal orientation of its fibrous fibers. The lateral portions of the longus capitis muscles (LoCM) lie at the lateral boundary of the corridor. PhR, pharyngeal raphe (sectioned).

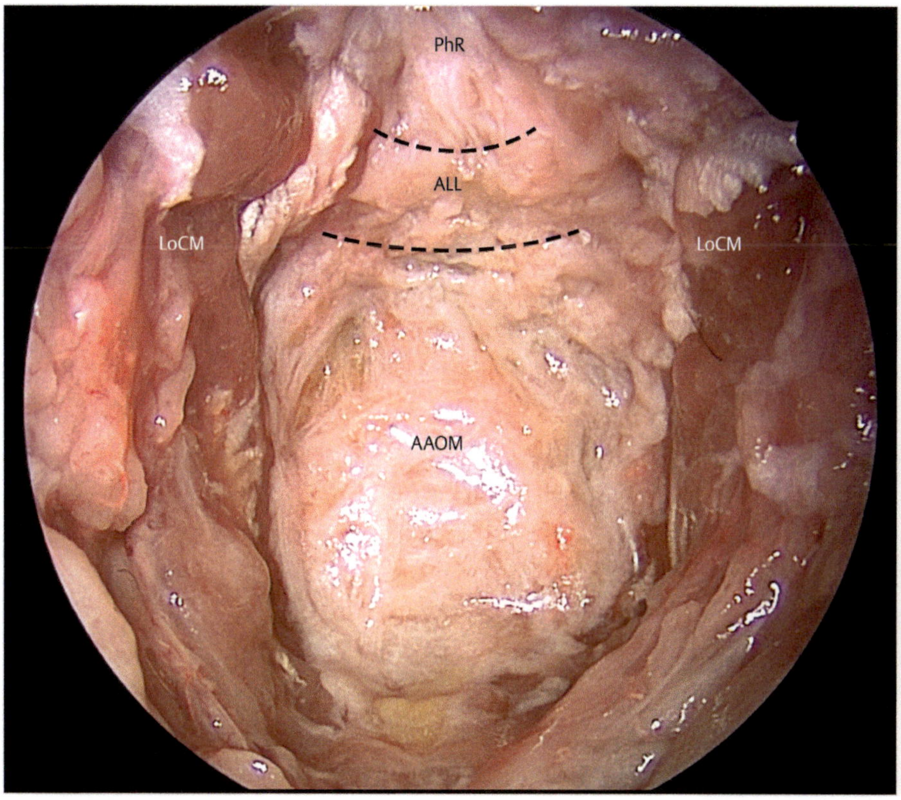

Fig. 13.12 Step 4. The anterior longitudinal ligament (ALL) is removed to expose the anterior atlanto-occipital membrane (AAOM). This can be distinguished from the anterior longitudinal ligament because its fibrous fibers are not craniocaudally oriented. (*Black dashed lines*: lines separating the areas of superior insertions of the pharyngeal raphe and anterior longitudinal ligament.) LoCM, longus capitis muscle; PhR, pharyngeal raphe (sectioned).

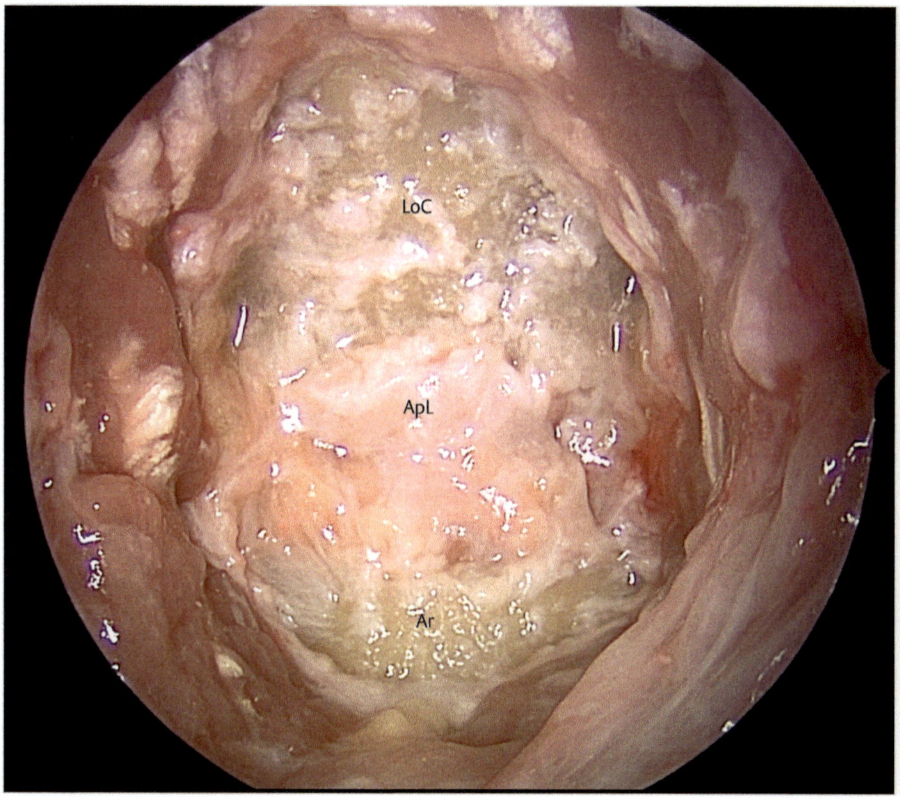

Fig. 13.13 Step 5. The anterior atlanto-occipital membrane is removed to expose the lower third of the clivus superiorly (LoC) and the anterior arch of the atlas (Ar) inferiorly. In this way, the clival insertion of the apical ligament (ApL) is identified. The inferior portion of the ligament is covered by a smooth tissue attached to the superior border of the anterior arch of the atlas.

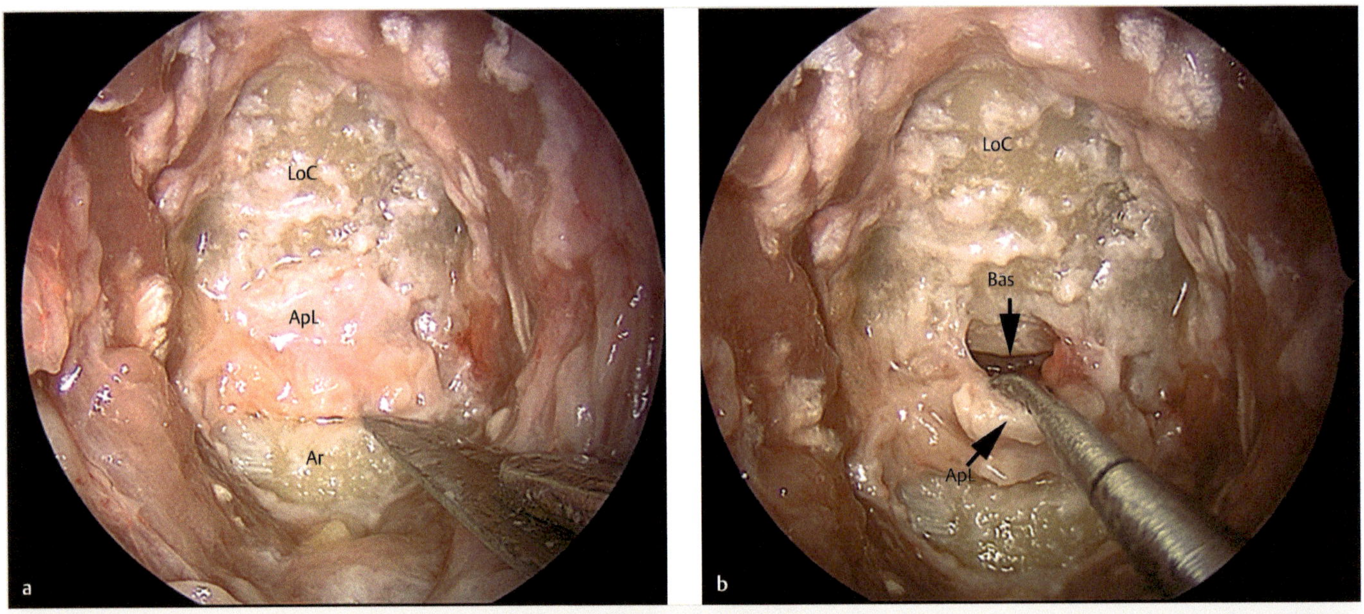

Fig. 13.14 (a, b) Step 6. The apical ligament (ApL) is removed to expose the basion (Bas), which is the most anterior portion of the foramen magnum. Ar, anterior arch of the atlas; LoC, lower clivus.

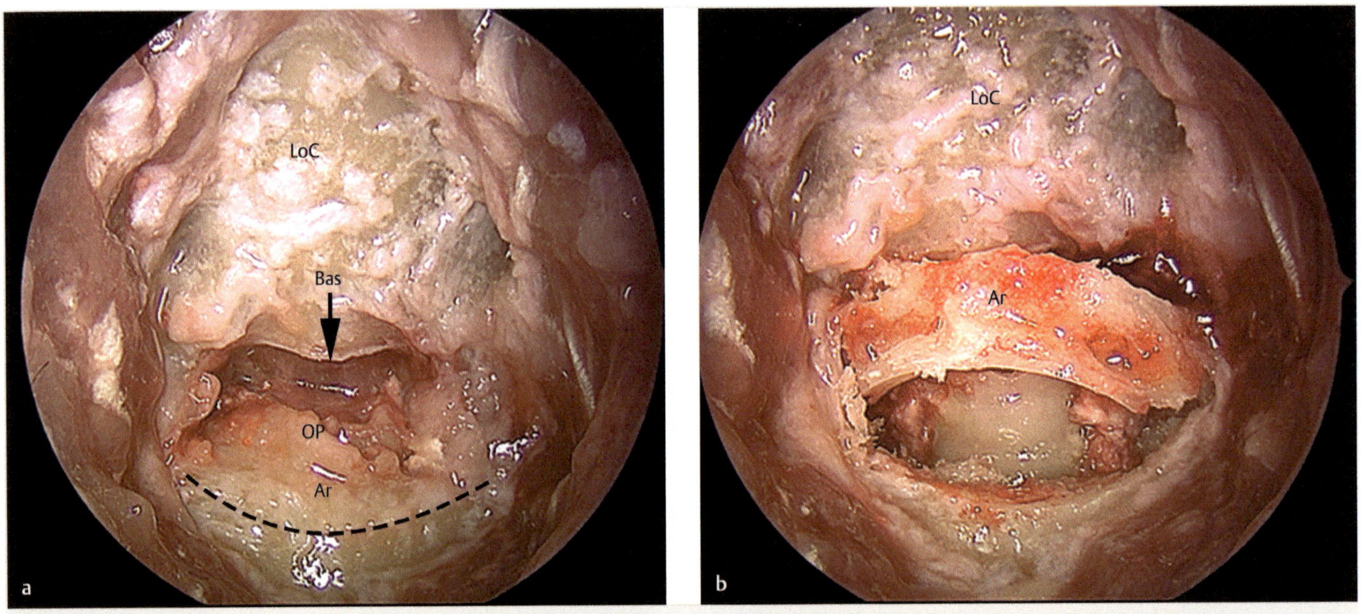

Fig. 13.15 (a, b) Step 7. After removing the apical ligament, the most cranial portion of the odontoid process (OP) is identified behind the anterior arch of the atlas (Ar). A curvilinear osteotomy (*black dashed line*) of the superior portion of the anterior arch of the atlas is made. Bas, basion; LoC, lower clivus.

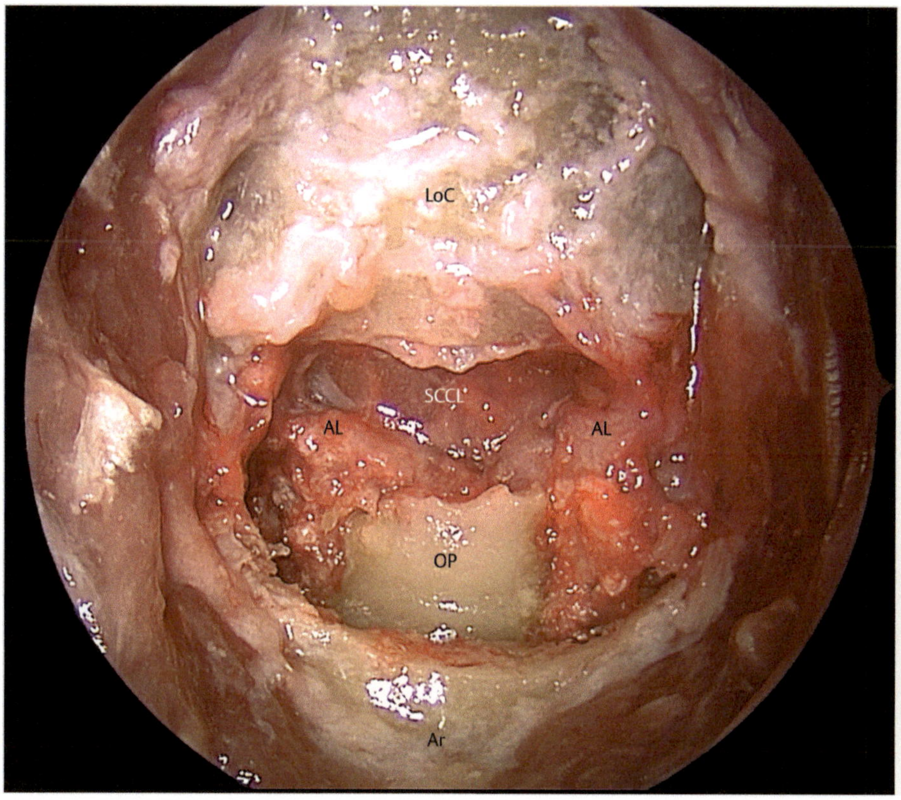

Fig. 13.16 The odontoid process. The odontoid process (OP), which lies behind the anterior arch of the atlas (Ar), serves for lower insertion of the apical and alar ligaments (AL). The alar ligaments and the apical ligament reach the lower third of the clivus (LoC) laterally and on the midline, respectively. More posteriorly, the superior crus of the cruciform ligament (SCCL) separates the alar ligaments from the tectorial membrane.

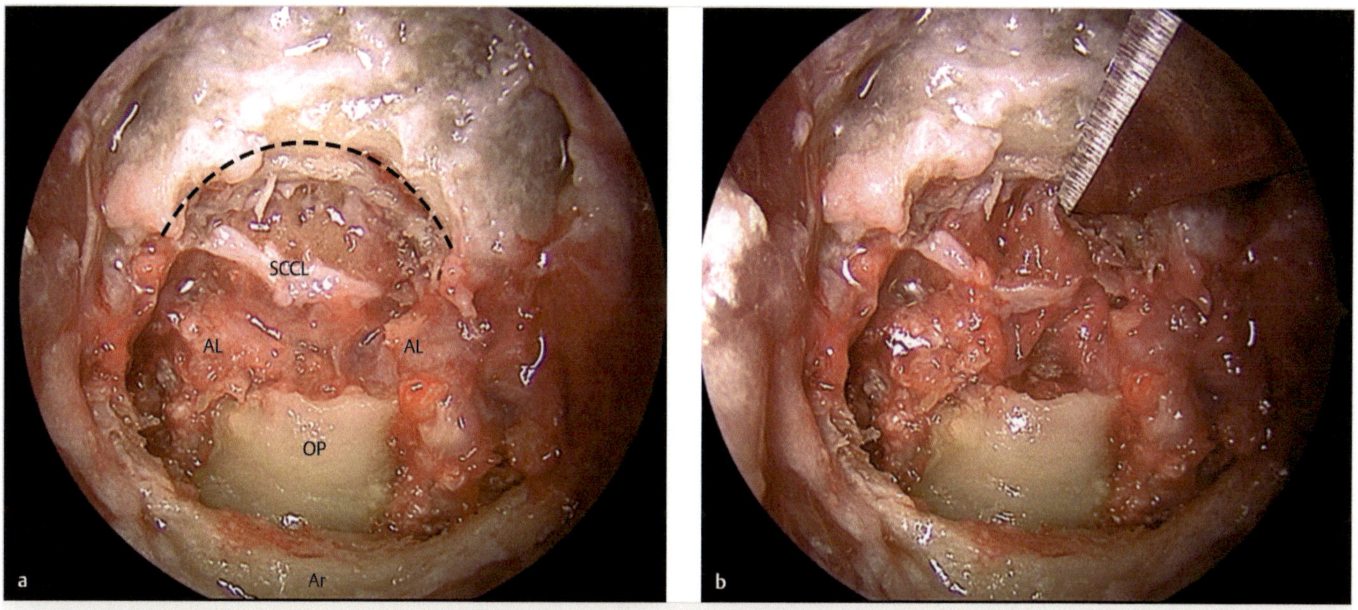

Fig. 13.17 (a, b) Step 8. A small osteotomy of the caudal part of the lower third of the clivus (*black dashed line*) is made and the superior crus of the cruciform ligament (SCCL) removed. AL, alar ligaments; Ar, anterior arch of the atlas; OP, odontoid process.

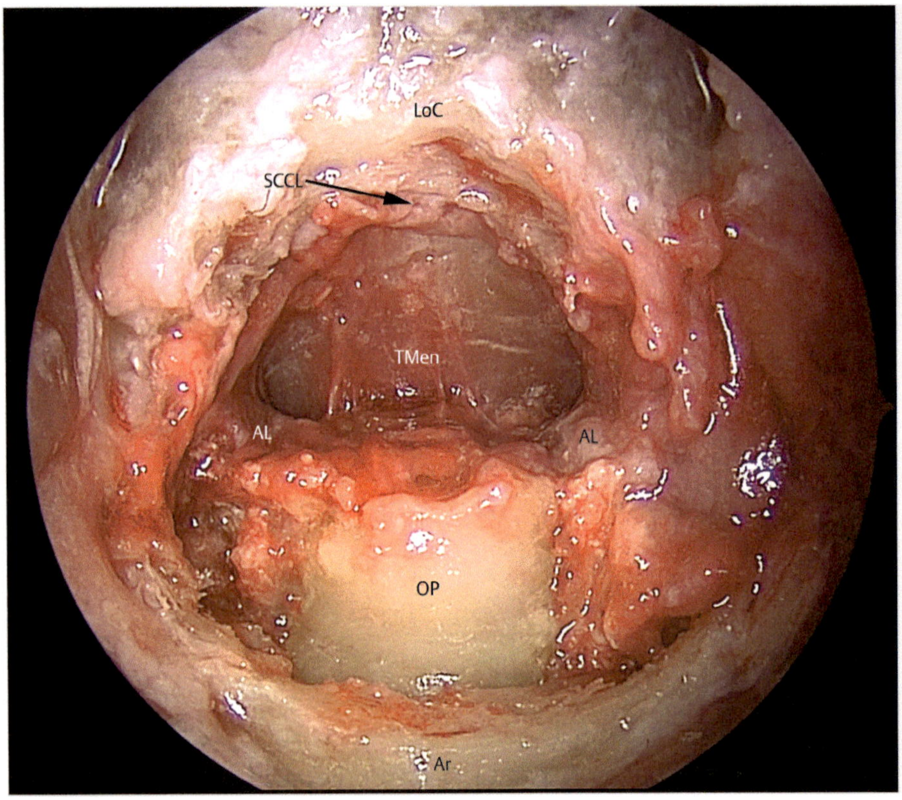

Fig. 13.18 The tectorial membrane. After removing the superior crus of the cruciform ligament (SCCL), the tectorial membrane (TMen) comes in to view. AL, alar ligament; Ar, anterior arch of the atlas; LoC, lower clivus; OP, odontoid process.

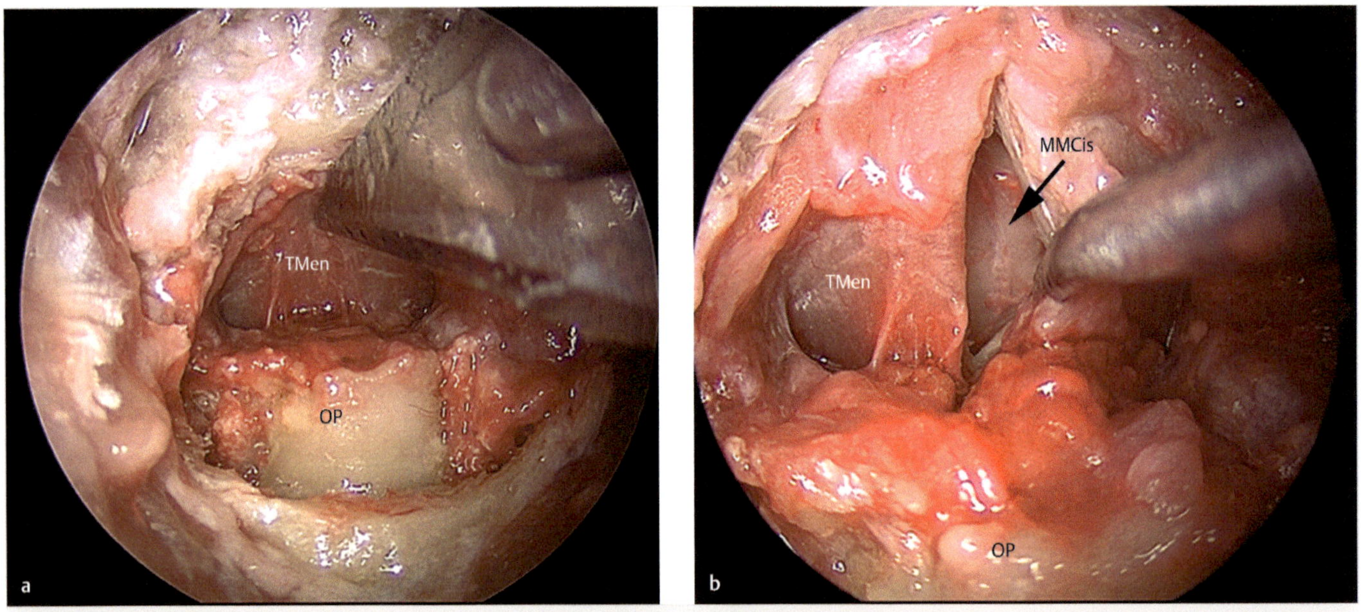

Fig. 13.19 (a, b) Step 9. A vertical median incision is made on the tectorial membrane (TMen) to enter the median medullary cistern (MMCis). Then, the tectorial membrane is displaced, without damaging the medulla oblongata and the spinal cord.

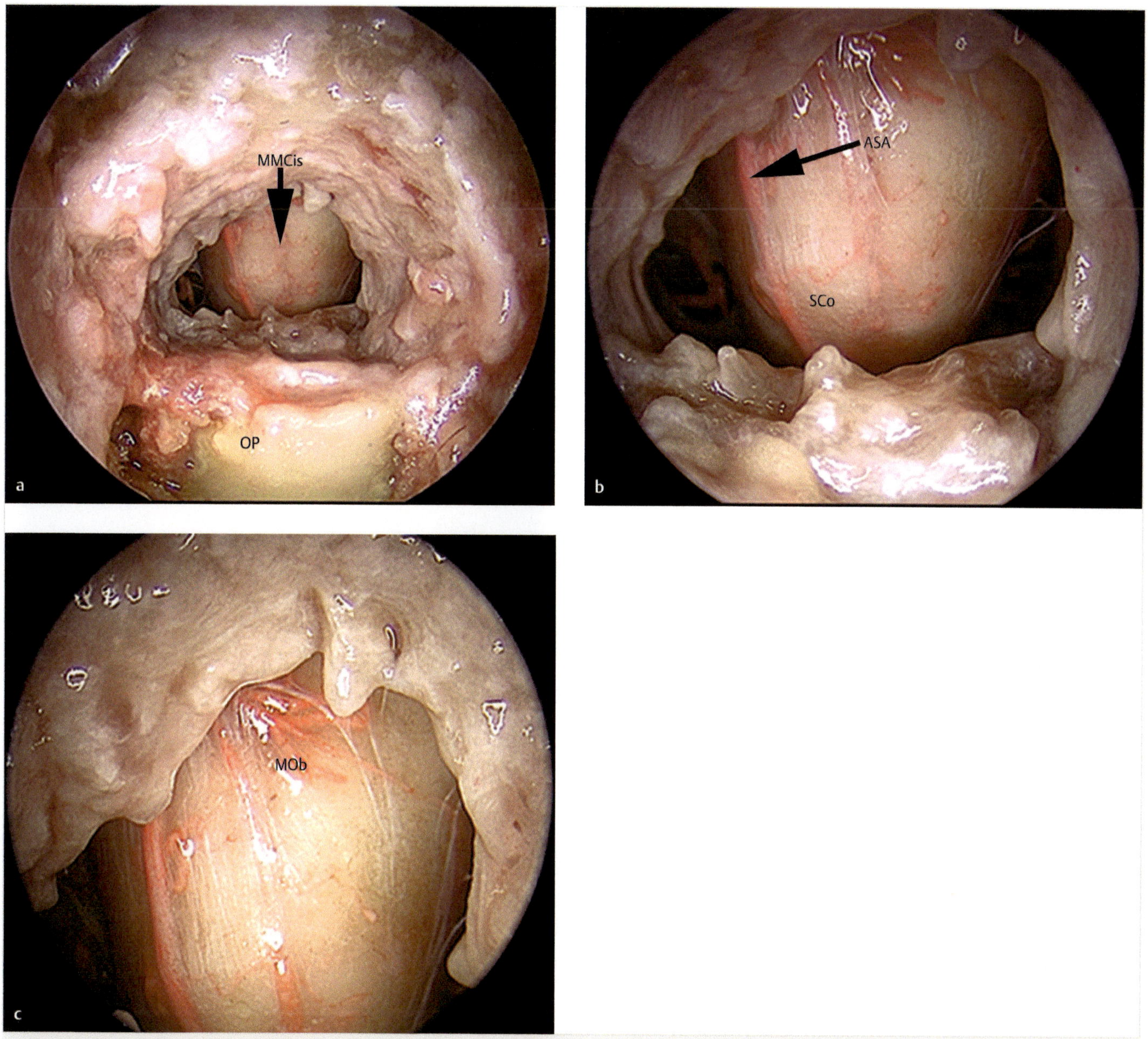

Fig. 13.20 (a–c) The median medullary cistern. After removing the tectorial membrane, the median medullary cistern (MMCis) is explored by positioning the endoscope above the odontoid process (OP). The junction between medulla oblongata (MOb) and the spinal cord (SCo) can be reached with straight instrumentation through this corridor. The anterior spinal artery (ASA) is also identified.

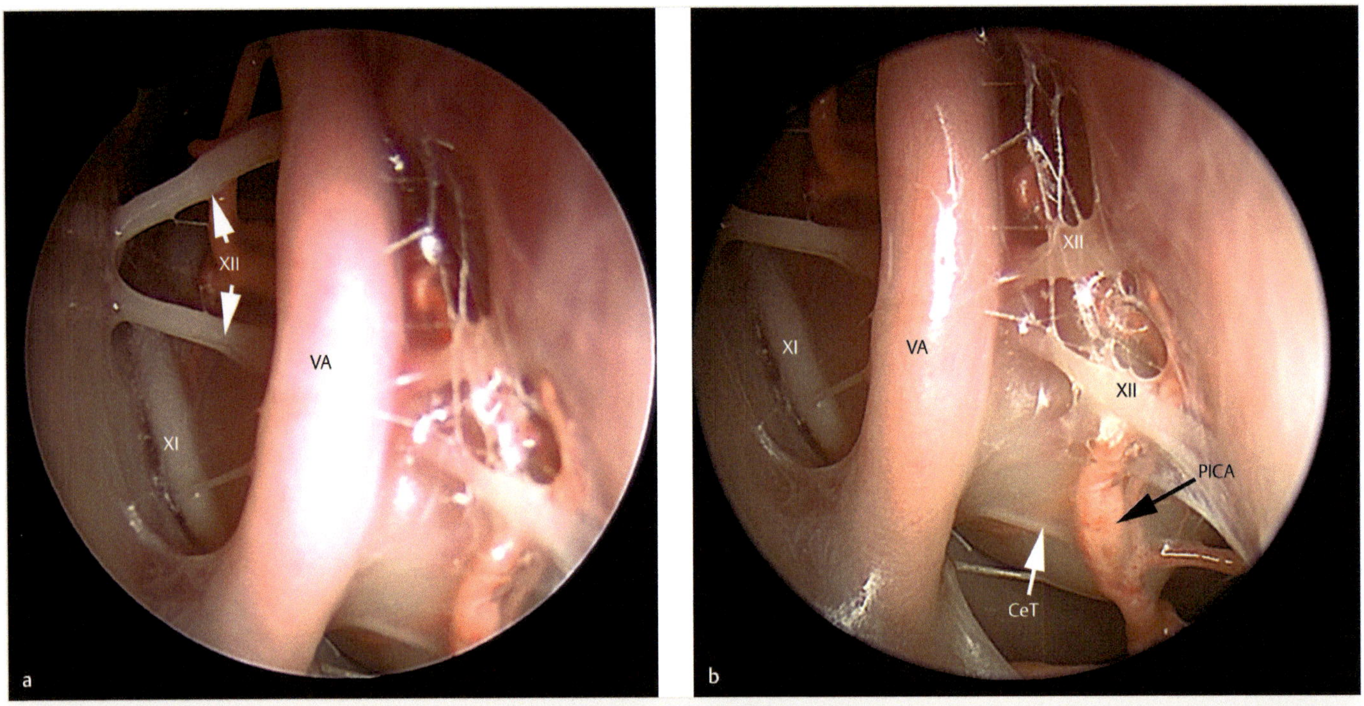

Fig. 13.21 (a, b) The hypoglossal nerve. With a 70-degree scope turned laterally (to the right side), the rootlets of the hypoglossal nerve (XII), which pass posterolaterally to the vertebral artery (VA), are identified. Posterolaterally to the hypoglossal rootlets, the spinal root of the accessory nerve (XI) runs from inferior to superior, in front of the cerebellar tonsil (CeT). The posterior inferior cerebellar artery (PICA) passes above the hypoglossal nerve and gives some branches that run posterolaterally to the rootlets of the same nerve.

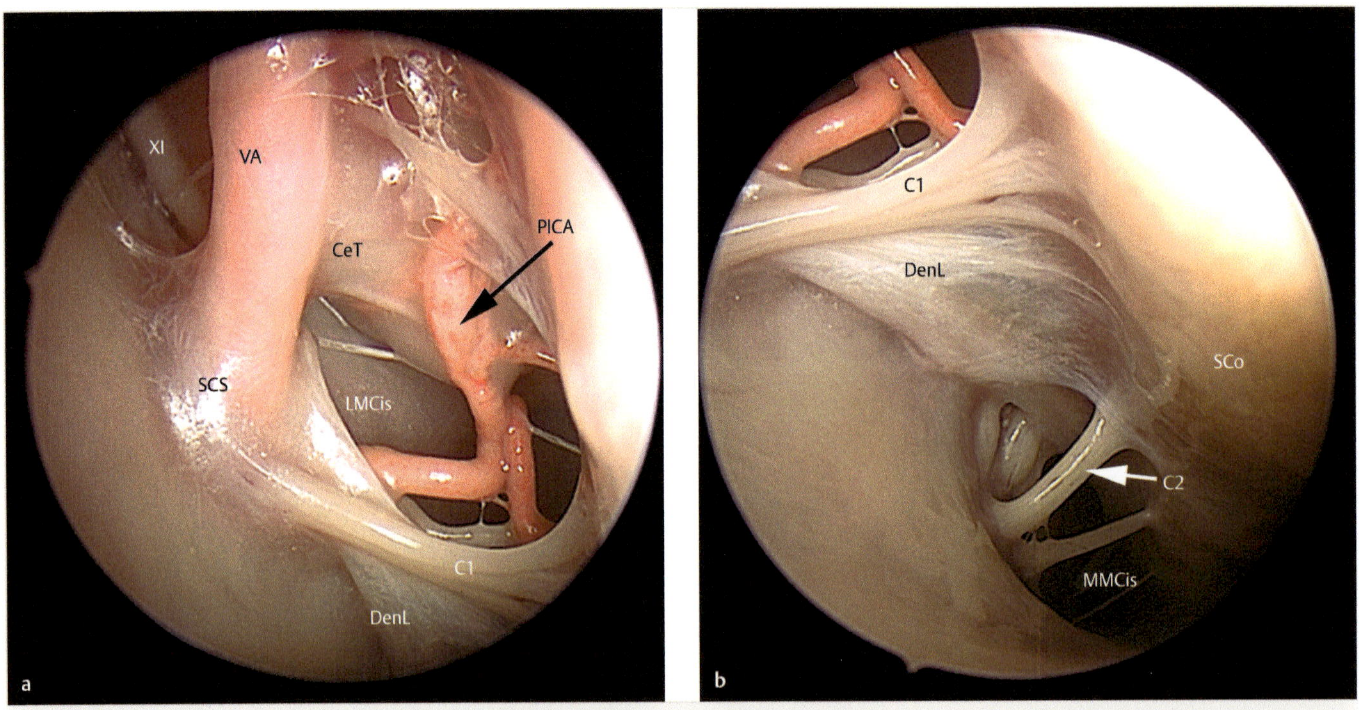

Fig. 13.22 (a, b) The first cervical nerve and the suboccipital cavernous sinus. The first cervical nerve (C1) passes anteroinferiorly to the vertebral artery (VA). Its cisternal tract ends where the vertebral artery enters the subarachnoid space. This area is formed by a venous plexus that is defined as the suboccipital cavernous sinus (SCS), in view of the similarity with the cavernous sinus with respect to the internal carotid artery. The ventral rootlets of the first cervical nerve lie in front of the first denticulate ligament (DenL), while the spinal root of the accessory nerve (XI) and the dorsal rootlets of the first cervical nerve run behind this ligament. The former goes superiorly toward the jugular foramen, while the latter overcome the upper edge of the denticulate ligament joining the ventral rootlets. The first denticulate ligament ends superiorly in the posterior portion of the suboccipital cavernous sinus. C2, second cervical nerve; CeT, cerebellar tonsil; LMCis, lateral medullary cistern; MMCis, median medullary cistern; PICA, posterior inferior cerebellar artery; SCo, spinal cord.

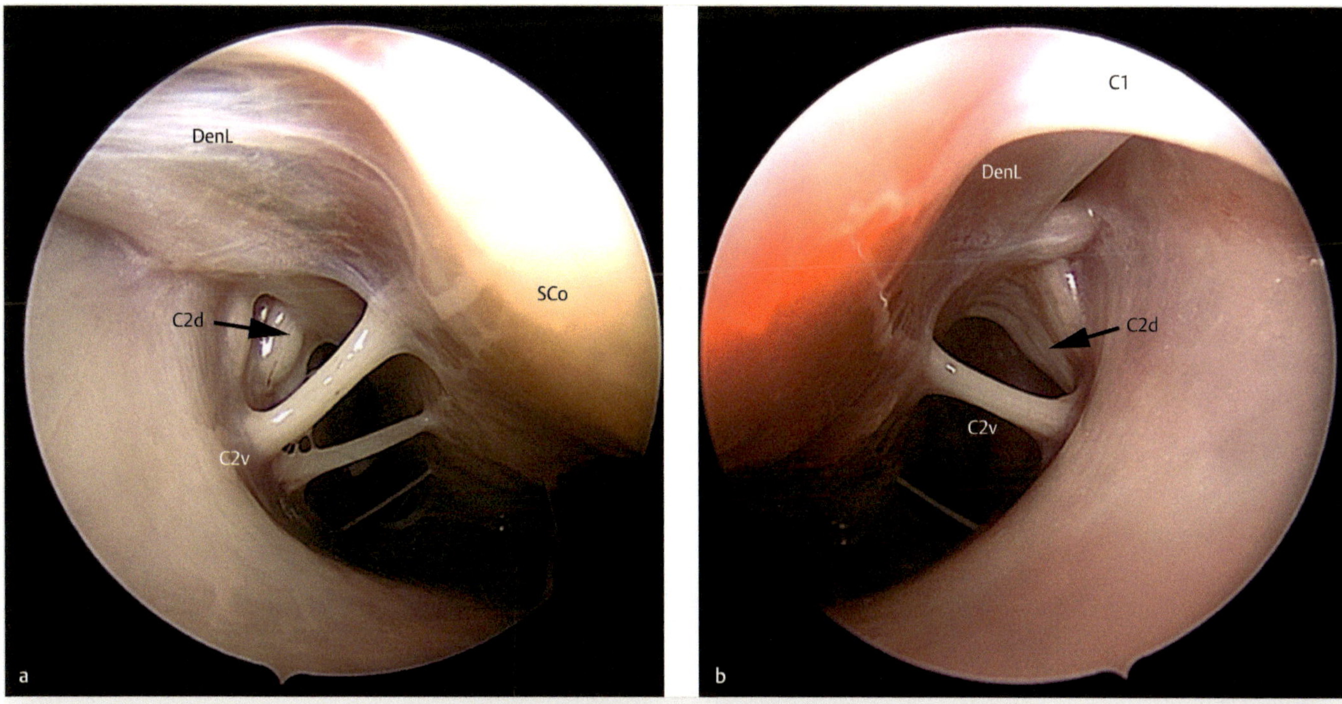

Fig. 13.23 (a, b) The second cervical nerve. The ventral rootlets of the second cervical nerve (C2v) lie in front of the first denticulate ligament (DenL). The dorsal rootlets (C2d) lie posteriorly and pass below the denticulate ligament. Therefore, the first denticulate ligament is interposed between the first (C1) and second cervical nerves. SCo, spinal cord.

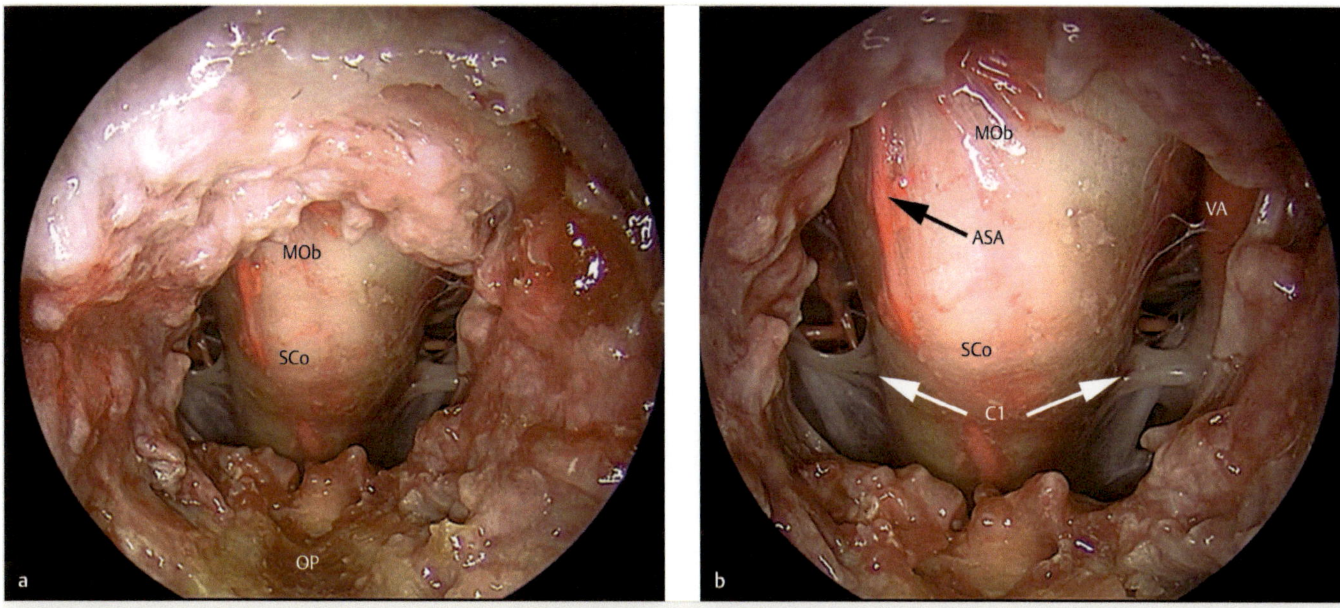

Fig. 13.24 (a, b) Step 10. The superior portion of the odontoid process (OP) is removed to expose the first cervical nerve (C1). ASA, anterior spinal artery; MOb, medulla oblongata; SCo, spinal cord; VA, vertebral artery.

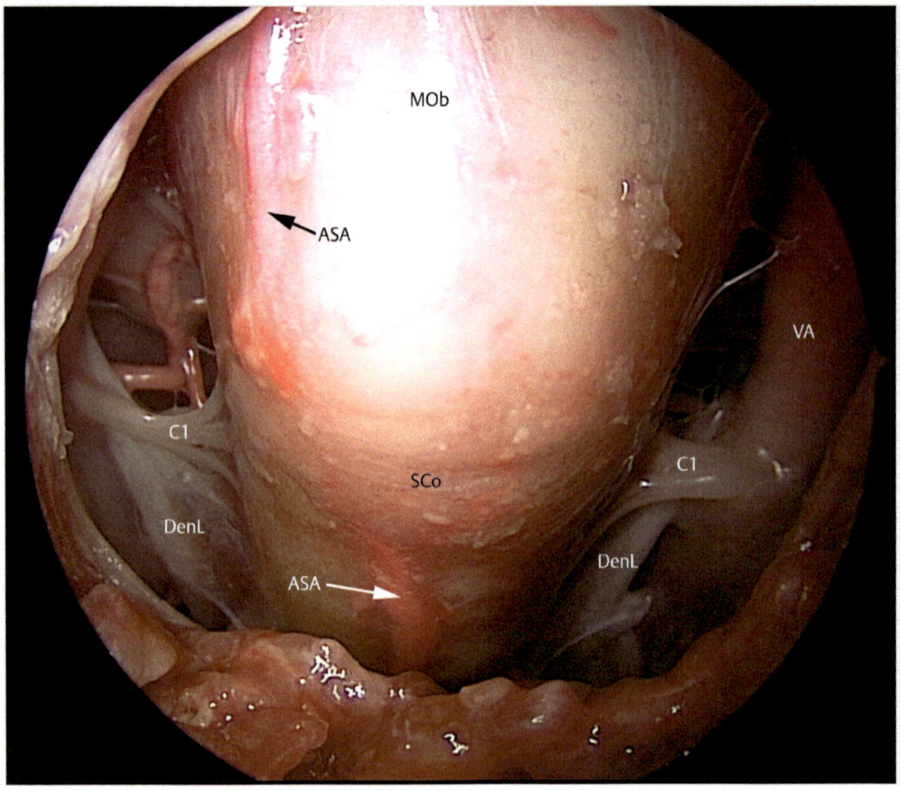

Fig. 13.25 Direct intradural view after superior odontoidectomy. After removing the superior portion of the odontoid process, the first cervical nerves (C1) are directly visible in front of the denticulate ligaments (DenL). ASA, anterior spinal artery; MOb, medulla oblongata; SCo, spinal cord; VA, vertebral artery.

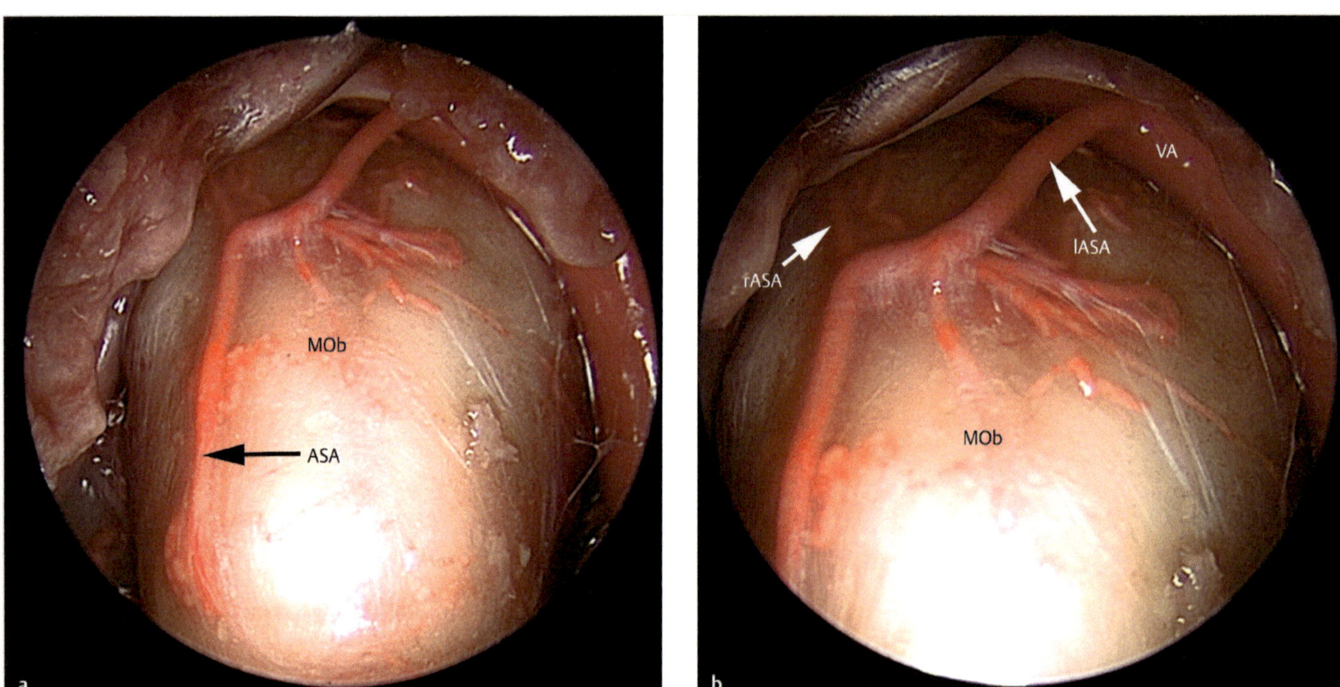

Fig. 13.26 (a, b) The anterior spinal artery. A 70-degree scope turned cranially is placed through the transodontoid corridor to analyze the entire course of the anterior spinal artery (ASA), which arises from the fusion of the left anterior spinal artery (lASA) and the right anterior spinal artery (rASA). They take origin from the inferomedial surface of the ipsilateral vertebral artery (VA). Then, the anterior spinal artery runs on the ventral surface of the medulla oblongata (MOb) and the spinal cord. The anterior spinal artery is more frequently median but can also be paramedian, as in this specimen.

Complete Transodontoid Approach

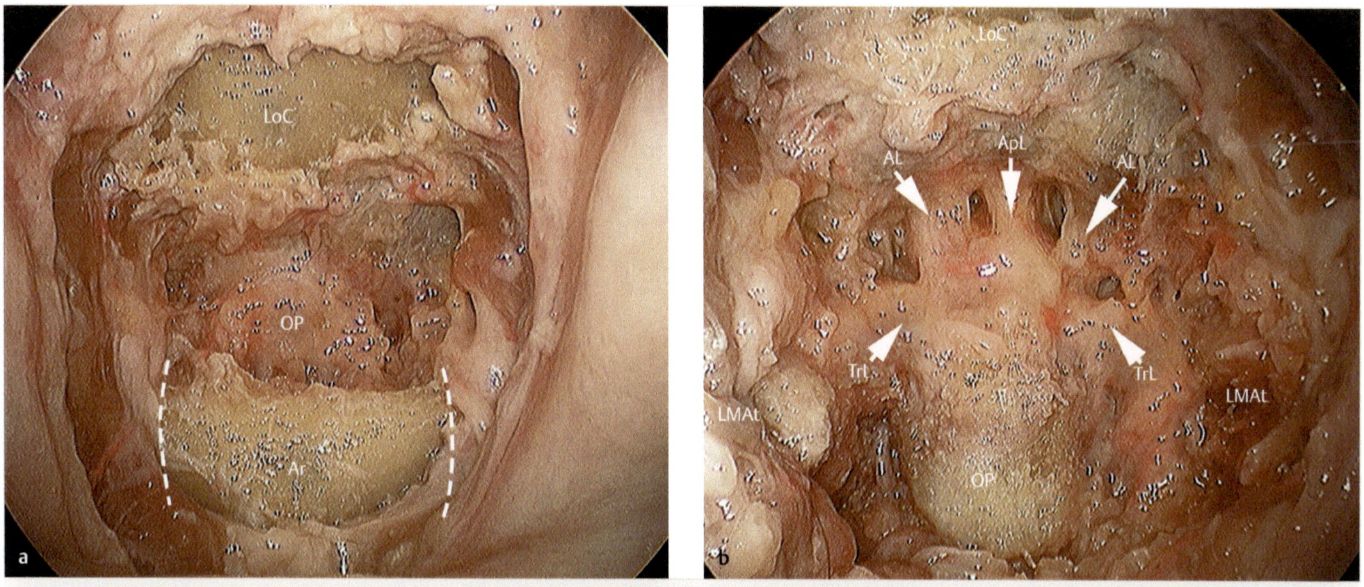

Fig. 13.27 (a, b) Step 11. The following steps can be performed starting from step 5. The anterior arch of the atlas (Ar) is completely removed by performing two osteotomies (*white dashed lines*) at the lateral masses of the atlas (LMAt). In this way, the odontoid process (OP) can be completely exposed. The transverse ligaments (TrL) arise from the dorsolateral surface of the odontoid process on both sides and insert on the lateral masses of the atlas. The alar ligaments (AL) and the apical ligament (ApL) arise from the tip of the odontoid process and reach the medial surface of the occipital condyles and lower clivus (LoC), respectively.

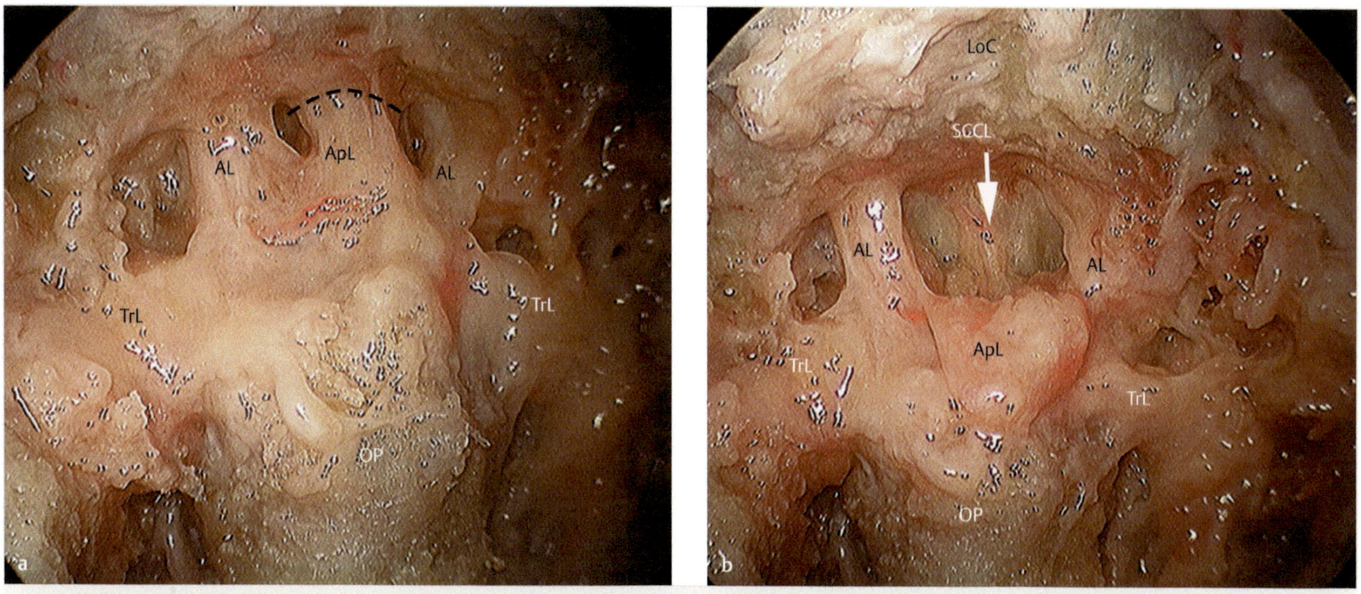

Fig. 13.28 (a, b) Ligaments of the odontoid process. The first layer of ligaments surrounding the odontoid process (OP) is formed by the transverse ligaments (TrL), alar ligaments (AL), and apical ligaments (ApL). After sectioning the apical ligament (*black dashed line*), the superior crus of the cruciform ligament (SCCL), which arises from the transverse ligament and reaches the lower clivus (LoC), comes into view.

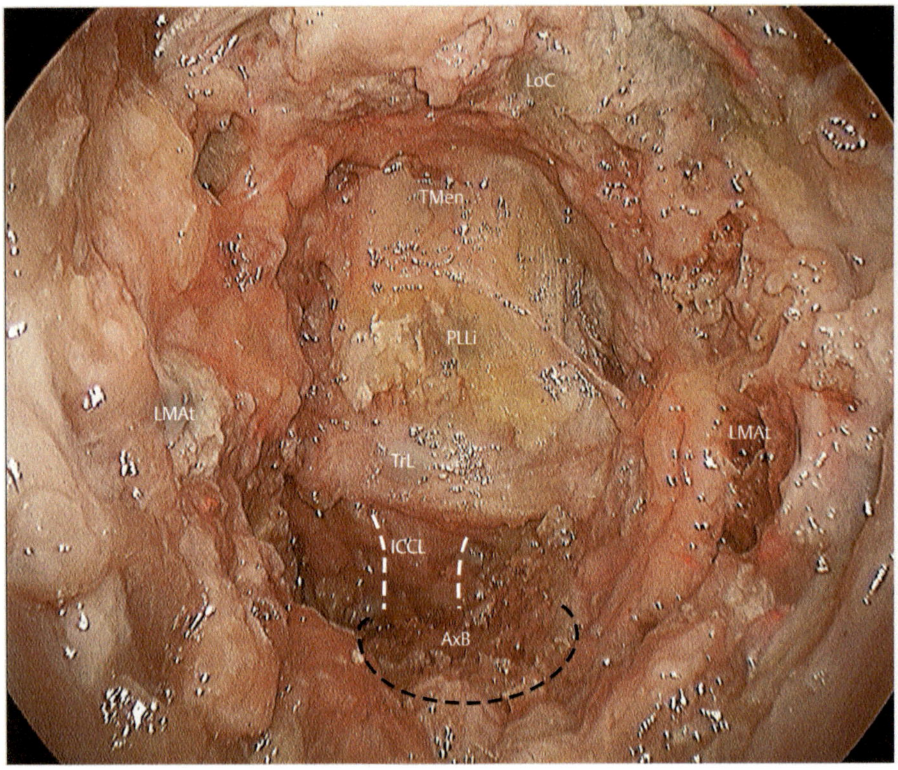

Fig. 13.29 Step 12. After sectioning the alar and apical ligaments, the odontoid process is completely removed, from its root (*black dashed line*) on the body of the axis (AxB) to the cranial apex. The transverse ligament (TrL) is entirely visible along with the inferior crus of the cruciform ligament (ICCL; *white dashed lines*), which extends from the transverse ligament to the body of the axis. The posterior longitudinal ligament (PLLi) is identified above and behind the transverse ligament. This ligament is posterior to the cruciform ligament. In the present specimen, some fibers of the PLLi arise from the transverse ligament. The tectorial membrane (TMen) results from a cranial thickening and widening of the posterior longitudinal ligament anteriorly. LMAt, lateral mass of the atlas; LoC, lower clivus.

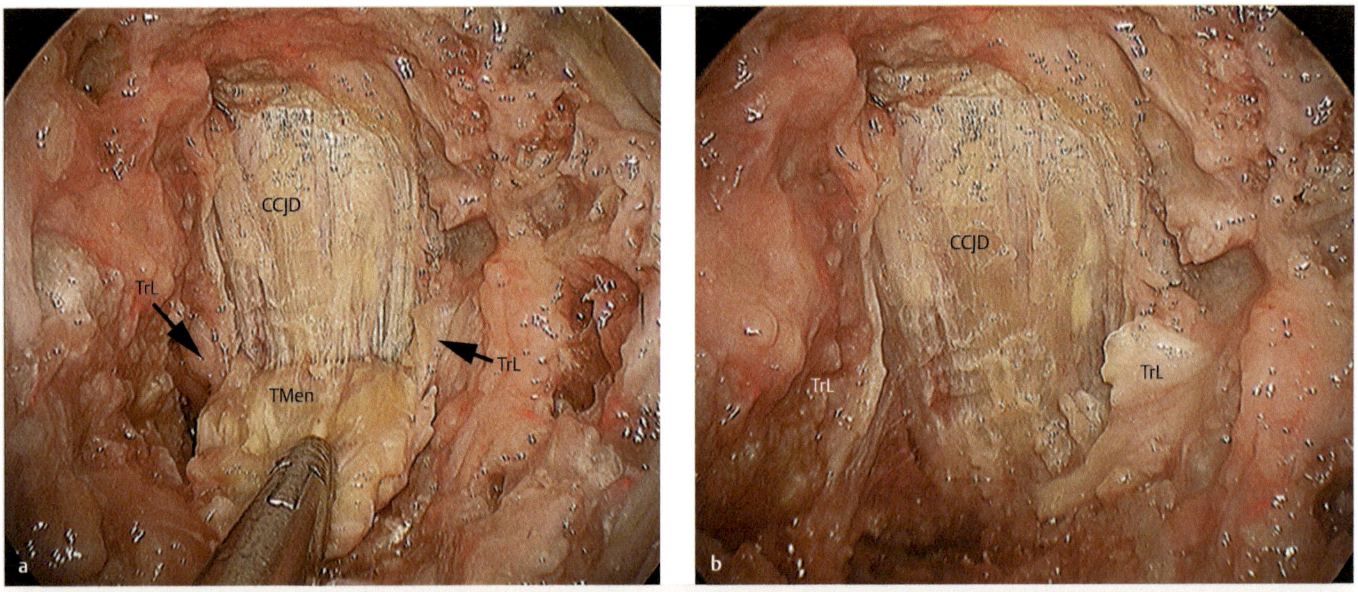

Fig. 13.30 (a, b) Step 13. The dura mater of the craniocervical junction (CCJD) is visible after removing the central part of the transverse ligament (TrL) and reflecting anteriorly the tectorial membrane (TMen).

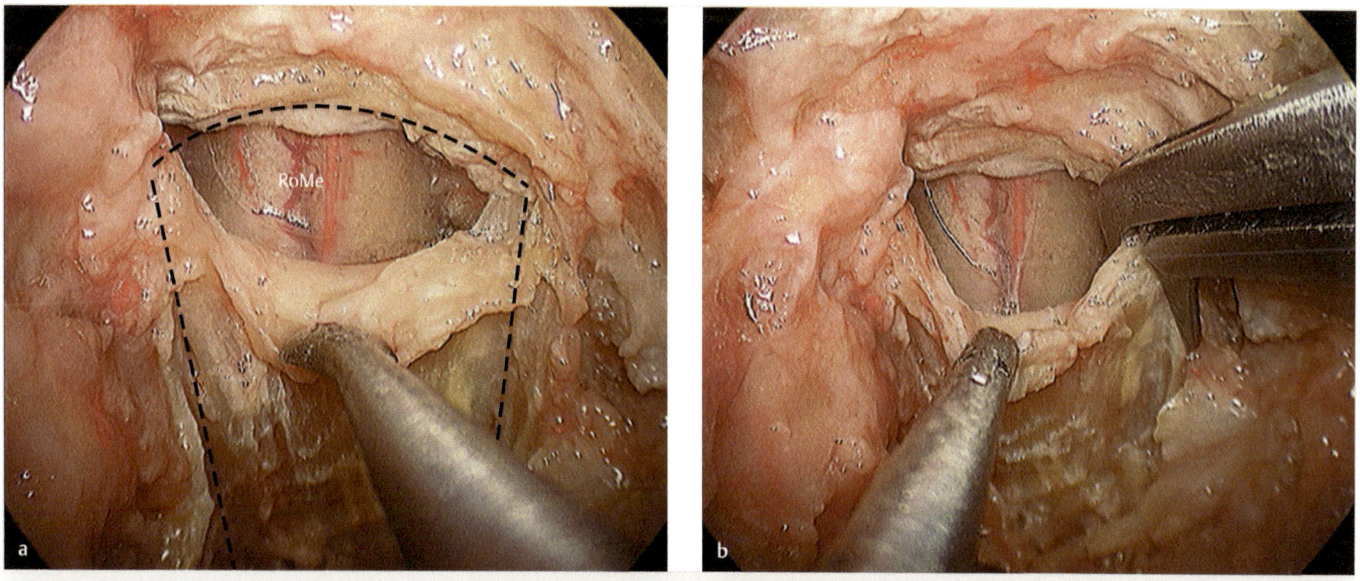

Fig. 13.31 (a, b) Step 14. A squared transdural window (*black dashed line*) is obtained by removing the dura of the craniocervical junction. RoMe, rhomboid membrane.

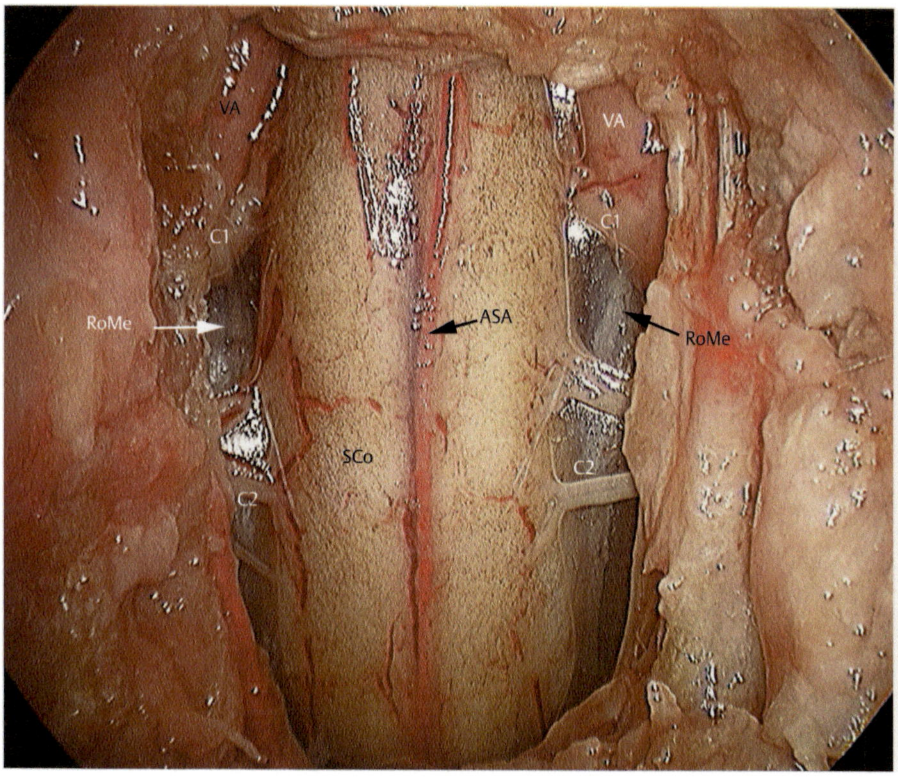

Fig. 13.32 The rhomboid membrane. After performing a wide opening of the dura mater, the premedullary cistern, where the rhomboid membrane (RoMe) is still visible, is accessed. The anatomical relationship between the vertebral arteries (VA) and the roots of the first cervical nerves (C1) are visible in the upper portion of the field of view. The roots of the second cervical nerves (C2) are also exposed. ASA, anterior spinal artery; SCo, spinal cord.

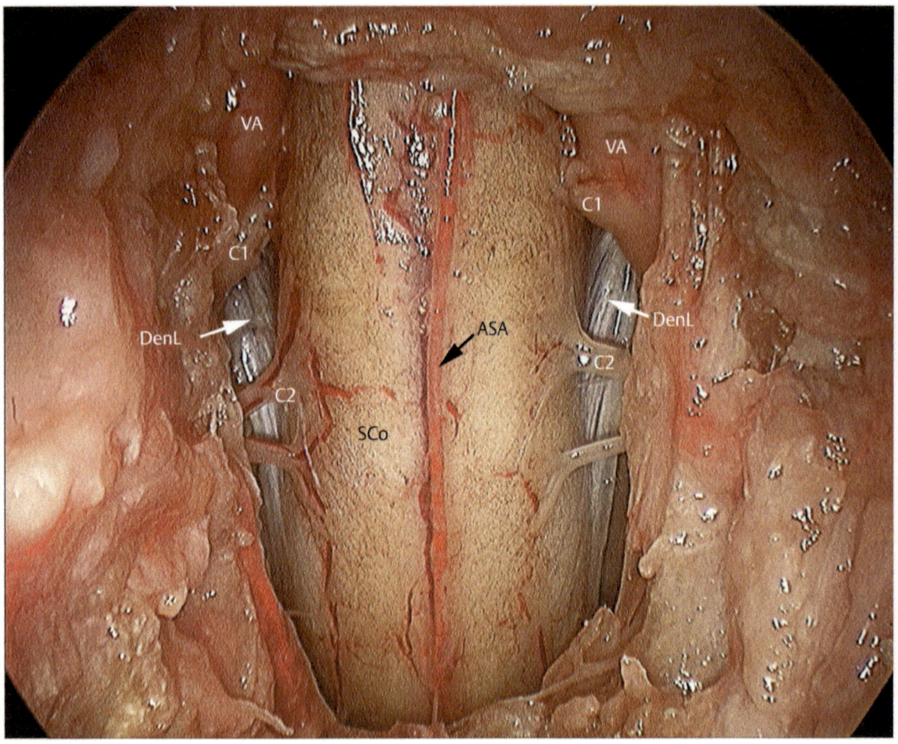

Fig. 13.33 Step 15. After removing the rhomboid membrane, the denticulate ligaments (DenL) are visible on both sides of the spinal cord (SCo). The roots of the second cervical nerves (C2) can be reached with a 0-degree scope and straight instruments only after performing a total odontoidectomy. ASA, anterior spinal artery; C1, first cervical nerve; VA, vertebral artery.

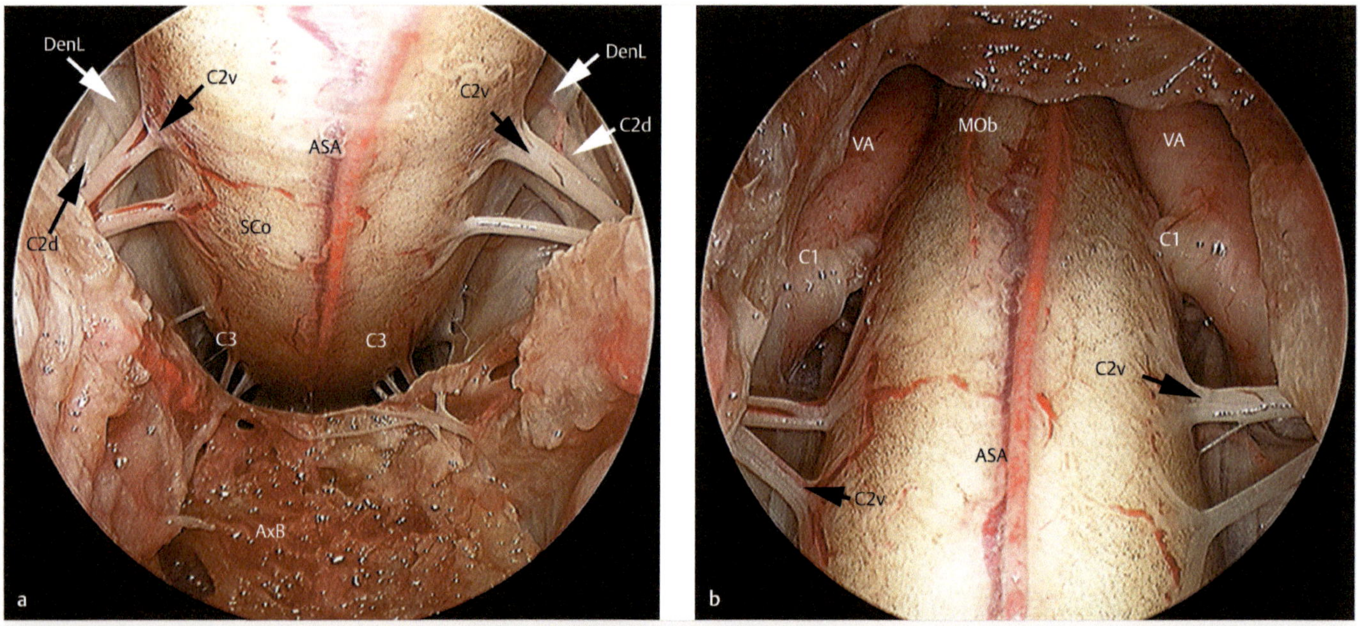

Fig. 13.34 (a, b) The spinal canal. A 70-degree endoscope is employed to watch below and above the level of the transodontoid window. Overcoming the body of the axis (AxB) with the scope turned inferiorly, the roots of the third cervical nerves (C3) are identified. By rotating the scope upward, the medulla oblongata (MOb) becomes visible between the vertebral arteries (VA). The angled view enables a better perspective of the ventral (C2v) and dorsal (C2d) roots of the second cervical nerves. ASA, anterior spinal artery; C1, first cervical nerve; DenL, denticulate ligament; SCo, spinal cord.

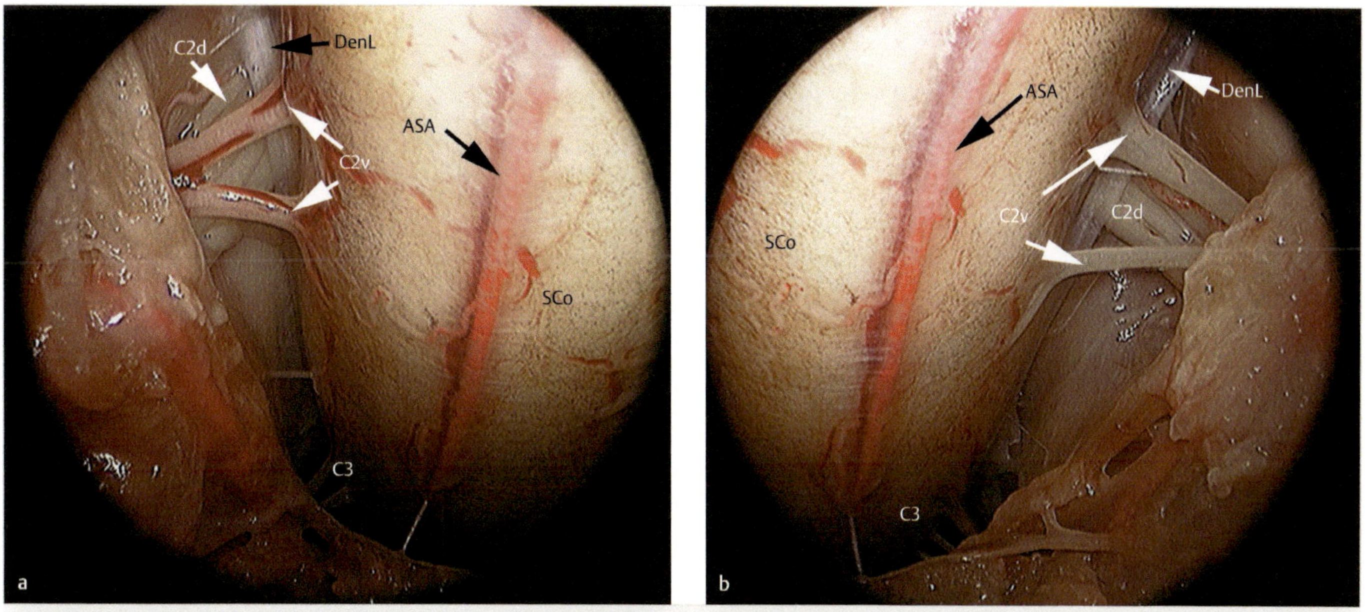

Fig. 13.35 (a, b) Roots of the cervical nerves. View with a 70-degree scope turned inferolaterally, and placed in front of the anterior spinal artery (ASA). The ventral (C2v) and dorsal roots of the second cervical nerve (C2d) can be seen while running anterior and posterior to the denticulate ligament (DenL), respectively. C3, third cervical nerve; SCo, spinal cord.

References

[1] de Almeida JR, Zanation AM, Snyderman CH, et al. Defining the nasopalatine line: the limit for endonasal surgery of the spine. Laryngoscope 2009;119(2):239–244

[2] Alfieri A, Jho HD, Tschabitscher M. Endoscopic endonasal approach to the ventral cranio-cervical junction: anatomical study. Acta Neurochir (Wien) 2002;144(3):219–225, discussion 225

[3] Lee A, Sommer D, Reddy K, Murty N, Gunnarsson T. Endoscopic transnasal approach to the craniocervical junction. Skull Base 2010;20(3):199–205

[4] Shkarubo AN, Andreev DN, Konovalov NA, et al. Surgical treatment of skull base tumors, extending to craniovertebral junction. World Neurosurg 2017;99:47–58

[5] Chibbaro S, Cebula H, Aldea S, et al. Endonasal endoscopic odontoidectomy in ventral diseases of the craniocervical junction: results of a multicenter experience. World Neurosurg 2017;106:382–393

[6] Liu JK, Patel J, Goldstein IM, Eloy JA. Endoscopic endonasal transclival transodontoid approach for ventral decompression of the craniovertebral junction: operative technique and nuances. Neurosurg Focus 2015;38(4):E17

[7] Morales-Valero SF, Serchi E, Zoli M, Mazzatenta D, Van Gompel JJ. Endoscopic endonasal approach for craniovertebral junction pathology: a review of the literature. Neurosurg Focus 2015;38(4):E15

[8] Gladi M, Iacoangeli M, Specchia N, et al. Endoscopic transnasal odontoid resection to decompress the bulbo-medullary junction: a reliable anterior minimally invasive technique without posterior fusion. Eur Spine J 2012;21(Suppl 1):S55–S60

[9] Iacoangeli M, Gladi M, Alvaro L, Di Rienzo A, Specchia N, Scerrati M. Endoscopic endonasal odontoidectomy with anterior C1 arch preservation in elderly patients affected by rheumatoid arthritis. Spine J 2013;13(5):542–548

[10] Iacoangeli M, Nasi D, Colasanti R, et al. Endoscopic endonasal odontoidectomy with anterior C1 arch preservation in rheumatoid arthritis: long-term follow-up and further technical improvement by anterior endoscopic C1-C2 screw fixation and fusion. World Neurosurg 2017;107:820–829

[11] Kooshkabadi A, Choi PA, Koutourousiou M, et al. Atlanto-occipital instability following endoscopic endonasal approach for lower clival lesions: experience with 212 cases. Neurosurgery 2015;77(6):888–897, discussion 897

[12] Re M, Iacoangeli M, Di Somma L, et al. Endoscopic endonasal approach to the craniocervical junction: the importance of anterior C1 arch preservation or its reconstruction. Acta Otorhinolaryngol Ital 2016;36(2):107–118

14 Orbital Decompression, Optic Decompression, Supraorbital Approach, and Transorbital Approach

Davide Mattavelli, Marco Ravanelli, Andrea Luigi Camillo Carobbio, Davide Lombardi

The sinonasal cavity can be used as a corridor toward the orbital cavity and the optic canal. In particular, the ethmoid complex and the maxillary sinus are adjacent to the medial and inferior orbital walls, respectively, while the optic canal can be reached at the junction between the lateral and superior walls of the sphenoid sinus. Consequently, transnasal endoscopic surgery is currently employed for performing orbital and optic decompression (mainly for Graves' disease and posttraumatic optic neuropathy),[1,2] repair of some fractures of the orbital walls,[3,4] and resecting selected orbital tumors and skull base lesions that compress the optic nerve.[5–8] Additionally, transnasal endoscopic surgery is an excellent approach to drain subperiosteal and orbital abscesses resulting from complicated acute rhinosinusitis.[9,10]

This chapter includes the description of four procedures: orbital decompression, optic decompression, supraorbital approach, and transorbital approach.

Orbital decompression is indicated when intraorbital pressure increases (causing exophthalmos, strabismus, and/or diplopia) as a result of dysthyroidism (especially Graves' disease) or infection (i.e., abscesses requiring surgical drainage), leading to impairment of the optic nerve function. The medial wall and the portion of the inferior one medial to the infraorbital nerve can be removed through a transnasal approach. Furthermore, periorbital incision and lysis of the intraorbital connective septa further decrease intraorbital pressure in cases of severe orbital hypertension.

Optic decompression is indicated when retrobulbar compressive optic neuropathy occurs as a consequence of trauma, dysthyroidism, or skull base tumors or tumor-like lesions (e.g., fibrous dysplasia). The main clinical manifestations leading to indicate an optic decompression are visual field/acuity impairment, dyschromatopsia, and alteration in visual evoked potentials. Decompression can be obtained by removing the medial wall of the optic canal, incising the optic periosteum, and sectioning the annulus of Zinn. While performing these maneuvers, particular attention should be paid to not damage the ophthalmic artery, which commonly runs in the inferomedial quadrant of the optic canal.

The transnasal supraorbital approach consists of a subperiosteal dissection along the inferior face of the orbital roof. This route can be adopted to address lesions or fluid collections (i.e., subperiosteal abscesses) located below the orbital roof or to expand the transcribriform or transplanum–transtuberculum approach in lesions with lateral extension. To reach the orbital roof via a subperiosteal plane, the ethmoidal arteries must be sectioned to have a full view of the dihedral corner between the lamina papyracea and the fovea ethmoidalis. Craniectomy of the lesser sphenoidal wing and removal of the optic strut are also possible through this approach, providing subtotal exposure of the paraclinoid tract of the internal carotid artery.

The transnasal transorbital approach allows access to the extraconal and intraconal compartments of the orbit passing through the periorbit. Removal of orbital tumors is usually performed by blunt dissection with the help of cottonoids gently pushed along the surface of the lesion; this minimizes the chance of injury to neurovascular structures. However, from cadaveric dissection aiming to acquire sound anatomical knowledge of the position and relationship of the most important orbital structures, it is suggested to meticulously remove the orbital fat and identify the nerves and vessels running within the orbit. The main landmarks guiding orbital dissection are the extrinsic orbital muscles, which can be adequately exposed by removing the extraconal fat. Schematically, three triangles between the skull

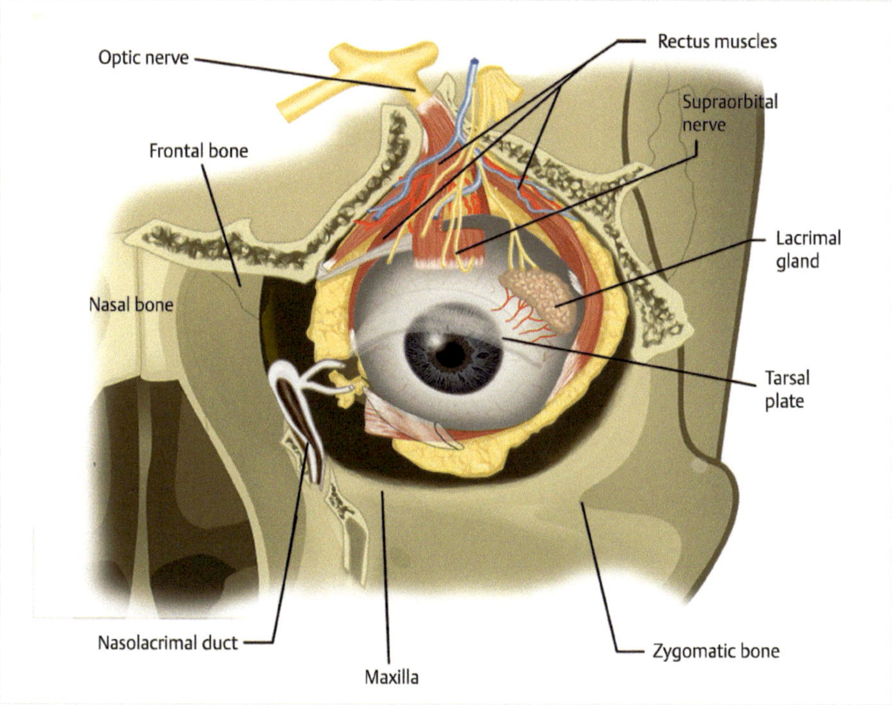

Fig. 14.1 Anterior view of the orbital cavity. This illustration shows the architecture of the left orbital cavity as seen from an anterior-to-posterior perspective.

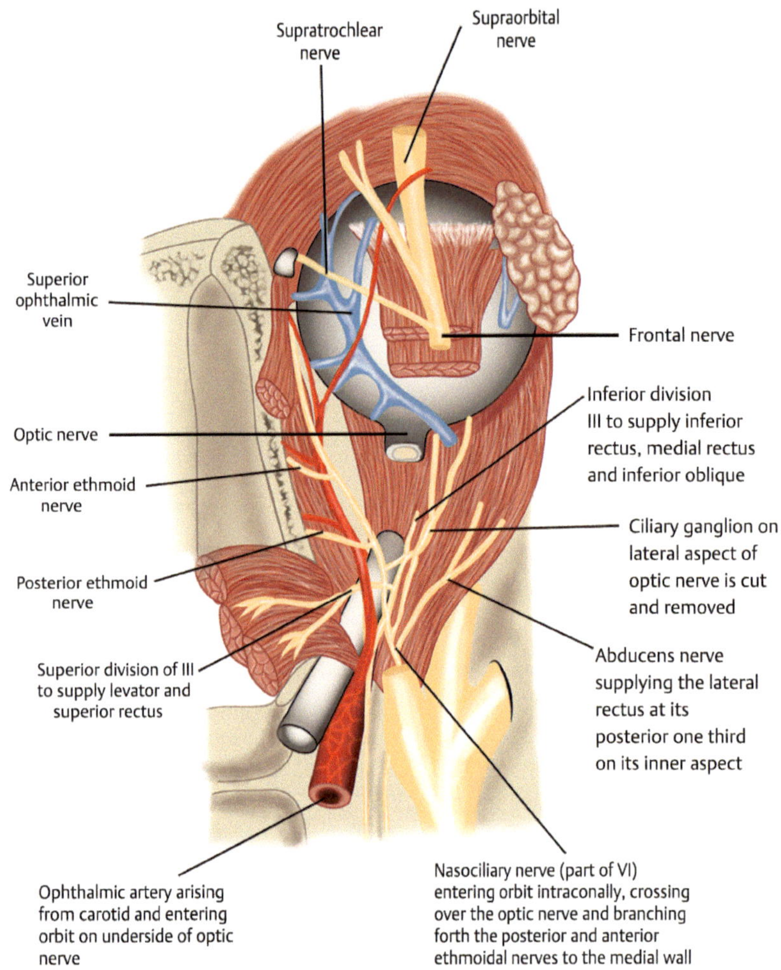

Fig. 14.2 Superior view of the orbital cavity. This illustration shows the architecture of the right orbital cavity as seen from a cranial-to-caudal perspective.

base, the medial rectus muscle, the inferior rectus muscle, and the orbital floor can be identified to access the intraconal orbital content.

In recent years, transorbital endoscopic approaches through eyelid skin and/or conjunctiva are gaining increasing popularity.[11–15] Although the step-by-step description of these techniques (i.e., superior eyelid crease approach, precaruncular approach, preseptal lower eyelid approach, and lateral retrocanthal approach) is beyond the purposes of the present atlas, it is of note that transorbital endoscopic approaches are progressively included in the toolkit of skull base surgeons, thus warranting dedicated study and training. Therefore, the reader is strongly recommended to acquire familiarity with these approaches and use a cadaver dissection setting to compare the different degrees of maneuverability and exposure provided by endoscopic transnasal and transconjunctival/transcutaneous transorbital approaches when targeting orbital compartments and related skull base areas.

252

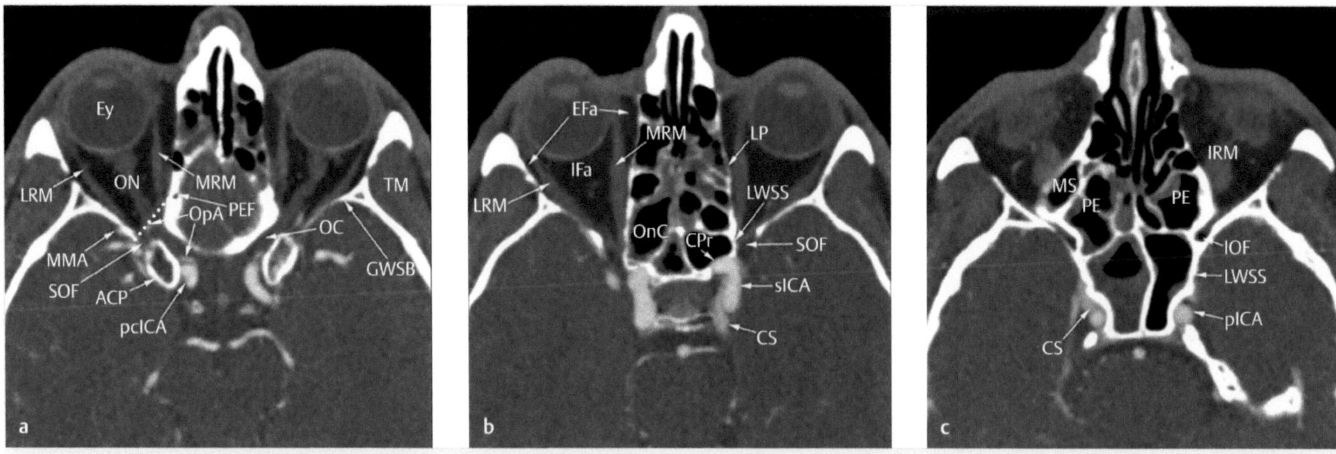

Fig. 14.3 Contrast-enhanced CT axial anatomy of the orbit and orbital apex. The panel shows three axial contrast-enhanced CT scans passing through the orbital cavity (**a** is the most cranial and **c** is the most caudal). The orbital cavity is separated from the ethmoidal compartments by the lamina papyracea (LP). The posterolateral orbital wall separates the orbital content from the temporal fossa anteriorly and middle cranial fossa posteriorly and is formed by the zygomatic bone anteriorly and the greater wing of the sphenoid bone (GWSB) posteriorly. The orbital apex can be defined as the portion of the orbital cavity and related canals/fissures that lies posterior to a plane (*white dotted line*) passing through the lateral border of the superior orbital fissure (SOF) and the posterior ethmoidal foramen (PEF). It includes the optic canal (OC) and the superior orbital fissure and is adjacent to the cranial portion of the lateral wall of the sphenoid sinus (LWSS). ACP, anterior clinoid process; CPr, carotid prominence; CS, cavernous sinus; EFA, extraconal fat; Ey, eyeball; LRM, lateral rectus muscle; IFa, intraconal fat; IOF, inferior orbital fissure; IRM, inferior rectus muscle; MMA, middle meningeal artery; MRM, medial rectus muscle; MS, maxillary sinus; ON, optic nerve; OnC, Onodi's cell; OpA, ophthalmic artery; pcICA, paraclinoid tract of the internal carotid artery; PE, posterior ethmoid; pICA, paraclival tract of the internal carotid artery; sICA, parasellar tract of the internal carotid artery; TM, temporal muscle.

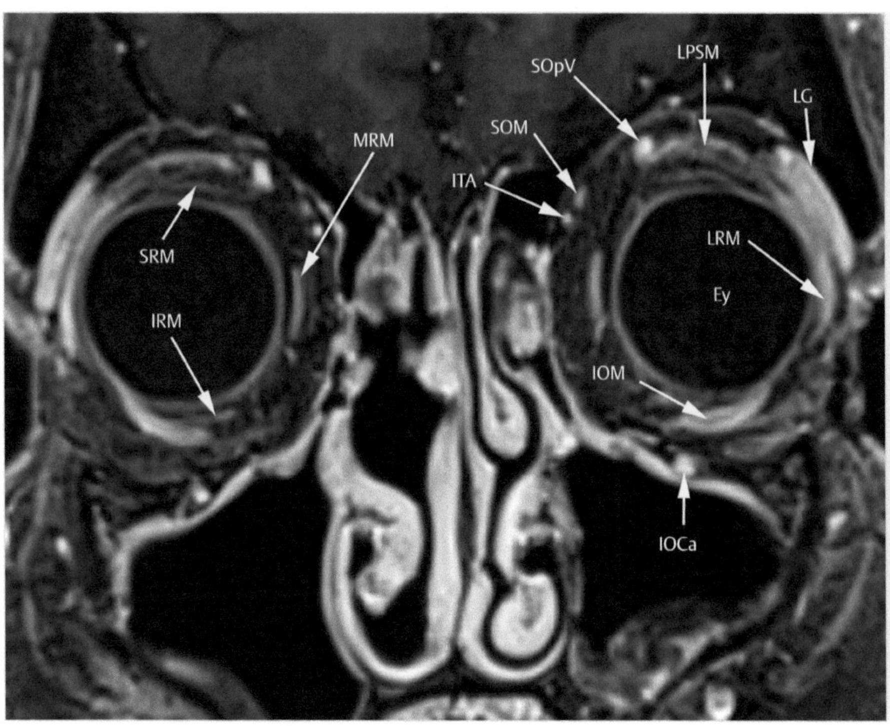

Fig. 14.4 Coronal MRI scan of the anterior orbital content. This contrast-enhanced T1-weighted MRI with fat saturation shows the anterior portion of the superior rectus muscle (SRM), medial rectus muscle (MRM), inferior rectus muscle (IRM), and lateral rectus muscle (LRM) few millimeters posterior to their insertion on the eyeball (Ey). The inferior oblique muscle (IOM) can be identified in the inferior portion of the orbital cavity. The superior oblique muscle (SOM) runs in a cranial position with respect to the infratrochlear artery (ITA), which is one of the terminal branches of the ophthalmic artery, and becomes thinner while getting close to the trochlea. The superior ophthalmic vein (SOpV) usually runs close to the medial border of the levator palpebrae superioris muscle (LPSM), anteriorly, and adjacent to the inferior surface of the muscle, posteriorly. IOCa, infraorbital canal; LG, lacrimal gland.

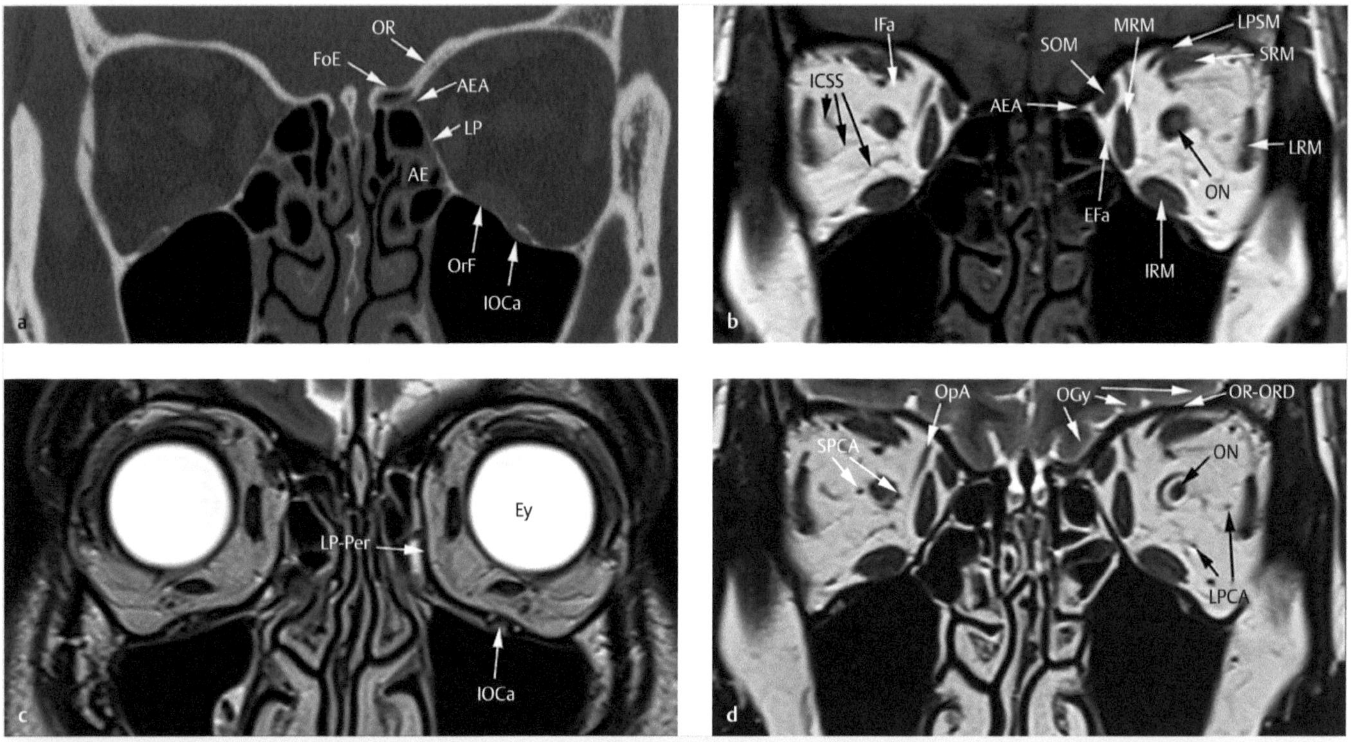

Fig. 14.5 CT and MRI coronal anatomy of the orbit. The coronal CT scan **(a)** shows the bony structures surrounding the orbital cavity. The lamina papyracea (LP) and the orbital floor (OrF) separate the orbital content from the anterior (AE) and posterior ethmoid compartments and from the maxillary sinus, respectively. The infraorbital canal (IOCa) runs within the orbital floor in a posterior-to-anterior direction. The ethmoidal canals run from the orbital cavity to the olfactory groove, housing the anterior, middle (when present), and posterior ethmoidal arteries. The orbital roof (OR) is a thick bony lamina, formed by the frontal bone anteriorly and the sphenoid bone posteriorly. This lamina tilts superiorly from the level of the fovea ethmoidalis (FoE), following the superior convexity of the orbital content. One T1-weighted **(b)** and two T2-weighted **(c, d)** MRI scans show the orbital content and adjacent structures. The orbital fat can be divided into extraconal orbital fat (EFa) and intraconal orbital fat (IFa) with respect to the cone formed by the medial (MRM), inferior (IRM), lateral (LRM), and superior (SRM) rectus muscles. The levator palpebrae superioris oblique muscle (LPSM), superior oblique muscle (SOM), and inferior oblique muscle lie within the extraconal compartment (i.e., between the muscular cone and the orbital walls) together with some neurovascular structures (e.g., supratrochlear, supraorbital, and lacrimal bundles). The optic nerve (ON), short posterior ciliary artery (SPCA), and long posterior ciliary artery (LPCA) run within the intraconal compartment. The ophthalmic artery (OpA) has a tortuous course within the orbital cavity: after exiting from the optic canal, it first turns laterally and superiorly around the optic nerve, then it runs in a borderline fashion between the intraconal and extraconal compartments, in the space between the superior rectus, the medial rectus, and the superior oblique muscle, and finally it moves close to the inferior border of the superior oblique muscle. The fat tissues of the intraconal and extraconal compartments are only partially separated from each other by the muscular cone. An intricate system of connective fibers, called intraorbital connective septal system (ICSS), connects the orbital compartments and their contents with the extrinsic muscles and the periorbit. As seen in the MRI scans, the planes formed by the periorbit and the lamina papyracea (LP-Per) medially and by the periorbit, orbital roof and related dura (OR-ORD) superiorly appear as hypointense lines between the hyperintense signals of orbital fat and ethmoidal mucosa/cerebrospinal fluid, respectively. Ey, eyeball; IOCa, infraorbital canal; OGy, orbital gyri.

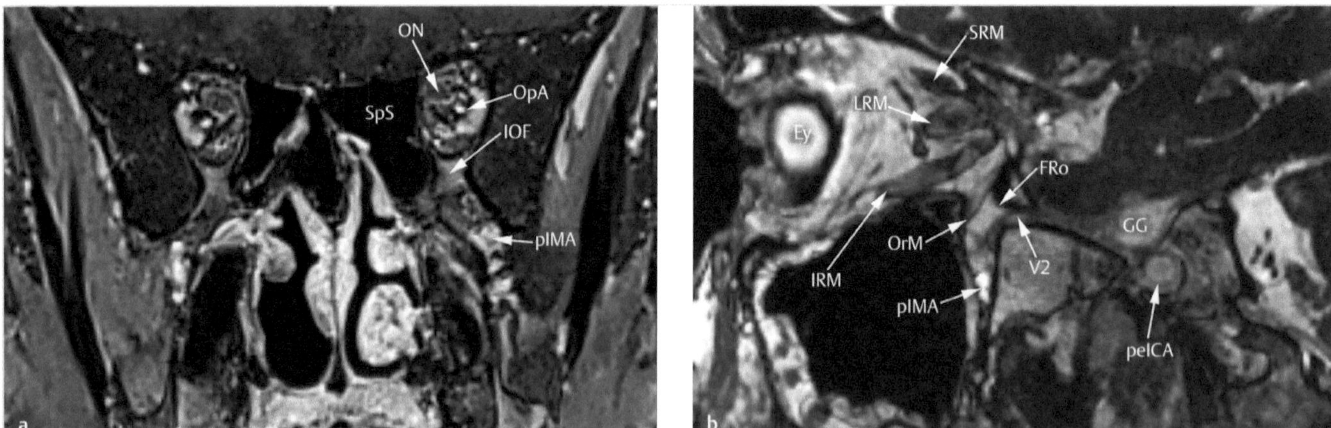

Fig. 14.6 Coronal and sagittal MRI anatomy of the orbital apex (anterior portion). The T1-weighted contrast-enhanced coronal MRI scan with fat saturation **(a)** shows the optic nerve (ON) and ophthalmic artery (OpA) few millimeters after the entrance within the orbital cavity. The inferior quadrant of the orbital apex is opened toward the pterygopalatine fossa via the inferior orbital fissure inferior orbital fissure. As shown in the sagittal contrast-enhanced CISS (constructive interference in steady state) MRI **(b)**, the inferior orbital fissure is interrupted by the orbitalis muscle (OrM; also called Müller's muscle), which appears as a thin hypointense structure located anterosuperiorly with respect to the foramen rotundum (FRo). V2, maxillary nerve; Ey, eyeball; GG, gasserian ganglion; IRM, inferior rectus muscle; LRM, lateral rectus muscle; peICA, petrous tract of the internal carotid artery; pIMA, pterygopalatine tract of the internal maxillary artery; SpS, sphenoid sinus; SRM, superior rectus muscle.

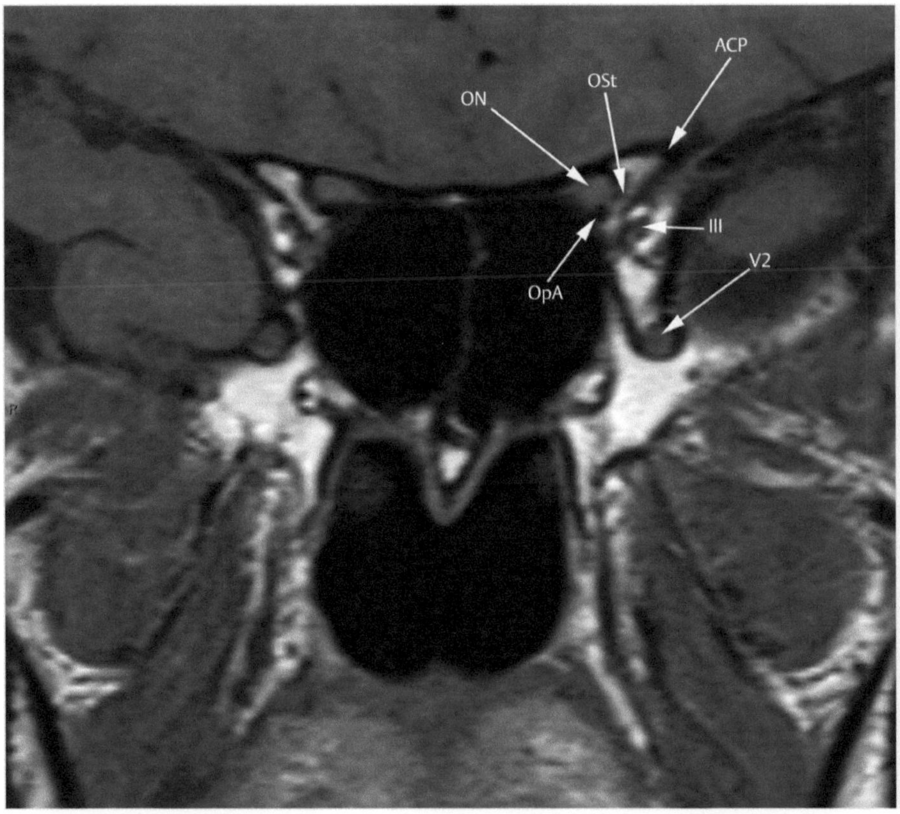

Fig. 14.7 Coronal MRI anatomy of the orbital apex (middle portion). This T1-weighted coronal MRI scan shows the optic nerve (ON) and the ophthalmic artery (OpA) within the optic canal, being separated from the superior orbital fissure by the optic strut (OSt). The oculomotor nerve (III) can be identified within the superior orbital fissure, surrounded by hyperintense fat tissue. V2, maxillary nerve; ACP, anterior clinoid process.

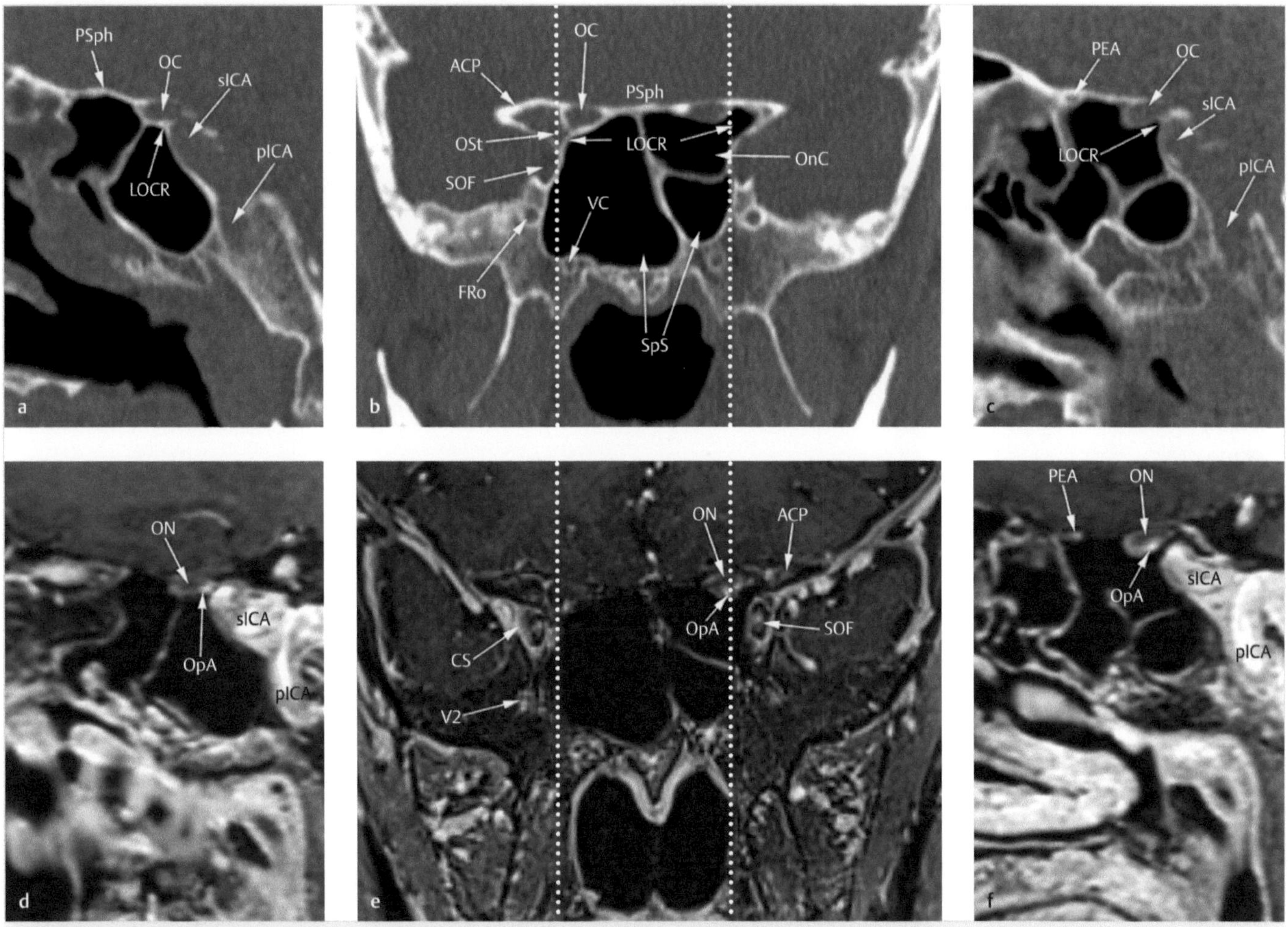

Fig. 14.8 (a–f) Coronal and sagittal CT and MRI anatomy of the orbital apex (posterior portion). The panel shows two coronal scans (CT, upper images; contrast-enhanced T1-weighted MRI with fat saturation, lower images) in the middle and four sagittal scans corresponding to *white dotted lines* The optic strut (OSt) serves as root for the anterior clinoid process (ACP) and separates the optic canal (OC) from the superior orbital fissure and cavernous sinus (CS). This bony structure can be variably pneumatized by the lateral optic–carotid recess (LOCR) of the sphenoid sinus (SpS) or Onodi's cell (OC). V2, maxillary nerve; FRo, foramen rotundum; OpA, ophthalmic artery; pICA, paraclival tract of the internal carotid artery; PEA, posterior ethmoidal artery; PSph, planum sphenoidale; sICA, parasellar tract of the internal carotid artery; SOF, superior orbital fissure; VC, vidian canal.

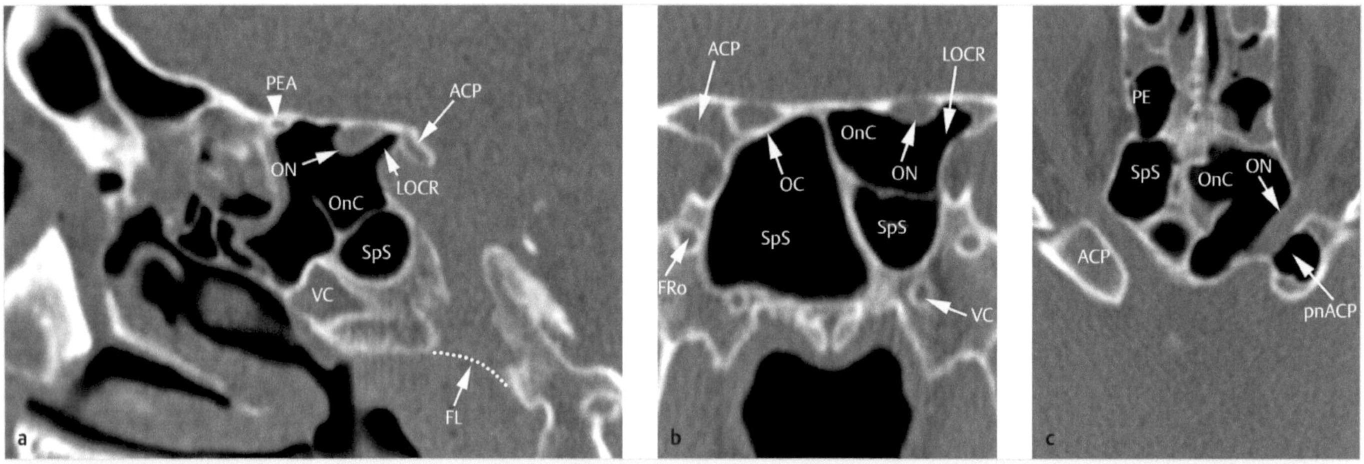

Fig. 14.9 (a–c) Multiplanar CT anatomy of the orbital apex (posterior portion). The posterior ethmoidal artery (PEA) runs approximately 7 mm anterior to the optic canal (OC). Pneumatization of the optic strut through the lateral optic–carotid recess (LOCR) can reach the anterior clinoid process (ACP) following the inferolateral surface of the optic nerve (ON). (*White dotted line*: foramen lacerum.) FL, foramen lacerum; FRo, foramen rotundum; OnC, Onodi's cell; PE, posterior ethmoid compartment; pnACP, pneumatized anterior clinoid process; SpS, sphenoid sinus; VC, vidian canal.

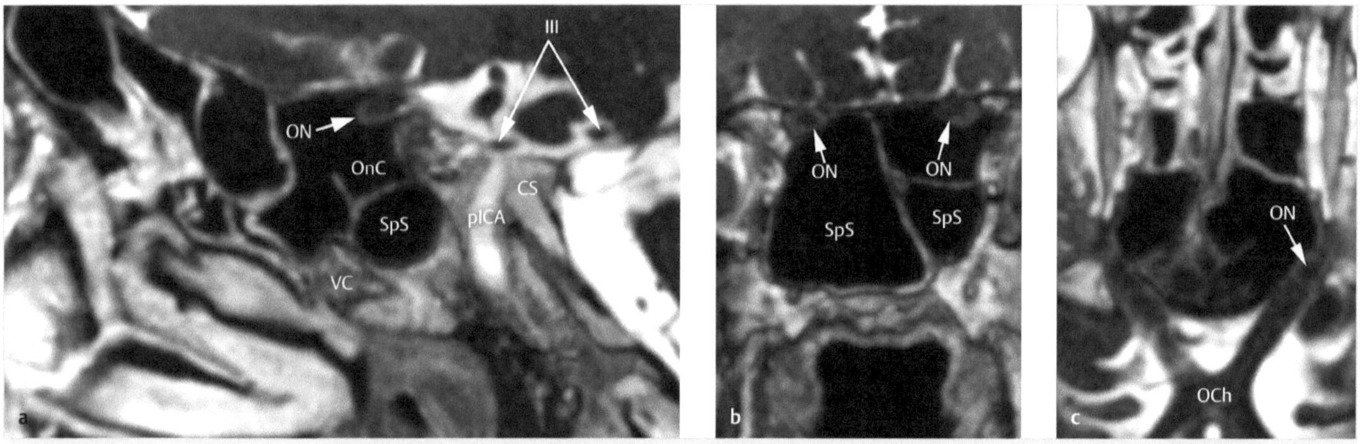

Fig. 14.10 (a–c) Multiplanar constructive interference in steady state (CISS) MRI anatomy of the orbital apex (posterior portion). Multiplanar CISS reconstruction provides the complete view of the optic apparatus, including optic tracts, optic chiasm (OCh), and optic nerve (ON). III, oculomotor nerve; CS, cavernous sinus; OnC, Onodi's cell; pICA, paraclival tract of the internal carotid artery; SpS, sphenoid sinus; VC, vidian canal.

Endoscopic Dissection

Nasal Phase

- Total uncinectomy.
- Anterior ethmoidectomy.
- Posterior ethmoidectomy.
- Type A endoscopic medial maxillectomy.
- Paraseptal sphenoidotomy.
- Transrostral sphenoidotomy.
- Expanded transrostral sphenoidotomy.
- Transethmoidal sphenoidotomy.
- Facultative: type B–D endoscopic medial maxillectomy.

Skull Base Phase

Two-Wall Orbital Decompression

- Step 1: Removal of the medial orbital wall.
- Step 2: Removal of the orbital floor medial to the infraorbital canal.

Optic Decompression

- Step 1: Removal of the inferomedial wall of the optic canal.
- Step 2: Incision of the periosteum of the optic canal.

Supraorbital Approach

- Step 1: Section of the ethmoidal arteries.
- Step 2: Subperiosteal dissection of the orbital roof.
- Step 3: Partial craniectomy of the orbital roof and exposure of the paraclinoid carotid artery.
- Step 4: Removal of the optic strut.
- Step 5: Incision of the superior carotid ring.

Transorbital Approach

- Step 1: Removal of the periorbit.
- Step 2: Lysis of the intraorbital connective septal system.
- Step 3: Removal of the extraconal fat.
- Step 4: Removal of the intraconal fat.

Two-Wall Orbital Decompression

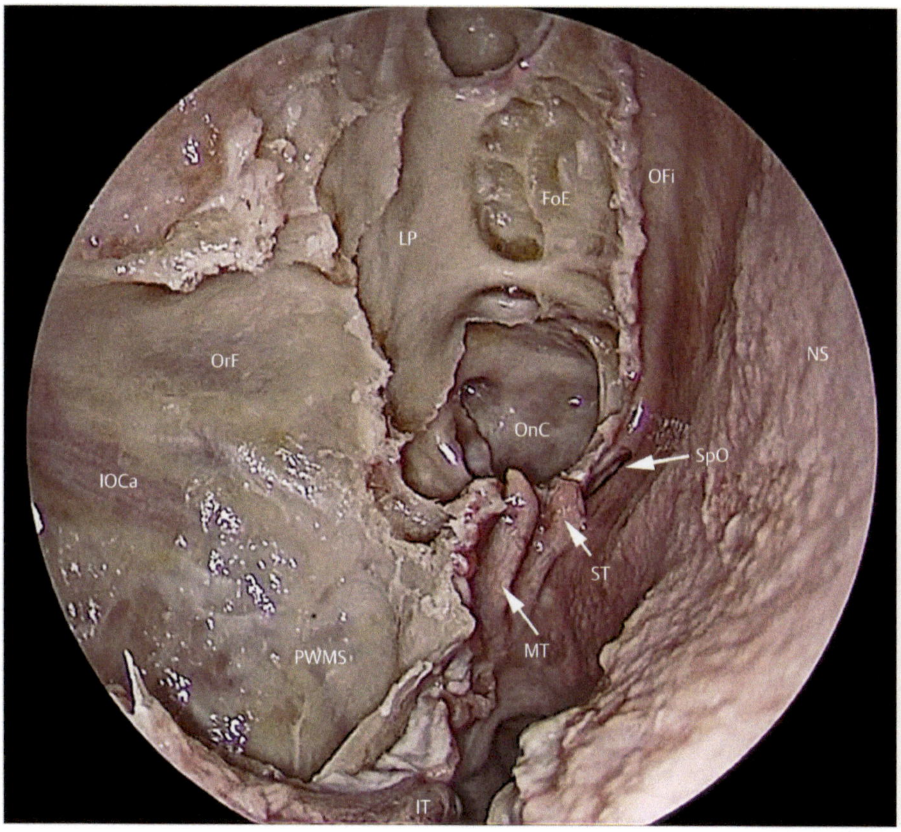

Fig. 14.11 Surgical field before orbital decompression. After performing a complete ethmoidectomy with the middle and superior turbinectomy and type A endoscopic medial maxillectomy, the dihedral angle between the lamina papyracea (LP) and the orbital floor (OrF) is exposed. The posterior wall of the maxillary sinus (PWMS) and the infraorbital canal (IOCa) can be identified through the endoscopic medial maxillectomy. The tails of the middle turbinate (MT) and the superior turbinate (ST) mark the position of the sphenopalatine foramen and the inferior orbital fissure. The dihedral angle between the lamina papyracea and the fovea ethmoidalis (FoE) is also identified by removing the most cranial ethmoid lamellae. A wide opening of the sphenoid sinus and Onodi's cell (OnC), when present, is also useful to expose further bony landmarks. IT, inferior turbinate; NS, nasal septum; OFi, olfactory fissure; SpO, sphenoidal ostium.

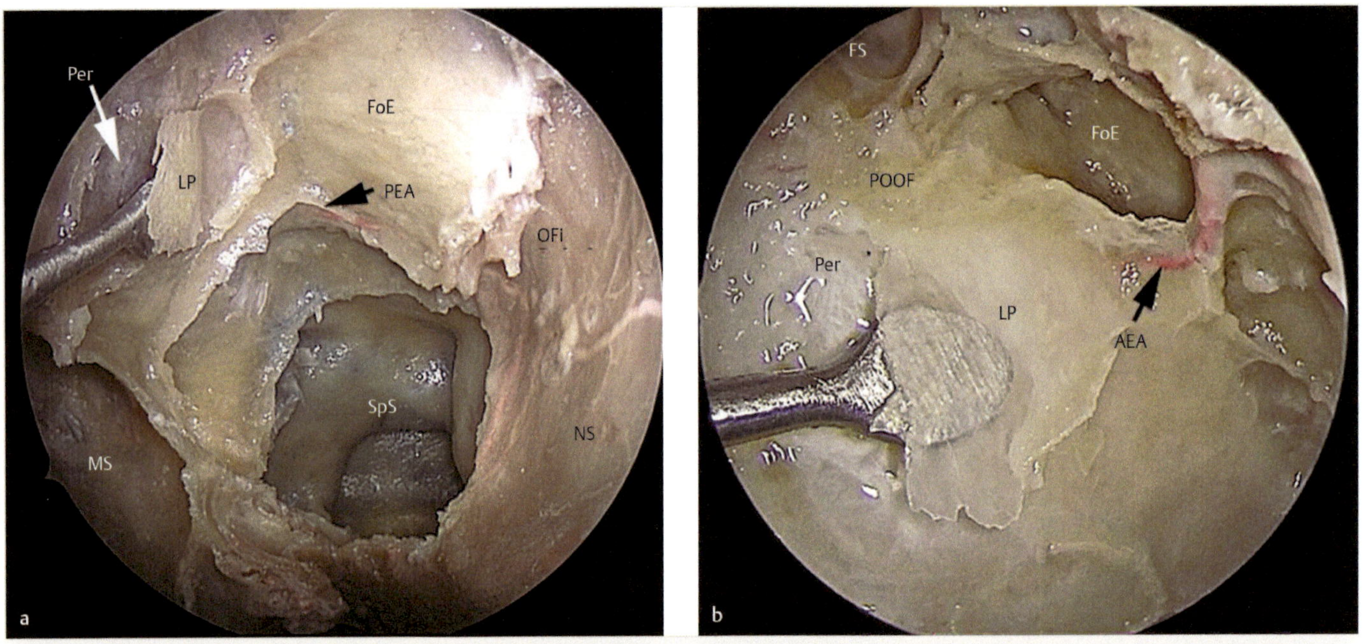

Fig. 14.12 (a, b) Step 1 (part 1). The lamina papyracea (LP) is gently entered and a dissector is placed in the plane between the bone and the periorbit (Per), which is laterally displaced before fracturing the bony lamina in a medial direction. This procedure must be carried out paying attention not to damage the anterior (AEA) or posterior ethmoidal arteries (PEA), which run from the lamina papyracea toward the olfactory fissure (OFi), parallel to the fovea ethmoidalis (FoE). During decompression, a 45-degree scope turned laterally can be used to better assess the variable thickness of the lamina papyracea, the pars orbitalis ossis frontalis (POOF), and the fovea ethmoidalis, which both belong to the frontal bone. FS, frontal sinus; MS, maxillary sinus; SpS, sphenoid sinus.

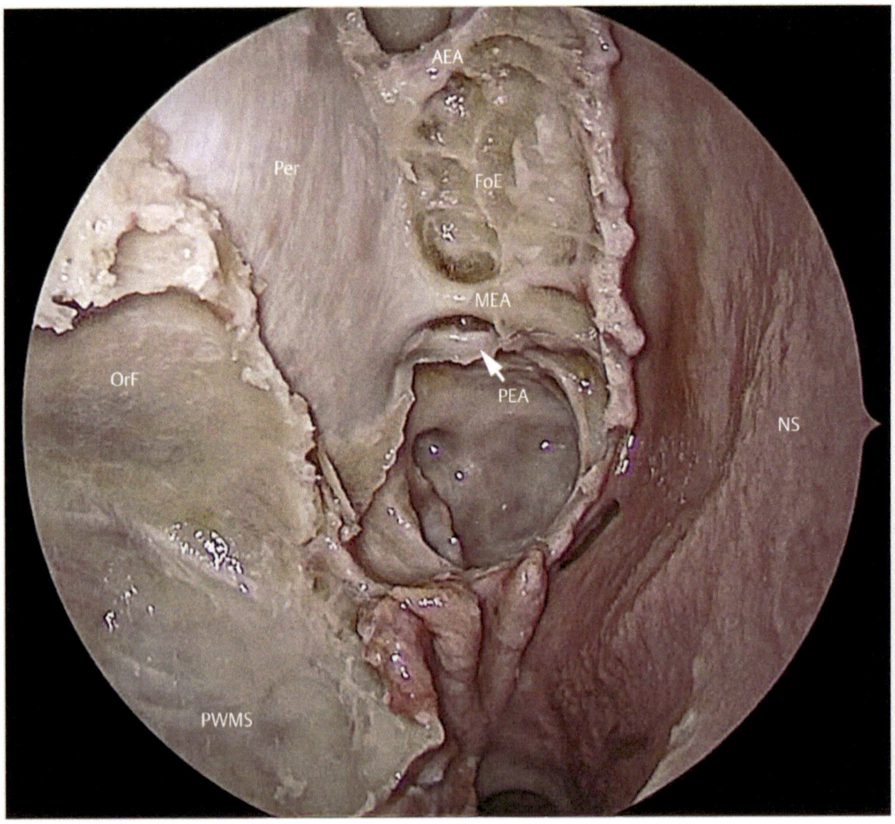

Fig. 14.13 Step 1 (part 2). The removal of the medial orbital wall is completed. Note that the periorbit (Per) continues into the periosteum that surrounds the anterior (AEA), middle (MEA), and posterior (PEA) ethmoidal arteries. The MEA can be found in 25 to 30% of subjects. FoE, fovea ethmoidalis; NS, nasal septum; OrF, orbital floor; PWMS, posterior wall of the maxillary sinus.

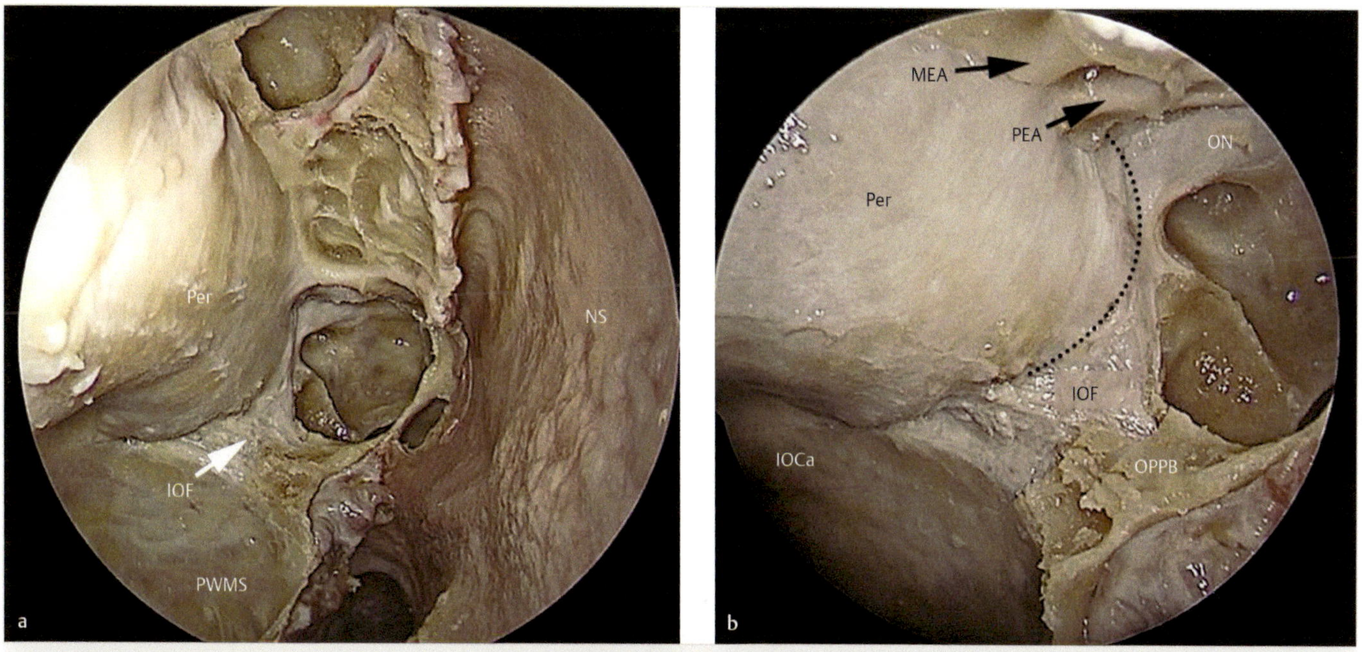

Fig. 14.14 (a, b) Step 2. The orbital floor up to the inferior orbital fissure (IOF) posteriorly and to the infraorbital canal (IOCa) medially has been removed. The inferior orbital fissure can be better exposed by removing the superomedial portion of the posterior wall of the maxillary sinus (PWMS) and the orbital process of the palatine bone (OPPB). The position of the annulus of Zinn (*black dotted line*) can be identified by a curved line in front of the optic nerve (ON) and cranial to the inferior orbital fissure. The periorbit (Per) can be incised to increase the effect of decompression (see Transorbital approach). MEA, middle ethmoidal artery; NS, nasal septum; PEA, posterior ethmoidal artery.

Optic Decompression

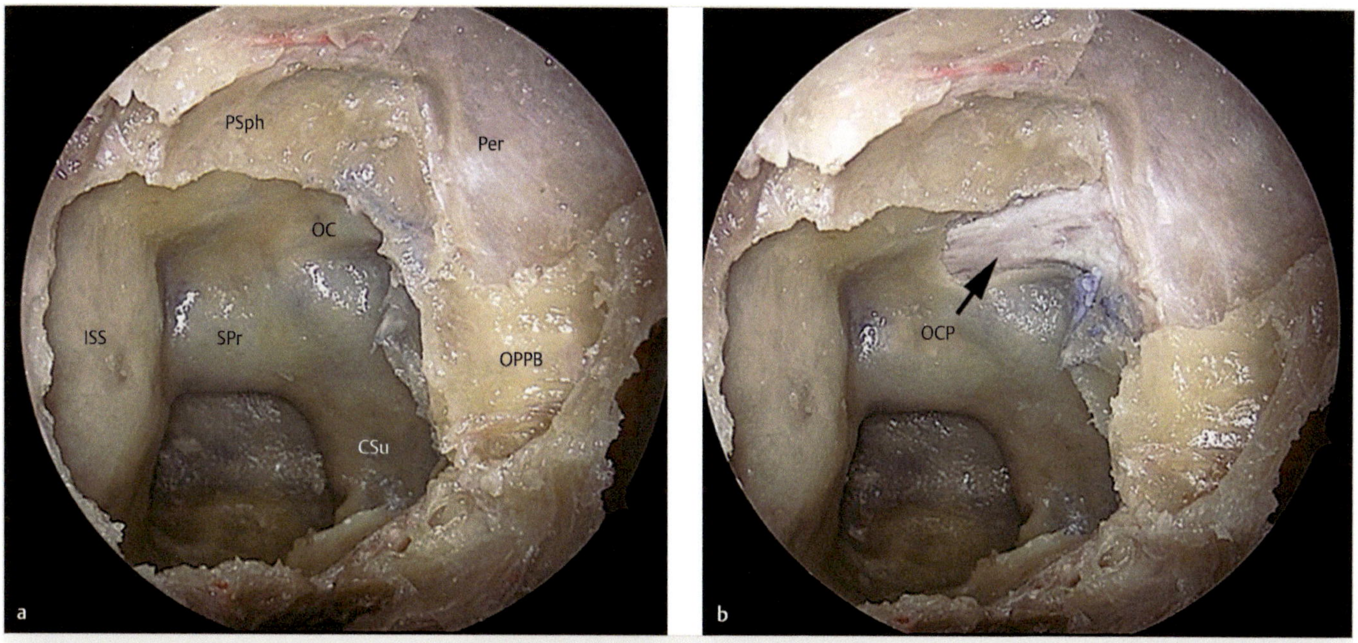

Fig. 14.15 (a, b) Step 1. Through transethmoidal sphenoidotomy, the principal bony landmarks surrounding the prominence of the optic canal (OC) can be identified: sellar prominence (SPr), planum sphenoidale (PSph), carotid sulcus (CSu), and carotid prominence. Removal from anterior to posterior of the medial-inferior wall of the optic canal leads to exposure of the corresponding periosteum (OCP), which anteriorly continues into the periorbit (Per). ISS, inter-sphenoid sinus septum; OPPB, orbital process of the palatine bone.

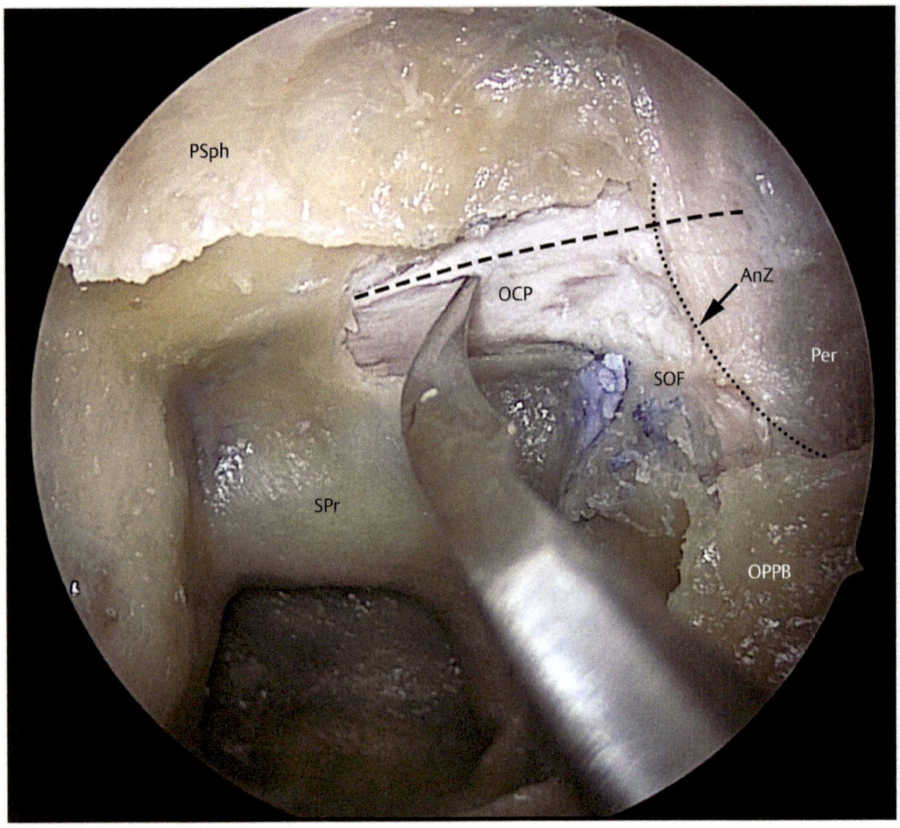

Fig. 14.16 Step 2 (part 1). A horizontal incision (*black dashed line*) along the upper border of optic canal periosteum (OCP) is performed with the intent to not injure the ophthalmic artery (OpA), the medial rectus muscle, and the structures running in the superior orbital fissure (SOF). The incision must include the annulus of Zinn (AnZ; *black dotted line*) and the posterior portion of the periorbit (Per) in order to optimize the decompression. As an alternative, incision of the periosteum of the optic canal can be performed in an anterior-to-posterior fashion, starting from the annulus of Zinn. OPPB, orbital process of the palatine bone; PSph, planum sphenoidale; SPr, sellar prominence.

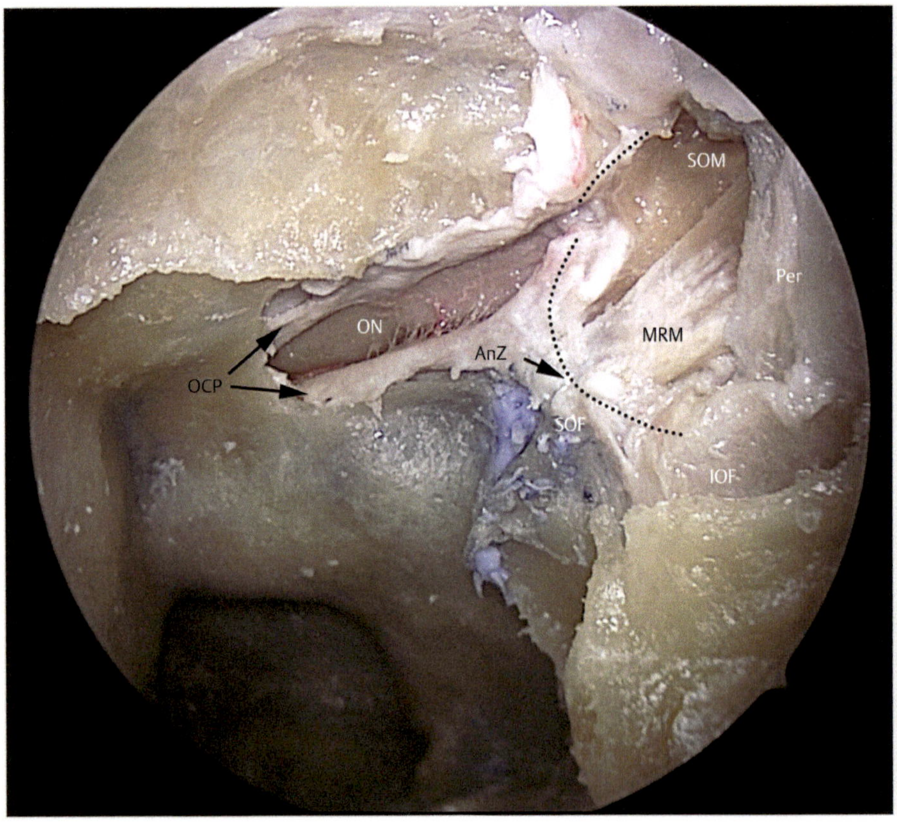

Fig. 14.17 Step 2 (part 2). After cutting the periosteum of the optic canal (OCP), the annulus of Zinn (AnZ; *black dotted line*), and the periorbit (Per), the periosteal flaps are displaced to identify the optic nerve (ON), the superior oblique muscle (SOM), and the medial rectus muscle (MRM). SOF, superior orbital fissure; IOF, inferior orbital fissure.

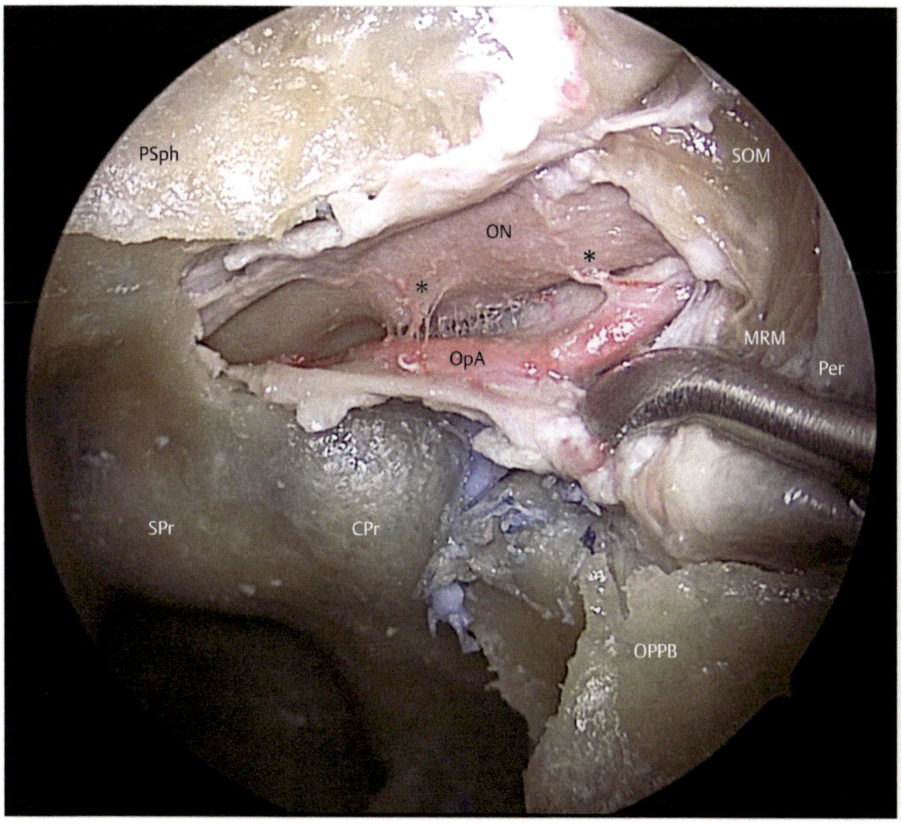

Fig. 14.18 The ophthalmic artery. With the help of a dissector, the inferior periosteal flap of the optic canal is displaced inferiorly to show the anatomical relationship between the optic nerve (ON) and the ophthalmic artery (OpA). The artery gives several branches toward the optic nerve (*black asterisks*), the largest being the central retinal artery. Both the optic nerve and the ophthalmic artery enter the annulus of Zinn, which can be recognized based on the posterior insertion of the superior oblique muscle (SOM) and the medial rectus muscle (MRM). CPr, carotid prominence; OPPB, orbital process of the palatine bone; PSph, planum sphenoidale; SPr, sellar prominence.

Supraorbital Approach

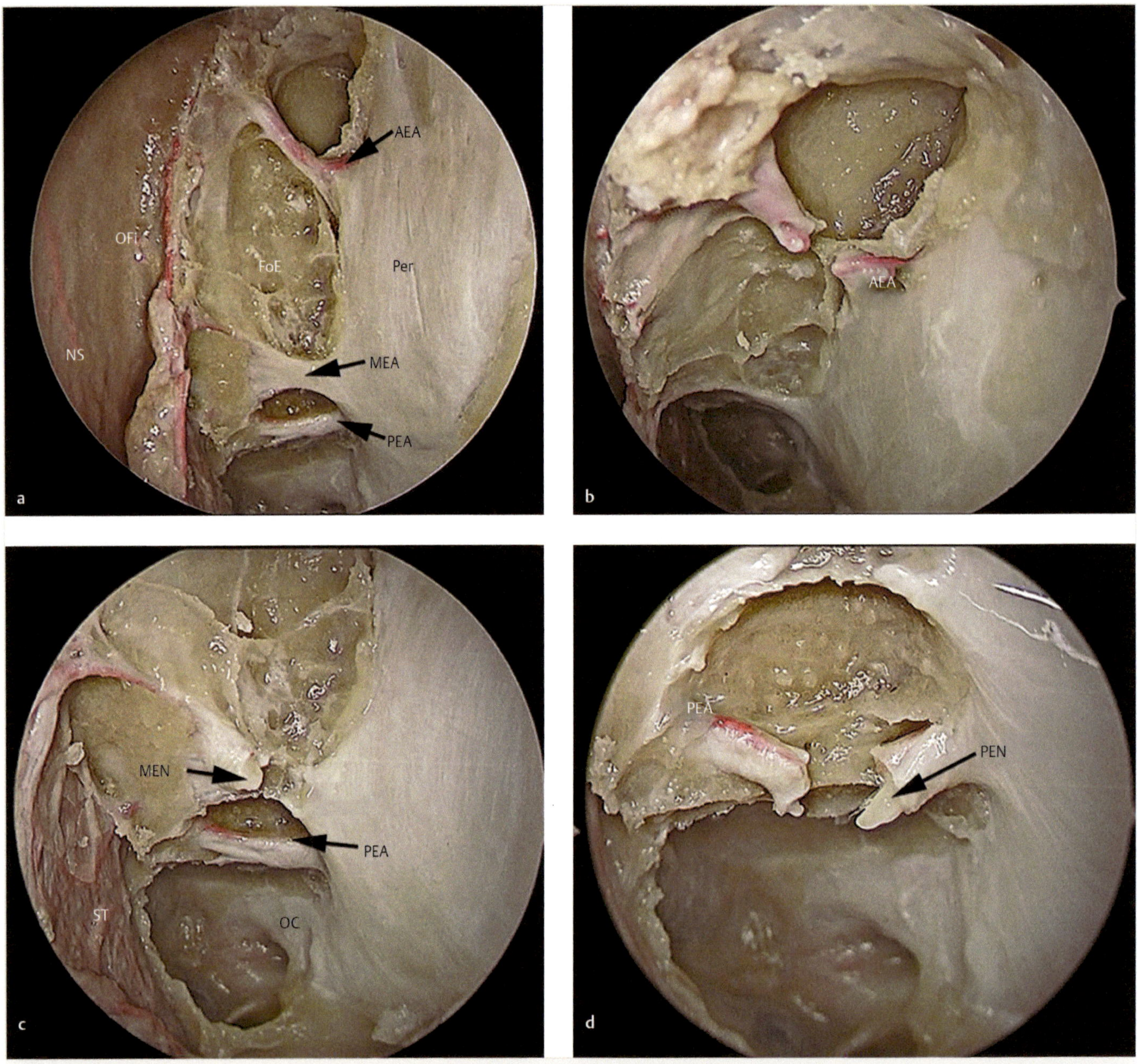

Fig. 14.19 (a–d) Step 1. After removing the inferior portion of the ethmoidal bony canals, an overview of the fovea ethmoidalis (FoE) and the anterior ethmoidal artery (AEA), the middle ethmoidal artery (MEA), and the posterior ethmoidal artery (PEA) is obtained with a 70-degree scope turned upward. The anterior ethmoidal nerve, the middle ethmoidal nerve (MEN), and the posterior ethmoidal nerve (PEN) can be identified parallel to the respective arteries. The ethmoidal bundles are commonly cut in the midpoint of the bony canal to avert their stumps to slip away into the orbit. OC, optic canal; NS, nasal septum; OFi, olfactory fissure; ST, superior turbinate.

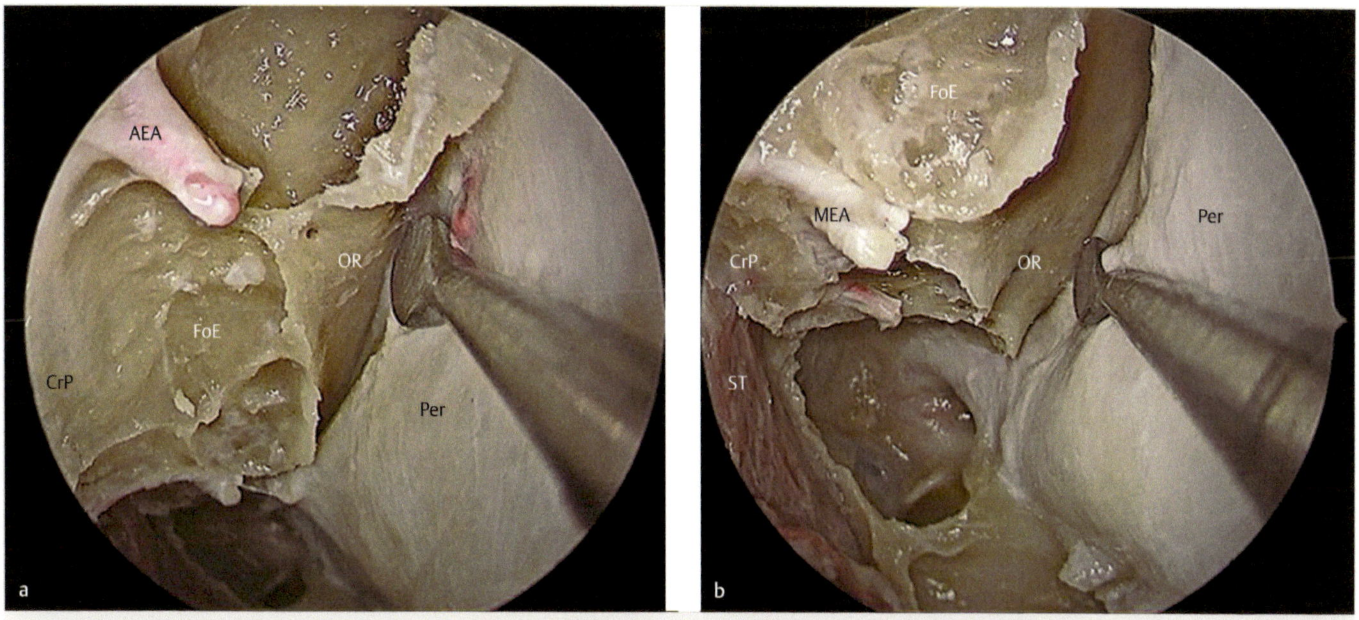

Fig. 14.20 (a, b) Step 2 (part 1). With a dissector, the periorbit (Per) is gently separated from the bony orbital roof (OR) starting from the point where the ethmoidal arteries have been sectioned and proceeding laterally. AEA, anterior ethmoidal artery; CrP, cribriform plate; FoE, fovea ethmoidalis; MEA, medial ethmoidal artery; ST, superior turbinate.

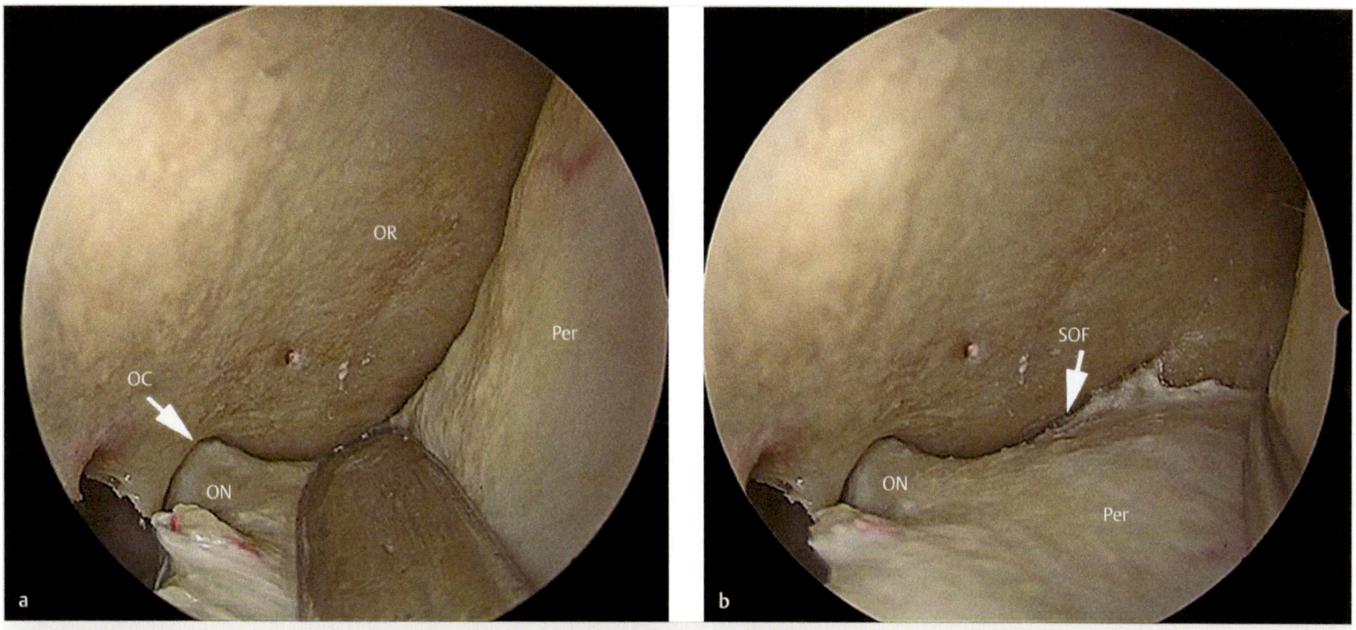

Fig. 14.21 (a, b) Step 2 (part 2). The subperiosteal dissection is performed following a medial-to-lateral and anterior-to-posterior trajectory: the orbital roof (OR) up to the optic canal (OC) and the superior orbital fissure (SOF) posteromedially and posterolaterally, respectively, are exposed. Note that a remarkable displacement of the periorbit (Per) is required to expose the superior orbital fissure (SOF). ON, optic nerve.

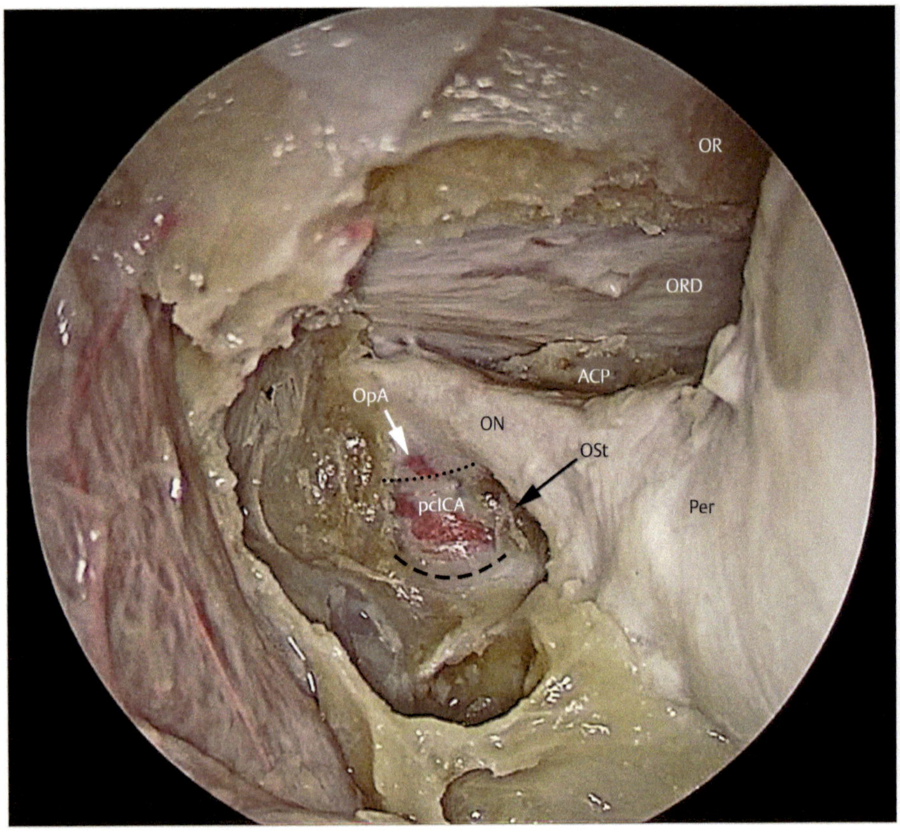

Fig. 14.22 Step 3. Partial removal of the orbital roof (OR) allows exposure of the dura of the orbital roof (ORD). Optic decompression and removal of the superior portion of the carotid prominence is performed to expose the paraclinoid tract of the internal carotid artery (pclCA), which lies between the inferior (*black dashed line*) and superior carotid ring (*black dotted line*), also called Perneczky's ring. In this way, the optic strut (OSt) is completely isolated from the surrounding bones except for the anterior clinoid process (ACP). The ophthalmic artery (OpA) enters the optic canal with the optic nerve (ON) passing superiorly to the superior carotid ring. The artery usually originates from paraclinoid/intracranial internal carotid artery. Per, periorbit.

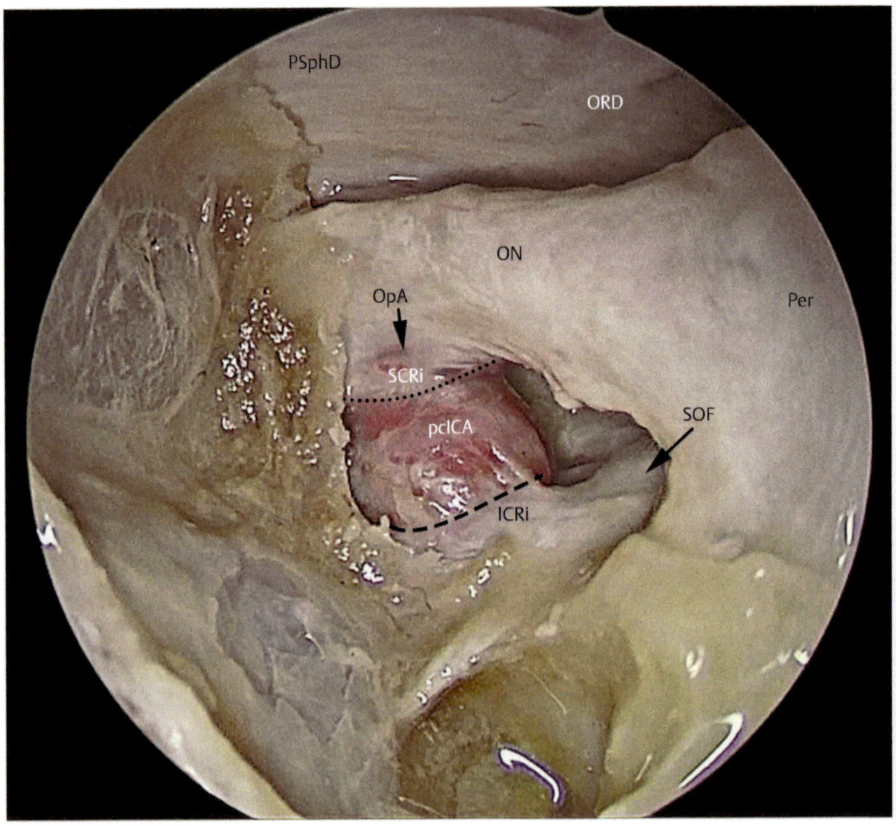

Fig. 14.23 Step 4. Removal of the optic strut leads to complete exposure of the optic nerve (ON) and identification of the medial portion of the superior orbital fissure (SOF). Note that the superior carotid ring (SCRi; *black dotted line*) and the inferior carotid ring (ICRi; *black dashed line*) continue laterally into the periosteum that surrounds the ON and the superior orbital fissure, respectively. The paraclinoid tract of the internal carotid artery (pclCA) is enclosed between the inferior carotid ring proximally and the superior carotid ring distally. OpA, ophthalmic artery; ORD, dura of the orbital roof; Per, periorbit; PSphD, dura of the planum sphenoidale.

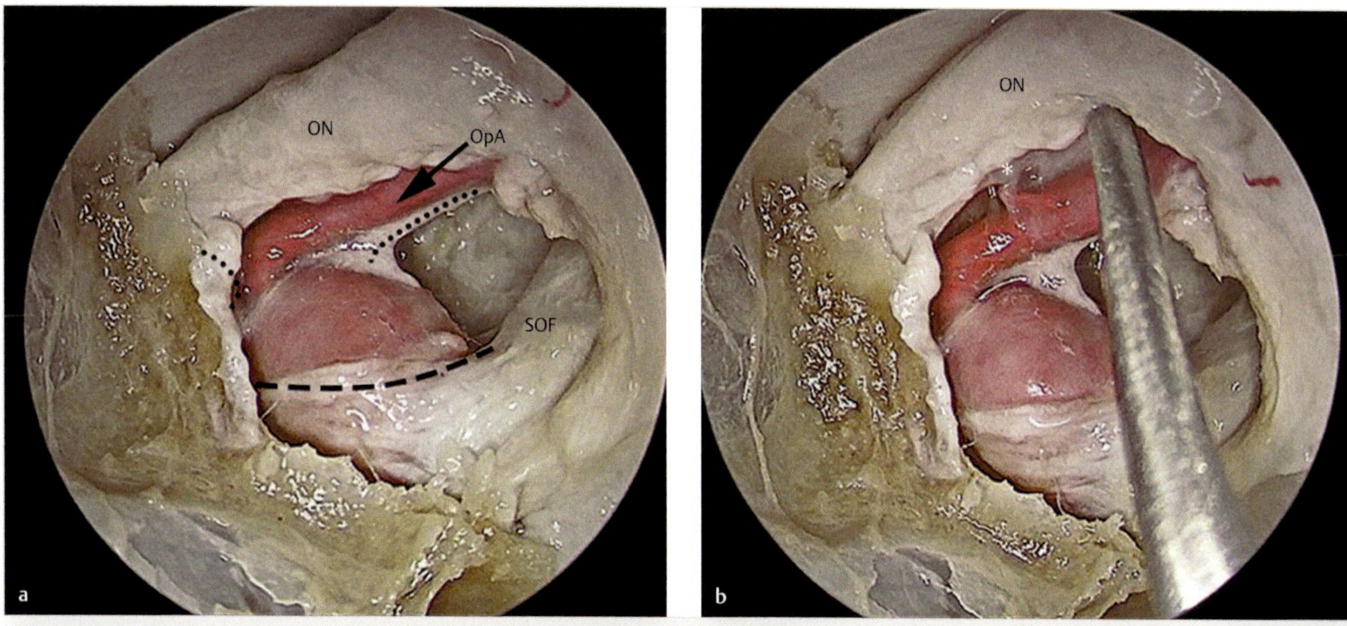

Fig. 14.24 (a, b) Step 5. The superior carotid ring (*black dotted line*) is incised to expose the ophthalmic artery and its branches (*white asterisk*) for the optic nerve (ON). (*Black dashed line*: inferior carotid ring.) SOF, superior orbital fissure.

Transorbital Approach

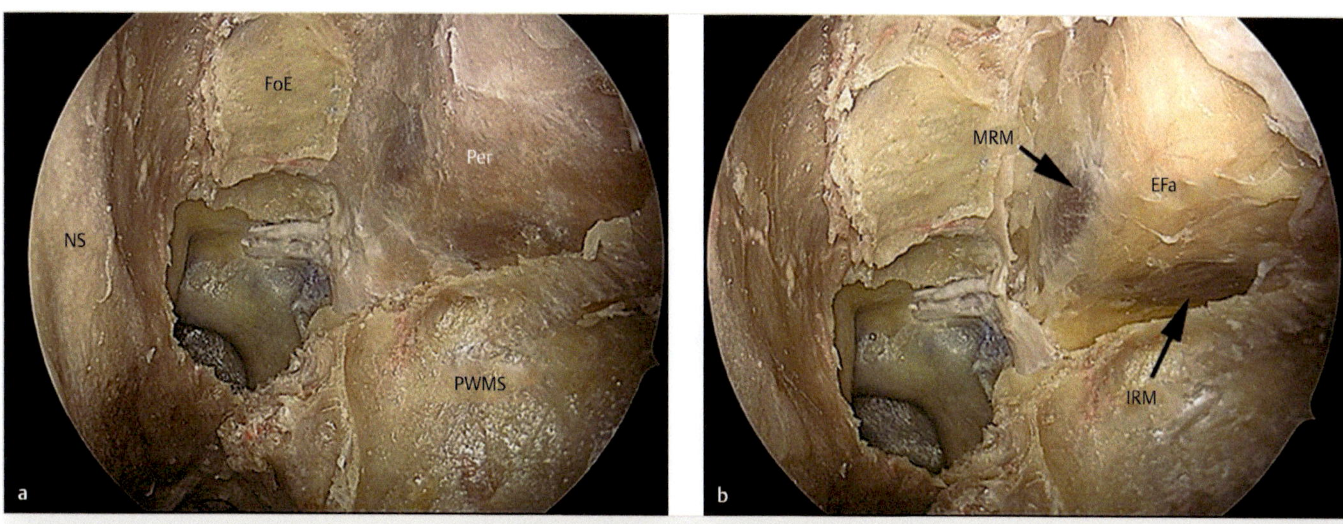

Fig. 14.25 (a, b) Step 1. After completing a two-wall orbital decompression, the periorbit is removed to expose the extraconal fat (EFa) together with the medial rectus muscle (MRM) and the inferior rectus muscle (IRM). FoE, fovea ethmoidalis; NS, nasal septum; PWMS, posterior wall of the maxillary sinus.

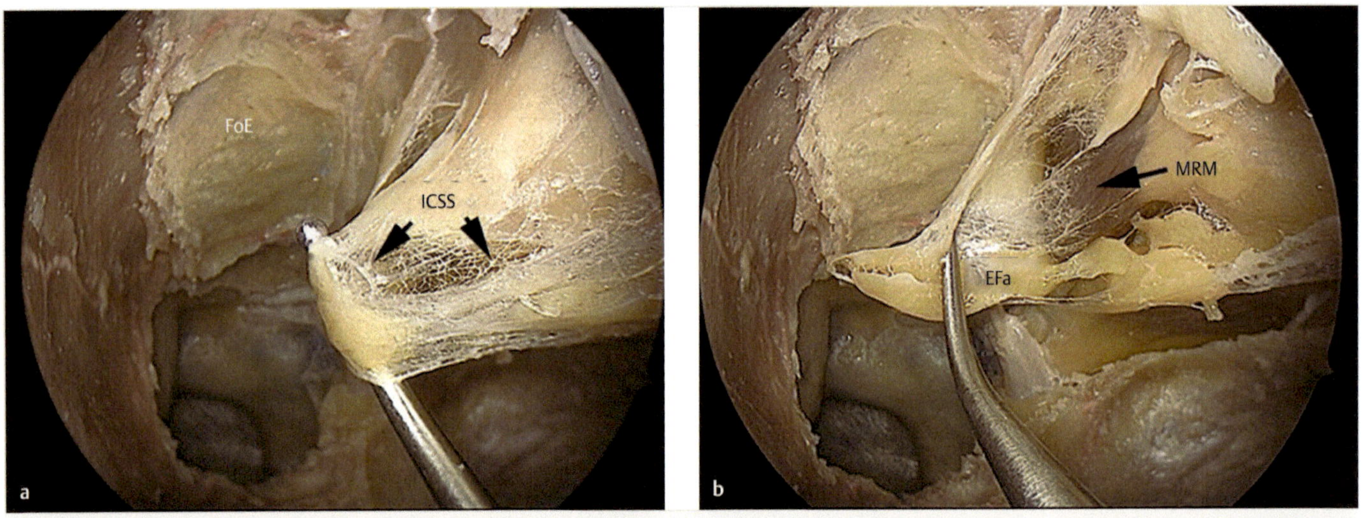

Fig. 14.26 (a, b) Step 2. Using a ball probe placed within the extraconal fat (EFa), the intraorbital connective septal system (ICSS) is stretched and fragmented. This connective system is formed by an intricate web of septa attaching to the orbital structures. FoE, fovea ethmoidalis; MRM, medial rectus muscle.

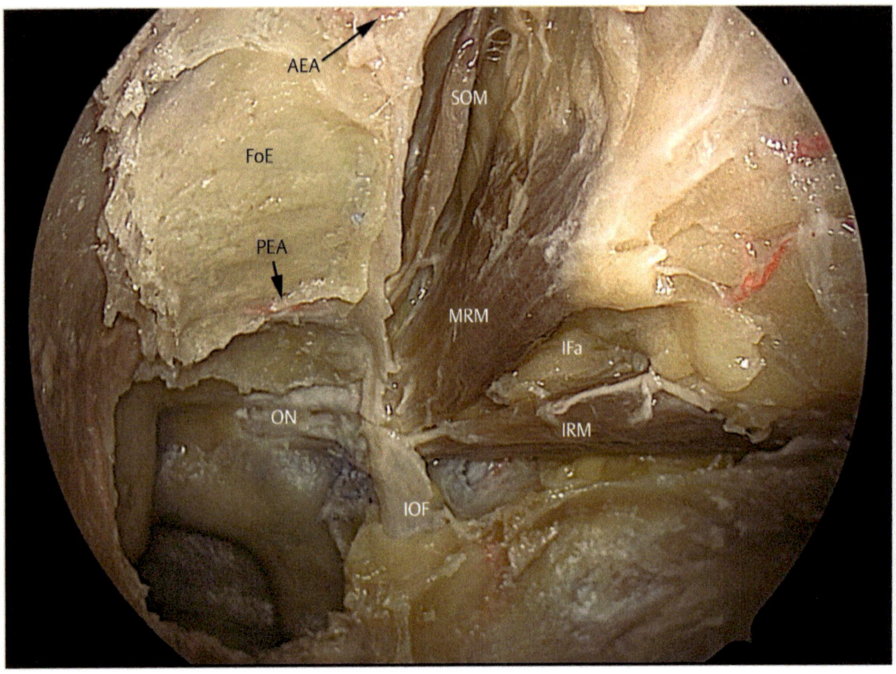

Fig. 14.27 Step 3. All the extraconal fat is removed to visualize the extraocular muscles connecting the eyeball with the orbital apex. The superior oblique muscle (SOM), the medial rectus muscle (MRM), and the inferior rectus muscle (IRM) are identified from cranial to caudal. The intraconal fat (IFa) becomes visible through the triangular spaces between the muscles. AEA, anterior ethmoidal artery FoE, fovea ethmoidalis; IOF, inferior orbital fissure; ON, optic nerve; PEA, posterior ethmoidal artery.

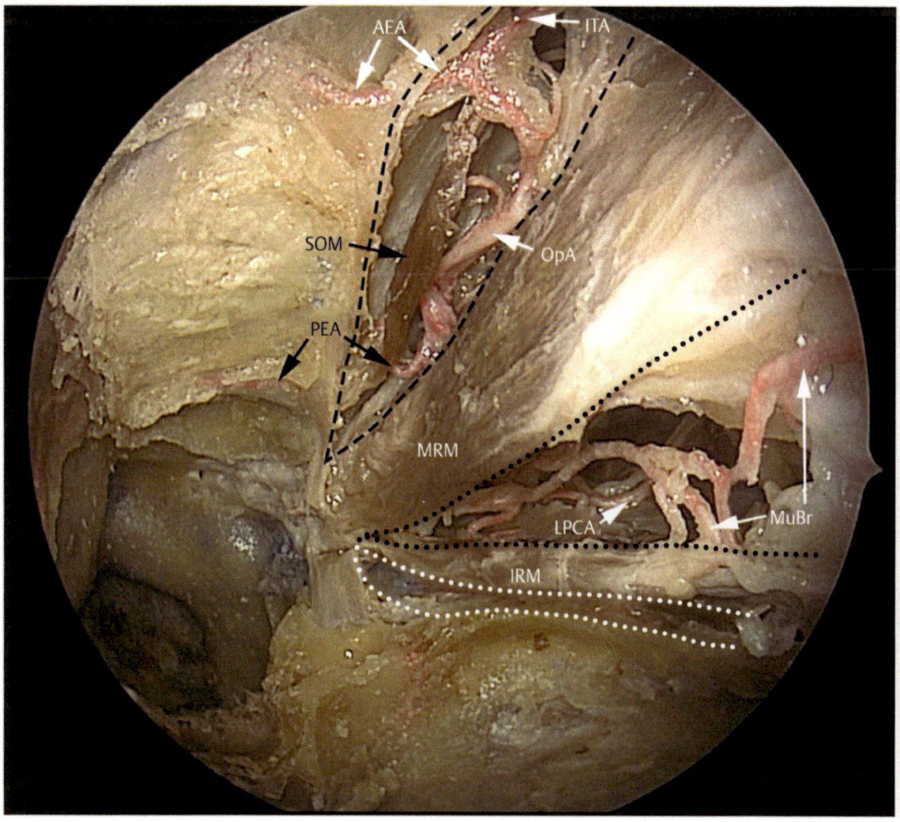

Fig. 14.28 Step 4. The intraconal fat is removed preserving the neurovascular structures of the orbit. Three triangles to access the intraconal space can be identified. The cranial triangle (*black dashed line*), which is enclosed between the skull base and the medial rectus muscle (MRM), provides access to the superior oblique muscle (SOM), the ophthalmic artery (OpA), the infratrochlear artery (ITA), and the intraorbital tract of the anterior ethmoidal artery (AEA) and the posterior ethmoidal artery (PEA). The intermediate triangle (*black dotted line*) is bounded by the medial rectus muscle and the inferior rectus muscle (IRM) and gives access to the long posterior ciliary artery (LPCA) and the muscular branches (MuBr) of the ophthalmic artery. The caudal triangle (*white dotted line*) is enclosed between the inferior rectus muscle and the orbital floor and gives access to the proximal portion of the infraorbital bundle and the inferior ophthalmic vein.

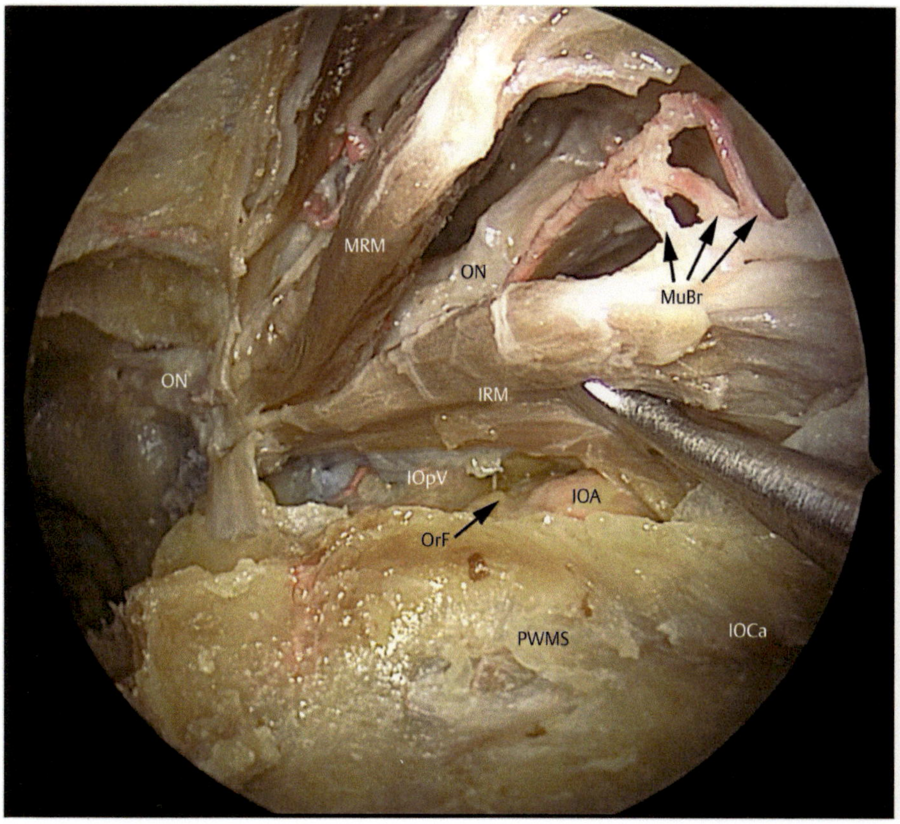

Fig. 14.29 The caudal triangle. Using a dissector, the inferior rectus muscle (IRM) is displaced superiorly to explore the caudal triangle. The inferior ophthalmic vein (IOpV) and the infraorbital artery (IOA) come into view. IOCa, infraorbital canal; ON, optic nerve; OrF, orbital floor; MRM, medial rectus muscle; MuBr, muscular branches of the ophthalmic artery; PWMS, posterior wall of the maxillary sinus.

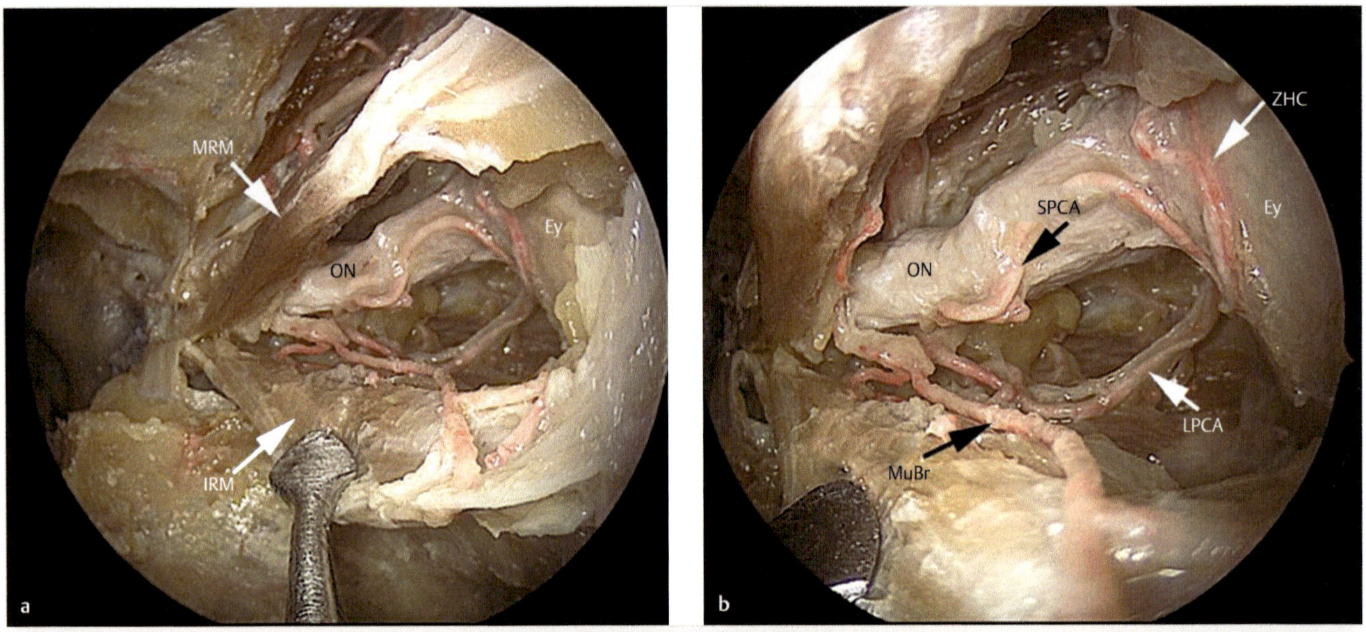

Fig. 14.30 (a, b) The intermediate triangle (part 1). The inferior rectus muscle (IRM) is pushed inferiorly to explore the intermediate triangle. The course of the optic nerve (ON) from the orbital apex to the eyeball (Ey), parallel to the long posterior ciliary artery (LPCA) and the short posterior ciliary artery (SPCA), can be seen. These arteries form an arterial circle, called Zinn–Haller circle (ZHC), around the area where the ON enters the eyeball. MRM, medial rectus muscle; MuBr, muscular branches of the ophthalmic artery.

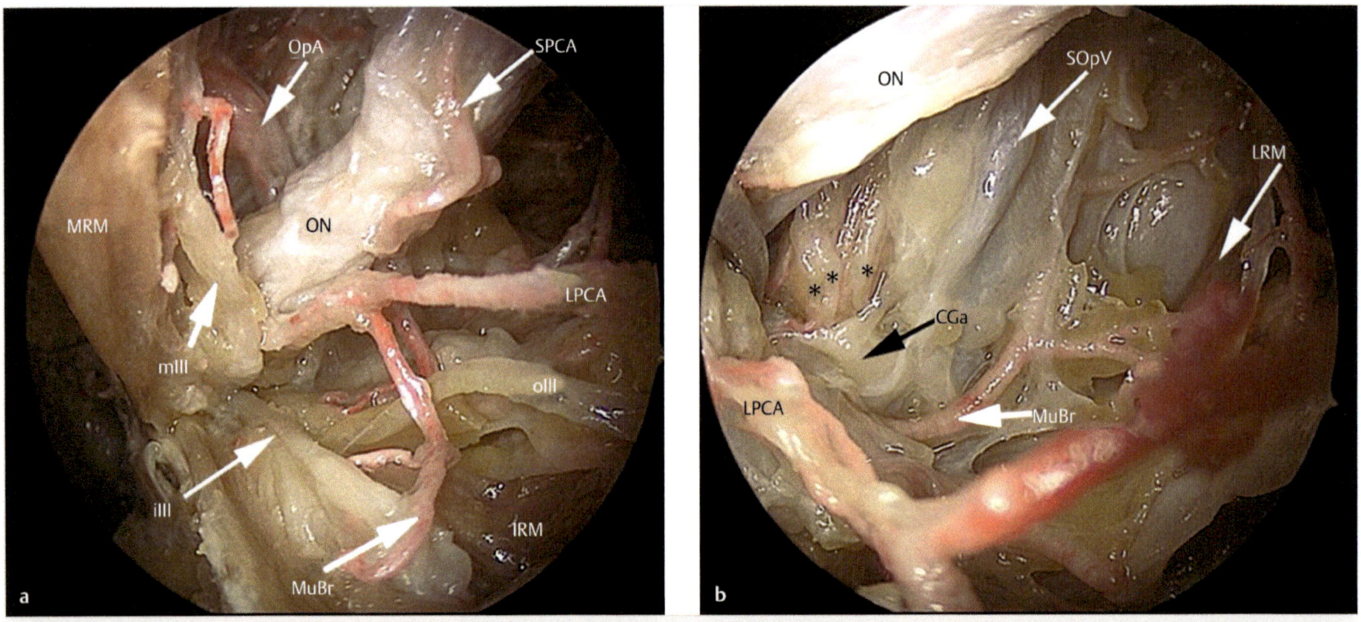

Fig. 14.31 (a, b) The intermediate triangle (part 2). With a 45-degree scope turned toward the orbital apex, the intermediate triangle is explored. The branches of the oculomotor nerve (mIII, iIII, oIII) for the medial rectus muscle (MRM), the inferior rectus muscle (IRM), and the inferior oblique muscle can be identified below the optic nerve (ON). The ophthalmic artery (OpA) runs superiorly to the optic nerve. The superior ophthalmic vein (SOpV) and the ciliary ganglion (CGa) with its efferent branches (*black asterisks*) can be identified lateral to the optic nerve. LPCA, long posterior ciliary artery; LRM, lateral rectus muscle; MuBr, muscular branches of the ophthalmic artery; SPCA, short posterior ciliary artery.

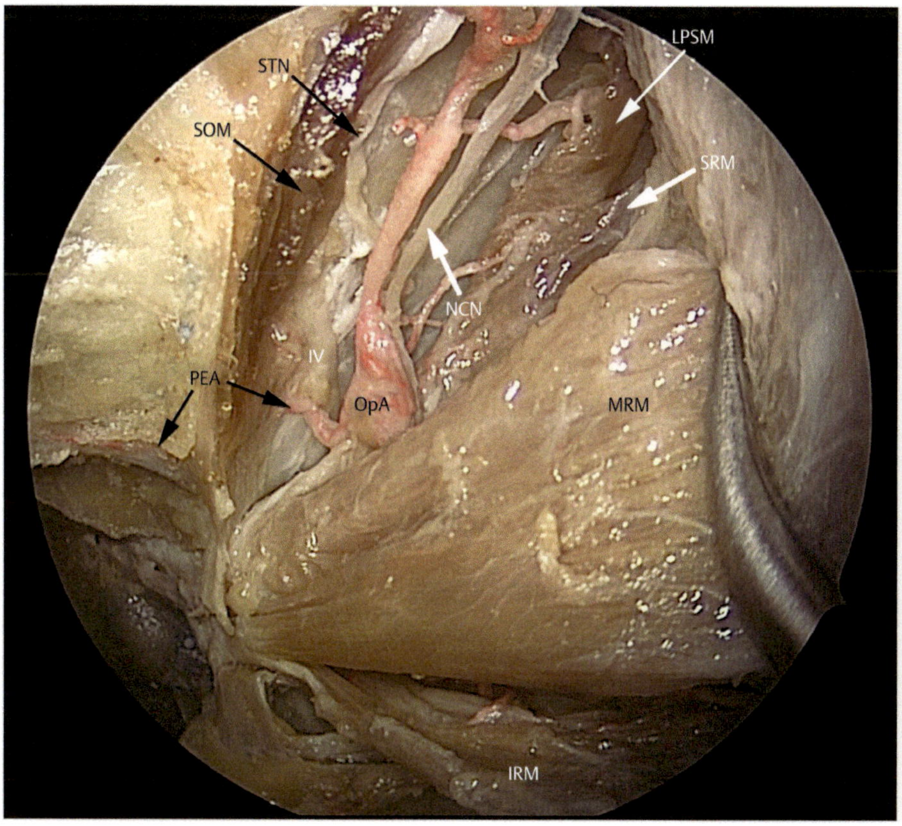

Fig. 14.32 The cranial triangle (part 1). The medial rectus muscle (MRM) is displaced laterally to expose the cranial triangle. The ophthalmic artery (OpA) runs from posterior to anterior and from lateral to medial passing inferiorly to the levator palpebrae superioris muscle (LPSM) and the superior rectus muscle (SRM). The nasociliary nerve (NCN) runs parallel to the ophthalmic artery in the intraconal space, whereas the supratrochlear nerve (STN) and the supraorbital nerve run in the extraconal space along the orbital roof. The trochlear nerve (IV) reaches the superior oblique muscle (SOM) almost where it crosses the posterior ethmoidal artery (PEA).

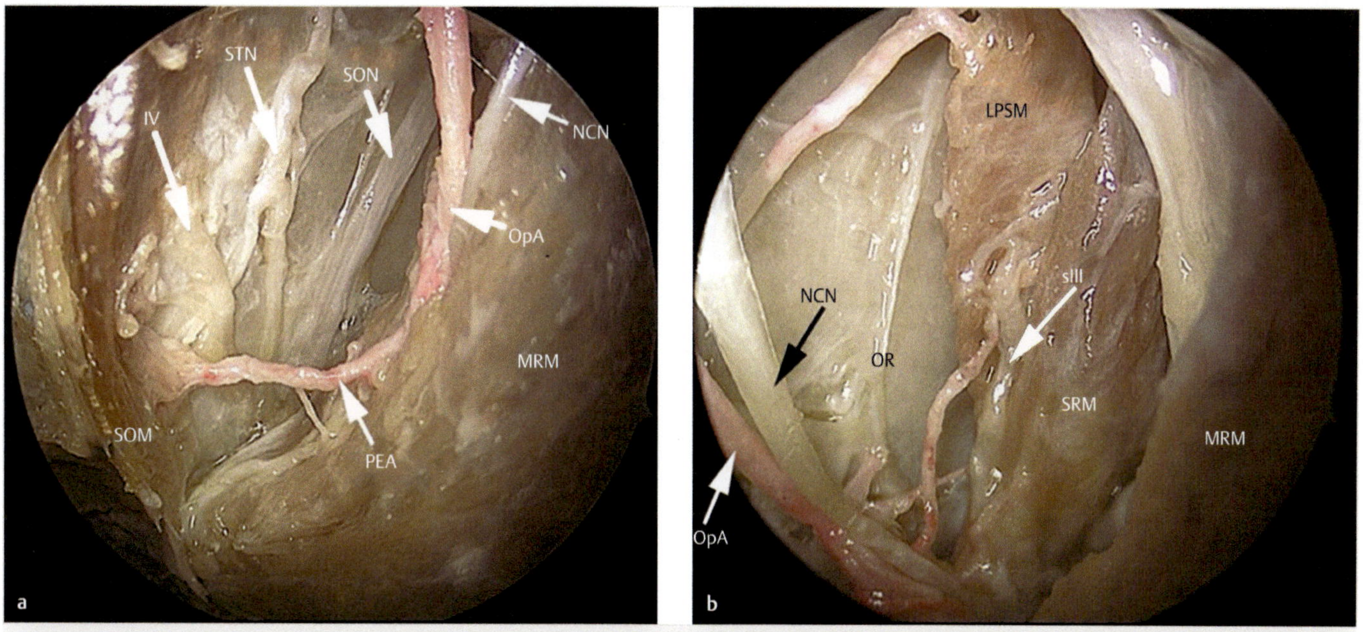

Fig. 14.33 (a, b) The cranial triangle (part 2). Moving the scope toward the orbital roof (OR), the supratrochlear nerve (STN) and the supraorbital nerve (SON) can be identified medially to the levator palpebrae superioris (LPSM) and the superior rectus muscle (SRM). These muscles are supplied by a branch of the oculomotor nerve (sIII). IV, trochlear nerve; MRM, medial rectus muscle; NCN, nasociliary nerve; OpA, ophthalmic artery; PEA, posterior ethmoidal artery; SOM, superior oblique muscle.

References

[1] Boboridis KG, Uddin J, Mikropoulos DG, et al. Critical appraisal on orbital decompression for thyroid eye disease: a systematic review and literature search. Adv Ther 2015;32(7):595–611

[2] Emanuelli E, Bignami M, Digilio E, Fusetti S, Volo T, Castelnuovo P. Post-traumatic optic neuropathy: our surgical and medical protocol. Eur Arch Otorhinolaryngol 2015;272(11):3301-3309

[3] Colletti G, Saibene AM, Giannini L, et al. Endoscopic endonasal repair with polyethylene implants in medial orbital wall fractures: a prospective study on 25 cases. J Craniomaxillofac Surg 2018;46(2):274–282

[4] Kuhnel T, Jagle H, Hosemann W, Weber R, Vielsmeier V. Orbital floor fracture repair: the endonasal approach. Rhinology 2017;55(4):348–354

[5] Bleier BS, Castelnuovo P, Battaglia P, et al. Endoscopic endonasal orbital cavernous hemangioma resection: global experience in techniques and outcomes. Int Forum Allergy Rhinol 2016;6(2):156–161

[6] Castelnuovo P, Turri-Zanoni M, Battaglia P, Locatelli D, Dallan I. Endoscopic endonasal management of orbital pathologies. Neurosurg Clin N Am 2015;26(3):463–472

[7] Berhouma M, Jacquesson T, Abouaf L, Vighetto A, Jouanneau E. Endoscopic endonasal optic nerve and orbital apex decompression for nontraumatic optic neuropathy: surgical nuances and review of the literature. Neurosurg Focus 2014;37(4):E19

[8] Stokken J, Gumber D, Antisdel J, Sindwani R. Endoscopic surgery of the orbital apex: outcomes and emerging techniques. Laryngoscope 2016;126(1):20–24

[9] Teinzer F, Stammberger H, Tomazic PV. Transnasal endoscopic treatment of orbital complications of acute sinusitis: the Graz concept. Ann Otol Rhinol Laryngol 2015;124(5):368–373

[10] Gavriel H, Jabrin B, Eviatar E. Management of superior subperiosteal orbital abscess. Eur Arch Otorhinolaryngol 2016;273(1):145–150

[11] Balakrishnan K, Moe KS. Applications and outcomes of orbital and transorbital endoscopic surgery. Otolaryngol Head Neck Surg 2011;144(5):815–820

[12] Locatelli D, Pozzi F, Turri-Zanoni M, et al. Transorbital endoscopic approaches to the skull base: current concepts and future perspectives. J Neurosurg Sci 2016;60(4):514–525

[13] Moe KS, Bergeron CM, Ellenbogen RG. Transorbital neuroendoscopic surgery. Neurosurgery 2010;67(3, Suppl Operative):ons16–ons28

[14] Ramakrishna R, Kim LJ, Bly RA, Moe K, Ferreira M Jr. Transorbital neuroendoscopic surgery for the treatment of skull base lesions. J Clin Neurosci 2016;24:99–104

[15] Ferrari M, Schreiber A, Mattavelli D, et al. The inferolateral transorbital endoscopic approach: a preclinical anatomic study. World Neurosurg 2016;90:403–413

15 Transpterygomaxillary Approach

Piero Nicolai, Alberto Schreiber, Marco Ravanelli, Davide Mattavelli, Alberto Deganello

The pterygopalatine fossa is a narrow space bounded by the pterygoid process posteriorly, maxillary sinus anterolaterally, and perpendicular process of the palatine bone anteromedially. This space is the watershed between the sinonasal cavity, infratemporal fossa, and orbital cavity, and houses several neurovascular structures, including the maxillary nerve and the pterygopalatine ganglion with their branches together with the pterygopalatine tract of the internal maxillary artery with its collateral vessels. In view of its supposed origin at the base of the pterygoid process, juvenile angiofibroma is particularly prone to extend within the pterygopalatine fossa and toward adjacent compartments.[1] Furthermore, sinonasal or nasopharyngeal tumors can reach the pterygopalatine fossa passing through the sphenopalatine foramen or invading its bony boundaries. More rarely, primary neurogenic, vascular, or other lesions can be found in this area. The transnasal endoscopic approach to the pterygopalatine fossa has been employed to resect juvenile angiofibromas,[2] vidian and maxillary nerve schwannomas,[3–6] fibro-osseous lesions,[7] hemangiomas,[7] sinonasal or nasopharyngeal malignancies with lateral extension,[7] and other rarer lesions.

The pterygopalatine fossa can be dissected through the maxillary sinus in a layer-by-layer fashion. The most important bony landmarks are the infraorbital canal, which marks the position of the pterygomaxillary fissure (i.e., the transition between the infratemporal fossa and the pterygopalatine fossa),[8] and the sphenopalatine foramen, which serves as the starting point to remove the perpendicular process of the palatine bone and the posterior maxillary wall. This step is preferably performed keeping the periosteum intact to protect the neurovascular structures of the pterygopalatine fossa. Inferomedially, the subperiosteal dissection demarcates a triangular area that corresponds to the pterygomaxillary junction, where the maxilla fuses with the pterygoid process. The periosteum is then incised and the underlying fat is meticulously removed to expose the neurovascular structures. After skeletonizing the pterygopalatine tract of the internal maxillary artery and

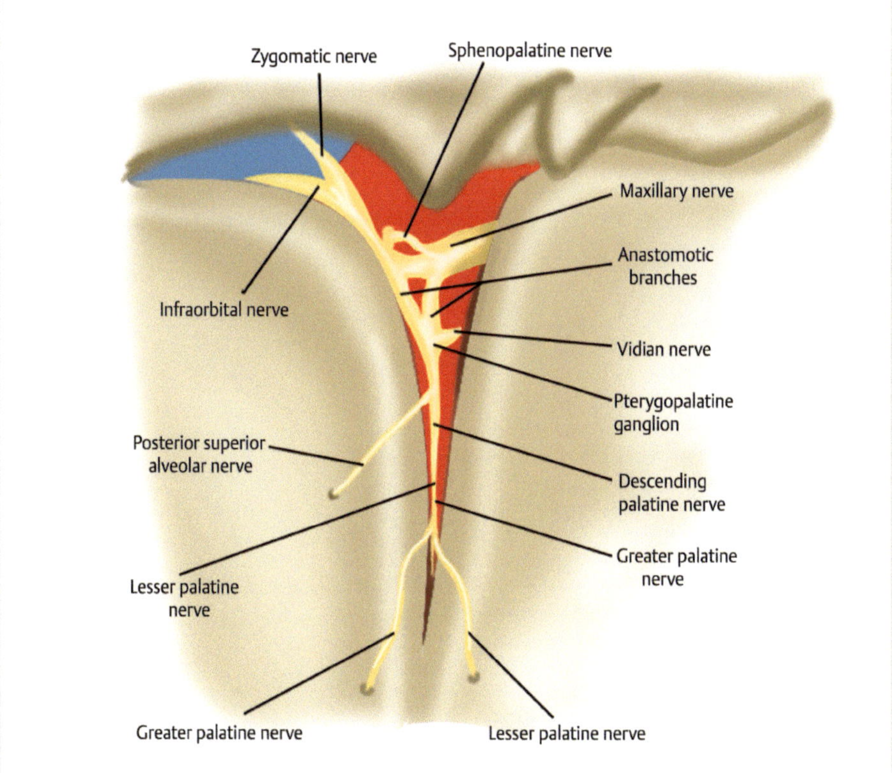

Fig. 15.1 Lateral to medial view of the pterygopalatine fossa as seen from the pterygomaxillary fissure. The drawing shows the left pterygopalatine fossa (*red area*), inferior orbital fissure (*blue area*), and their nervous content.

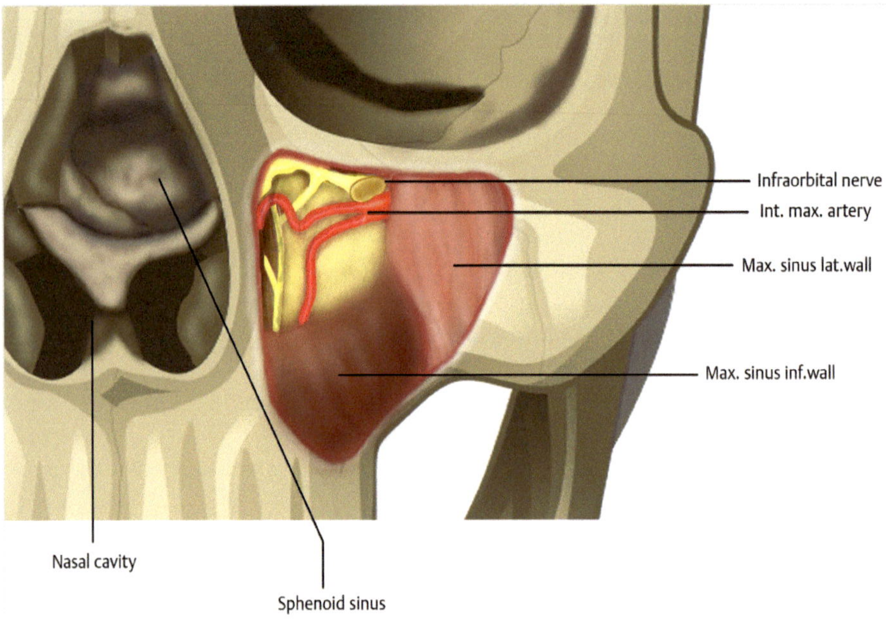

Fig. 15.2 Position of the pterygopalatine fossa as seen through the transantral window.

its collaterals, they are removed to analyze the nervous structures, which lie in front of the pterygoid process and cranial insertion of the lateral pterygoid muscle.

The complete removal of fat and neurovascular structures allows identification of the different pathways of communication of the pterygopalatine fossa with adjacent compartments. Specifically, the vidian canal, foramen rotundum, inferior orbital fissure, and pterygomaxillary fissure connect the pterygopalatine fossa with the foramen lacerum, middle cranial fossa, orbital cavity, and infratemporal fossa, respectively.

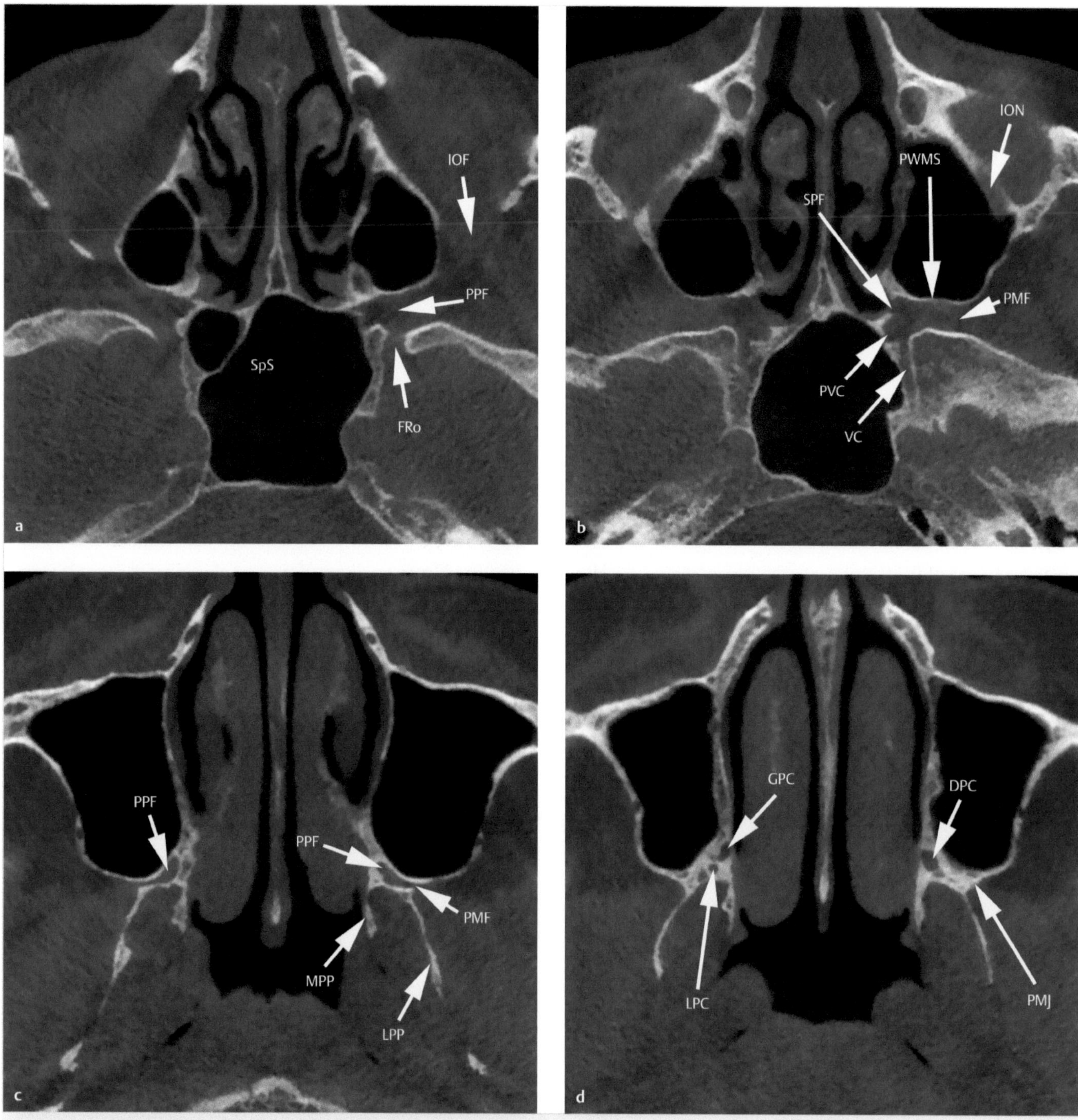

Fig. 15.3 (a–d) Axial CT anatomy of the pterygopalatine fossa. The panel includes four axial CT scans passing through the pterygopalatine fossa (PPF). The pterygopalatine fossa lies between the posterior wall of the maxillary sinus (PWMS) anteriorly and the pterygoid process posteriorly. The base of the pterygoid process houses the foramen rotundum (FRo) and the vidian canal (VC), while the caudal portion is formed by the medial pterygoid plate (MPP) and the lateral pterygoid plate (LPP). The pterygopalatine fossa is a crossroad region, which is connected with the nasal cavity, orbital cavity, and infratemporal fossa through the sphenopalatine foramen (SPF), inferior orbital fissure (IOF), and pterygomaxillary fissure (PMF), respectively. Caudally, the pterygopalatine fossa ends blindly with the pterygomaxillary junction (PMJ). DPC, descending palatine canal; GPC, greater palatine canal; ION, infraorbital nerve; LPC, lesser palatine canal; PVC, palatovaginal canal; SpS, sphenoid sinus.

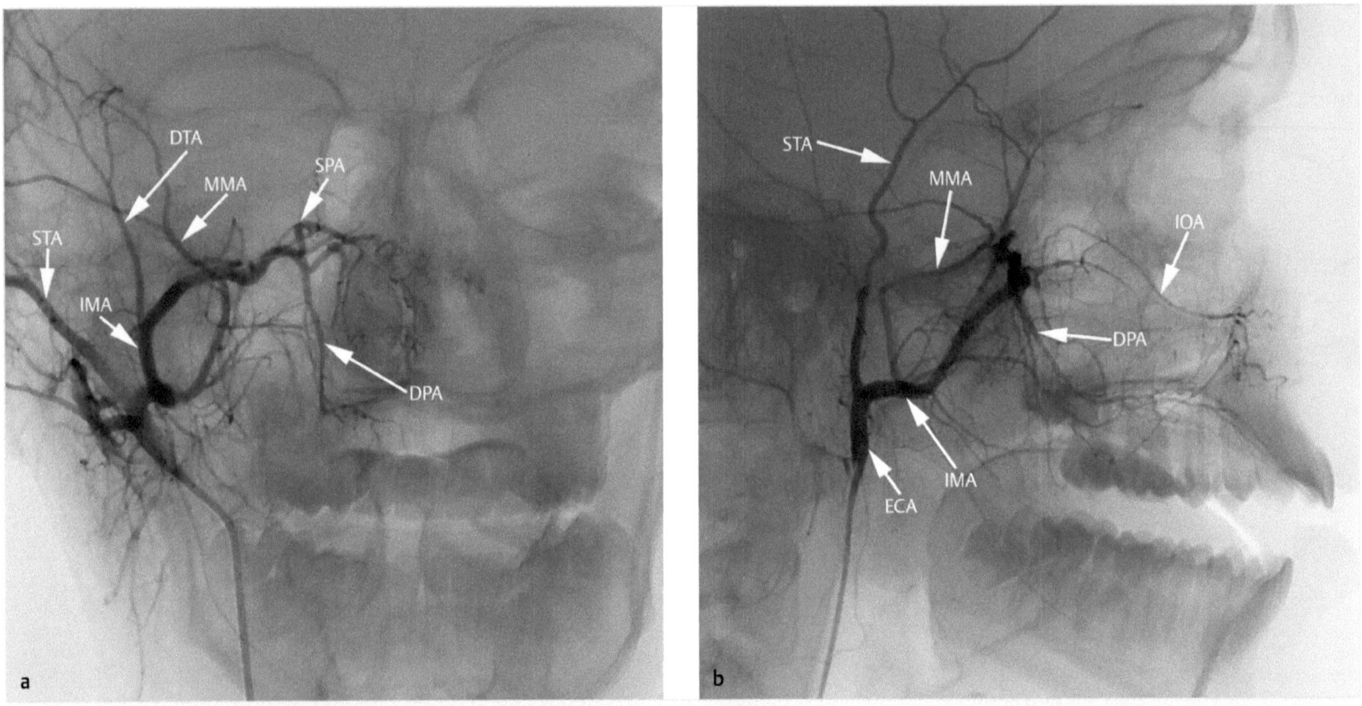

Fig. 15.4 Angiography of the internal maxillary artery. The panel includes an anterior-to-posterior **(a)** and lateral-to-medial angiograms **(b)** of the right internal maxillary artery (IMA). The terminal branches of the external carotid artery (ECA) are the superficial temporal artery (STA) and the internal maxillary artery, which is formed by the condylar, infratemporal, and pterygopalatine tracts. The internal maxillary artery gives origin to the middle meningeal artery (MMA) and other collateral branches before ending with the sphenopalatine artery (SPA) and descending palatine artery (DPA). DTA, deep temporal artery; IOA, infraorbital artery.

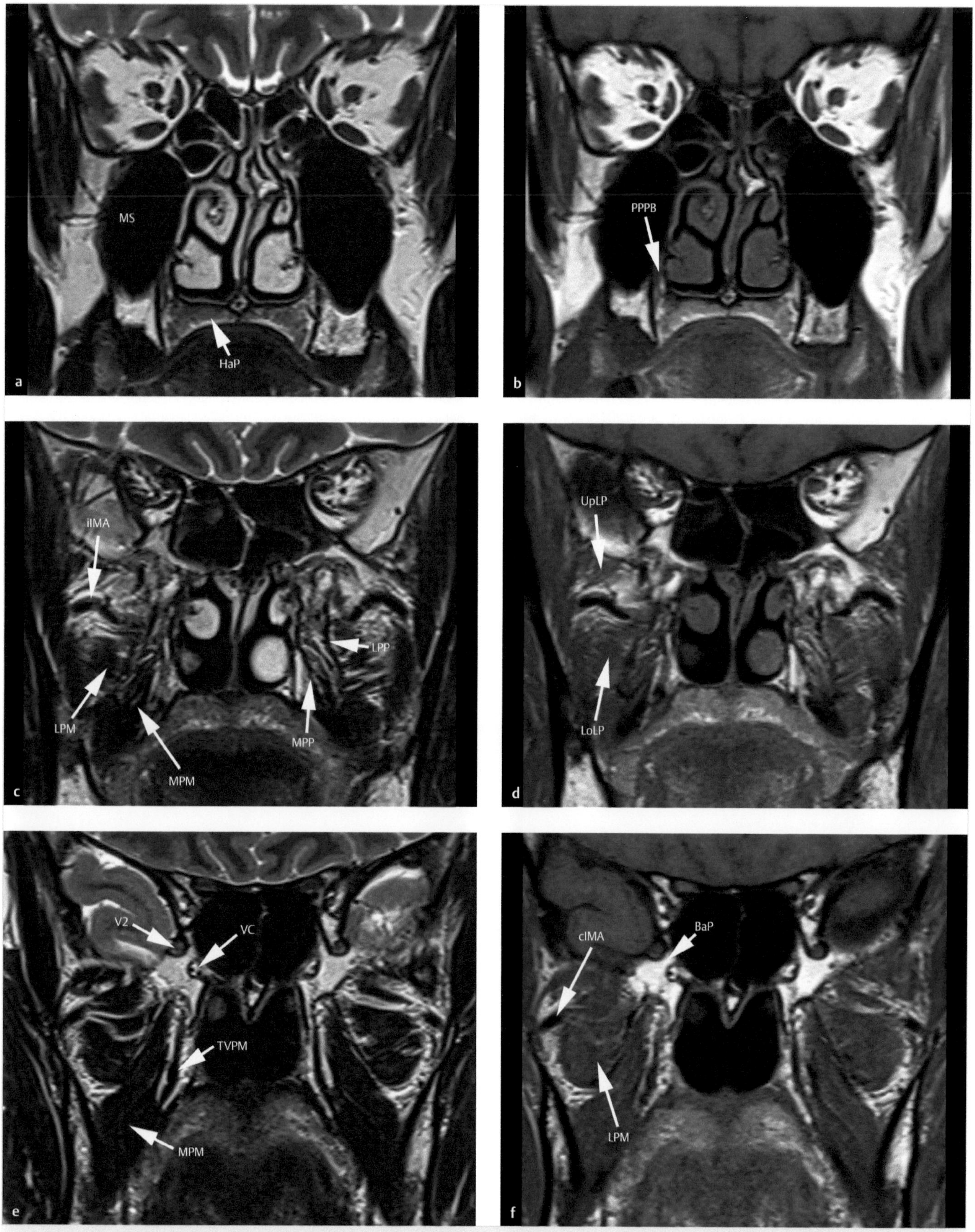

Fig. 15.5 Coronal MRI anatomy of the pterygopalatine fossa and adjacent areas. The panel includes two series of T2-weighted **(a, c, e)** and T1-weighted **(b, d, f)** MRI images, from anterior (upper images) to posterior (lower images). The position of the images composing this panel is showed in ▶Fig. 15.7: the upper, middle, and lower images correspond to A, B, and C, respectively. The pterygopalatine fossa is a narrow space enclosed between the maxillary sinus (MS) and the perpendicular process of the palatine bone (PPPB) anteriorly and pterygoid process posteriorly. The pterygoid process, which is formed by the base (BaP) along with the medial pterygoid plate (MPP) and the lateral medial pterygoid plate (LPP), serves as the cranial insertion of the medial pterygoid muscle (MPM) and the lateral pterygoid muscle (LPM). The condylar tract of the internal maxillary artery (cIMA) runs around to the mandibular condyle, whereas the infratemporal tract (iIMA) passes between the upper head of the lateral pterygoid muscle (UpLP) and the lower head of the lateral pterygoid muscle (LoLP). V2, maxillary nerve; HaP, hard palate; TVPM, tensor veli palatini muscle; VC, vidian canal.

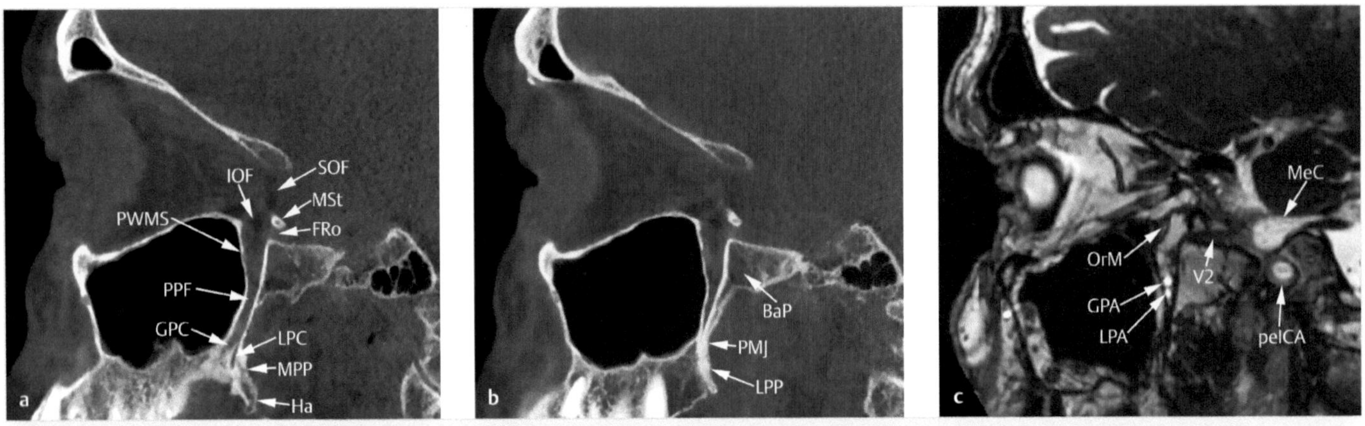

Fig. 15.6 Sagittal CT and MRI anatomy of the pterygopalatine fossa. The panel includes two sagittal CT scans **(a, b)** and a constructive interference in steady state (CISS) MRI scan passing through the pterygopalatine fossa (PPF) **(c)**. The position of the images composing this panel is showed in ▶Fig. 15.7: **a** corresponds to D, whereas the **b** and **c** to E. The foramen rotundum (FRo) ends anteriorly in the cranial portion of the pterygopalatine fossa and is separated from the superior orbital fissure (SOF) by a bony bridge called the maxillary strut (MSt). Cranially, the pterygopalatine fossa continues into the orbital cavity through the inferior orbital fissure (IOF), which is transversally closed to the orbitalis muscle (OrM), also called Müller's muscle. In the caudal portion, the pterygopalatine fossa ends with the greater palatine canal (GPC) and the lesser palatine canal (LPC) medially and the pterygomaxillary junction (PMJ) laterally. V2, maxillary nerve; BaP, base of the pterygoid process; GPA, greater palatine artery; Ha, hamulus; LPA, lesser palatine artery; LPP, lateral pterygoid plate; MeC, Meckel's cave; MPP, medial pterygoid plate; peICA, petrous tract of the internal carotid artery; PWMS, posterior wall of the maxillary sinus.

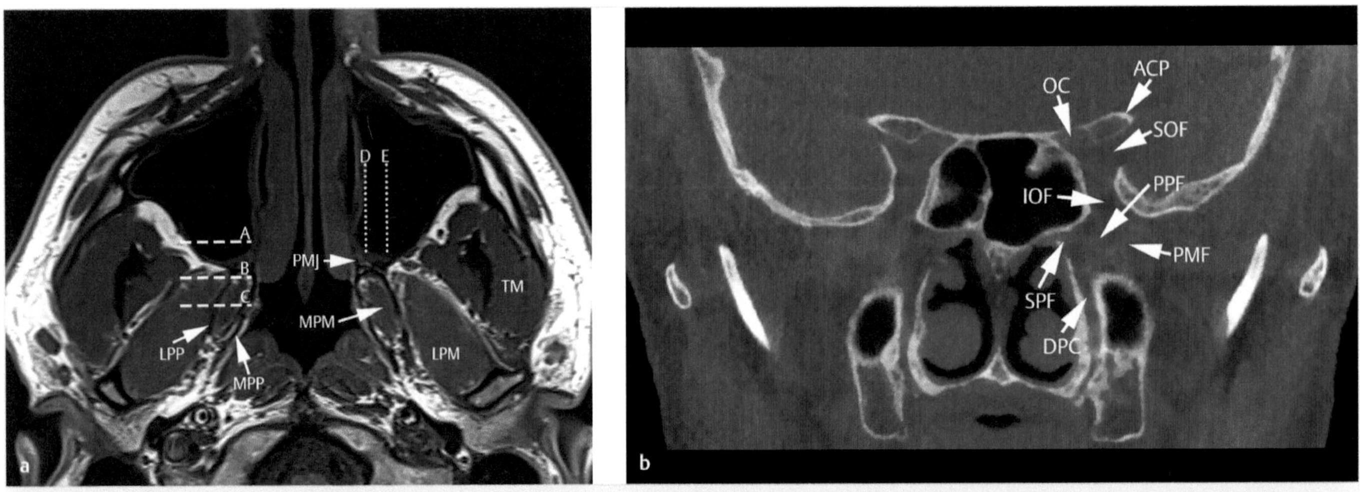

Fig. 15.7 (a, b) Axial and coronal MRI and CT anatomy of the areas adjacent to the pterygopalatine fossa. In the axial T1-weighted MRI scan **(a)**, the *white dashed lines* (A–C) depict the position of images composing ▶Fig. 15.5, while the *white dotted lines* (D, E) depict the position of the images composing ▶Fig. 15.6. The pterygopalatine fossa (PPF) is surrounded by a number of anatomical areas. It is adjacent to the maxillary sinus anteriorly, infratemporal fossa posteriorly and laterally, sinonasal tract medially, orbital apex superiorly, and palate inferiorly. ACP, anterior clinoid process; DPC, descending palatine canal; IOF, inferior orbital fissure; LPM, lateral pterygoid muscle; LPP, lateral pterygoid plate; MPM, medial pterygoid muscle; MPP, medial pterygoid plate; OC, optic canal; PMF, pterygomaxillary fissure; PMJ, pterygomaxillary junction; SOF, superior orbital fissure; SPF, sphenopalatine foramen; TM, temporal muscle.

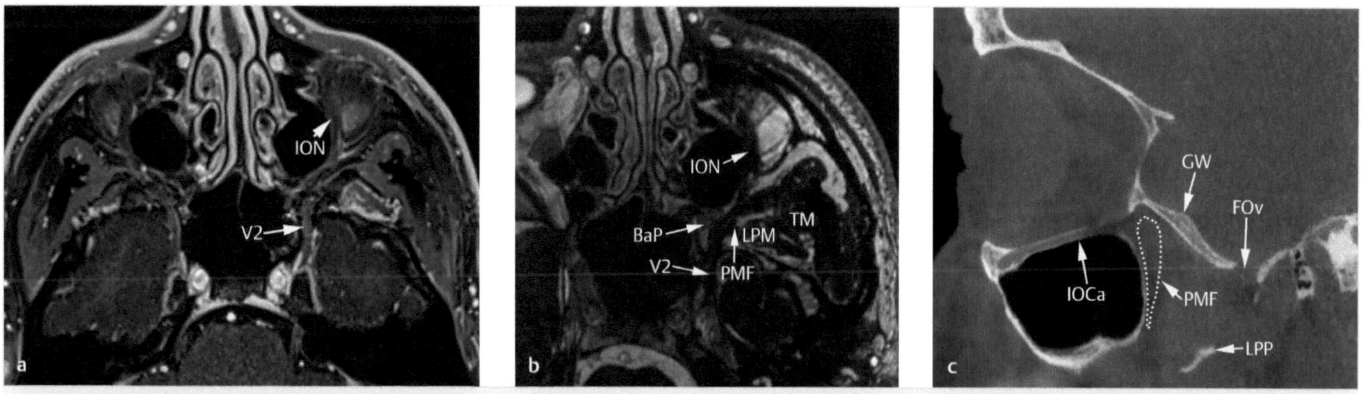

Fig. 15.8 Axial and sagittal MRI and CT anatomy of the infraorbital nerve. The panel includes an axial T1-weighted contrast-enhanced fat-saturated MRI **(a)**, a curved CISS (constructive interference in steady state) MRI **(b)**, and a sagittal CT scan **(c)**. After arising from the maxillary nerve (V2), the infraorbital nerve (ION) tilts laterally and enters the infraorbital canal (IOCa), forming the shape of a bayonet. The medial edge of the posterior end of the infraorbital canal mostly corresponds to the level of the pterygomaxillary fissure (PMF; *white dotted line*), thus serving as a guide to distinguish the limit between the pterygopalatine fossa and the infratemporal fossa. BaP, base of the pterygoid process; FOv, foramen ovale; GW, greater wing of the sphenoid bone; LPM, lateral pterygoid muscle; LPP, lateral pterygoid plate; TM, temporal muscle.

Endoscopic Dissection

Nasal Phase

- Horizontal uncinectomy.
- Type A–B endoscopic medial maxillectomy.
- Facultative: Type C–D endoscopic medial maxillectomy.
- Facultative: Vertical uncinectomy.
- Facultative: Anterior ethmoidectomy.
- Facultative: Posterior ethmoidectomy.
- Facultative: Middle turbinectomy.
- Facultative: Septectomy.

Skull Base Phase

- Step 1: Removal of the mucosa of the maxillary sinus.
- Step 2: Exposure of the descending palatine canal.
- Step 3: Removal of the posterior wall of the maxillary sinus.
- Step 4: Removal of the anterior periosteum of the pterygopalatine fossa.
- Step 5: Removal of the fat of the pterygopalatine fossa.
- Step 6: Partial removal of the vascular compartment.
- Step 7: Complete removal of the vascular compartment.

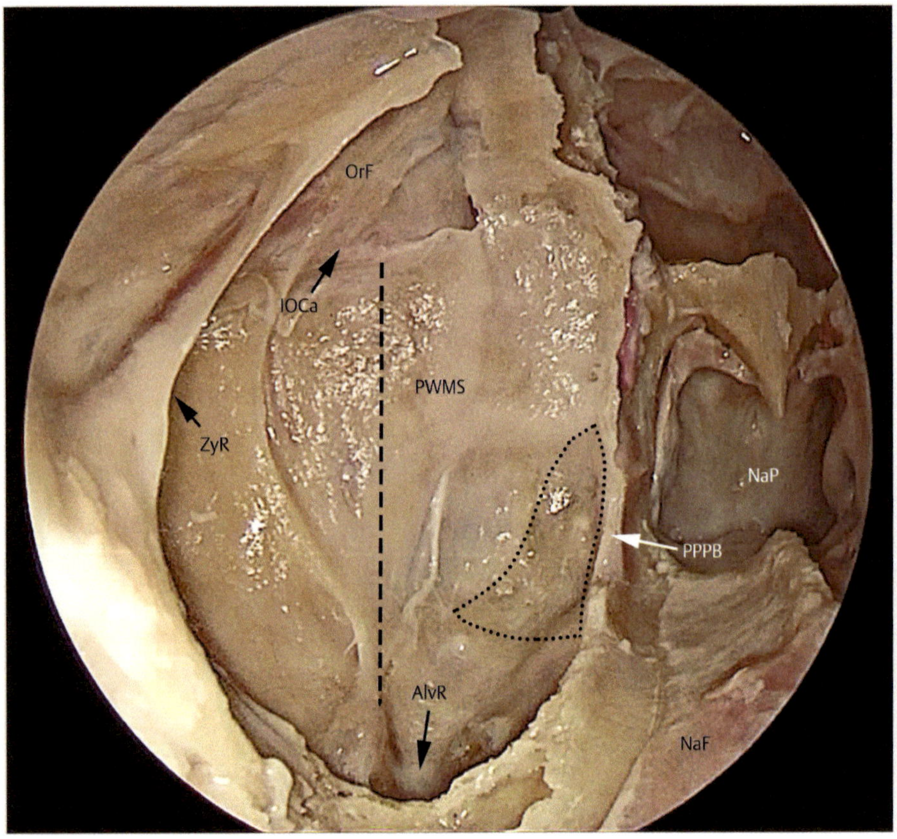

Fig. 15.9 Step 1. After completing a type C endoscopic medial maxillectomy, the mucosa of the maxillary sinus is removed to obtain an overview of bony landmarks: the orbital floor (OrF) superiorly, the zygomatic recess (ZyR) laterally, the posterior wall of the maxillary sinus (PWMS) posteriorly, and the alveolar recess (AlvR) inferiorly. The perpendicular process of the palatine bone (PPPB) is identified posteromedially and the infraorbital canal (IOCa) superolaterally. The pterygopalatine fossa lies behind the posterior wall of the maxillary sinus, between the perpendicular process of the palatine bone and the inferior projection of the posteromedial end of the infraorbital canal (*black dashed line*). The area of thick bone that is identified in the posterior wall of the maxillary sinus (*black dotted line*) corresponds to the pterygomaxillary junction, which anchors the maxilla to the pterygoid process. NaF, nasal floor; NaP, nasopharyngeal posterior wall.

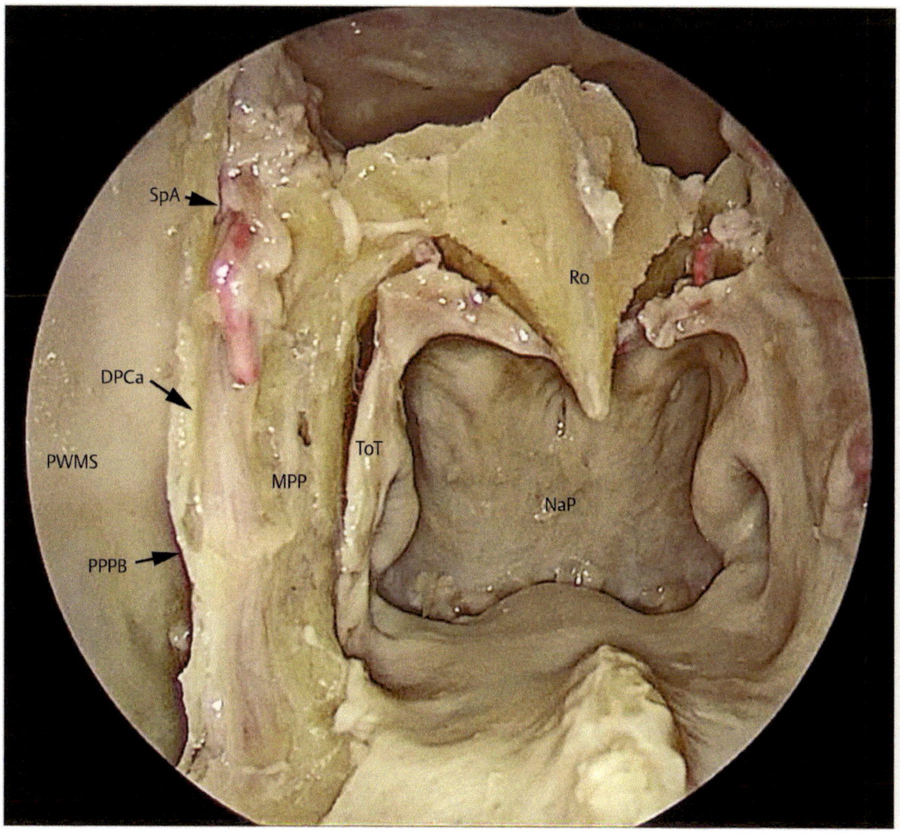

Fig. 15.10 Step 2. The perpendicular process of the palatine bone (PPPB) is gently removed to expose the descending palatine artery and nerve within their bony canal (DPCa). This canal runs between the perpendicular process of the palatine bone and the pterygoid process of the sphenoid. Following the medial pterygoid plate (MPP) posteriorly, the torus tubarius (ToT) is identified. NaP, nasopharyngeal posterior wall; PWMS, posterior wall of the maxillary sinus; Ro, sphenoidal rostrum; SpA, sphenopalatine artery.

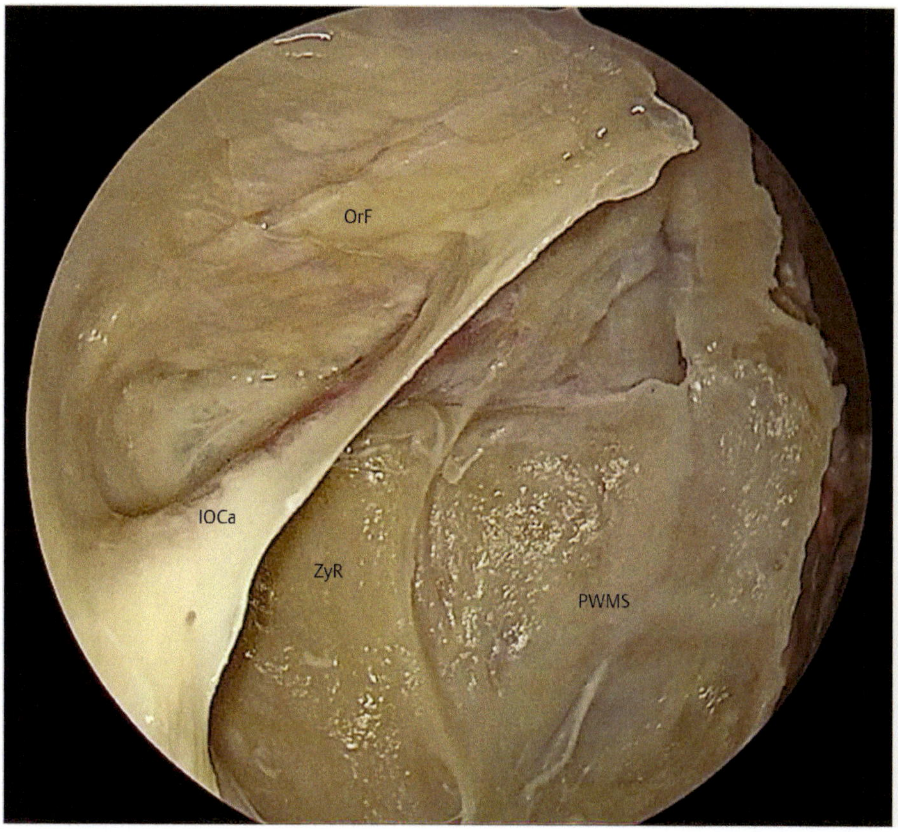

Fig. 15.11 The infraorbital canal and the zygomatic recess. With a 70-degree scope turned laterally, the zygomatic recess (ZyR) and the anterior portion of the infraorbital canal (IOCa) are visualized. OrF, orbital floor; PWMS, posterior wall of the maxillary sinus.

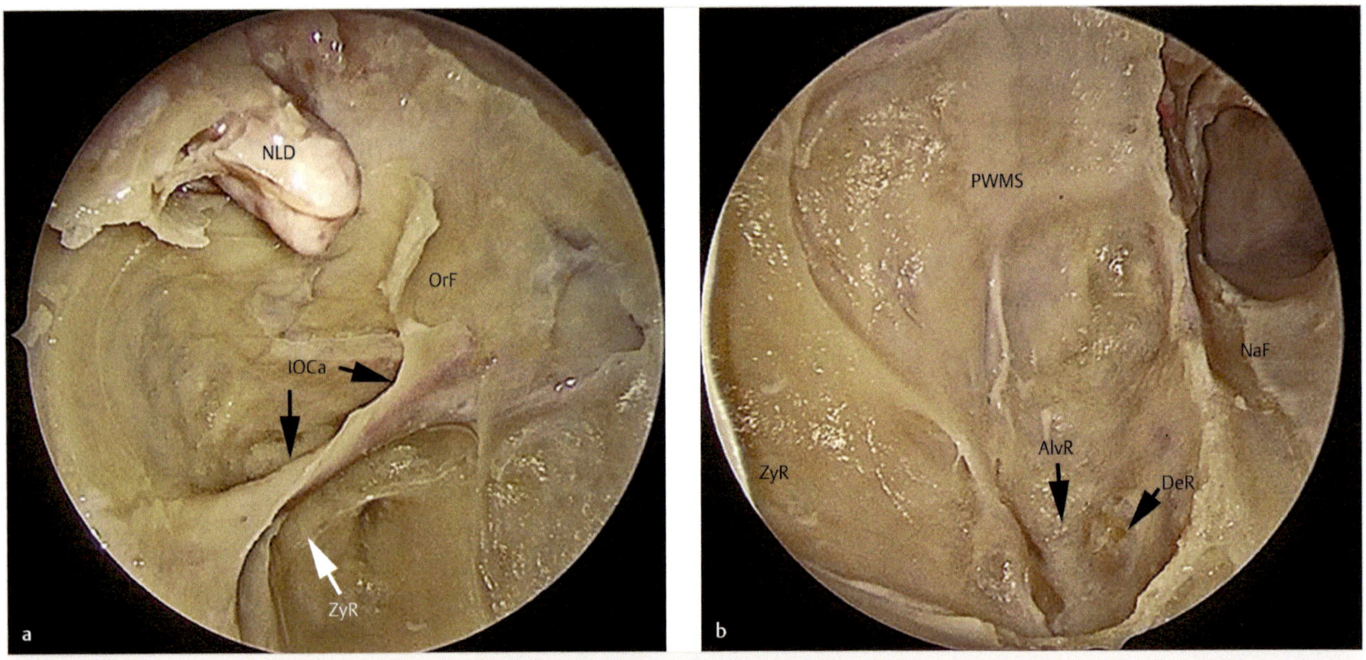

Fig. 15.12 The nasolacrimal duct and the alveolar recess. With a 70-degree scope turned superolaterally **(a)** and inferiorly **(b)**, the highest portion of the nasolacrimal duct (NLD) within its bony canal and the alveolar recess (AlvR), respectively, are identified. The apical portion of the dental roots (DeR) can be seen in the alveolar recess. IOCa, infraorbital canal; NaF, nasal floor; OrF, orbital floor; PWMS, posterior wall of the maxillary sinus; ZyR, zygomatic recess.

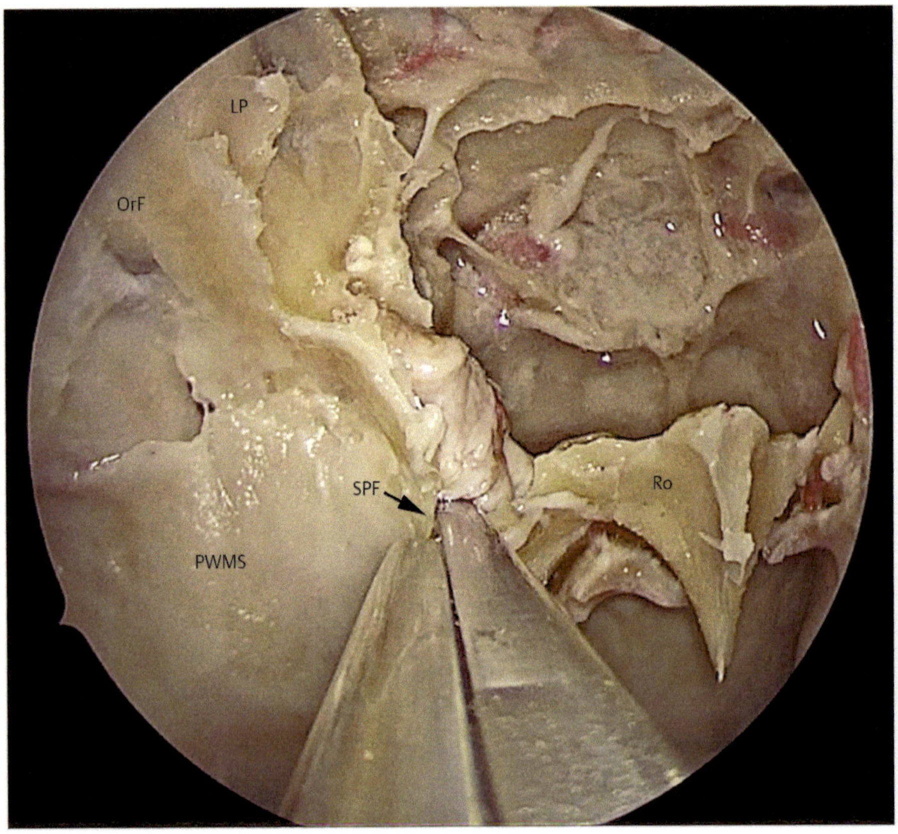

Fig. 15.13 Step 3 (part 1). Starting from the sphenopalatine foramen (SPF), the posterior wall of the maxillary sinus (PWMS) is progressively removed following the subperiosteal plane. LP, lamina papyracea; OrF, orbital floor; Ro, rostrum.

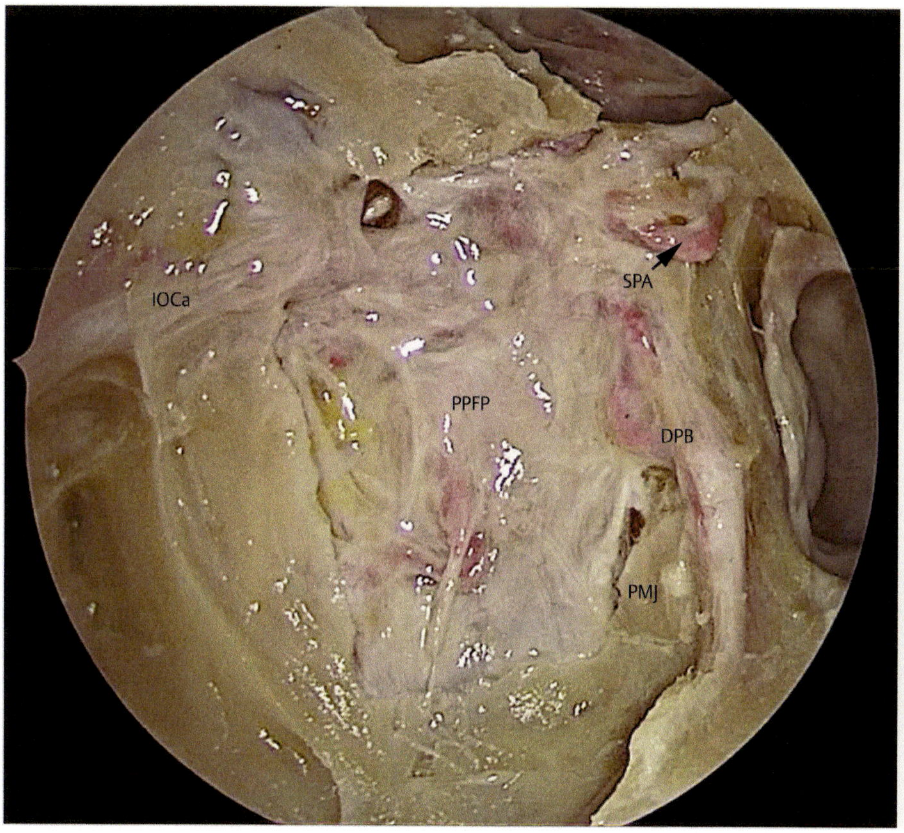

Fig. 15.14 Step 3 (part 2). The posterior wall of the maxillary sinus is removed to expose the periosteum of the pterygopalatine fossa (PPFP). This step provides a clear view of the main pedicles coming from the pterygopalatine fossa: the pedicle within the infraorbital canal (IOCa), the sphenopalatine artery (SPA), and the descending palatine bundle (DPB). Being formed by thick bone attached to the pterygoid process, the pterygomaxillary junction (PMJ) is usually left in the inferomedial corner of the bony window.

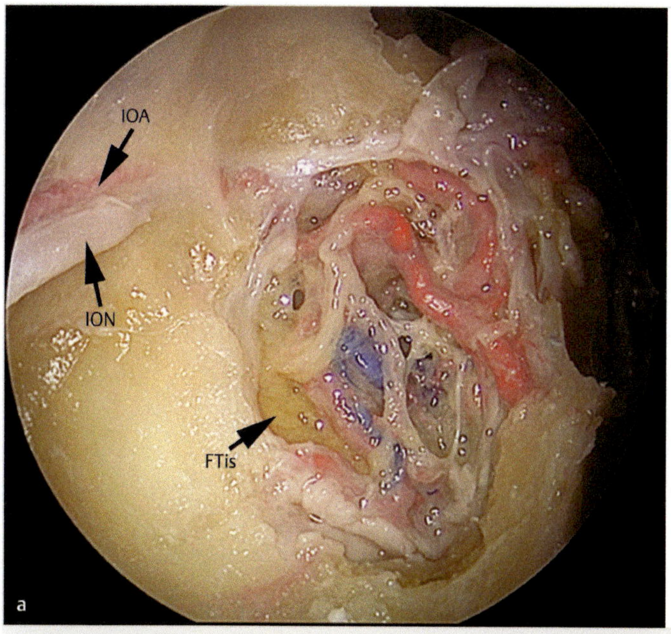

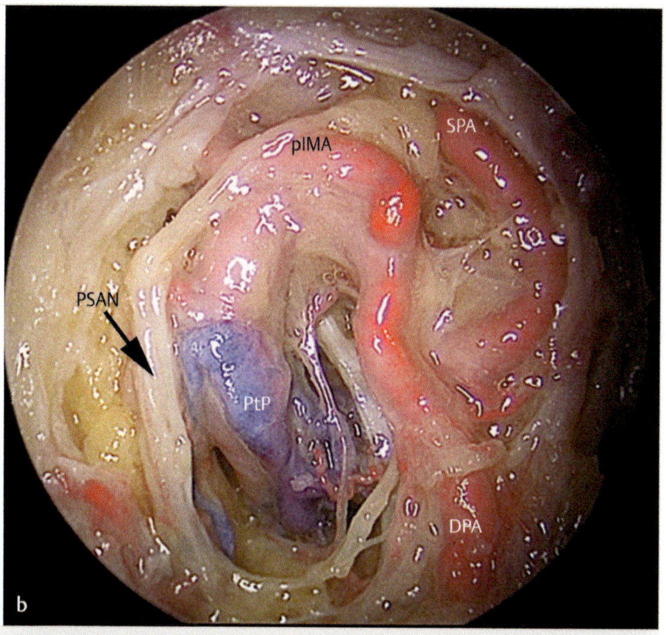

Fig. 15.15 (a, b) Step 4. The anterior periosteum of the pterygopalatine fossa is removed to identify the fat tissue (FTis) that fills this space and surrounds the neurovascular structures. The veins of this specimen were injected with blue silicon to show how the pterygoid plexus (PtP) also reaches the pterygopalatine fossa. The posterior superior alveolar nerve (PSAN), which can pass either anterior or posterior to the pterygopalatine tract of the internal maxillary artery (pIMA), is usually the first nerve that crosses diagonally the anterior portion of the pterygopalatine fossa. DPA, descending palatine artery; IOA, infraorbital artery; ION, infraorbital nerve; SPA, sphenopalatine artery.

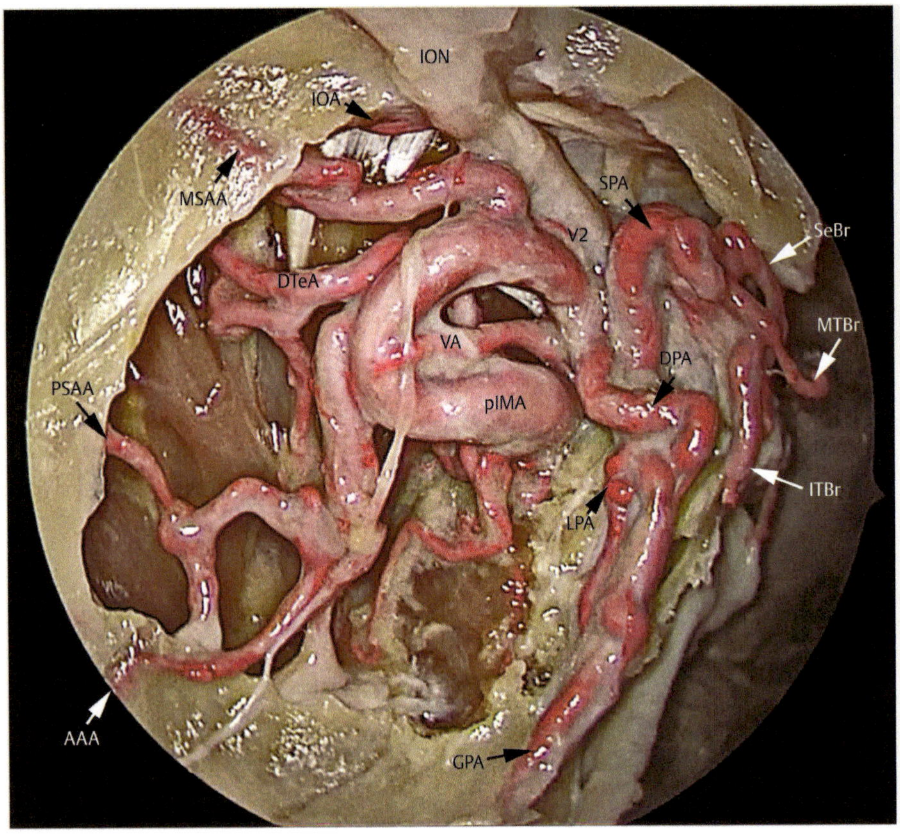

Fig. 15.16 Step 5. The fat tissue is removed to identify the anterior portion of the pterygopalatine fossa, which is also called the vascular compartment. The pterygopalatine tract of the internal maxillary artery (pIMA) ends with the sphenopalatine artery (SPA) and the descending palatine artery (DPA). The sphenopalatine artery divides into the septal branch (SeBr), the middle turbinate branch (MTBr), and the inferior turbinate branch (ITBr). The descending palatine artery divides into the lesser palatine artery (LPA) and the greater palatine artery (GPA). The internal maxillary artery also gives several collateral branches including the vidian artery (VA), infraorbital artery (IOA), deep temporal artery (DTeA), posterior superior alveolar artery (PSAA), and alveolar antral artery (AAA). The infraorbital artery gives origin to the middle superior alveolar artery (MSAA). The maxillary nerve (V2) lies above the last portion of the internal maxillary artery and continues into the infraorbital nerve (ION).

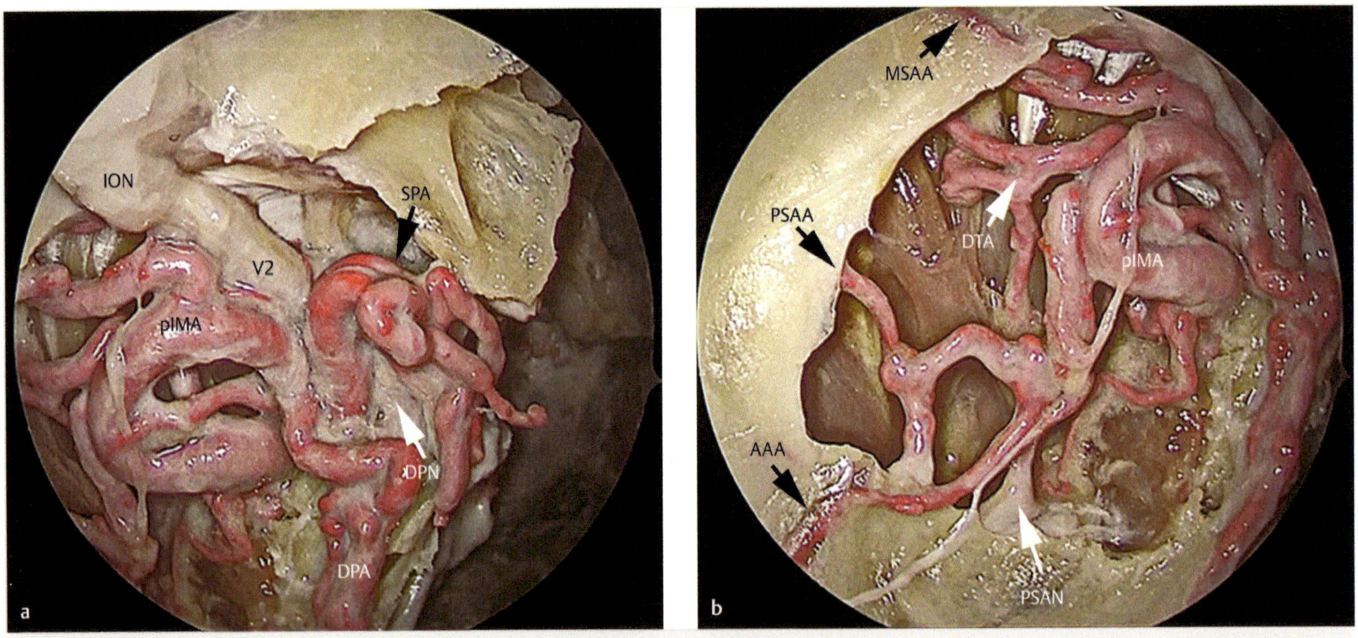

Fig. 15.17 (a, b) Vascular compartment. The bifurcation of the pterygopalatine tract of the internal maxillary artery (pIMA) lies in the superomedial portion of this region. The sphenopalatine artery (SPA) goes medially toward the sphenopalatine foramen, passing anteriorly and medially to the maxillary nerve (V2). The descending palatine artery (DPA) goes inferiorly toward the descending palatine canal, running anteriorly to the descending palatine nerve (DPN). Most of the collateral branches lie in the inferolateral portion of the pterygopalatine fossa. The posterior superior alveolar artery (PSAA) and the alveolar antral artery (AAA) run on the external and internal surfaces of the lateral maxillary wall, respectively. DTA, deep temporal artery; ION, infraorbital nerve; MSAA, middle superior alveolar artery; PSAN, posterior superior alveolar nerve.

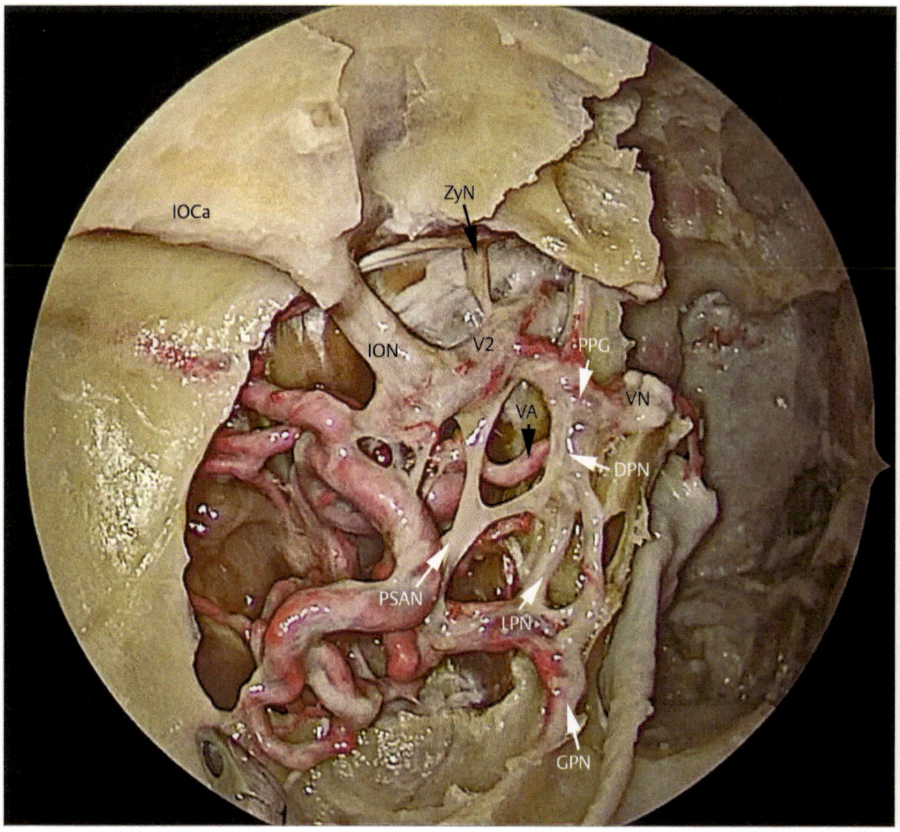

Fig. 15.18 Nervous compartment. Displacing anteriorly and inferiorly the internal maxillary artery, the nervous compartment comes into view. The maxillary nerve (V2) ends with the infraorbital nerve (ION), which enters the infraorbital canal (IOCa), and the descending palatine nerve (DPN), which further divides into the lesser palatine nerve (LPN) and the greater palatine nerve (GPN). The pterygopalatine ganglion (PPG), where the vidian nerve (VN) ends, is located in the superomedial portion of the pterygopalatine fossa. The vidian artery (VA), which arises at the junction between the infratemporal and the pterygopalatine tract of the internal maxillary artery, is the only artery of this region running across the nervous compartment to reach the vidian canal. The other main branches of the maxillary nerve are the zygomatic nerve (ZyN), which reaches the orbit through the inferior orbital fissure, and the posterior superior alveolar nerve (PSAN), which crosses in a diagonal fashion the vascular compartment.

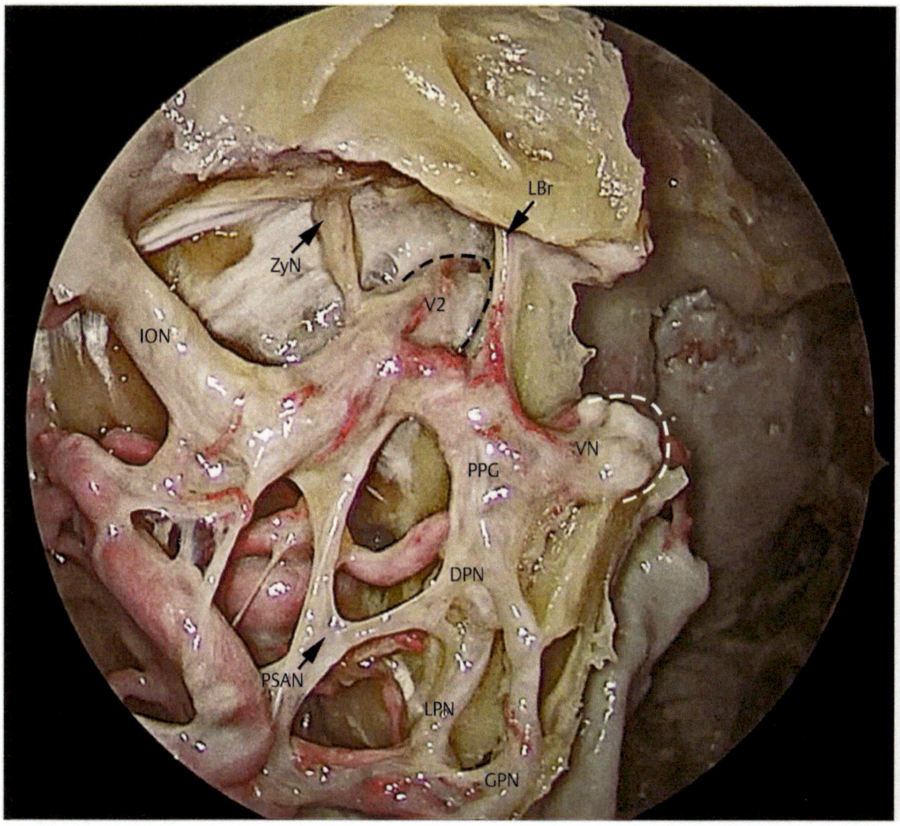

Fig. 15.19 The base of the pterygoid process. The base of the pterygoid process is a cuboid portion of the sphenoid bone that houses the vidian canal (*white dashed line*) inferomedially and the foramen rotundum (*black dashed line*) superolaterally. The vidian nerve (VN) and the maxillary nerve (V2) run in these bony canals, respectively. The VN ends into the pterygopalatine ganglion (PPG), which gives a lacrimal branch (LBr) fusing with the zygomatic nerve (ZyN) and provides the nerve supply for the lacrimal gland. Moreover, the pterygopalatine ganglion gives several branches to almost all the nerves of the pterygopalatine fossa. DPN, descending palatine nerve; GPN, greater palatine nerve; LPN, lesser palatine nerve; PSAN, posterior superior alveolar nerve.

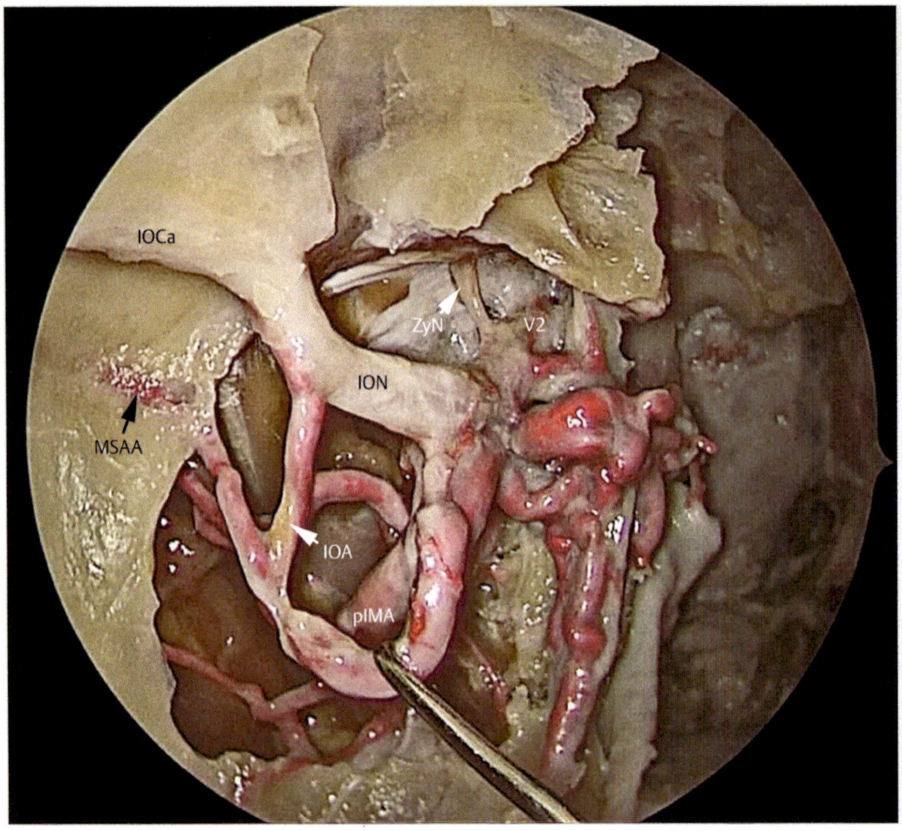

Fig. 15.20 The infraorbital nerve and the infraorbital artery. The infraorbital artery and the middle superior alveolar artery (MSAA) arise from a common branch of the pterygopalatine tract of the internal maxillary artery (pIMA). The infraorbital artery reaches the infraorbital nerve (ION) before its entrance into the infraorbital canal (IOCa). V2, maxillary nerve; ZyN, zygomatic nerve.

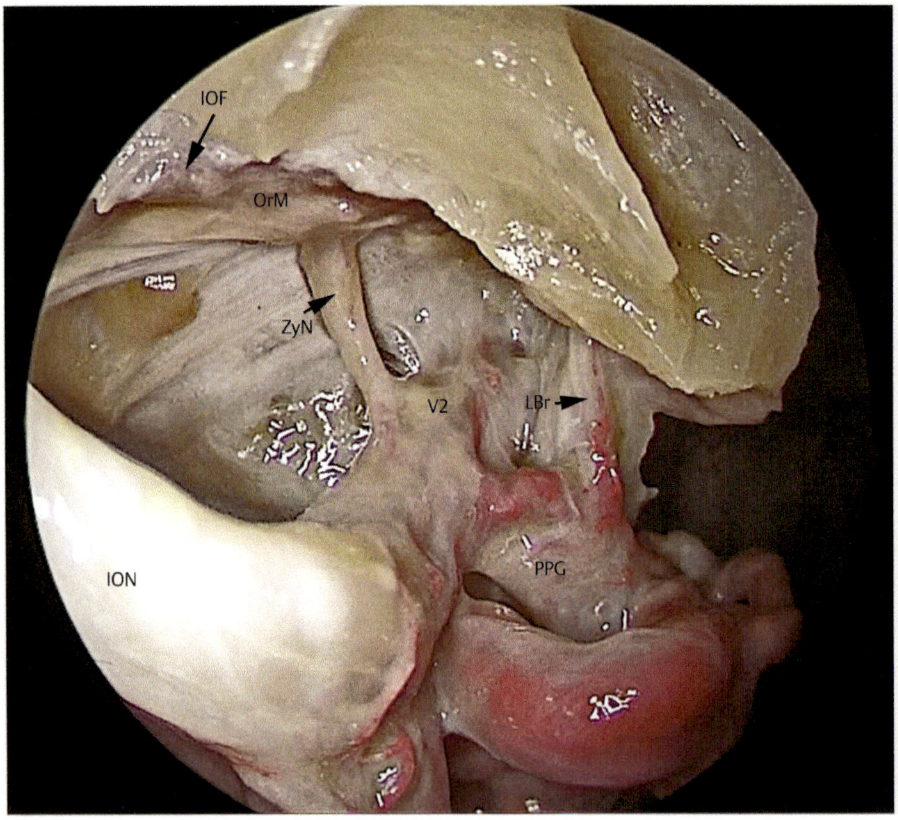

Fig. 15.21 The maxillary nerve. After passing through the foramen rotundum, the maxillary nerve (V2) gives off superiorly the zygomatic nerve (ZyN), which runs into the inferior orbital fissure (IOF) crossing the orbitalis muscle (OrM), also called Müller's muscle. The maxillary nerve runs within the pterygopalatine fossa with a bayonet shape and bifurcates into the infraorbital nerve (ION), which continues anteriorly, and the descending palatine nerve, which descends inferomedially. The pterygopalatine ganglion (PPG) lies medially to the maxillary nerve. LBr, lacrimal branch of the pterygopalatine ganglion.

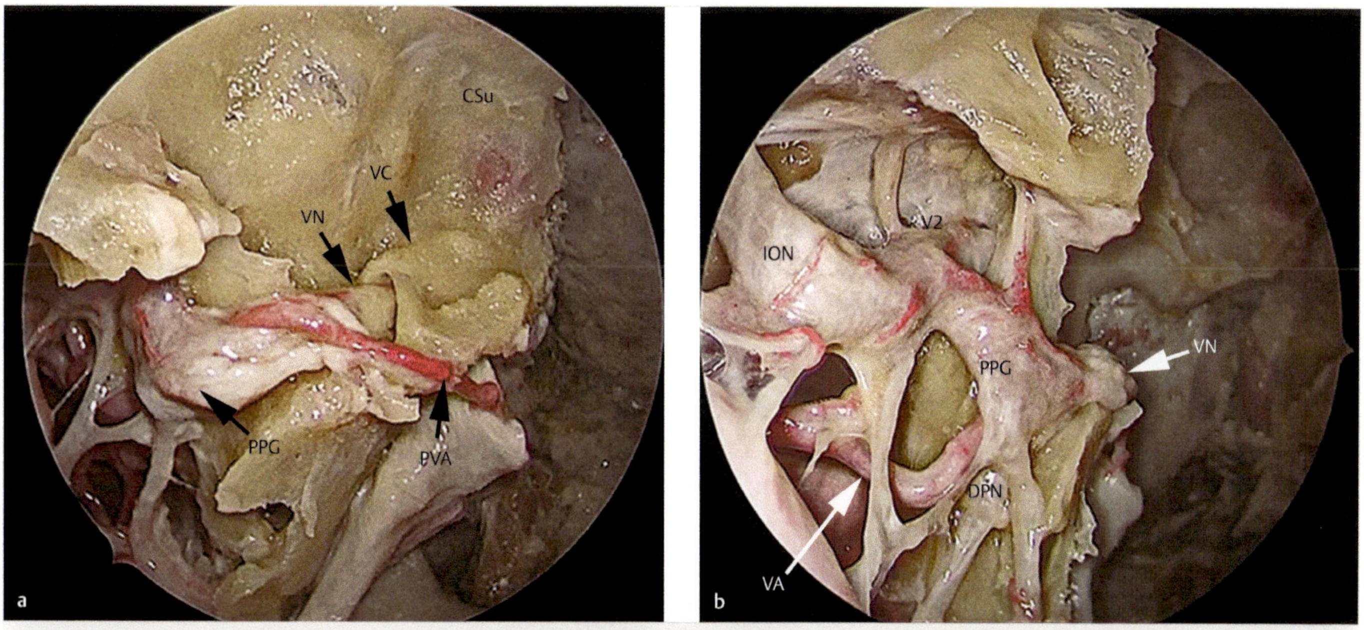

Fig. 15.22 (a, b) The vidian nerve. The vidian nerve (VN) is visualized with a 70-degree scope turned inferolaterally (left image) and a 0-degree scope centered on the pterygopalatine ganglion (PPG) (right image). The vidian nerve runs within the vidian canal (VC), which begins at the inferior portion of the carotid sulcus (CSu), along the anterior edge of the foramen lacerum. For this reason, the vidian nerve and its canal are used as a landmark toward the anterior genu between the petrous and the paraclival tract of the internal carotid artery. The palatovaginal artery (PVA) is a collateral branch of the vidian artery that runs in the sulcus in between the perpendicular portion of the palatine bone and the vaginal process of the sphenoid bone, called palatovaginal canal. The maxillary nerve (V2) runs from Meckel's cave to the pterygopalatine fossa within the foramen rotundum, which has a slightly different direction compared to the vidian canal: the former runs from posterolateral to anteromedial, and the latter from posteromedial to anterolateral. DPN, descending palatine nerve; ION, infraorbital nerve; PPG, pterygopalatine ganglion.

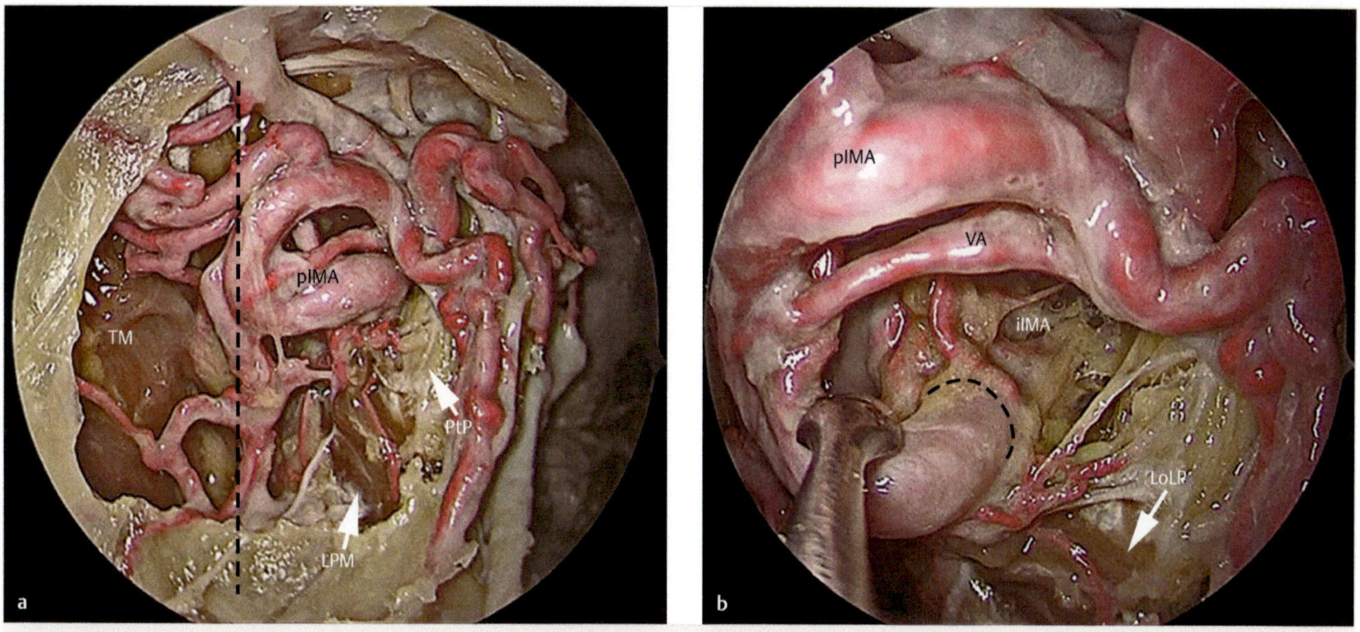

Fig. 15.23 (a, b) The internal maxillary artery. The pterygopalatine tract of the internal maxillary artery (pIMA) lies medially to the inferior projection of the posterior end of the infraorbital canal (*vertical black dashed line*). The deep muscular boundary of this area is formed by the temporal muscle (TM) laterally and the lateral pterygoid muscle (LPM) medially. The limit (*curved black dashed line*) between the infratemporal tract of the internal maxillary artery (iIMA) and the pterygopalatine tract of the internal maxillary artery is found above the lower head of the lateral pterygoid muscle (LoLP). The vidian artery (VA) arises a few millimeters after this point and runs horizontally toward the base of the pterygoid process. PtP, pterygoid process.

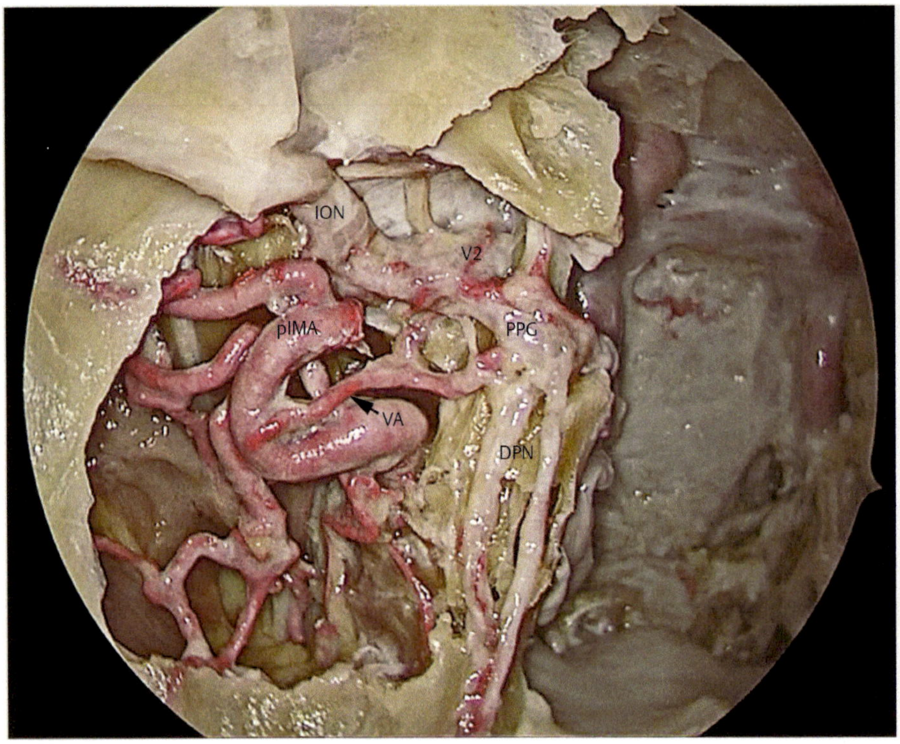

Fig. 15.24 Step 6 (part 1). The distal portion of the pterygopalatine tract of the internal maxillary artery (pIMA) is removed to completely expose the nervous compartment. V2, maxillary nerve; DPN, descending palatine artery; ION, infraorbital nerve; PPG, pterygopalatine nerve; VA, vidian artery.

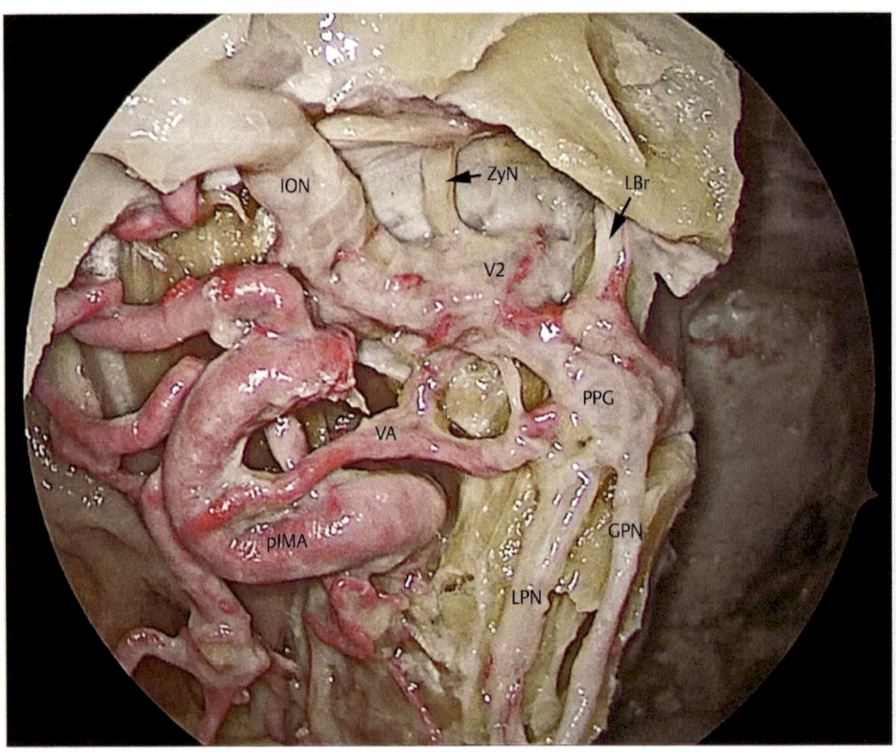

Fig. 15.25 Step 6 (part 2). The maxillary nerve (V2) continues into the infraorbital nerve (ION) via a bayonet-shape tract into the upper portion of the pterygopalatine fossa. The lesser palatine nerve (LPN) and the greater palatine nerve (GPN) arise from the maxillary nerve with a perpendicular descending trajectory. LBr, lacrimal branch of the pterygopalatine ganglion; pIMA, pterygopalatine tract of the internal maxillary artery; PPG, pterygopalatine ganglion; VA, vidian artery; ZyN, zygomatic nerve.

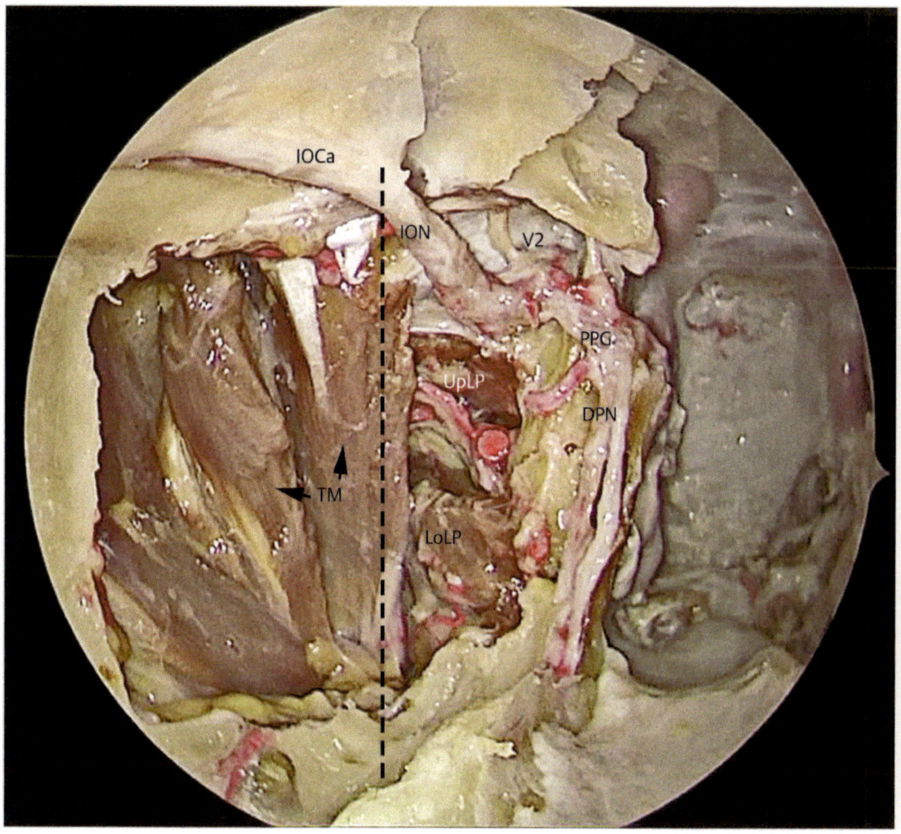

Fig. 15.26 Step 7. The remaining portion of the vascular compartment is removed to entirely expose the muscular plane. The temporal muscle (TM) lies laterally to the inferior projection (*black dashed line*) of the posterior end of the infraorbital canal (IOCa). The lateral pterygoid muscle, which is formed by the upper (UpLP) and lower (LoLP) heads, lies medially to the above-mentioned projection. V2, maxillary nerve; DPN, descending palatine nerve; ION, infraorbital nerve; PPG, pterygopalatine ganglion.

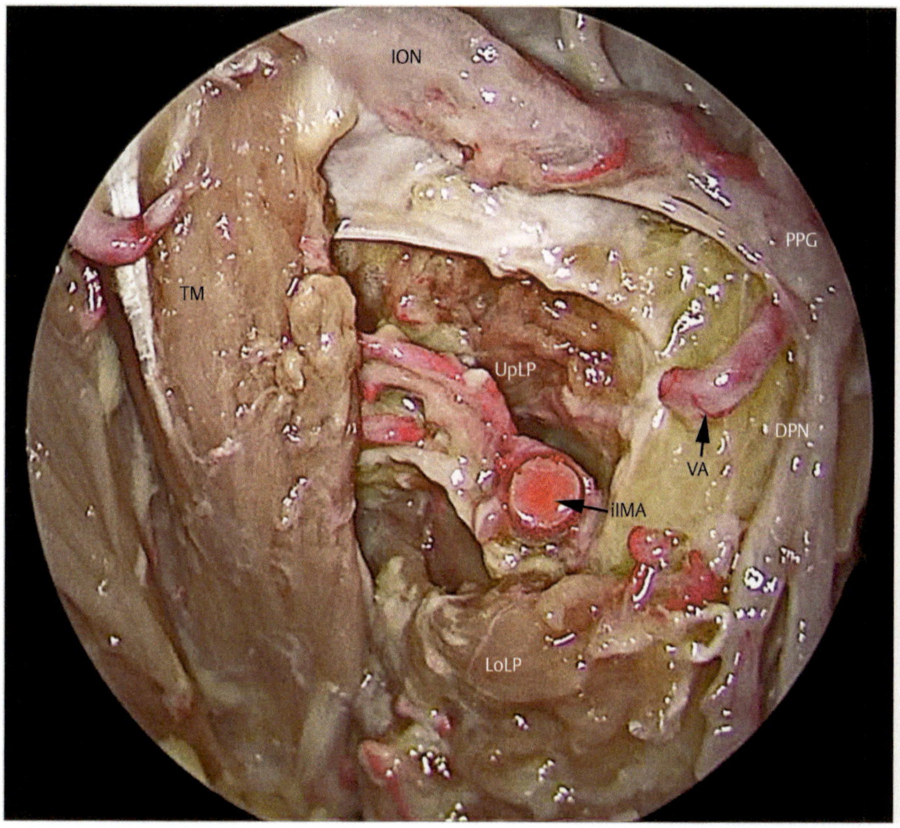

Fig. 15.27 Access to the infratemporal fossa. The infratemporal tract of the internal maxillary artery (iIMA) passes through a squared window that is formed by the descending palatine nerve (DPN) and the pterygoid process medially, the temporal muscle (TM) laterally, the infraorbital nerve (ION) and the upper head of the lateral pterygoid muscle (UpLP) superiorly, and the lower head of the lateral pterygoid muscle (LoLP) inferiorly. PPG, pterygopalatine ganglion; VA, vidian artery.

References

[1] Bertazzoni G, Schreiber A, Ferrari M, et al. Contemporary management of juvenile angiofibroma. Curr Opin Otolaryngol Head Neck Surg 2018

[2] Langdon C, Herman P, Verillaud B, et al. Expanded endoscopic endonasal surgery for advanced stage juvenile angiofibromas: a retrospective multi-center study. Rhinology 2016;54(3):239–246

[3] Karligkiotis A, Turri-Zanoni M, Sica E, et al. Role of endoscopic surgery in the management of sinonasal and skull base schwannomas. Head Neck 2016;38(Suppl 1):E2074–E2082

[4] Shi J, Chen J, Chen T, et al. Neuroendoscopic resection of trigeminal schwannoma in the pterygopalatine/infratemporal fossa via the transnasal perpendicular plate palatine bone or transnasal maxillary sinus approach. World Neurosurg 2018;120:e1011–e1016

[5] Yang L, Hu L, Zhao W, Zhang H, Liu Q, Wang D. Endoscopic endonasal approach for trigeminal schwannomas: our experience of 39 patients in 10 years. Eur Arch Otorhinolaryngol 2018;275(3):735–741

[6] Zhou B, Huang Q, Shen PH, et al. The intranasal endoscopic removal of schwannoma of the pterygopalatine and infratemporal fossae via the prelacrimal recess approach. J Neurosurg 2016;124(4):1068–1073

[7] Battaglia P, Turri-Zanoni M, Lepera D, et al. Endoscopic transnasal approaches to pterygopalatine fossa tumors. Head Neck 2016;38(Suppl 1):E214–E220

[8] Elhadi AM, Zaidi HA, Yagmurlu K, et al. Infraorbital nerve: a surgically relevant landmark for the pterygopalatine fossa, cavernous sinus, and anterolateral skull base in endoscopic transmaxillary approaches. J Neurosurg 2016;125(6):1460–1468

16 Infratemporal Fossa Approach

Alberto Schreiber, Marco Ravanelli, Marco Ferrari, Vittorio Rampinelli

The infratemporal fossa is a deep space of the upper neck that lies inferiorly to the middle cranial fossa, medially, and the zygomatic arch and temporal fossa, laterally. It is bounded by the posterolateral maxillary wall (also called maxillary tuberosity) anteriorly, the greater wing of the sphenoid bone and squamous portion of the temporal bone superiorly, the lateral pterygoid plate medially, the mandibular ramus laterally, and the upper parapharyngeal space posteriorly. Inferiorly, the infratemporal fossa narrows progressively and ends at the medial surface of the mandibular angle, following the direction of the medial pterygoid muscle. The masticatory space, which is the space including the masticatory muscles, is enveloped in the doubling of the superficial sheet of the deep cervical fascia in the masseteric and deep temporal fascial laterally, and the interpterygoid fascia medially. Consequently, the infratemporal fossa contains the deep portion of the masticatory space, which includes the pterygoid muscles, and the caudal portion of the temporal muscle along with several neurovascular structures. The infratemporal fossa communicates medially with the pterygopalatine fossa through the pterygomaxillary fissure, which is in continuity with the inferior orbital fissure, cranially.[1,2]

Several lesions can primarily originate in the infratemporal fossa, which can also be invaded by tumors arising from contiguous compartments (i.e., parapharyngeal space, sinonasal tract, skull base). Primary lesions can have either a slow, expansive pattern of growth (e.g., schwannomas and juvenile angiofibromas) or an aggressive, infiltrative behavior like malignant tumors (e.g., adenoid cystic carcinomas, adenocarcinomas, chondrosarcomas, and soft-tissue sarcomas).[3] The transnasal endoscopic infratemporal fossa approach has been employed as sole access or in combination with other transnasal or extranasal corridors to manage juvenile angiofibromas,[4–6] schwannomas,[4,5,7–9] maxillary/nasopharyngeal tumors with posterolateral extension,[4,5,10] meningiomas,[4,11] and other rare lesions affecting the retromaxillary areas.[4,5]

The first step of the transnasal endoscopic approach to infratemporal fossa consists of exposing the posterolateral wall of the maxillary sinus. To obtain an adequate exposure of the retromaxillary areas, an endoscopic medial maxillectomy, which is detailed in Chapter 5, is therefore required. The removal of structures making up the medial and anterior maxillary walls can be modulated based on the need for mediolateral and craniocaudal exposure.[12] Performing posterior septectomy or creating a transseptal window can be of some use when approaching the infratemporal fossa, enabling a diagonal trajectory of dissection that facilitates the exposure of far lateral structures.[13–15] A thorough knowledge of bony landmarks within the maxillary sinus is of utmost importance to adequately tailor the removal of the posterolateral bony wall. In particular, the

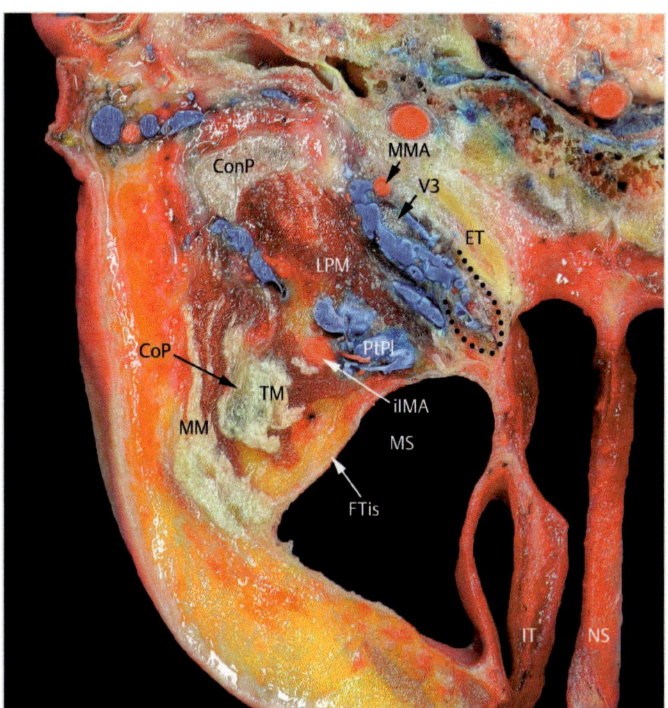

Fig. 16.1 Axial view of the infratemporal fossa. This axial cadaver cut shows the content of the infratemporal fossa and its relationship with the maxillary sinus (MS). V3, mandibular nerve; ConP, condylar process of the mandible; CoP, coronoid process of the mandible; ET, eustachian tube; FTis, fat tissue; iIMA, infratemporal tract of the internal maxillary artery; LPM, lateral pterygoid muscle; MM, masseter muscle; MMA, middle meningeal artery; PtPl, pterygoid plexus; TM, temporal muscle. (*Black dotted line*, pterygoid plates.)

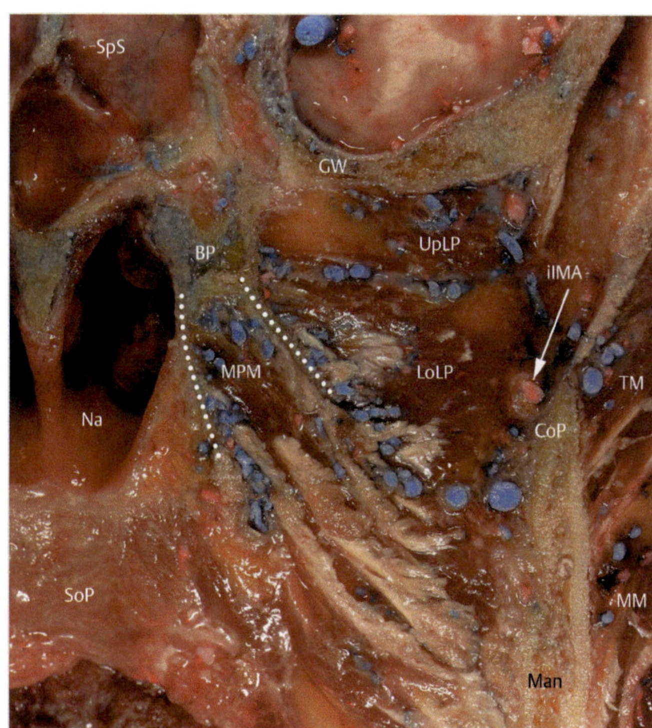

Fig. 16.2 Coronal view of the infratemporal fossa. This coronal cadaver cut shows the content of the infratemporal fossa. BP, base of the pterygoid process; CoP, coronoid process of the mandible; GW, greater wing of the sphenoid bone; iIMA, infratemporal tract of the internal maxillary artery; LoLP, lower head of the lateral pterygoid muscle; Man, mandible (ramus); MM, masseteric muscle; MPM, medial pterygoid muscle; Na, nasopharynx; SoP, soft palate; SpS, sphenoid sinus; TM, temporal muscle; UpLP, upper head of the lateral pterygoid muscle. (*White dotted lines*, pterygoid plates.)

infraorbital nerve can be adopted as the main reference to guide the resection of the posterolateral wall. The cross that is formed by the horizontal line parallel to the infraorbital canal and the vertical line passing at the posterior end of the canal can be used to schematize transmaxillary approaches. Considering this imaginary landmark, the lower lateral quadrant can be considered the door toward the infratemporal fossa, while the upper medial, lower medial, and upper lateral quadrants lead to the middle cranial fossa, pterygopalatine fossa, and orbital cavity, respectively.

In this chapter, three corridors of dissection within the infratemporal fossa are presented.[16] The first (lateral) corridor exposes the coronoid process, passing through the temporal muscle. The second (middle) corridor reaches the anterior aspect of the temporomandibular joint exploiting the connective space between the temporal and lateral pterygoid muscles, where the internal maxillary artery runs. The third (medial) corridor exposes the mandibular nerve, middle meningeal artery, and the posterior aspect of the temporomandibular joint via the space that is obtained detaching the lateral pterygoid muscle from the lateral pterygoid plate. Therefore, the most important structure that guides the dissection through the infratemporal fossa is the lateral pterygoid muscle, whose medial and lateral surfaces lead to the most important neurovascular structures of this area.

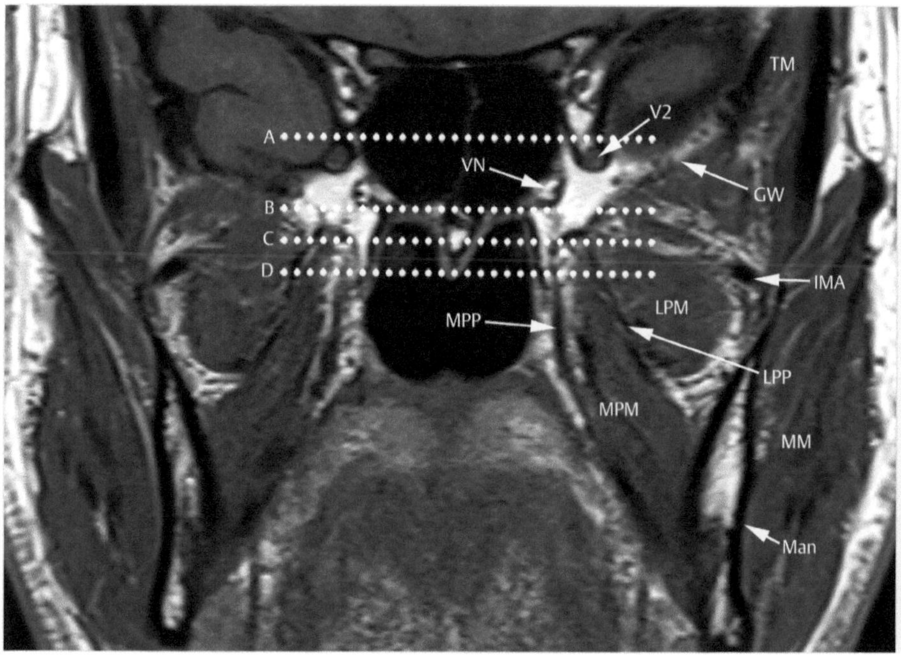

Fig. 16.3 Coronal MRI anatomy of the infratemporal fossa. This T1-weighted MRI coronal image passing through the pterygoid process shows an overview of the anatomy of the infratemporal fossa and depicts the position of images composing ▶Fig. 16.4 and ▶Fig. 16.5 with *white dotted lines* (A–D). The infratemporal fossa lies below the greater wing of the sphenoid bone (GW) and medial to the mandible (Man). It corresponds to the deep portion of the masticatory space and includes the medial pterygoid muscle (MPM) and the lateral pterygoid muscle (LPM) along with the caudal insertion of the temporal muscle (TM). On the contrary, the masseter muscle (MM) lies lateral to the mandible. The queen vascular structure of the infratemporal fossa is the internal maxillary artery (IMA), which runs from posterolateral to anteromedial and reaches the pterygopalatine fossa. V2, maxillary nerve; LPP, lateral pterygoid plate; MPP, medial pterygoid plate; VN, vidian nerve.

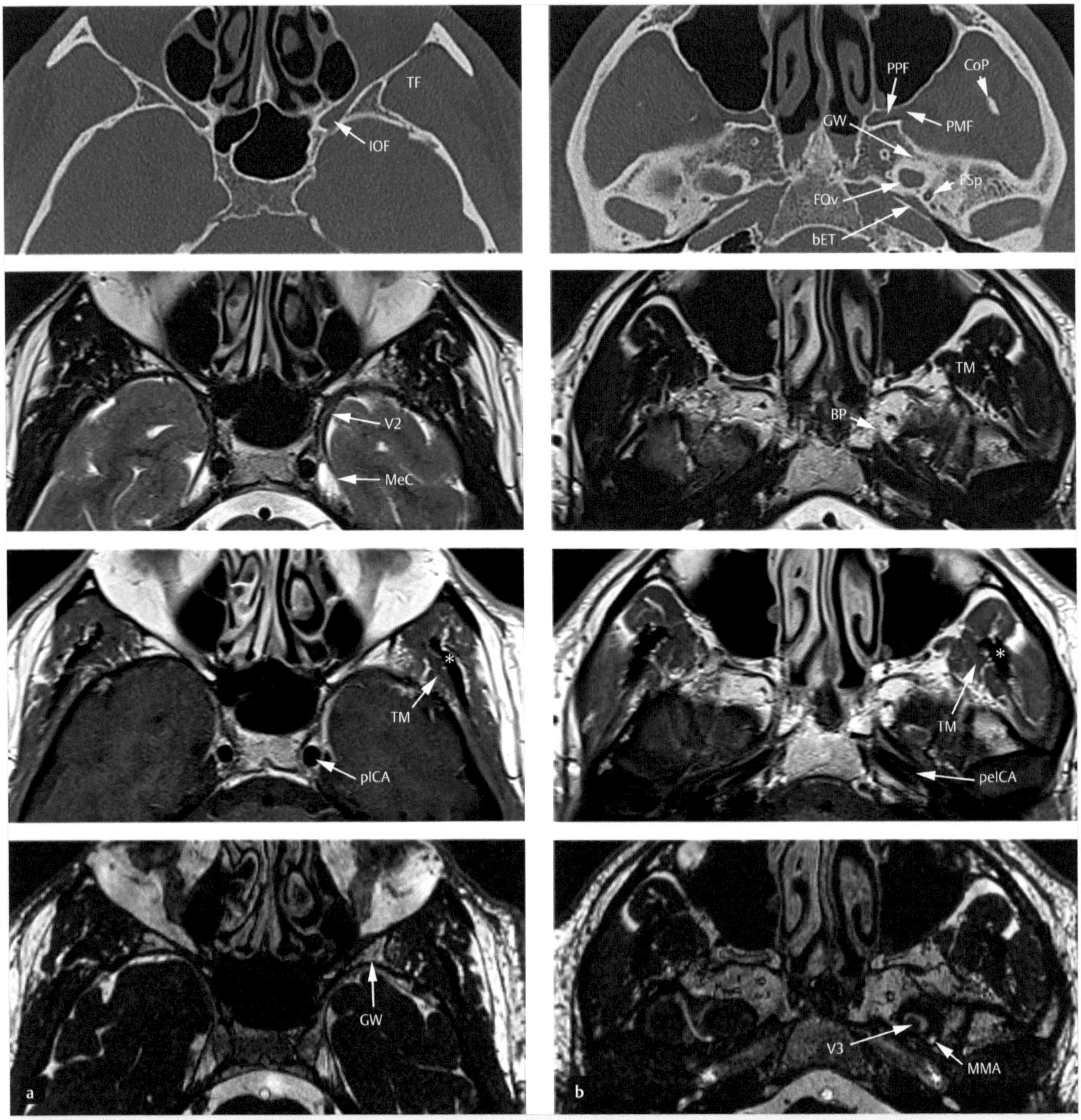

Fig. 16.4 Axial anatomy of the infratemporal fossa (part 1). The panel includes, from above to below, CT, T2-weighted, contrast-enhanced T1-weighted, and contrast-enhanced CISS (constructive interference in steady state) MRI axial images passing through the infratemporal fossa. The planes of images of columns a and b are depicted in ▶Fig. 16.3. The infratemporal fossa lies inferior to both the skull base, medially, and the temporal fossa (TF), laterally. The bony roof of the medial portion of the infratemporal fossa consists of the horizontal portion of the greater wing of the sphenoid bone (GW). This bony structure includes the foramina ovale (FOv) and spinosum (FSp), where the mandibular nerve (V3) and middle meningeal artery (MMA) cross the skull base, and includes also a vertical part separating the middle cranial fossa, orbital cavity, and temporal fossa. Both the foramina are located anterior to the bony portion of the eustachian tube (bET) and petrous tract of the internal carotid artery (peICA). The infratemporal fossa continues into the pterygopalatine fossa (PPF) through the pterygomaxillary fissure (PMF). The lateral portion of the infratemporal fossa houses the temporal muscle (TM), which consists of several muscular fibers reaching a single, central tendinous structure (*white asterisk*). V2, maxillary nerve; BaP, base of the pterygoid process; CoP, condylar process; IOF, inferior orbital fissure; MeC, Meckel's cave; pICA, paraclival tract of the internal carotid artery.

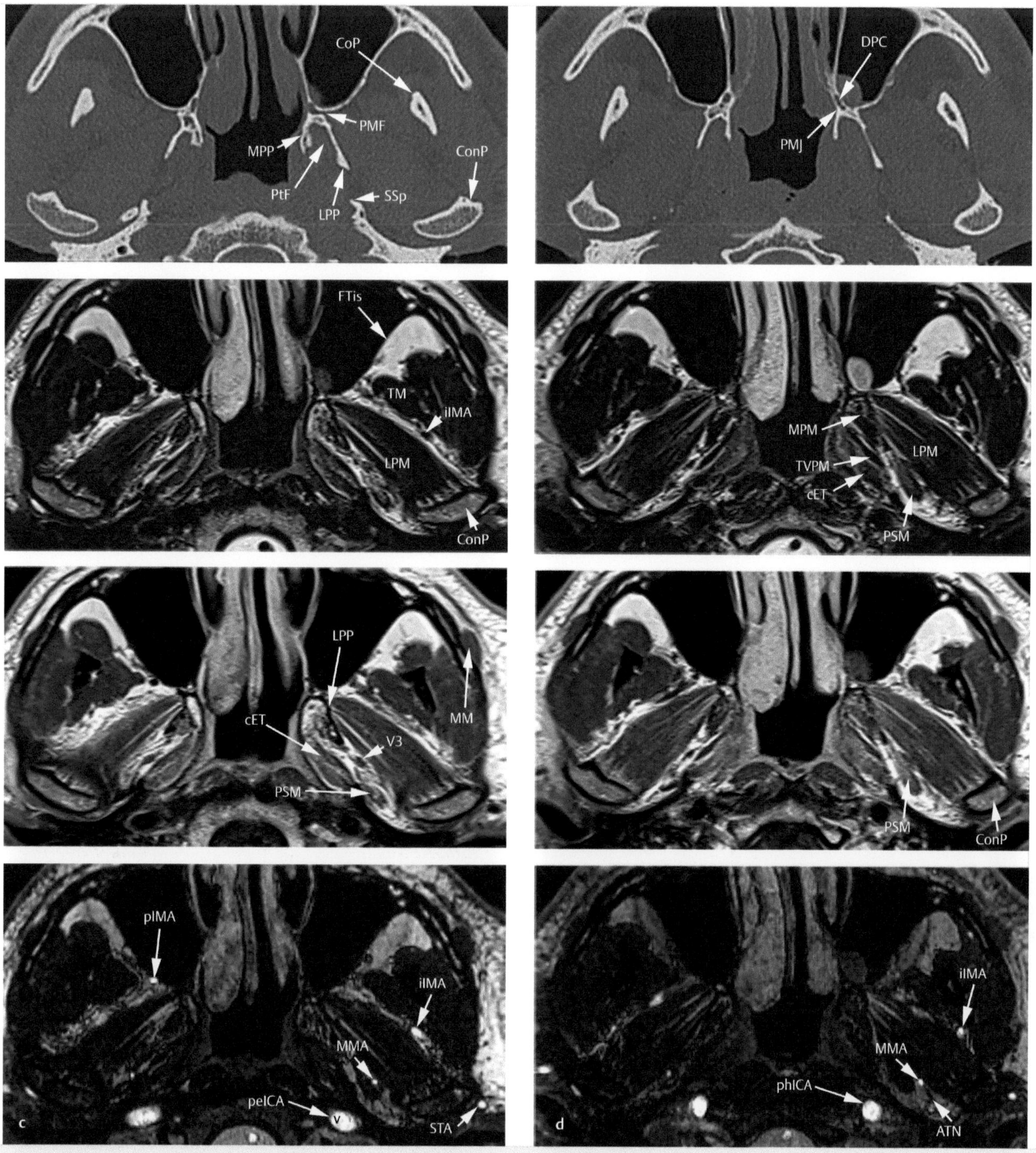

Fig. 16.5 Axial anatomy of the infratemporal fossa (part 2). The panel includes, from above to below, CT, T2-weighted, contrast-enhanced T1-weighted, and contrast-enhanced CISS (constructive interference in steady state) MRI axial images passing through the infratemporal fossa. The planes of images of columns c and d are depicted in ▶Fig. 16.3. The lateral pterygoid muscle (LPM) and the medial pterygoid muscle (MPM) lie caudally to the greater wing of the sphenoid bone and base of the pterygoid process, respectively. The lateral pterygoid muscle has a horizontal trajectory, from the lateral pterygoid plate (LPP) and greater wing of the sphenoid, anteromedially, to the condylar process (ConP) of the mandible and articular disk of the temporomandibular joint, posterolaterally. The medial pterygoid muscle has a more vertical orientation (from cranial-medial to caudal-lateral), from the pterygoid fossa (PfF), superomedially, to the inner surface of the mandibular angle, inferolaterally. These axial images summarize the three main corridors of the transnasal infratemporal approach through the posterolateral maxillary wall. The first corridor is directed toward the coronoid process of the mandible (CoP) and passes through a thick layer of fat tissue (FTis) of the infratemporal fossa. The second corridor lies between the temporal muscle (TM) and the lateral pterygoid muscle; this pathway follows the course of the infratemporal tract of the internal maxillary artery (iIMA) and guides toward the anteromedial aspect of the temporomandibular joint. The third corridor is located on the posterolateral surface of the lateral pterygoid muscle and follows the direction of the lateral pterygoid plate; this trajectory is directed toward the posteromedial aspect of the temporomandibular joint and crosses the mandibular nerve (V3), its branches, and the middle meningeal artery (MMA). In this case, an anatomical variant was present on the left side: the pterygospinosus muscle (PSM) can be found between the spina sphenoidalis (SSp) and the lateral pterygoid plate. This structure can also be identified as ligamentous or ossified (Civinini's bar) and usually separates the anterior and posterior divisions of the mandibular nerve. ATN, auriculotemporal nerve; cET, cartilaginous portion of the eustachian tube; DPC, descending palatine canal; MM, masseter muscle; MPP, medial pterygoid plate; peICA, petrous tract of the internal carotid artery; phICA, parapharyngeal tract of the internal carotid artery; pIMA, pterygopalatine tract of the internal maxillary artery; PMF, pterygomaxillary fissure; PMJ, pterygomaxillary junction; STA, superficial temporal artery; TVPM, tensor veli palatini muscle; v, vertical portion of the petrous internal carotid artery.

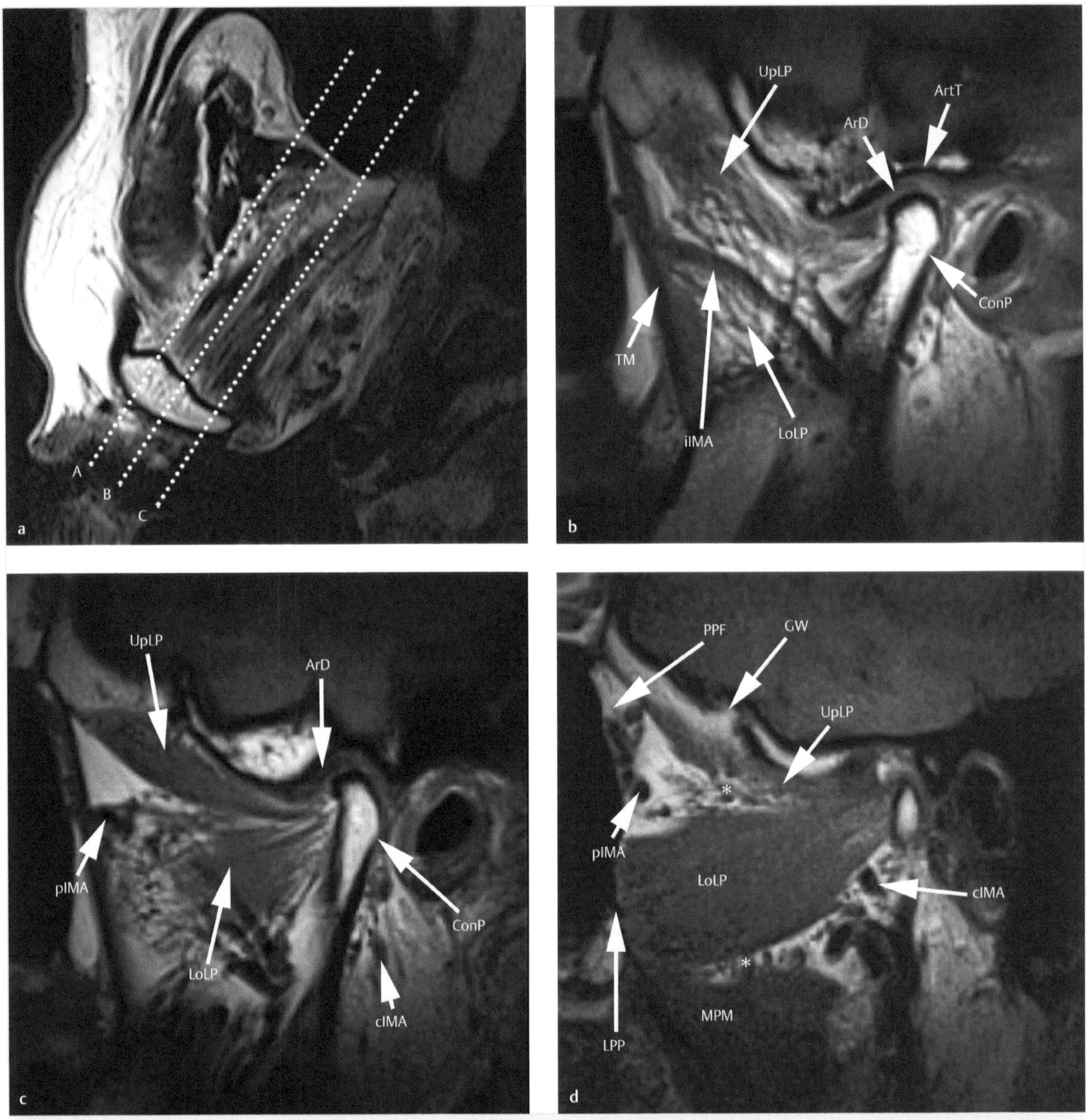

Fig. 16.6 Parasagittal anatomy of the infratemporal fossa and the temporomandibular joint. The panel includes an axial image **(a)** depicting the position of three parasagittal T1-weighted MRI images **(b–d)**. The internal maxillary artery has three tracts: the condylar tract (cIMA) crosses the posterior aspect of the condylar process (ConP) of the mandible; the infratemporal tract runs on the lateral surface of the lateral pterygoid muscle and then passes between its upper (UpLP) and lower (LoLP) bellies; the pterygopalatine tract (pIMA) enters the pterygomaxillary fissure and runs into the pterygopalatine fossa (PPF). The upper belly of the lateral pterygoid muscle inserts on the greater wing of the sphenoid bone (GW), anteromedially, and onto the articular disk (ArD) of the temporomandibular joint, posterolaterally. The lower belly of the same muscle is attached to the lateral pterygoid plate (LPP), anteromedially, and the condylar process of the mandible, posterolaterally. Notably, the lateral pterygoid muscle is entirely surrounded by the pterygoid venous plexus (*white asterisks*), which fills the adipose portions of the infratemporal fossa. ArtT, articular tubercle of the temporal bone; TM, temporal muscle.

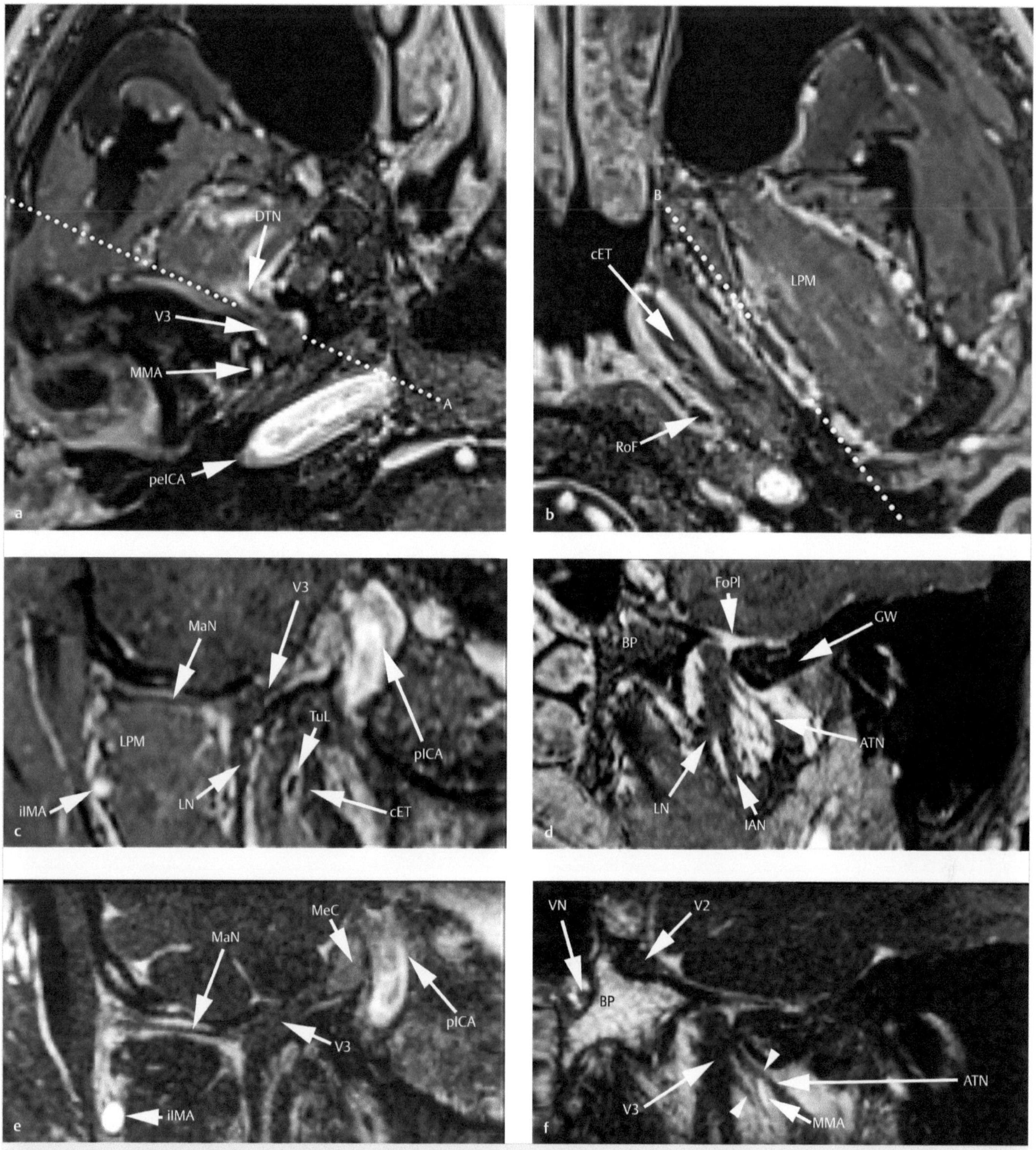

Fig. 16.7 (a–f) MRI anatomy of the mandibular nerve. The panel includes two axial images **(a, b)** depicting the position of two couples of paracoronal (A) and parasagittal (B) contrast-enhanced, fat-suppressed T1-weighted and contrast-enhanced CISS (constructive interference in steady state) MRI images. The anterior division of the mandibular nerve (V3) includes several motor branches and one sensitive branch, which is the buccal nerve. Among the motor branches, the masseteric nerve (MaN) runs parallel to the skull base and passes through the mandibular notch to provide the nerve supply for the masseter muscle. The posterior division of the mandibular nerve mostly consists of sensitive branches, with the exception of the mylohyoid nerve. The lingual nerve (LN) and inferior alveolar nerve (IAN) run in a vertical fashion and are surrounded by the foraminal plexus (FoPl) and pterygoid plexus in their upper portion. The auriculotemporal nerve (ATN) runs with a posterolateral direction crossing the middle meningeal artery (MMA) and sometimes forming a loop around the vessel (*white arrowheads*), as in the present case. V2, maxillary nerve; BP, base of the pterygoid process; cET, cartilaginous portion of the eustachian tube; GW, greater wing of the sphenoid bone; iIMA, infratemporal tract of the internal carotid artery; LPM, lateral pterygoid muscle; MeC, Meckel's cave; peICA, petrous tract of the internal carotid artery; pICA, paraclival tract of the internal carotid artery; TuL, tubal lumen.

Endoscopic Dissection

Nasal Phase

- Vertical and horizontal uncinectomy.
- Type C or D endoscopic medial maxillectomy.
- Facultative: Middle turbinectomy.
- Facultative: Septectomy.

Skull Base Phase

- Step 1: Removal of the posterolateral wall of the maxillary sinus.
- Step 2: Removal of the fat tissue of the infratemporal fossa.
- Step 3: Exposure of the coronoid process (first corridor).
- Step 4: Dissection between the temporal muscle and the lateral pterygoid muscle (second corridor).
- Step 5: Dissection between the lateral pterygoid muscle and the lateral pterygoid plate (third corridor).
- Step 6: Removal of the upper head of the lateral pterygoid muscle.
- Step 7: Removal of the lower head of the lateral pterygoid muscle.
- Step 8: Removal of the insertion of the lower head of the lateral pterygoid muscle.
- Step 9: Removal of the insertion of the upper head of the lateral pterygoid muscle.

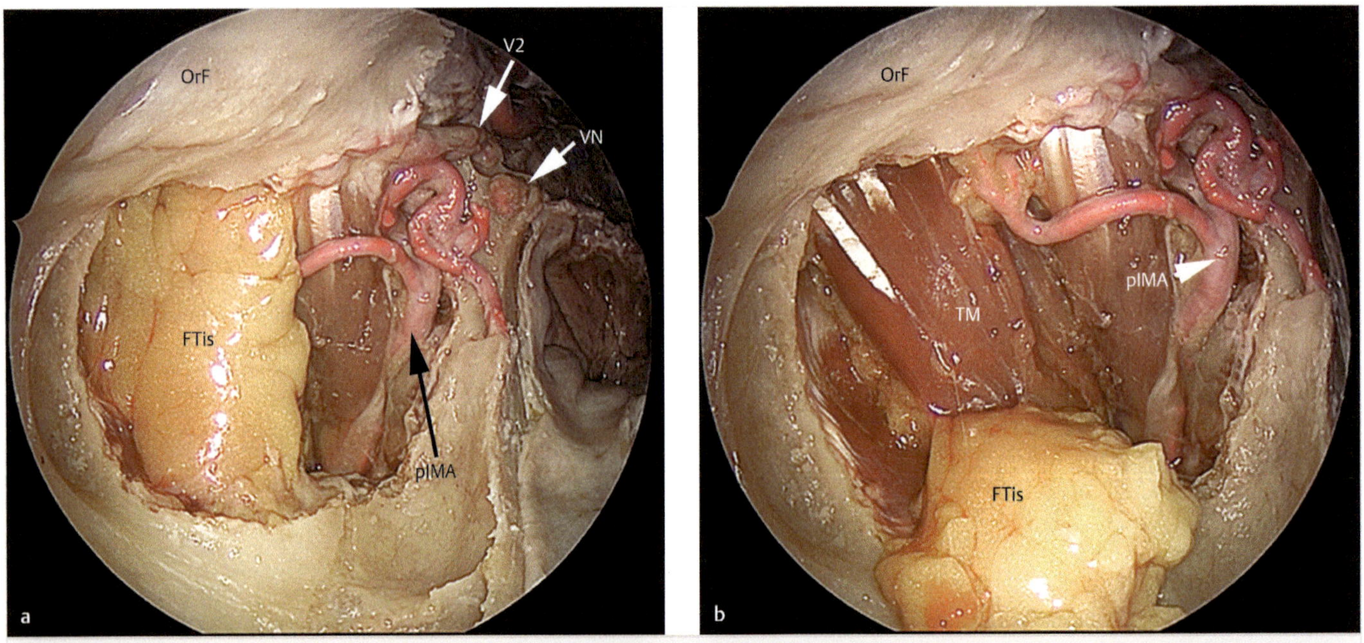

Fig. 16.8 (a, b) Steps 1 and 2. The posterolateral wall of the maxillary sinus is removed up to the orbital floor (OrF), superiorly, and the alveolar recess, inferiorly. In this way, the pterygopalatine and infratemporal fossae are exposed. After removing the periosteum and fat of the pterygopalatine fossa, the thick layer of fat tissue (FTis) of the infratemporal fossa is detached from the temporal muscle (TM). V2, maxillary nerve; pIMA, pterygopalatine tract of the internal maxillary artery; VN, vidian nerve.

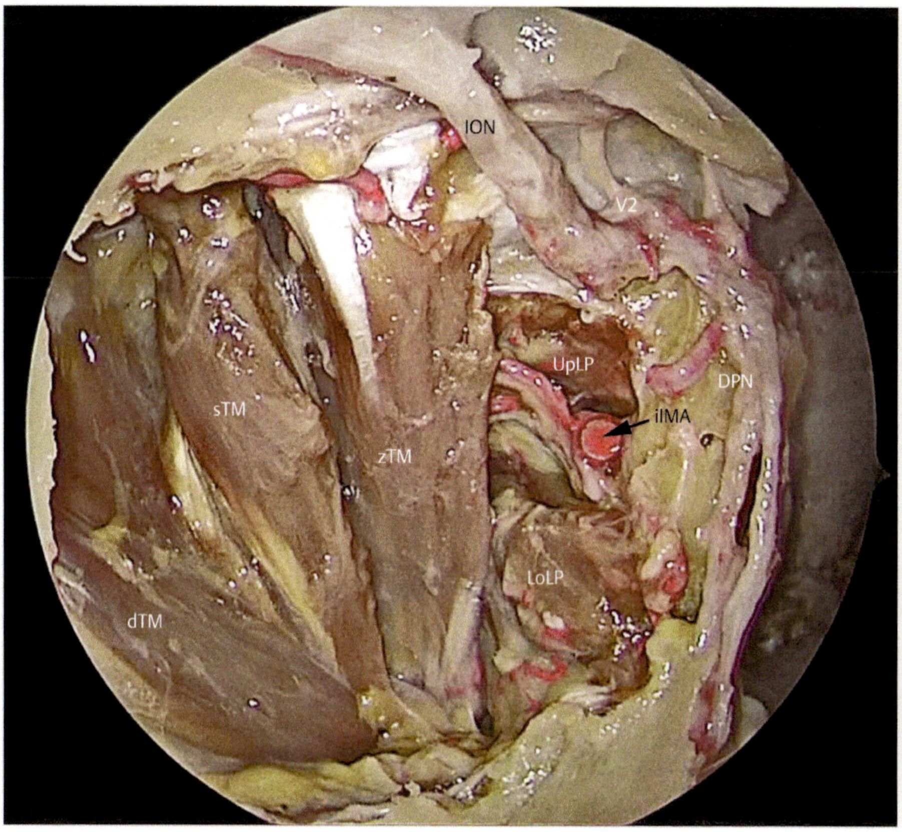

Fig. 16.9 The temporal muscle. The temporal muscle is formed by three portions: the deep portion (dTM) arises from the central part of the temporal fossa, the superficial portion (sTM) from the peripheral part, and the zygomatic part (zTM) from the inferomedial surface of the zygomatic arch and the greater sphenoidal wing. V2, maxillary nerve; DPN, descending palatine artery; iIMA, infratemporal tract of the internal maxillary artery; ION, infraorbital nerve; LoLP, lower head of the lateral pterygoid muscle; UpLP, upper head of the lateral pterygoid muscle.

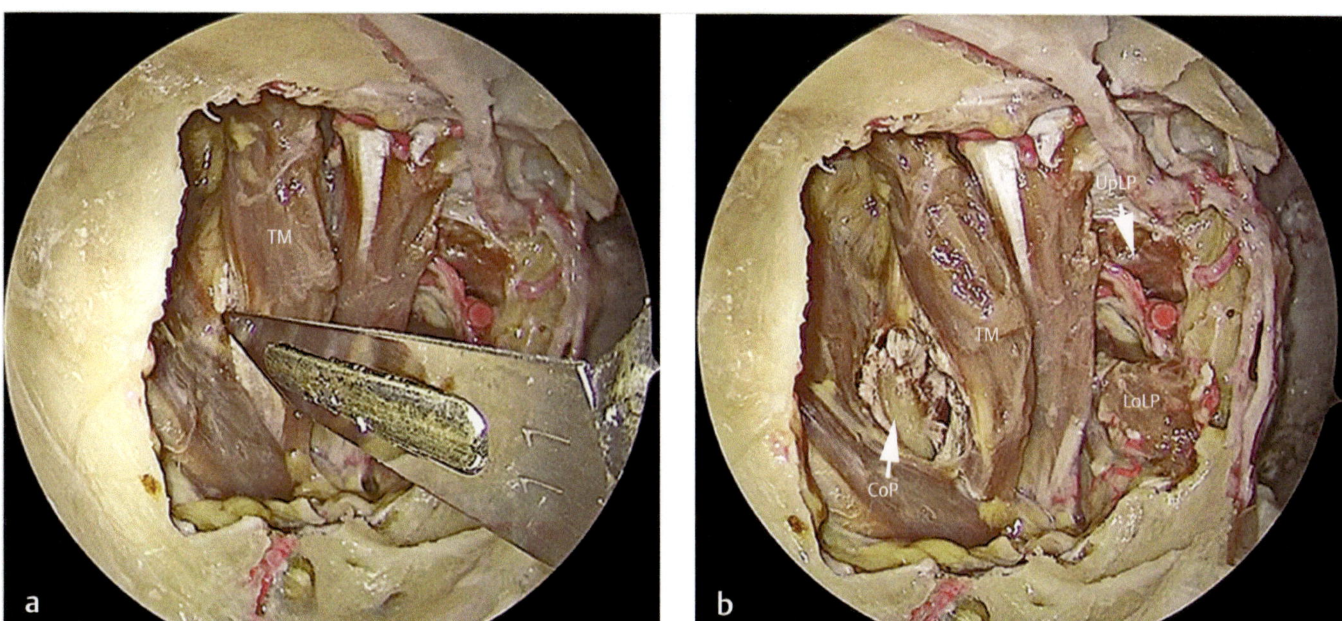

Fig. 16.10 (a, b) Step 3. With a blunt instrument, the temporal muscle (TM) is palpated to identify the coronoid process (CoP). Then, a vertical incision of the muscle is made to expose the coronoid process of the mandible. LoLP, lower head of the lateral pterygoid muscle; UpLP, upper head of the lateral pterygoid muscle.

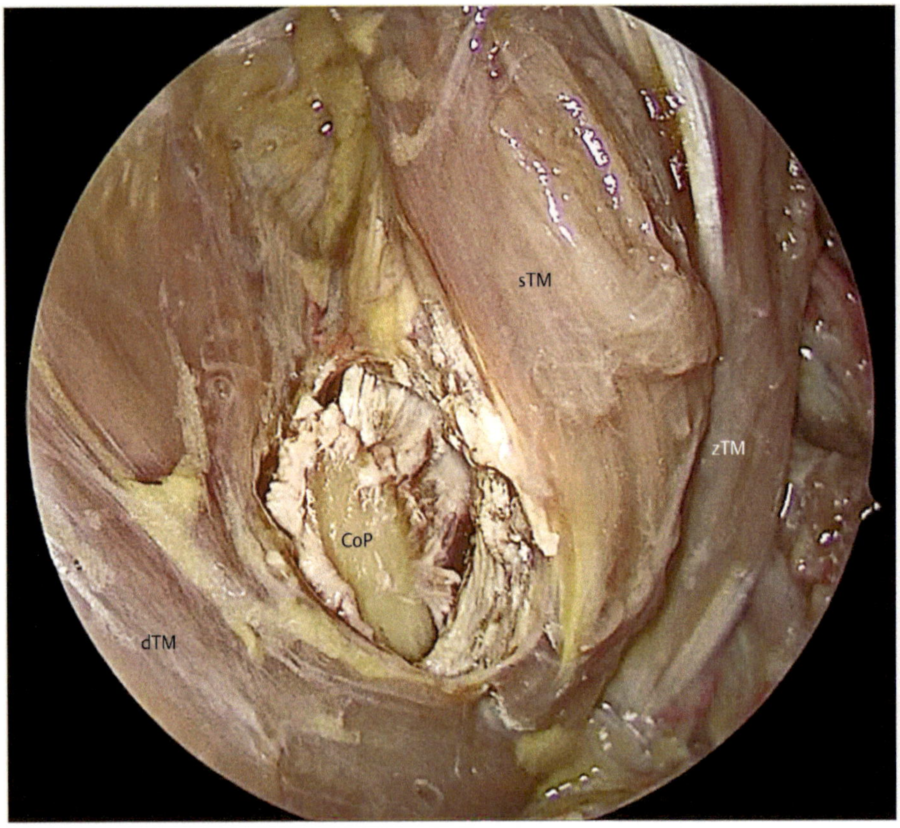

Fig. 16.11 The first corridor. The coronoid process (CoP) is found between the deep (dTM) and superficial (sTM) portions of the temporal muscle. The deep, superficial, and zygomatic (zTM) portions of the temporal muscle insert on the anterior, middle, and posterior portions of the coronoid process, respectively.

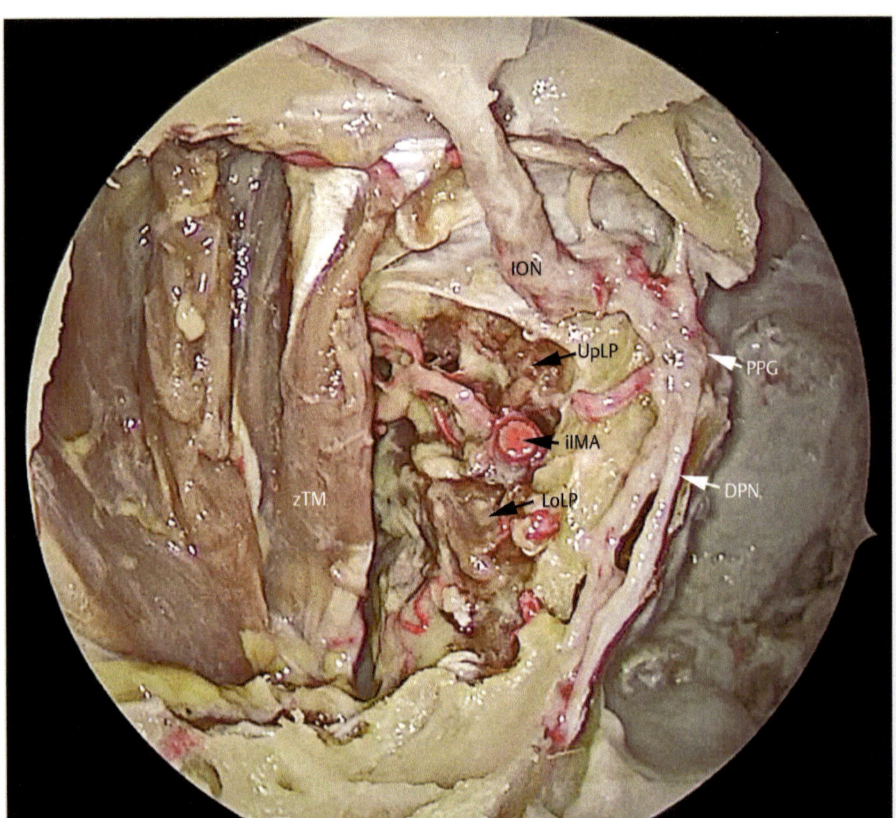

Fig. 16.12 The second corridor. The plane between the zygomatic portion of the temporal muscle (zTM) and the lower (LoLP) and upper (UpLP) heads of the lateral pterygoid muscle is fully identified. The infratemporal tract of the internal maxillary artery passes between the two heads of the lateral pterygoid muscle. DPN, descending palatine nerve; ION, infraorbital nerve; PPG, pterygopalatine ganglion.

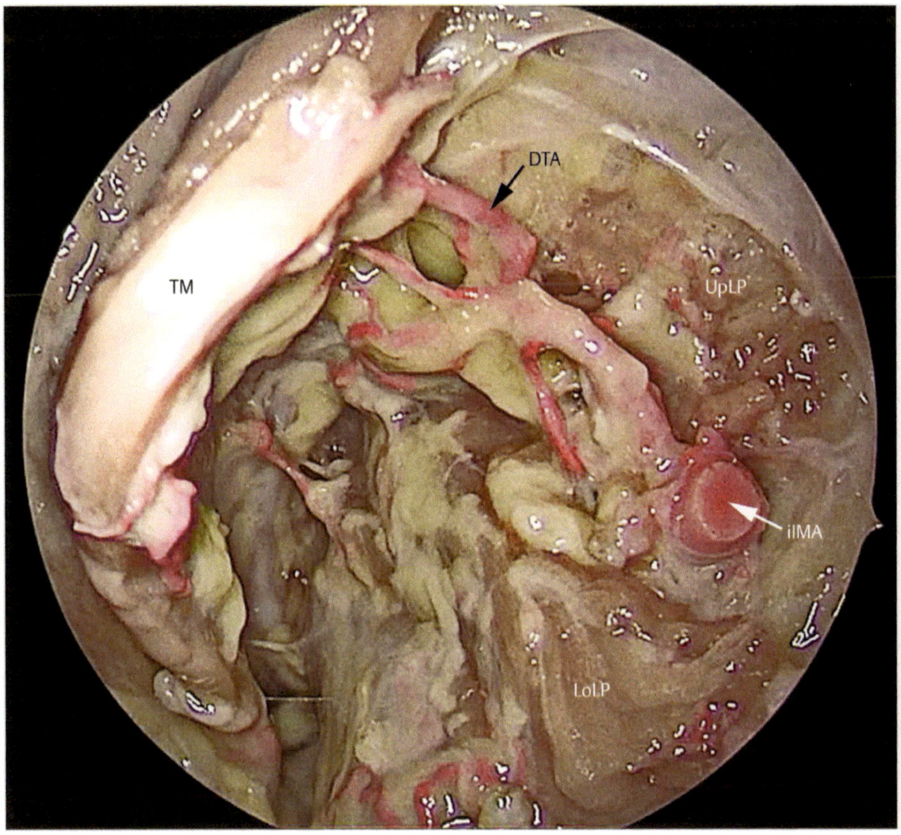

Fig. 16.13 Step 4 (part 1). The lateral pterygoid muscle (LPM) and the zygomatic part of the temporal muscle (zTM) are progressively separated to enlarge the second corridor. In this space, one or more deep temporal arteries (DTA) run toward the temporal muscle. Furthermore, several muscular arteries cross this corridor going from the internal maxillary artery to the other masticatory muscles.

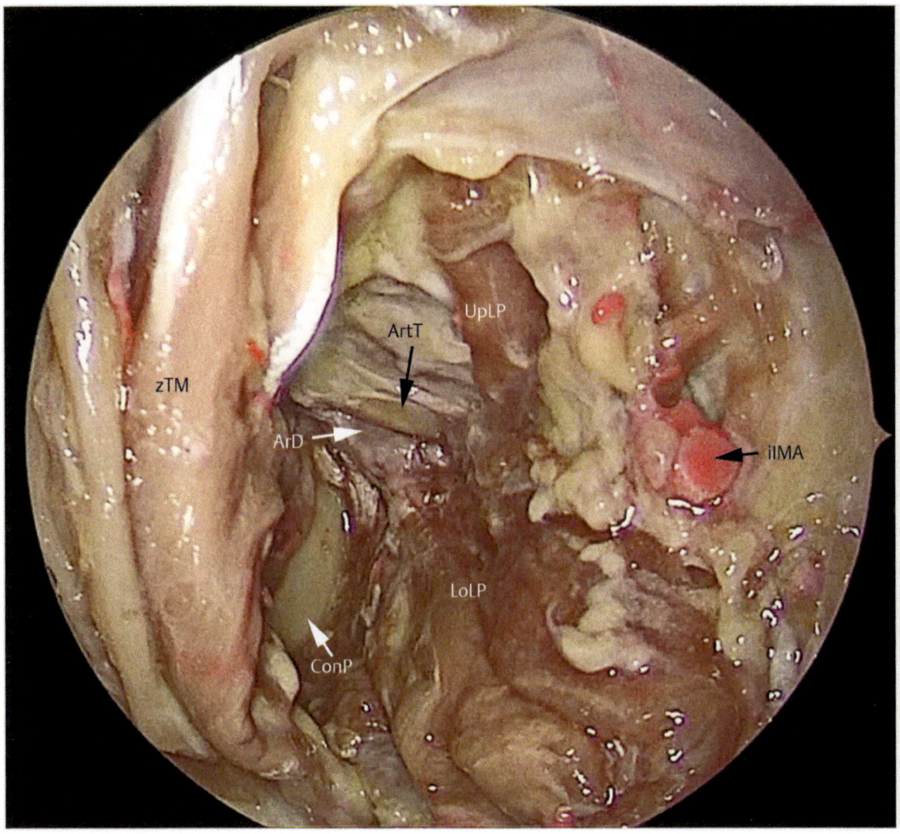

Fig. 16.14 Step 4 (part 2). The dissection along the second corridor is continued until the anteromedial portion of the temporomandibular joint is exposed. The condylar process (ConP), the articular disk (ArD), and the articular tubercle (ArtT) are the posterior limit of the second corridor. iIMA, infratemporal portion of the internal maxillary artery; LoLP, lower head of the lateral pterygoid muscle; UpLP, upper head of the lateral pterygoid muscle; zTM, zygomatic portion of the temporal muscle.

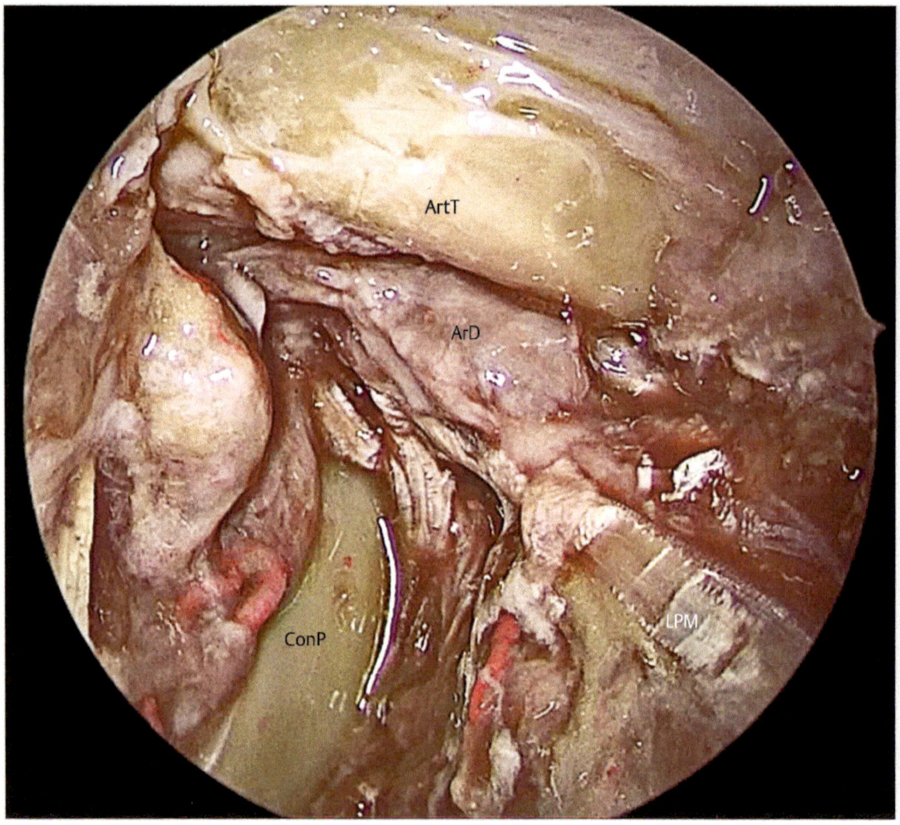

Fig. 16.15 The anteromedial portion of the temporomandibular joint. Superiorly, the temporomandibular joint is formed by the glenoid fossa, which is anteriorly limited by the articular tubercle of the temporal bone (ArtT). Inferiorly, the temporomandibular joint is formed by the condylar process (ConP) of the mandible. Between these bony structures, the articular disk (ArD) fills most of the temporomandibular joint and also serves as insertion for some fibers of the lateral pterygoid muscle (LPM).

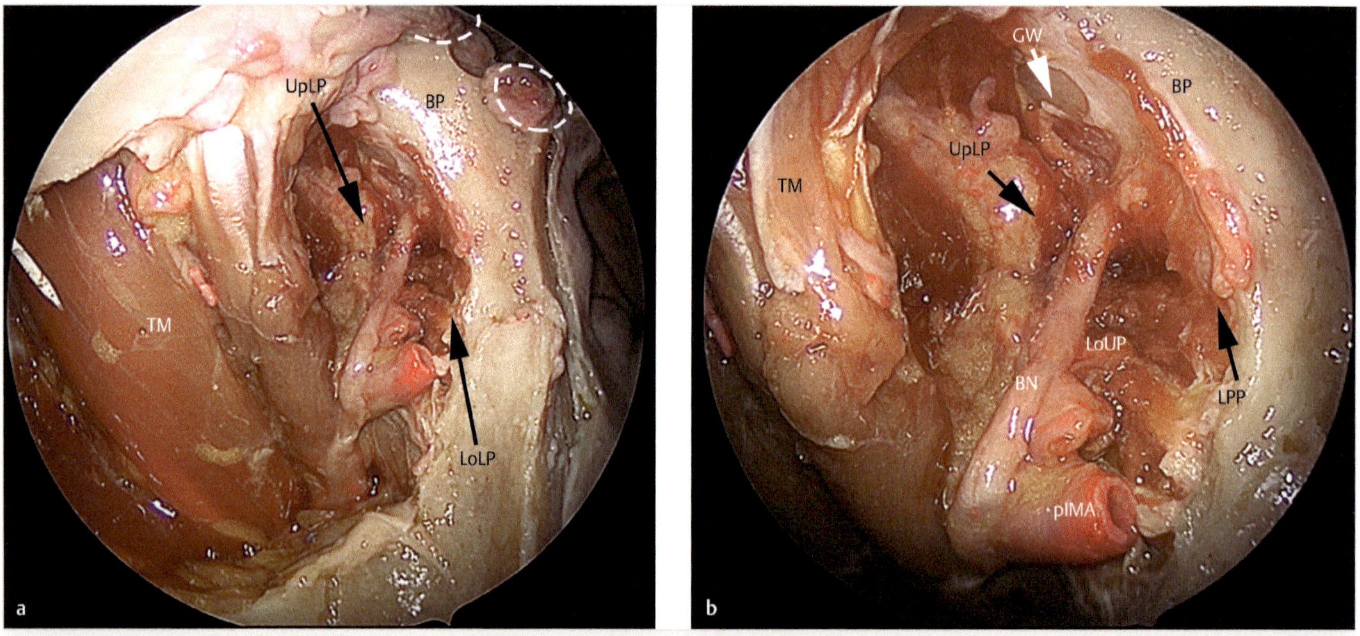

Fig. 16.16 (a, b) Step 5. The third corridor is found between the lower (LoLP) and upper (UpLP) heads of the lateral pterygoid muscle laterally, and the lateral pterygoid plate (LPP), basipterygoid (BP), and greater wing of the sphenoid bone (GW) medially and superiorly. The buccal nerve (BN) is usually found between the fibers of the lateral pterygoid muscle, across the passage from the infratemporal to the pterygopalatine (pIMA) tracts of the internal maxillary artery. This nerve reaches the vertical fibers of the temporal muscle (TM) and then runs downward to reach the buccal mucosa. (*White dashed lines*: Positions of the foramen rotundum [laterally] and the vidian canal [medially].)

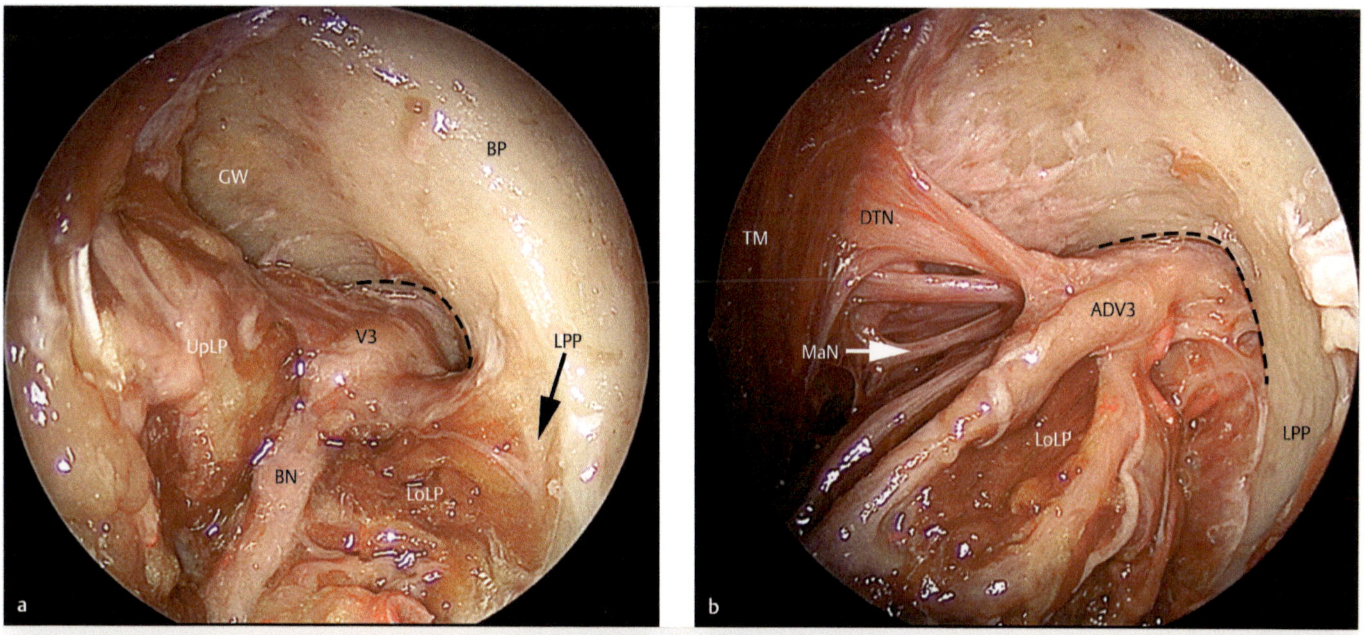

Fig. 16.17 (a, b) Step 6. In order to expose the foramen ovale (*black dashed line*) and the mandibular nerve (V3), the upper head of the lateral pterygoid muscle (UpLP) is dissected from the lateral pterygoid plate (LPP), the greater wing of the sphenoid bone (GW), and the basipterygoid (BP). The anterior division of the mandibular nerve (ADV3) and deep temporal (DTN) and masseteric (MaN) nerves come into view after removing the upper head of the lateral pterygoid muscle. LoLP, lower head of the lateral pterygoid muscle; TM, temporal muscle.

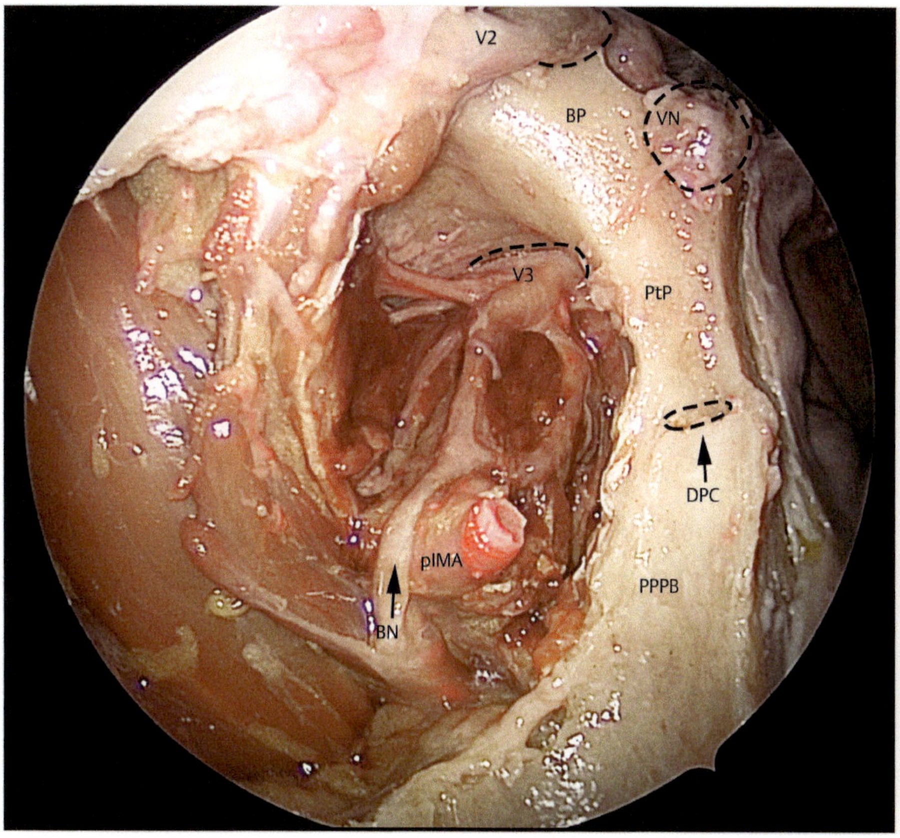

Fig. 16.18 Overview of the third corridor after removing the upper head of the lateral pterygoid muscle. The maxillary (V2) and vidian (VN) nerves cross the basipterygoid (BP) passing through the foramen rotundum and the vidian canal (*black dashed lines*), respectively. The descending palatine canal (DPC) lies (*black dashed line*) between the pterygoid process (PtP) and the perpendicular process of the palatine bone (PPPB). The mandibular nerve (V3) passes through the foramen ovale (*black dashed line*). BN, buccal nerve; pIMA, pterygopalatine tract of the internal maxillary artery.

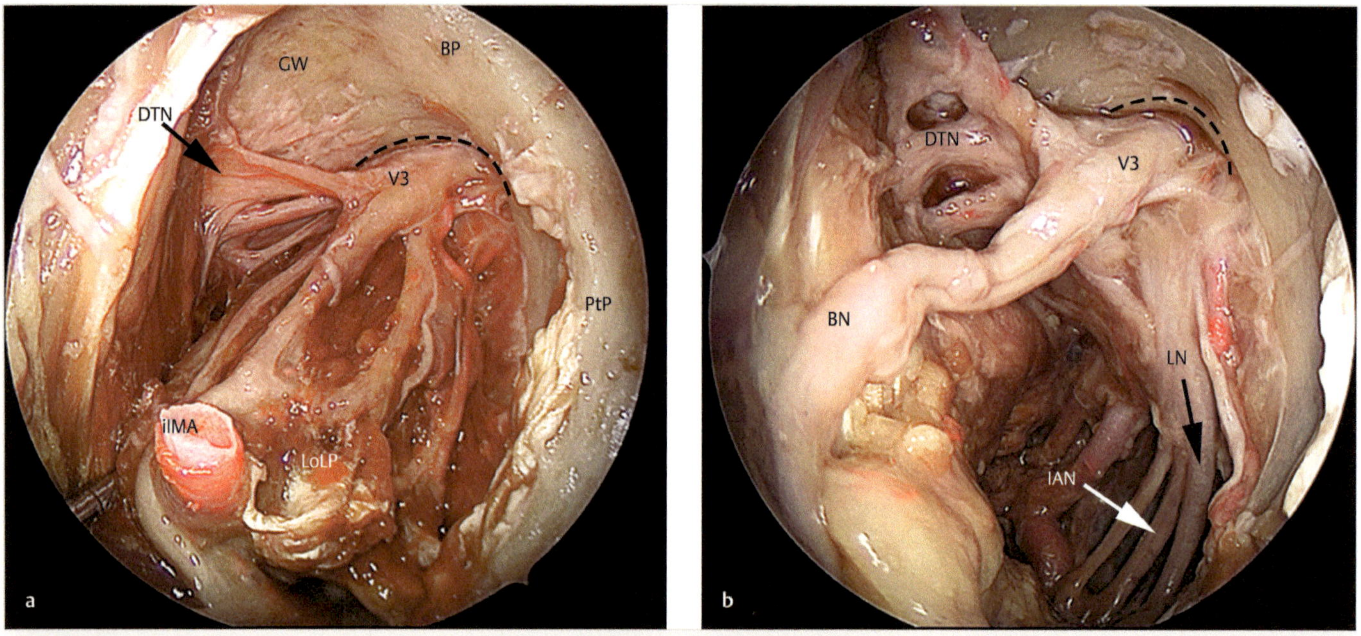

Fig. 16.19 (a, b) Step 7. The lower head of the lateral pterygoid muscle (LoLP) is removed to expose the lingual nerve (LN) and inferior alveolar nerve (IAN). (*Black dashed line*: Foramen ovale.) V3, mandibular nerve; BN, buccal nerve; BP, basipterygoid; DTN, deep temporal nerves; GW, greater wing of the sphenoid bone; iIMA, infratemporal tract of the internal maxillary artery; PtP, pterygoid process.

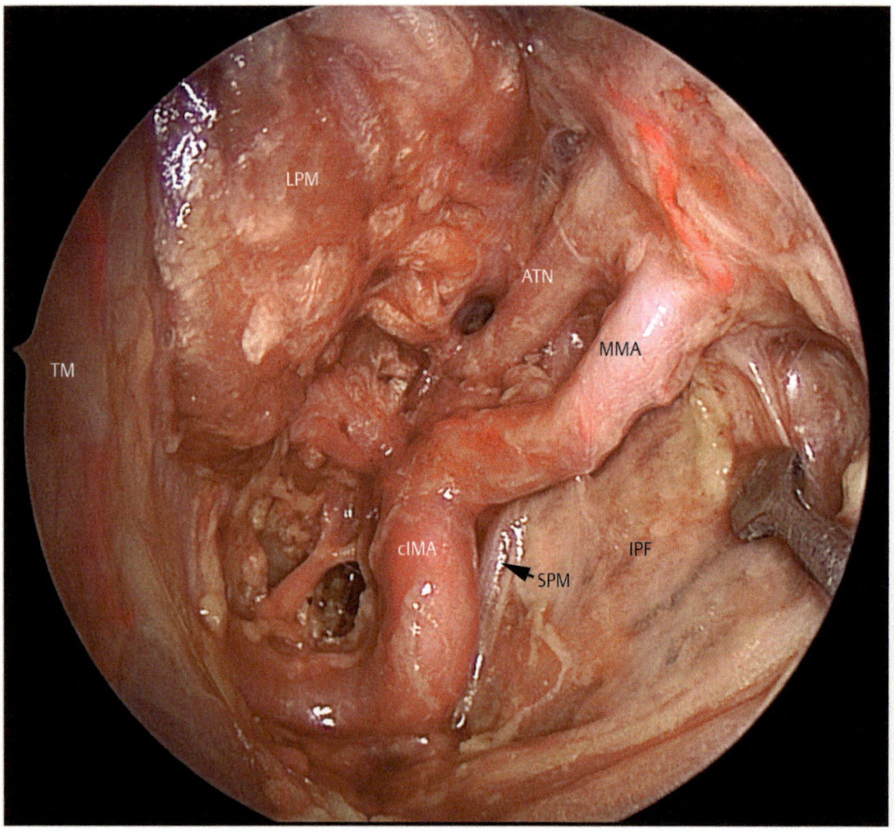

Fig. 16.20 The middle meningeal artery. Moving the scope posteriorly along the third corridor and lateral to the mandibular nerve, the condylar tract of the internal maxillary artery (cIMA) is identified together with the middle meningeal artery (MMA) and the auriculotemporal nerve (ATN). The insertion of the lower head of the lateral pterygoid muscle (LPM) covers the inferior and distal portions of the corridor. The cranial insertion of the stylopharyngeal muscle (SPM) can be seen through the interpterygoid fascia (IPF), which is the upper medial prolongation of the superficial sheet of the deep cervical fascia and represents the posterior boundary of the infratemporal fossa. TM, temporal muscle.

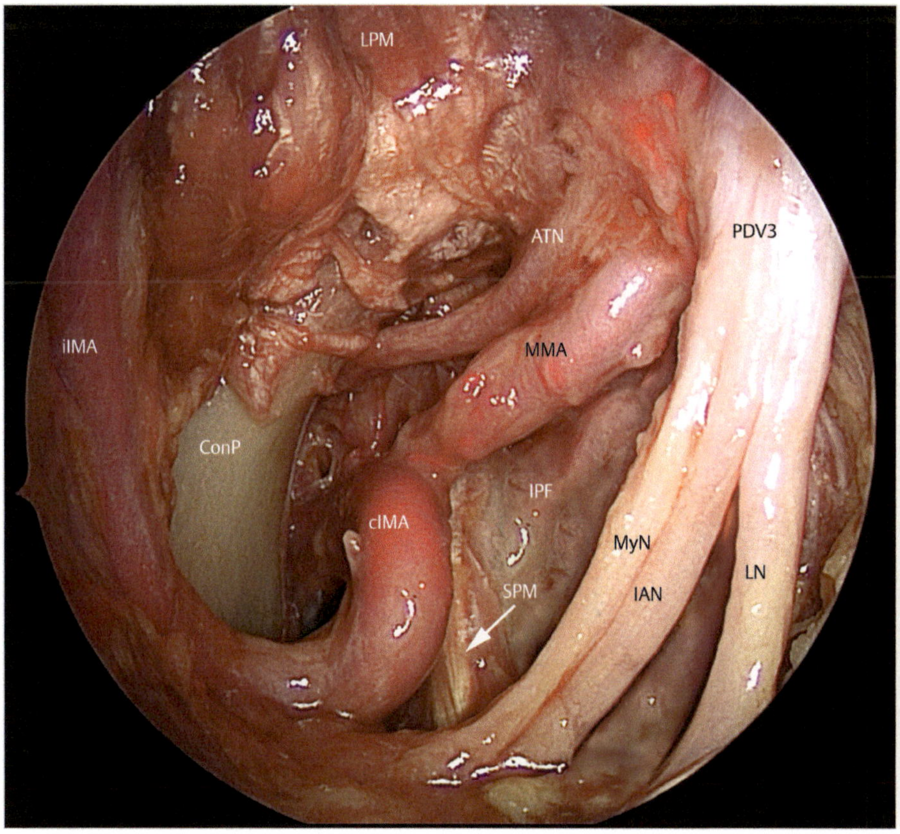

Fig. 16.21 Step 8. The insertion of the lower head of the lateral pterygoid muscle is removed to expose the condylar process (ConP) of the mandible. The auriculotemporal nerve (ATN) turns posterolaterally and passes behind the temporomandibular joint. cIMA, condylar tract of the internal maxillary artery; iIMA, infratemporal tract of the internal maxillary artery; IPF, interpterygoid fascia; LN, lingual nerve; LPM, lateral pterygoid muscle; MMA, middle meningeal artery; MyN, mylohyoid nerve; PDV3, posterior division of the mandibular nerve; SPM, stylopharyngeal muscle.

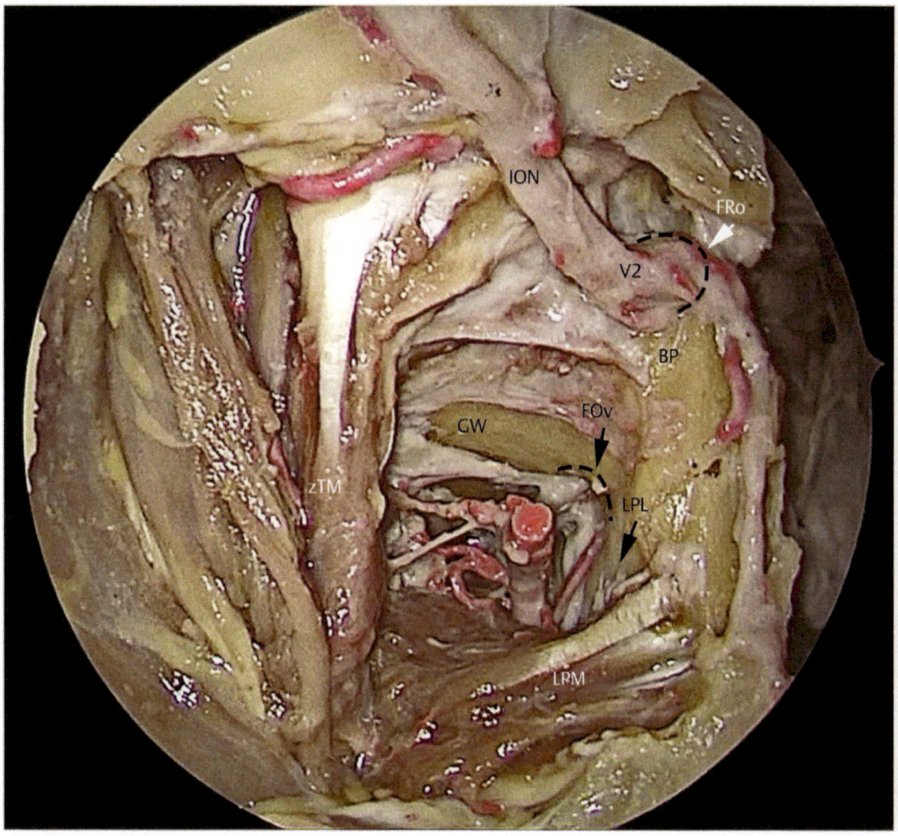

Fig. 16.22 Dissection of the mandibular nerve (part 1). All the connective tissue filling the squared window enclosed between the basipterygoid (BP) and lateral pterygoid plate (LPP) medially, the zygomatic portion of the temporal muscle (zTM) laterally, the maxillary (V2) and infraorbital (ION) nerves and greater wing of the sphenoid bone (GW) superiorly, and the lower head of the lateral pterygoid muscle (LPM) inferiorly is removed to completely expose the area of the foramen ovale. (*Black dashed lines*: Foramina rotundum and ovale.) FOv, foramen ovale; FRo, foramen rotundum.

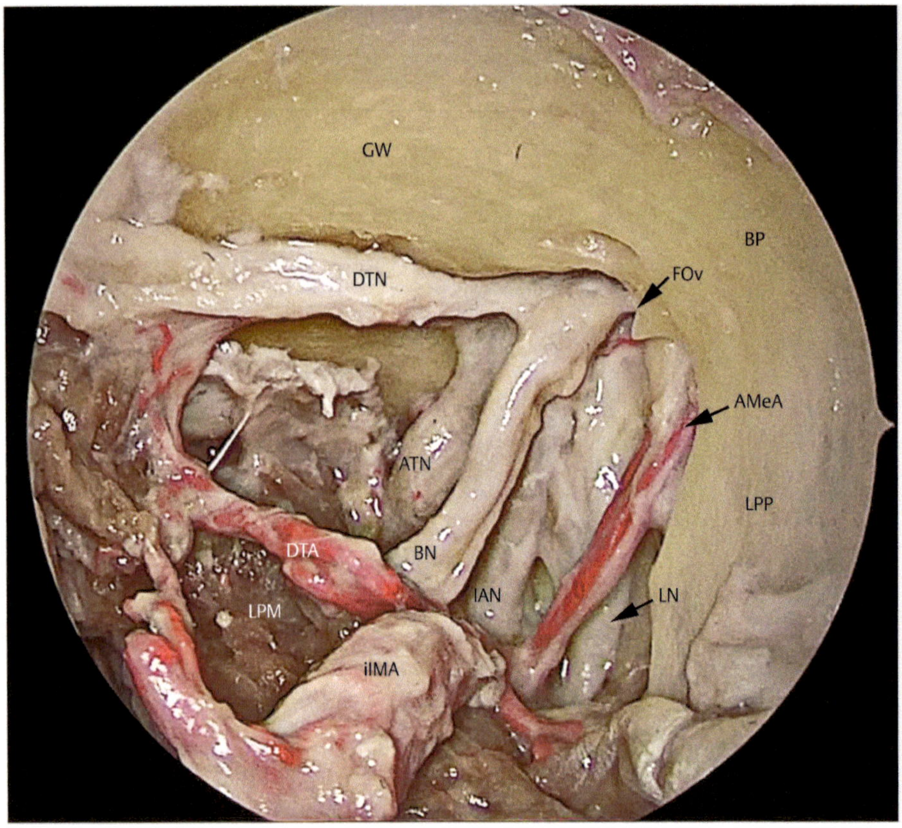

Fig. 16.23 Dissection of the mandibular nerve (part 2). The deep temporal nerves (DTN) run laterally along the inferior surface of the greater wing of the sphenoid bone (GW). The buccal nerve (BN) courses anteriorly, inferiorly, and laterally toward the buccal mucosa. The auriculotemporal nerve (ATN) runs with a posterolateral direction to reach the parotid space. The inferior alveolar (IAN) and lingual (LN) nerves run in a caudal fashion toward the mandible and the tongue, respectively. The accessory meningeal artery (AMeA) passes through the foramen ovale (FOv) together with the mandibular nerve. BP, basipterygoid; DTA, deep temporal artery; iIMA, infratemporal tract of the internal maxillary artery; LPM, lateral pterygoid muscle; LPP, lateral pterygoid plate.

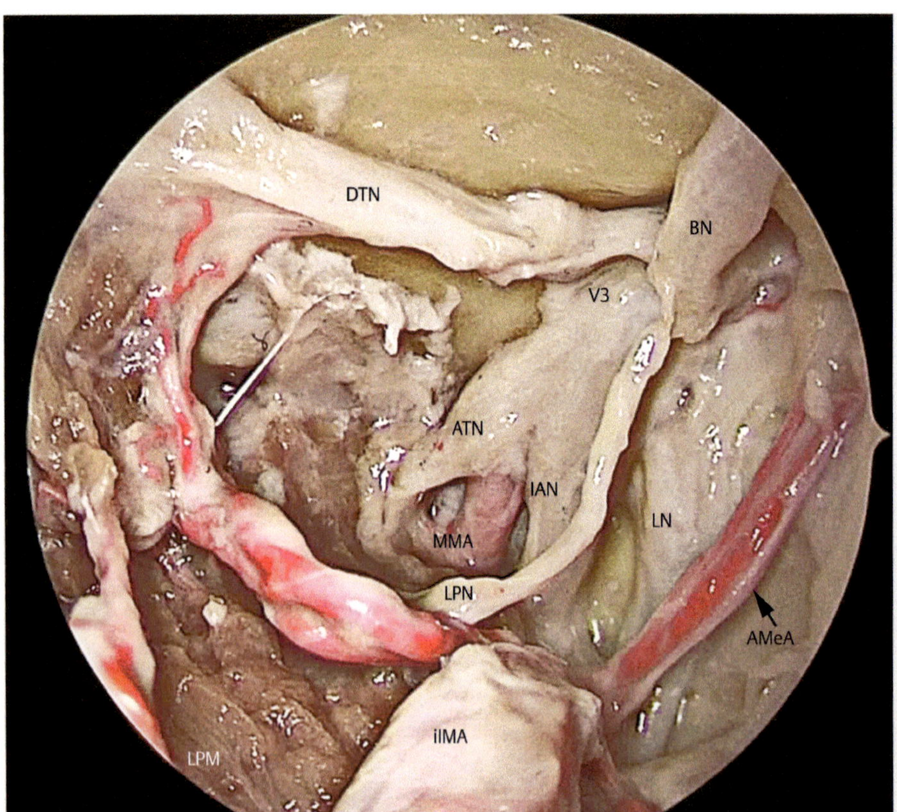

Fig. 16.24 Step 9. The posterolateral insertion of the upper head of the lateral pterygoid muscle is progressively removed. The buccal (BN), deep temporal (DTN), lateral pterygoid (LPN), medial pterygoid, and masseteric nerves are the main anterior branches of the mandibular nerve (V3). The auriculotemporal (ATN), inferior alveolar (IAN), and lingual (LN) nerves are the main posterior branches. The lower head of the lateral pterygoid muscle (LPM) can be left intact. The middle meningeal artery (MMA) lies posteromedially to the auriculotemporal nerve, which can also form a loop around the vessel. An accessory meningeal artery (AMeA) is usually found in front of the lingual nerve and behind the buccal nerve. iIMA, infratemporal tract of the internal maxillary artery.

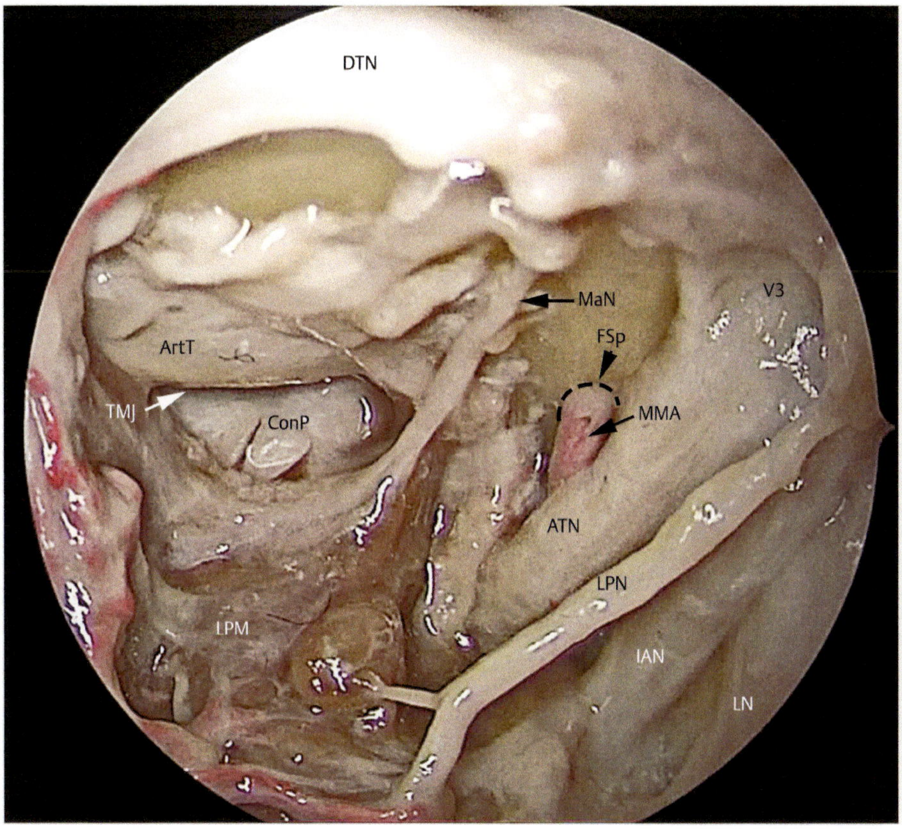

Fig. 16.25 The posteromedial portion of the temporomandibular joint. The masseteric nerve (MaN) runs anteriorly to the condylar process (ConP) of the mandible and the temporomandibular joint (TMJ), while the auriculotemporal nerve (ATN) moves behind them after crossing the middle meningeal artery (MMA). (*Black dashed line*: Foramen spinosum.) V3, mandibular nerve; ArtT, articular tubercle; DTN, deep temporal nerve; FSp, foramen spinosum; IAN, inferior alveolar nerve; LN, lingual nerve; LPM, lateral pterygoid muscle; LPN, lateral pterygoid nerve.

References

[1] Stambuk HE, Patel SG. Imaging of the parapharyngeal space. Otolaryngol Clin North Am 2008;41(1):77–101, vi

[2] Dallan I, Lenzi R, Bignami M, et al. Endoscopic transnasal anatomy of the infratemporal fossa and upper parapharyngeal regions: correlations with traditional perspectives and surgical implications. Minim Invasive Neurosurg 2010;53(5–6):261–269

[3] Ohue S, Fukushima T, Kumon Y, Ohnishi T, Friedman AH. Preauricular transzygomatic anterior infratemporal fossa approach for tumors in or around infratemporal fossa lesions. Neurosurg Rev 2012;35(4):583–592, discussion 592

[4] Battaglia P, Turri-Zanoni M, Dallan I, et al. Endoscopic endonasal transpterygoid transmaxillary approach to the infratemporal and upper parapharyngeal tumors. Otolaryngol Head Neck Surg 2014;150(4):696–702

[5] Taylor RJ, Patel MR, Wheless SA, et al. Endoscopic endonasal approaches to infratemporal fossa tumors: a classification system and case series. Laryngoscope 2014;124(11):2443–2450

[6] Langdon C, Herman P, Verillaud B, et al. Expanded endoscopic endonasal surgery for advanced stage juvenile angiofibromas: a retrospective multi-center study. Rhinology 2016;54(3):239–246

[7] Yang L, Hu L, Zhao W, Zhang H, Liu Q, Wang D. Endoscopic endonasal approach for trigeminal schwannomas: our experience of 39 patients in 10 years. Eur Arch Otorhinolaryngol 2018;275(3):735–741

[8] Zhou B, Huang Q, Shen PH, et al. The intranasal endoscopic removal of schwannoma of the pterygopalatine and infratemporal fossae via the prelacrimal recess approach. J Neurosurg 2016;124(4):1068–1073

[9] Raza SM, Amine MA, Anand V, Schwartz TH. Endoscopic endonasal resection of trigeminal schwannomas. Neurosurg Clin N Am 2015;26(3):473–479

[10] Lee JT, Suh JD, Carrau RL, Chu MW, Chiu AG. Endoscopic Denker's approach for resection of lesions involving the anteroinferior maxillary sinus and infratemporal fossa. Laryngoscope 2017;127(3):556–560

[11] Shin M, Shojima M, Kondo K, et al. Endoscopic endonasal craniofacial surgery for recurrent skull base meningiomas involving the pterygopalatine fossa, the infratemporal fossa, the orbit, and the paranasal sinus. World Neurosurg 2018;112:e302–e312

[12] Schreiber A, Ferrari M, Rampinelli V, et al. Modular endoscopic medial maxillectomies: quantitative analysis of surgical exposure in a preclinical setting. World Neurosurg 2017;100:44–55

[13] Harvey RJ, Sheehan PO, Debnath NI, Schlosser RJ. Transseptal approach for extended endoscopic resections of the maxilla and infratemporal fossa. Am J Rhinol Allergy 2009;23(4):426–432

[14] Ramakrishnan VR, Suh JD, Chiu AG, Palmer JN. Septal dislocation for endoscopic access of the anterolateral maxillary sinus and infratemporal fossa. Am J Rhinol Allergy 2011;25(2):128–130

[15] Upadhyay S, Dolci RL, Buohliqah L, et al. Effect of incremental endoscopic maxillectomy on surgical exposure of the pterygopalatine and infratemporal fossae. J Neurol Surg B Skull Base 2016;77(1):66–74

[16] Hosseini SM, Razfar A, Carrau RL, et al. Endonasal transpterygoid approach to the infratemporal fossa: correlation of endoscopic and multiplanar CT anatomy. Head Neck 2012;34(3):313–320

17 Medial Transcavernous Approach

Marco Ferrari, Marco Ravanelli, Davide Lancini, Francesco Belotti, Francesco Doglietto

The cavernous sinus is a venous dural sinus that is located in the cranial portion of the parasellar region and houses a number of neurovascular structures that are partially or totally immersed in venous blood. Due to the density of relevant structures, Parkinson and Dolenc defined this area as "anatomic jewel box."[1] From a topographic standpoint, the cavernous sinus can be considered boat-shaped (i.e., like a prism), with the keel oriented anteroinferiorly.[2] Therefore, it has five walls: the anterior wall faces the sphenoid sinus and the superior orbital fissure, the posterior wall is adjacent to the posterior cranial fossa, the medial wall separates the venous sinus from the sellar region, the lateral wall neighbors the Meckel cave and the middle cranial fossa, and the roof is intimately related to the anterior clinoid process and the petroclinoid folds of the tentorium cerebri.

The paraclival and parasellar tracts of the internal carotid artery are located within the cavernous sinus along with the oculomotor, trochlear, ophthalmic, abducens, and maxillary nerves. In greater detail, only the internal carotid artery and the abducens nerve are actually free within the sinus, whereas the remaining structures are included within one or more of the above-mentioned walls. The cavernous portion of the internal carotid artery can be used to define four main compartments, which can be variably invaded by tumors of this area[3]: the inferior compartment lies between the anterior and inferior aspects of the parasellar carotid artery and the anterior wall of the cavernous sinus; the superior compartment is located between the superior face of the horizontal parasellar carotid artery and the roof of the cavernous sinus; the posterior compartment is enclosed between the paraclival tract of the internal carotid artery and the posterior wall of the cavernous sinus; the lateral compartment is situated between the cavernous carotid artery and the lateral wall of the cavernous sinus. Additionally, some other minor structures can be found in the cavernous sinus, namely, the sympathetic branch tended from the internal carotid artery to the abducens nerve, the meningohypophyseal and inferolateral trunks, and a complex system of dural ligaments, which only recently has been systematically described.[4]

Given the dense network of critical structures, the cavernous sinus has been historically considered to be an unapproachable area when invaded by tumors. With the increasing experience, implementation, and refinement of hemostatic materials and neurophysiological monitoring, and evolution of anatomical knowledge of the cavernous sinus, its surgical clearance in well-selected cases is no longer considered a heresy.[5-7] Consistently with this trend, the morbidity of approaching the cavernous sinus in adequately selected cases has been widely resized.[8]

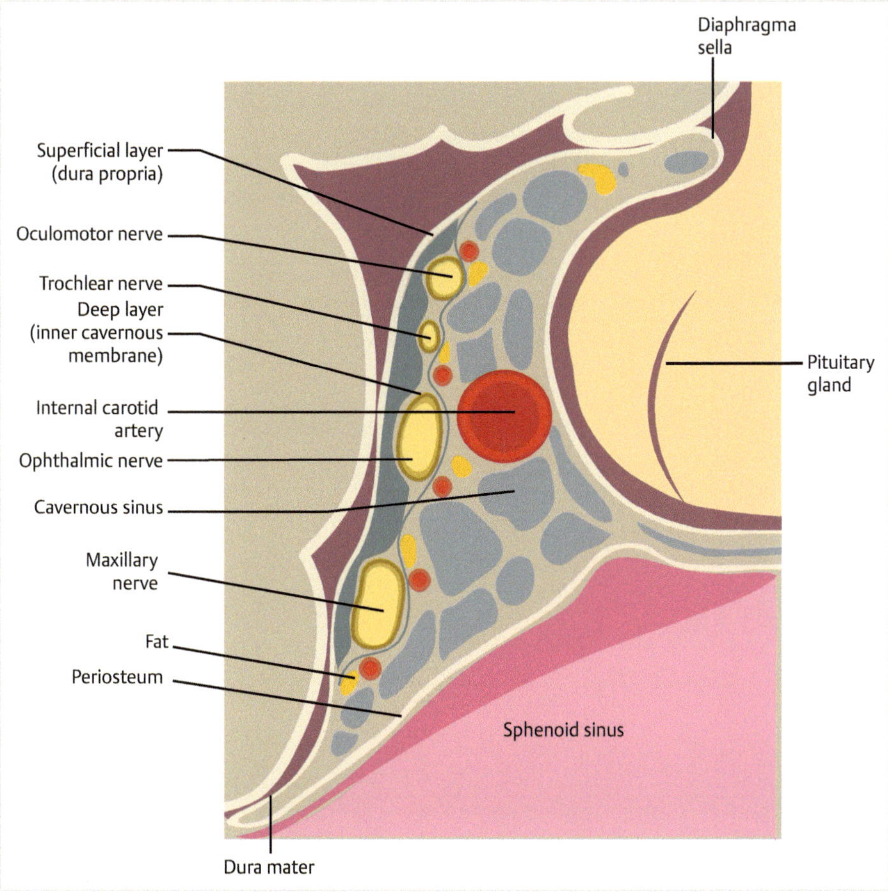

Fig. 17.1 Coronal view of the cavernous sinus. This coronal illustration shows architecture of the cavernous sinus and its relationship with intracranial spaces and sphenoid sinus.

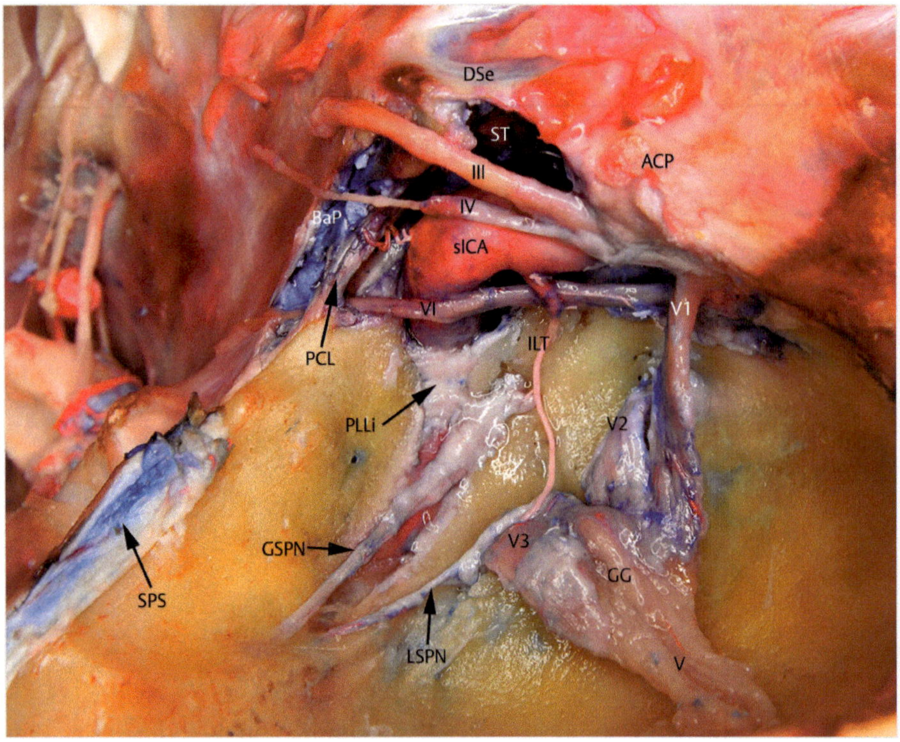

Fig. 17.2 Intracranial view of the cavernous sinus. This cadaver picture shows with a superolateral-to-inferomedial perspective the right parasellar area. The gasserian ganglion (GG) and related trigeminal branches have been displaced anteriorly. III, oculomotor nerve; IV, trochlear nerve; VI, abducens nerve; V, trigeminal stem; V1, ophthalmic nerve; V2, maxillary nerve; V3, mandibular nerve; VI, abducens nerve; ACP, anterior clinoid process; BaP, basilar plexus; DSe, dorsum sellae; GSPN, greater superficial petrosal nerve; ILT, inferolateral trunk; LSPN, lesser superficial petrosal nerve; PCL, petroclinoid (Gruber's) ligament; PLLi, petrolingual ligament; sICA, parasellar tract of the internal carotid artery; SPS, superior petrosal sinus; ST, sella turcica.

Two main transnasal endoscopic approaches to the cavernous sinus can be identified with respect to the internal carotid artery: the medial transcavernous approach, which will be described in this chapter, and the lateral transcavernous approach, illustrated in Chapter 18. Both approaches pass through the anterior wall of the cavernous sinus, which is exposed underneath the carotid prominence and carotid sulcus. Further details on the borderline area between the lateral portion of the cavernous sinus and Meckel's cave are reported in Chapter 21.

The medial transcavernous approach, which was first developed to treat sellar lesions extending to the cavernous sinus, is employed to manage the inferior compartment and to a lesser extent to reach the superior and posterior compartments. This approach has been mostly adopted for the treatment of nonfunctioning pituitary adenomas with resectable extension to the cavernous sinus.[9,10] Its role in the removal of functioning and/or nonresectable adenomas is more controversial due to the difficulty to fully control symptoms, although subtotal or partial reduction of tumor volume could facilitate adjuvant stereotactic radiotherapy or Gamma Knife radiosurgery.[11-18] Meningiomas of the cavernous sinus pose more serious concerns due to the higher rate of complications following endoscopic resection.[19] Consequently, stereotactic radiotherapy or Gamma Knife radiosurgery, alone or following endoscopic subtotal resection, is emerging as a valuable alternative to aggressive surgery.[20] Finally, a large number of nonadenomatous, nonmeningeal tumors (metastases, chordomas, chondrosarcomas, hemangiomas, lymphomas, craniopharyngiomas, schwannomas), and tumor-like lesions (sarcoidosis, fungal infection, thrombophlebitis complicating acute rhinosinusitis) of the cavernous sinus have been approached endoscopically to obtain a histological/microbiological diagnosis and/or to remove the lesion.[19,21-23]

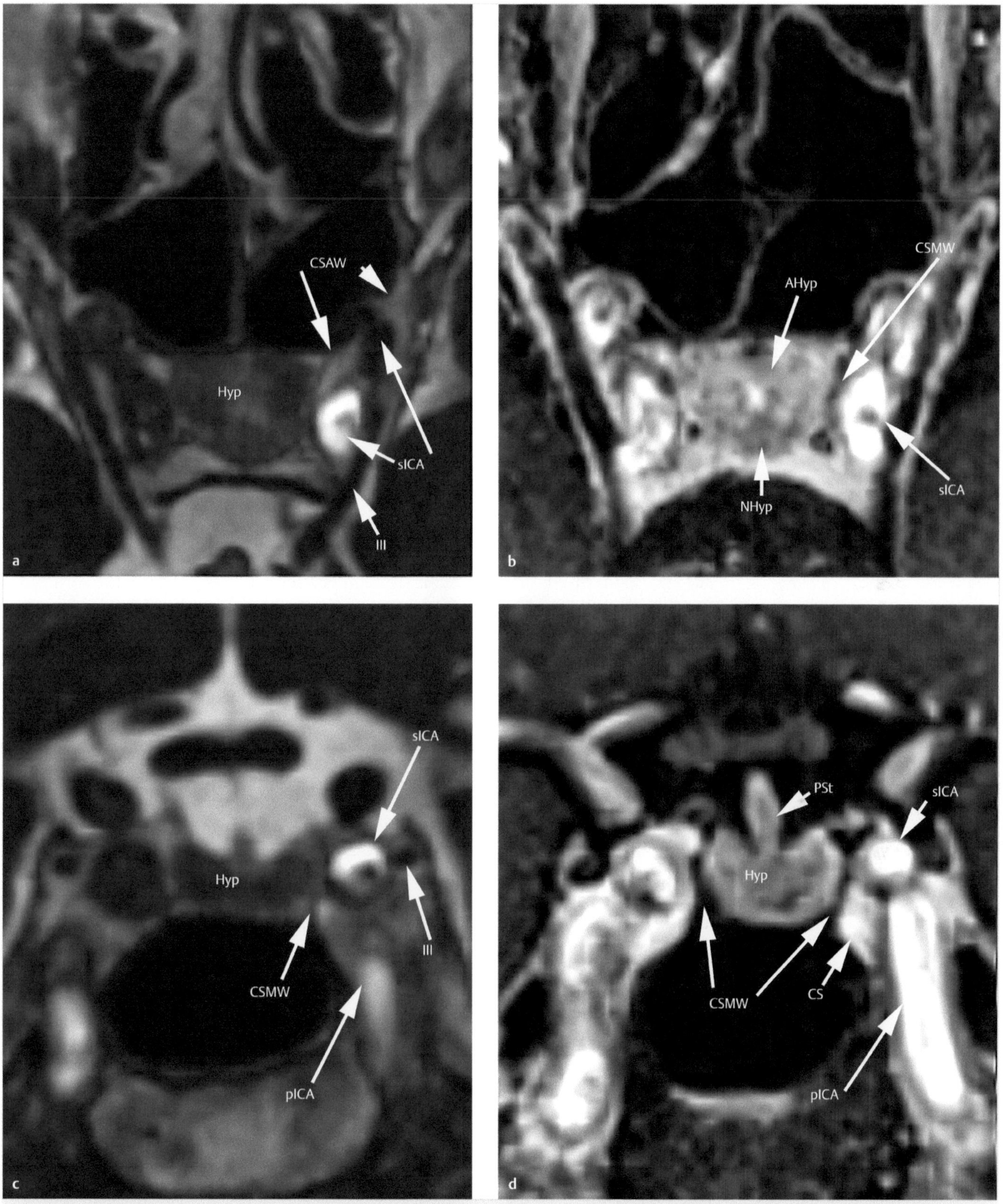

Fig. 17.3 (a–d) Axial and coronal MRI anatomy of the medial portion of the cavernous sinus. Axial (upper images) and coronal (lower images) CISS (constructive interference in steady state) MRI (left column) and T1-weighted contrast-enhanced, fat-saturated MRI images (right column). The medial transcavernous approach is located in the small niche between the parasellar (sICA) and paraclival tracts of the internal carotid artery (pICA) laterally and the hypophysis (Hyp) and sphenoid sinus (SpS) medially. This area is accessed through the anterior wall of the cavernous sinus (CSAW). The medial wall of the cavernous sinus (CSMW) is a thin and sometimes incomplete barrier separating the sella from the cavernous sinus (CS). III, oculomotor nerve; AHyp, adenohypophysis; NHyp, neurohypophysis; PSt, pituitary stalk.

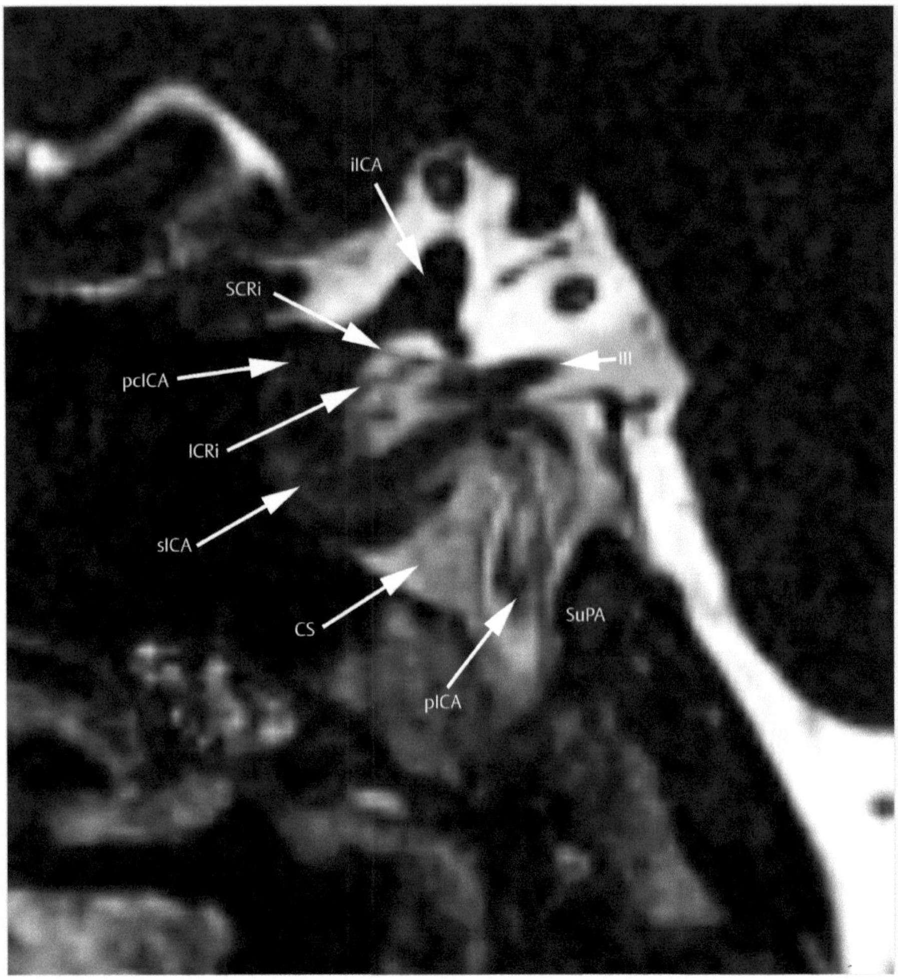

Fig. 17.4 Sagittal MRI anatomy of the medial portion of the cavernous sinus. Sagittal CISS (constructive interference in steady state) MRI image passing through the paraclival (pICA), parasellar (sICA), paraclinoid (pclCA), and intracranial tract of the internal carotid artery (iICA). The paraclival and parasellar tracts of the vessel form the cavernous portion of the internal carotid artery, which is surrounded by the venous blood of the cavernous sinus (CS). The paraclinoid tract is delimited by the inferior carotid ring (ICRi) and the superior carotid ring (SCRi), which form the anterior portion of the roof of the cavernous sinus. The oculomotor nerve (III) pierces the posterior half of the roof of the cavernous sinus to enter its lateral wall. SuPA, superior petrous apex.

Endoscopic Dissection

Nasal Phase

- Paraseptal sphenoidotomy.
- Transrostral sphenoidotomy.
- Expanded transrostral sphenoidotomy.
- Vertical uncinectomy.
- Anterior ethmoidectomy.
- Posterior ethmoidectomy.
- Transethmoidal sphenoidotomy.
- Middle and superior turbinectomy.

Skull Base Phase

- Facultative: Transsellar approach.
- Step 1: Removal of the sellar prominence and partial removal of the carotid prominence.
- Step 2: Incision of the anterior wall of the cavernous sinus.
- Step 3: Removal of the inferior parasellar ligament and fat tissue within the cavernous sinus.
- Step 4: Dissection of the superior compartment of the cavernous sinus.
- Step 5: Removal of the midclivus, carotid sulcus, and lateral portion of the carotid prominence.
- Step 6: Inferomedial extension of the periosteal incision.

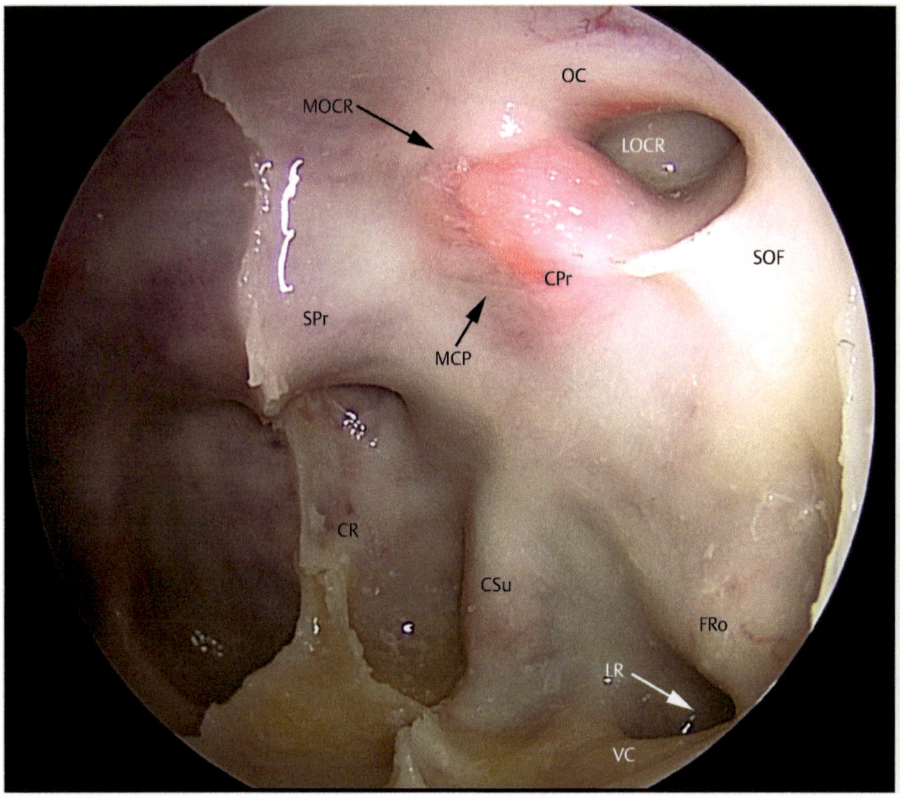

Fig. 17.5 Bony landmarks. The bony projection of the medial portion of the cavernous sinus lies in between the sellar prominence (SPr) and the clival recess (CR), medially, and the carotid prominence (CPr) and the carotid sulcus (CSu), laterally. When the sphenoid is poorly pneumatized, the carotid sulcus can be found by following the vidian canal (VC). FRo, foramen rotundum; LOCR, lateral optic-carotid recess; MCP, middle clinoid process; MOCR, medial optic-carotid recess; LR, lateral recess; OC, optic canal; SOF, superior orbital fissure.

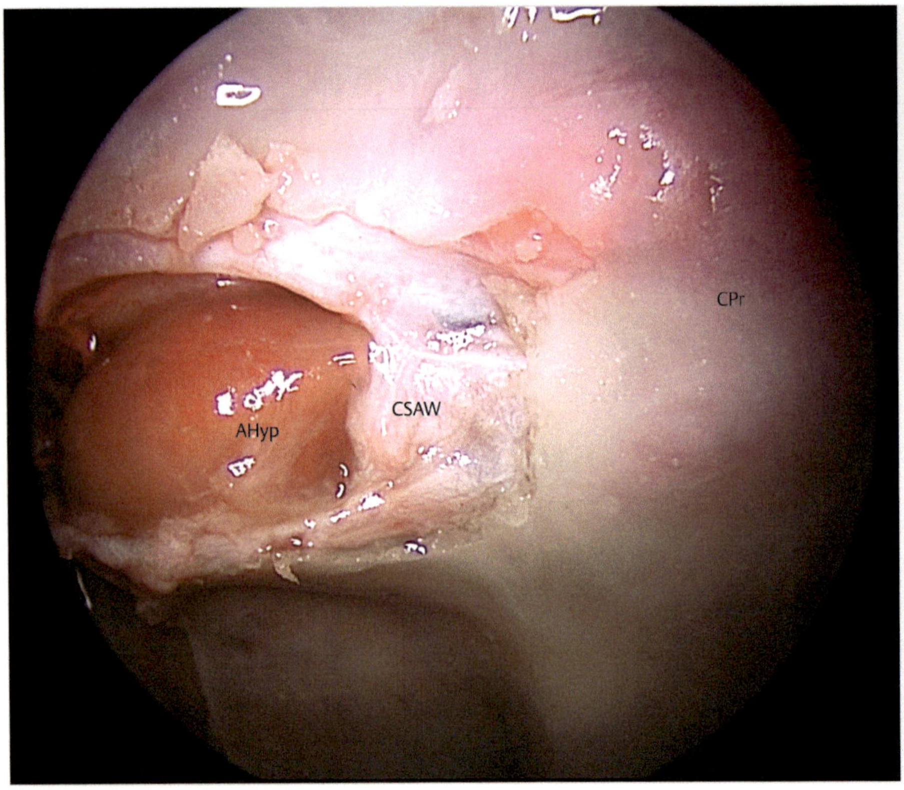

Fig. 17.6 Step 1. The sellar prominence and the medial portion of the carotid prominence (CPr) are removed to expose the anterior wall of the cavernous sinus (CSAW). AHyp, adenohypophysis.

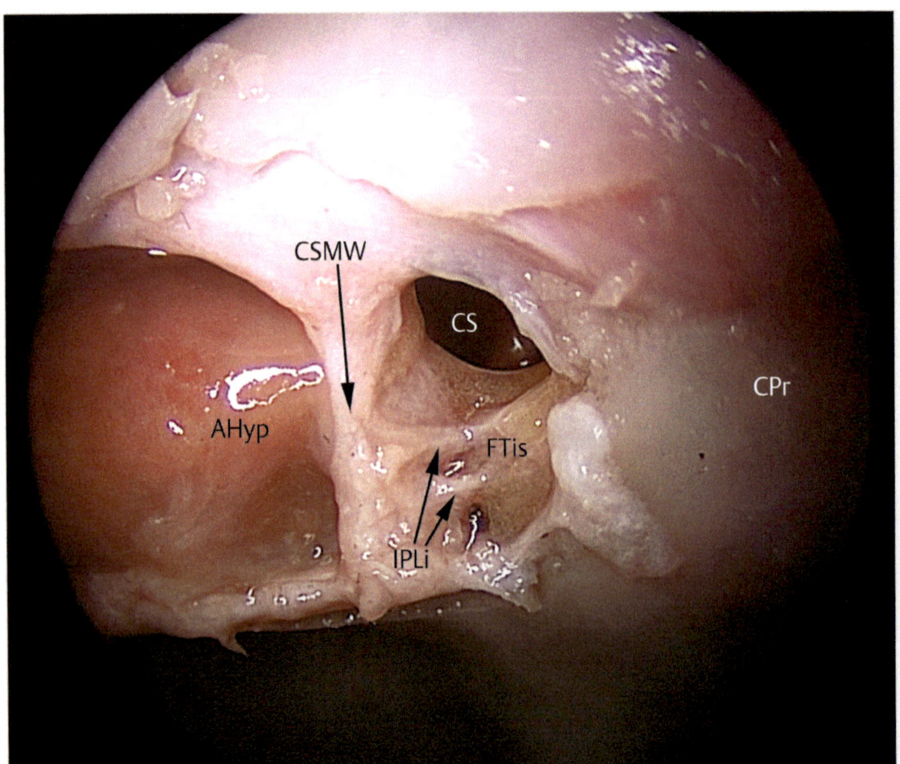

Fig. 17.7 Step 2. A vertical incision on the anterior wall of the cavernous sinus is made to expose the inferior parasellar ligament(s) (IPLi). This ligament is frequently surrounded by fat tissue (FTis) and anchors the medial wall of the cavernous sinus (CSMW) to the anterior wall. AHyp, adenohypophysis; CPr, carotid prominence; CS, cavernous sinus (lumen).

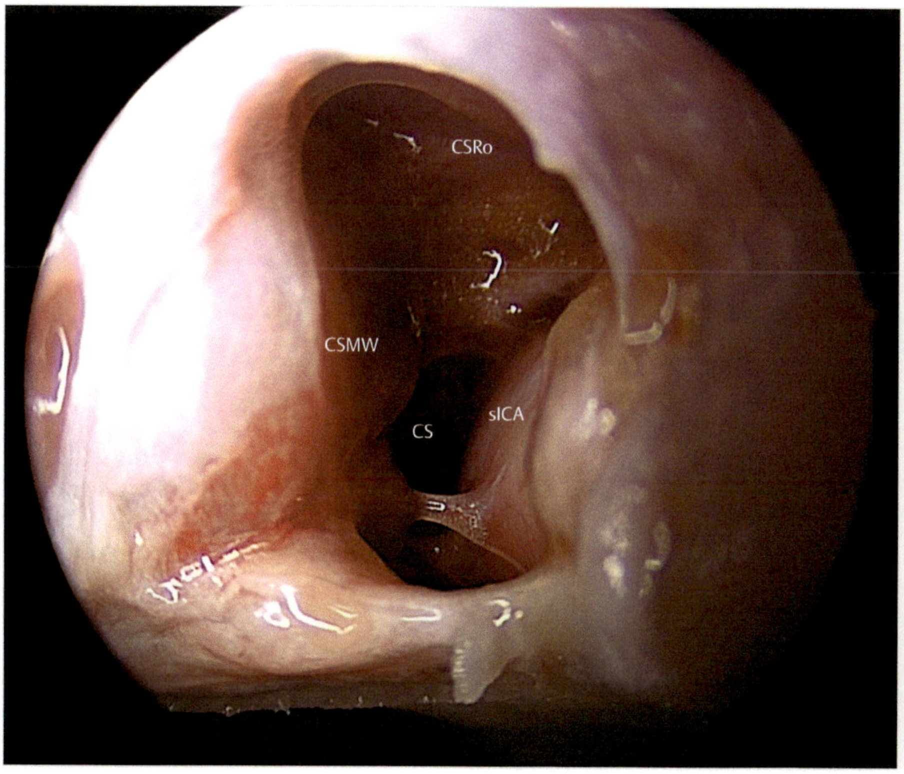

Fig. 17.8 Step 3. After removing the inferior parasellar ligament and adjacent fat tissue, the anterior half of the roof (CSRo) and medial wall (CSMW) of the cavernous sinus come into view along with the parasellar tract of the internal carotid artery (sICA). The anterior half of the roof of the cavernous sinus represents the inferior periosteal lining of the anterior clinoid process. The oculomotor triangle can be found following posteriorly the roof of the cavernous sinus. CS, cavernous sinus (lumen).

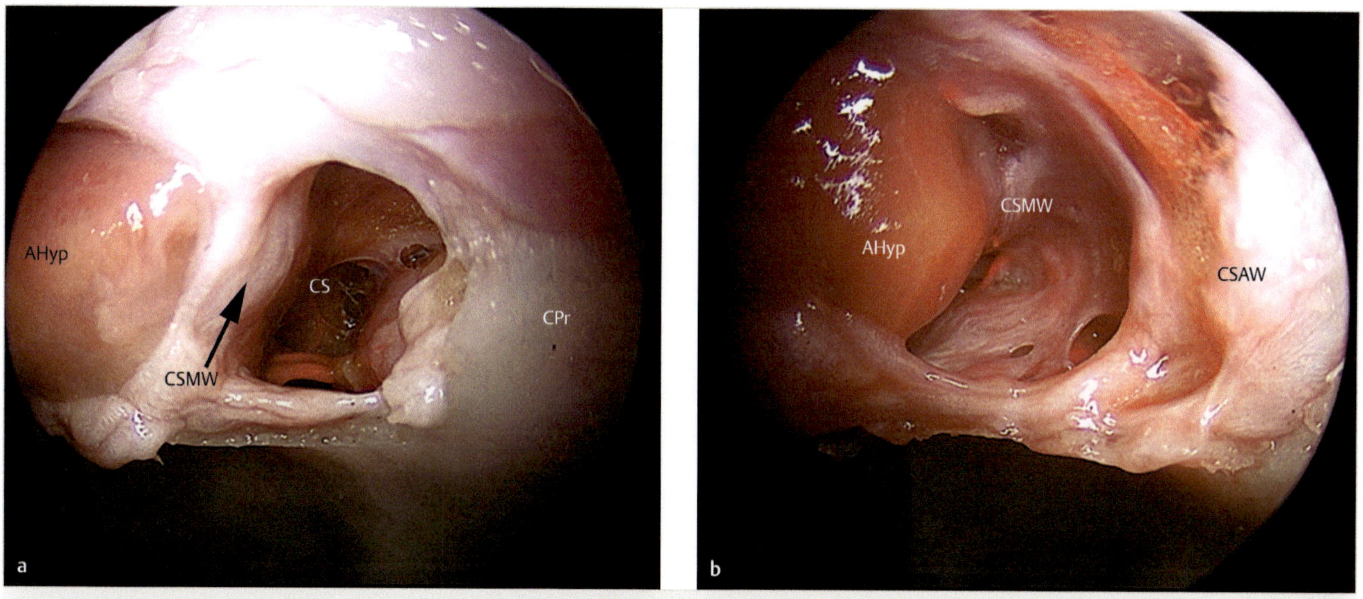

Fig. 17.9 (a, b) Medial wall of the cavernous sinus. The transsellar approach is performed together with the medial transcavernous approach to expose the medial and lateral side of the medial wall of the cavernous sinus (CSMW), respectively. AHyp, adenohypophysis; CPr, carotid prominence; CS, cavernous sinus (lumen); CSAW, anterior wall of the cavernous sinus.

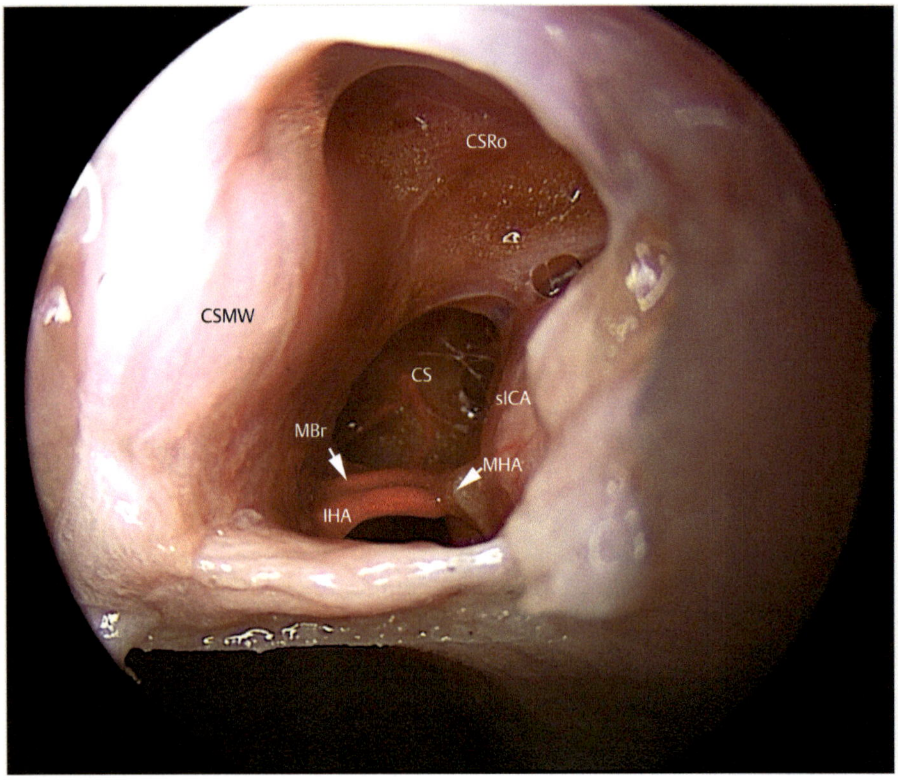

Fig. 17.10 Meningohypophyseal artery. The meningohypophyseal artery (MHA) arises from the medial aspect of the parasellar tract of the internal carotid artery (sICA). This arterial trunk early bifurcates forming the inferior hypophyseal artery (IHA) and a meningeal branch (MBr). Both arteries pass through the medial wall of the cavernous sinus (CSMW) to reach the pituitary gland and surrounding meninges, respectively. CS, cavernous sinus (lumen); CSRo, roof of the cavernous sinus.

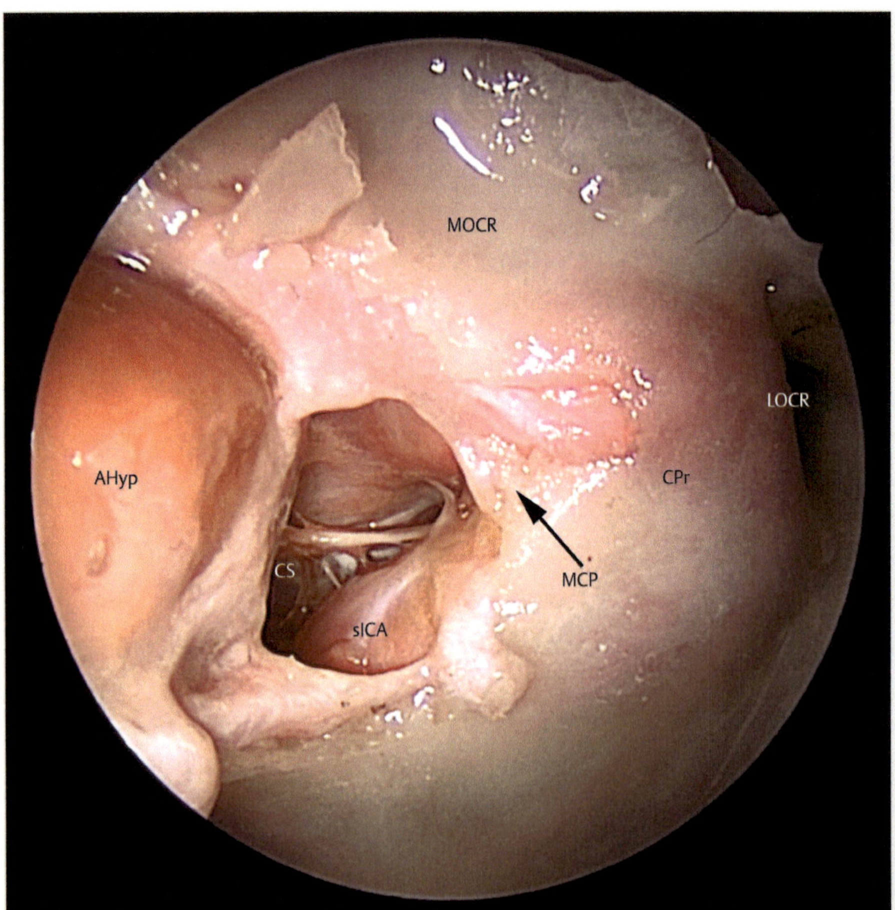

Fig. 17.11 Parasellar tract of the internal carotid artery and related bony landmarks. With a 70-degree scope turned superolaterally, the relationship between the Parasellar tract of the internal carotid artery (sICA), carotid prominence (CPr), medial (MOCR) and lateral optic-carotid recess (LOCR), and middle clinoid process (MCP) is assessed. Of note, the medial optic–carotid recess is rarely pneumatized and represents the lateral end of the tuberculum sellae; the lateral optic–carotid recess is the pneumatization of the optic strut, which separates the internal carotid artery, optic nerve, and superior orbital fissure; the middle clinoid process is found in around one-third of subjects and is located inferomedially to the passage from the parasellar to paraclinoid tract of the internal carotid artery. AHyp, adenohypophysis; CS, cavernous sinus (lumen).

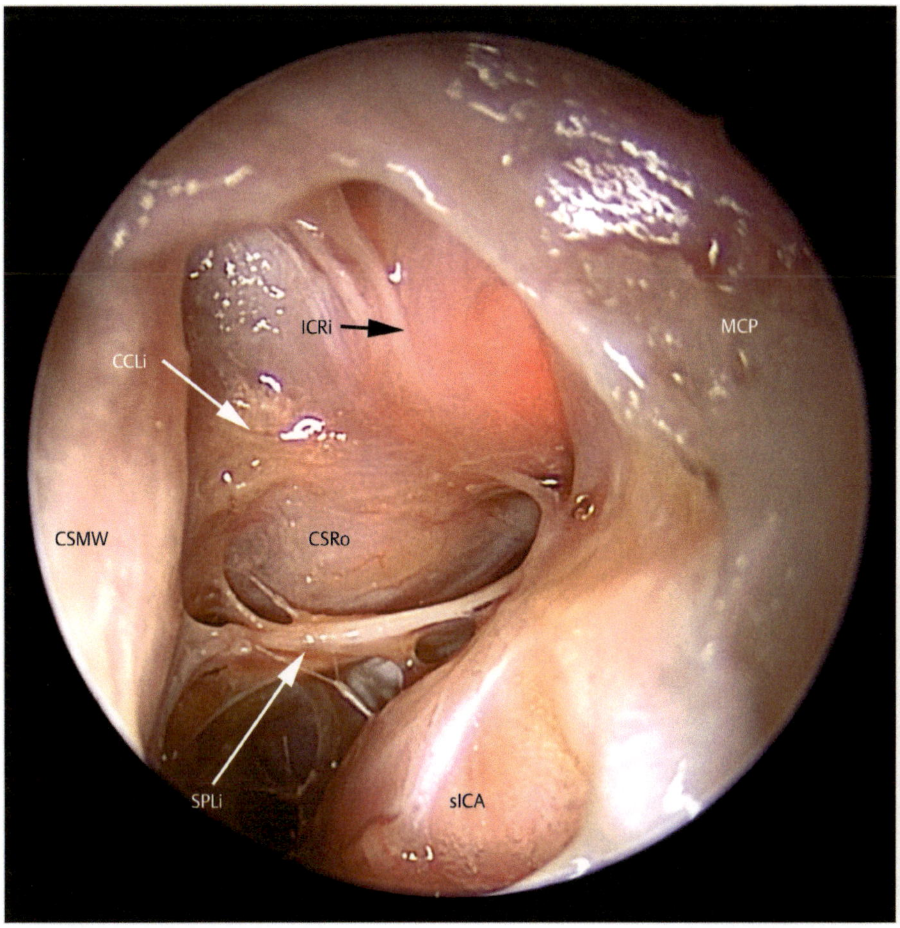

Fig. 17.12 Step 4. A 70-degre scope turned superolaterally is placed through the opening in the anterior wall of the cavernous sinus. The area where the parasellar tract of the internal carotid artery (sICA) passes through the roof of the cavernous sinus (CSRo), which is defined as inferior carotid ring (ICRi), comes into view. The caroticoclinoid ligament (CCLi) connects the inferior carotid ring with the medial wall of the cavernous sinus (CSMW), contributing to form the roof of the cavernous sinus (CSRo). The anterior clinoid process lies superiorly and laterally to the inferior carotid ring. The fibrous trabecula that arises from the medial wall of the cavernous sinus and reaches the parasellar carotid artery is called the superior parasellar ligament (SPLi). The latter structure also reaches the middle clinoid process (MCP), when present.

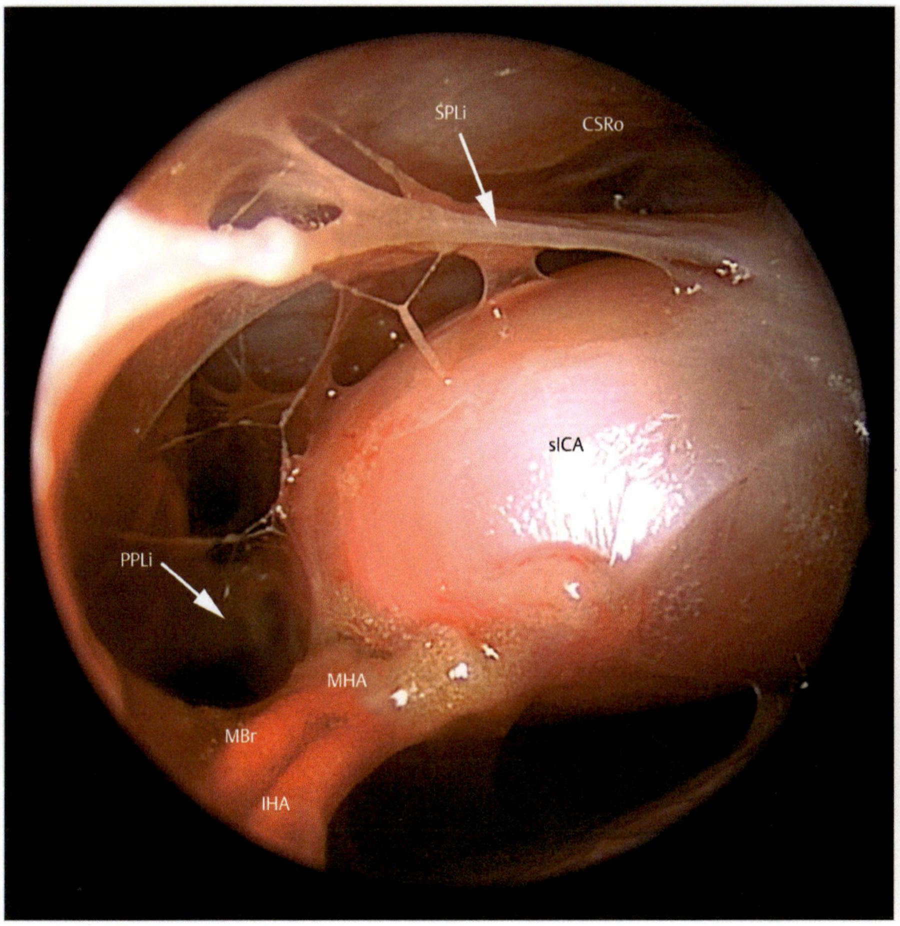

Fig. 17.13 Parasellar tract of the internal carotid artery and the posterior parasellar ligament. A 70-degree scope is turned laterally and moved posteriorly within the cavernous sinus. The posterior portion of the parasellar tract of the internal carotid artery comes into view along with the posterior parasellar ligament (PPLi), which connects the internal carotid artery with the medial and posterior walls of the cavernous sinus. The meningohypophyseal artery (MHA), hypophyseal artery (IHA), and meningeal branch (MBr) are seen from a medial-to-lateral perspective. CSRo, roof of the cavernous sinus.

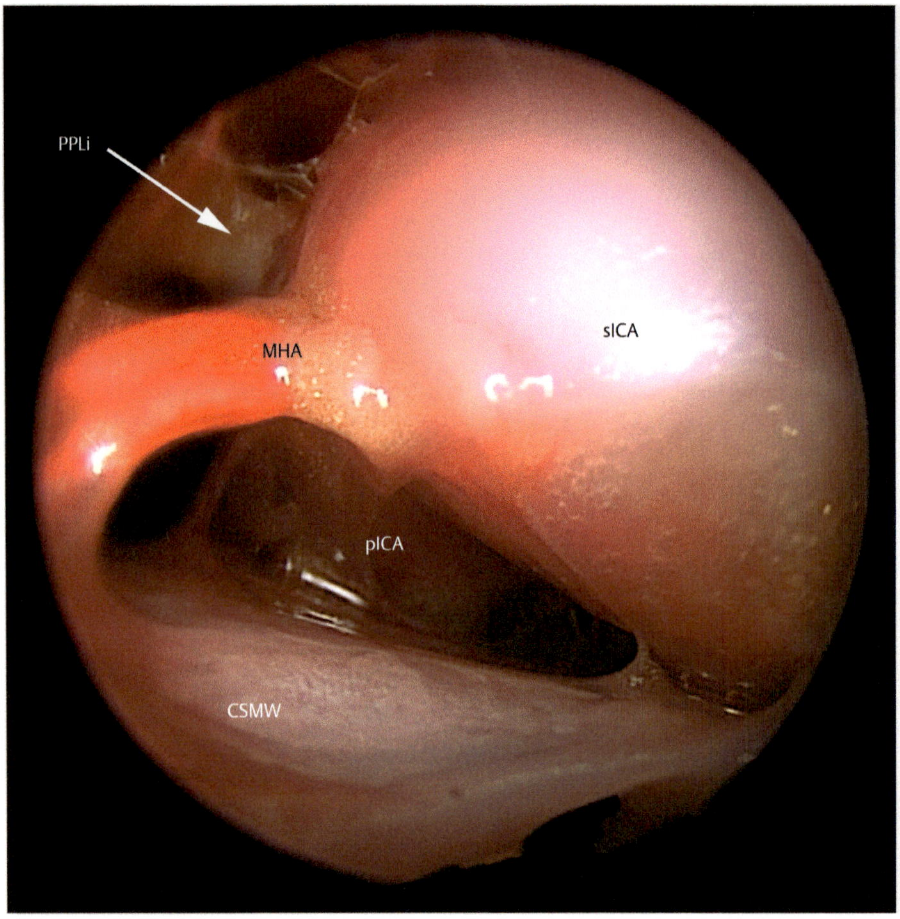

Fig. 17.14 Paraclival tract of the internal carotid artery and the posterior parasellar ligament. A 70-degree scope is turned inferolaterally to identify the paraclival tract of the internal carotid artery (pICA). This perspective allows the understanding of the three-dimensional relationships among the parasellar (sICA) and paraclival tracts of the internal carotid artery, meningohypophyseal artery (MHA), and posterior parasellar ligament (PPLi). CSMW, medial wall of the cavernous sinus.

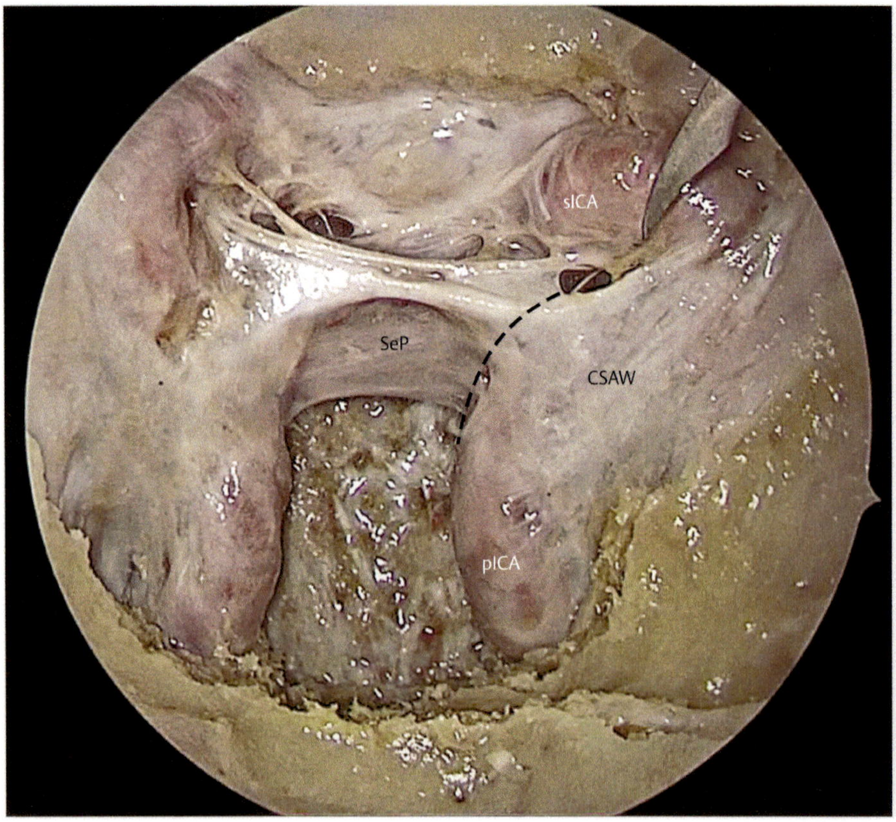

Fig. 17.15 Steps 5 and 6 (part 1). The carotid prominence, carotid sulcus, and midclivus are entirely removed. The paraclival tract of the internal carotid artery (pICA) is completely exposed and the small aperture of the anterior wall of the cavernous sinus (CSAW) is extended inferiorly (*black dashed line*), staying medially to the internal carotid artery. SeP, parasellar periosteum; sICA, parasellar tract of the internal carotid artery.

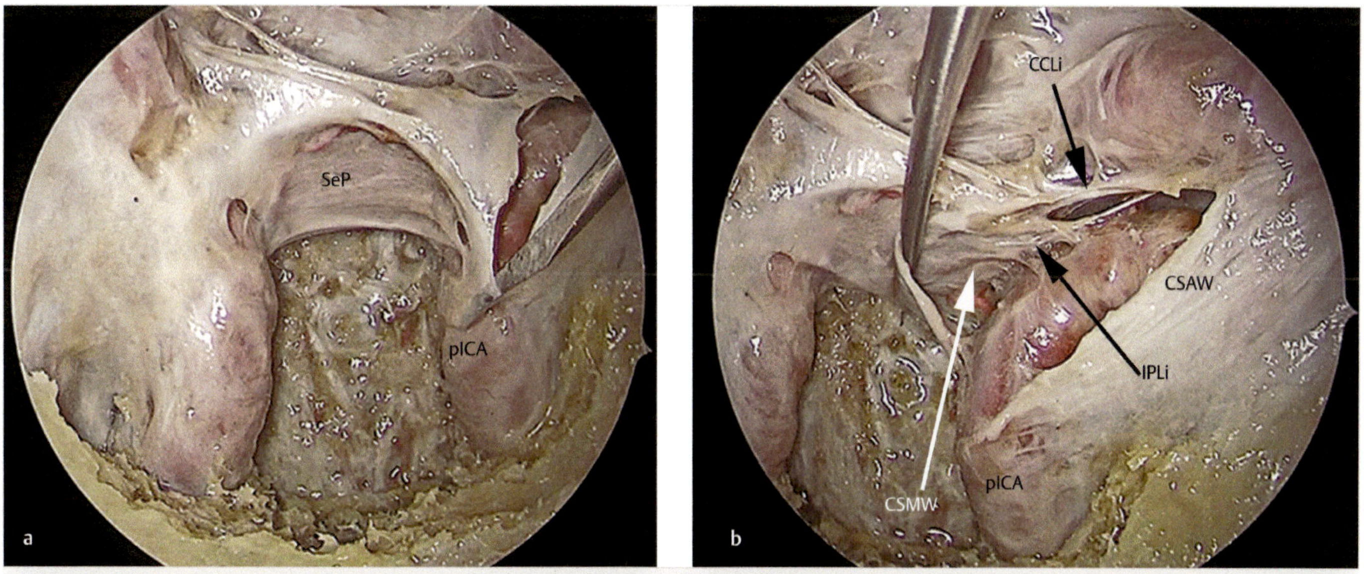

Fig. 17.16 (a, b) Steps 5 and 6 (part 2). The periosteal incision of the anterior wall of the cavernous sinus (CSAW) is extended along the medial surface of the paraclival tract of the internal carotid artery (pICA) to expose the inferior part of the medial portion of the cavernous sinus. CCLi, caroticoclinoid ligament; CSMW, medial wall of the cavernous sinus; IPLi, inferior parasellar ligament; SeP, sellar periosteum.

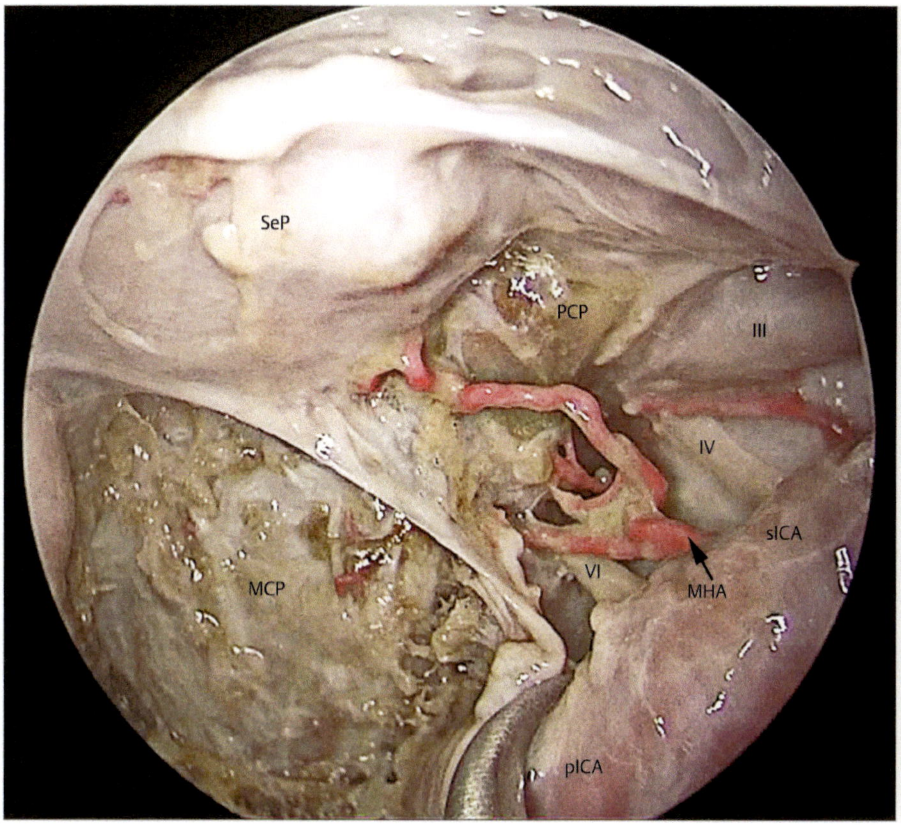

Fig. 17.17 Posterior clinoid process. The paraclival (pICA) and parasellar tracts of the internal carotid artery (sICA) are displaced laterally to entirely show the meningohypophyseal artery (MHA) and its branches. Most branches run behind the posterior clinoid process (PCP), while those reaching the pituitary gland are located anteriorly. The abducens (VI), trochlear (IV), and oculomotor (III) nerves enter the cavernous sinus inferiorly and laterally to the posterior clinoid process. MCP, midclivus periosteum; SeP, sellar periosteum.

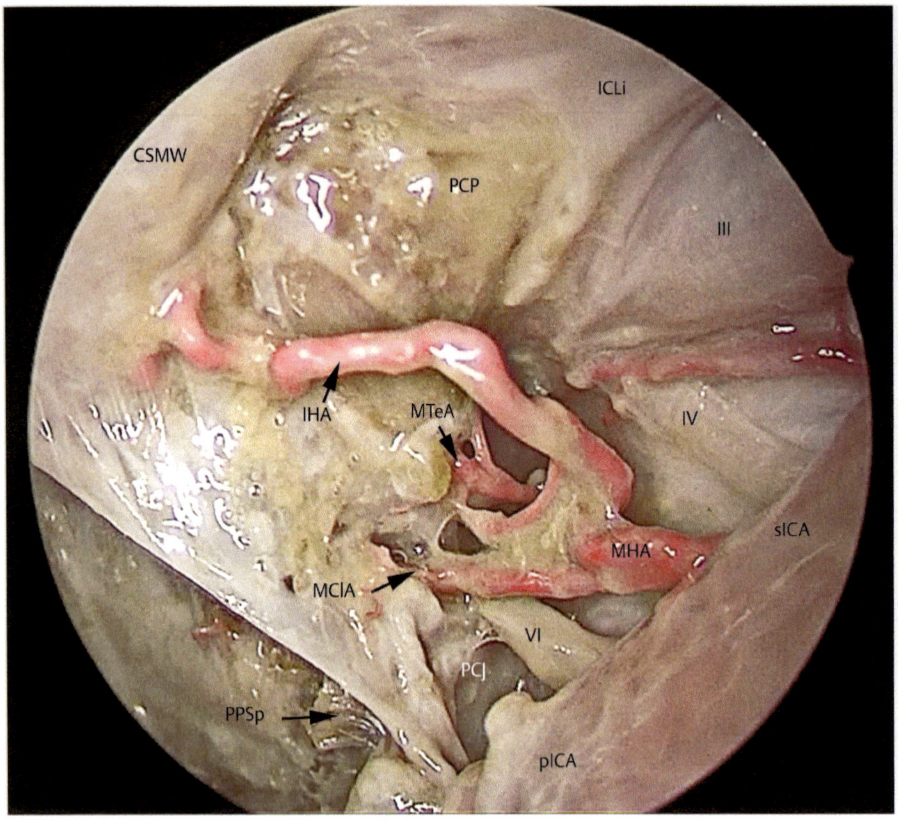

Fig. 17.18 Medial branches of the meningohypophyseal artery. The meningohypophyseal artery ends with the inferior hypophyseal artery (IHA) and several meningeal branches characterized by variable branching patterns. The medial branches can be seen from this perspective: the medial clival artery (MClA) runs behind the posterior clinoid process (PCP), reaching the midclivus superoposteriorly to the petrous process of the sphenoid bone (PPSp); the medial tentorial artery (MTeA) runs laterally to the middle portion of the posterior clinoid process and reaches the posterior petroclinoid fold. III, oculomotor nerve; IV, trochlear nerve; VI, abducens nerve; ICLi, interclinoid ligament; PCJ, petroclival junction; pICA, paraclival tract of the internal carotid artery; sICA, parasellar tract of the internal carotid artery; SeP, sellar periosteum.

Reference

[1] Parkinson D. Carotid cavernous fistula. History and anatomy. In: Dolenc VV, ed. The Cavernous Sinus: A Multidisciplinary Approach to Vascular and Tumorous Lesions. Wien: Springer-Verlag; 1987:3–29

[2] Rhoton ALJ. The middle cranial base and cavernous sinus. In: Dolenc VV, Rogers L, eds. Cavernous Sinus Developments and Future Perspectives. Wien: Springer-Verlag; 2009:3–25

[3] Fernandez-Miranda JC, Zwagerman NT, Abhinav K, et al. Cavernous sinus compartments from the endoscopic endonasal approach: anatomical considerations and surgical relevance to adenoma surgery. J Neurosurg 2018;129(2):430–441

[4] Truong HQ, Lieber S, Najera E, Alves-Belo JT, Gardner PA, Fernandez-Miranda JC. The medial wall of the cavernous sinus. Part 1: surgical anatomy, ligaments, and surgical technique for its mobilization and/or resection. J Neurosurg 2018:1–9

[5] Krayenbühl N, Hafez A, Hernesniemi JA, Krisht AF. Taming the cavernous sinus: technique of hemostasis using fibrin glue. Neurosurgery 2007;61(3, Suppl):E52–, discussion E52

[6] Stokken JK, Halderman A, Recinos PF, Woodard TD, Sindwani R. Strategies for improving visualization during endoscopic skull base surgery. Otolaryngol Clin North Am 2016;49(1):131–140

[7] Shkarubo AN, Chernov IV, Ogurtsova AA, et al. Neurophysiological identification of cranial nerves during endoscopic endonasal surgery of skull base tumors: pilot study technical report. World Neurosurg 2017;98:230–238

[8] Dhandapani S, Singh H, Negm HM, Cohen S, Anand VK, Schwartz TH. Cavernous sinus invasion in pituitary adenomas: systematic review and pooled data meta-analysis of radiologic criteria and comparison of endoscopic and microscopic surgery. World Neurosurg 2016;96:36–46

[9] Toda M, Kosugi K, Ozawa H, Ogawa K, Yoshida K. Surgical treatment of cavernous sinus lesion in patients with nonfunctioning pituitary adenomas via the endoscopic endonasal approach. J Neurol Surg B Skull Base 2018;79(Suppl 4):S311–S315

[10] Ferreli F, Turri-Zanoni M, Canevari FR, et al. Endoscopic endonasal management of non-functioning pituitary adenomas with cavernous sinus invasion: a 10-year experience. Rhinology 2015;53(4):308–316

[11] Elshazly K, Kshettry VR, Farrell CJ, Nyquist G, Rosen M, Evans JJ. Clinical outcomes after endoscopic endonasal resection of giant pituitary adenomas. World Neurosurg 2018;114:e447–e456

[12] Ajlan A, Achrol AS, Albakr A, et al. Cavernous sinus involvement by pituitary adenomas: clinical implications and outcomes of endoscopic endonasal resection. J Neurol Surg B Skull Base 2017;78(3):273–282

[13] Cohen-Cohen S, Gardner PA, Alves-Belo JT, et al. The medial wall of the cavernous sinus. Part 2: selective medial wall resection in 50 pituitary adenoma patients. J Neurosurg 2018:1–10

[14] Hwang J, Seol HJ, Nam DH, Lee JI, Lee MH, Kong DS. Therapeutic strategy for cavernous sinus-invading non-functioning pituitary adenomas based on the modified knosp grading system. Brain Tumor Res Treat 2016;4(2):63–69

[15] Woodworth GF, Patel KS, Shin B, et al. Surgical outcomes using a medial-to-lateral endonasal endoscopic approach to pituitary adenomas invading the cavernous sinus. J Neurosurg 2014;120(5):1086–1094

[16] Park HH, Kim EH, Ku CR, Lee EJ, Kim SH. Outcomes of aggressive surgical resection in growth hormone-secreting pituitary adenomas with cavernous sinus invasion. World Neurosurg 2018;117:e280–e289

[17] Zoli M, Milanese L, Bonfatti R, et al. Cavernous sinus invasion by pituitary adenomas: role of endoscopic endonasal surgery. J Neurosurg Sci 2016;60(4):485–494

[18] Trevisi G, Vigo V, Morena MG, et al. Comparison of endoscopic versus microsurgical resection of pituitary adenomas with parasellar extension and evaluation of the predictive value of a simple 4-quadrant radiologic classification. World Neurosurg 2019;121:e769–e774

[19] Koutourousiou M, Vaz Guimaraes Filho F, Fernandez-Miranda JC, et al. Endoscopic endonasal surgery for tumors of the cavernous sinus: a series of 234 patients. World Neurosurg 2017;103:713–732

[20] Park KJ, Kano H, Iyer A, et al. Gamma Knife stereotactic radiosurgery for cavernous sinus meningioma: long-term follow-up in 200 patients. J Neurosurg 2018:1–10

[21] Patrona A, Patel KS, Bander ED, et al. Endoscopic endonasal surgery for nonadenomatous, nonmeningeal pathology involving the cavernous sinus. J Neurosurg 2017;126(3):880–888

[22] Hughes JD, Kapurch J, Van Gompel JJ, et al. Diagnosis and outcome of biopsies of indeterminate lesions of the cavernous sinus and Meckel's cave: a retrospective case series in 85 patients. Neurosurgery 2018;83(3):529–539

[23] Kou YF, Killeen D, Whittemore B, et al. Intracranial complications of acute sinusitis in children: the role of endoscopic sinus surgery. Int J Pediatr Otorhinolaryngol 2018;110:147–151

18 Lateral Transcavernous Approach

Marco Ferrari, Marco Ravanelli, Francesco Belotti, Alberto Schreiber, Roberto Maroldi

The lateral compartment of the cavernous sinus is located between the cavernous portion of the internal carotid artery and the lateral wall of the cavernous sinus.[1] The mediolateral extension of sellar lesions invading the cavernous sinus is classified in four grades according to Micko et al[2]: grades 1 to 3 are defined in relation to three lines connecting the cross-sectional parasellar and intracranial internal carotid artery (grade 3 is further divided into 3A or 3B when the tumor grows cranially or caudally to the parasellar internal carotid artery, respectively). Namely, the medial tangent, the line through the cross-sectional centers, and the lateral tangent permit definition of the incremental medial-to-lateral extension of pituitary adenomas with parasellar growth. In grade 4, the parasellar tract of the internal carotid artery is encased by the tumor. Meningiomas of the parasellar area frequently involve the lateral compartment of the cavernous sinus by following the meningeal framework.[3] As a consequence of the lateral position of neural structures within the cavernous sinus, parasellar schwannomas tend to arise from the lateral compartment. Similarly, hemangiomas and epidermoid cysts frequently invade the lateral portion of the cavernous sinus.[4–10] Thus, both neurogenic and meningeal lesions of the parasellar area pose similar, if not greater, problems to grade 3 and 4 pituitary adenomas.

The lateral transcavernous approach passes laterally to the parasellar tract of the internal carotid artery, from the anterior wall to the roof and posterior wall of the cavernous sinus.[11] When far posterior extension to the interpeduncular/parapeduncular area is needed, the medial and lateral transcavernous sinus corridors can be merged and/or further extended posteriorly with the transdorsal or transoculomotor triangle approaches (see interdural hypophysiopexy, as shown in Chapter 10).[12,13] Given its wider lateral extension compared to the medial transcavernous approach, a superior transpterygoid approach can be helpful, though not strictly necessary, to adequately expose the inferolateral portion of cavernous

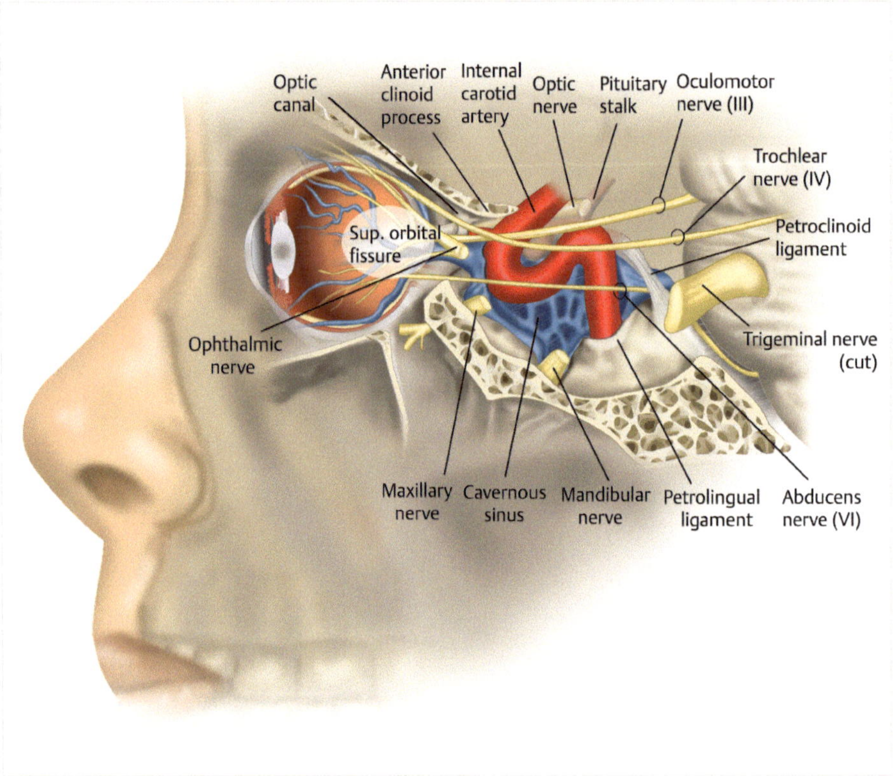

Fig. 18.1 Sagittal view of the cavernous sinus. This sagittal illustration shows the main structures of the lateral portion of the cavernous sinus.

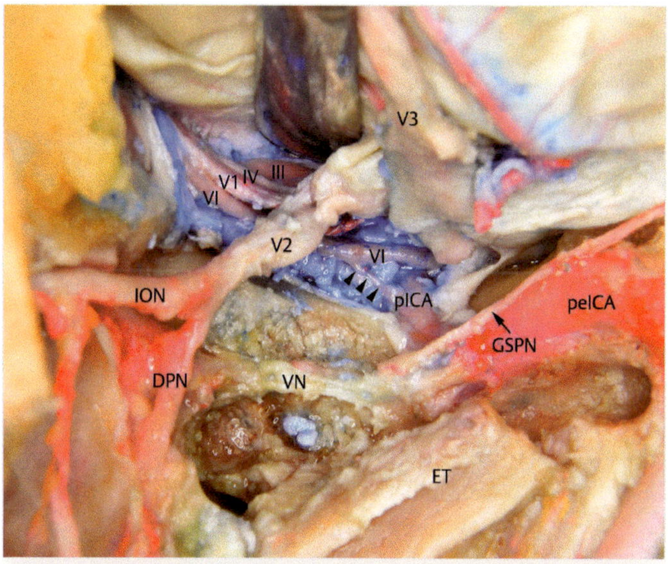

Fig. 18.2 Subtemporal lateral-to-medial view of the cavernous sinus. This cadaver picture shows with a lateral-to-medial epidural perspective the lateral portion of the left cavernous sinus. The mandibular nerve (V3) has been sectioned and displaced to properly expose the cavernous sinus. III, oculomotor nerve; IV, trochlear nerve; V1, ophthalmic nerve; V2, maxillary nerve; VI, abducens nerve; DPN, descending palatine nerve; ET, eustachian tube; GSPN, greater superficial petrosal nerve; ION, infraorbital nerve; peICA, petrous tract of the internal carotid artery; pICA, paraclival tract of the internal carotid artery; VN, vidian nerve. (*Black arrowheads*, sympathetic branch for the abducens nerve.)

sinus (see also Chapter 21). The lateral transcavernous approach crosses the trajectory of the nerves of the lateral wall of the cavernous sinus and Meckel's cave, which are therefore exposed to the risk of being damaged. Considering the benign behavior of most diseases involving this area, there is general consensus that their management should be discussed by a multidisciplinary team and tailored on a case-by-case basis. The current trend consists of achieving the most complete resection while minimizing the risk of postoperative complications. In line with this philosophy, stereotactic radiotherapy or Gamma Knife radiosurgery should be kept in consideration to manage critical and/or residual extensions of the lesion rather than with aggressive surgery.

This chapter illustrates in a step-by-step fashion the dissection of the lateral transcavernous approach, and provides several anatomical details on the vascularization of the lateral portion of the cavernous sinus. Interestingly, the identification of structures within the cavernous sinus will entail meticulous removal of fat tissue that can be variably found within the dural sinus, and especially nearby neurovascular structures.[14,15] Given their strict relationship, the lateral transcavernous approach and suprapetrous approach to Meckel's cave share several anatomical details. Therefore, reading of Chapter 21 is strongly recommended before starting dissection of the lateral compartment of the cavernous sinus.

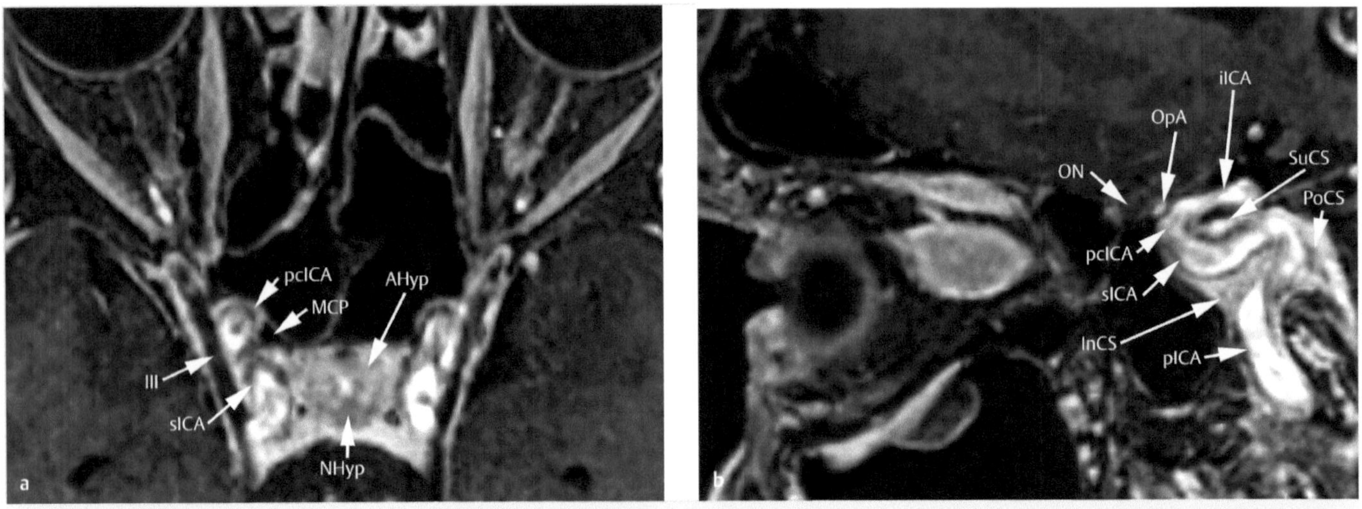

Fig. 18.3 Axial and sagittal MRI anatomy of the cavernous sinus. Axial **(a)** and sagittal **(b)** T1-weighted contrast-enhanced fat-saturated images passing through the cavernous sinus. The cavernous sinus is formed by four compartments: the inferior compartment (InCS) is located anterior and inferior to the paraclival (pICA) and parasellar tracts of the internal carotid artery (sICA). The superior compartment (SuCS) lies between the parasellar carotid artery and the roof of the cavernous sinus. The posterior compartment (PoCS) is located posterior to the internal carotid artery and anterior to the posterior wall of the cavernous sinus. The lateral compartment, which is shown in ▶Fig. 18.4, lies between the internal carotid artery and the lateral wall of the cavernous sinus. III, oculomotor nerve; AHyp, adenohypophysis; iICA, intracranial tract of the internal carotid artery; MCP, middle clinoid process; NHyp, neurohypophysis; ON, optic nerve; OpA, ophthalmic artery; pcICA, paraclinoid tract of the internal carotid artery.

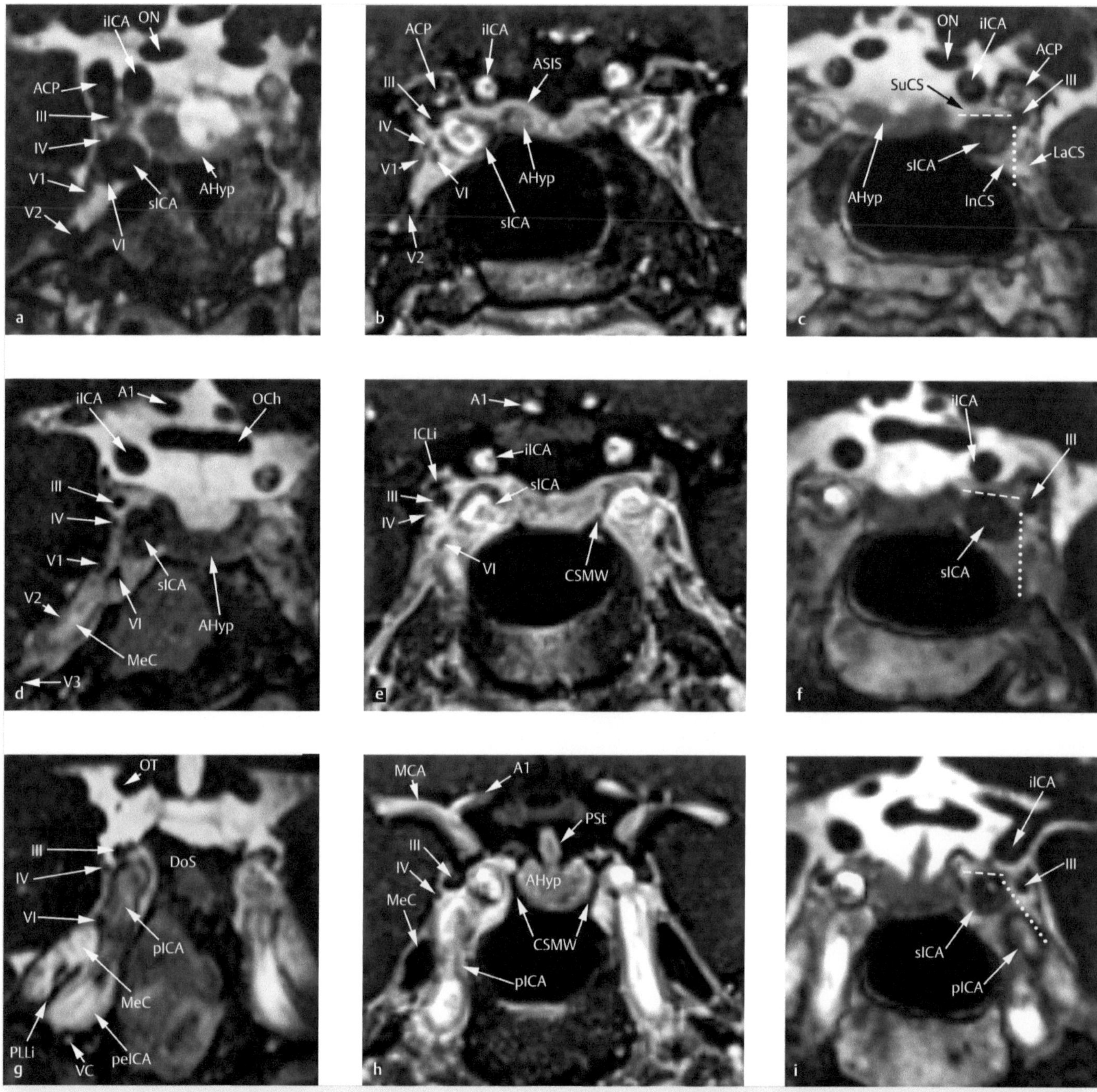

Fig. 18.4 (a–i) Coronal MRI anatomy of the cavernous sinus. The panel includes six CISS (constructive interference in steady state) MRI (left and right columns) and three T1-weighted contrast-enhanced fat-saturated images (central column) passing through the anterior (upper row), middle (middle row), and posterior portions of the cavernous sinus (lower row). The lateral compartment of the cavernous sinus (LaCS) is located laterally to the virtual plane (*white dotted line*) tangent to the lateral surface of the paraclival (pICA) and parasellar tracts of the internal carotid artery (sICA). The superior compartment (SuCS) lies between the plane passing through the superior aspect of the parasellar carotid artery (*white dashed line*) and the roof of the cavernous sinus and the anterior clinoid process (ACP). The lateral compartment houses several cranial nerves, namely, the oculomotor nerve (III), which runs in a borderline position close to the superior compartment, the trochlear (IV), abducens (VI), ophthalmic (V1), and maxillary nerves (V2). Moreover, the lateral compartment is adjacent to Meckel's cave (MeC). V3, mandibular nerve; A1, precommunicating tract of the anterior cerebral artery; AHyp, adenohypophysis; ASIS, anterosuperior cavernous sinus; CSMW, medial wall of the cavernous sinus; DoS, dorsum sellae; ICLi, interclinoid ligament; iICA, intracranial tract of the internal carotid artery; MCA, middle cerebral artery; OCh, optic chiasm; ON, optic nerve; OT, optic tract; peICA, petrous tract of the internal carotid artery; PLLi, petrolingual ligament; PSt, pituitary stalk; VC, vidian canal.

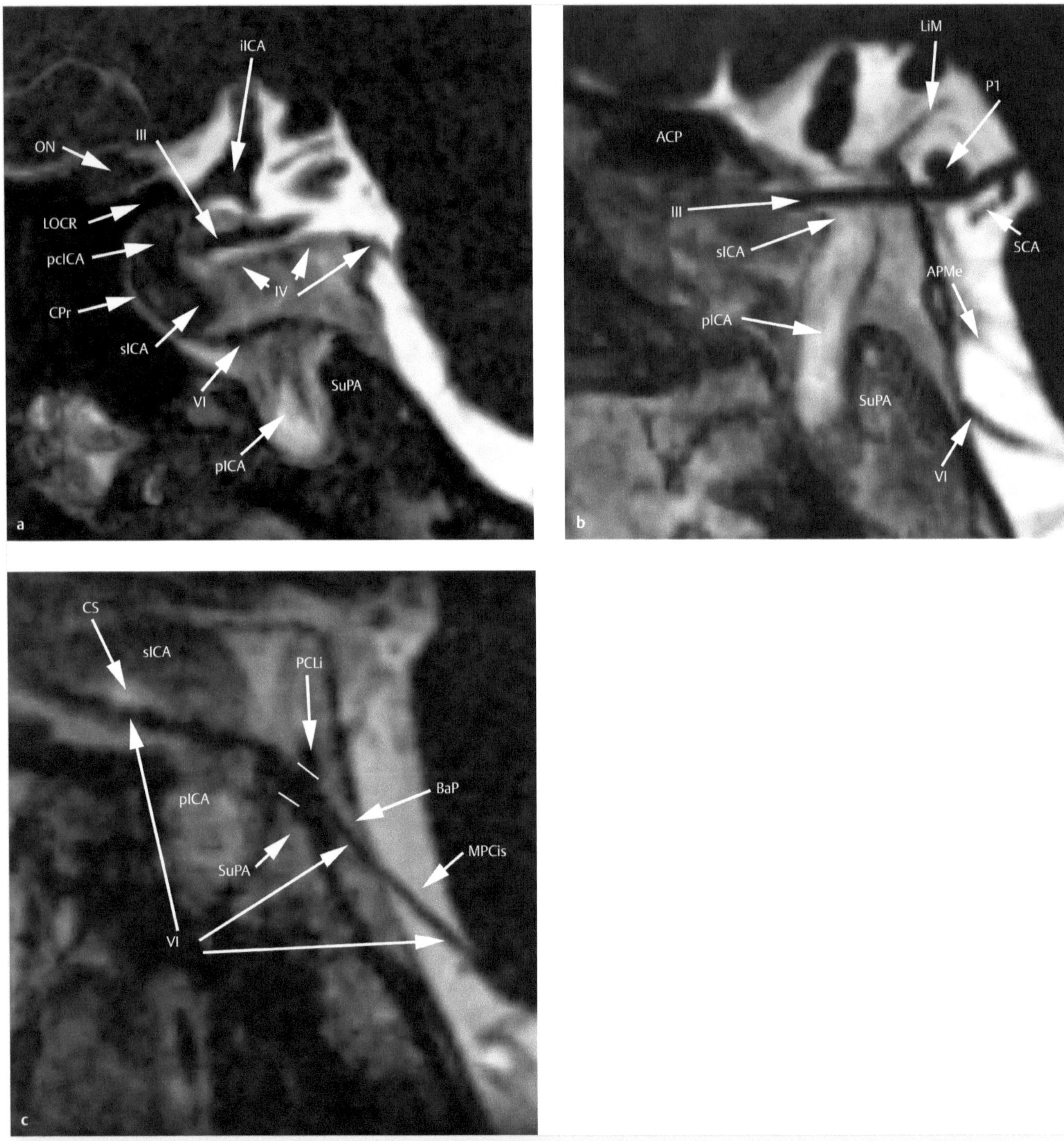

Fig. 18.5 Sagittal and parasagittal MRI of the oculomotor, trochlear, and abducens nerves. The panel includes one sagittal **(a)** and two parasagittal **(b, c)** CISS (constructive interference in steady state) MRI depicting the anatomy of the oculomotor (III), trochlear (IV), and abducens nerves (VI). The oculomotor nerve arises from the mesencephalon and passes between the precommunicating tract of the posterior cerebral artery (P1) and the superior cerebellar artery (SCA). Then, it reaches the cavernous sinus (CS) by piercing the posterior half of its roof. Finally, it runs within the lateral wall of the cavernous sinus while coursing adjacently to the inferior aspect of the anterior clinoid process (ACP). The trochlear nerve reaches the cavernous sinus below the oculomotor nerve, passing through the anterior insertion of the tentorium. The abducens nerve arises from the bulbopontine sulcus and runs within the median prepontine cistern (MPCis). Thereafter, it enters the basilar plexus (BaP) and reaches Dorello's canal (between the two *white bars*), which is formed by the petroclival junction and the superior petrous apex (SuPA) inferiorly and the petroclinoid (or Gruber's) ligament (PCLi) superiorly. The abducens nerve runs inside the cavernous sinus through Dorello's canal, where it sharply acquires a more horizontal trajectory compared to the previous tracts. APMe, anterior pontine membrane; CPr, carotid prominence; iICA, intracranial tract of the internal carotid artery; LiM, Liliequist's membrane; LOCR, lateral optic–carotid recess; ON, optic nerve; pcICA, paraclinoid tract of the internal carotid artery; pICA, paraclival tract of the internal carotid artery; sICA, parasellar tract of the internal carotid artery.

Endoscopic Dissection

Nasal Phase

- Paraseptal sphenoidotomy.
- Transrostral sphenoidotomy.
- Expanded transrostral sphenoidotomy.
- Vertical uncinectomy.
- Horizontal uncinectomy.
- Anterior ethmoidectomy.
- Posterior ethmoidectomy.
- Transethmoidal sphenoidotomy.
- Middle and superior turbinectomy.
- Type A endoscopic medial maxillectomy.
- Facultative: Type B–D endoscopic medial maxillectomy.

Skull Base Phase

- Facultative: Transsellar approach.
- Facultative: Transcavernous (medial) approach.
- Facultative: Transclival (midclivus) approach.
- Facultative: Optic and orbital decompression.
- Facultative: Superior transpterygoid approach.
- Step 1: Removal of the carotid prominence and lateral wall of the sphenoid sinus.
- Step 2: Removal of the optic strut.
- Step 3: Removal of the carotid sulcus and partial removal of the midclivus.
- Step 4: Removal of the lingual process.
- Step 5: Incision of the anterior wall of the cavernous sinus.
- Step 6: Medialization of the sellar portion of the internal carotid artery.
- Step 7: Dissection of the lateral compartment of the cavernous sinus.
- Step 8: Section of the inferolateral trunk.
- Step 9: Dissection of the posterior compartment of the cavernous sinus.
- Step 10: Dissection of the inferior compartment of the cavernous sinus.

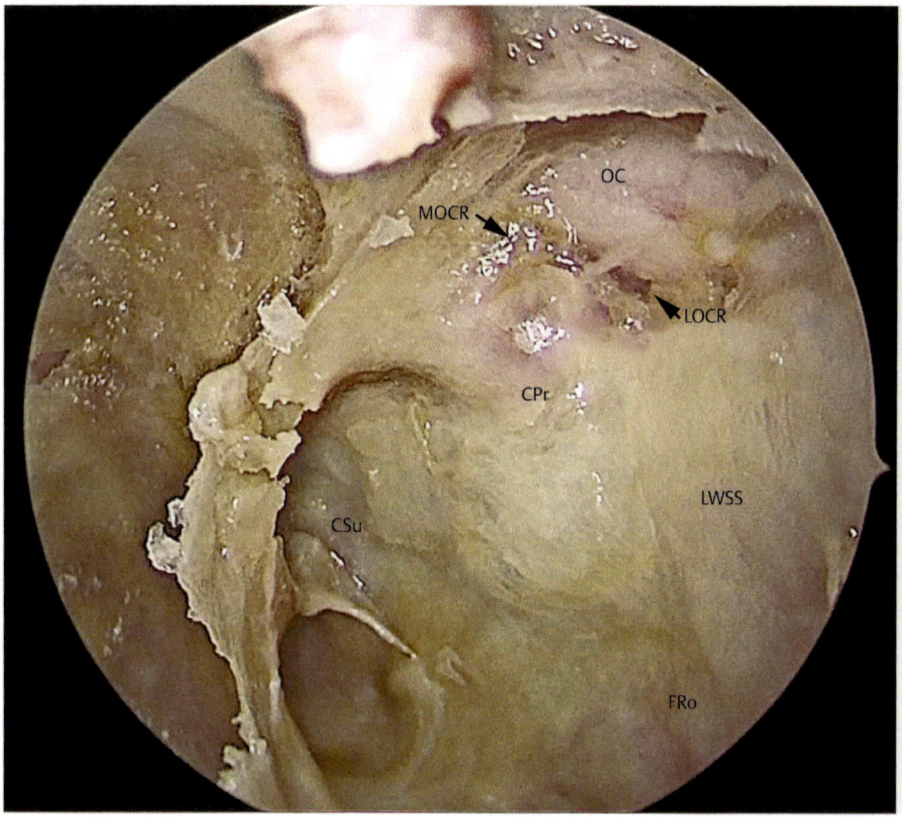

Fig. 18.6 Bony landmarks. The anterior projection of the lateral compartment of the cavernous sinus corresponds to the junction between the carotid prominence (CPr) and the lateral wall of the sphenoid sinus (LWSS). This dihedral angle is located below the lateral optic–carotid recess (LOCR). CSu, carotid sulcus; FRo, foramen rotundum; MOCR, medial optic–carotid recess; OC, optic canal.

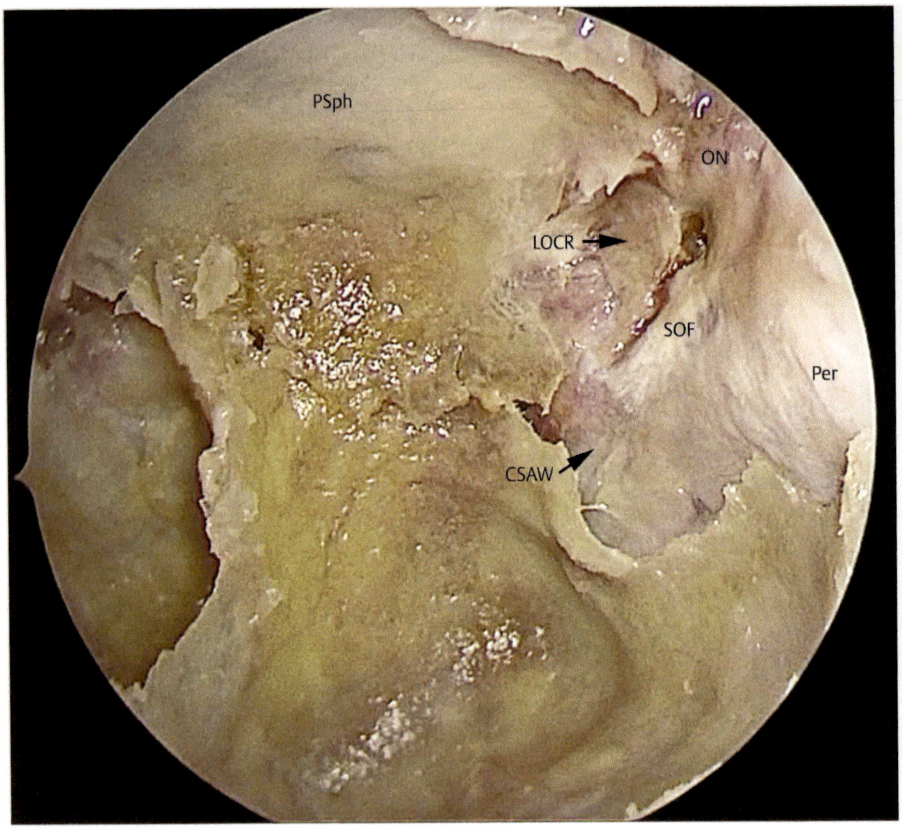

Fig. 18.7 Step 1. The carotid prominence and the lateral wall of the sphenoid sinus are removed to expose the anterior wall of the cavernous sinus (CSAW) and the superior orbital fissure (SOF). The lateral optic–carotid recess (LOCR) corresponds to the optic strut, which can be variably pneumatized and serves as the inferomedial root of the anterior clinoid process. The two remaining roots are the medial end of the lesser wing of sphenoid bone and the lateral end of the planum sphenoidale (PSph). ON, optic nerve; Per, periorbit.

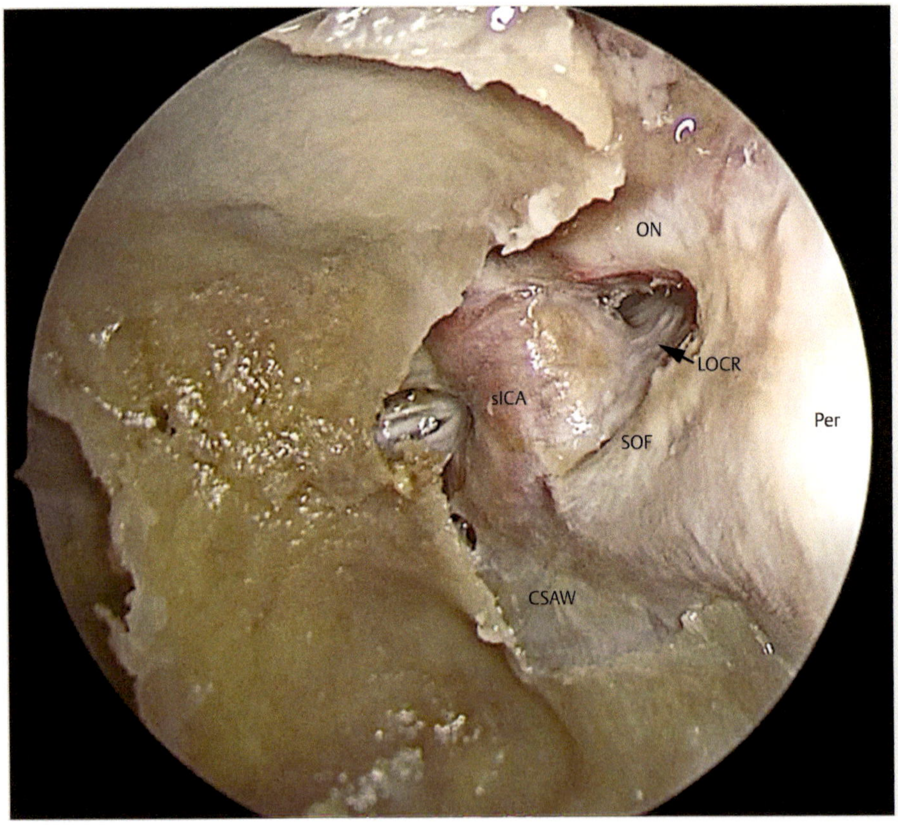

Fig. 18.8 Step 2. The optic strut is removed to show that the lateral optic–carotid recess (LOCR) is surrounded by noble structures including the parasellar (sICA) and paraclinoid tracts of the internal carotid artery, the superior orbital fissure (SOF), and the optic nerve (ON). After these steps, the superior portion of the anterior wall of the cavernous sinus (CSAW) is completely exposed. Per, periorbit.

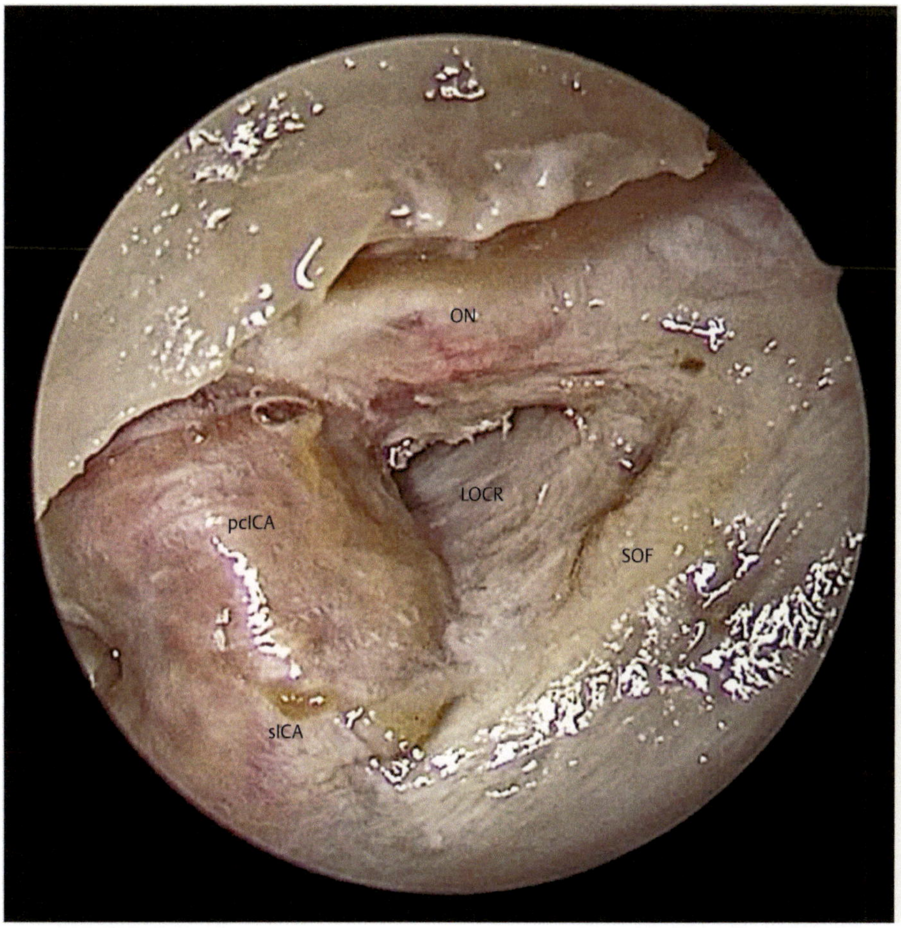

Fig. 18.9 The triangle of the lateral optic–carotid recess. The dural tunnel covering the optic strut has a triangular section formed by the optic nerve (ON) superiorly, the superior orbital fissure (SOF) antero-latero-inferiorly, and the parasellar (sICA) and paraclinoid (pcICA) tracts of the internal carotid artery postero-medio-inferiorly. LOCR, position of the lateral optic–carotid recess.

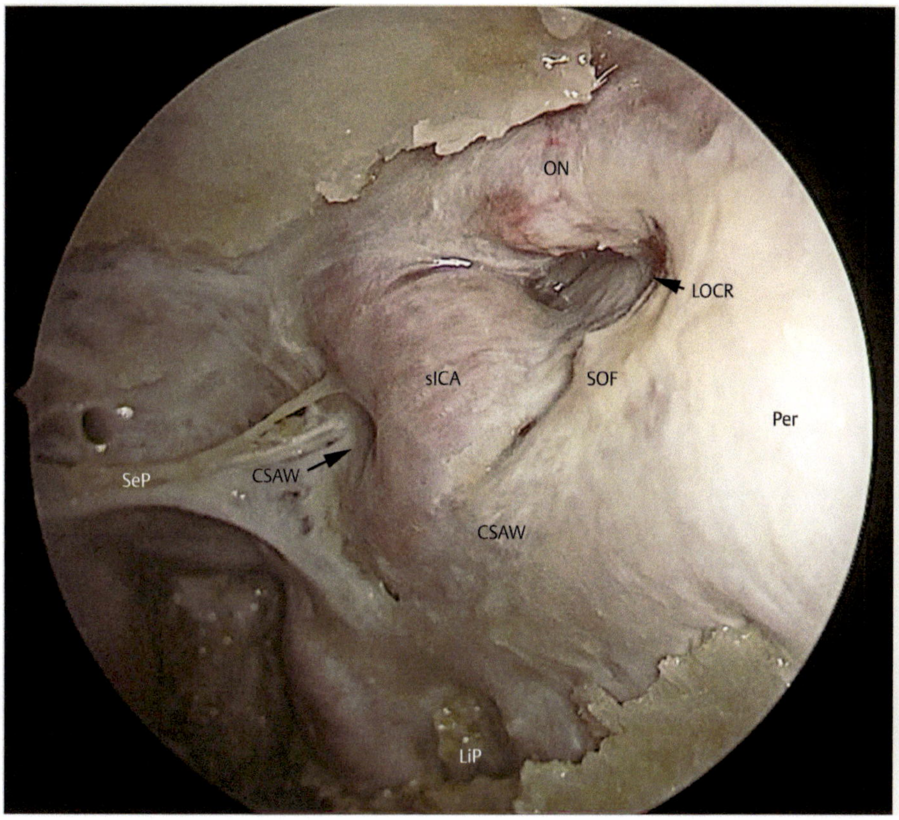

Fig. 18.10 Step 3 (part 1). The anterior wall of the cavernous sinus (CSAW) is entirely exposed by removing the carotid sulcus and the inferior portion of the lateral wall of the sphenoid sinus. The sellar prominence and the midclivus are removed to allow medialization of the internal carotid artery during the next dissection steps. LiP, lingual process; LOCR, lateral optic–carotid recess; Per, periorbit; SeP, sellar periosteum; sICA, parasellar tract of the internal carotid artery.

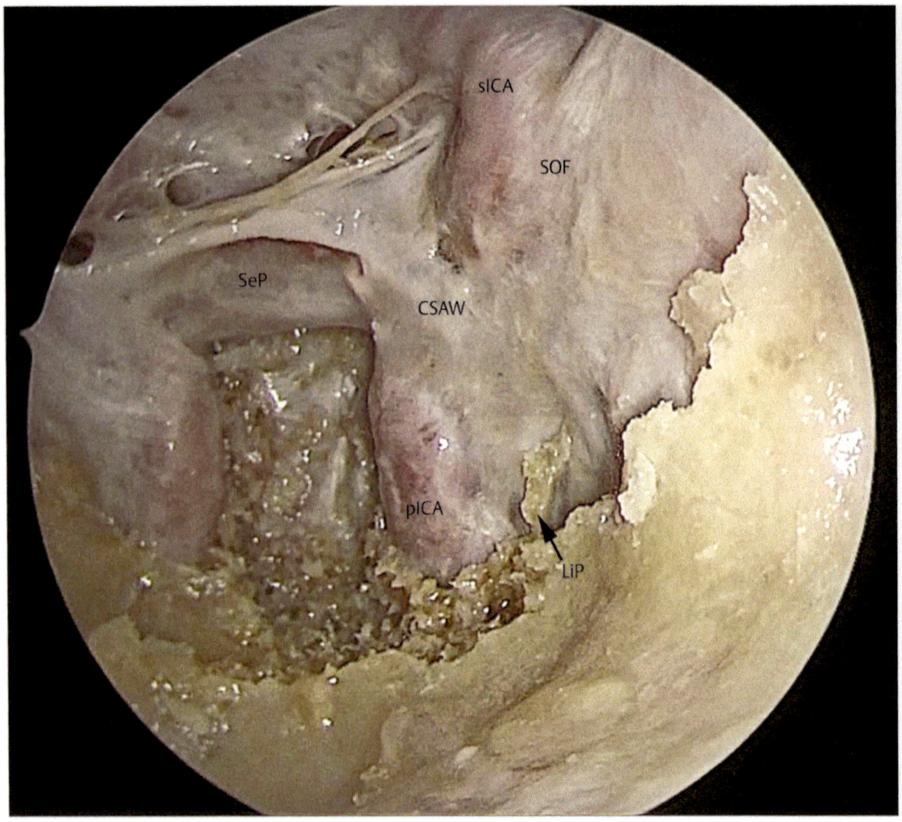

Fig. 18.11 Step 3 (part 2). The lingual process of the sphenoid sinus (LiP) is found at the inferolateral aspect of the paraclival tract of the internal carotid artery (pICA). This bony landmark marks the passage from the cavernous sinus, medially, to Meckel's cave, laterally. CSAW, anterior wall of the cavernous sinus; SOF, superior orbital fissure; SeP, sellar periosteum; sICA, parasellar tract of the internal carotid artery.

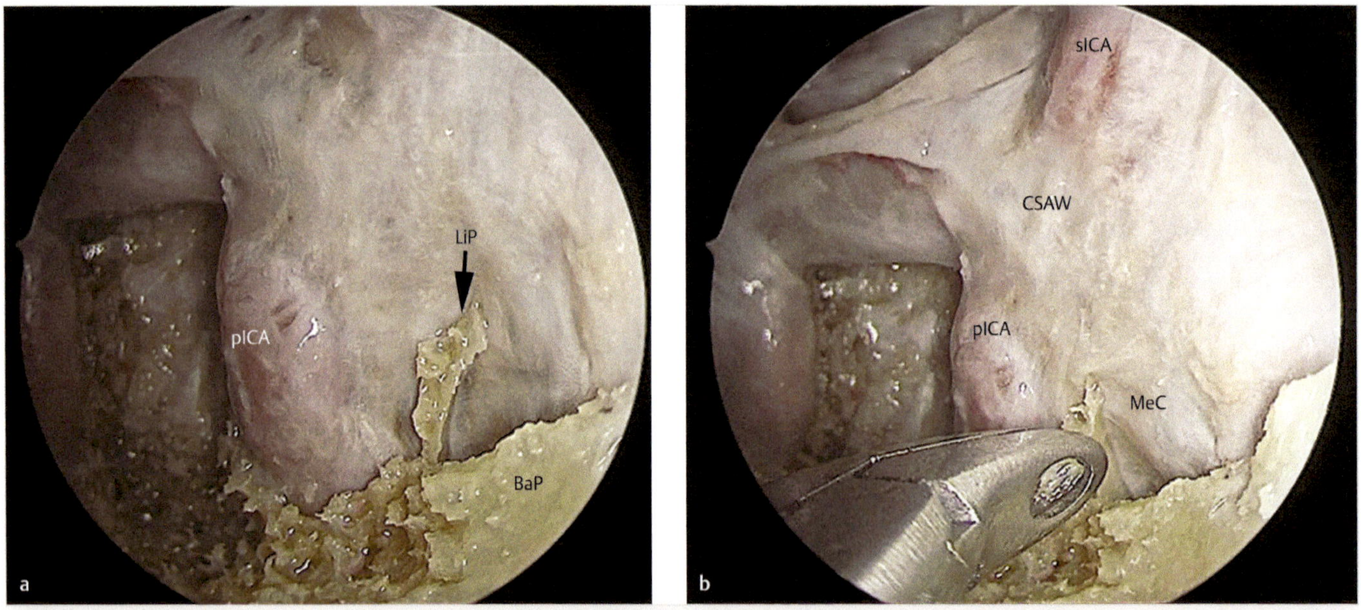

Fig. 18.12 (a, b) Step 4. The periosteum of the anterior wall of the cavernous sinus (CSAW) and Meckel's cave (MeC) are dissected from the lingual process (LiP), which is subsequently removed. BaP, base of the pterygoid process; pICA, paraclival tract of the internal carotid artery; CSAW, anterior wall of the cavernous sinus; sICA, parasellar tract of the internal carotid artery.

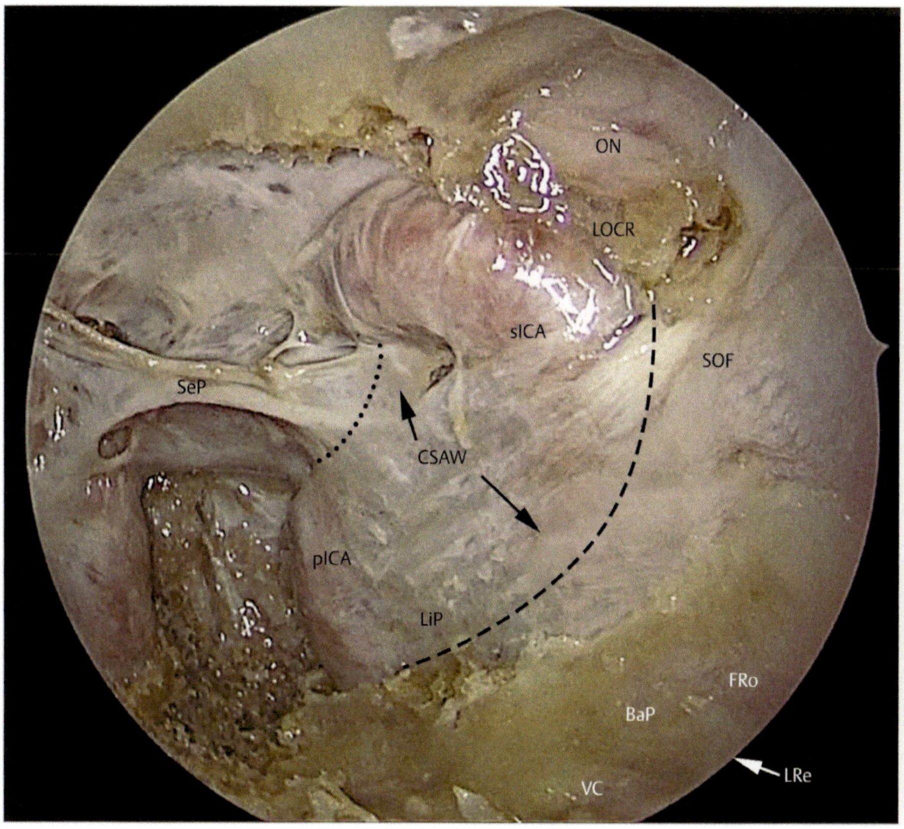

Fig. 18.13 Overview of periosteal incisions for transcavernous approaches. The cavernous sinus can be accessed through its anterior wall (CSAW) via two approaches. In the medial transcavernous approach, the periosteal incision (*black dotted line*) is made between the sellar periosteum (SeP) and the paraclival (pICA) and parasellar (sICA) tracts of the internal carotid artery. In the lateral transcavernous approach, the periosteum is incised (*black dashed line*) from the lingual process (LiP) to the lateral optic–carotid recess (LOCR), staying laterally to the internal carotid artery, medially to the superior orbital fissure (SOF), and superiorly to the base of the pterygoid process (BaP). FRo, foramen rotundum; LRe, lateral recess of the sphenoid sinus; ON, optic nerve; VC, vidian canal.

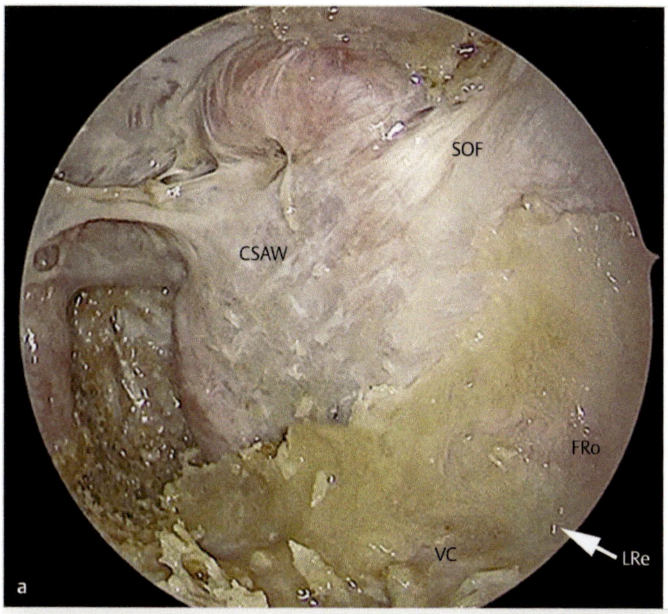

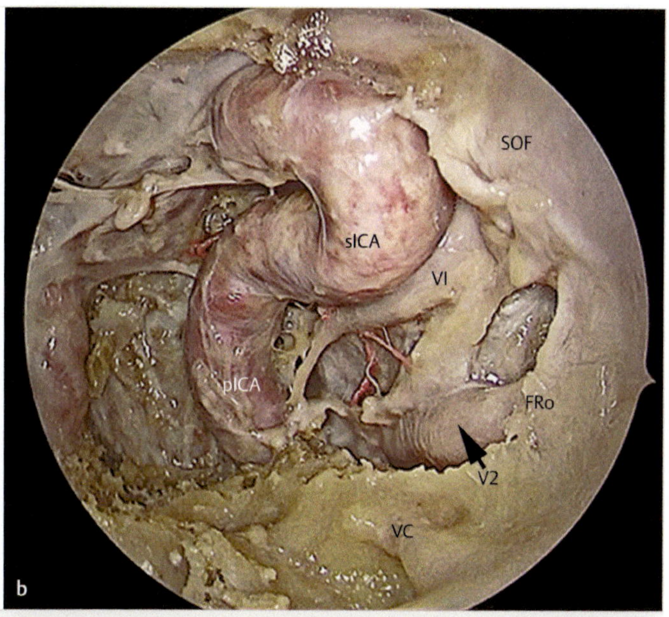

Fig. 18.14 (a, b) Step 5. The anterior wall of the cavernous sinus (CSAW) is removed and the abduces nerve (VI) comes into view while running toward the superior orbital fissure (SOF). The maxillary nerve (V2) is seen before it enters the foramen rotundum (FRo). LRe, lateral recess of the sphenoid sinus; sICA, parasellar tract of the internal carotid artery; VC, vidian canal.

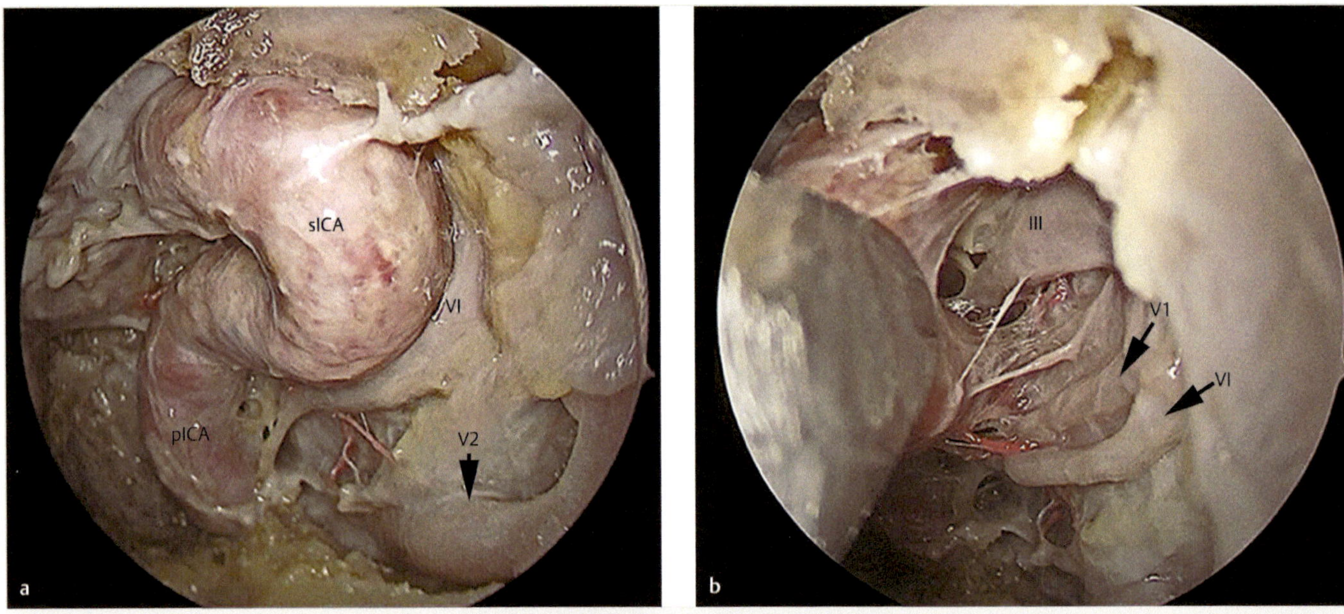

Fig. 18.15 (a, b) Step 6. A dissector is placed between the parasellar tract of the internal carotid artery (sICA) and the abducens nerve (VI) to medialize the artery. In this way, the oculomotor (III) and ophthalmic (V1) nerves come into view. V2, maxillary nerve; pICA, paraclival tract of the internal carotid artery.

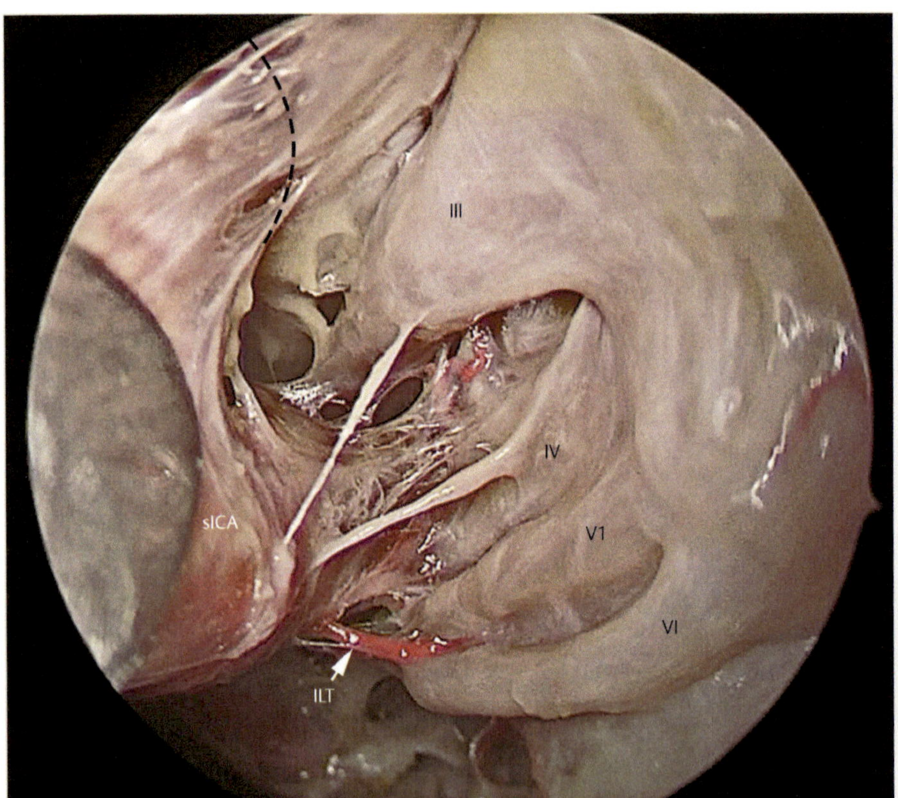

Fig. 18.16 Step 7. From this step, a three-hand dissection is recommended. The lateral compartment of the cavernous sinus is gently dissected sparing the neurovascular structures located lateral to the parasellar tract of the internal carotid artery (sICA). The oculomotor (III), trochlear (IV), ophthalmic (V1), and abducens (VI) nerves are identified along the lateral wall of the cavernous sinus. Of note, given the parallel course of the abducens and ophthalmic nerves, the former usually has to be dislocated cranially or caudally (as in this image) to identify both. The inferolateral trunk (ILT) comes into view while horizontally crossing the trajectory of dissection. This arterial trunk usually passes between the ophthalmic and abducens nerves and provides several branches for nerves and dura of the cavernous sinus and Meckel's cave. Superiorly, the superior carotid ring (*black dashed line*) is identified medial to the oculomotor nerve.

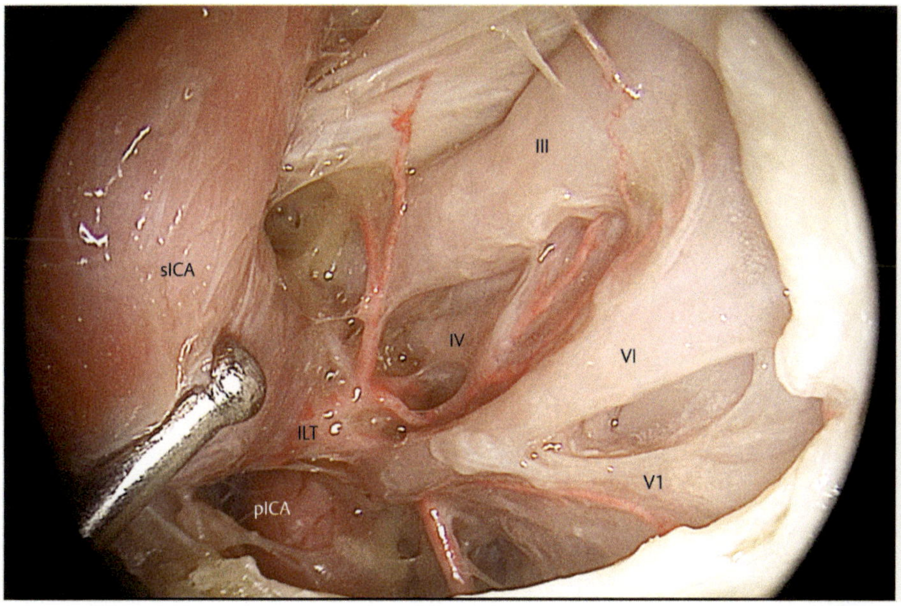

Fig. 18.17 The inferolateral trunk. The inferolateral trunk (ILT) arises from the lateral surface of the parasellar tract of the internal carotid artery (sICA) and branches early into several small arteries for the nerves of the cavernous sinus and Meckel's cave. In this specimen, five main branches can be recognized from cranial to caudal: the superior branch for the oculomotor nerve (III), the posterior branch toward the tentorium, two horizontal branches for the trochlear nerve (IV), abducens (VI), and ophthalmic (V1) nerves, and the inferior branch reaching the foramina rotundum and ovale and supplying the maxillary and mandibular nerves, respectively. The main branch of the inferolateral trunk passes between the abducens and ophthalmic nerves. pICA, paraclival tract of the internal carotid artery.

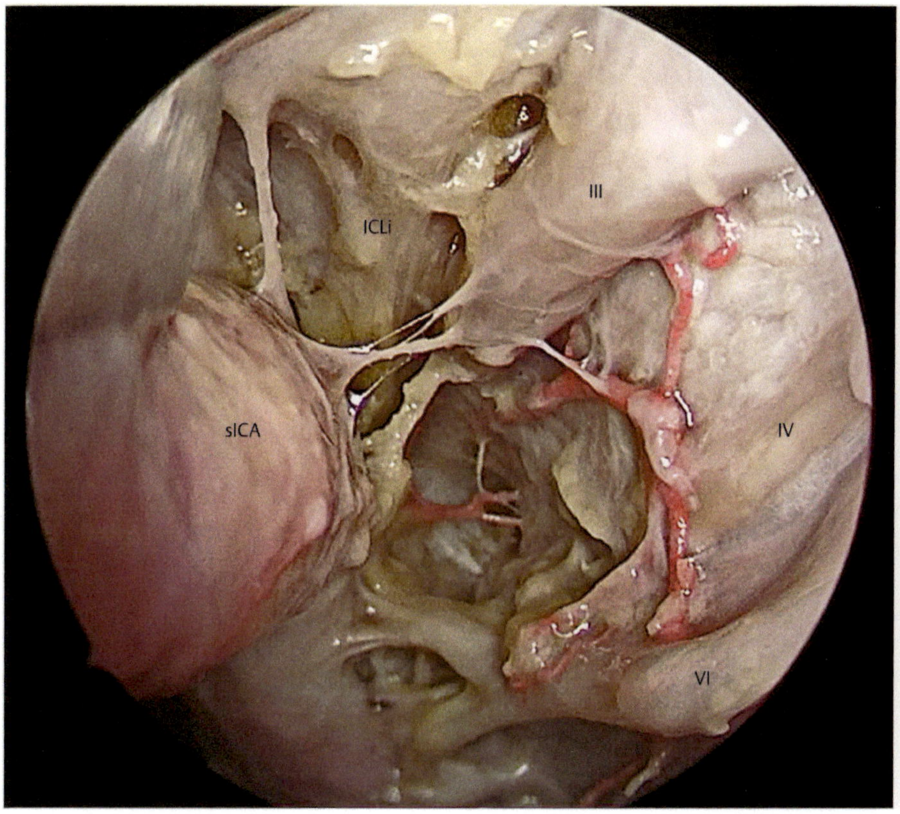

Fig. 18.18 Step 8. The inferolateral trunk is cut to create a corridor toward the posterior compartment of the cavernous sinus. The fat tissue of the superior compartment located medially to the oculomotor nerve (III) is removed to identify the interclinoid ligament (ICLi), which represents the medial boundary of the oculomotor triangle. This ligament is attached to the inferior carotidring anteriorly and caroticoclinoid ligament anteromedially. IV, trochlear nerve; VI, abducens nerve; sICA, parasellar tract of the internal carotid artery.

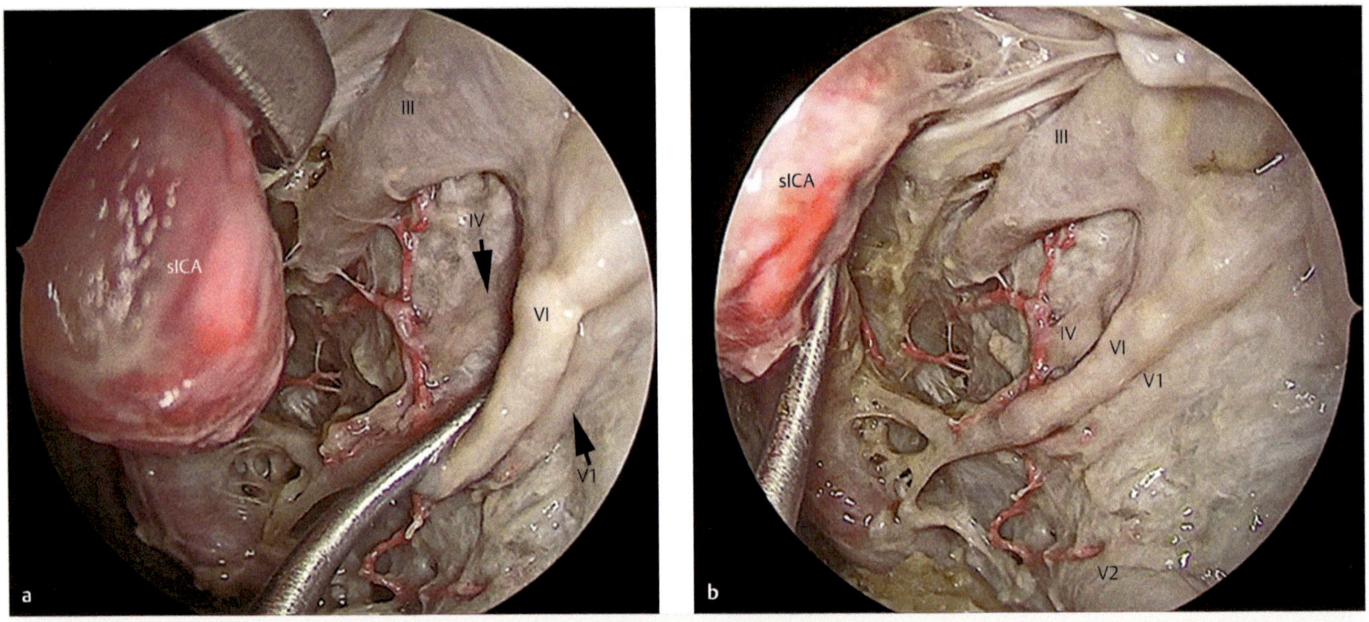

Fig. 18.19 (a, b) Overview of the lateral wall of the cavernous sinus. After completely removing the fat tissue in the lateral and posterior compartments of the cavernous sinus, a full view of the lateral wall is obtained. III, oculomotor nerve; IV, trochlear nerve; V1, ophthalmic nerve; V2, maxillary nerve; VI, abducens nerve; sICA, parasellar tract of the internal carotid artery.

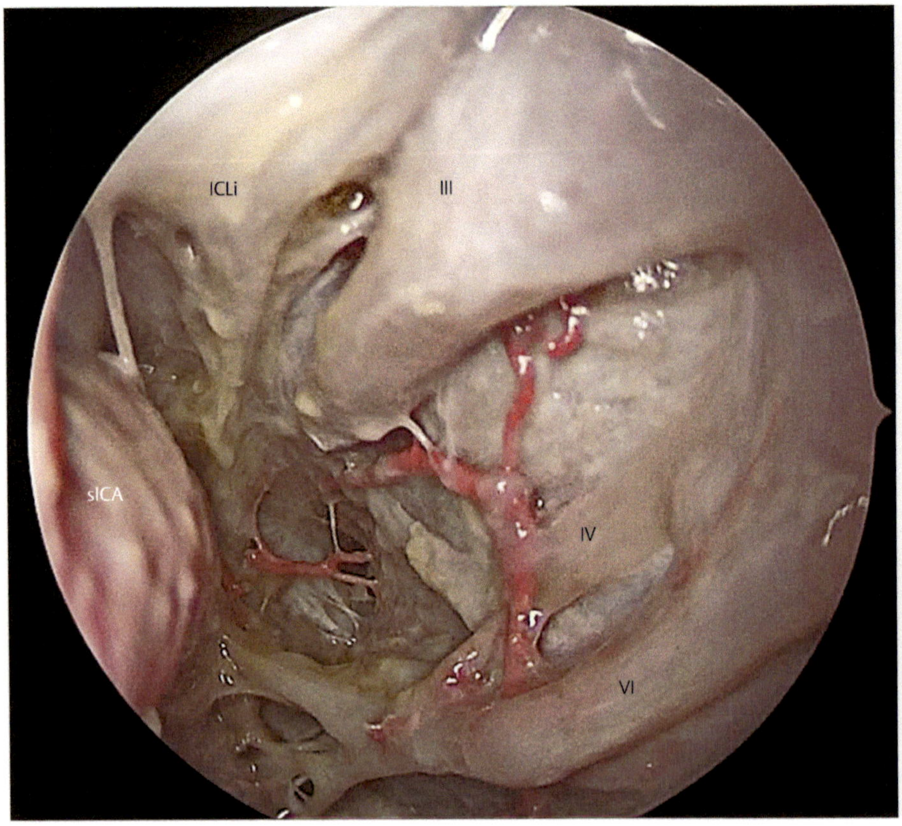

Fig. 18.20 Relationship between the superior and lateral compartments of the cavernous sinus. A 0-degree scope is placed between the parasellar tract of the internal carotid artery (sICA) and the oculomotor nerve (III). The passage from the superior to the lateral compartment is approximately marked by a virtual sagittal plane passing through the interclinoid ligament (ICLi). IV, trochlear nerve; VI, abducens nerve.

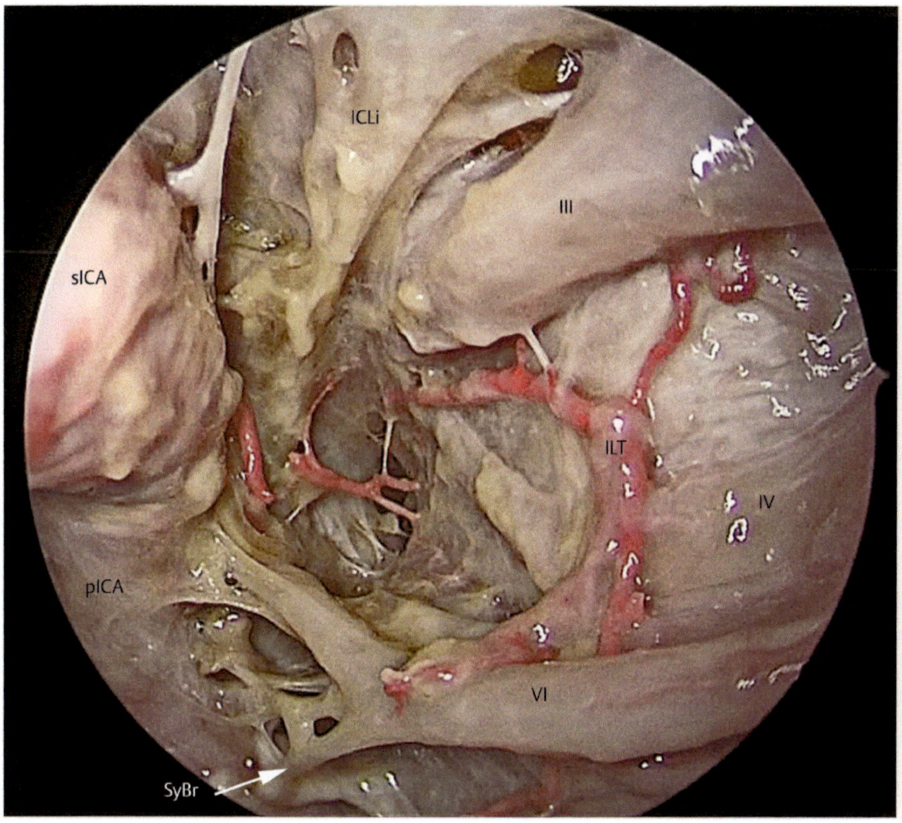

Fig. 18.21 Relationship between the inferior and lateral compartments of the cavernous sinus. A 0-degree scope is placed between the parasellar tract of the internal carotid artery (sICA) and the abducens nerve (VI). The passage from the lateral to the inferior compartment is located along a virtual plane passing tangent to the lateral aspect of the paraclival (pICA) and parasellar tract of the internal carotid artery (sICA). Of note, being free within the lumen of the cavernous sinus, the abducens nerve (VI) is the structure located closest to this virtual plane. III, oculomotor nerve; IV, trochlear nerve; ICLi, interclinoid ligament; ILT, inferolateral trunk; SyBr, sympathetic branch for the abducens nerve.

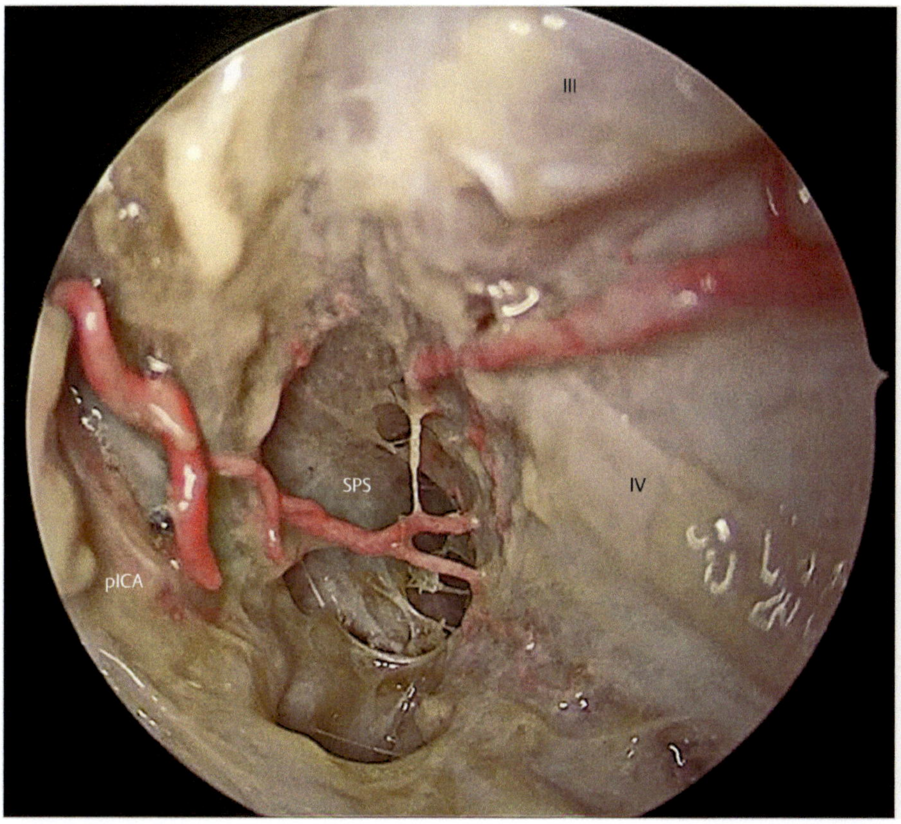

Fig. 18.22 The superior petrosal sinus. A 0-degree scope is moved posteriorly following the direction of the oculomotor (III) and trochlear (IV) nerves. The area where the superior petrosal sinus (SPS) communicates with the cavernous sinus is identified lateral to the paraclival tract of the internal carotid artery (pICA).

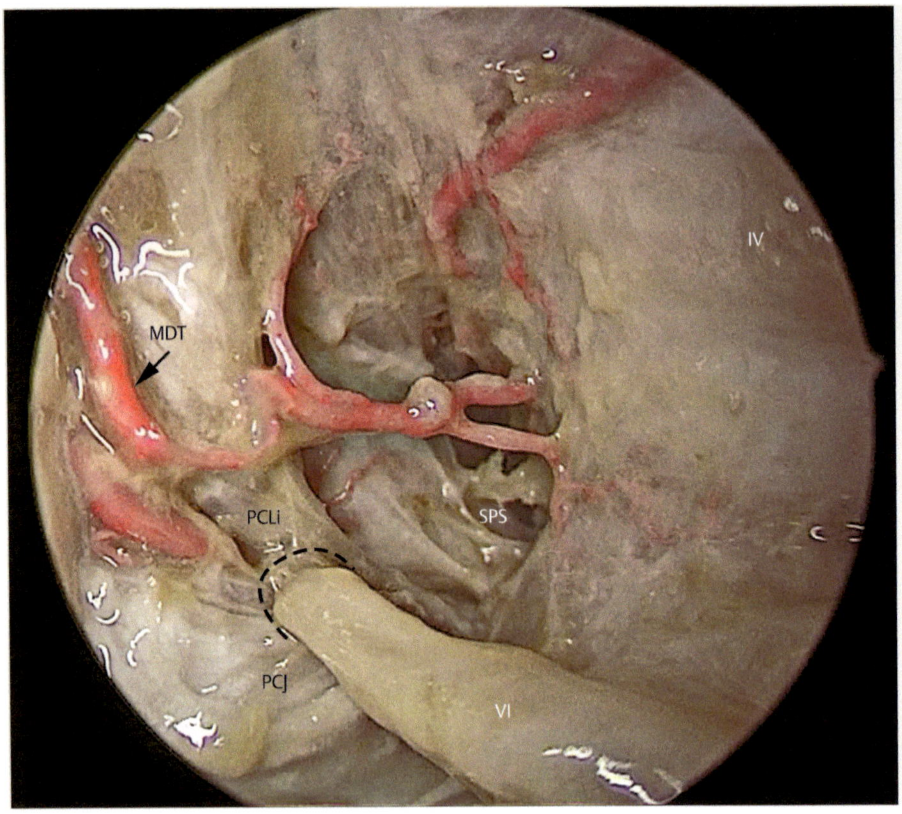

Fig. 18.23 Step 9. The fat tissue within the posterior compartment of the cavernous sinus is completely removed to identify the point where the abducens nerve (VI) enters the cavernous sinus. This short passage is called Dorello's canal (*black dashed line*) and is enclosed between the petroclinoid ligament (PCLi; also called Gruber's ligament) cranially and the petroclival junction (PCJ) caudally. Dorello's canal lies medially to the superior petrosal sinus (SPS) and inferior to the meningeal branches arising from the meningohypophyseal trunk. In this specimen, the arterial branches for the tentorium cerebri, clivus, and dorsum sellae arise from a common trunk called the meningodorsal trunk (MDT). IV, trochlear nerve.

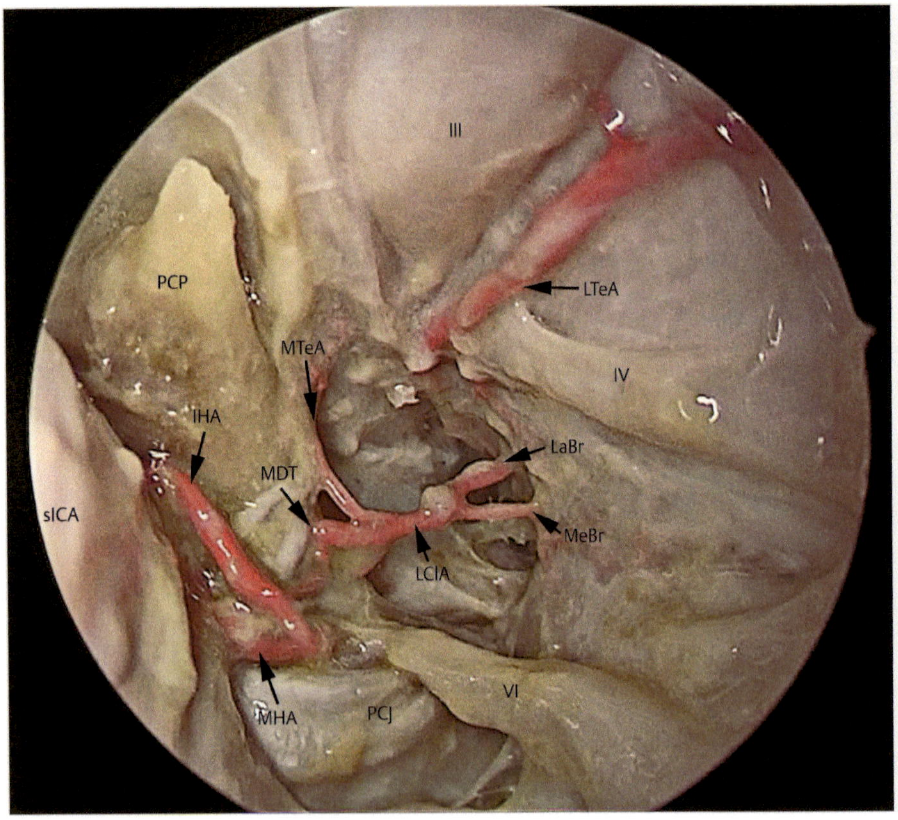

Fig. 18.24 Lateral branches of the meningohypophyseal artery. The meningohypophyseal artery (MHA) usually arises from the medial surface of the parasellar tract of the internal carotid artery (sICA). It bifurcates early into the inferior hypophyseal artery (IHA) and several meningeal branches that can have a common origin from the so-called meningodorsal trunk (MDT): the medial tentorial artery (MTeA), also called the Bernasconi–Cassinari artery, passes behind the posterior clinoid process (PCP) and runs superiorly toward the anterior petroclinoid fold; the medial clival artery goes inferiorly and medially toward the midclivus; the lateral clival artery (LClA) goes laterally and divides early into the lateral branch (LaBr), which runs parallel to the superior petrosal sinus, and the medial branch (MeBr), which runs parallel to the inferior petrosal sinus. The latter branches pass below the trochlear nerve (IV), while the lateral tentorial artery (LTeA), which can variably arise from the inferolateral trunk (as in this specimen) or from the meningohypophyseal trunk, runs between the trochlear and oculomotor (III) nerves. VI, abducens nerve; PCJ, petroclival junction.

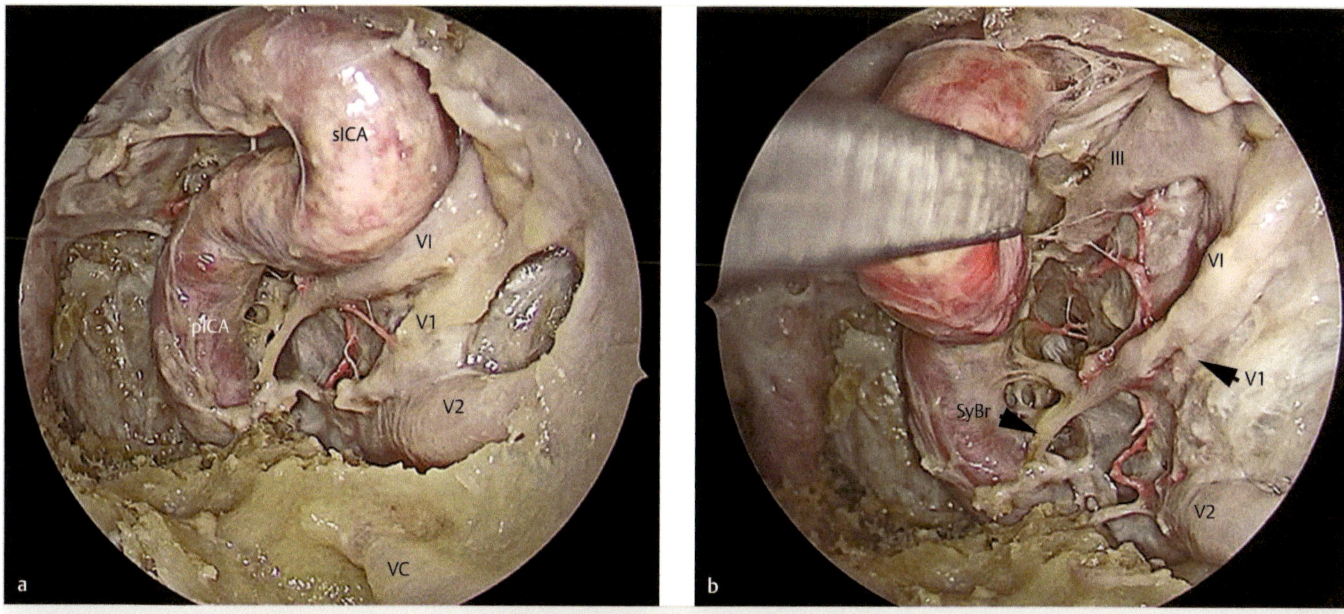

Fig. 18.25 (a, b) Overview of the inferior compartment of the cavernous sinus. A 0-degree scope is placed above the vidian canal (VC), and the parasellar (sICA) and paraclival tracts of the internal carotid artery (pICA) are displaced medially to have an overview of the inferior compartment of the cavernous sinus. III, oculomotor nerve; V1, ophthalmic nerve; V2, maxillary nerve; VI, abducens nerve; SyBr, sympathetic branch for the abducens nerve.

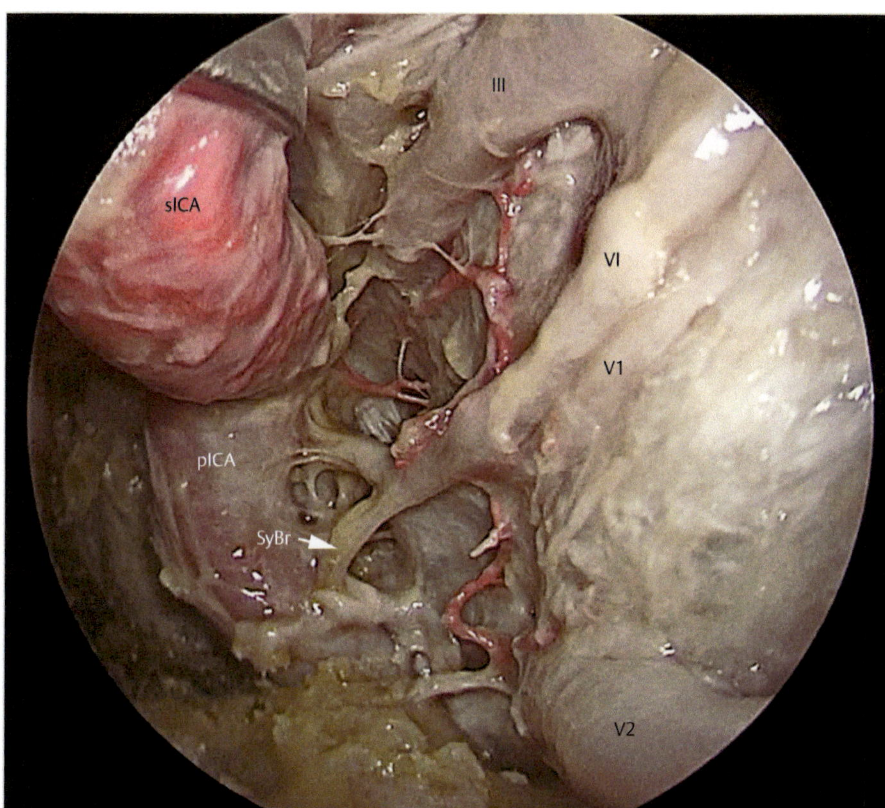

Fig. 18.26 Step 10. The fat tissue in the inferior compartment is completely removed. The sympathetic branch (SyBr) for the abducens nerve (VI) arises from the internal carotid plexus of the paraclival tract of the internal carotid artery (pICA). Compared to the cavernous tract of the abducens nerve, which runs with a horizontal trajectory, the sympathetic branch has a more vertical orientation. III, oculomotor nerve; V1, ophthalmic nerve; V2, maxillary nerve; sICA, parasellar tract of the internal carotid artery.

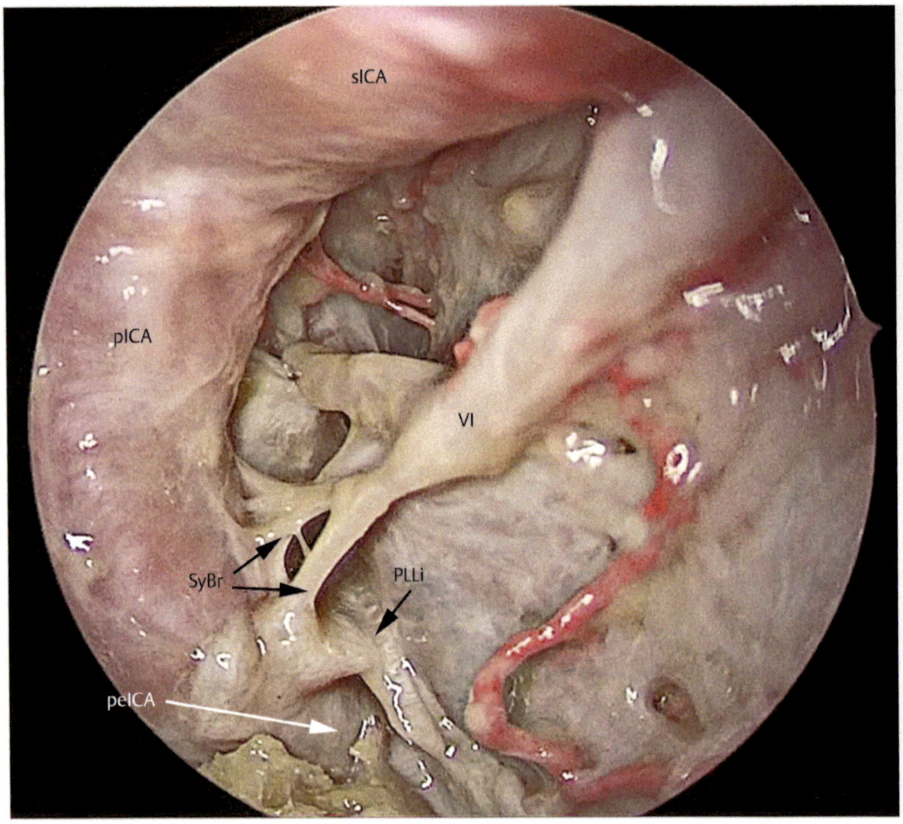

Fig. 18.27 The petrolingual ligament. The petrolingual ligament (PLLi) comes into view in the inferior portion of the inferior compartment of the cavernous sinus. This ligament is tended from the petrous apex posterosuperiorly to the lingual process of the sphenoid bone inferoanteriorly, and marks the passage from the cavernous sinus, medially, to Meckel's cave, laterally. It covers the most medial portion of the petrous tract of the internal carotid artery (peICA), just lateral to the point where the vessel turns superiorly to form the paraclival tract (pICA). VI, abducens nerve; sICA, parasellar tract of the internal carotid artery; SyBr, sympathetic branch for the abducens nerve.

References

[1] Fernandez-Miranda JC, Zwagerman NT, Abhinav K, et al. Cavernous sinus compartments from the endoscopic endonasal approach: anatomical considerations and surgical relevance to adenoma surgery. J Neurosurg 2018;129(2):430–441

[2] Micko AS, Wöhrer A, Wolfsberger S, Knosp E. Invasion of the cavernous sinus space in pituitary adenomas: endoscopic verification and its correlation with an MRI-based classification. J Neurosurg 2015;122(4):803–811

[3] Lobo B, Zhang X, Barkhoudarian G, Griffiths CF, Kelly DF. Endonasal endoscopic management of parasellar and cavernous sinus meningiomas. Neurosurg Clin N Am 2015;26(3):389–401

[4] Hardesty DA, Montaser AS, Carrau RL, Prevedello DM. Limits of endoscopic endonasal transpterygoid approach to cavernous sinus and Meckel's cave. J Neurosurg Sci 2018;62(3):332–338

[5] Pamir MN, Kilic T, Ozek MM, Ozduman K, Türe U. Non-meningeal tumours of the cavernous sinus: a surgical analysis. J Clin Neurosci 2006;13(6):626–635

[6] el-Kalliny M, van Loveren H, Keller JT, Tew JM Jr. Tumors of the lateral wall of the cavernous sinus. J Neurosurg 1992;77(4):508–514

[7] Fraser JF, Mass AY, Brown S, Anand VK, Schwartz TH. Transnasal endoscopic resection of a cavernous sinus hemangioma: technical note and review of the literature. Skull Base 2008;18(5):309–315

[8] Zhou LF, Mao Y, Chen L. Diagnosis and surgical treatment of cavernous sinus hemangiomas: an experience of 20 cases. Surg Neurol 2003;60(1):31–36, discussion 36–37

[9] Noblett DA, Chang J, Toussi A, Dublin A, Shahlaie K. Hemangioma of the cavernous sinus: a case series. J Neurol Surg Rep 2018;79(2):e26–e30

[10] Patrona A, Patel KS, Bander ED, et al. Endoscopic endonasal surgery for nonadenomatous, nonmeningeal pathology involving the cavernous sinus. J Neurosurg 2017;126(3):880–888

[11] Koutourousiou M, Vaz Guimaraes Filho F, Fernandez-Miranda JC, et al. Endoscopic endonasal surgery for tumors of the cavernous sinus: a series of 234 patients. World Neurosurg 2017;103:713–732

[12] Fernandez-Miranda JC, Gardner PA, Rastelli MM Jr, et al. Endoscopic endonasal transcavernous posterior clinoidectomy with interdural pituitary transposition. J Neurosurg 2014;121(1):91–99

[13] Ferrareze Nunes C, Lieber S, Truong HQ, et al. Endoscopic endonasal transoculomotor triangle approach for adenomas invading the parapeduncular space: surgical anatomy, technical nuances, and case series. J Neurosurg 2018:1–11

[14] Hosoya T, Kera M, Suzuki T, Yamaguchi K. Fat in the normal cavernous sinus. Neuroradiology 1986;28(3):264–266

[15] Tokiguchi S, Kurashima A, Ito J, Takahashi H, Shimbo Y. Fat in the dural sinus: CT and anatomical correlations. Neuroradiology 1988;30(1):78–80

19 Medial Petrous Apex Approach

Vittorio Rampinelli, Marco Ravanelli, Andrea Bolzoni Villaret, Francesco Doglietto

The petrous apex, a complex bony area located between the middle and posterior cranial fossa, is surrounded by a number of important neurovascular structures, including the petrous and paraclival tract of the internal carotid artery, trigeminal nerve, Gasserian ganglion, abducens nerve, acoustic-facial bundle, and all the vessels and nerves of the jugular foramen. Topographically, the petrous apex is the anteromedial portion of the petrous bone and is enclosed between the internal acoustic meatus and the petroclival junction. The petrous apex can be schematically divided into three subunits, which can be variably exposed through the transnasal routes. The superior portion lies above the axial plane passing through the superior surface of the petrous horizontal tract of the internal carotid artery. The anteroinferior and posteroinferior portions lie below the aforementioned plane, anteromedially and posterolaterally to the vertical portion of the petrous internal carotid artery, respectively.[1]

Several endoscopic transnasal surgical routes have been designed to reach the petrous apex, namely, the medial petrous apex approach, the infrapetrous approach, and the suprapetrous (Meckel's cave) approach. The medial petrous apex approach exploits the transclival pathway through the midclivus to reach the medial segment of the superior and anteroinferior portions of the petrous apex.[2,3] This approach has been employed either alone or as lateral extension of the middle transclival approach to manage several diseases of the petroclival area, including fluid-containing lesions requiring surgical drainage such as cholesterol granuloma and petrous apicitis,[2–5] as well as solid tumors such as chondrosarcomas,[3,6] chordomas,[3,7,8] and meningiomas.[9,10] The infrapetrous and suprapetrous corridors are described in Chapters 20 and 21, respectively. Skull base teams treating lesions of the petroclival area should master both the transnasal and the lateral transcranial/transpetrosal surgical techniques, which are selected or combined depending on the extension and nature of the disease.

From an anatomical–topographical perspective, the medial petrous apex approach exploits the narrow bony area (called "carotid-clival window") between the paraclival internal carotid artery, anteriorly, and the periosteum of the posterior cranial fossa, posteriorly.[11,12] This area corresponds to the petroclival junction, thus being the floor of Dorello's canal, where the abducens nerve runs below the petroclinoid ligament (also called petrosphenoidal or Gruber's ligament), passing from the basilar plexus to the cavernous sinus. In addition, the tract of the nerve passing through the basilar plexus runs with an ascending trajectory immediately behind the petroclival junction. As a consequence, the dissection of this anatomical space should be performed carefully to avoid damaging the abducens nerve.[13] In cases requiring a large exposure, the paraclival tract of the internal carotid artery can be uncovered from the surrounding bone and subsequently lateralized to widen the window of the medial petrous apex approach.[3]

The network of dural sinuses and plexuses between the periosteum and the dura of this anatomic area is exceedingly intricate, including the basilar plexus, the inferior and superior petrosal sinus, and the cavernous sinus. Therefore, intense venous bleeding should be expected when the petroclival periosteum is entered.

Laboratory dissection including all three transnasal routes toward the petrous apex is strongly recommended to fully understand potentials and limitations of these pathways.

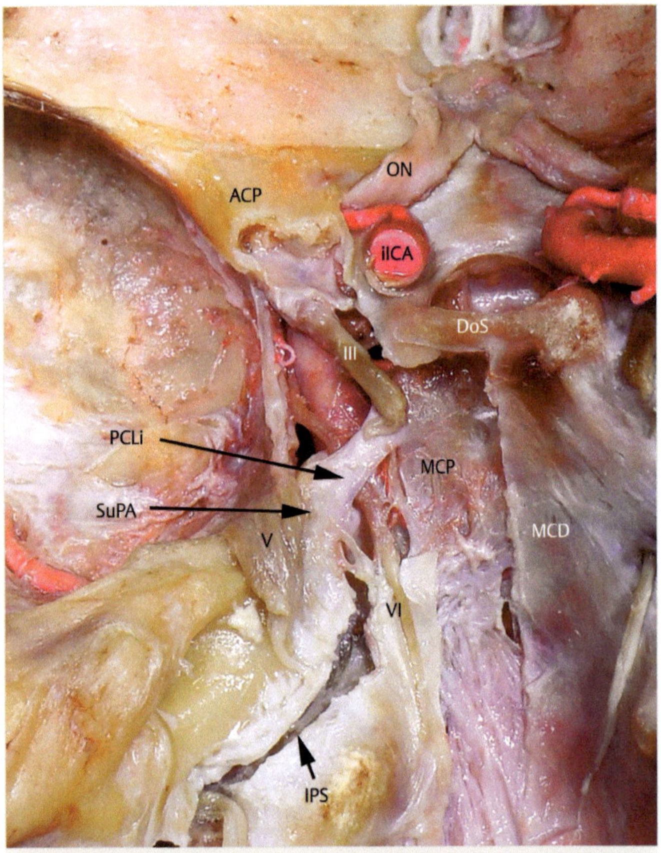

Fig. 19.1 Intracranial view of the superior petrous apex. This cadaver picture show the anatomy of the superior petrous apex (SuPA) as seen from posterosuperior to anteroinferior. III, oculomotor nerve; V, trigeminal stem; VI, abducens nerve; ACP, anterior clinoid process; DoS, dorsum sellae; iICA, intracranial tract of the internal carotid artery; IPS, inferior petrosal sinus; MCD, dura of the midclivus; MCP, periosteum of the midclivus; ON, optic nerve; PCLi, petroclinoid ligament; SuPA, superior petrous apex.

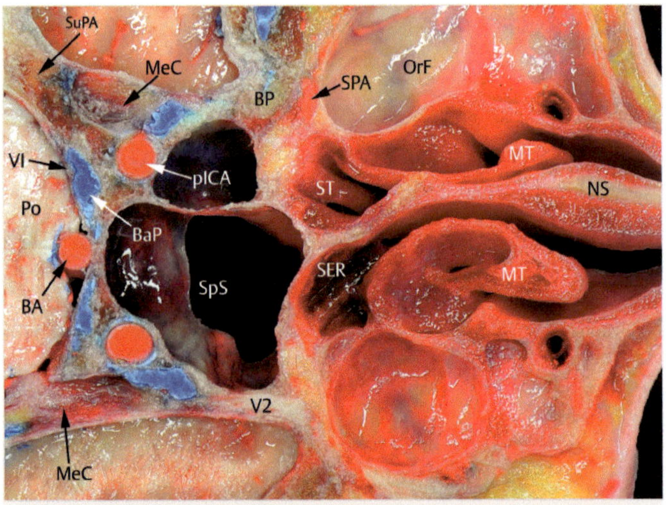

Fig. 19.2 Axial view of the superior petrous apex. This axial cadaver cut shows with a cranial-to-caudal perspective the corridor toward the superior portion of the petrous apex (SuPA). V2, maxillary nerve; VI, abducens nerve; BA, basilar artery; BaP, basilar plexus; BP, base of the pterygoid process; MeC, Meckel's cave; MT, middle turbinate; NS, nasal septum; OrF, orbital floor; pICA, paraclival tract of the internal carotid artery; Po, pons; SER, sphenoethmoidal recess; SPA, sphenopalatine artery; SpS, sphenoid sinus; ST, superior turbinate.

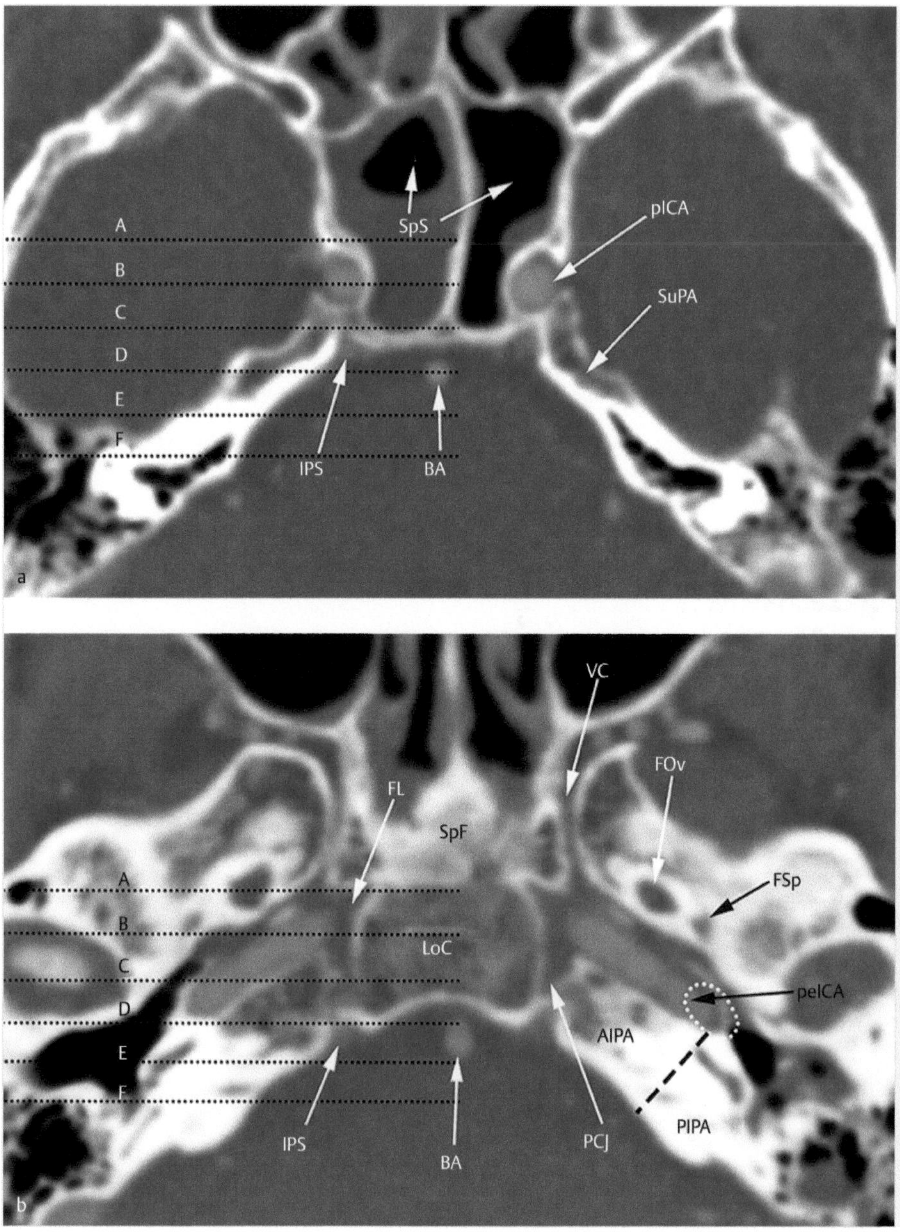

Fig. 19.3 CT axial anatomy of the petrous apex and surrounding structures. The panel shows two contrast-enhanced axial CT scans: **(a)** the first scan passes through the superior petrous apex (SuPA), whereas **(b)** the second scan passes through the anterior (AIPA) and posterior portions of the inferior petrous apex (PIPA), which are separated by a virtual plane (*black dashed line*) passing between the external carotid foramen (*white dotted circle*) and reaching the posterior cranial fossa. The superior petrous apex is closely adjacent to paraclival tract of the internal carotid artery (pICA) and the midclivus. The anteroinferior petrous apex is strictly related to the petrous tract of the internal carotid artery (peICA) and the lower clivus (LoC). The posteroinferior petrous apex is adjacent to the jugular foramen. The *black dotted lines* (A–F) refer to the positions of coronal scans of ▶ Fig. 19.4. BA, basilar artery; FL, foramen lacerum; FOv, foramen ovale; FSp, foramen spinosum; IPS, inferior petrosal sinus; PCJ, petroclival junction; SpF, sphenoidal floor; SpS, sphenoid sinus; VC, vidian canal.

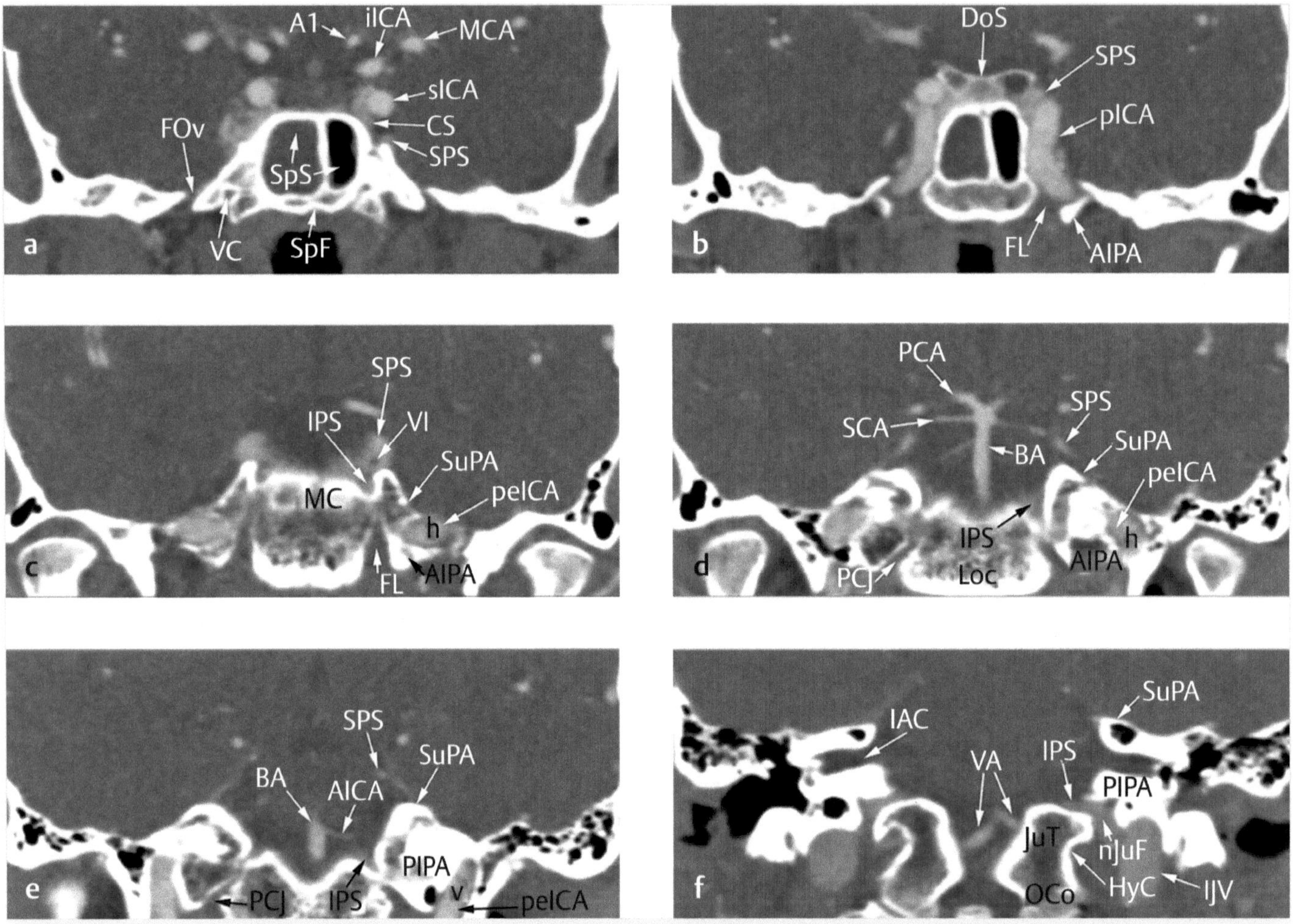

Fig. 19.4 (a–f) Coronal CT anatomy of the petrous apex and surrounding structures. This panel of contrast-enhanced coronal CT scans (A–F; as depicted in ▶Fig. 19.3) shows a number of bony and vascular structures of the petroclival area (six images from anterior to posterior, from **a** to **f**). The superior petrous apex (SuPA) lies lateral to the midclivus (MC), foramen lacerum (FL), and petroclival junction (PCJ). This area is intimately related to the abducens nerve (VI), inferior petrosal sinus (IPS), and superior petrosal sinus (SPS). The foramen lacerum is located between the anteroinferior petrous apex (AIPA), laterally, and the lower clivus (LoC), medially, and serves as bed for the anterior genu of the internal carotid artery, which is the passage from the horizontal (h) portion of the petrous tract (peICA) to the paraclival tract of the internal carotid artery (pICA). The posteroinferior petrous apex (PIPA) is closely related to the vertical (v) portion of the petrous internal carotid artery and to the nervous compartment of the jugular foramen (nJuF). A1, precommunicating tract of the anterior cerebral artery; AICA, anterior inferior cerebellar artery; BA, basilar artery; CS, cavernous sinus; DoS, dorsum sellae; FOv, foramen ovale; HyC, hypoglossal canal; IAC, internal acoustic canal; IJV, internal jugular vein; iICA, intracranial tract of the internal carotid artery; JuT, jugular tuberculum; MCA, middle cerebral artery; OCo, occipital condyle; PCA, posterior cerebral artery; SCA, superior cerebellar artery; sICA, parasellar tract of the internal carotid artery; SpF, sphenoidal floor; SpS, sphenoid sinus; VA, vertebral arteries; VC, vidian canal.

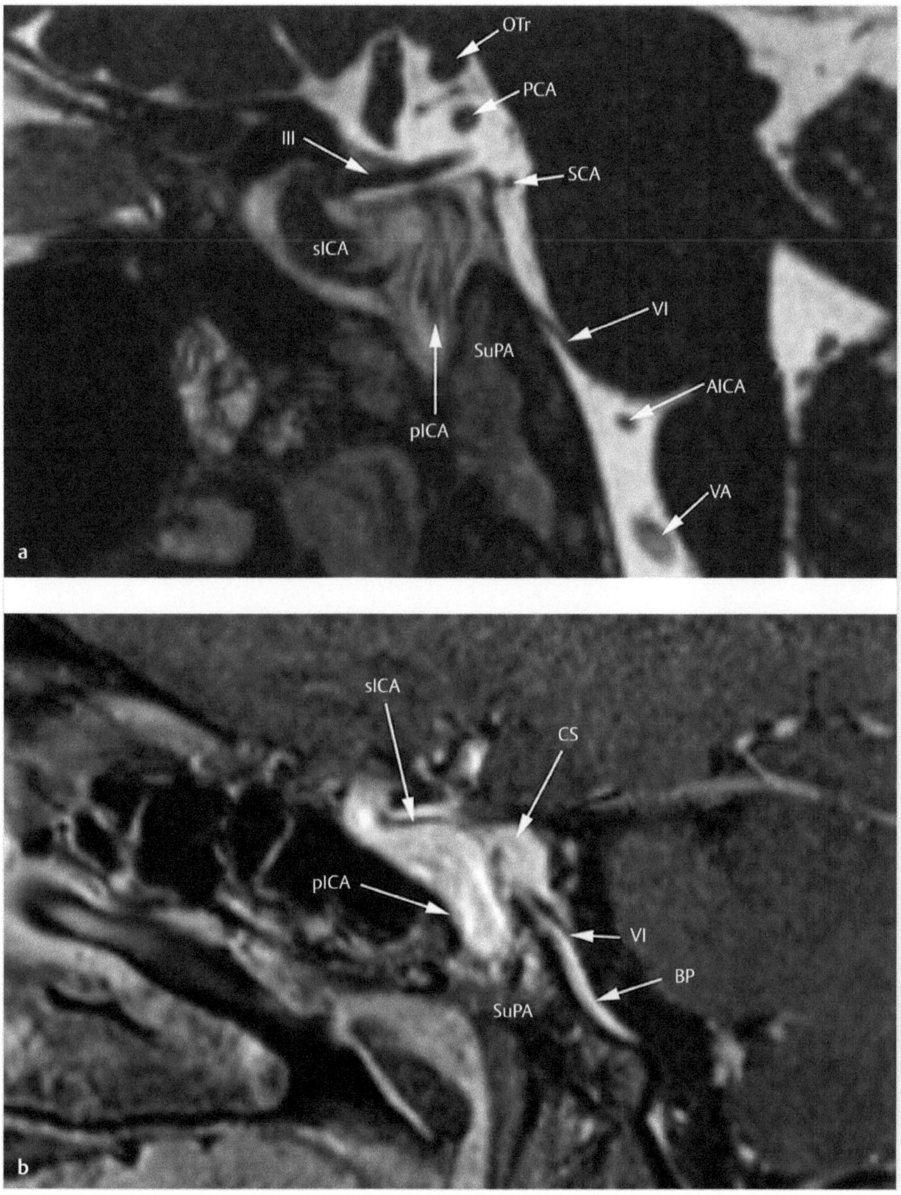

Fig. 19.5 MRI sagittal anatomy of the abducens nerve. The panel shows two sagittal MRI scans, a CISS (constructive interference in steady state) scan **(a)** and a contrast-enhanced T1-weighted scan **(b)**. The abducens nerve (VI) runs with an ascending trajectory within the prepontine cistern and through the basilar plexus (BP). During its course, the nerve passes above the superior petrous apex (SuPA) and lateral to the paraclival (pICA) and sellar tracts of the internal carotid artery (sICA). III, oculomotor nerve; AICA, anterior inferior cerebellar artery; CS, cavernous sinus; OTr, optic tract; PCA, posterior cerebral artery; SCA, superior cerebellar artery; VA, vertebral artery.

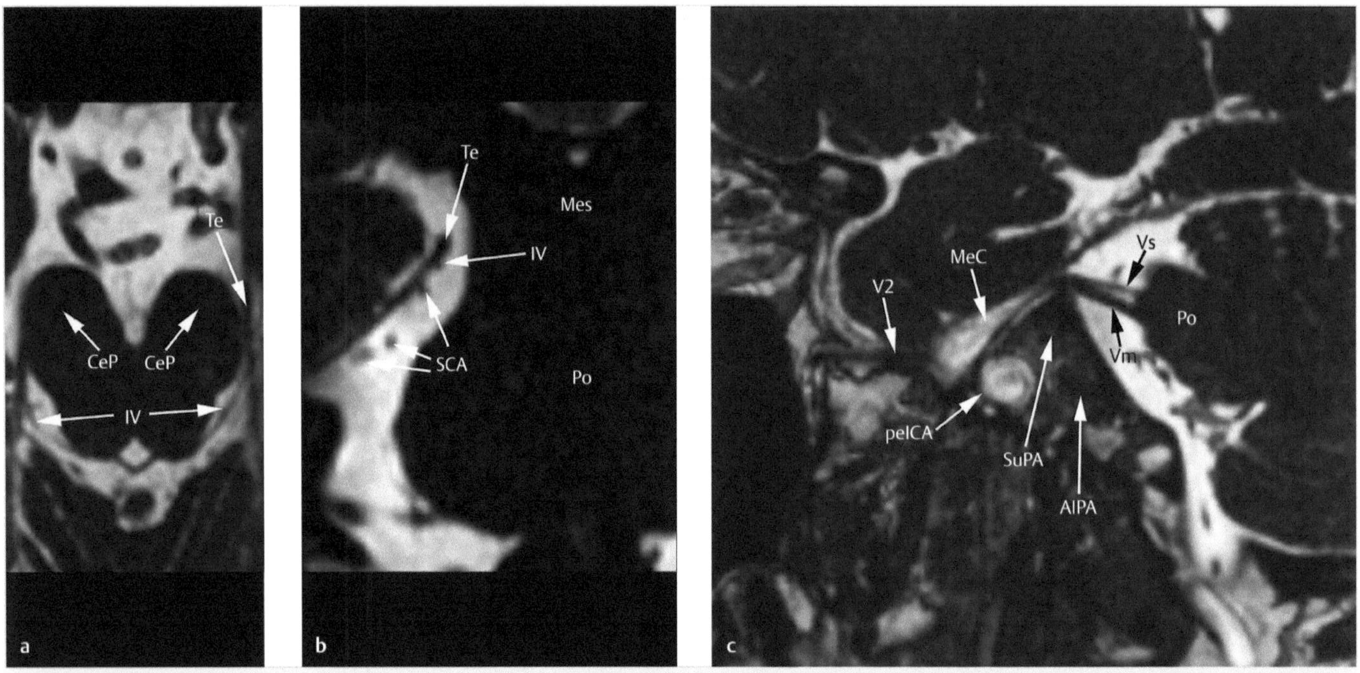

Fig. 19.6 MRI anatomy of the trochlear and trigeminal nerves. The panel shows an axial **(a)**, a coronal **(b)**, and a sagittal **(c)** CISS (constructive interference in steady state) MRI depicting the trochlear nerve (IV) and the trigeminal stem (V). The trochlear nerve arises from the dorsal portion of the mesencephalon (Mes), turns around the cerebral pedicle (CeP), and finally pierces the tentorium (Te) to reach the cavernous sinus. When running along the inferior surface of the tentorium, the trochlear nerve is parallel to the branches of the superior cerebellar artery (SCA). The trigeminal stem (V) arises from the pons (Po) and reaches the trigeminal porus, which lies between the tentorium and the petrous ridge. The sensitive (Vs) and motor (Vm) roots can be differentiated. V2, maxillary nerve; AIPA, anteroinferior petrous apex; MeC, Meckel's cave; peICA, petrous tract of the internal carotid artery; SuPA, superior petrous apex.

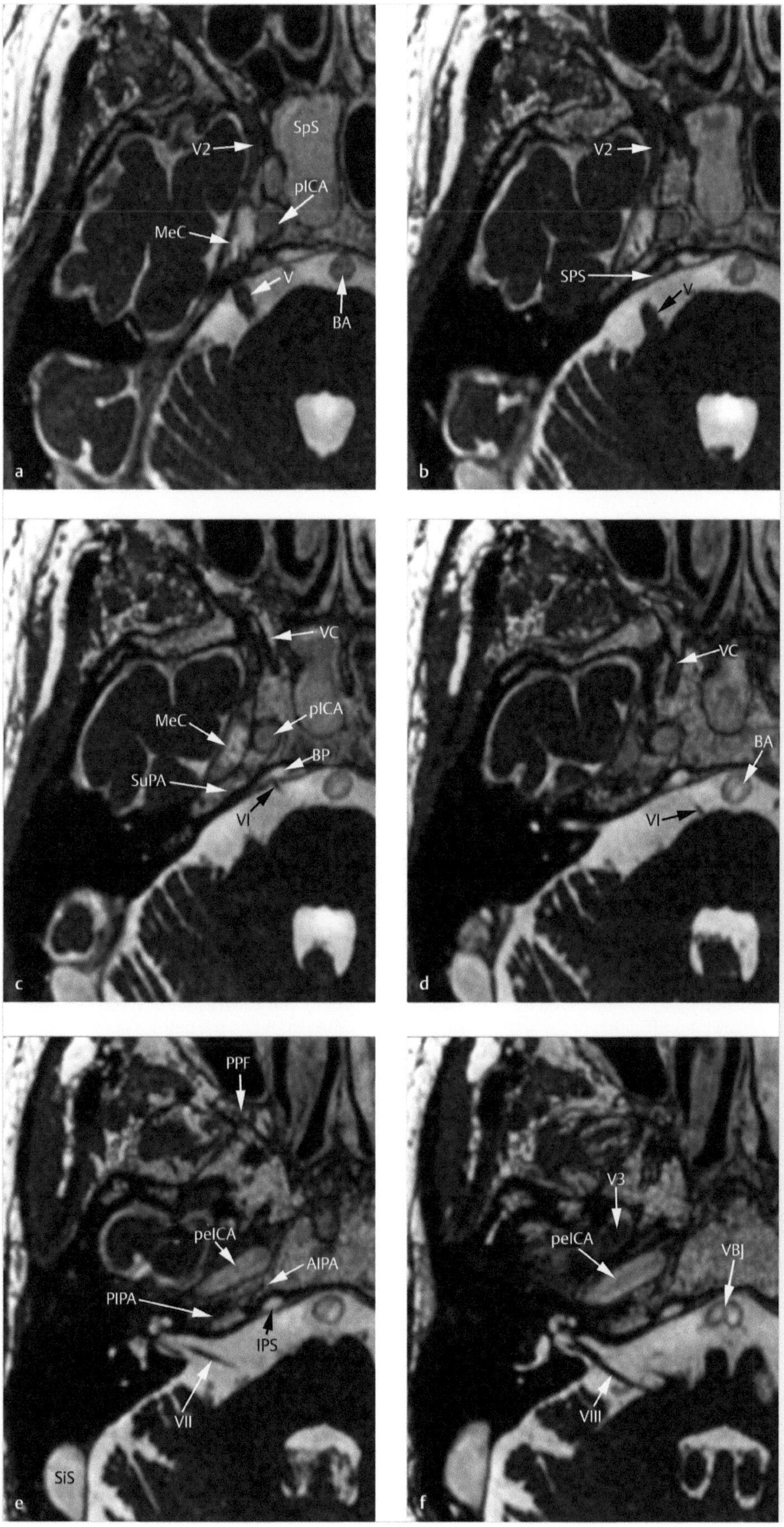

Fig. 19.7 (a–f) Constructive interference in steady state (CISS) MRI axial anatomy of the petrous apex and surrounding structures. This sequential panel of axial CISS sequences precisely depicts the craniocaudal disposition of several skull base and cisternal structures in the petroclival area (six images from cranial to caudal, from **a** to **f**). From cranial to caudal, the cisternal compartment houses the trigeminal stem (V), abducens nerve (VI), facial nerve (VII), and vestibulocochlear nerve (VIII); with the same perspective, the skull base compartment includes Meckel's cave (MeC), superior petrosal sinus (SPS), superior petrous apex (SuPA), inferior petrosal sinus (IPS), and anteroinferior (AIPA) and posteroinferior petrous apex (PIPA). The superior and inferior portions of the petrous apex are intimately related to the paraclival (pICA) and petrous tracts of the internal carotid artery (peICA), respectively. V2, mandibular nerve; V3, mandibular nerve; BA, basilar artery; BP, basilar plexus; PPF, pterygopalatine fossa; SiS, sigmoid sinus; SpS, sphenoid sinus; VBJ, vertebrobasilar junction; VC, vidian canal.

Endoscopic Dissection

Nasal Phase

- Paraseptal sphenoidotomy.
- Transrostral sphenoidotomy.
- Expanded transrostral sphenoidotomy.
- Type A endoscopic medial maxillectomy.
- Facultative: Vertical uncinectomy.
- Facultative: Anterior ethmoidectomy.
- Facultative: Posterior ethmoidectomy.
- Facultative: Transethmoidal sphenoidotomy.
- Facultative: Middle and superior turbinectomy.
- Facultative: Type B–D endoscopic medial maxillectomy.

Skull Base Phase

- Facultative: Transsellar approach.
- Facultative: Transclival (midclivus) approach.
- Facultative: Transclival (lower clivus) approach.
- Facultative: Transcavernous (medial) approach.
- Facultative: Transcavernous (lateral) approach.
- Step 1: Removal of the ipsilateral half of the sphenoid sinus floor and of the anterior cortical bone of the midclivus.
- Step 2: Removal of the anterior portion of the ipsilateral carotid sulcus (this step can be performed after Step 6 to better understand the anatomy of the paraclival internal carotid artery).
- Step 3: Removal of the ipsilateral half of the posterior cortical bone of the midclivus.
- Step 4: Removal of the posterior portion of the carotid sulcus.
- Step 5: Removal of the middle clival periosteum.
- Steps
- 6: Removal of the ipsilateral petrous process of the sphenoid.
- Step 7: Removal of the lingual process of the sphenoid and the inferior part of the lateral wall of the sphenoid sinus, including part of the greater wing of the sphenoid.
- Step 8: Incision of the middle clival dura.

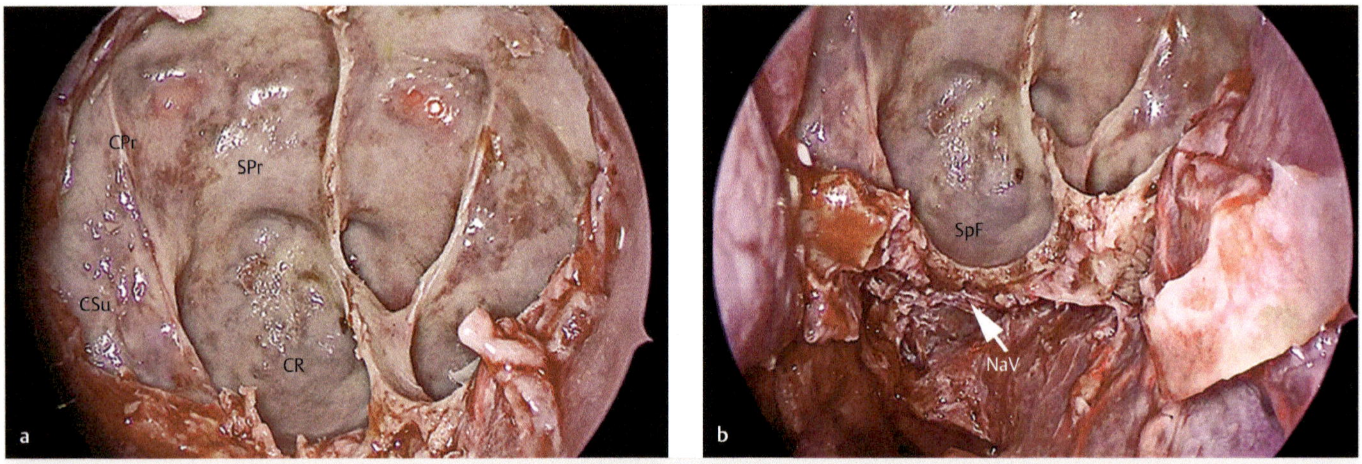

Fig. 19.8 (a, b) Exposure of the sphenoid sinus after completing the extended transrostral sphenoidotomy. The visualization of the anatomical landmarks of the posterior wall of the sphenoid sinus allows identification of the limits of the approach. When targeting the petrous apex, it is necessary to determine the position of the ipsilateral carotid prominence (CPr) and the carotid sulcus (CSu). Medial to them, the clival recess (CR) can be visible below the sellar prominence (SPr) according to sphenoid sinus pneumatization. The floor of the sphenoid sinus (SpF), which corresponds to the nasopharyngeal vault (NaV), separates the middle and lower clivus.

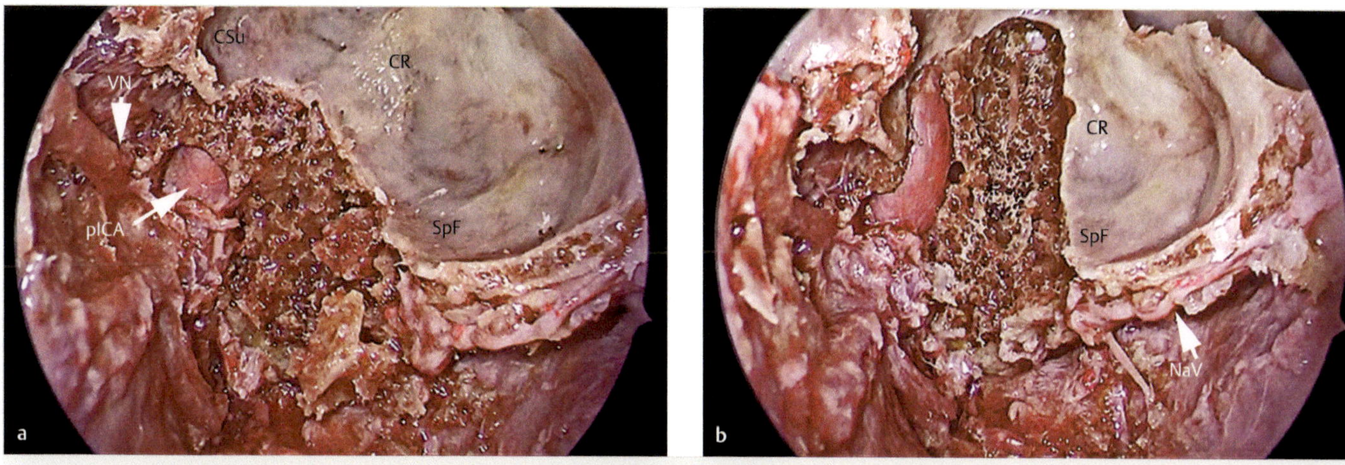

Fig. 19.9 (a, b) Steps 1 and 2. The bone of the ipsilateral half of the floor of the sphenoid sinus (SpF) and the anterior cortical bone of the middle clivus, namely, the clival recess (CR), are removed. After identifying the vidian nerve (VN) at the lateral end of the sphenoid sinus floor, it is tracked back to the anterior genu of the internal carotid artery and bony removal is extended to the anterior portion of the carotid sulcus (CSu) until the paraclival internal carotid artery (pICA) comes into view (this maneuver can be postponed after Step 6). NaV, nasopharyngeal vault.

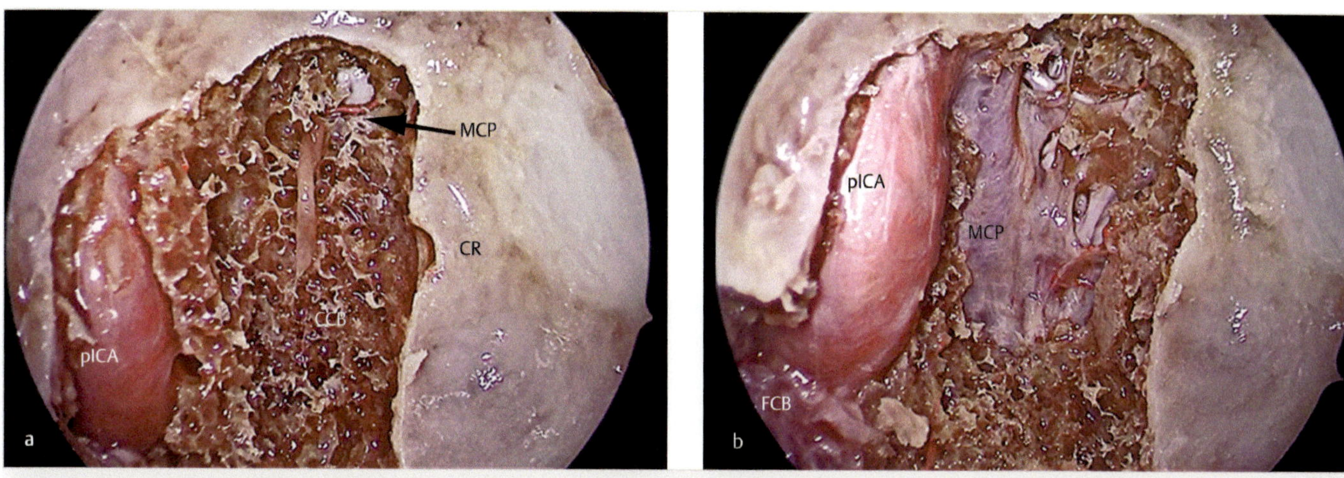

Fig. 19.10 (a, b) Step 3. After removing the medullary bone of the middle clivus, the posterior clivus cortical bone (CCB) is removed to complete the exposure of the midclivus periosteum (MCP). CR, clival recess; FCB, fibrocartilago basalis; pICA, paraclival tract of the internal carotid artery.

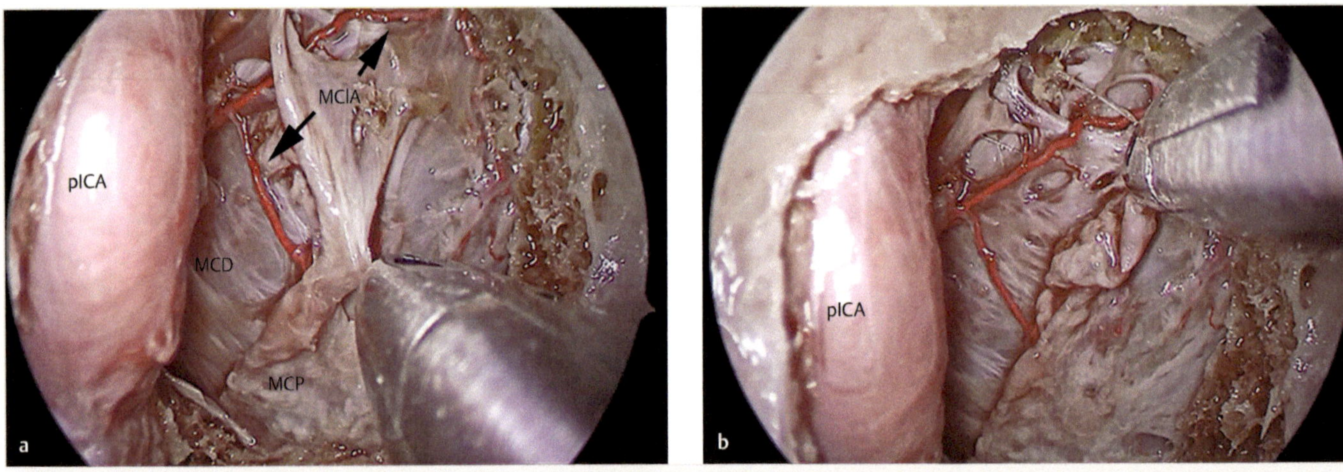

Fig. 19.11 (a, b) Steps 4 and 5. After removing the posterior portion of the carotid sulcus, the periosteum of the midclivus (MCP) is incised and gently removed to expose the dura mater of the midclivus (MCD). The medial clival artery (MClA) runs between the dura and the periosteum; however, some of its branches may perforate the periosteum to reach the midclivus bone. pICA, paraclival tract of the internal carotid artery.

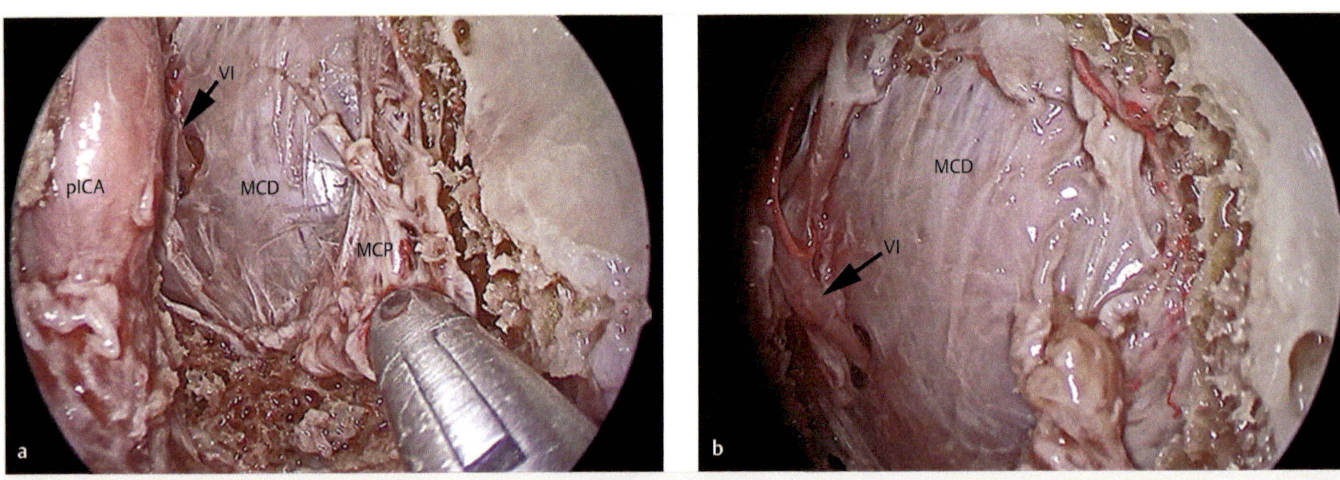

Fig. 19.12 (a, b) Step 5. The periosteum of the midclivus (MCP) is completely removed. The space between the periosteum and the dura of the midclivus (MCD) corresponds to the basilar venous plexus. The point where the abducens nerve (VI) pierces the dura mater of the midclivus can be identified. The nerve runs with an anterior–superior–lateral trajectory and crosses the paraclival portion of the internal carotid artery (pICA) on its posterolateral surface.

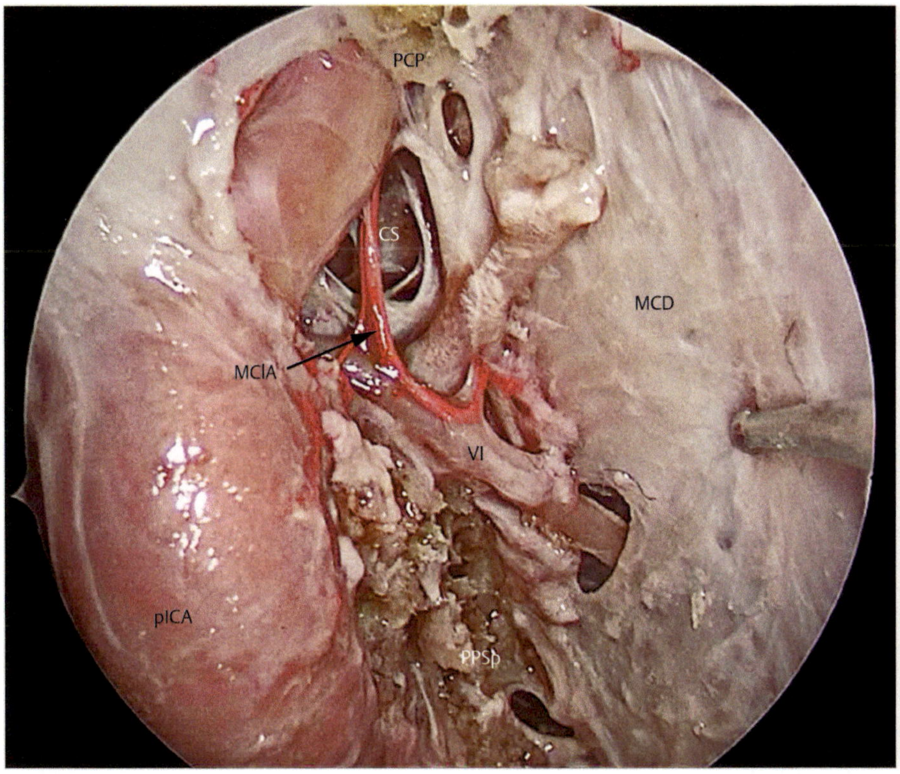

Fig. 19.13 Detailed view (with a 70-degree endoscope) of the relationship between the paraclival portion of the internal carotid artery and the abducens nerve. The abducens nerve (VI) passes behind and lateral to the paraclival portion of the internal carotid artery (pICA) to reach the cavernous sinus. Branches of the medial clival artery (MClA) descend from the cavernous sinus (CS) and reach the abducens nerve. The nerve passes above the petrous process of the sphenoid bone (PPSp). MCD, dura mater of the midclivus; PCP, posterior clinoid process.

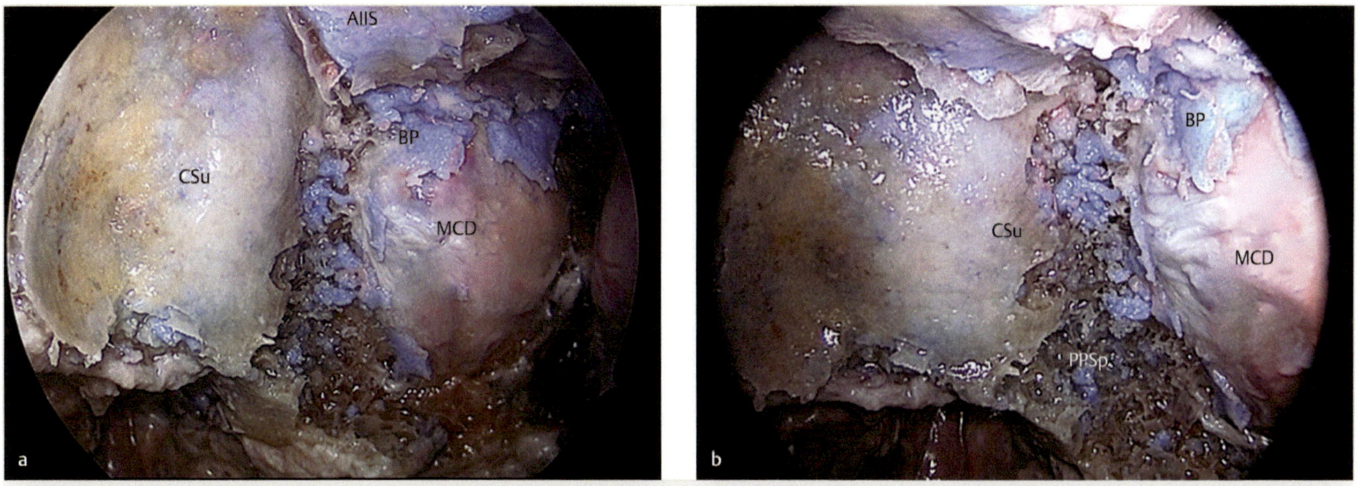

Fig. 19.14 (a, b) Procedure repeated on a specimen with venous injection. The dura mater of the midclivus (MCD) is exposed. The anterior part of the inferior intercavernous sinus (AIIS) is visible at the superior border of the surgical corridor. The basilar plexus (BP) is visible in the space between the periosteum and the dura mater of the midclivus. Notably, only the posterior portion of the carotid sulcus (CSu) needs to be removed to expose the petrous apex. However, leaving the anterior portion of this bony structure hampers full visualization of the paraclival tract of the internal carotid artery and prevents its lateralization. The petroclival area is better visualized using an angled (70-degree) endoscope (right image) compared to a 0-degree endoscope (left image). PPSp, petrous process of the sphenoid bone.

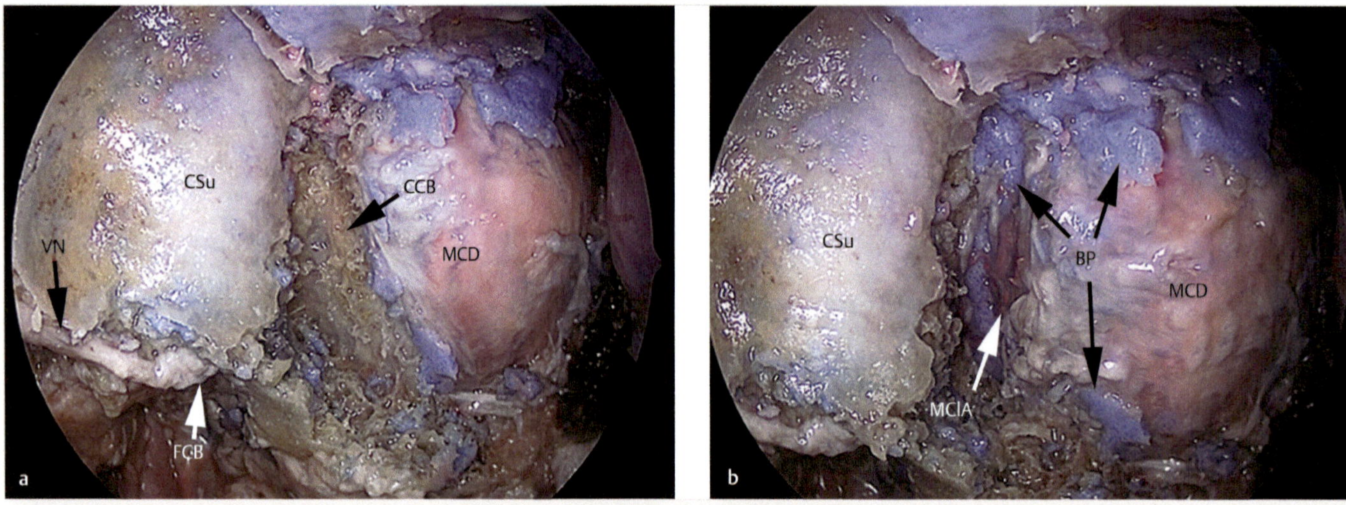

Fig. 19.15 (a, b) Step 4. The vidian nerve (VN) is followed to expose the fibrocartilago basalis (FCB). The posterior portion of the carotid sulcus (Csu) is removed starting from the posterior clival cortical bone (CCB), enabling the view of the medial clival artery (MClA). BP, basilar plexus; MCD, dura mater of the midclivus.

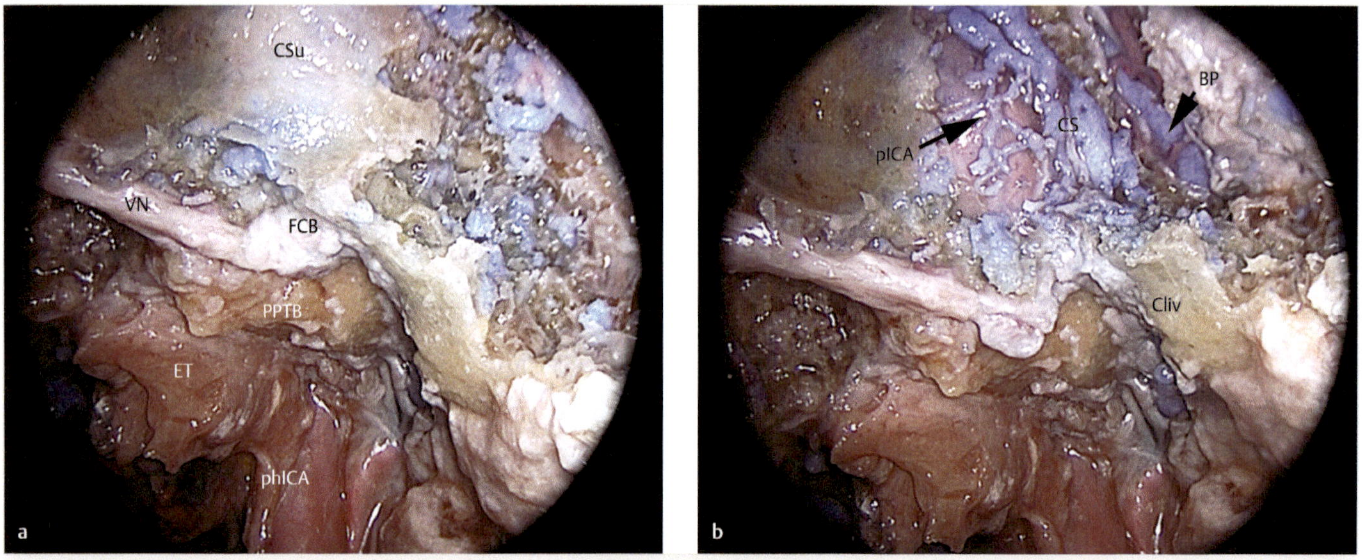

Fig. 19.16 (a, b) Removal of the carotid sulcus and overview of anatomical relationships between the petrous apex and the upper parapharyngeal space. The paraclival portion of the internal carotid artery (pICA) is exposed by removing the carotid sulcus (CSu). The vidian nerve (VN) and the fibrocartilago basalis (FCB) can be identified below the anterior genu of the internal carotid artery. The petrous portion of the temporal bone (PPTB) comes into view posterolateral to the fibrocartilago basalis when a medial parapharyngeal space approach is added. The sectioned eustachian tube (ET) and the parapharyngeal portion of the internal carotid artery (phICA) are also visible. These spatial relationships are better appreciated with a 70-degree endoscope. BP, basilar plexus; Cliv, lower clivus; CS, cavernous sinus.

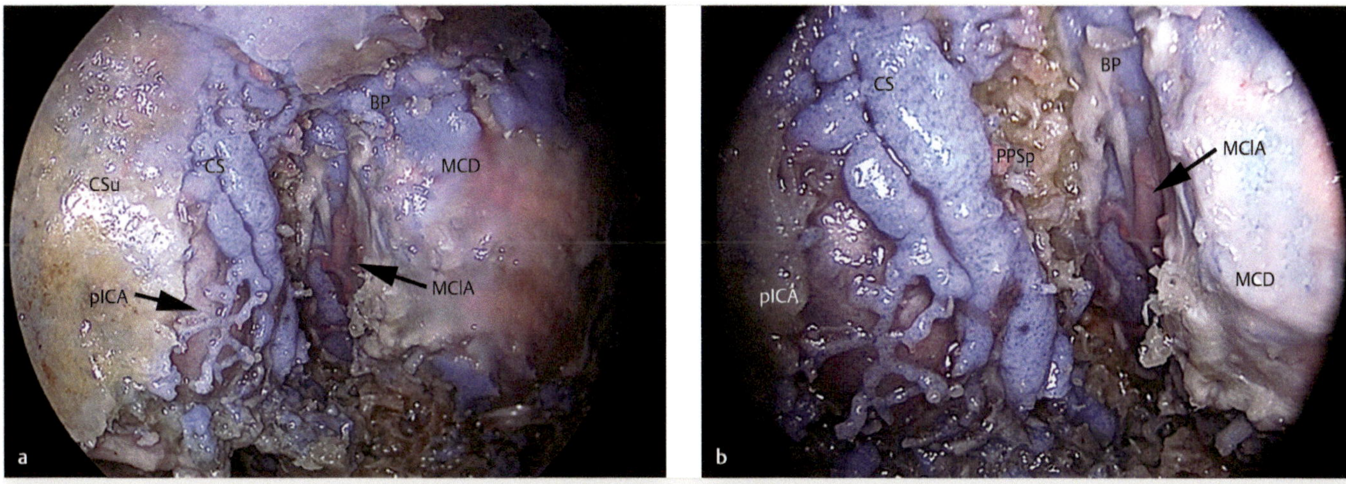

Fig. 19.17 (a, b) The petrous process of the sphenoid bone. The anterior and posterior boundaries of the petrous process of the sphenoid bone (PPSp) are the cavernous sinus (CS) and the basilar plexus (BP), respectively. It is easier to see this relationship using a 45-degree endoscope (right image) compared to a 0-degree scope endoscope (left image). The cavernous sinus surrounds the paraclival portion of the internal carotid artery (pICA), whereas the basilar plexus contains branches from the medial clival artery (MClA). CSu, carotid sulcus; MCD, dura mater of the midclivus.

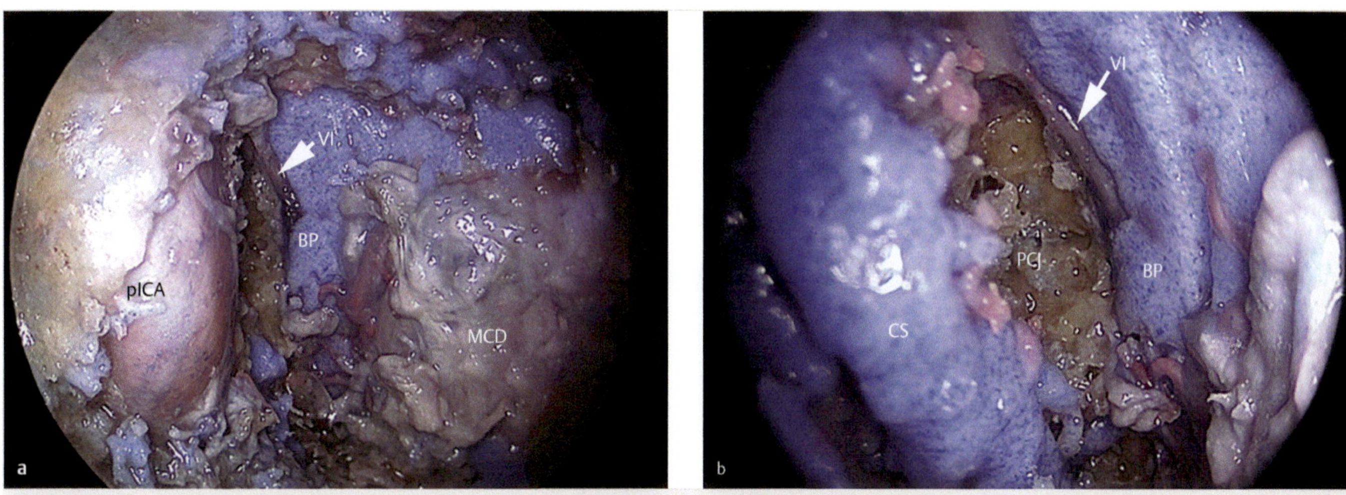

Fig. 19.18 (a, b) Abducens nerve. The petrous process of the sphenoid bone constitutes the medial portion of the petroclival junction (PCJ). The abducens nerve (VI) runs first through the basilar plexus (BP) and then reaches the cavernous sinus (CS) via Dorello's canal, which is a small passage bounded by the petroclival junction, inferiorly, and the petroclinoid (or Gruber's) ligament, superiorly. This anatomical relationship can be better analyzed with a 70-degree endoscope (right image). MCD, dura mater of the midclivus; pICA, paraclival portion of the internal carotid artery.

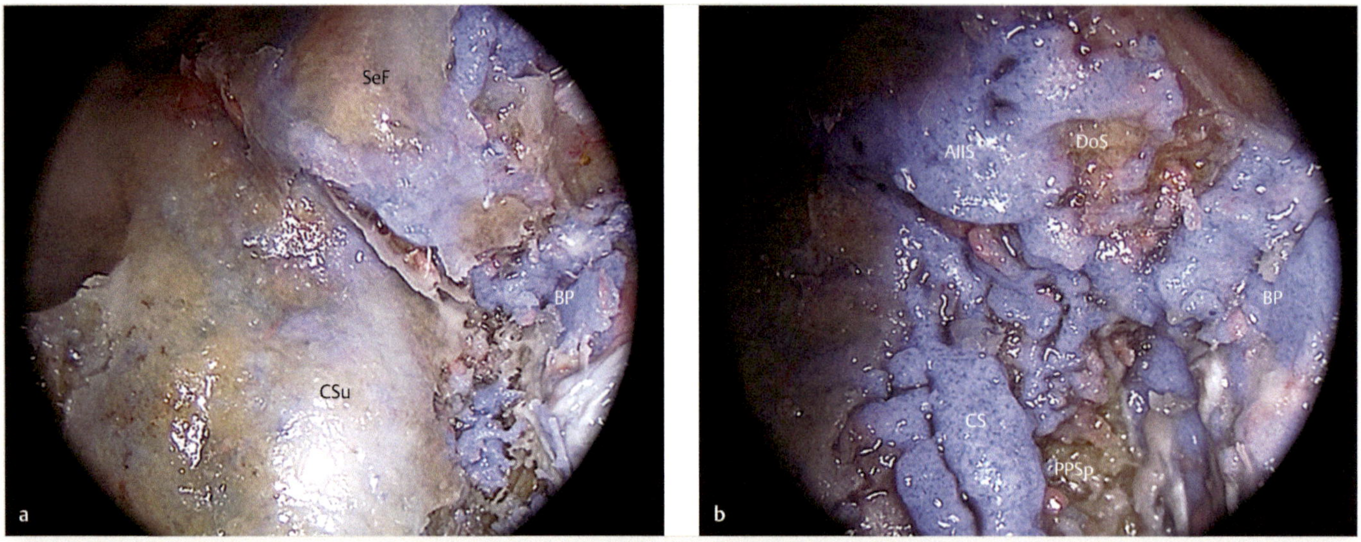

Fig. 19.19 (a, b) Upper boundaries of the medial petrous apex approach as seen with a 70-degree endoscope. The carotid sulcus (CSu) lies inferiorly, anteriorly, and laterally to the sellar floor (SeF). After removing both these bony structures, the intricate venous network formed by the basilar plexus (BP), the anterior part of the inferior intercavernous sinus (AIIS), and the cavernous sinus (CS) can be identified. DoS, dorsum sellae; PPSp, petrous process of the sphenoid bone.

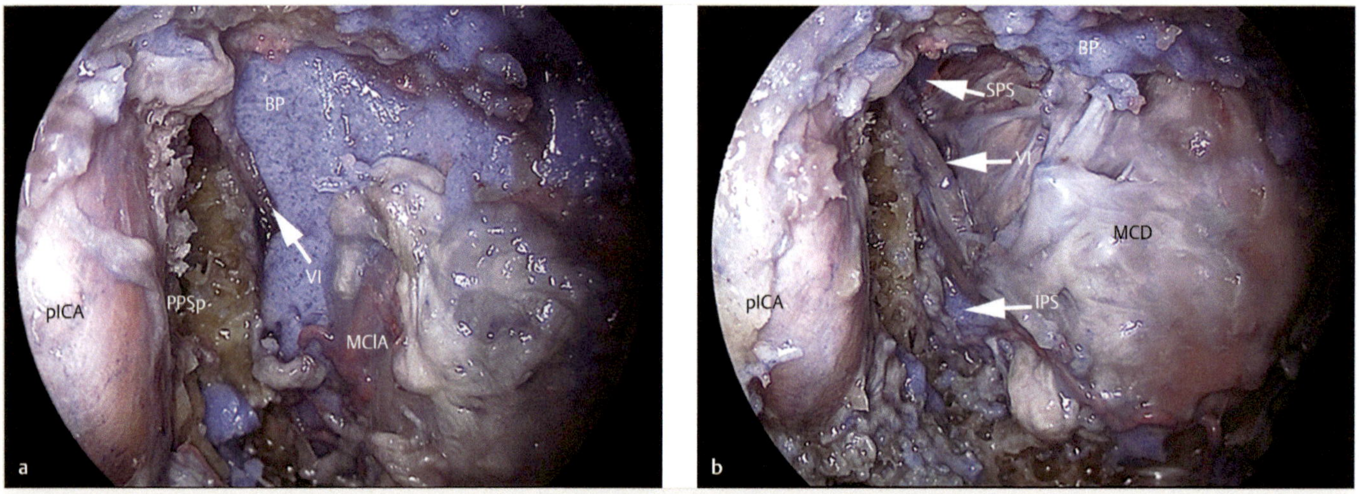

Fig. 19.20 (a, b) Dural sinuses surrounding the abducens nerve as seen from the contralateral nostril. The abducens nerve (VI) exits the basilar plexus (BP) to reach the cavernous sinus passing above the petrous process of the sphenoid bone (PPSp). The superior petrosal sinus (SPS) communicates with the posterolateral end of the cavernous sinus, above the abducens nerve (VI). The anteromedial end of the inferior petrosal sinus (IPS) communicates with the basilar plexus and runs below the abducens nerve. MCD, dura mater of the midclivus; MCIA, medial clival artery; pICA, paraclival portion of the internal carotid artery.

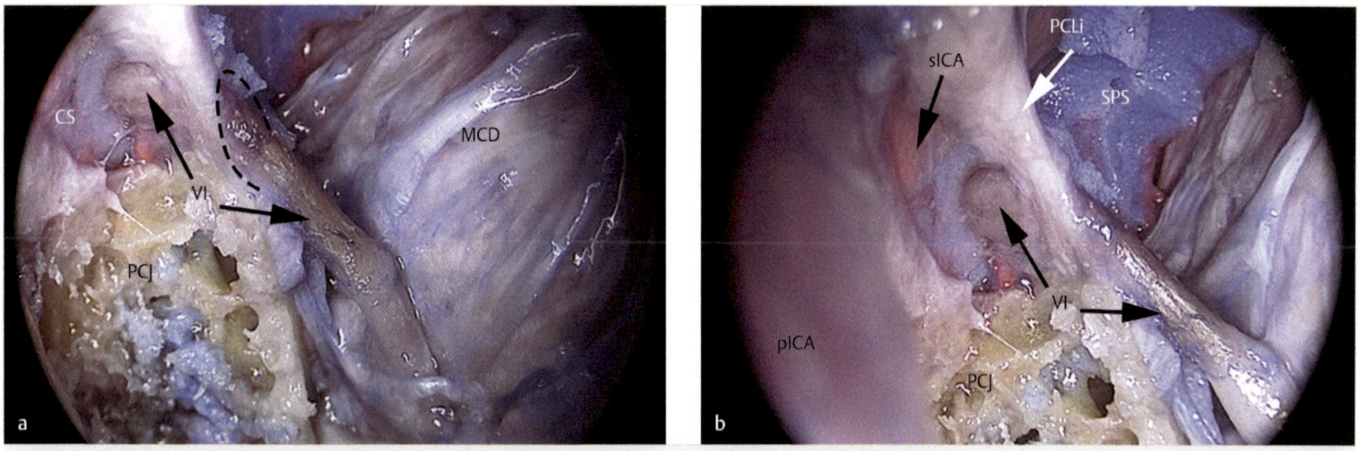

Fig. 19.21 (a, b) Dorello's canal. The petroclinoid (or Gruber's) ligament (PCLi) extends from the petrous apex to the dorsum sellae, passing above the abducens nerve (VI) and the petroclival junction (PCJ). Dorello's canal (*black dashed line*) is formed by the bone of the petroclival junction, inferiorly, and the petroclinoid ligament, superiorly. When the abducens nerve reaches the cavernous sinus (CS), it crosses the parasellar portion of the internal carotid artery (sICA) in a posteromedial-to-anterolateral direction. MCD, dura mater of the midclivus; pICA, paraclival portion of the internal carotid artery; SPS, superior petrosal sinus.

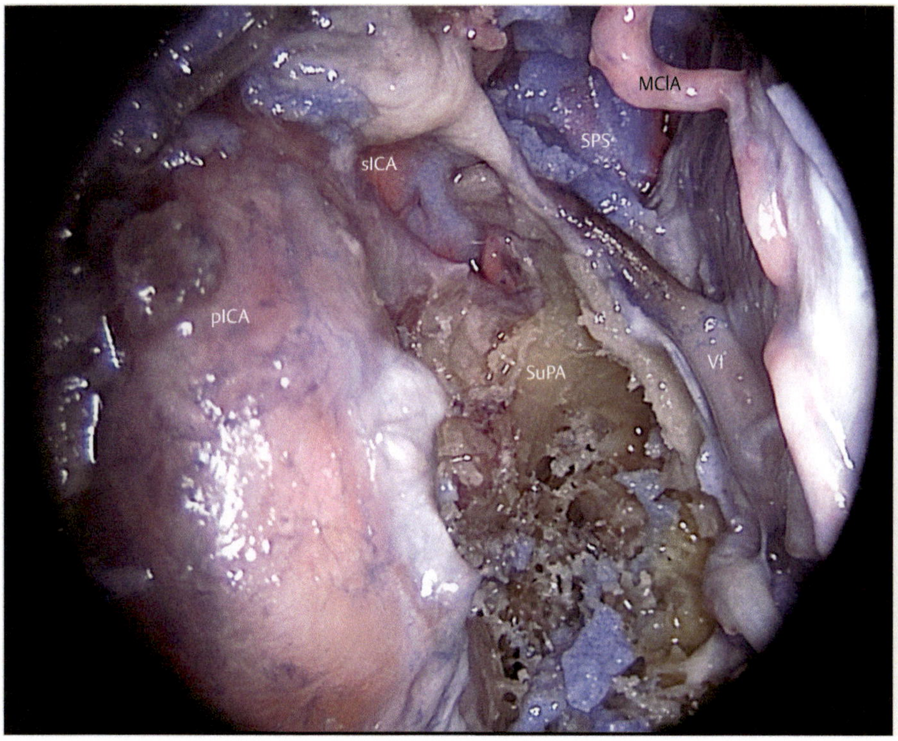

Fig. 19.22 Step 6. Employing a 70-degree endoscope turned superolaterally, the petrous process of the sphenoid bone lying behind the paraclival portion of the internal carotid artery (pICA) is progressively removed to expose the superior petrous apex (SuPA). VI, abducens nerve; MClA, medial clival artery; sICA, parasellar portion of the internal carotid artery; SPS, superior petrosal sinus.

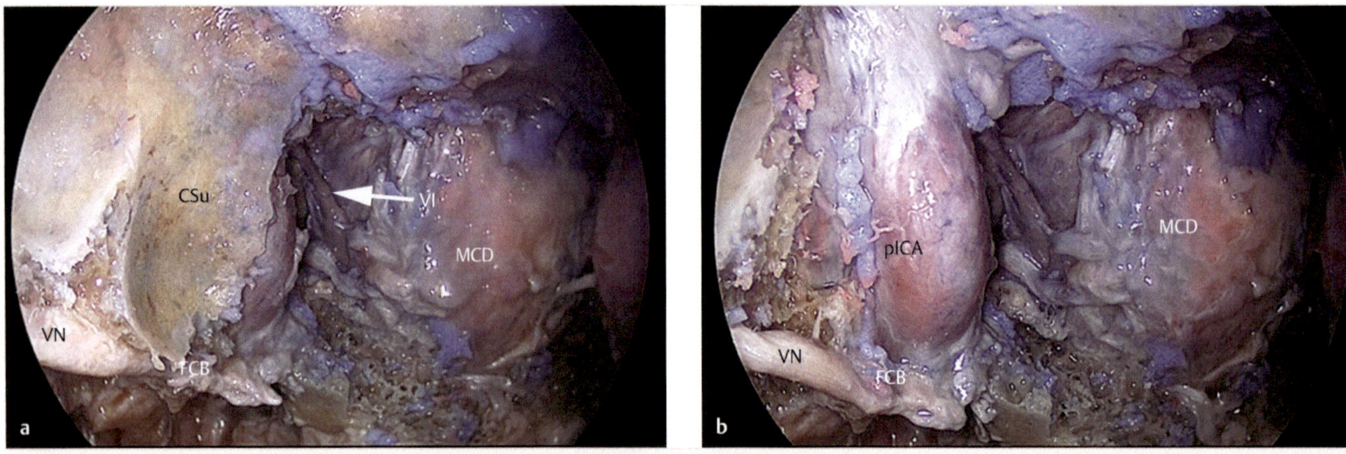

Fig. 19.23 (a, b) The paraclival tract of the internal carotid artery. Completing the removal of the carotid sulcus (CSu), as described for Step 2, allows for understanding the relationship between the paraclival tract of the internal carotid artery (pICA), abducens nerve (VI), and petrous apex. FCP, fibrocartilago basalis; MCD, dura mater of the midclivus; VN, vidian nerve.

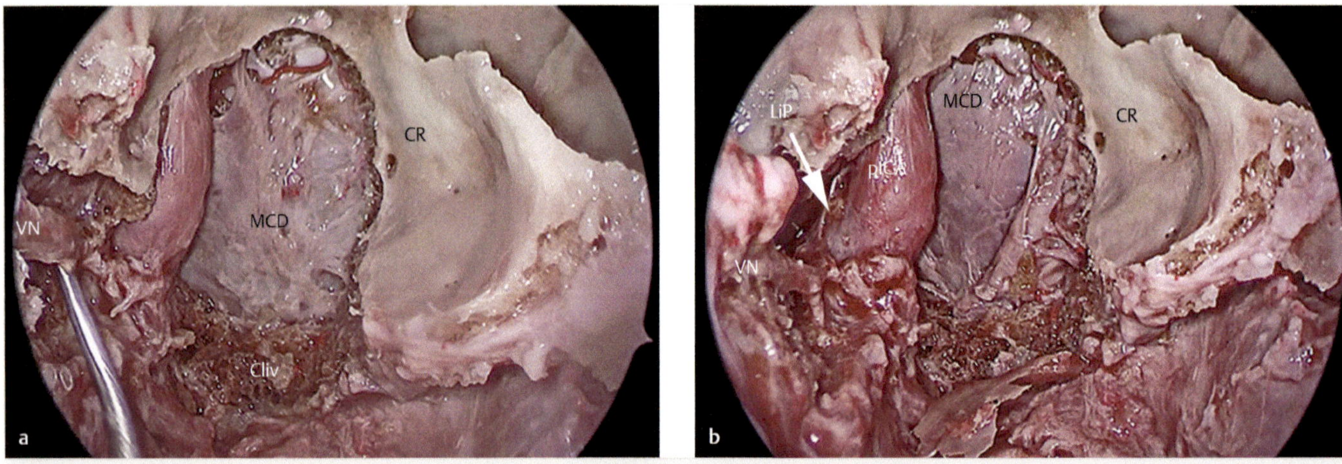

Fig. 19.24 (a, b) The anterolateral portion of the carotid sulcus and lingual process. By removing the anterolateral portion of the carotid sulcus, the lingual process (LiP) of the sphenoid bone, which covers laterally the lower paraclival internal carotid artery (pICA), comes into view. Cliv, lower clivus; CR, clival recess; MCD, dura mater of the midclivus; VN, vidian nerve.

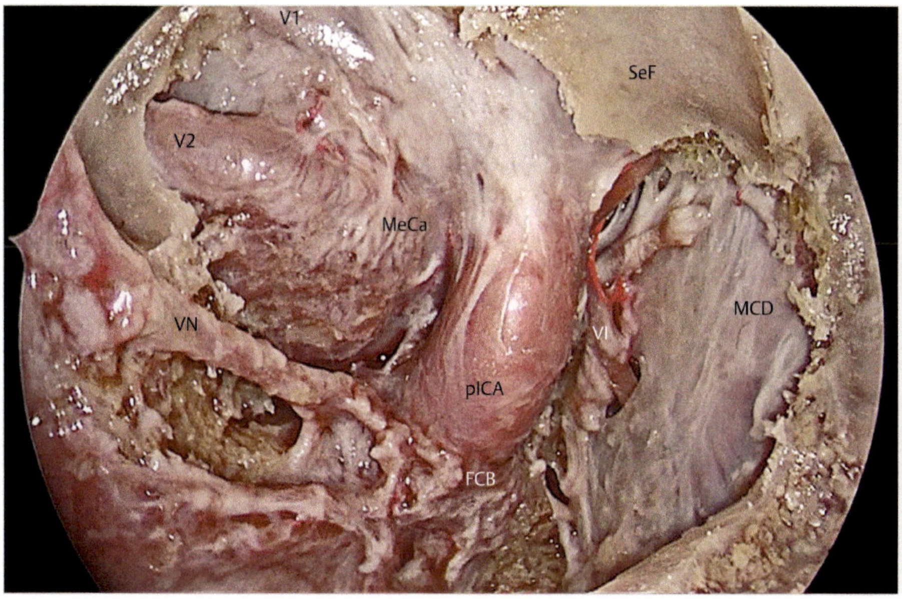

Fig. 19.25 Exploring the anatomical relationships with Meckel's cave. After removing the lateral wall of the sphenoid sinus, Meckel's cave (MeCa) is visualized with a 70-degree endoscope to understand its anatomical relationships with the medial petrous apex and the paraclival portion of the internal carotid artery (pICA). V1, ophthalmic nerve; V2, maxillary nerve; VI, abducens nerve FCB, fibrocartilago basalis; MCD, dura mater of the midclivus; SeF, sellar floor; VN, vidian nerve.

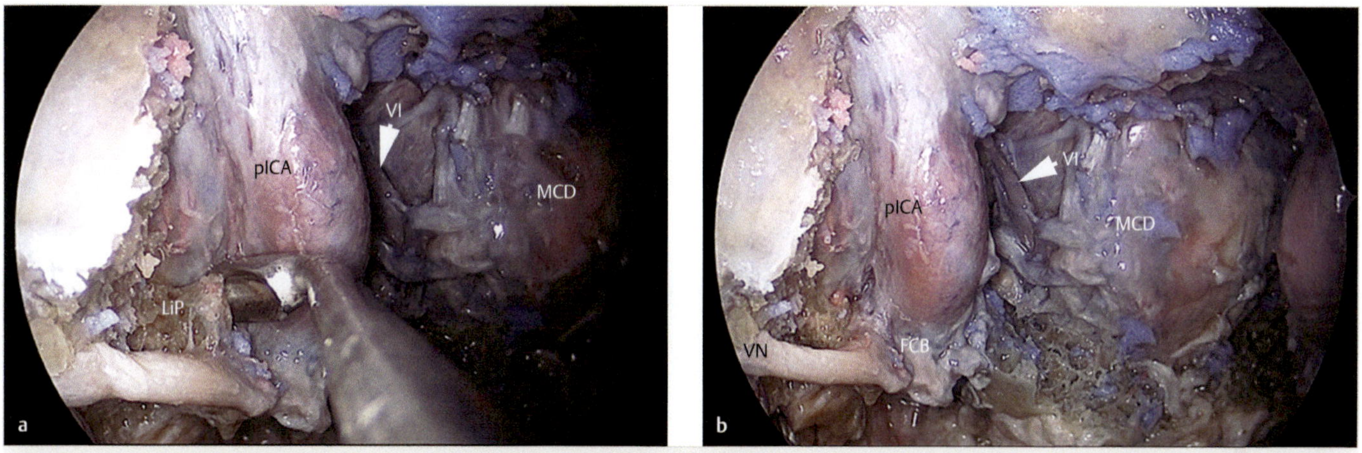

Fig. 19.26 (a, b) Step 7. The lingual process of the sphenoid (LiP), which is located between the paraclival portion of the internal carotid artery (pICA) and Meckel's cave, is removed. VI, abducens nerve; CSAW, cavernous sinus anterior wall; FCB, fibrocartilago basalis; MCD, dura mater of the midclivus; VN, vidian nerve.

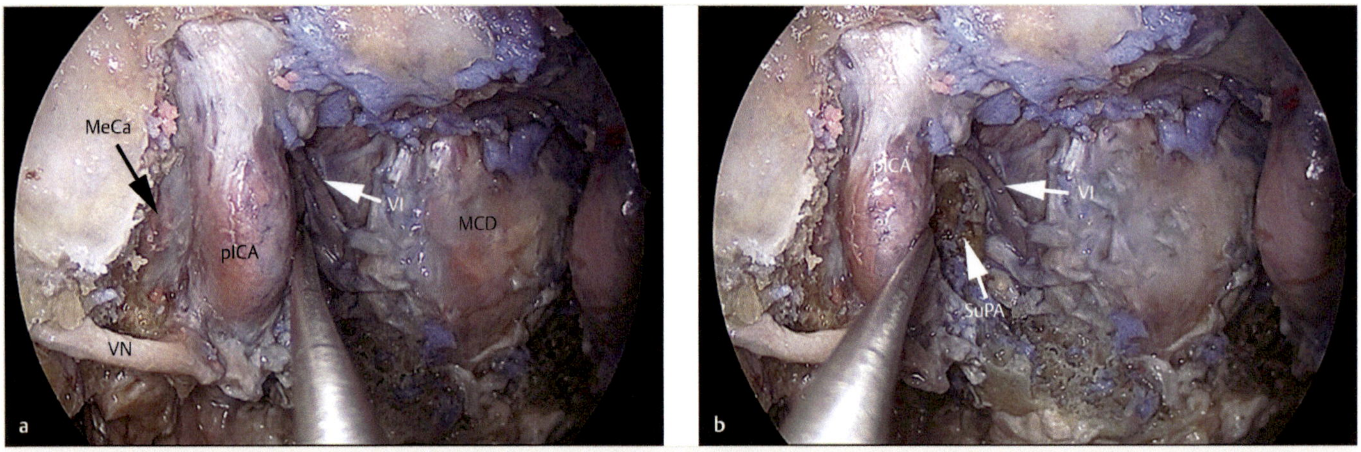

Fig. 19.27 (a, b) Lateralization of the paraclival portion of the internal carotid artery. After removal of the lingual process of the sphenoid bone, the paraclival portion of the internal carotid artery (pICA) can be gently pushed laterally toward Meckel's cave (MeCa) to achieve better visualization of the superior petrous apex (SuPA) with a 0-degree endoscope positioned through the contralateral nostril. VI, abducens nerve; MCD, dura mater of the midclivus; VN, vidian nerve.

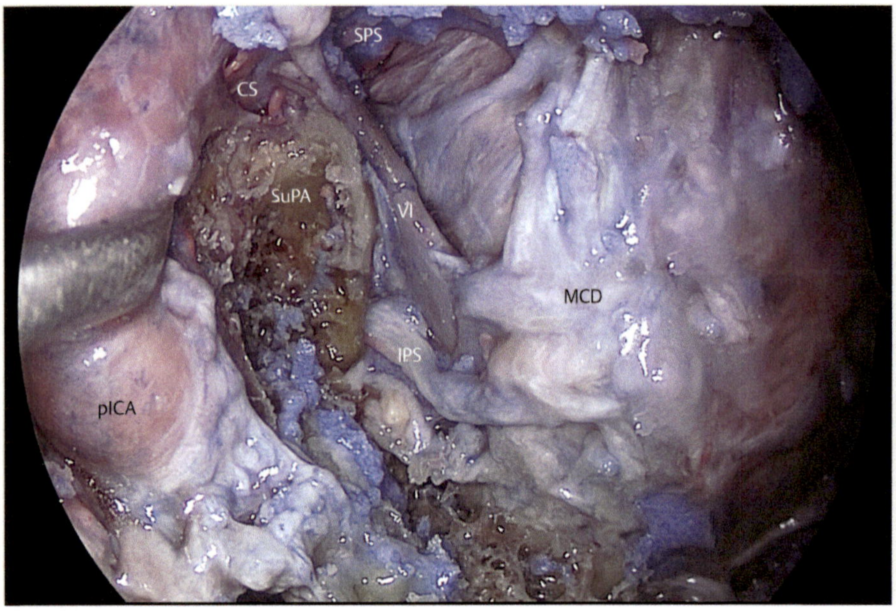

Fig. 19.28 Close view of the petrous apex with lateralization of the paraclival portion of the internal carotid artery. The anatomical structures surrounding the superior petrous apex (SuPA) include the following: the cavernous sinus (CS), which is located anterosuperiorly to the petrous apex; the anteromedial end of the superior petrosal sinus (SPS); the abducens nerve (VI), which runs between the petrous apex and the inferior petrosal sinus (IPS), anteroinferiorly, and superior petrosal sinus, posterosuperiorly. MCD, dura mater of the midclivus.

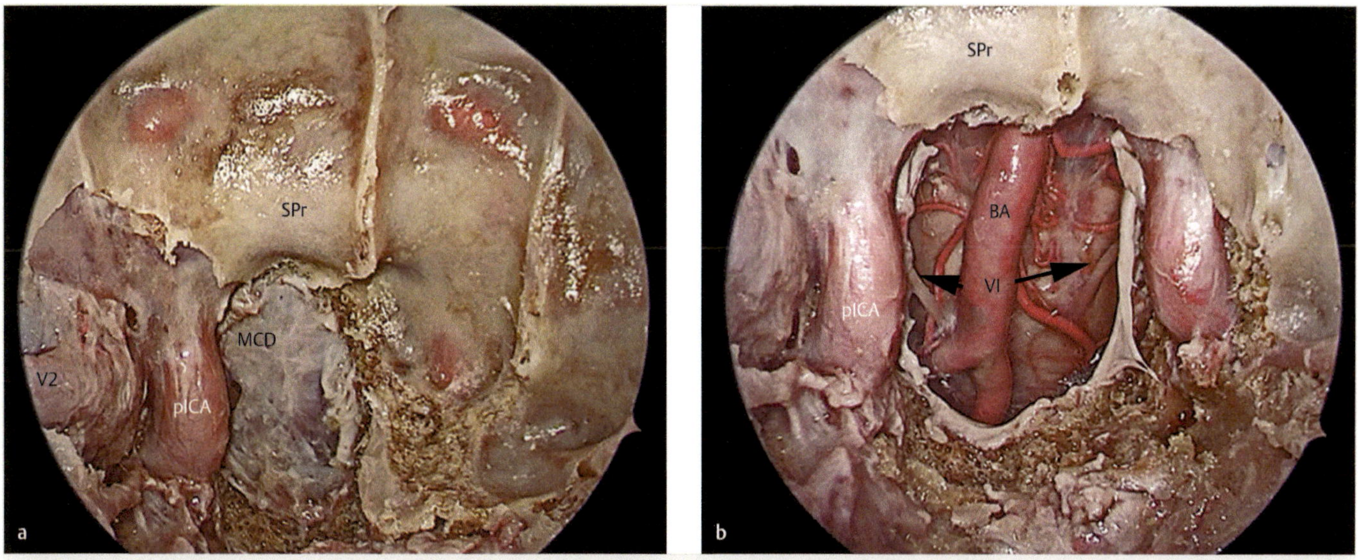

Fig. 19.29 (a, b) Step 8. The dura mater of the midclivus (MCD) is opened. As an alternative, the transclival midclivus approach module can be added to expose the basilar artery (BA) and both abducens nerves (VI). V2, maxillary nerve; pICA, paraclival portion of the internal carotid artery; SPr, sellar prominence.

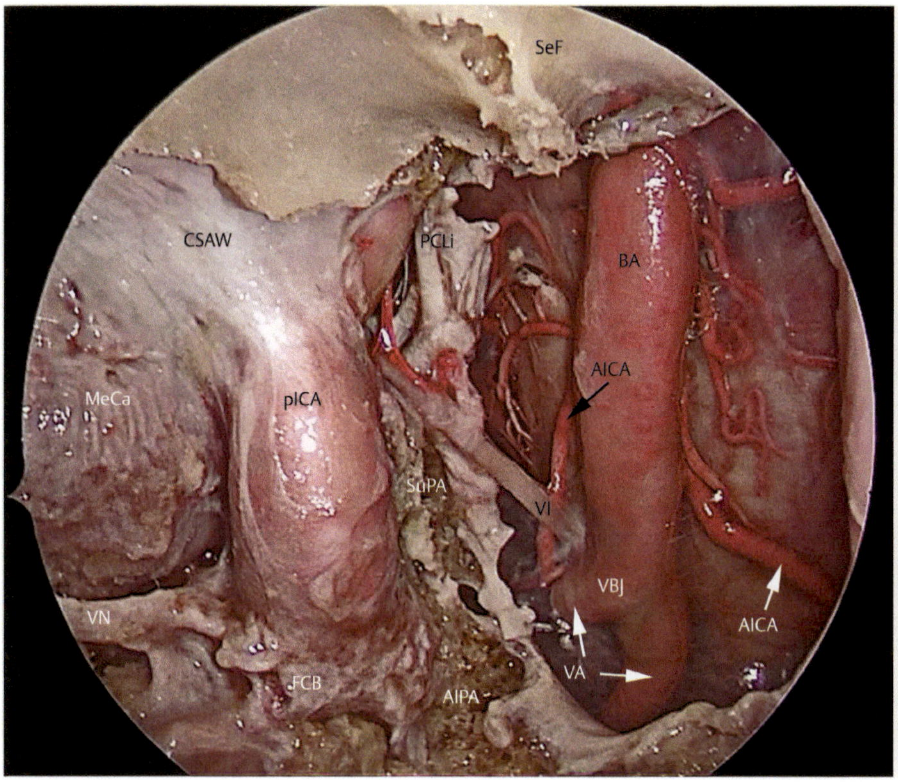

Fig. 19.30 Intradural anatomy of the abducens nerve as seen with a 70-degree endoscope. The abducens nerve (VI) arises from the pontomedullary junction and runs below the anterior inferior cerebellar artery (AICA), which branches from the basilar artery (BA). Then, the abducens nerve enters the basilar plexus. AIPA, anterior inferior petrous apex; CSAW, cavernous sinus anterior wall; FCB, fibrocartilago basalis; MeCa, Meckel's cave; pICA, paraclival portion of the internal carotid artery; PCLi, petroclival, or Gruber's, ligament; SeF, sellar floor; SuPA, superior petrous apex; VA, vertebral artery; VBJ, vertebrobasilar junction; VN, vidian nerve.

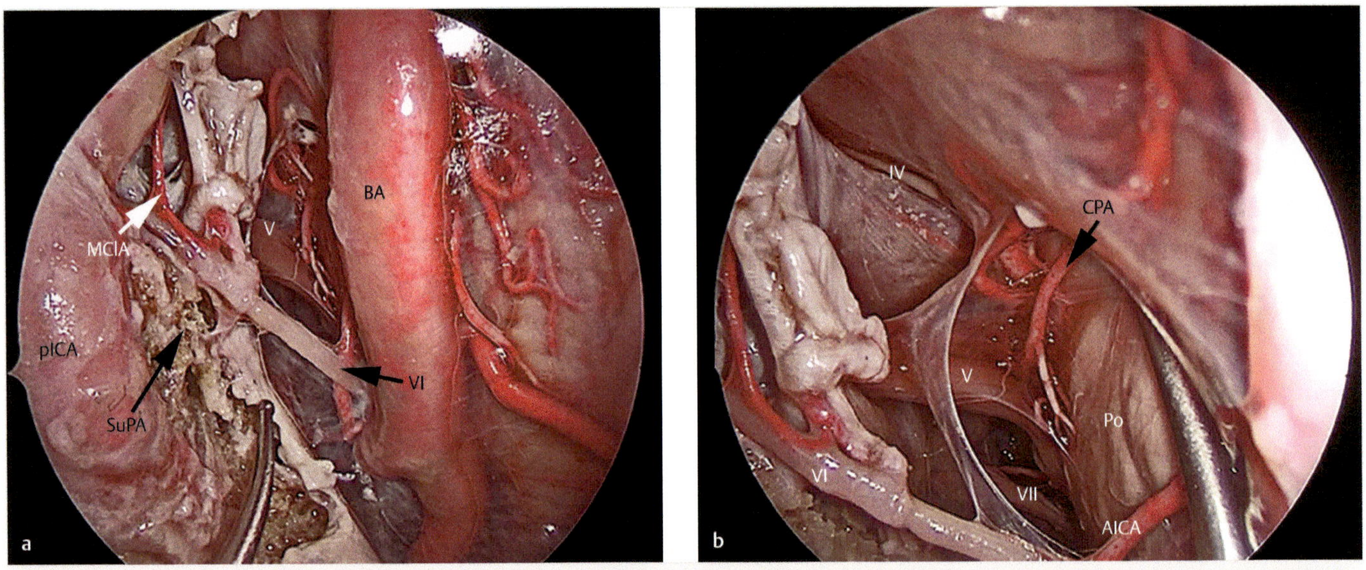

Fig. 19.31 (a, b) The trigeminal stem. The trigeminal stem (V), which arises from the pons (Po), can be identified lateral to the abducens nerve (VI) with a 70-degree endoscope. The facial nerve (VII) comes into view further laterally. The trochlear nerve (IV) is also visible while entering the cerebellar tentorium in the upper part of the visual field. One or more circumferential pontine arteries can be seen (CPA) running toward the area where the trigeminal stem arises. VI, abducens nerve; AICA, anterior inferior cerebellar artery; MClA, medial clival artery; PA, petrous apex; pICA, paraclival tract of the internal carotid artery; SuPA, superior petrous apex.

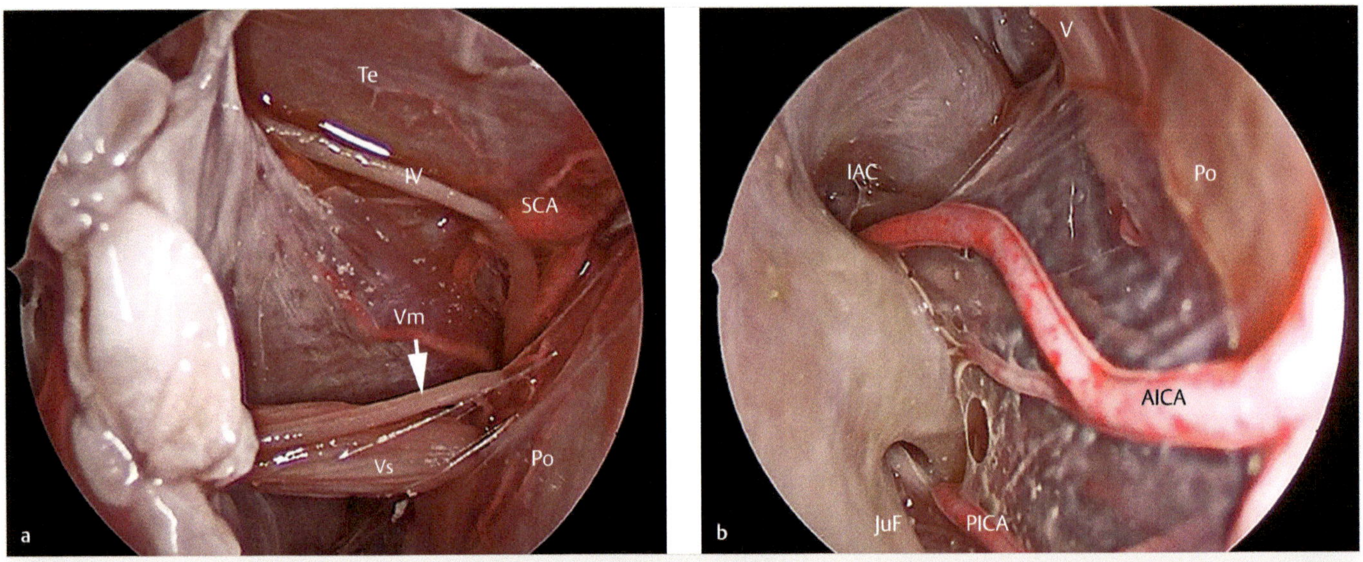

Fig. 19.32 (a, b) Intradural anatomy of the posterior surface of the petrous part of the temporal bone. With a 70-degree scope turned laterally, the posterior cranial fossa is visible around the corner corresponding to the petroclival region. The cerebellar tentorium (Te) is identified as the upper boundary of this area. The cisternal portion of the trochlear nerve (IV) is visible below the tentorium. More anteriorly, the trochlear nerve pierces the free edge of the tentorium to enter the cavernous sinus. The superior cerebellar artery (SCA) is the main vessel encroaching the trigeminal stem (V). This nerve is composed of a motor root (Vm) and a sensory root (Vs), which are strictly adjacent. The other two main arteries of the posterior cranial fossa vasculature are the anterior inferior cerebellar artery (AICA) and the posterior inferior cerebellar artery (PICA). These arteries have strict relationships with the nerves entering the internal auditory canal (IAC) and the jugular foramen (JuF), respectively. In this specimen, the anterior inferior cerebellar artery forms a loop within the internal acoustic meatus. Po, pons.

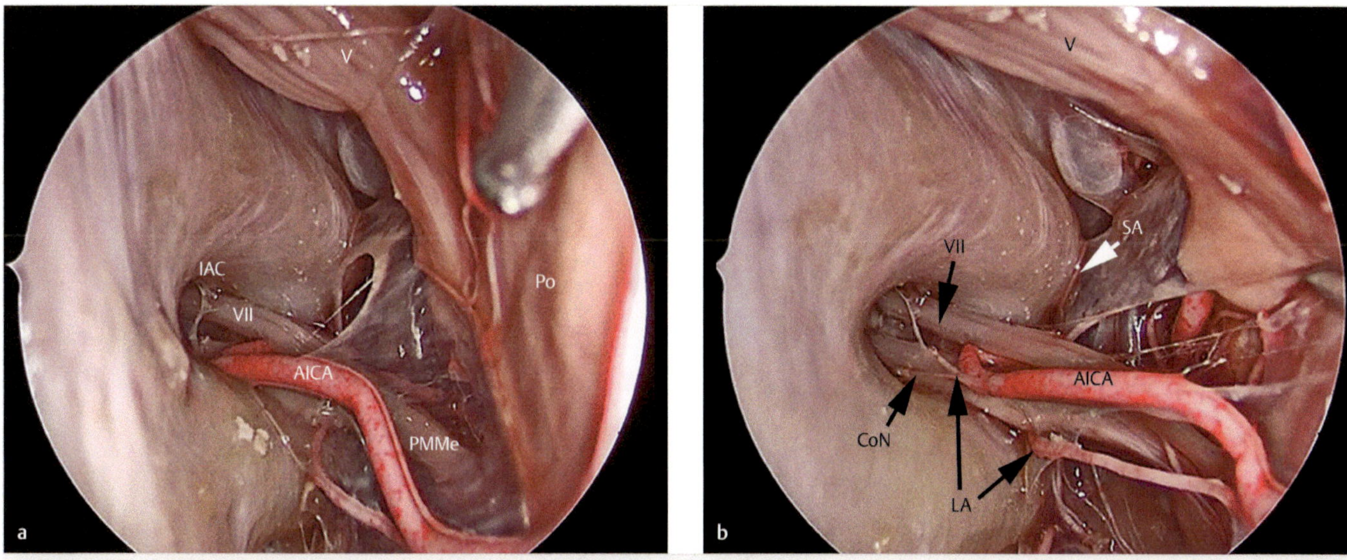

Fig. 19.33 (a, b) The internal auditory canal. With a 70-degree endoscope directed inferolaterally toward the internal auditory canal (IAC), the relationship between the anterior inferior cerebellar artery (AICA) and the facial nerve (VII) can be clearly visualized. The facial (VII) and cochlear nerve (CoN) can be distinguished by moving the scope close to the internal auditory canal. The anterior inferior cerebellar artery commonly passes between the facial and cochlear nerves, as in this case. Furthermore, two collateral branches of the anterior inferior cerebellar artery, namely, the labyrinthine arteries (LA) and the subarcuate artery (SA), can be seen. PMMe, pontomesencephalic membrane.

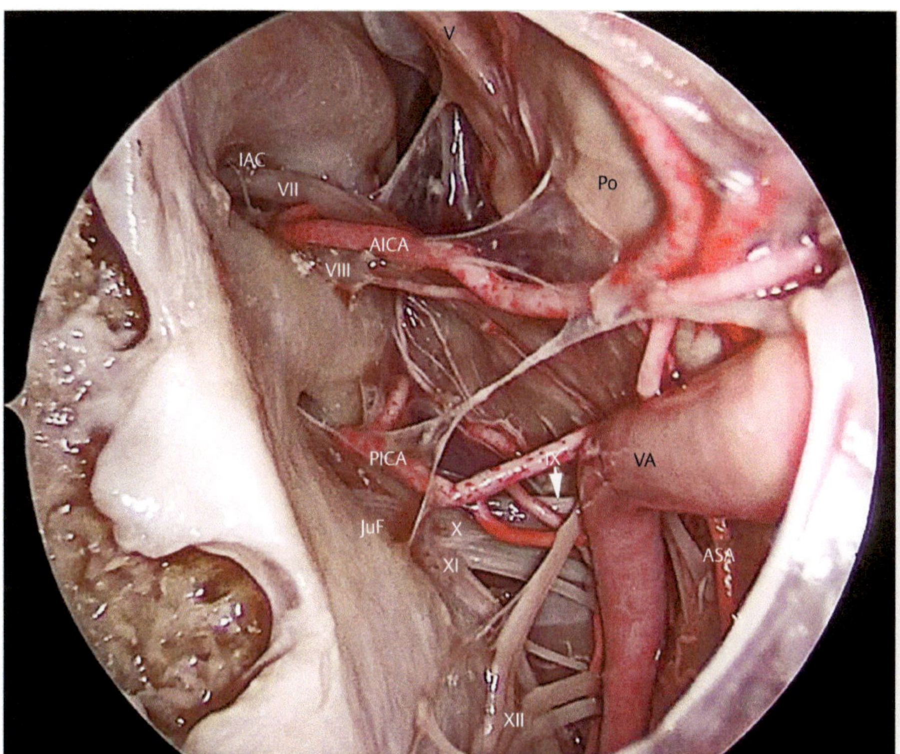

Fig. 19.34 Intradural anatomy of the jugular foramen. Turning the 70-degree endoscope more inferiorly, medial visualization of several neurovascular structures is obtained. The facial nerve (VII), the anterior inferior nerve (VIII), and the anteroinferior cerebellar artery (AICA) can be identified in the superior portion of the visual field. The posterior inferior cerebellar artery (PICA), vertebral artery (VA), hypoglossal nerve (XII), glossopharyngeal nerve (IX), vagus nerve (X), spinal accessory nerve (XI), and anterior spinal artery (ASA) are located in the inferior portion of the visual field. IAC, internal auditory canal; JuF, jugular foramen; Po, pons; V, trigeminal nerve.

References

[1] Scopel TF, Fernandez-Miranda JC, Pinheiro-Neto CD, et al. Petrous apex cholesterol granulomas: endonasal versus infracochlear approach. Laryngoscope 2012;122(4):751–761

[2] Presutti L, Villari D, Marchioni D. Petrous apex cholesterol granuloma: transsphenoid endoscopic approach. J Laryngol Otol 2006;120(6):e20

[3] Zanation AM, Snyderman CH, Carrau RL, Gardner PA, Prevedello DM, Kassam AB. Endoscopic endonasal surgery for petrous apex lesions. Laryngoscope 2009;119(1):19–25

[4] Georgalas C, Kania R, Guichard JP, Sauvaget E, Tran Ba Huy P, Herman P. Endoscopic transsphenoidal surgery for cholesterol granulomas involving the petrous apex. Clin Otolaryngol 2008;33(1):38–42

[5] Paluzzi A, Gardner P, Fernandez-Miranda JC, et al. Endoscopic endonasal approach to cholesterol granulomas of the petrous apex: a series of 17 patients: clinical article. J Neurosurg 2012;116(4):792–798

[6] Carlson ML, O'Connell BP, Breen JT, et al. Petroclival chondrosarcoma: a multicenter review of 55 cases and new staging system. Otol Neurotol 2016;37(7):940–950

[7] Mohyeldin A, Prevedello DM, Jamshidi AO, Ditzel Filho LF, Carrau RL. Nuances in the treatment of malignant tumors of the clival and petroclival region. Int Arch Otorhinolaryngol 2014;18(Suppl 2):S157–S172

[8] Koutourousiou M, Gardner PA, Tormenti MJ, et al. Endoscopic endonasal approach for resection of cranial base chordomas: outcomes and learning curve. Neurosurgery 2012;71(3):614–624, discussion 624–625

[9] Koutourousiou M, Fernandez-Miranda JC, Vaz-Guimaraes Filho F, et al. Outcomes of endonasal and lateral approaches to petroclival meningiomas. World Neurosurg 2017;99:500–517

[10] Beer-Furlan A, Abi-Hachem R, Jamshidi AO, Carrau RL, Prevedello DM. Endoscopic trans-sphenoidal surgery for petroclival and clival meningiomas. J Neurosurg Sci 2016;60(4):495–502

[11] Simal-Julián JA, Miranda-Lloret P, Botella-Asunción C, Kassam A. Full endoscopic endonasal expanded approach to the petroclival region: optimizing the carotid-clival window. Acta Neurochir (Wien) 2014;156(8):1627–1629

[12] Chatrath P, Nouraei SA, De Cordova J, Patel M, Saleh HA. Endonasal endoscopic approach to the petrous apex: an image-guided quantitative anatomical study. Clin Otolaryngol 2007;32(4):255–260

[13] Barges-Coll J, Fernandez-Miranda JC, Prevedello DM, et al. Avoiding injury to the abducens nerve during expanded endonasal endoscopic surgery: anatomic and clinical case studies. Neurosurgery 2010;67(1):144–154, discussion 154

20 Infrapetrous Approach

Davide Lancini, Marco Ravanelli, Marco Ferrari, Alberto Schreiber

According to the topographical classification of the petrous apex into three segments (superior, anteroinferior, and posteroinferior), the transnasal infrapetrous pathway leads to the anteroinferior portion.[1] A general overview on endoscopic transnasal approaches to the petrous apex is reported in Chapter 19 together with details on the topography of this skull base area.

The infrapetrous route exploits the space below the horizontal tract of the petrous internal carotid artery to expose the anteroinferior portion of the petrous apex and adjacent structures. This narrow pathway is laterally bounded by the lateral pterygoid plate, the mandibular nerve, and the parapharyngeal internal carotid artery and crosses the area of the basipterygoid and the foramen lacerum, which is composed of a dense tissue called fibrocartilago basalis. Depending on the need for exposure and freedom of movement, the corridor can be harvested by either removing (as explained in Chapters 23 and 24) or displacing the eustachian tube inferiorly.[2] This chapter includes the description of the infrapetrous approach both as an extension of the medial petrous apex (described in Chapter 19) or the medial parapharyngeal approach (described in Chapter 23) and as independent route to the petrous apex with eustachian tube transposition via the lower transpterygoid approach. The trajectory of the infrapetrous approach leads to the area of the hypoglossal canal and neighboring neurovascular structures, serving as midway corridor between the transcondylar/transjugular tuberculum "far medial" approach (described in Chapter 22) medially, the lateral parapharyngeal approach (described in Chapter 24) laterally, and the suprapetrous approach to Meckel's cave (described in Chapter 21) superiorly.

The infrapetrous route has been employed either alone or in combination with other transnasal corridors to manage lesions of the inferior portion of petroclival area, mostly cholesterol granulomas[3] or extradural tumors such as chordomas and chondrosarcomas.[4–6] As mentioned in the previous chapter, the role of transnasal endoscopic routes toward the petrous apex should be seen in the wide context of other corridors, including classical transcranial and newly emerging transorbital and contralateral transmaxillary approaches.[7–11]

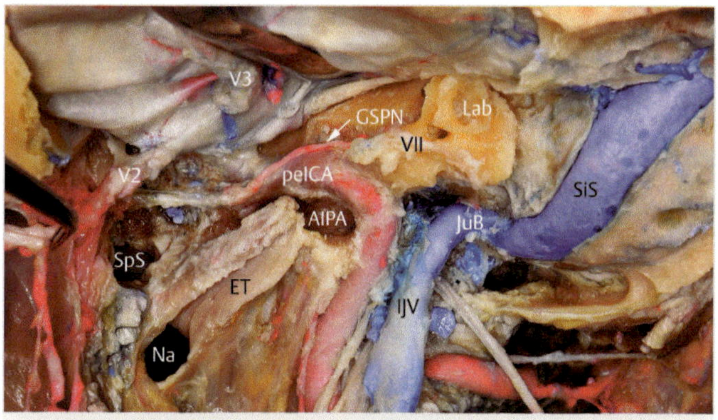

Fig. 20.1 Subtemporal lateral-to-medial view of the transnasal route toward the anteroinferior petrous apex. This cadaver picture shows with a lateral-to-medial epidural perspective left middle cranial fossa and carotid canal. V2, maxillary nerve; V3, mandibular nerve; VII, facial nerve (tympanic tract); AIPA, anteroinferior petrous apex; ET, eustachian tube; GSPN, greater superficial petrosal nerve; IJV, internal jugular vein; JuB, jugular bulb; Lab, labyrinth; Na, nasopharynx; peICA, petrous tract of the internal carotid artery; SiS, sigmoid sinus; SpS, sphenoid sinus; VN, vidian nerve.

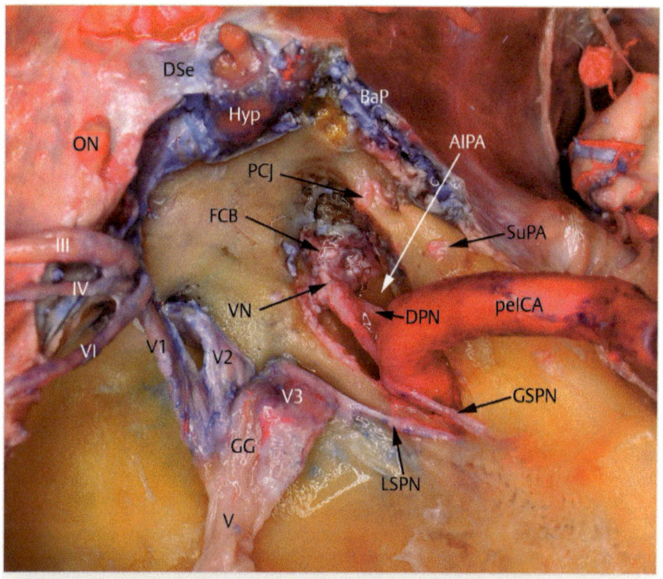

Fig. 20.2 Intracranial superolateral-to-inferomedial view of the petroclival area. This cadaver picture shows with a superolateral-to-inferomedial intracranial perspective the left petroclival area. The oculomotor (III), trochlear (IV), abducens (VI), ophthalmic (V1), maxillary (V2), and mandibular nerve (V3) have been displaced along with the gasserian ganglion (GG), trigeminal stem (V), and internal carotid artery. AIPA, anteroinferior petrous apex; BaP, basilar plexus; DPN, deep petrosal nerve; DSe, dorsum sellae; FCB, fibrocartilago basalis; GSPN, greater superficial petrosal nerve; Hyp, hypophysis; LSPN, lesser superficial petrosal nerve; ON, optic nerve; PCJ, petroclival junction; peICA, petrous tract of the internal carotid artery; SuPA, superior petrous apex; VN, vidian nerve.

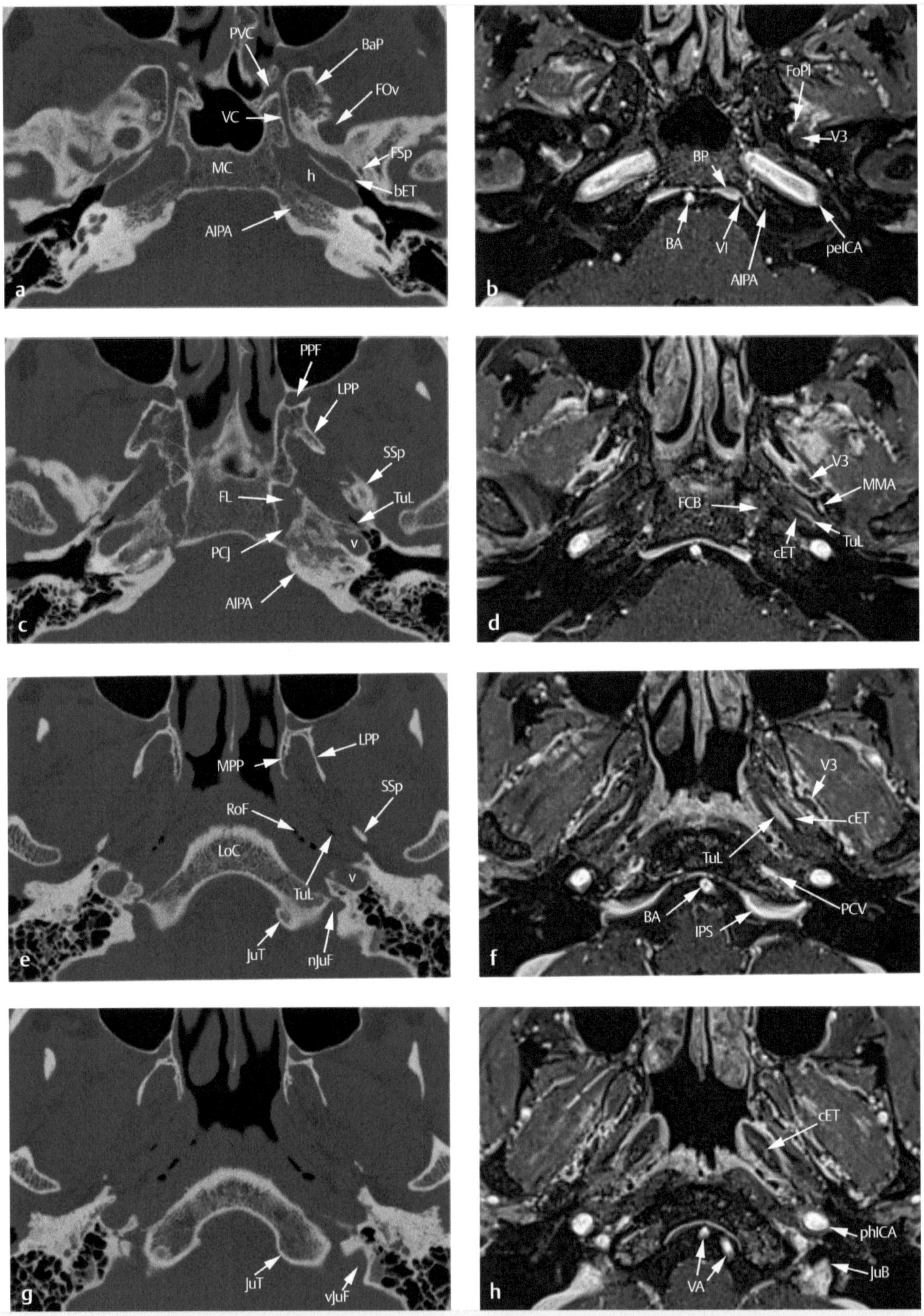

Fig. 20.3 (a–h) Axial CT and MRI anatomy of the foramen lacerum and the petrous apex. The panel includes four CT and four contrast-enhanced T1-weighted MRI axial images passing through the vidian nerves cranially (upper images) and the jugular foramen (lower images) caudally. The anteroinferior petrous apex (AIPA) lies posterior to the horizontal portion (h) of the petrous tract of the internal carotid artery (peICA) and is enclosed between the midclivus (MC), medially, and the internal acoustic meatus and inner ear, laterally. The basilar plexus (BP) and the abducens nerve (VI) are located in a medial position with respect to the anteroinferior petrous apex, which is adjacent to several venous vessels including the petroclival vein (PCV), anteriorly, and the inferior petrosal sinus (IPS), posteriorly. Anteromedially to the petrous apex, the foramen lacerum (FL), which is filled by the fibrocartilago basalis (FCB), serves as a bed for the anterior genu of the internal carotid artery, namely, the passage between the petrous and paraclival tracts of the vessel. V3, mandibular nerve; BA, basilar artery; BaP, basipterygoid; bET, bony portion of the eustachian tube; cET, cartilaginous portion of the Eustachian tube; FOv, foramen ovale; FoPl, foraminal plexus; FSp, foramen spinosum; JuB, jugular bulb; JuT, jugular tubercle; LoC, lower clivus; LPP, lateral pterygoid plate; MMA, middle meningeal artery; MPP, medial pterygoid plate; nJuF, nervous compartment of the jugular foramen; PCJ, petroclival junction; phICA, parapharyngeal tract of the internal carotid artery; PPF, pterygopalatine fossa; PVC, palatovaginal canal; RoF, Rosemüller's fossa; SSp, spina sphenoidalis; TuL, tubal lumen; v, vertical portion of the petrous tract of the internal carotid artery; VA, vertebral artery; VC, vidian canal; vJuF, vascular compartment of the jugular foramen.

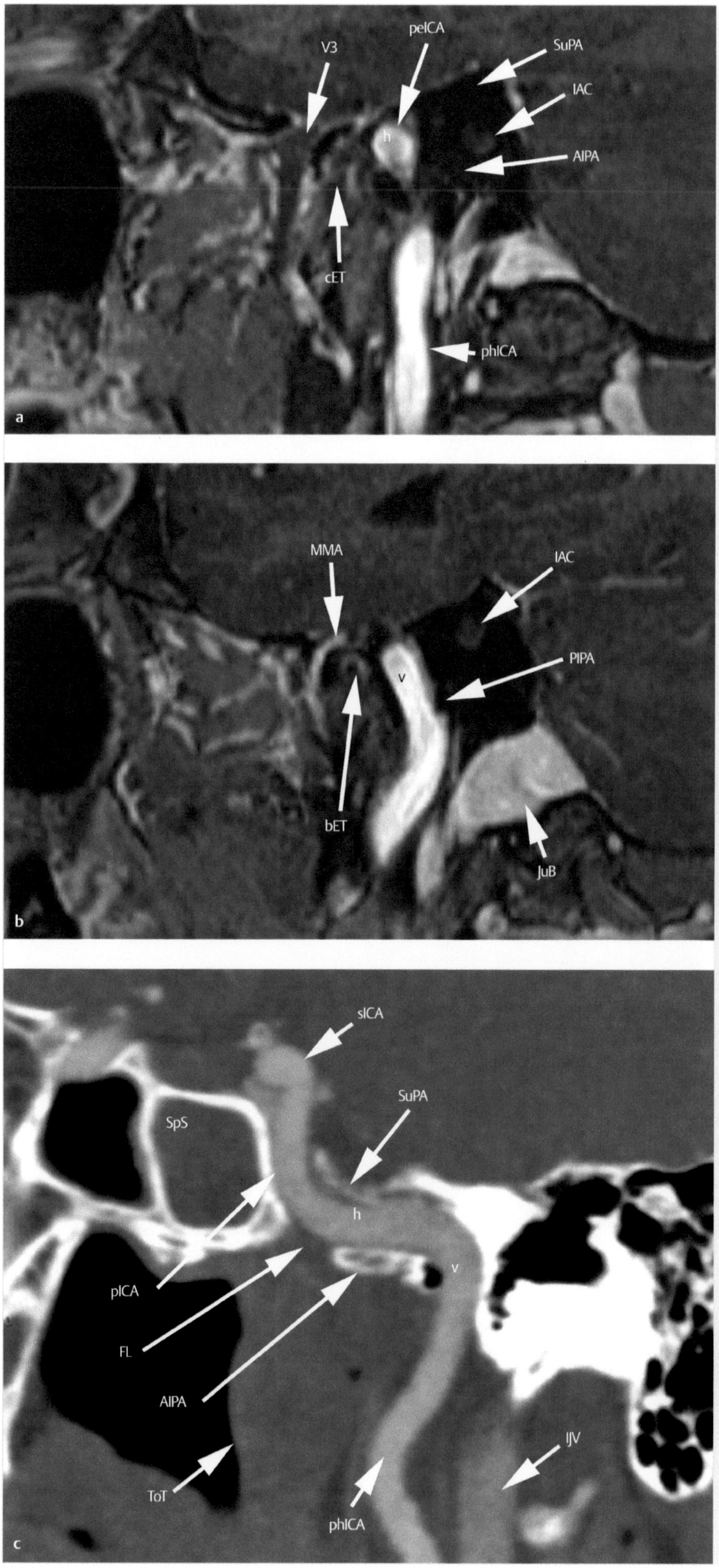

Fig. 20.4 (a–c) Sagittal and paracoronal anatomy of the petrous apex. The panel includes two sagittal contrast-enhanced T1-weighted images **(a, b)** and one paracoronal contrast-enhanced CT image **(c)** passing through the petrous apex. The orientation of the CT image is parallel to the petrous tract of the internal carotid artery. The horizontal tract (h) of the petrous segment of the internal carotid artery (peICA) lies posterior to the mandibular nerve (V3) and the cartilaginous portion of the eustachian tube (cET) and anterior to the anteroinferior petrous apex (AIPA), whereas the vertical tract (v) is located posterior to the middle meningeal artery (MMA) and the bony portion of the tube (bET) and anterior to the posteroinferior petrous apex (PIPA). The internal acoustic meatus (IAC) passes nearby both the anteroinferior and the posteroinferior portions of the petrous apex with a horizontal path, which is orthogonally cut in sagittal images. As seen in the paracoronal CT image, the anteroinferior petrous apex lies posterolaterally to the foramen lacerum (FL). IJV, internal jugular vein; JuB, jugular bulb; phICA, parapharyngeal tract of the internal carotid artery; pICA, paraclival tract of the internal carotid artery; sICA, parasellar tract of the internal carotid artery; SpS, sphenoid sinus; SuPA, superior portion of the petrous apex; ToT, torus tubarius.

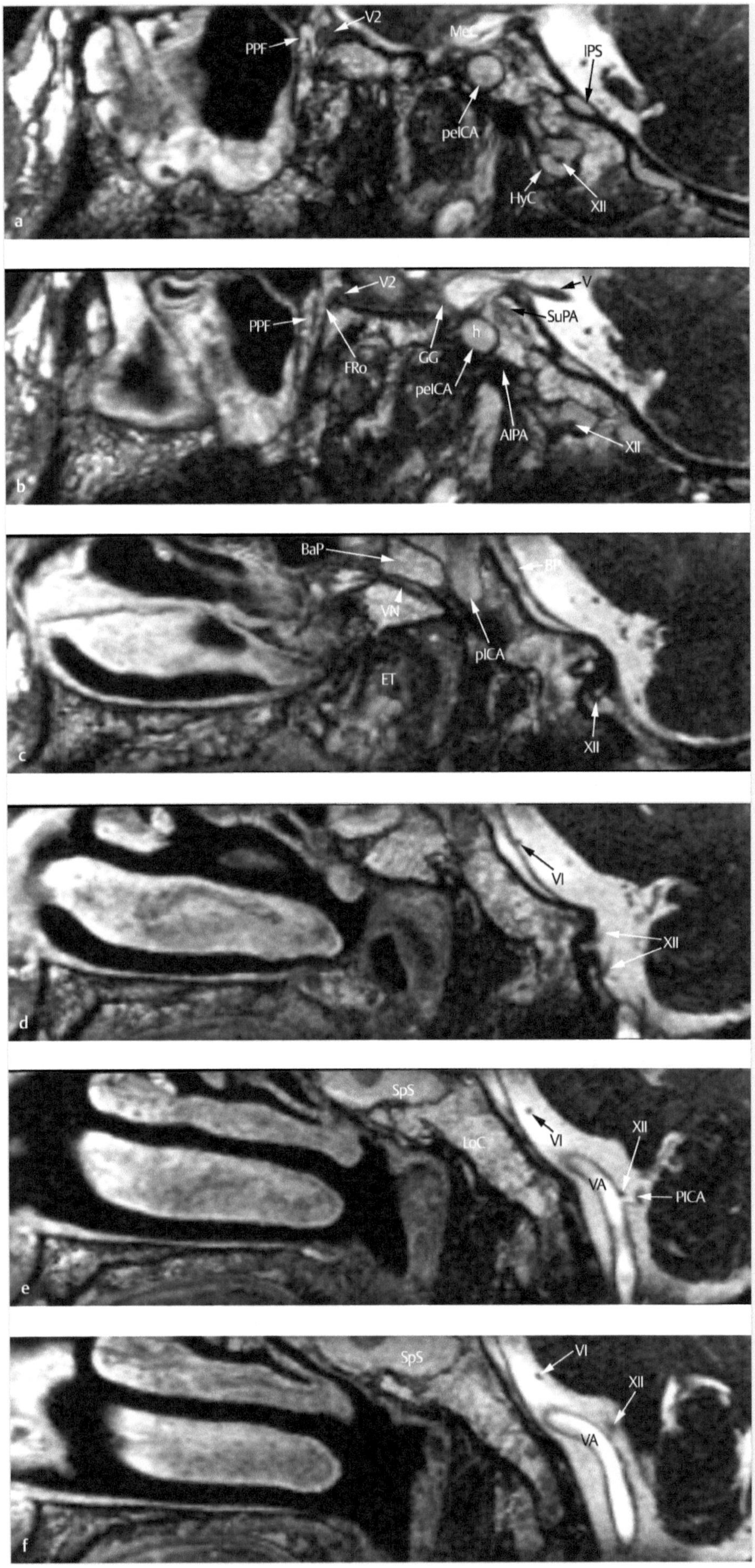

Fig. 20.5 (a–f) Sagittal MRI anatomy of the petrous apex. The panel contains six sagittal CISS (constructive interference in steady state) MRI images passing through the medial portion of the petrous apex, from lateral **(a)** to medial **(f)**. The anteroinferior petrous apex (AIPA) can be exposed by passing through the pterygopalatine fossa (PPF) and the basipterygoid (BaP), below the petrous tract of the internal carotid artery (peICA). The inferior petrosal sinus (IPS) and the hypoglossal canal (HyC) are, respectively, located posterior and posteroinferior to the anteroinferior petrous apex. V2, maxillary nerve; VI, abducens nerve; XII, hypoglossal nerve; BP, basilar plexus; ET, eustachian tube; FRo, foramen rotundum; GG, gasserian ganglion; LoC, lower clivus; MeC, Meckel's cave; PICA, posterior inferior cerebellar artery; pICA, paraclival tract of the internal carotid artery; SpS, sphenoid sinus; VA, vertebral artery; VN, vidian nerve.

Endoscopic Dissection

Nasal Phase

- Anterior and posterior ethmoidectomy.
- Transethmoidal sphenoidotomy.
- Removal of the sphenoid sinus floor (only for the infrapetrous extension of the medial parapharyngeal and medial petrous apex approach).
- Type B, C, or D endoscopic medial maxillectomy.

Skull Base Phase

Infrapetrous Extension of the Medial Parapharyngeal and Medial Petrous Apex Approach

- Medial parapharyngeal approach.
- Facultative: Medial petrous apex approach.
- Step 1: Exposure of the anteroinferior petrous apex.
- Step 2: Drilling of the anteroinferior petrous apex.
- Step 3: Drilling of the petroclival junction.

Infrapetrous Approach with Eustachian Tube Transposition

- Transpterygomaxillary approach.
- Step 1: Removal of the medial pterygoid plate.
- Step 2: Exposure of the fibrocartilago basalis.
- Step 3: Incision of the nasopharynx.
- Step 4: Inferior transposition of the eustachian tube.
- Step 5: Dissection of the fibrocartilago basalis.
- Step 6: Removal of the fibrocartilago basalis.
- Step 7: Posteroinferior septectomy and drilling of the lower clivus.
- Step 8: Removal of the cortical bone of the lower clivus.
- Step 9: Incision of the dura of the lower clivus.

Infrapetrous Extension of the Medial Parapharyngeal and the Medial Petrous Apex Approach

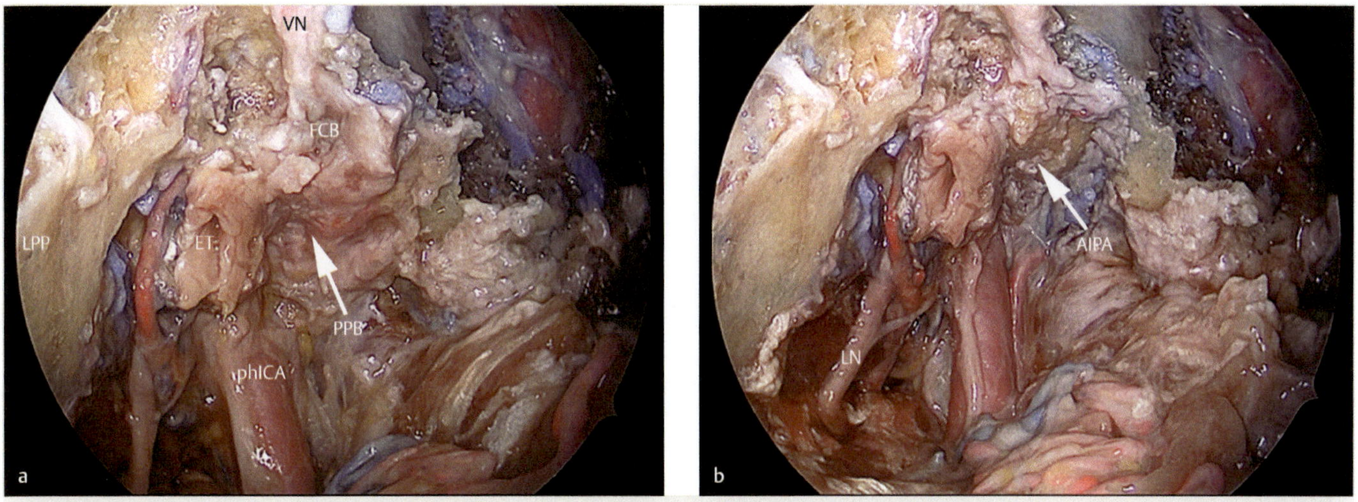

Fig. 20.6 (a, b) Step 1. After completing the medial parapharyngeal and medial petrous apex approaches, the anteroinferior petrous apex (AIPA) is uncovered from the periosteum of the petrous bone (PPB). This subunit of the petrous apex is enclosed between the axial plane passing through the foramen lacerum, cranially, and the external carotid foramen, caudally. It is divided from the posteroinferior petrous apex by a plane passing through the medial border of the external carotid foramen and crossing the posterior surface of the petrous bone. The foramen lacerum is filled by the fibrocartilago basalis (FCB). LN, lingual nerve; LPP, lateral pterygoid plate; phICA, parapharyngeal tract of the internal carotid artery; VN, vidian nerve.

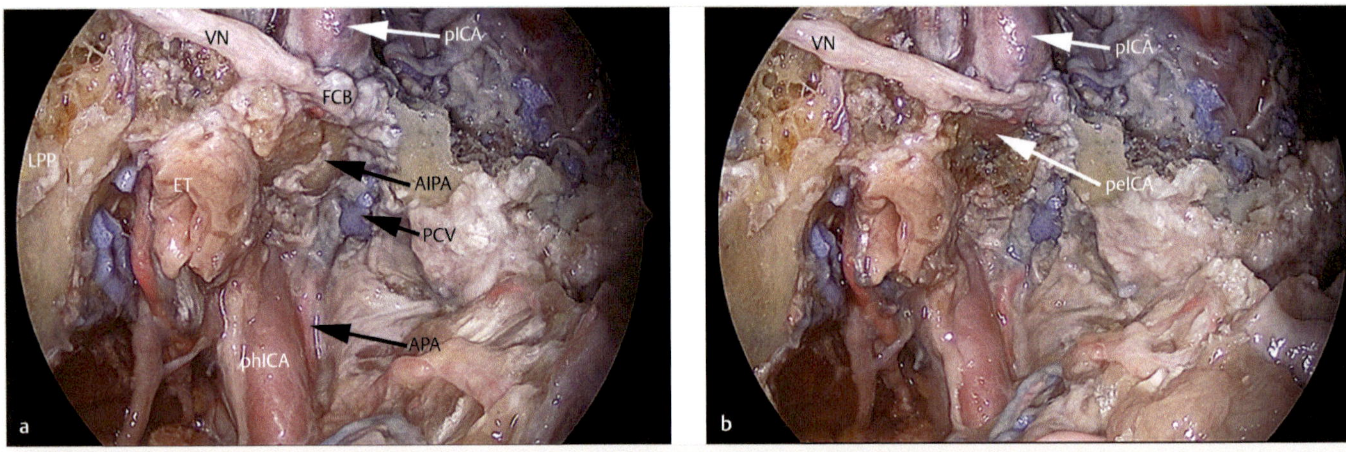

Fig. 20.7 (a, b) Step 2 (part 1). The dissection is easily carried out with a 0-degree scope placed through the contralateral nostril. The anteroinferior petrous apex (AIPA) is removed in the area between the sectioned eustachian tube (ET) anteriorly, the vidian nerve (VN) and the fibrocartilago basalis (FCB) medially, the petroclival vein (PCV) posteriorly, and the parapharyngeal tract of the internal carotid artery (phICA) laterally. This procedure uncovers the inferior surface of the petrous tract of the internal carotid artery (peICA). APA, ascending pharyngeal artery; LPP, lateral pterygoid process; pICA, paraclival tract of the internal carotid artery.

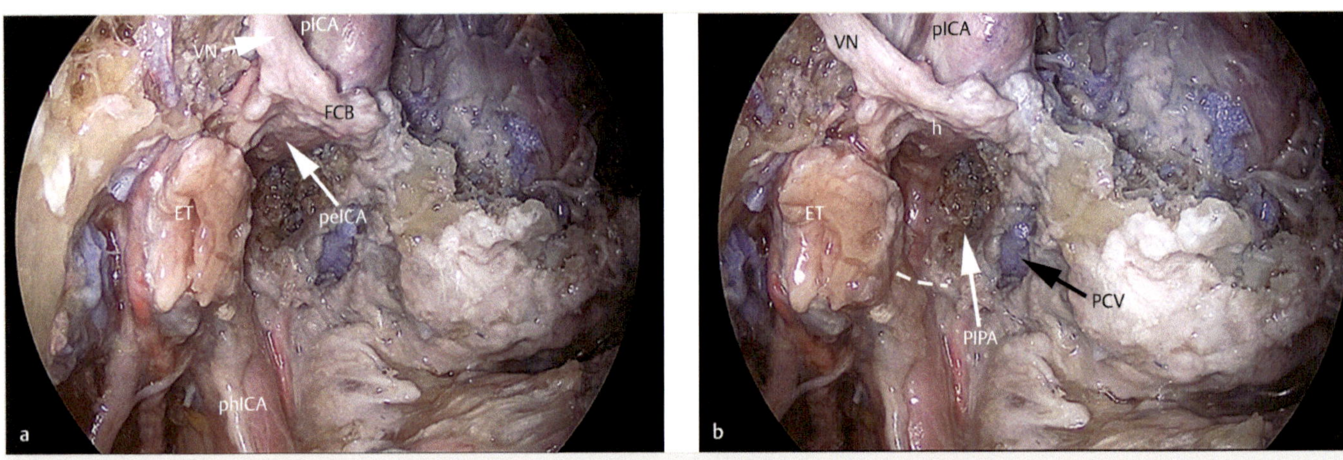

Fig. 20.8 (a, b) Step 2 (part 2). After completing removal of the anteroinferior petrous apex, the vertical (v) and horizontal (h) portions of the petrous tract of the internal carotid artery (peICA) are exposed, from the external carotid foramen (*white dashed line*), posterolaterally, to the fibrocartilago basalis (FCB), anteromedially. The posteroinferior petrous apex (PIPA) comes into view posterior to the vertical portion of the petrous internal carotid artery and laterally to the petroclival vein (PCV), which runs along the extracranial side of the petroclival suture and shows several connecting venous branches with the inferior petrosal sinus. ET, eustachian tube [sectioned]; pICA, paraclival tract of the internal carotid artery; phICA, parapharyngeal tract of the internal carotid artery; VN, vidian nerve.

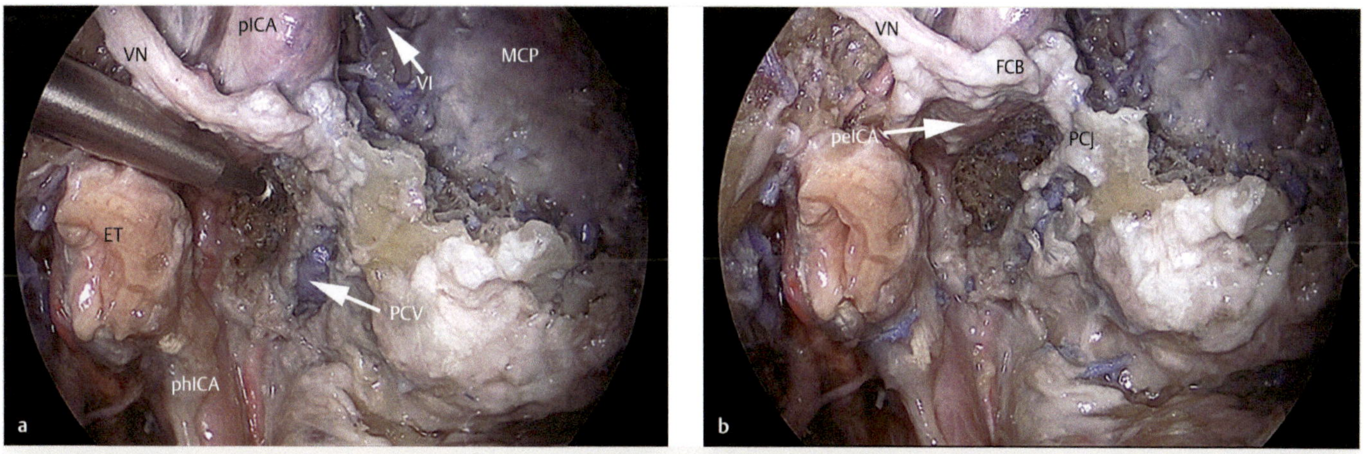

Fig. 20.9 (a, b) Step 3. The bone lying inferior and medial to the petrous (peICA) and paraclival (pICA) tracts of the internal carotid artery is drilled out. This procedure allows removal of the petroclival junction (PCJ) and merges the infrapetrous and medial petrous apex routes. VI, abducens nerve; ET, eustachian tube [sectioned]; FCB, fibrocartilago basalis; MCP, periosteum of the midclivus; PCV, petroclival vein; phICA, parapharyngeal tract of the internal carotid artery; VN, vidian nerve.

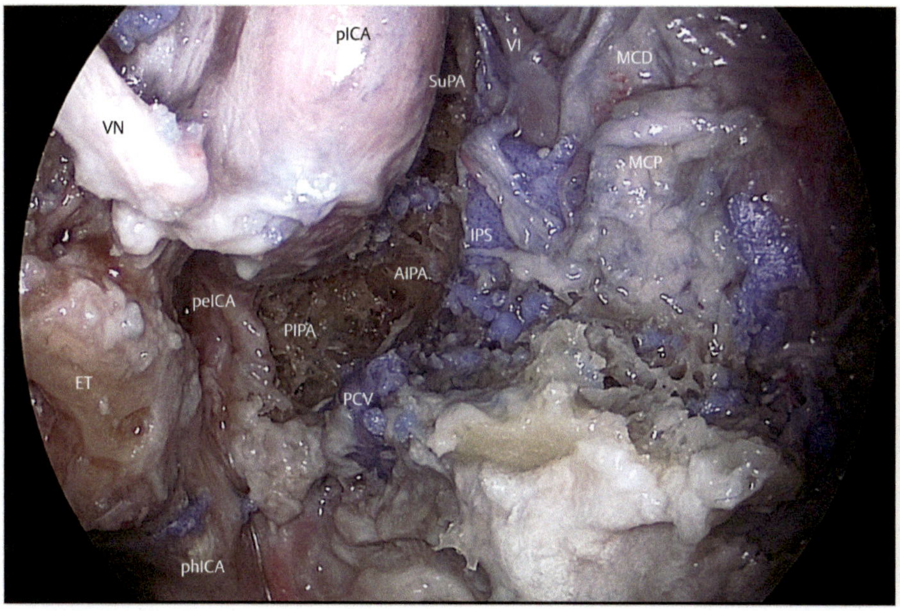

Fig. 20.10 Full exposure of the petrous apex. By combining the infrapetrous approach with the medial petrous apex approach, full exposure of the posteroinferior (PIPA), anteroinferior (AIPA), and superior (SuPA) subunits of the petrous apex is obtained. After removing the medial portion of the petroclival junction (PCJ), the connections between the petroclival vein (PCV) and the inferior petrosal sinus (IPS) come into view. VI, abducens nerve; ET, eustachian tube [sectioned]; MCD, dura of the midclivus; MCP, periosteum of the midclivus; pICA, paraclival tract of the internal carotid artery; peICA, petrous tract of the internal carotid artery; phICA, parapharyngeal tract of the internal carotid artery; VN, vidian nerve.

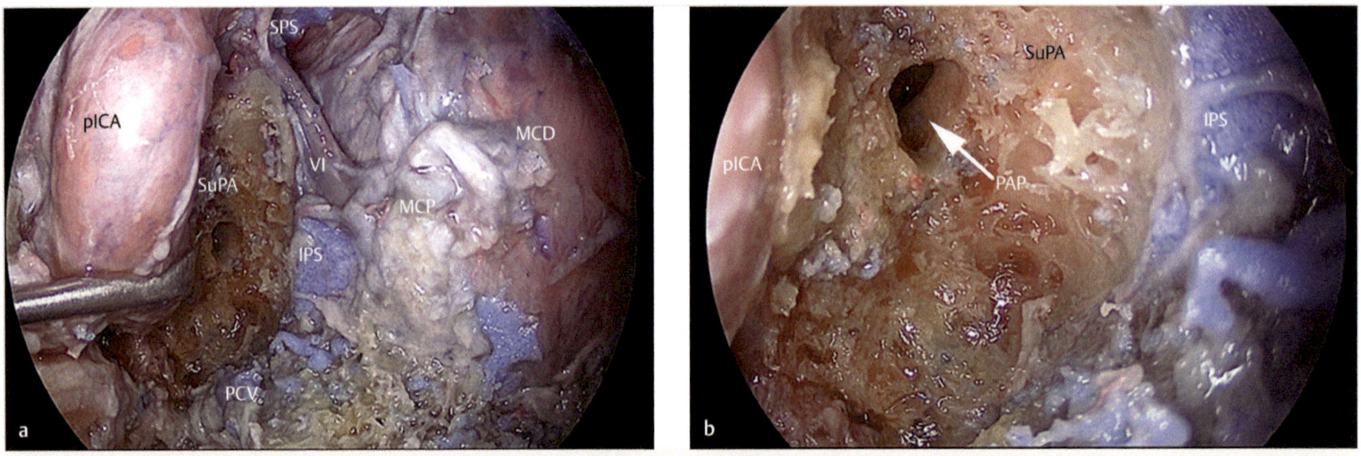

Fig. 20.11 (a, b) Pneumatization of the petrous apex. Petrous apex pneumatization (PAP) can be observed in each subunit. In this case, it was located in the superior subunit (SuPA). VI, abducens nerve; IPS, inferior petrosal sinus; MCD, dura of the midclivus; MCP, periosteum of the midclivus; PCV, petroclival vein; pICA, paraclival tract of the internal carotid artery; SPS, superior petrosal sinus.

Lower Transpterygoid Approach

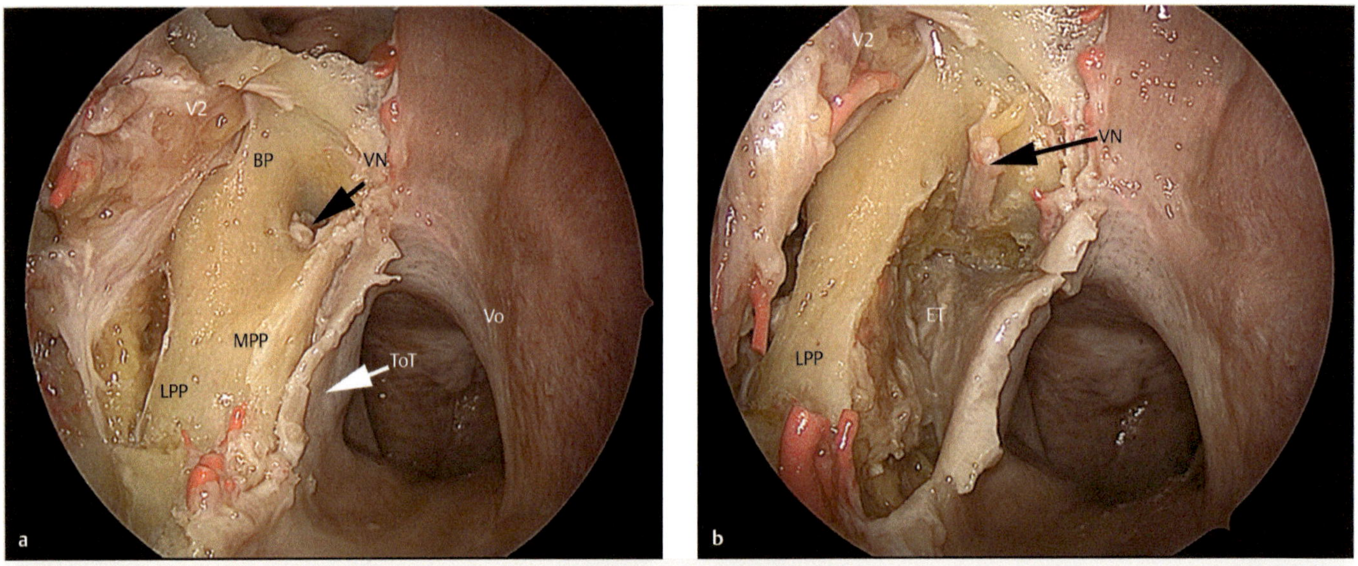

Fig. 20.12 (a, b) Step 1. After performing a type B (or more extended) endoscopic medial maxillectomy, the perpendicular process of the palatine bone is removed to expose the three subunits of the pterygoid process, which are the base of the pterygoid process (BP), the medial pterygoid plate (MPP), and the lateral pterygoid plate (LPP). In the base of the pterygoid process, the vidian nerve (VN) is identified and sectioned to expose the foramen rotundum and maxillary nerve (V2). The medial pterygoid plate is removed below the vidian nerve to expose the eustachian tube (ET), whose position can be identified at the beginning of the dissection using the torus tubarius (ToT) as a landmark. Vo, vomer.

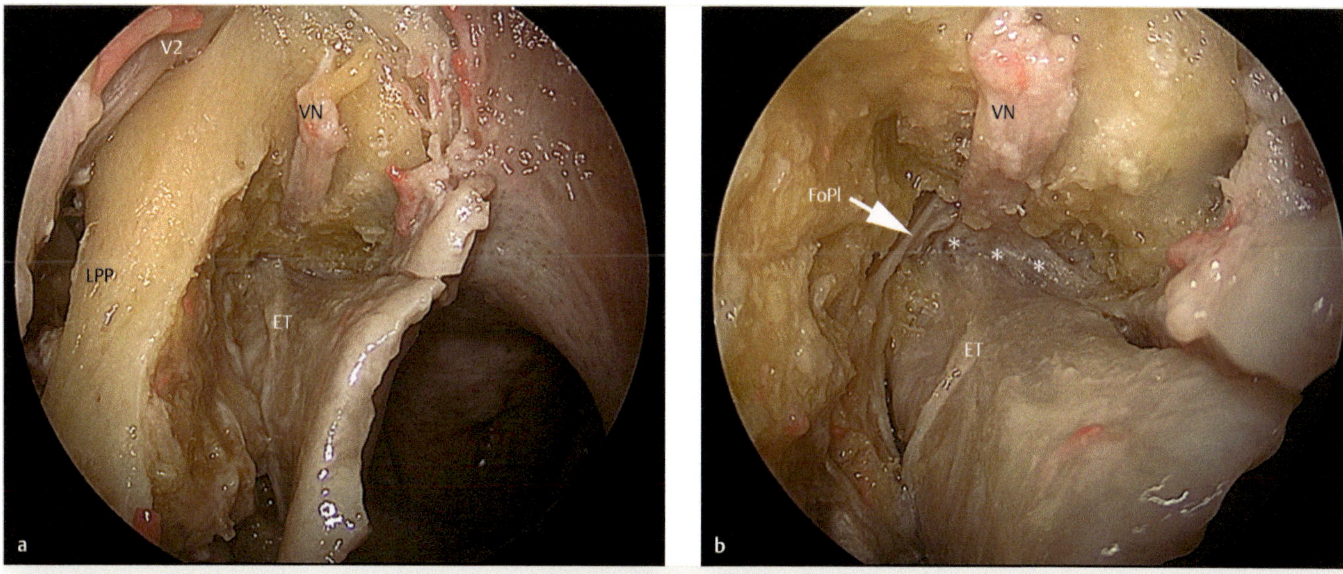

Fig. 20.13 (a, b) Step 2. The bone under the vidian nerve (VN) is removed to expose the fibrous connections (*white asterisks*) between the cartilaginous portion of the eustachian tube (ET) and the fibrocartilago basalis. The foraminal plexus (FoPl) surrounding the mandibular nerve can be exposed. V2, maxillary nerve; LPP, lateral pterygoid plate.

Infrapetrous Approach with Eustachian Tube Transposition

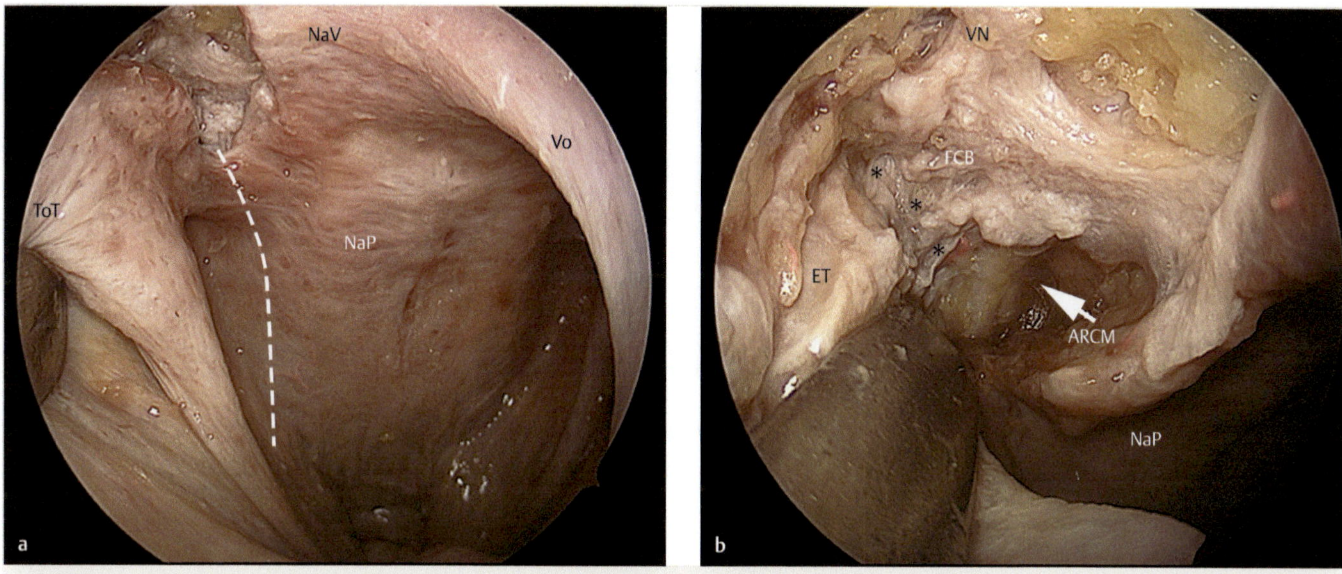

Fig. 20.14 (a, b) Step 3. A vertical mucosal incision (*white dashed line*) on the posterior wall of the nasopharynx (NaP) and the nasopharyngeal vault (NaV), medial to the Rosenmüller fossa, is performed. This incision allows us to laterally displace the torus tubarius (ToT) and the eustachian tube (ET), stretching the connections (*black asterisks*) between the cartilaginous tube and the fibrocartilago basalis (FCB). ARCM, anterior rectus capitis muscle; VN, vidian nerve; Vo, vomer.

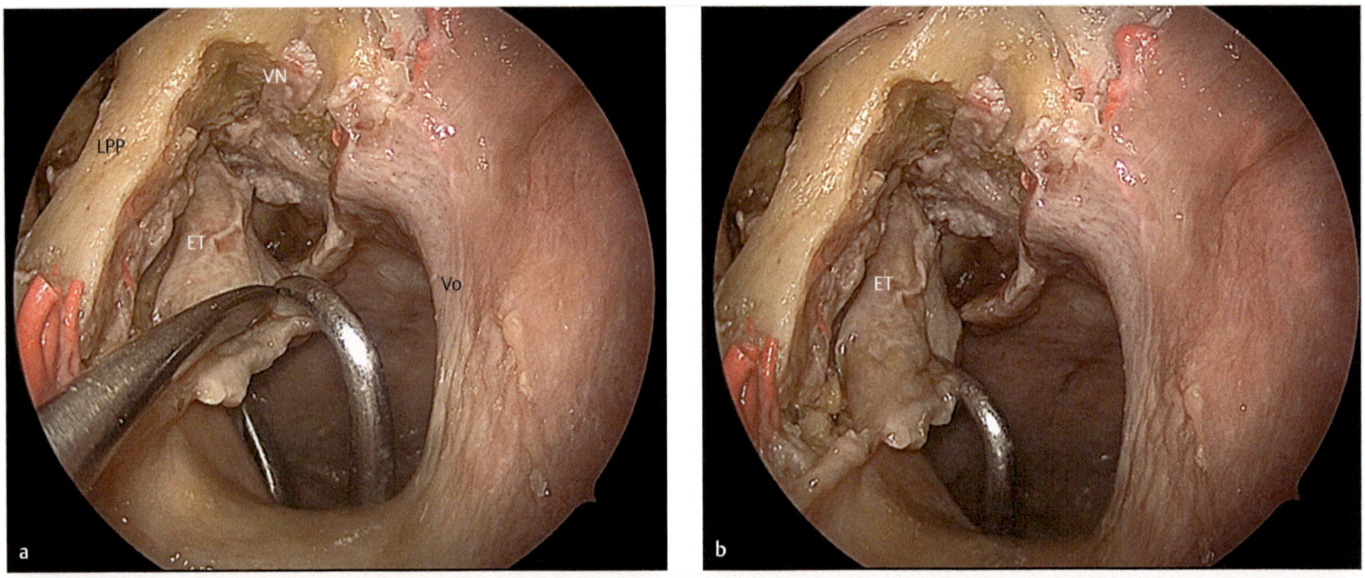

Fig. 20.15 (a, b) Step 4. Passing through the oral cavity and the oropharynx, the eustachian tube (ET) is grasped and displaced inferiorly. LPP, lateral pterygoid plate; VN, vidian nerve; Vo, vomer.

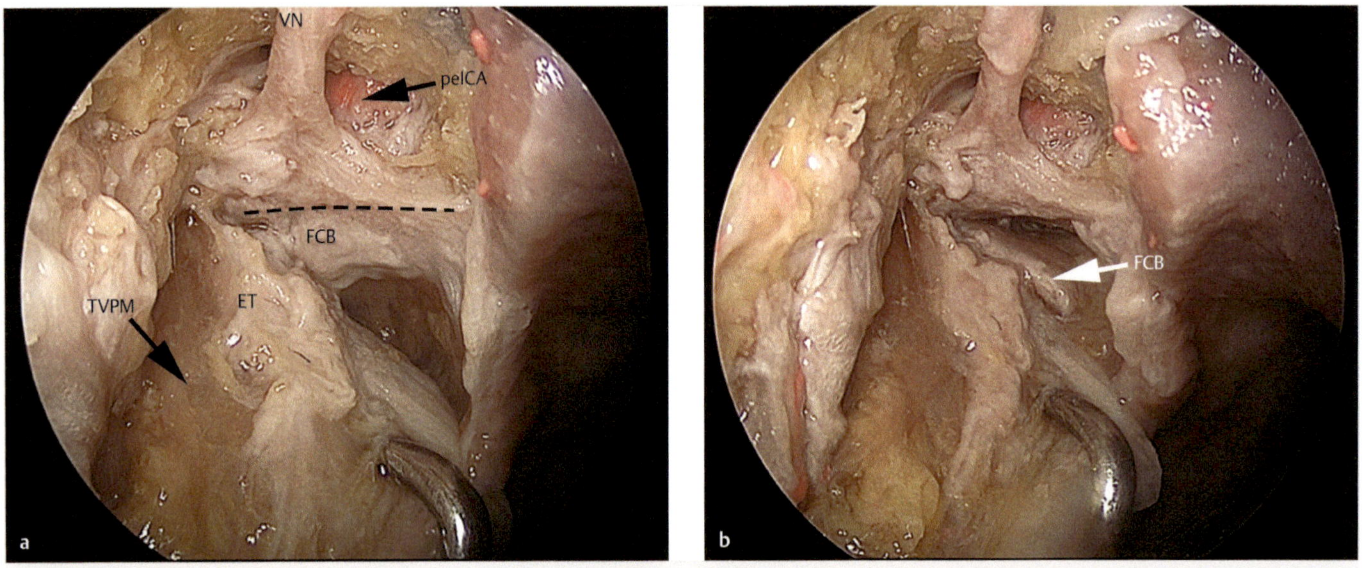

Fig. 20.16 (a, b) Step 5. A horizontal incision (*black dashed line*) is made below the vidian nerve (VN) and the fibrocartilago basalis (FCB) is dissected from the petrous tract of the internal carotid artery (peICA). ET, eustachian tube; TVPM, tensor veli palatine muscle.

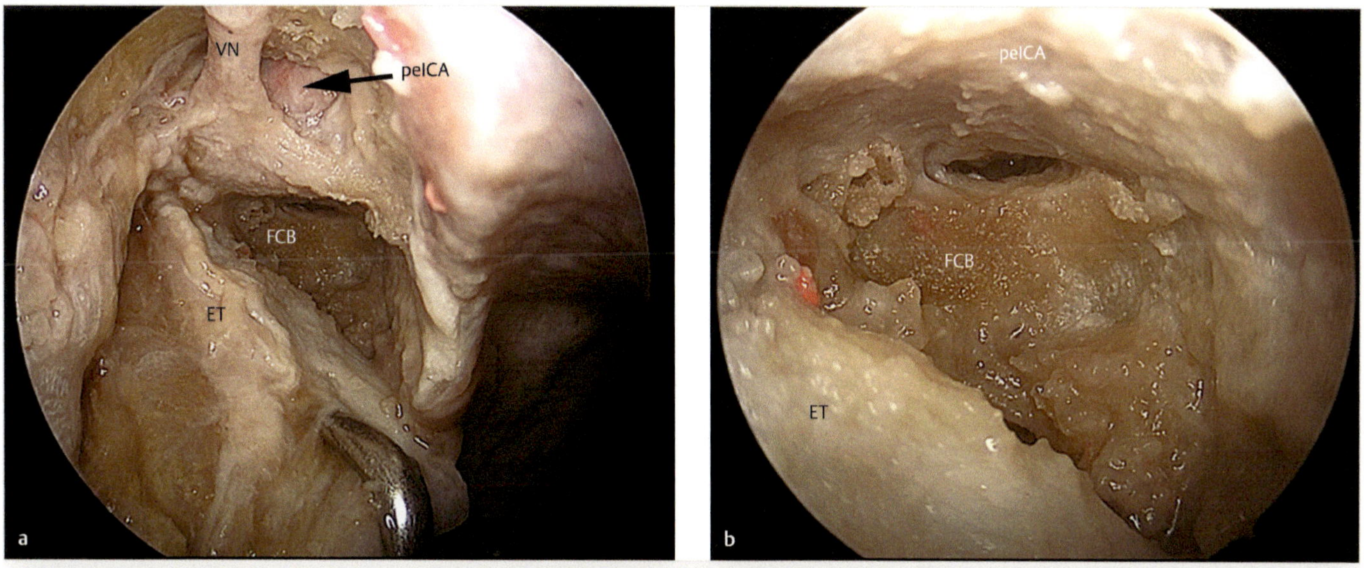

Fig. 20.17 (a, b) Step 6 (part 1). The fibrocartilago basalis (FCB) is progressively removed proceeding from anterior to posterior between the eustachian tube (ET) inferiorly and the petrous tract of the internal carotid artery (peICA) superiorly. VN, vidian nerve.

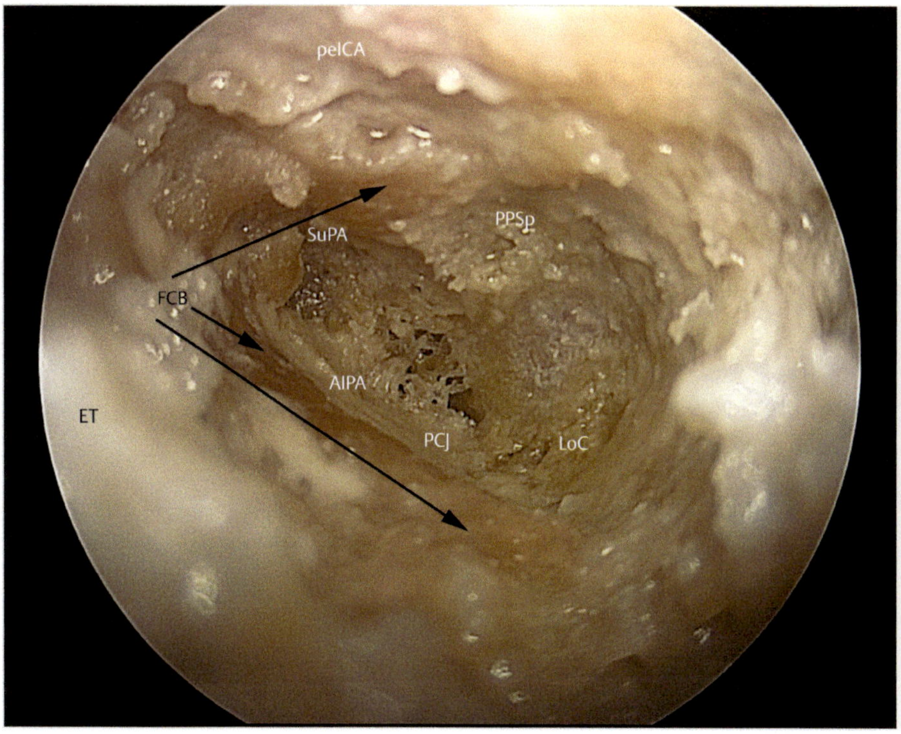

Fig. 20.18 Step 6 (part 2). After completing the removal of the fibrocartilago basalis (FCB), the superior (SuPA) and anteroinferior (AIPA) subunits of the petrous apex are exposed together with the petrous process of the sphenoid bone (PPSp), the lower clivus (LoC), and the petroclival junction (PCJ). ET, eustachian tube; peICA, petrous tract of the internal carotid artery.

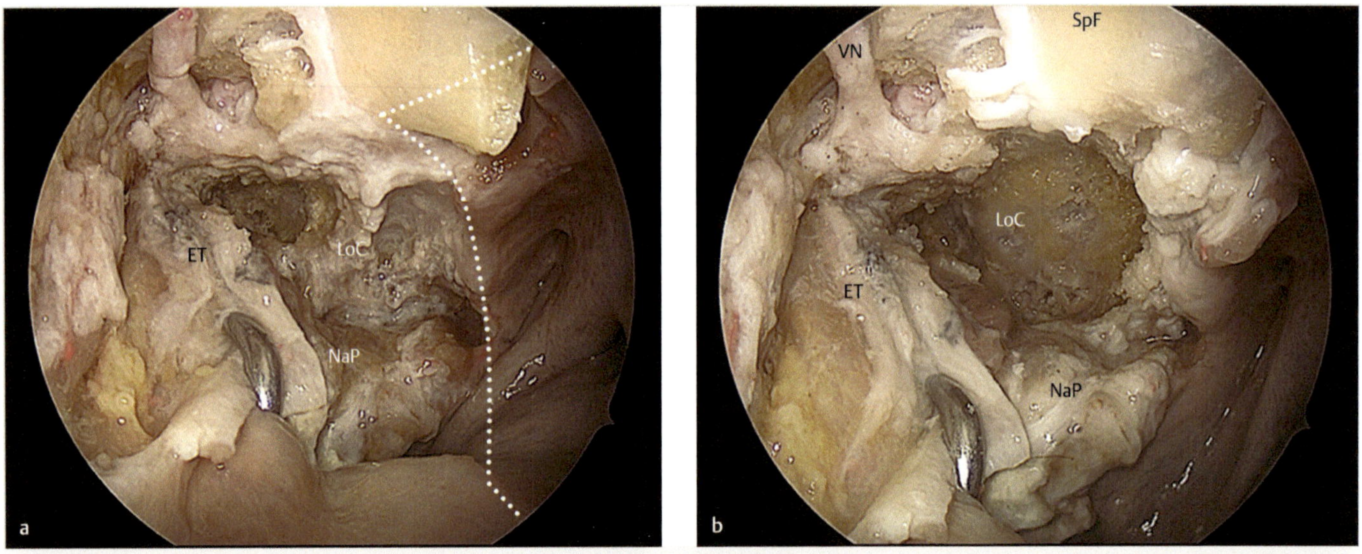

Fig. 20.19 Step 7. A posteroinferior septectomy is performed (*white dotted line*) and the posterior wall of the nasopharynx (NaP) is dissected from the lower clivus (LoC). The lower clivus is drilled exposing the inner cortical bone. ET, eustachian tube; SpF, sphenoidal floor; VN, vidian nerve.

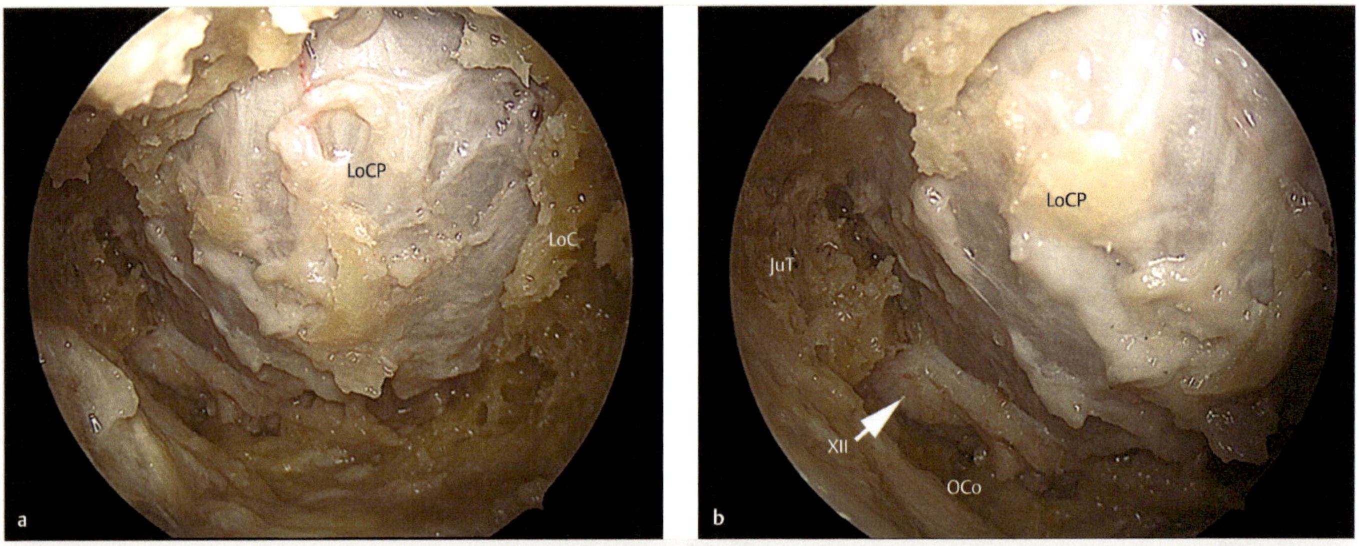

Fig. 20.20 (a, b) Step 8. By removing the cortical bone of the lower clivus (LoC), the periosteum of the lower clivus (LoCP) and the hypoglossal nerve (XII) are exposed. The nerve is identified between the jugular tubercle (JuT) superiorly and the occipital condyle (OCo) inferiorly.

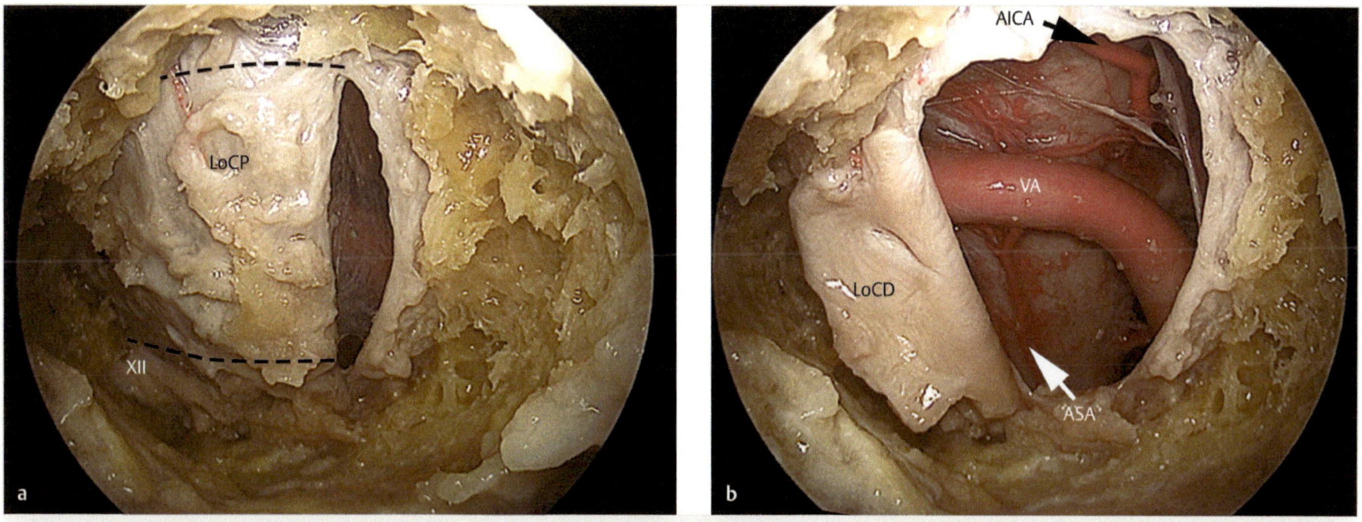

Fig. 20.21 (a, b) Step 9. A vertical midline and two parallel horizontal incisions (*horizontal black dashed lines*) of the periosteum (LoCP) and dura (LoCD) of the lower clivus are made, thus creating a transdural window above the hypoglossal nerve (XII). The anterior spinal artery (ASA), left vertebral artery (VA), and anterior inferior cerebellar artery (AICA) are identified in front of the spinal cord and the medulla oblongata.

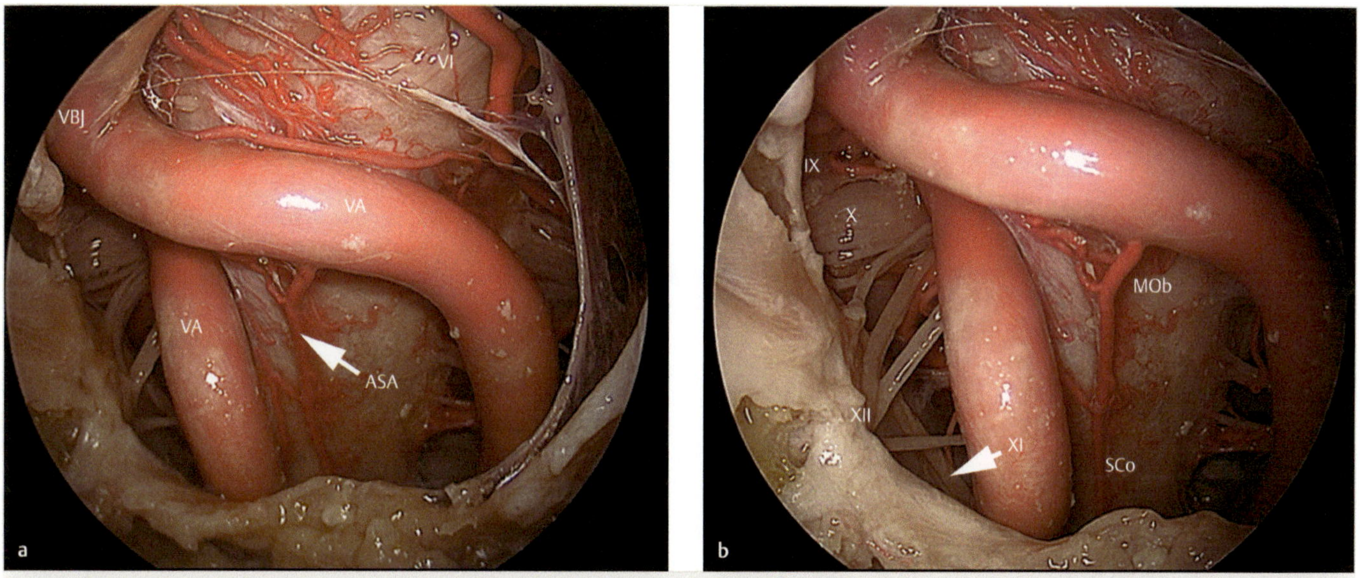

Fig. 20.22 (a, b) The premedullary and prepontine cisterns. The arachnoid of the premedullary and prepontine cisterns is removed to identify their content. The two vertebral arteries (VA) can be identified on the lateral side of the medulla oblongata (MOb) and the spinal cord (SCo). These arteries give a small medial branch each, which merge forming the anterior spinal artery (ASA). While running in a cranial direction, the vertebral arteries show a variable grade of tortuosity and fuse in the vertebrobasilar junction (VBJ). The lower cranial nerves can be identified lateral to the vertebral artery using a 45-degree scope: the glossopharyngeal (IX), vagus (X), and spinal accessory (XI) nerves run toward the jugular foramen; the hypoglossal nerve (XII) runs with a more posterior-to-anterior direction toward its bony canal, passing anterior to the spinal accessory nerve. VI, abducens nerve.

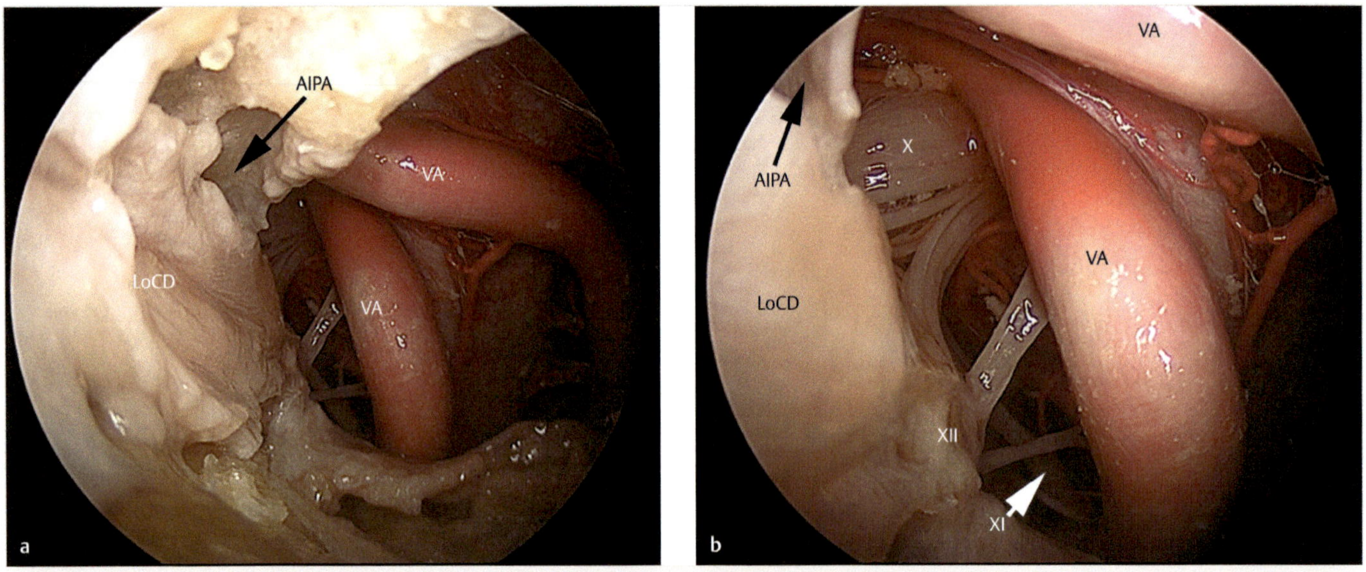

Fig. 20.23 (a, b) Relationships with the anteroinferior petrous apex. With a 70-degree scope turned laterally, the relationships of neurovascular structures with the anteroinferior petrous apex (AIPA) can be seen. The hypoglossal nerve (XII) runs caudal to the petrous apex. The glossopharyngeal, vagus (X), and spinal accessory (XI) nerves are located posteriorly to both the anteroinferior and the posteroinferior petrous apex. LoCD, dura of the lower clivus; VA, vertebral artery.

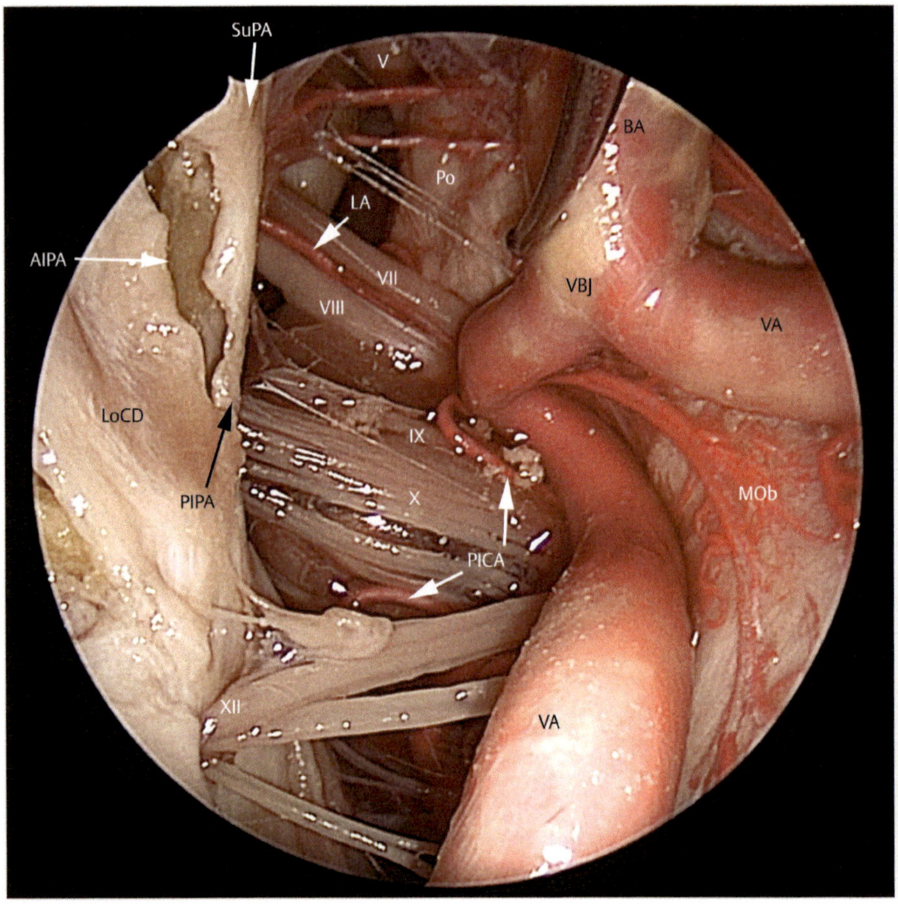

Fig. 20.24 Overview of the intracranial structures adjacent to the petrous apex. Endoscopic view with a 70-degree scope turned superolaterally and placed at the inferior border of the transdural window. A number of neurovascular structures can be identified all around the area of the petrous apex. The trigeminal stem (V) runs from the pons (Po) to the trigeminal impression, which lies cranially to the superior petrous apex (SuPA). The facial (VII) and vestibulocochlear (VIII) nerves, together with the labyrinthine artery (LA), reach the internal acoustic canal, which lies posterolaterally to the petrous apex. The glossopharyngeal (IX), vagus (X), and spinal accessory nerves run toward the jugular foramen, which lies lateral to the posteroinferior petrous apex (PIPA). The rootlets of the hypoglossal nerve (XII) merge and run toward the jugular tubercle and the occipital condyle, which are located inferior to the anteroinferior petrous apex (AIPA). BA, basilar artery; LoCD, dura of the lower clivus; MOb, medulla oblongata; PICA, posterior inferior cerebellar artery; Po, pons; VA, vertebral artery; VBJ, vertebrobasilar junction.

References

[1] Scopel TF, Fernandez-Miranda JC, Pinheiro-Neto CD, et al. Petrous apex cholesterol granulomas: endonasal versus infracochlear approach. Laryngoscope 2012;122(4):751–761

[2] Simal-Julián JA, Miranda-Lloret P, Beltrán-Giner A, Plaza-Ramirez E, Botella-Asunción C. Full endoscopic endonasal extreme far-medial approach: eustachian tube transposition. J Neurosurg Pediatr 2013;11(5):584–590

[3] McLaughlin N, Kelly DF, Prevedello DM, Shahlaie K, Carrau RL, Kassam AB. Endoscopic endonasal management of recurrent petrous apex cholesterol granuloma. J Neurol Surg B Skull Base 2012;73(3):190–196

[4] Taniguchi M, Akutsu N, Mizukawa K, Kohta M, Kimura H, Kohmura E. Endoscopic endonasal translacerum approach to the inferior petrous apex. J Neurosurg 2016;124(4):1032–1038

[5] Shin M, Kondo K, Hanakita S, et al. Endoscopic transsphenoidal anterior petrosal approach for locally aggressive tumors involving the internal auditory canal, jugular fossa, and cavernous sinus. J Neurosurg 2017;126(1):212–221

[6] Maurer AJ, Bonney PA, Iser CR, Ali R, Sanclement JA, Sughrue ME. Endoscopic endonasal infrapetrous transpterygoid approach to the petroclival junction for petrous apex chondrosarcoma: technical report. J Neurol Surg Rep 2015;76(1):e113–e116

[7] Van Gompel JJ, Alikhani P, Tabor MH, et al. Anterior inferior petrosectomy: defining the role of endonasal endoscopic techniques for petrous apex approaches. J Neurosurg 2014;120(6):1321–1325

[8] Jacquesson T, Berhouma M, Tringali S, Simon E, Jouanneau E. Which routes for petroclival tumors? A comparison bBetween the anterior expanded endoscopic endonasal approach and lateral or posterior routes. World Neurosurg 2015;83(6):929–936

[9] Jacquesson T, Simon E, Berhouma M, Jouanneau E. Anatomic comparison of anterior petrosectomy versus the expanded endoscopic endonasal approach: interest in petroclival tumors surgery. Surg Radiol Anat 2015;37(10): 1199–1207

[10] Di Somma A, Andaluz N, Cavallo LM, et al. Endoscopic transorbital route to the petrous apex: a feasibility anatomic study. Acta Neurochir (Wien) 2018;160(4):707–720

[11] Patel CR, Wang EW, Fernandez-Miranda JC, et al. Contralateral transmaxillary corridor: an augmented endoscopic approach to the petrous apex. J Neurosurg 2018; 129(1):211–219

21 The Suprapetrous (Meckel's Cave) Approach

Vittorio Rampinelli, Marco Ravanelli, Marco Ferrari, Davide Lancini, Alberto Schreiber

Meckel's cave is a cisternal space bounded by the dura and the periosteum that is located in the inferolateral portion of the parasellar area, which corresponds to the medial portion of the middle cranial fossa. It neighbors the cavernous and sphenoid sinuses medially, temporal lobe of the brain superolaterally, middle cranial fossa inferolaterally, and petrous tract of the internal carotid artery inferiorly. Meckel's cave houses several neural fibers running within the cerebrospinal fluid and merging to form the gasserian ganglion, which is also called the semilunar ganglion due to its crescent shape. The ophthalmic, maxillary, and mandibular nerves arise from the gasserian ganglion and run toward the superior orbital fissure, foramen rotundum, and foramen ovale, respectively.

As a natural consequence of its preeminent content in neural structures, Meckel's cave and adjacent areas mostly harbor neurogenic lesions, especially schwannomas and malignant peripheral nerve sheath tumors, the latter being exceedingly rare.[1–10] Secondarily, this area can be involved by several diseases that are located at the borderline between the lateral portion of the cavernous sinus and Meckel's cave, including sinonasal/nasopharyngeal malignancies (especially when exhibiting perineural spread like adenoid cystic carcinomas, squamous cell carcinomas, or nasopharyngeal carcinomas),[1,8,9,11] bone–cartilage-arising tumors (i.e., chordomas, chondrosarcomas),[1,2,5,9,12] meningiomas,[1,5,9] pituitary adenomas,[1,2] juvenile angiofibromas,[1,2,11] epidermoid, neuroenteric, or endodermal cysts,[1,2,5,13] metastases,[8–10,13] lymphomas,[8,9] neurosarcoidosis,[8,9] and other rare lesions.[1,9,14,15] The endoscopic transnasal approach has been adopted by some pioneering groups to remove or obtain a biopsy of these diseases.[1,3–8,10–12,14–16] More recently, the endoscopic

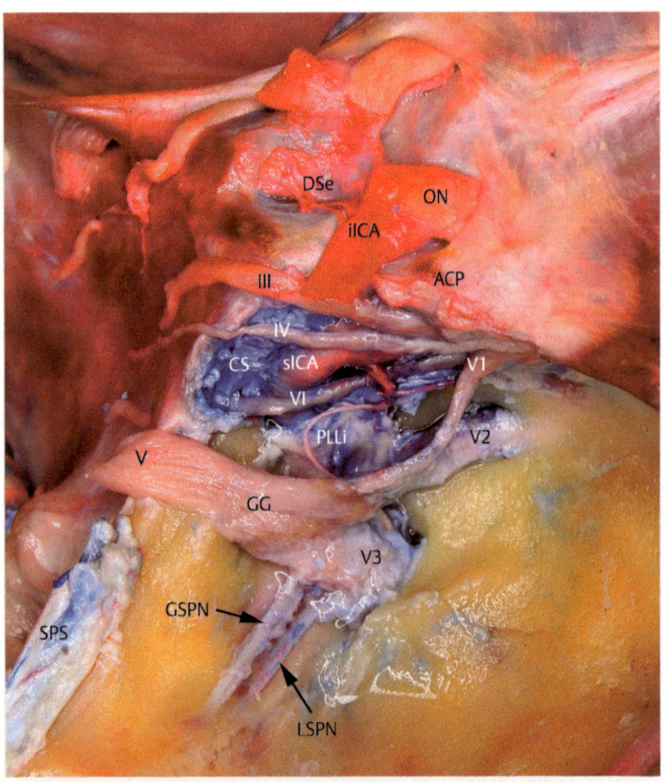

Fig. 21.1 Intracranial superolateral-to-inferomedial view of the parasellar area. This cadaver picture shows with a superolateral-to-inferomedial intracranial perspective the right parasellar area. III, oculomotor nerve; IV, trochlear nerve; V, trigeminal stem; V1, ophthalmic nerve; V2, maxillary nerve; V3, mandibular nerve; VI, abducens nerve; ACP, anterior clinoid process; CS, cavernous sinus; DSe, diaphragma sellae; GG, gasserian ganglion; GSPN, greater superficial petrosal nerve; iICA, intracranial tract of the internal carotid artery; LSPN, lesser superficial petrosal nerve; ON, optic nerve; PLLi, petrolingual ligament; sICA, parasellar tract of the internal carotid artery; SPS, superior petrosal sinus.

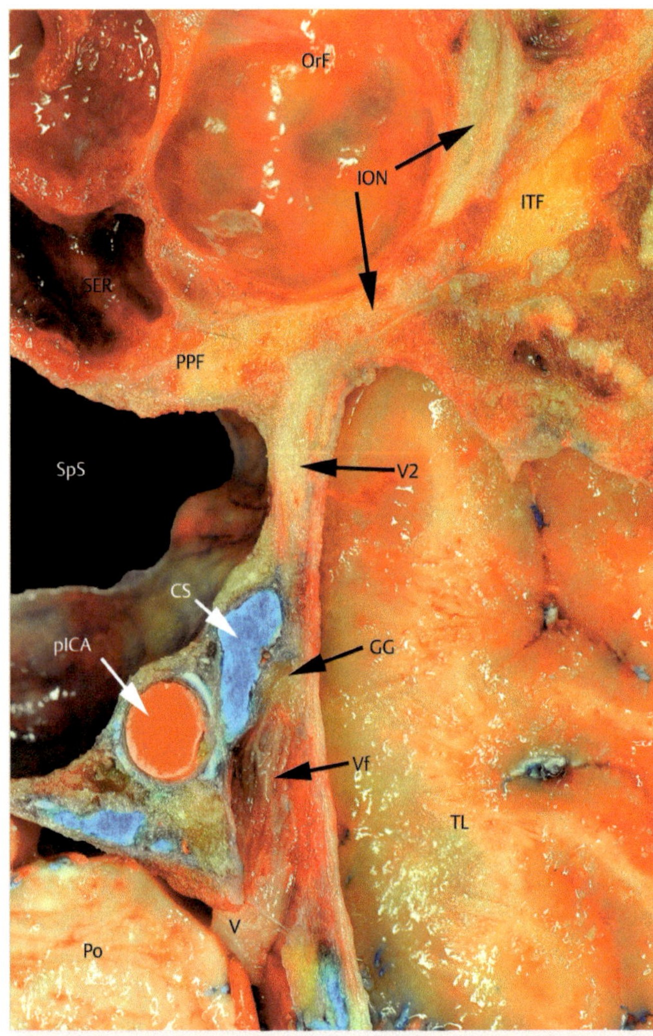

Fig. 21.2 Axial view of the Meckel's cave and adjacent areas. This axial cadaver cut shows with an inferior-to-superior perspective the left Meckel's cave. The cut has been performed through the trigeminal stem (V), trigeminal fibers within the Meckel's cave (Vf), gasserian ganglion (GG), maxillary nerve (V2), and infraorbital nerve (ION). CS, cavernous sinus; ITF, infratemporal fossa; OrF, orbital floor; pICA, paraclival tract of the internal carotid artery; Po, pons; PPF, pterygopalatine fossa; SER, sphenoethmoidal recess; SpS, sphenoid sinus; TL, temporal lobe of the brain.

transorbital corridor was also adopted as the sole or ancillary approach to manage some lesions involving the parasellar area and the middle cranial fossa.[17,18]

This chapter includes three modular extensions of the endoscopic transnasal approach to Meckel's cave: (1) the classic suprapetrous approach, formerly called the "front door to Meckel's cave," takes advantage of the quadrangular space defined by the petrous and paraclival tracts of the internal carotid artery caudally and medially, abducens nerve cranially, and maxillary nerve laterally[1,16,19]; (2) the extension through the superior transpterygoid approach takes advantage of the space gained by sectioning the inferior orbital fissure and allows exposure of the entirety of the mandibular nerve, from the gasserian ganglion to the infratemporal fossa[20,21]; and (3) the "transalisphenoid" approach includes partial removal of the greater sphenoidal wing, thereby providing wide access to the middle cranial fossa through the spaces between the trigeminal branches.[11]

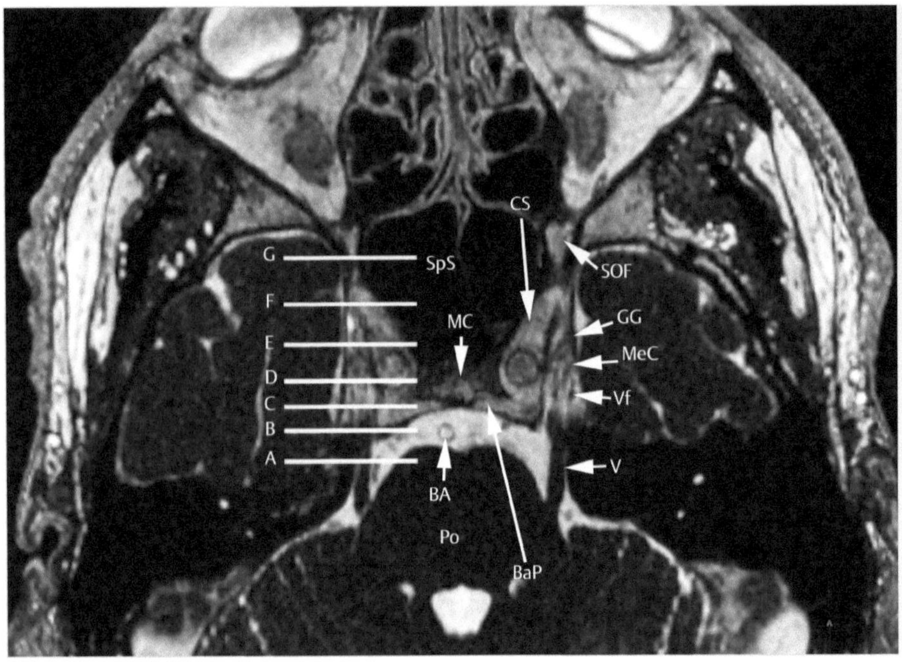

Fig. 21.3 Axial MRI anatomy of the trigeminal system. This axial CISS (constructive interference in steady state) MRI passes through the trigeminal stem (V), Meckel's cave (MeC), and superior orbital fissure (SOF). Meckel's cave lies between the cavernous sinus (CS) medially and the temporal lobe of the brain laterally. It is a cisternal space where the trigeminal fibers (Vf) run free within the cerebrospinal fluid before forming the gasserian ganglion (GG). These structures are aligned with the superior orbital fissure (SOF). *White lines* (A–G) show the position of images composing ▶Fig. 21.4. BA, basilar artery; BaP, basilar plexus; MC, midclivus; Po, pons; SpS, sphenoid sinus.

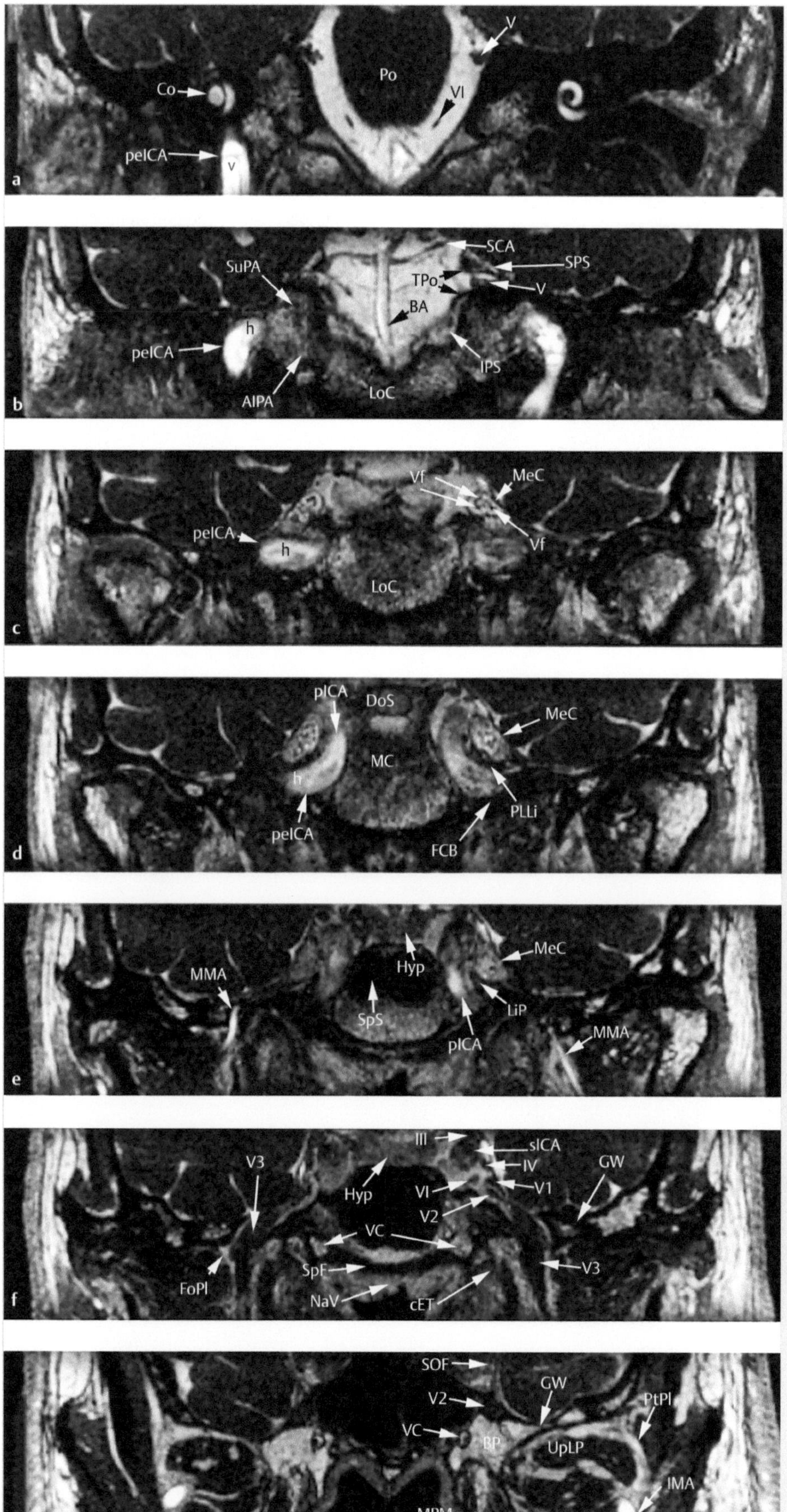

Fig. 21.4 (a–g) Coronal MRI anatomy of the trigeminal system and adjacent structures. The panel includes seven coronal CISS (constructive interference in steady state) MRI images passing through different portions of the trigeminal system, from posterior **(a)** to anterior **(g)**. The trigeminal stem (V) runs close to the superior cerebellar artery (SCA) in the prepontine cistern. Then, it enters Meckel's cave (MeC) passing through the trigeminal porus (TPo), which is a dural passage located between the superior (SPS) and inferior petrosal sinuses (IPS). Within Meckel's cave, the trigeminal stem splits into several fibers (Vf) that run free within the cerebrospinal fluid and merge anteriorly to form the gasserian ganglion. Finally, the gasserian ganglion gives the three branches of the trigeminal nerve, namely, the ophthalmic nerve (V1), the maxillary nerve (V2), and the mandibular nerve (V3). The ophthalmic nerve runs within the lateral wall of the cavernous sinus reaching the superior orbital fissure (SOF) together with the oculomotor (III), trochlear (IV), and abducens nerve (VI). The maxillary nerve runs within the base of the pterygoid process (BP) passing through the foramen rotundum. The mandibular nerve passes through the foramen ovale, where it is surrounded by the foraminal venous plexus (FoPl), and reaches the infratemporal fossa. AIPA, anteroinferior petrous apex; BA, basilar artery; cET, cartilaginous portion of the eustachian tube; Co, cochlea; DoS, dorsum sellae; FCB, fibrocartilago basalis; GW, greater wing of the sphenoid bone; h, horizontal portion of the petrous tract of the internal carotid artery; Hyp, hypophysis; IMA, internal maxillary artery; LiP, lingual process; LoC, lower clivus; LoLP, lower head of the lateral pterygoid muscle; MC, midclivus; MMA, middle meningeal artery; MPM, medial pterygoid muscle; NaV, nasopharyngeal vault; peICA, petrous tract of the internal carotid artery; pICA, paraclival tract of the internal carotid artery; PLLi, petrolingual ligament; Po, pons; PtPl, pterygoid plexus; sICA, parasellar tract of the internal carotid artery; SpF, sphenoidal floor; SpS, sphenoid sinus; SuPA, superior petrous apex; UpLP, upper head of the lateral pterygoid muscle; v, vertical portion of the petrous tract of the internal carotid artery; VC, vidian canal.

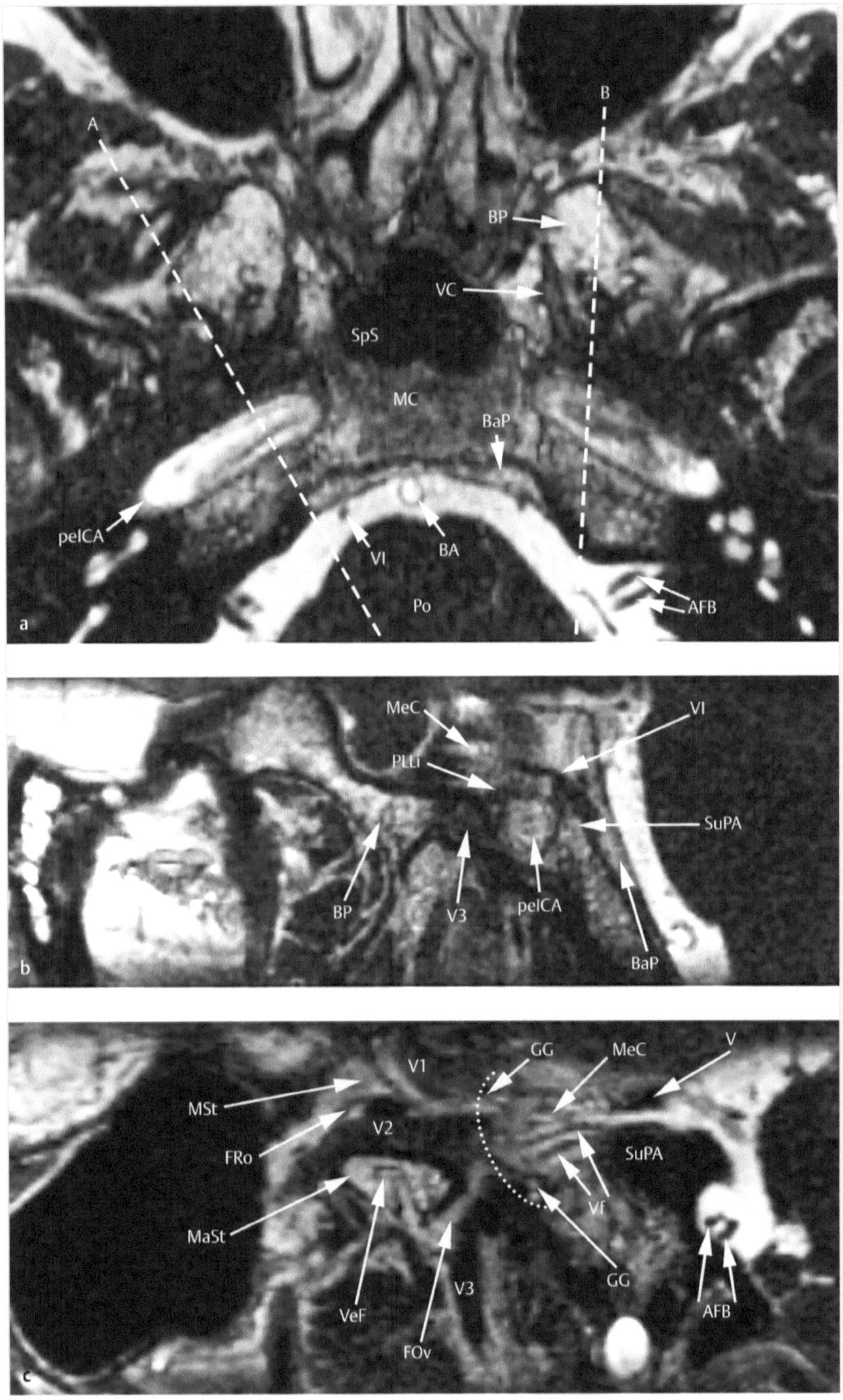

Fig. 21.5 Axial and parasagittal MRI anatomy of the trigeminal system and adjacent structures. The panel includes one axial **(a)** and two parasagittal **(b, c)** CISS (constructive interference in steady state) MRI images passing through the trigeminal system and adjacent structures. The *white dashed lines* (A and B) depict the orientation of the parasagittal images. The petrolingual ligament (PLLi) goes from the superior portion of the petrous apex (SuPA) to the lingual process of the sphenoid bone, passing above the petrous tract of the internal carotid artery (peICA), lateral to the paraclival tract of the internal carotid artery, and medial to Meckel's cave (MeC). This ligament is particularly important as it is intimately related to several important neurovascular structures, namely, the abducens nerve (VI), the gasserian ganglion (GG), the maxillary nerve (V2), and the mandibular nerve (V3). The gasserian ganglion is formed by several fibers (Vf) arising from the trigeminal stem (V). This ganglion is also called semilunar due to its crescent shape (*white dotted line*). The ophthalmic nerve (V1) runs from the gasserian ganglion to the superior orbital fissure, which is separated from the foramen rotundum (FRo) by the maxillary strut (MSt), a bony structure connecting the body of the sphenoid with the greater wing of the sphenoid. Similarly, the mandibular strut (MaSt) is a bony bridge connecting the base of the pterygoid process (BP) with the greater wing of the sphenoid and separating the foramen rotundum from the foramen ovale (FOv). The Vesalius foramen (VeF) is an inconstant bony canal, which contains a vein and passes through the mandibular strut. AFB, acoustic-facial bundle; BA, basilar artery; BaP, basilar plexus; MC, midclivus; Po, pons; SpS, sphenoid sinus; VC, vidian canal.

Endoscopic Dissection

Nasal Phase

- Paraseptal sphenoidotomy.
- Transrostral sphenoidotomy.
- Expanded transrostral sphenoidotomy.
- Total uncinectomy.
- Anterior ethmoidectomy.
- Posterior ethmoidectomy.
- Type A endoscopic medial maxillectomy.
- Facultative: optic and orbital decompression.
- Facultative: type B–D endoscopic medial maxillectomy.

Skull Base Phase

Suprapetrous Approach

- Facultative: Transsellar approach.
- Facultative: Transclival (midclivus) approach.
- Facultative: Transcavernous (lateral) approach.
- Step 1: Removal of the carotid prominence, lateral wall of the sphenoid sinus, and maxillary strut.
- Step 2: Partial exposure of the vidian canal and the foramen rotundum.
- Step 3: Incision of the quadrangular space.
- Step 4: Exposure of the petrous apex.

Superior Transpterygoid Approach

- Facultative: transpterygomaxillary approach.
- Step 5: Section of the sphenopalatine, palatovaginal, and vidian bundles.
- Step 6: Exposure of the foramen ovale.
- Step 7: Removal of the base of the pterygoid process.
- Step 8: Removal of the mandibular strut.

Transalisphenoid Approach

- Step 9: Removal of the bone of the foramen ovale.
- Step 10: Removal of the bone of the foramen spinosum.

Suprapetrous Approach

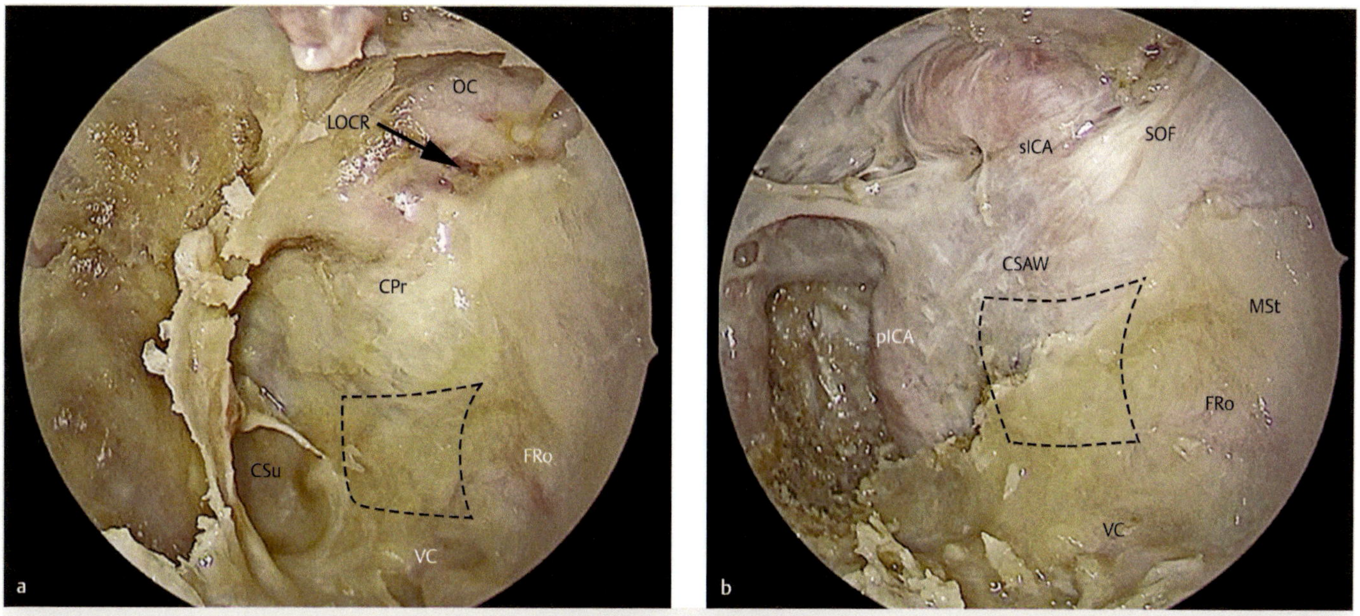

Fig. 21.6 (a, b) Step 1. The lateral optic–carotid recess (LOCR) is bounded by the optic canal (OC) superiorly, the carotid prominence (CPr) inferomedially, and the superior orbital fissure (SOF) inferolaterally. It corresponds to the anteromedial end of the optic strut, which separates the superior orbital fissure from the optic canal. More inferiorly, the maxillary strut (MSt) separates the foramen rotundum (FRo) from the superior orbital fissure. The carotid prominence and the lateral wall of the sphenoid sinus are progressively removed to expose the anterior wall of the cavernous sinus (CSAW) and harvest the access to Meckel's cave. (*Black dashed line:* Position of the quadrangular space.) CSu, carotid sulcus; pICA, paraclival tract of the internal carotid artery; sICA, parasellar tract of the internal carotid artery.

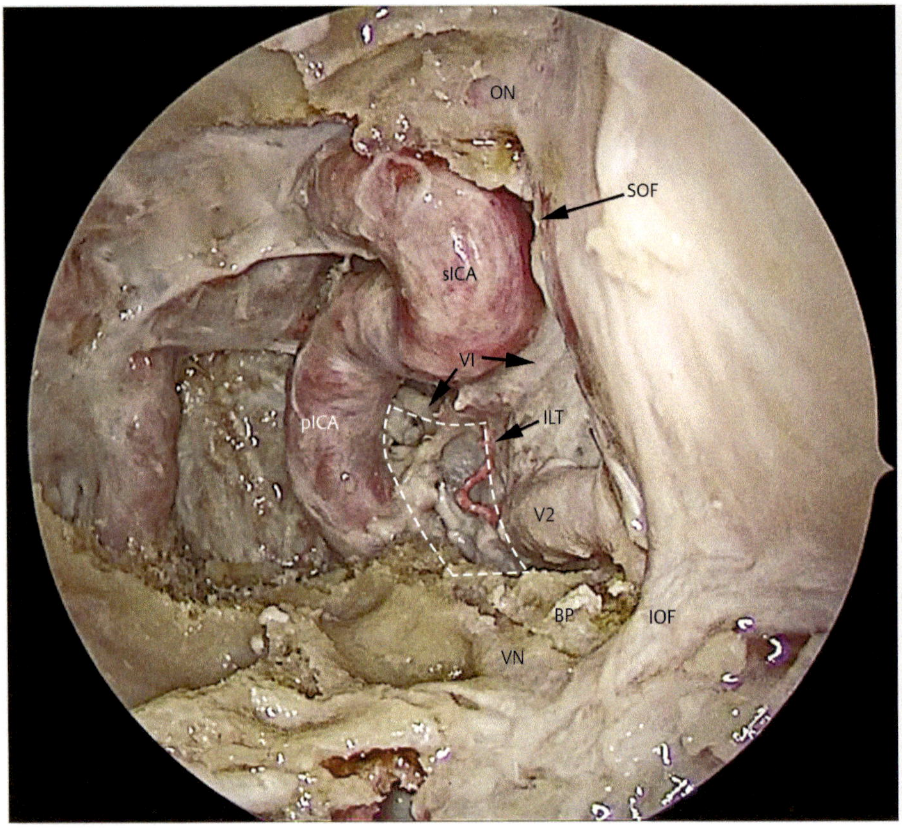

Fig. 21.7 Step 2. Removal of the lateral wall of the sphenoid sinus is completed including the maxillary strut and the cranial portion of the base of pterygoid process (BP). With this step, harvesting of the ethmoid–pterygoid–sphenoidal corridor to the parasellar area is completed. The quadrangular space (*white dashed line*) is identified between the paraclival tract of the internal carotid artery (pICA) medially, the maxillary nerve (V2) laterally, the petrous tract of the internal carotid artery inferiorly, and the abducens nerve (VI) superiorly. ILT, inferolateral trunk; IOF, inferior orbital fissure; sICA, parasellar tract of the internal carotid artery; SOF, superior orbital fissure; VN, vidian nerve.

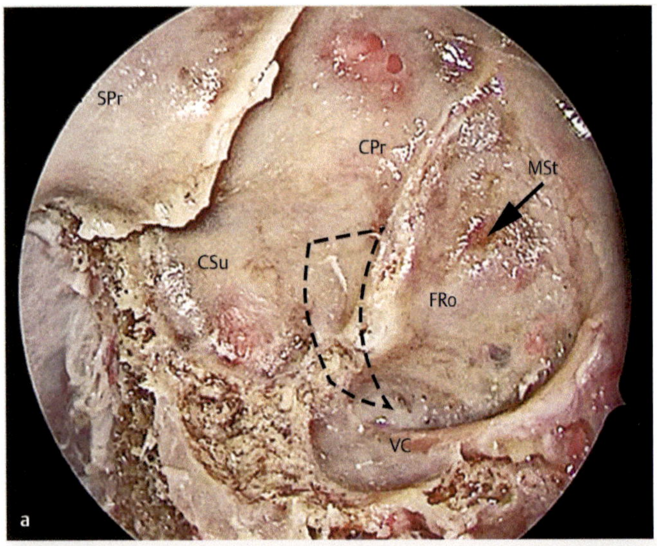

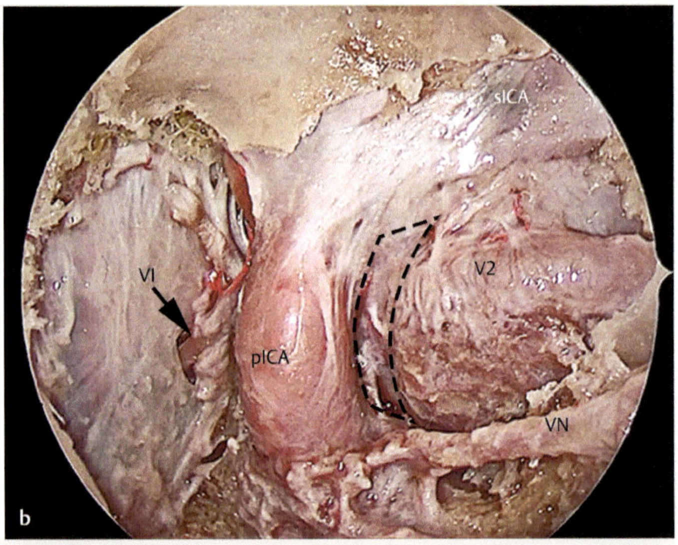

Fig. 21.8 The quadrangular space. A 70-degree scope turned laterally is used before **(a)** and after (right image) **(b)** removing the bone overlying the quadrangular space *(black dashed line)*. This perspective allows a three-dimensional understanding of the position of the quadrangular space with relevant surrounding structures. By performing a transclival midclivus approach (see Chapter 11), the spatial relationships between the midline posterior cranial fossa and quadrangular space can also be assessed. V2, maxillary nerve; VI, abducens nerve; CPr, carotid prominence; CSu, carotid sulcus; MSt, maxillary strut; pICA, paraclival tract of the internal carotid artery; sICA, parasellar tract of the internal carotid artery; SPr, sellar prominence; FRo, foramen rotundum; VC, vidian canal; VN, vidian nerve.

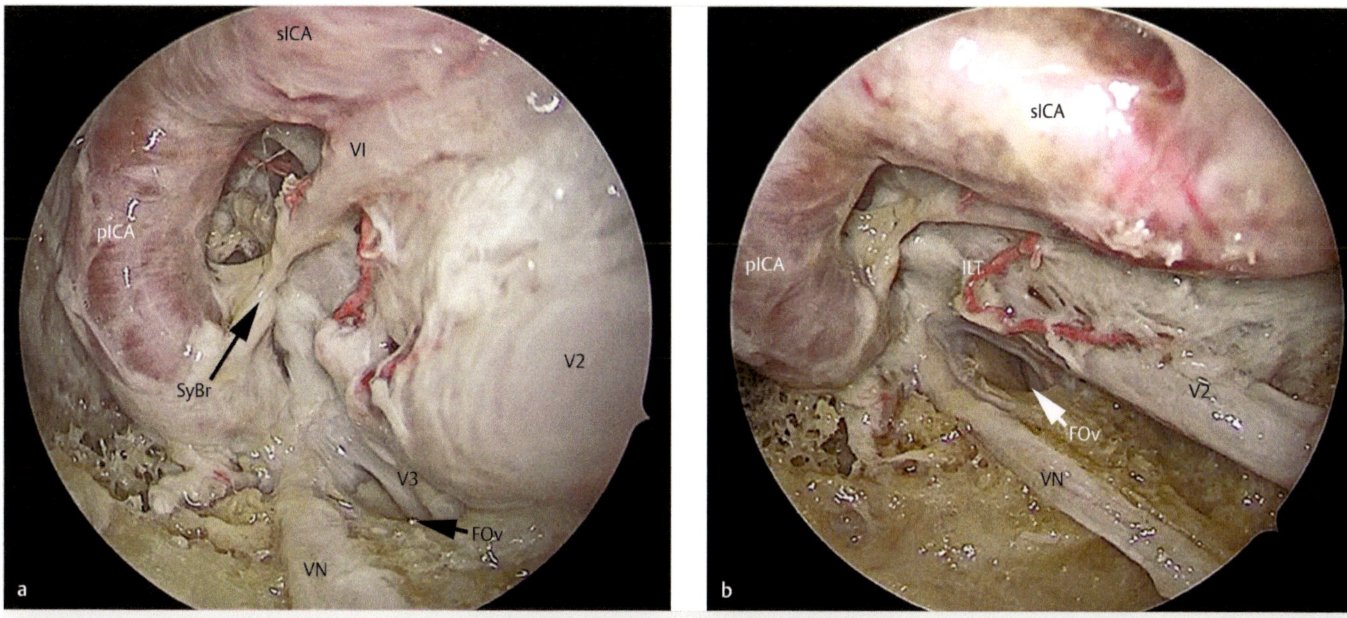

Fig. 21.9 (a, b) Identification of the foramen ovale. The foramen ovale (FOv) and the mandibular nerve (V3) are identified by dissecting the area between the maxillary nerve (V2), superolaterally, and the vidian nerve (VN), inferomedially. The sympathetic branch (SyBr) is found in the superomedial corner of the quadrangular space, where it runs from the paraclival tract of the internal carotid artery (pICA) to the abducens nerve (VI). The inferolateral trunk (ILT) is a branch of the parasellar tract of internal carotid artery (sICA); some of its branches reach Meckel's cave after turning around the abducens nerve (see also Chapter 18). With a 70-degree scope turned inferolaterally (right image), the three-dimensional relationship between vidian, maxillary, and mandibular nerves can be better conceived.

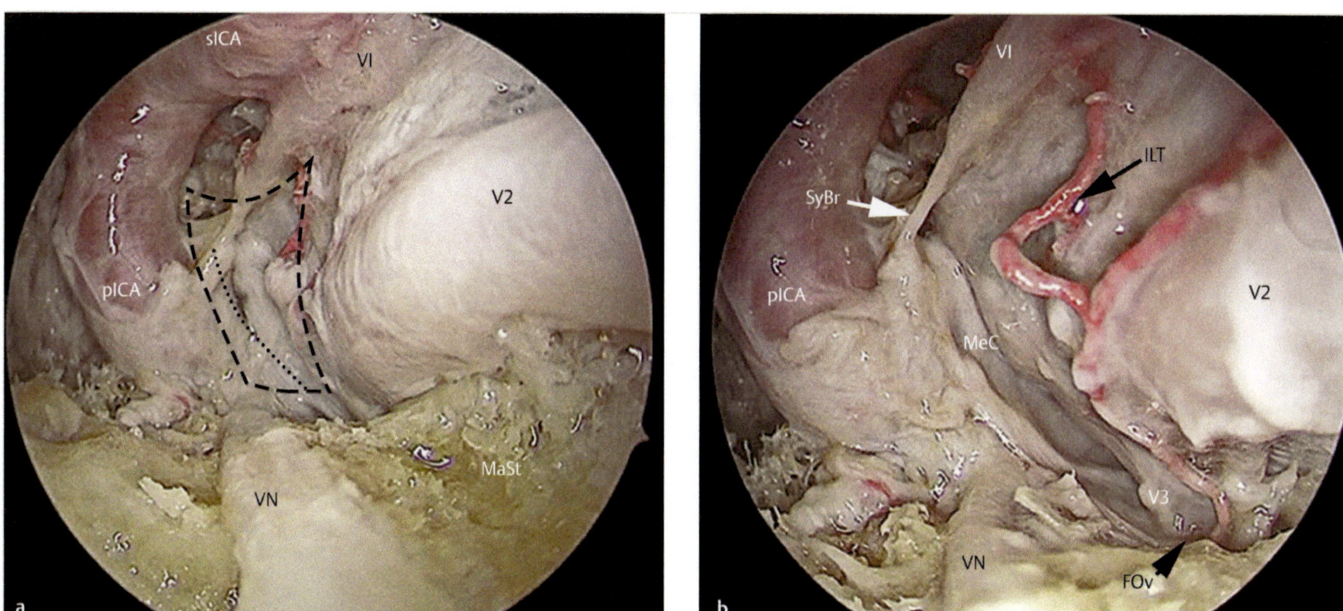

Fig. 21.10 (a, b) Step 3. A diagonal periosteal incision (*black dotted line*) following the shape of the anterior genu of the internal carotid artery is made from the sympathetic branch (SyBr) to the foramen ovale (FOv) to enter the area of Meckel's cave (MeC). The bone located between the posterior portion of the vidian nerve (VN) and the maxillary nerve (V2), which is defined mandibular strut (MaSt), separates the foramen rotundum from the foramen ovale. (*Black dashed line*: Quadrangular space.) V3, mandibular nerve; VI, abducens nerve; ILT, inferolateral trunk; pICA, paraclival tract of the internal carotid artery; sICA, parasellar tract of the internal carotid artery; SyBr, sympathetic branch.

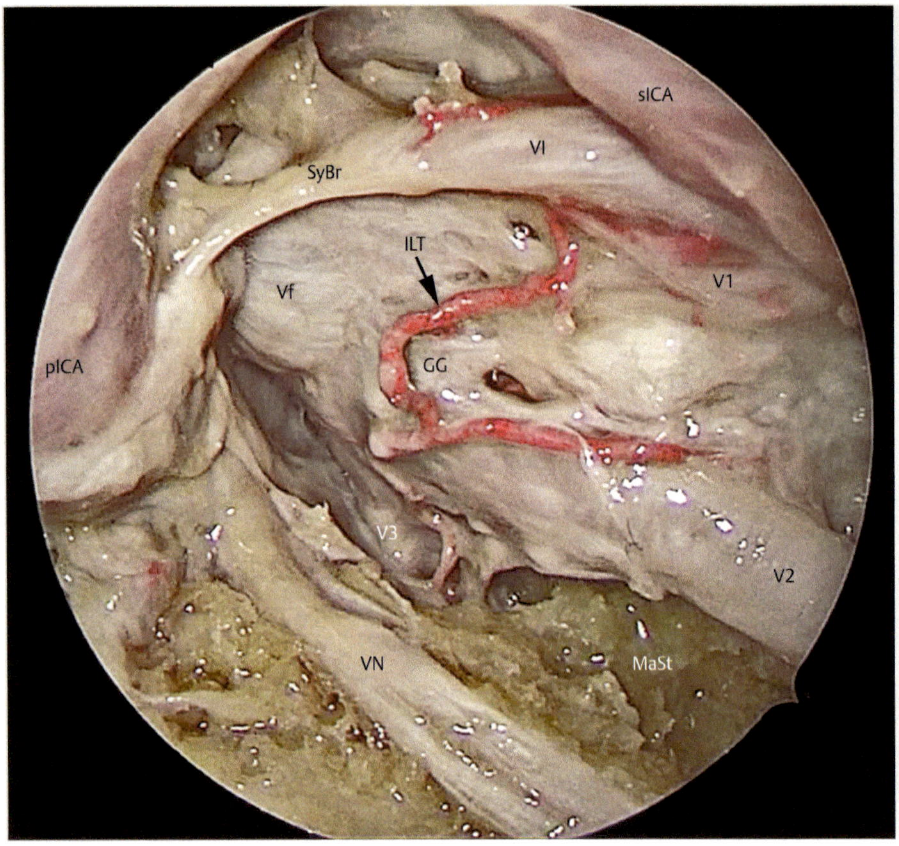

Fig. 21.11 The gasserian ganglion. With a 70-degree scope oriented inferolaterally, an overview of the trigeminal system, including the trigeminal fibers (Vf) glimpsed through the medial meningeal wall of Meckel's cave, the gasserian ganglion (GG), and the ophthalmic (V1), maxillary (V2), and mandibular nerves (V3) is obtained. Of note, this perspective allows understanding the different trajectories of the maxillary and vidian nerves (VN) compared to the mandibular and ophthalmic nerves. The ophthalmic nerve runs close to the abducens nerve (VI) toward the superior orbital fissure. ILT, inferolateral trunk; MaSt, mandibular strut; pICA, paraclival tract of the internal carotid artery; sICA, parasellar tract of the internal carotid artery; SyBr, sympathetic branch.

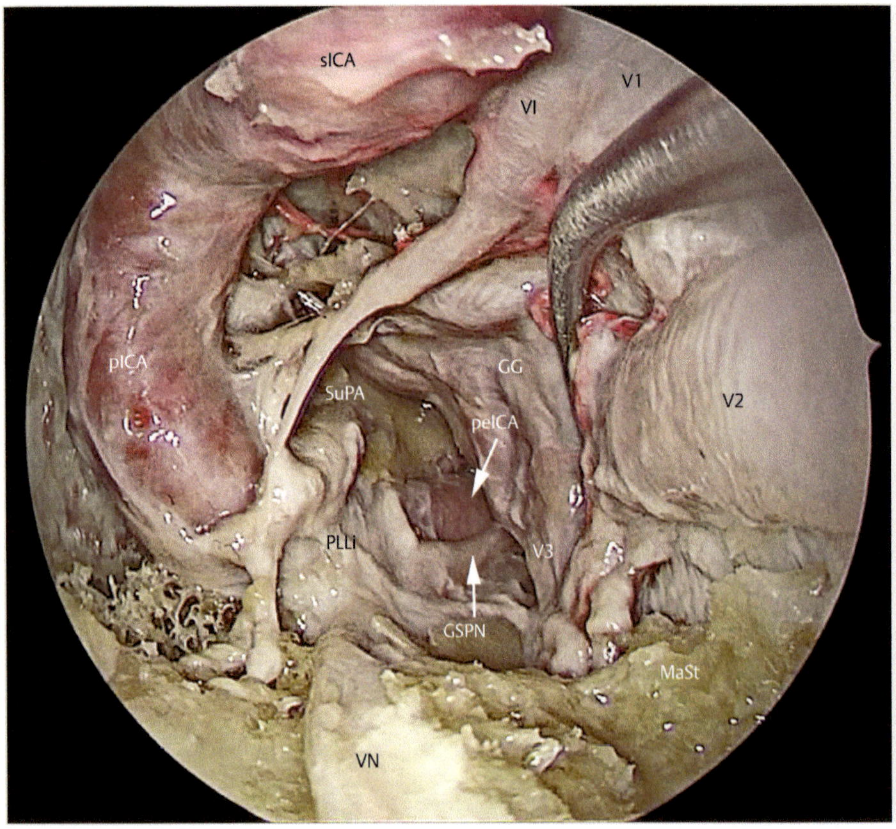

Fig. 21.12 Step 4. The gasserian ganglion (GG) is displaced laterally and a subperiosteal dissection is performed in an anterior-to-posterior direction to expose the petrous tract of the internal carotid artery (peICA), the petrolingual ligament (PLLi), and the superior petrous apex (SuPA). The petrolingual ligament covers superolaterally the angle between the paraclival (pICA) and petrous tracts of the internal carotid artery; its fibrous fibers continue into those of the fibrocartilago basalis. The greater superficial petrosal nerve (GSPN) runs above the petrous tract of the internal carotid artery toward the foramen lacerum, where it joins the deep petrosal nerve (from the internal sympathetic carotid plexus), forming the vidian nerve (VN). V1, ophthalmic nerve; V2, maxillary nerve; V3, mandibular nerve; VI, abducens nerve; MaSt, mandibular strut; sICA, parasellar tract of the internal carotid artery.

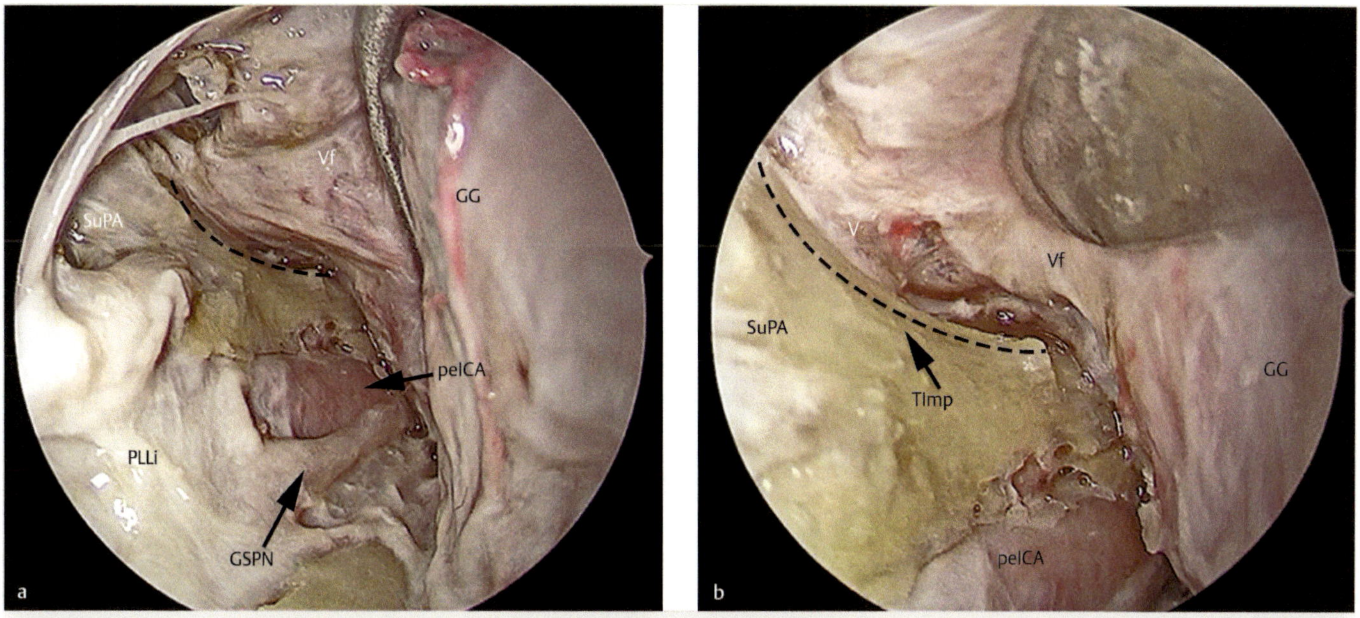

Fig. 21.13 (a, b) The trigeminal impression. The trigeminal impression (TImp) is a depression of the petrous ridge (*black dashed line*) located where the trigeminal nerve (V) passes from the posterior to the middle cranial fossa. It lies posterolaterally to the superior petrous apex (SuPA). Vf, trigeminal fibers within the Meckel's cave; GG, gasserian ganglion; GSPN, great superficial petrosal nerve; peICA, petrous tract of the internal carotid artery; PLLi, petrolingual ligament.

Upper Transpterygoid Approach

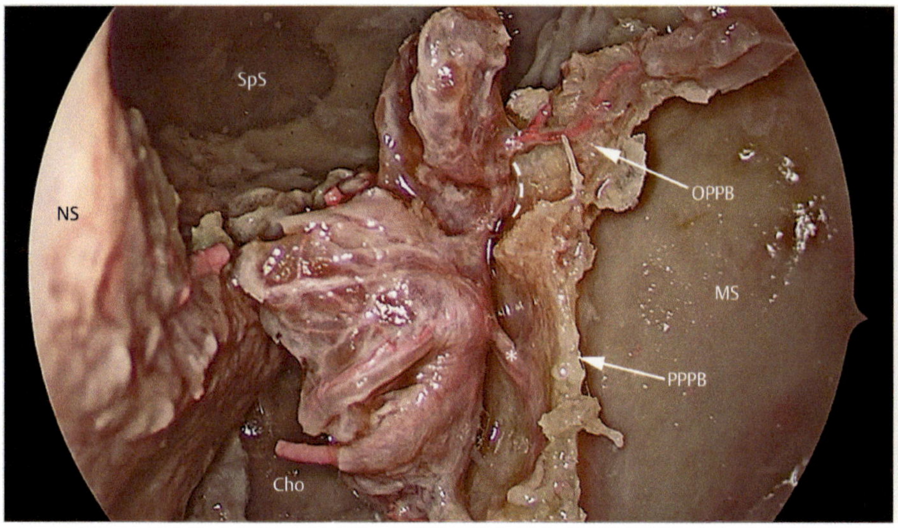

Fig. 21.14 The sphenopalatine foramen. After completing a type B endoscopic medial maxillectomy, the sphenopalatine foramen (*white dashed line*) is identified in the interface between the sphenoid sinus (SpS), the choana (Cho), and the maxillary sinus (MS). The anterior border of the sphenopalatine foramen is formed by the orbital process of the palatine bone (OPPB), which arises from the perpendicular process of the palatine bone (PPPB). Frequently, a small branch (*white asterisk*) of the descending palatine artery pierces the palatine bone and reaches the mucosa of the lateral nasal wall and the inferior turbinate. NS, nasal septum.

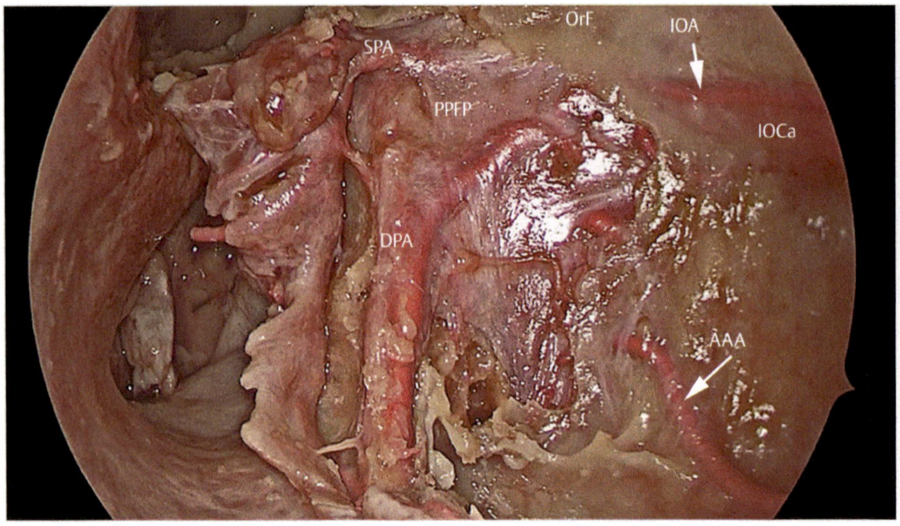

Fig. 21.15 Dissection of the pterygopalatine fossa (part 1). The perpendicular process of the palatine bone and the posterior wall of the maxillary sinus are removed to expose the descending palatine artery (DPA), sphenopalatine artery (SPA), and periosteum of the pterygopalatine fossa (PPFP). AAA, alveolar antral artery; IOA, infraorbital artery; IOCa, infraorbital canal; OrF, orbital floor.

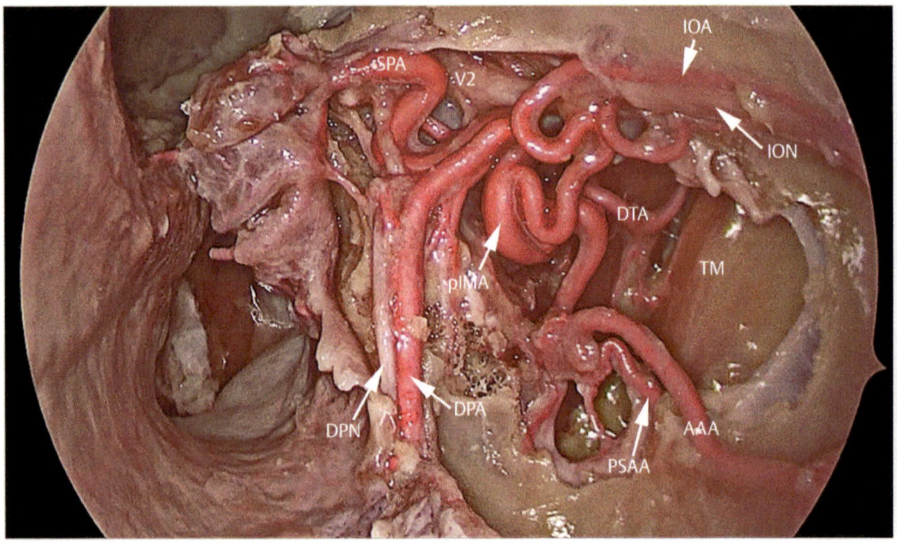

Fig. 21.16 Dissection of the pterygopalatine fossa (part 2). The fat tissue of the pterygopalatine and infratemporal fossae is removed to expose their neurovascular and muscular contents. The pterygopalatine fossa is formed by a vascular compartment (anterior) and a nervous compartment (posterior). The upper transpterygoid approach passes through the superior and medial portions of the pterygopalatine fossa. V2, maxillary nerve; AAA, alveolar antral artery; DPA, descending palatine artery; DPN, descending palatine nerve; DTA, deep temporal artery; IOA, infraorbital artery; ION, infraorbital nerve; pIMA, pterygopalatine tract of the internal maxillary artery; PSAA, posterior superior alveolar artery; SPA, sphenopalatine artery; TM, temporal muscle.

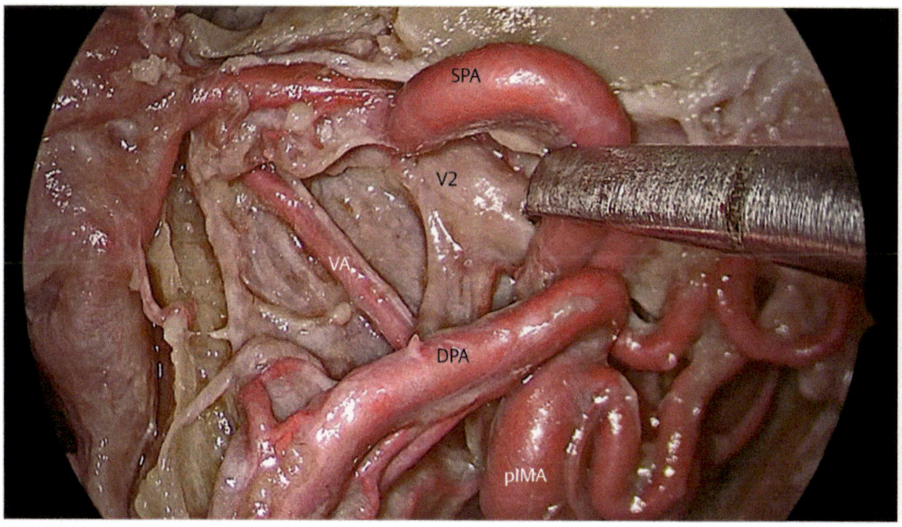

Fig. 21.17 The vidian artery. The vidian artery (VA), when present, arises from the pterygopalatine tract of the internal maxillary artery (pIMA) and can be found displacing laterally the sphenopalatine (SPA) and descending palatine (DPA) arteries. This artery runs along the portion of the pterygoid process that must be removed to harvest the upper transpterygoid corridor. V2, maxillary nerve.

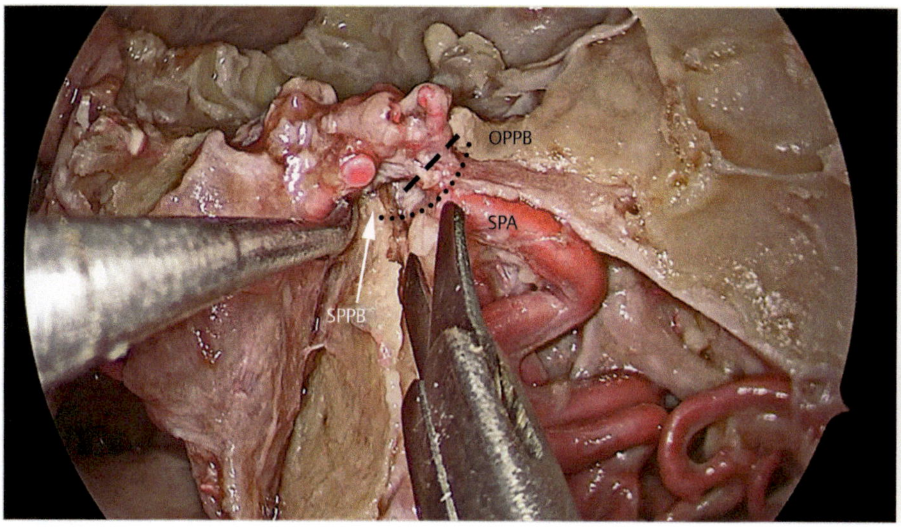

Fig. 21.18 Step 5 (part 1). The sphenopalatine bundle is cut (*black dashed line*) to completely expose the sphenoidal process of the palatine bone (SPPB), which is the posterior boundary of the sphenopalatine foramen. (*Black dotted line*: Position of the anterior boundary of the sphenopalatine foramen.) OPPB, orbital process of the palatine bone (subtotally removed); SPA, sphenopalatine artery.

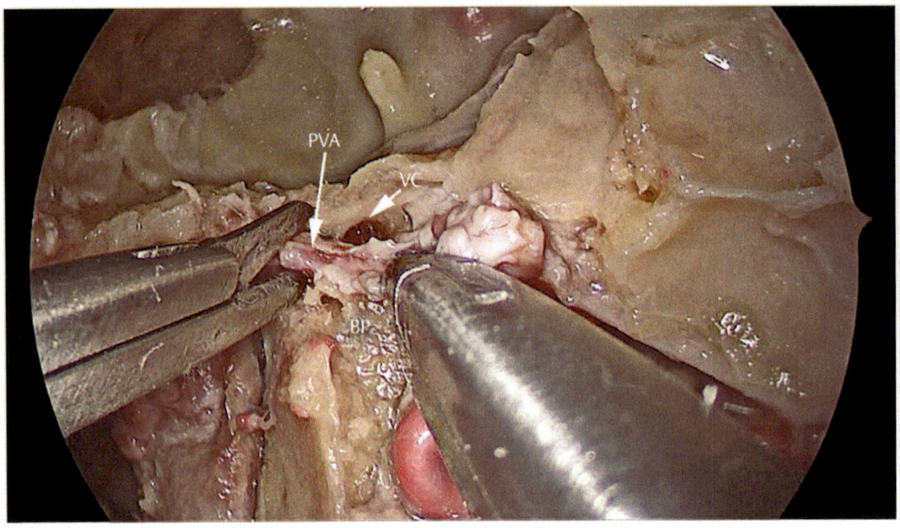

Fig. 21.19 Step 5 (part 2). The palatovaginal artery (PVA) and the vidian bundle are sequentially cut close to the anterior end of the vidian canal (VC) to complete the exposure of the base of the pterygoid process (BP).

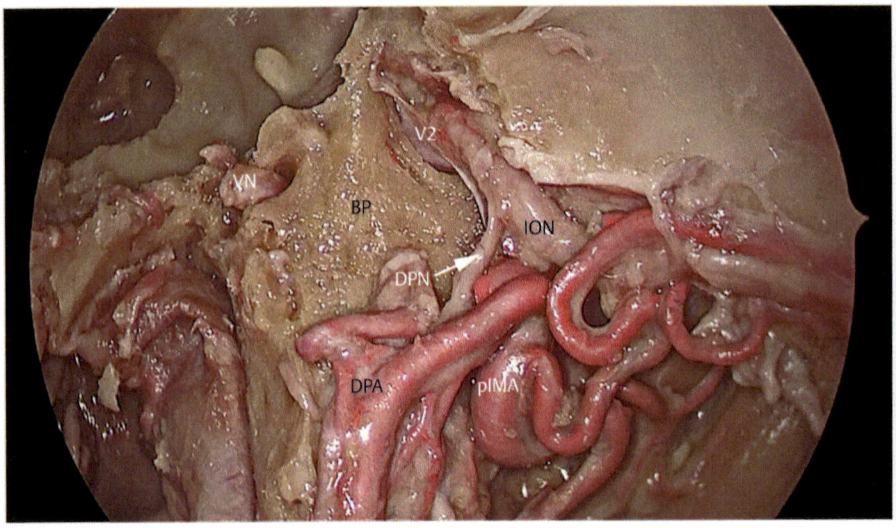

Fig. 21.20 The base of the pterygoid process. The base of the pterygoid process (BP) (or basipterygoid) is the crossroad between the sphenoidal floor medially, greater wing of the sphenoid bone laterally, and pterygoid plates inferiorly. The vidian (VN) and maxillary (V2) nerves run within the basipterygoid. The caudal portion of the basipterygoid can be partially covered by the descending palatine artery (DPA) and the descending palatine nerve (DPN), which can be cut to optimize exposure. ION, infraorbital nerve; pIMA, pterygopalatine tract of the internal maxillary artery.

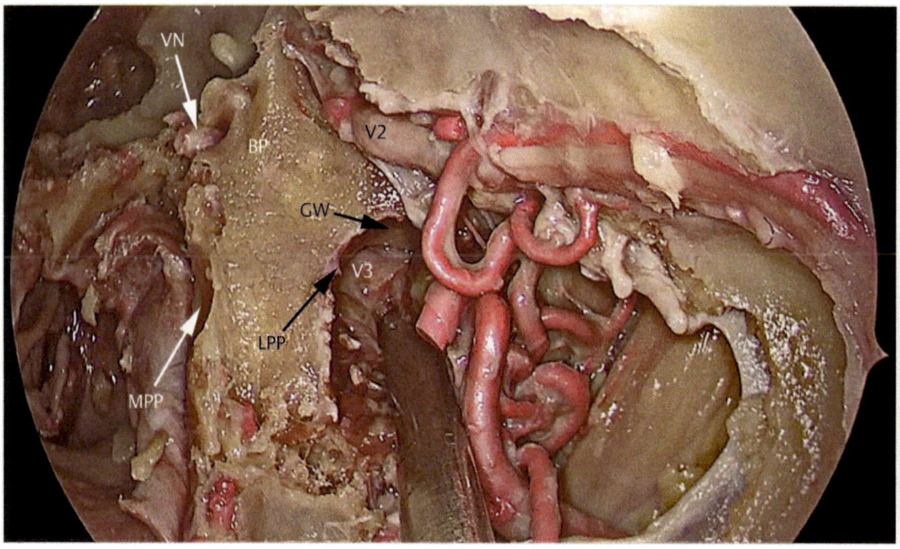

Fig. 21.21 Step 6. The foramen ovale and the extracranial portion of the mandibular nerve (V3) are exposed by performing a subperiosteal dissection along the junction between the lateral pterygoid plate (LPP) and the greater wing of the sphenoid bone (GW). V2, maxillary nerve; BP, base of the pterygoid process; MPP, medial pterygoid plate; VN, vidian nerve.

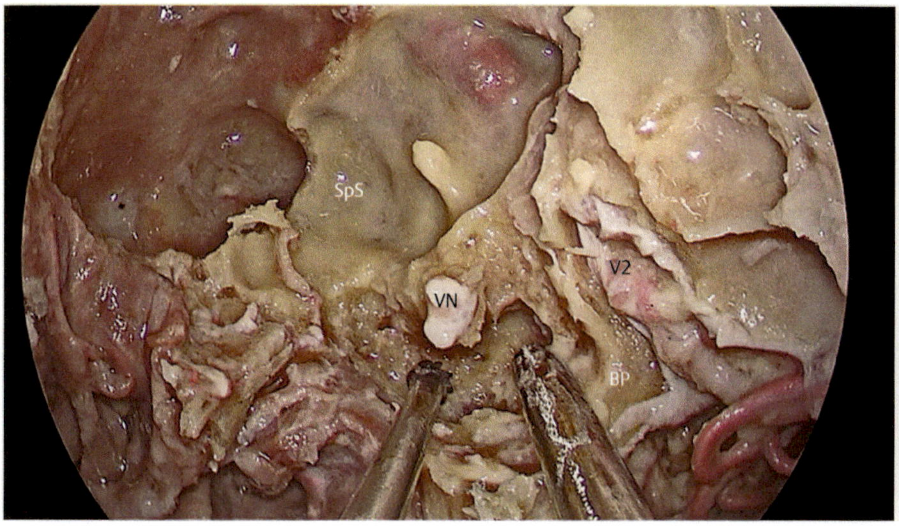

Fig. 21.22 Step 7 (part 1). The base of the pterygoid process (BP) is progressively removed. Bony removal is performed staying between the vidian nerve (VN) and the maxillary nerve (V2) and inferior to the VN. SpS, sphenoid sinus.

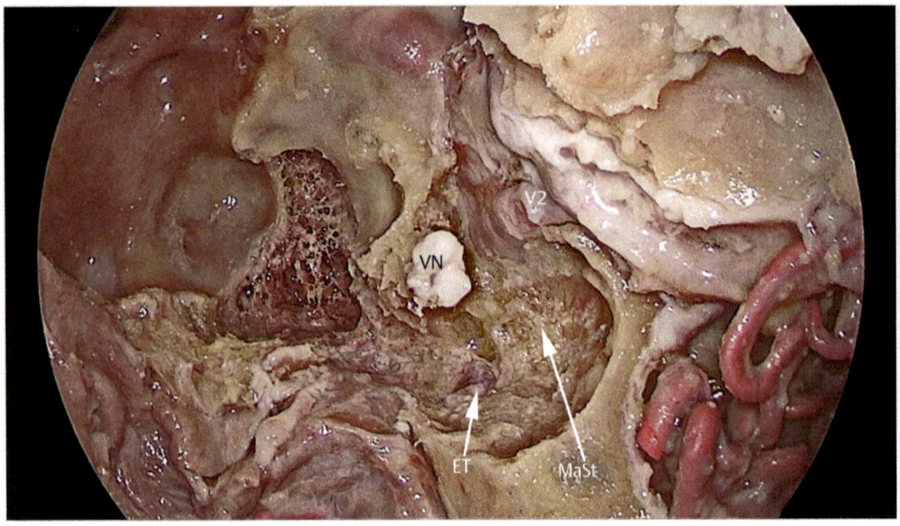

Fig. 21.23 Step 7 (part 2). After subtotal removal of the base of the pterygoid process, the mandibular strut (MaSt) is identified between the maxillary nerve (V2) superolaterally and the eustachian tube (ET) inferomedially. This bony bridge connects the base of the pterygoid process with the greater wing of the sphenoid process and separates the foramina rotundum and ovale. VN, vidian nerve.

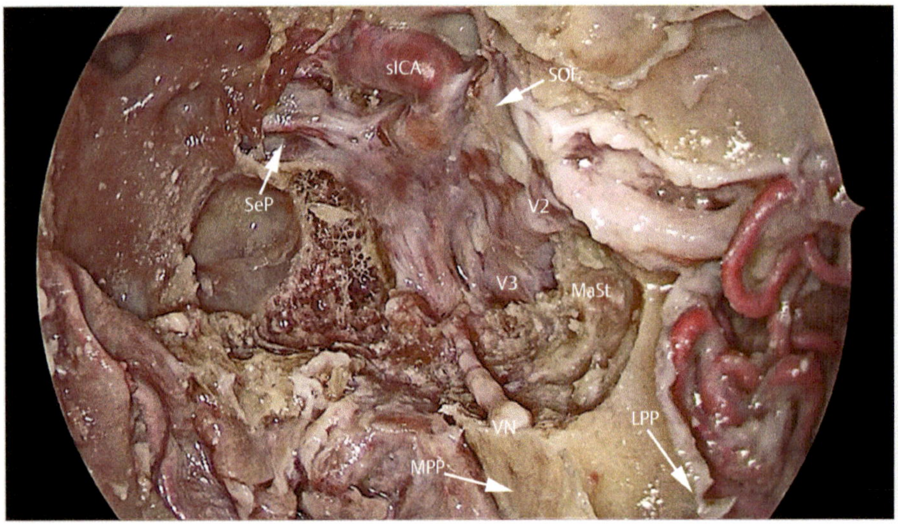

Fig. 21.24 Full exposure of the parasellar area. The upper transpterygoid approach provides a complete exposure of the parasellar area, from the sellar periosteum (SeP) and midclivus medially to the superior orbital fissure (SOF), maxillary nerve (V2), and mandibular nerve (V3) laterally. LPP, lateral pterygoid process; MaSt, mandibular strut; MPP, medial pterygoid process; sICA, parasellar tract of the internal carotid artery; VN, vidian nerve.

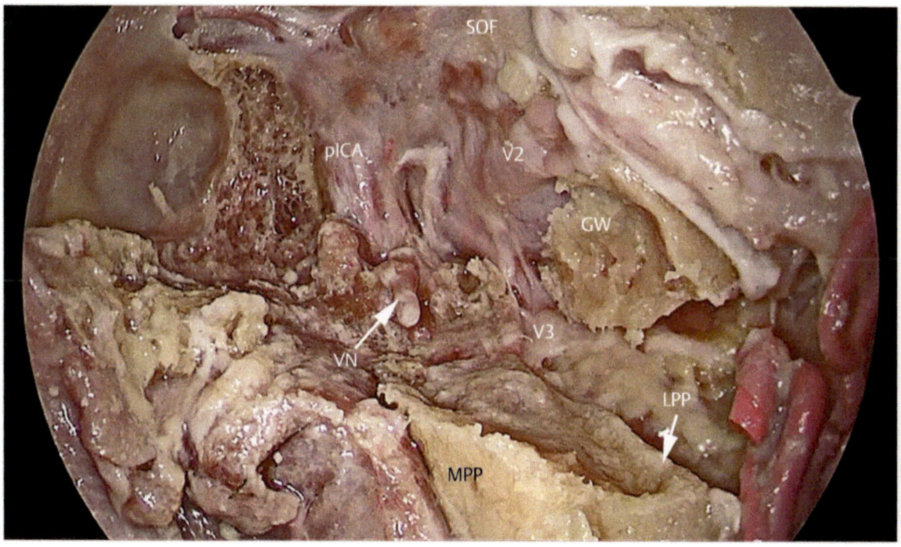

Fig. 21.25 Step 8. The maxillary strut is removed to obtain a full exposure of the mandibular nerve (V3), which is identified between the greater wing of the sphenoid bone (GW) superolaterally and the medial (MPP) and lateral (LPP) pterygoid plates inferomedially. V2, maxillary nerve; pICA, paraclival tract of the internal carotid artery; SOF, superior orbital fissure; VN, vidian nerve.

Transalisphenoid Approach

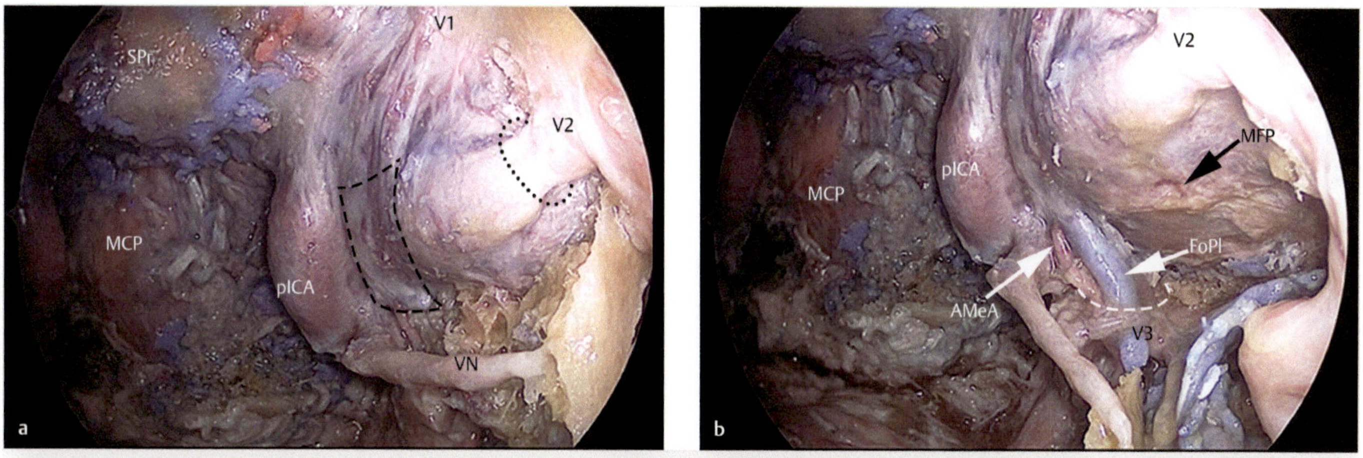

Fig. 21.26 (a, b) Step 9. After completing the suprapetrous and upper transpterygoid approaches, the greater wing of the sphenoid bone is removed to completely expose the structures of the foramen ovale (*white dashed line*), which are the mandibular nerve (V3), the accessory meningeal artery (AMeA), and the foraminal plexus (FoPl). This corridor allows access to the periosteum of the middle cranial fossa (MFP) through two windows: the cranial window is enclosed between the ophthalmic (V1) and maxillary nerves (V2), whereas the caudal window is located lateral to the maxillary nerve. (*Black dashed line*: Quadrangular space; *Black dotted line*: Position of the foramen rotundum.) MCP, midclivus periosteum; pICA, paraclival tract of the internal carotid artery; SPr, sellar prominence; VN, vidian nerve.

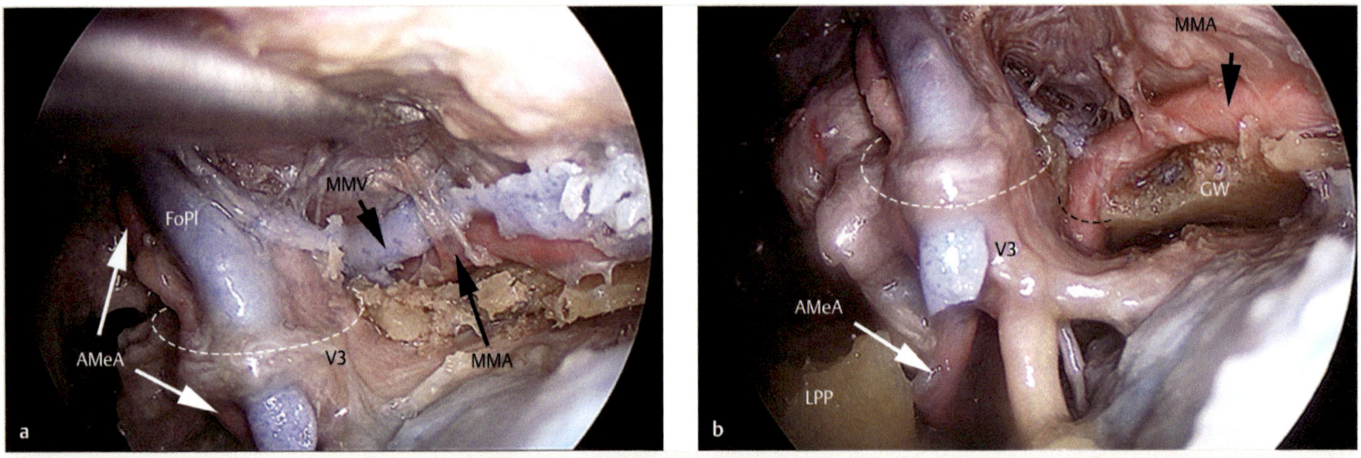

Fig. 21.27 (a, b) Step 10. Following the periosteum of the middle cranial fossa along the caudal window, the middle meningeal artery (MMA) can be exposed by removing the bone of the greater wing of the sphenoid bone (GW) that surrounds the foramen spinosum (*black dashed line*). The middle meningeal vein (MMV) can usually be found close to the middle meningeal artery while joining with the foraminal plexus (FoPl). (*White dashed line:* Foramen ovale.) V3, mandibular nerve; AMeA, accessory meningeal artery; LPP, lateral pterygoid plate.

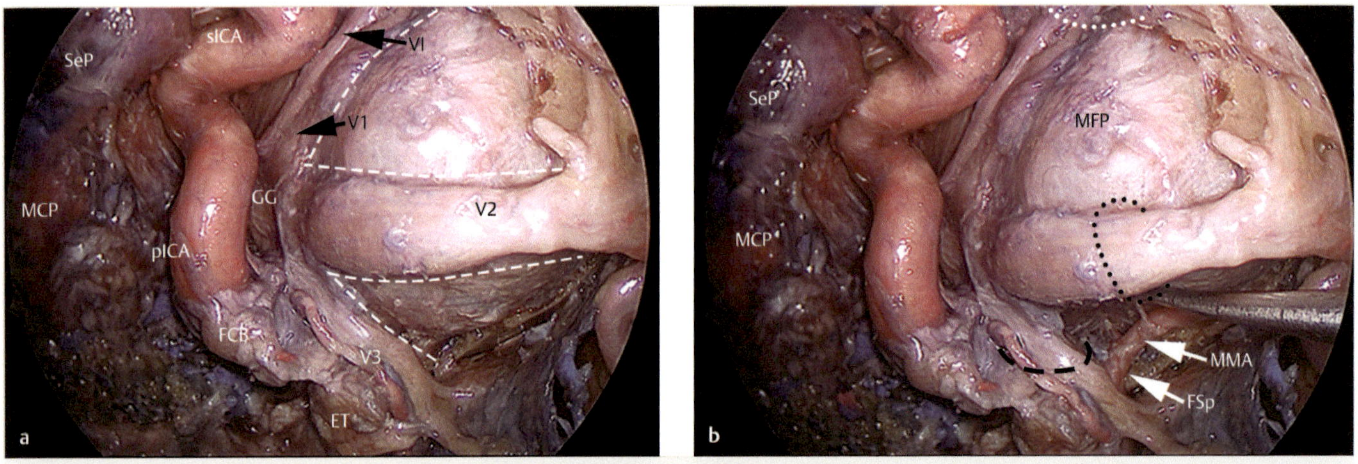

Fig. 21.28 (a, b) Overview of the windows toward the middle cranial fossa. An overview of the two windows providing access to the middle cranial fossa (*white dashed lines*) is obtained with a 70-degree scope oriented laterally. (*Black dashed line:* Foramen ovale; *Black dotted line:* Foramen rotundum; *White dotted line:* Superior orbital fissure.) V1, ophthalmic nerve; V2, maxillary nerve; V3, mandibular nerve; VI, abducens nerve; ET, eustachian tube; FCB, fibrocartilago basalis; FSp, foramen spinosum; GG, gasserian ganglion; MCP, midclivus periosteum; MFP, periosteum of the middle cranial fossa; pICA, paraclival tract of the internal carotid artery; SeP, sellar periosteum; sICA, parasellar tract of the internal carotid artery.

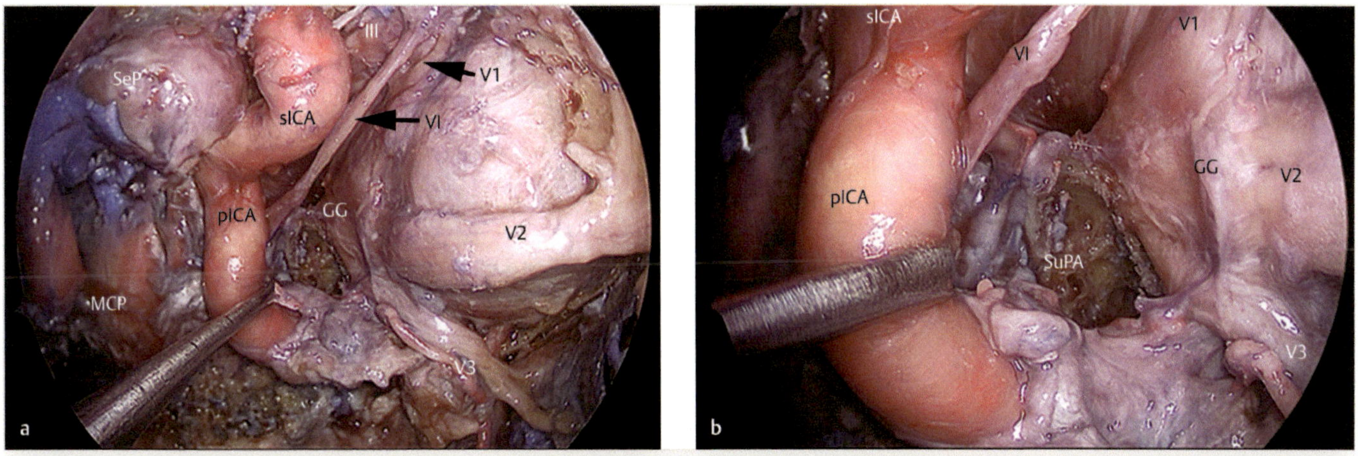

Fig. 21.29 (a, b) Overview of Meckel's cave and surrounding structures. The paraclival tract of the internal carotid artery (pICA) is displaced medially to expose the superior portion of the petrous apex (SuPA). Meckel's cave and its contents lie superolaterally to this portion of the petrous apex. III, oculomotor nerve; V1, ophthalmic nerve; V2, maxillary nerve; V3, mandibular nerve; VI, abducens nerve; ET, eustachian tube; FCB, fibrocartilago basalis; GG, gasserian ganglion; MCP, midclivus periosteum; pICA, paraclival tract of the internal carotid artery; SeP, parasellar periosteum; sICA, sellar tract of the internal carotid artery.

References

[1] Kassam AB, Prevedello DM, Carrau RL, et al. The front door to Meckel's cave: an anteromedial corridor via expanded endoscopic endonasal approach- technical considerations and clinical series. Neurosurgery 2009;64(3, Suppl):ons71–ons82, discussion ons82–ons83

[2] Pamir MN, Kilic T, Ozek MM, Ozduman K, Türe U. Non-meningeal tumours of the cavernous sinus: a surgical analysis. J Clin Neurosci 2006;13(6):626–635

[3] Hardesty DA, Montaser AS, Carrau RL, Prevedello DM. Limits of endoscopic endonasal transpterygoid approach to cavernous sinus and Meckel's cave. J Neurosurg Sci 2018;62(3):332–338

[4] Raza SM, Donaldson AM, Mehta A, Tsiouris AJ, Anand VK, Schwartz TH. Surgical management of trigeminal schwannomas: defining the role for endoscopic endonasal approaches. Neurosurg Focus 2014;37(4):E17

[5] Zoli M, Ratti S, Guaraldi F, et al. Endoscopic endonasal approach to primitive Meckel's cave tumors: a clinical series. Acta Neurochir (Wien) 2018;160(12):2349–2361

[6] Zhang Q, Feng K, Ge C, Hongchuan G, Mingchu L. Endoscopic endonasal management of trigeminal schwannomas extending into the infratemporal fossa. J Clin Neurosci 2012;19(6):862–865

[7] Taylor RJ, Patel MR, Wheless SA, et al. Endoscopic endonasal approaches to infratemporal fossa tumors: a classification system and case series. Laryngoscope 2014;124(11):2443–2450

[8] Palejwala SK, Zhao F, Lanker KC, et al. Imaging-ambiguous lesions of Meckel's cave-utility of endoscopic endonasal transpterygoid biopsy. World Neurosurg 2018;118:e346–e355

[9] Hughes JD, Kapurch J, Van Gompel JJ, et al. Diagnosis and outcome of biopsies of indeterminate lesions of the cavernous sinus and Meckel's cave: a retrospective case series in 85 patients. Neurosurgery 2018;83(3):529–539

[10] Wang X, Zhang X, Hu F, et al. Image-guided endoscopic endonasal transmaxillary transpterygoid approach to Meckel's cave. Turk Neurosurg 2016;26(2):309–314

[11] Truong HQ, Sun X, Celtikci E, et al. Endoscopic anterior transmaxillary "transalisphenoid" approach to Meckel's cave and the middle cranial fossa: an anatomical study and clinical application. J Neurosurg 2018;130(1):227–237

[12] Akay A, Göde S, Çağli MS. Neuronavigation-guided endoscopic endonasal excision of schwannoma-like chordoma of the Meckel's cave: a case report. Turk Neurosurg 2017

[13] el-Kalliny M, van Loveren H, Keller JT, Tew JM Jr. Tumors of the lateral wall of the cavernous sinus. J Neurosurg 1992;77(4):508–514

[14] Alobaid A, Schaeffer T, Virojanapa J, Dehdashti AR. Rare cause of trigeminal neuralgia: Meckel's cave meningocele. Acta Neurochir (Wien) 2015;157(7):1183–1186

[15] Kasliwal MK, Anand VK, Lavi E, Schwartz TH. Endoscopic management of a rare case of nasal glioma in Meckel's cave in an adult: case report. Minim Invasive Neurosurg 2010;53(4):191–193

[16] Jouanneau E, Simon E, Jacquesson T, et al. The endoscopic endonasal approach to the Meckel's cave tumors: surgical technique and indications. World Neurosurg 2014;82(6, Suppl):S155–S161

[17] Jeon C, Hong CK, Woo KI, et al. Endoscopic transorbital surgery for Meckel's cave and middle cranial fossa tumors: surgical technique and early results. J Neurosurg 2018:1–10

[18] Dallan I, Castelnuovo P, Locatelli D, et al. Multiportal combined transorbital transnasal endoscopic approach for the management of selected skull base lesions: preliminary experience. World Neurosurg 2015;84(1):97–107

[19] Simal Julián JA, Miranda Lloret P, García Piñero A, Botella Asunción C. Full endoscopic endonasal suprapetrous approach to Meckel's cave. Acta Neurochir (Wien) 2014;156(8):1623–1626

[20] Zhang X, Tabani H, El-Sayed I, Russell M, Feng X, Benet A. The endoscopic endonasal transmaxillary approach to Meckel's cave through the inferior orbital fissure. Oper Neurosurg (Hagerstown) 2017;13(3):367–373

[21] Hanakita S, Chang WC, Watanabe K, et al. Endoscopic endonasal approach to the anteromedial temporal fossa and mobilization of the lateral wall of the cavernous sinus through the inferior orbital fissure and V1-V2 corridor: an anatomic study and clinical considerations. World Neurosurg 2018;116:e169–e178

22 Transcondylar/Transjugular Tuberculum ("Far-Medial") Approach

Marco Ferrari, Marco Ravanelli, Francesco Belotti, Francesco Doglietto

The transcondylar/transjugular tuberculum approach is the extreme lateral extension of the lower transclival approach.[1] It was developed to resect clival and petroclival lesions with lateral extension and has been currently employed to treat chordomas, chondrosarcomas, meningiomas, and other lesions located medial to the plane passing along lower cranial nerves and acoustic-facial bundle.[1,2] This approach has been called "far-medial" in relation to the possibility to reach the area of the jugular foramen through a medial transnasal perspective, as an alternative to classical neurosurgical routes such as the far-lateral approach. Skull base teams dealing with lesions of this area should master and eventually combine the far-medial and classical transcranial approaches.[3–5]

The far-medial approach consists in the combination of two pathways contiguous to the hypoglossal canal, the transcondylar and the transjugular tuberculum, which are created by removing the bone of the occipital condyle and the jugular tuberculum that lie immediately below and above the hypoglossal canal, respectively. The former route leads to the vertebral artery, posterior inferior cerebellar artery, and spinal root of the accessory nerve, whereas the latter one paves the way toward the anterior inferior cerebellar artery, lower cranial nerves (glossopharyngeal, vagus, and cranial root of the accessory nerve), and acoustic-facial bundle (facial and vestibulocochlear nerve). Of note, the corridor through this area of the skull base is bounded and crossed by several venous vessels and plexuses (i.e., inferior petrosal sinus, petroclival vein, plexus of the hypoglossal canal) converging toward the internal jugular vein.[2] Therefore, intense venous bleeding should be expected and properly managed.

In addition to the anatomical landmarks discussed for transclival and transodontoid approaches, the far-medial approach requires early identification of the position and orientation of the hypoglossal canal. This can be achieved by sequentially using the tail of the inferior turbinate, anterior rectus capitis muscle, and a bony depression in its cranial insertion (i.e., supracondylar groove) as landmarks for the external opening of the hypoglossal canal.[1] The internal end can be identified by performing a subperiosteal removal of the lateral edge of the lower clivus until a funnel-shaped dural fold comes into view, allowing the localization of the canal before to start the bone removal.

Being based on the removal of thick bony structures, the far-medial approach is particularly useful in bony-originated tumors, such as chordomas and chondrosarcomas, which arise from the clivus or the petroclival junction and grow predominantly within the bone. It is worth mentioning that the far-medial approach is a challenging route by virtue of several factors: (1) it exploits a deep and diagonal surgical corridor, which requires dedicated instruments, high expertise, and remarkable precision in endoscopic transnasal maneuvers; (2) it crosses a number of important

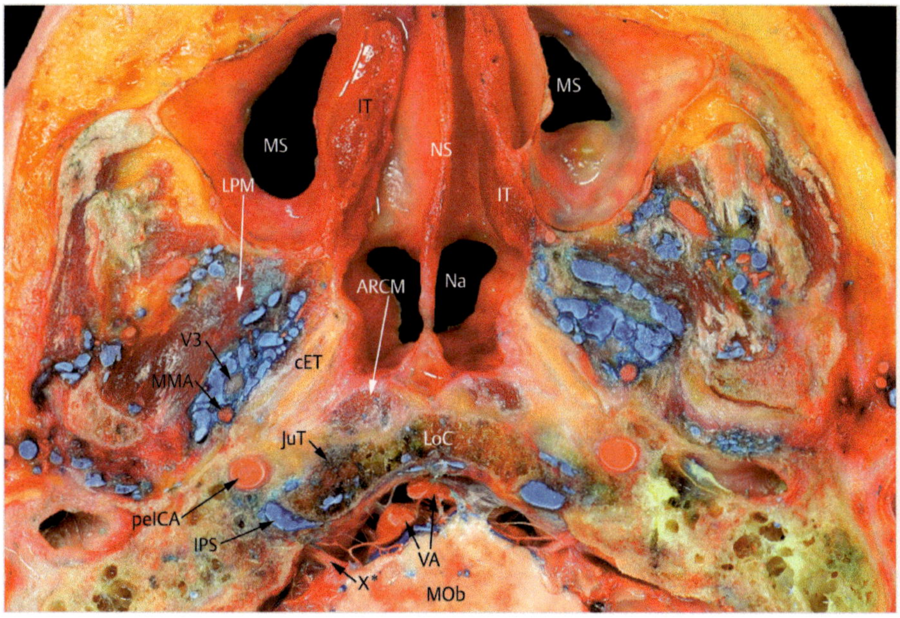

Fig. 22.1 Axial view of the jugular tuberculum and adjacent structures. This axial cadaver cut shows with a cranial-to-caudal perspective the jugular tuberculum (JuT) and adjacent structures. V3, mandibular nerve; X*, glossopharyngeal, vagus, and cranial accessory nerves; ARCM, anterior rectus capitis muscle; cET, cartilaginous portion of the eustachian tube; IPS, inferior petrosal sinus; IT, inferior turbinate; LoC, lower clivus; LPM, lateral pterygoid muscle; MMA, middle meningeal artery; MOb, medulla oblongata; MS, maxillary sinus; Na, nasopharynx; NS, nasal septum; peICA, petrous tract of the internal carotid artery; VA, vertebral artery.

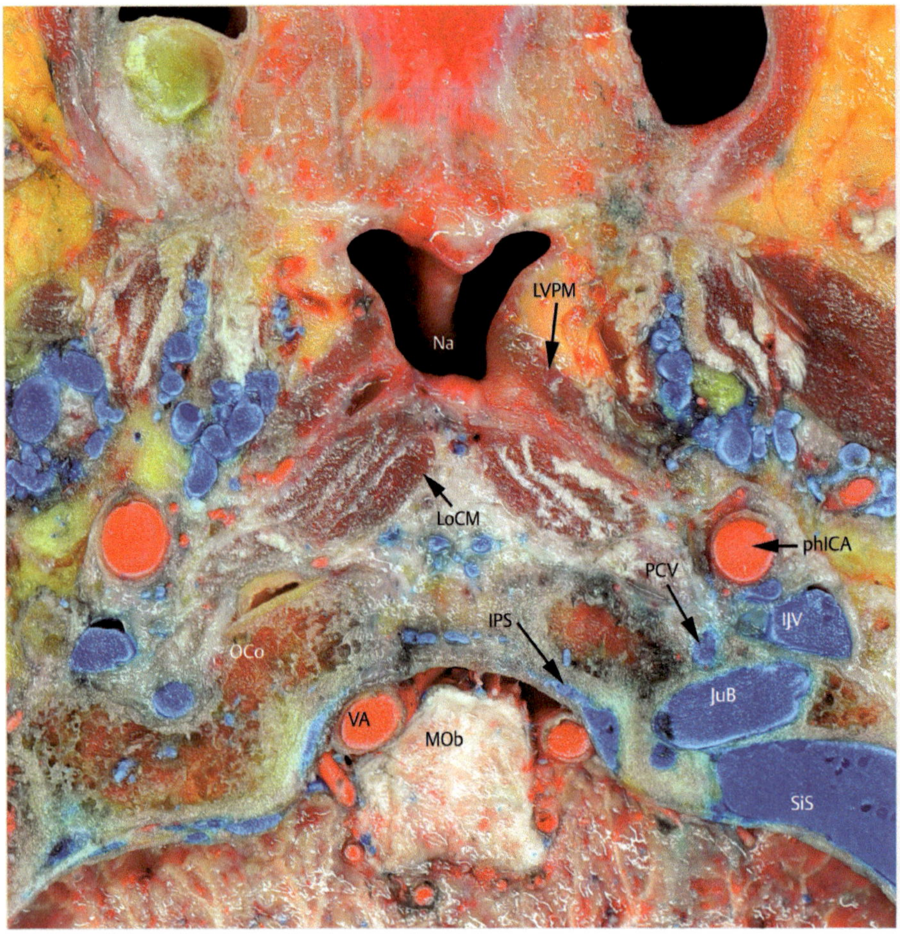

Fig. 22.2 Axial view of the occipital condyle and adjacent structures. This axial cadaver cut shows with a caudal-to-cranial perspective the occipital condyle (OCo). IJV, internal jugular vein; IPS, inferior petrosal sinus; JuB, jugular bulb; LoCM, longus capitis muscle; LVPM, levator veli palatini muscle; MOb, medulla oblongata; Na, nasopharynx; PCV, petroclival vein; phICA; parapharyngeal tract of the internal carotid artery; SiS, sigmoid sinus; VA, vertebral artery.

neurovascular structures, whose injury could lead to severe complications for the patient[1,2,6]; (3) it includes partial removal of the bony framework of the craniocervical junction, thus requiring careful assessment of the need for occipitocervical fusion[2]; (4) being an extension of the lower transclival approach, the difficulty to obtain a watertight closure of the dura is further remarked.

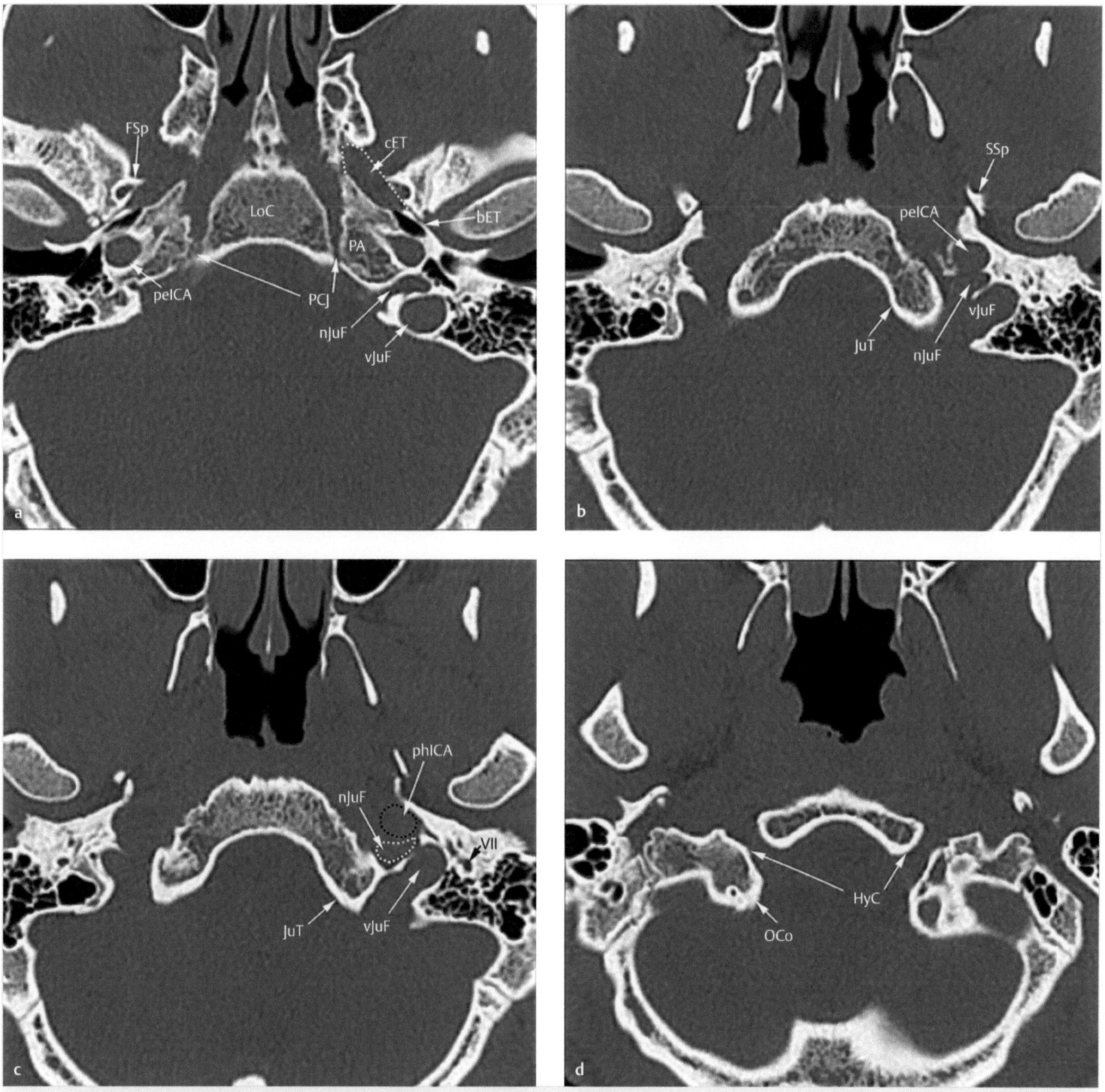

Fig. 22.3 (a–d) CT axial anatomy of the jugular foramen and surrounding structures. The panel shows four axial CT scans from a plane passing through the jugular tuberculum (JuT), cranially **(a)**, to a plane passing through the upper portion of occipital condyle (OCo), caudally **(d)**. The jugular tuberculum lies caudal to the petrous apex (PA) and the petroclival junction (PCJ), medial to the jugular foramen, which is formed by a vascular (vJuF) and a nervous (nJuF, *white dotted line*) compartment, lateral to the lower clivus (LoC), and cranial to the occipital condyle. The occipital condyle houses the hypoglossal canal (HyC), which runs from posteromedial to anterolateral. Other bony canals, which usually contain a vein with variable size and course, can be identified in the posterior portion of the occipital condyle. Of note, the petrous (peICA) and parapharyngeal (phICA, *black dotted line*) tracts of the internal carotid artery lie just anterior to the nervous compartment of the jugular foramen, while the vascular compartment is located medially to the mastoid tract of the facial nerve (VII). bET (*white dotted line*), bony portion of the eustachian tube; cET, cartilaginous portion of the eustachian tube; FSp, foramen spinosum; SSp, spina sphenoidalis.

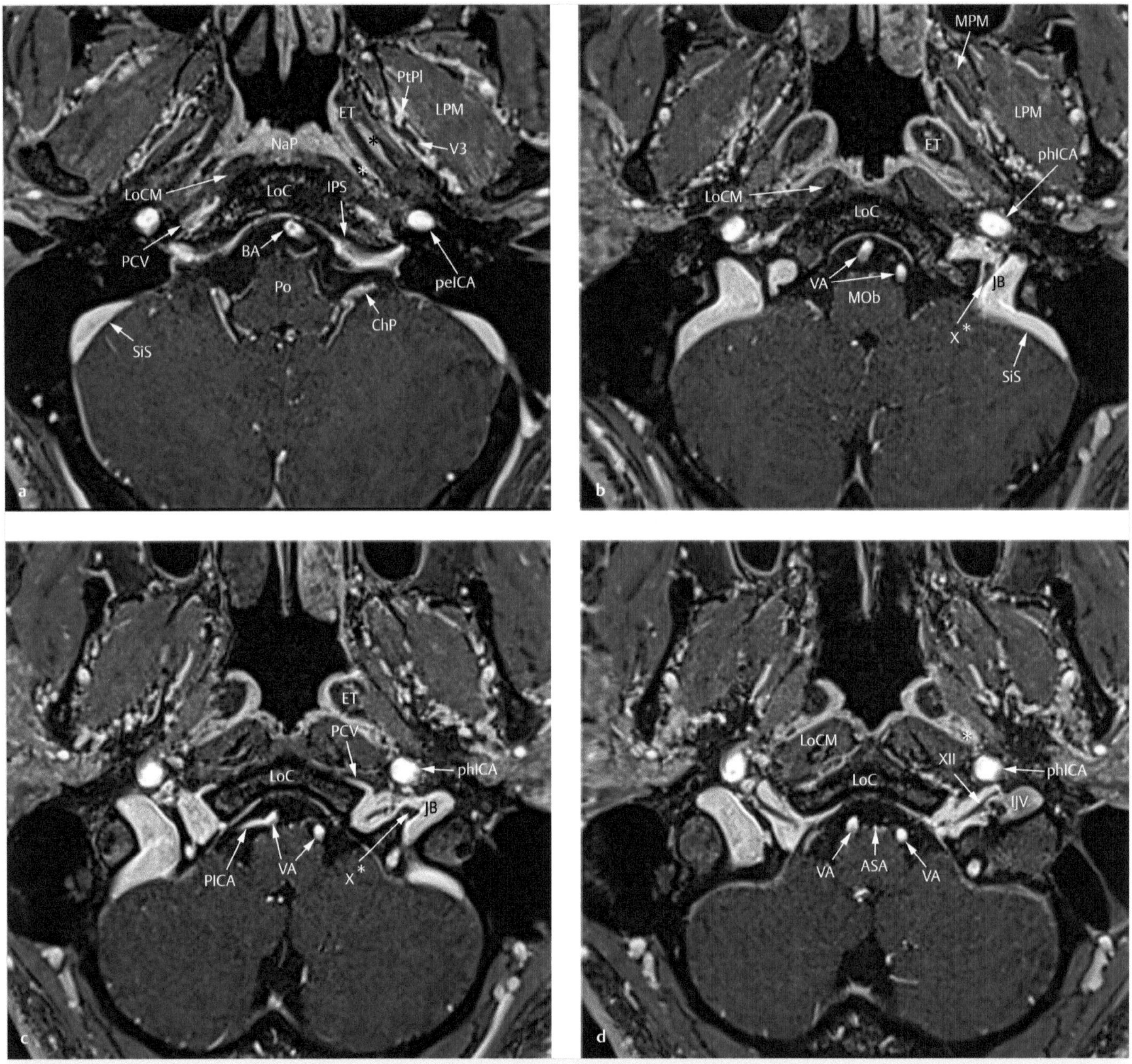

Fig. 22.4 (a–d) Axial MRI scan of the jugular foramen and hypoglossal canal regions. This panel of contrast-enhanced T1-weighted MRI scans with fat saturation shows several neurovascular structures of the area of the jugular foramen and the hypoglossal canal (four images from cranial to caudal, from **a** to **d**). The inferior petrosal sinus (IPS), sigmoid sinus (SiS), petroclival vein (PCV), and the venous plexus of the hypoglossal canal converge to form the jugular bulb (JB) and the internal jugular vein (IJV). Inferior petrosal sinus and petroclival vein run parallel along the intracranial and extracranial surfaces of the lower clivus (LoC), respectively. Due to contrast enhancement of the surrounding vascular structures, the intraforaminal and intracanalar tracts of the glossopharyngeal–vagus–accessory (X*) and hypoglossal (XII) nerves can be, respectively, identified. The vertebral arteries (VA), basilar artery (BA), anterior spinal artery (ASA), and cerebellar artery (PICA) can be identified in the cisternal space in front of the lower portion of the pons (Po), medulla oblongata (MOb), and cranial portion of the spinal cord. (*Black asterisk*: Contrast-enhanced mucosa of the eustachian tube; *White asterisk*: Rosenmüller's fossa or lateral nasopharyngeal recess.) V3, mandibular nerve; ChP, choroid plexus; ET, eustachian tube; LoCM, longus capitis muscle; LPM, lateral pterygoid muscle; MPM, medial pterygoid muscle; NaP, nasopharyngeal posterior wall; peICA, petrous tract of the internal carotid artery; phICA, parapharyngeal tract of the internal carotid artery; PtPl, pterygoid plexus.

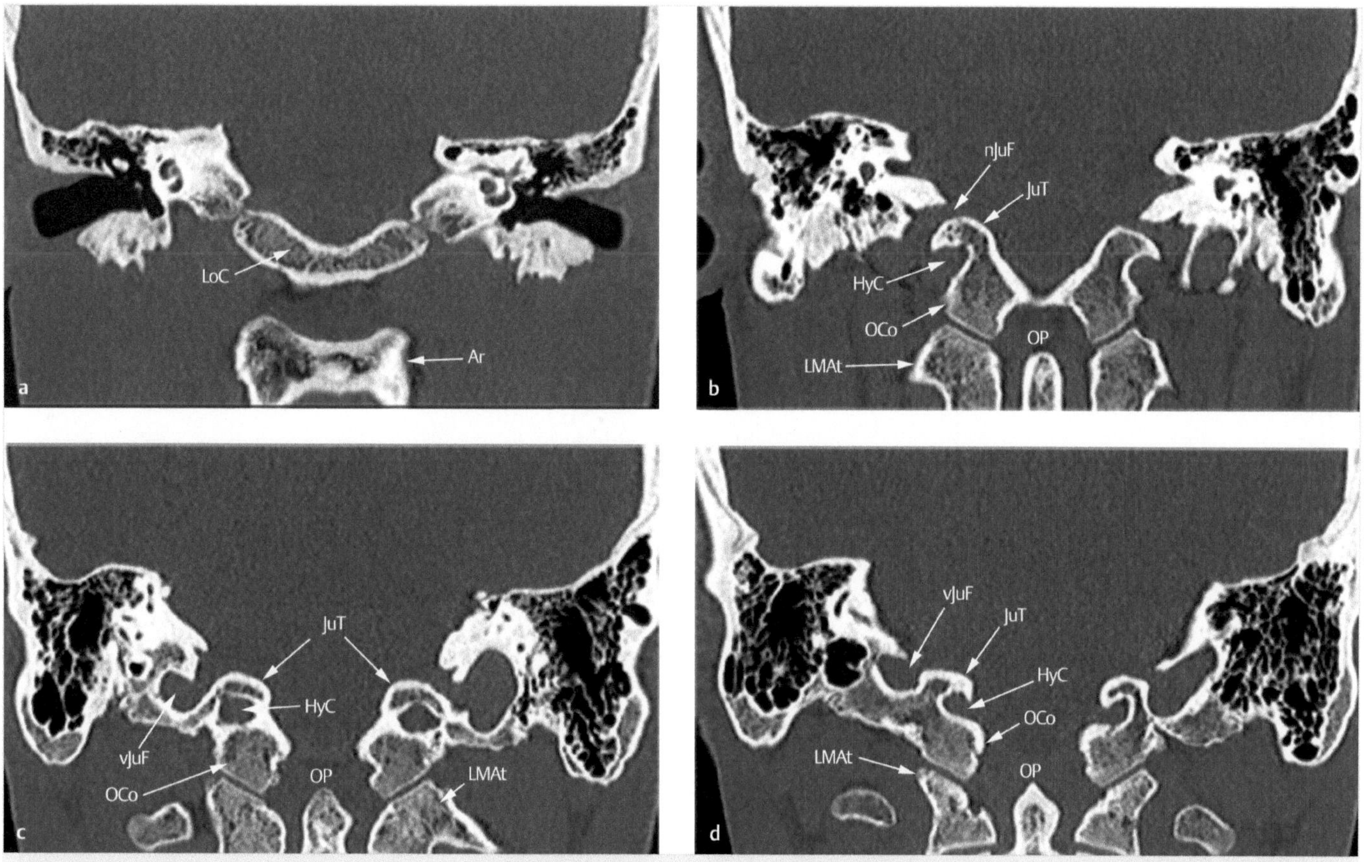

Fig. 22.5 (a–d) CT coronal anatomy of the jugular foramen and surrounding structures. The panel shows four coronal CT scans from a plane passing through the lower clivus (LoC), anteriorly **(a)**, to a plane passing through the posterior portion of hypoglossal canal (HyC), posteriorly (d). The hypoglossal canal run from posteromedial to anterolateral within the occipital condyle (OCo). The jugular tuberculum (JuT) separates the hypoglossal canal from the nervous compartment of the jugular foramen (nJuF), while the vascular compartment (vJuF) lies more posteriorly and laterally. Ar, anterior arch of the atlas; LMAt, lateral mass of the atlas; OP, odontoid process.

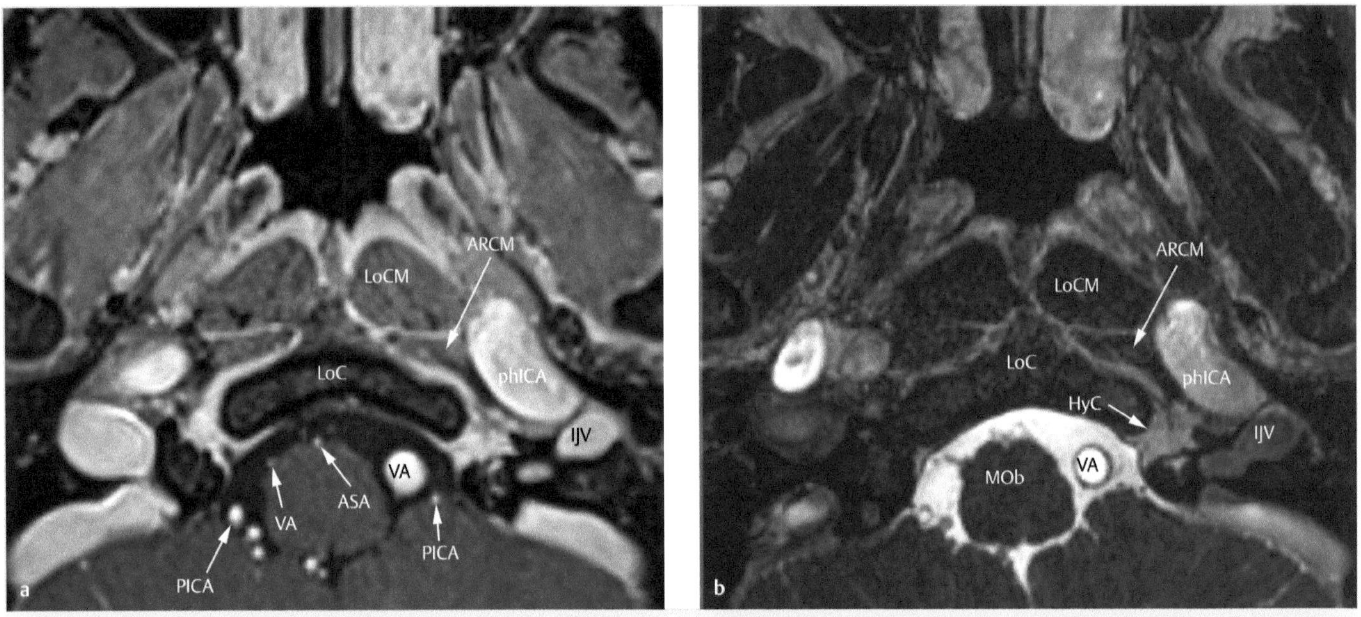

Fig. 22.6 MRI axial anatomy of the anterior rectus capitis muscle. The panel shows an axial contrast-enhanced T1-weighted MRI scan with fat saturation **(a)** and an axial CISS (constructive interference in steady state) MRI scan (right image) **(b)** passing through the longus capitis muscle (LoCM) and the anterior rectus capitis muscle (ARCM). The cranial insertion of the anterior rectus capitis muscle (also called the supracondylar groove) can be used as a landmark for the external end of the hypoglossal canal (HyC). Of note, in case of medial kinking of the parapharyngeal tract of the internal carotid artery (phICA), the dissection of the muscle should be performed carefully due to the adjacency of the artery. As shown in this case, the vertebral arteries (VA) can be remarkably asymmetric in terms of caliber and course; the right hypertrophic posterior inferior cerebellar artery (PICA) compensates for hypoplasia of vertebral artery on the same side. ASA, anterior spinal artery; IJV, internal jugular vein; LoC, lower clivus; MOb, medulla oblongata.

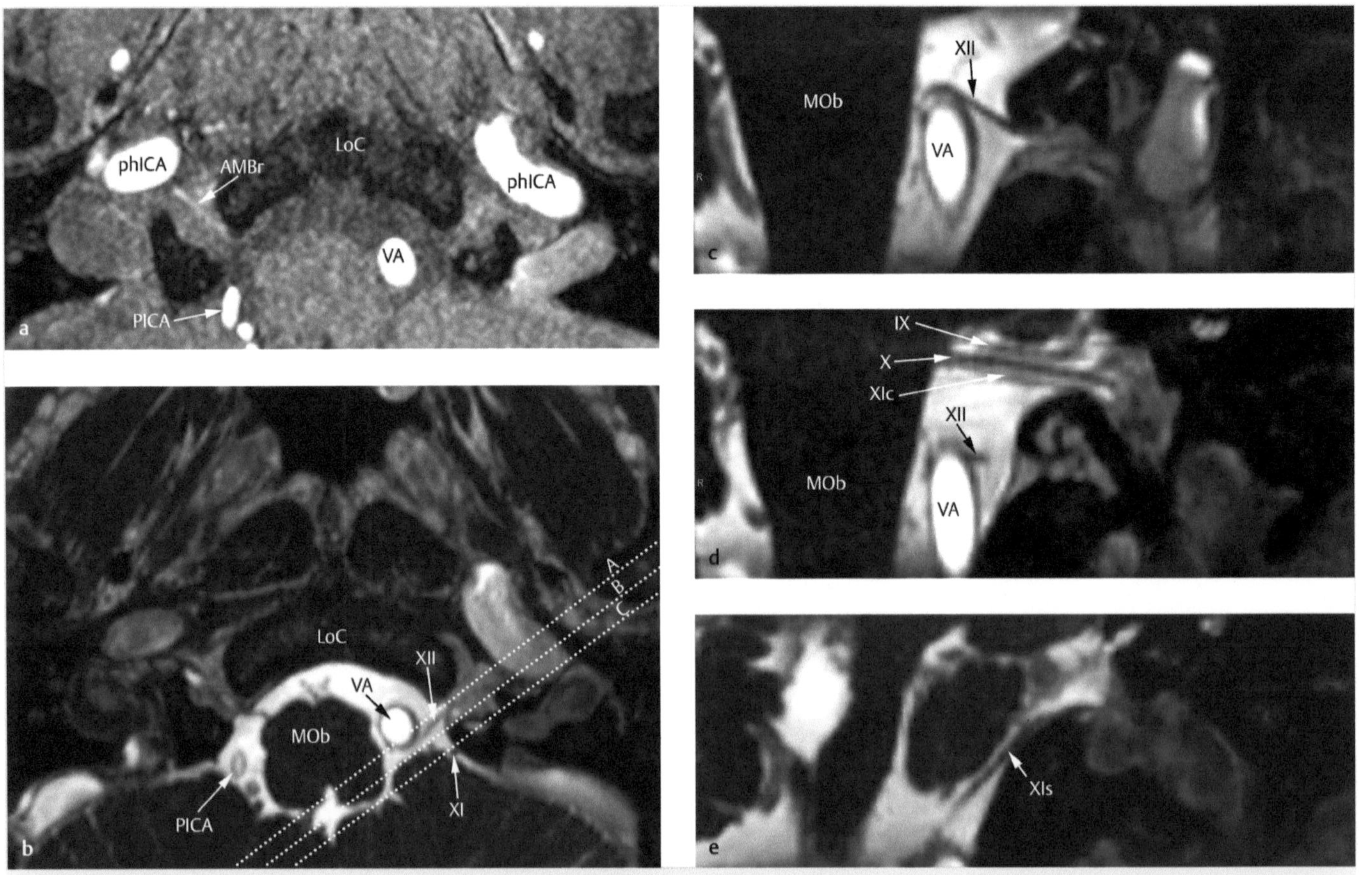

Fig. 22.7 MRI axial and paracoronal anatomy of the hypoglossal nerve. MRI angiography **(a)** shows the main arteries that run close to or within the hypoglossal canal: the vertebral artery (VA), the meningeal branch for the anterior condylar canal (AMBr) of the ascending pharyngeal artery, and the parapharyngeal tract of the internal carotid artery (phICA). Hypoplasia of the right vertebral artery is counterbalanced by the hypertrophic posterior inferior cerebellar artery (PICA). An axial **(b)** and three paracoronal CISS (constructive interference in steady state) MRI **(c–e)** depict the course and anatomic relationships of the cisternal tract of the glossopharyngeal (IX), vagus (X), cranial accessory (XIc), spinal accessory (XIs), and hypoglossal (XII) nerves. The *white dotted lines* mark the orientation of the paracoronal images. LoC, lower clivus; MOb, medulla oblongata.

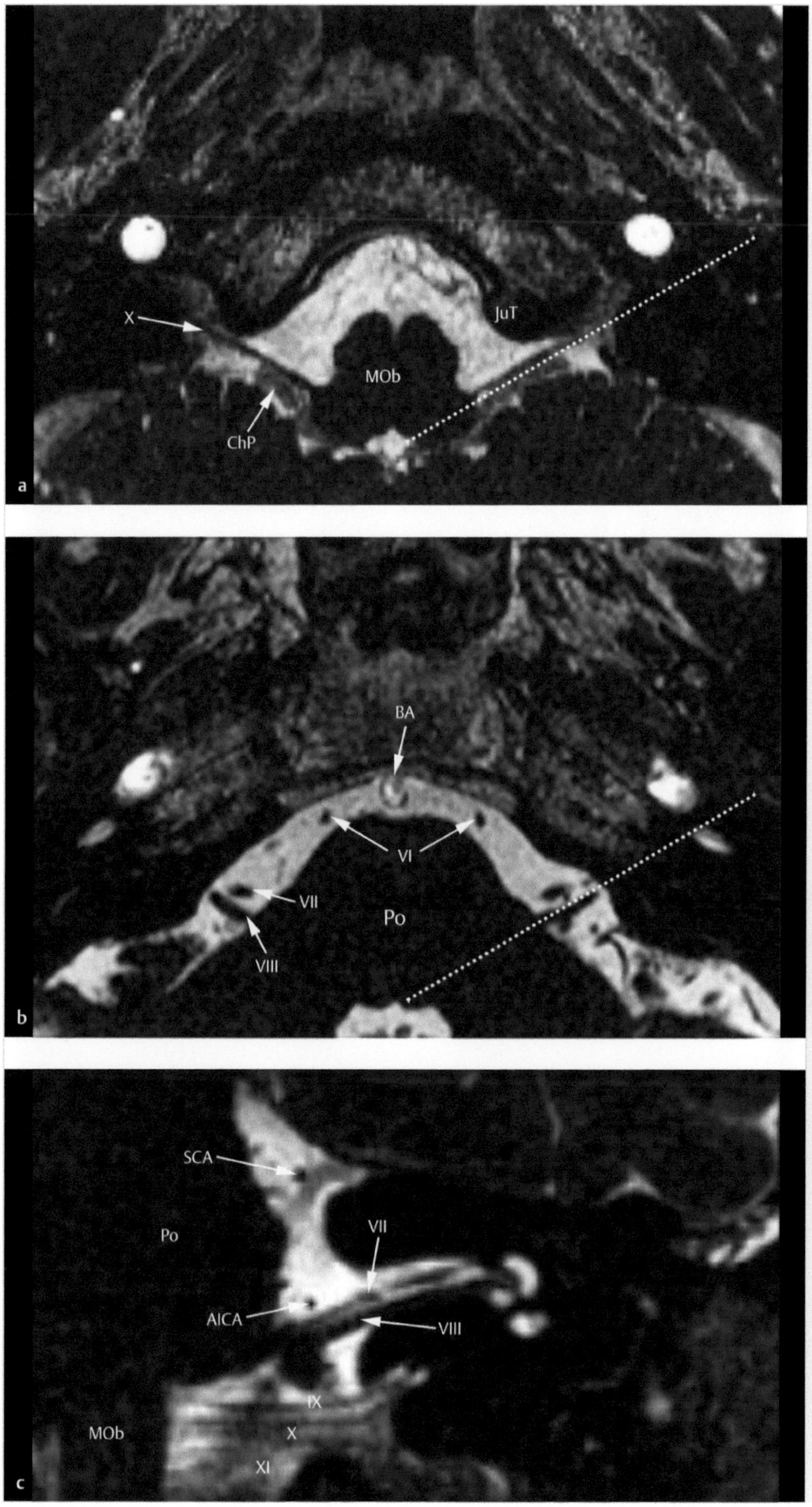

Fig. 22.8 MRI axial and paracoronal anatomy of the lower cranial nerves and the acoustic-facial bundle. Two axial constructive interference in steady state (CISS) MRI scans **(a, b)** and one paracoronal CISS MRI scan (lower image) **(c)**, whose orientation is marked by the *white dotted line*, summarize the cisternal anatomy of facial (VII), vestibulocochlear (VIII), glossopharyngeal (IX), vagus (X), and accessory (XI) nerve. Of note, the choroid plexus (ChP) lies between the acoustic-facial bundle, cranially, and the group of lower cranial nerves, caudally. VI, abducens nerves; AICA, anterior inferior cerebellar artery; BA, basilar artery; JuT, jugular tuberculum; MOb, medulla oblongata; Po, pons; SCA, superior cerebellar artery.

Endoscopic Dissection

Nasal Phase

- Paraseptal sphenoidotomy.
- Transrostral sphenoidotomy.
- Expanded transrostral sphenoidotomy.
- Vertical uncinectomy.
- Anterior ethmoidectomy.
- Posterior ethmoidectomy.
- Transethmoidal sphenoidotomy.
- Facultative: Horizontal uncinectomy.
- Facultative: Type A–D endoscopic medial maxillectomy.

Skull Base Phase

- Transclival (lower clivus) approach.
- Facultative: Transclival (midclivus) approach.
- Step 1: Removal of the anterior rectus capitis muscle.
- Step 2: Opening of the bony hypoglossal canal.
- Step 3: Opening of the periosteal sheath of the hypoglossal canal.
- Step 4: Medialization of the vertebral artery.
- Step 5: Partial removal of the jugular tuberculum.
- Step 6: Total removal of the jugular tuberculum.

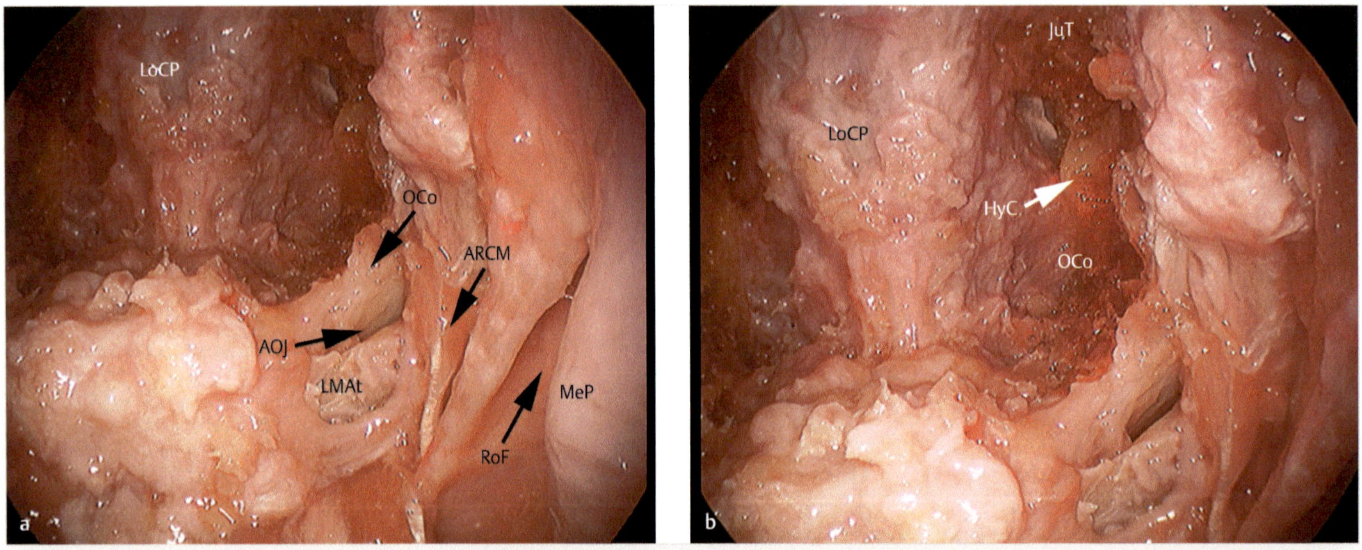

Fig. 22.9 (a, b) Landmarks for the hypoglossal canal. The hypoglossal canal (HyC) lies between the occipital condyle (OCo) inferiorly and the jugular tuberculum (JuT) superiorly. Together with the lateral mass of the atlas (LMAt), the occipital condyle forms the atlanto-occipital joint (AOJ). Both these bony structures are located deep to the anterior rectus capitis muscle (ARCM), which is just posterior to the fossa of Rosenmüller (RoF), medial plate of the torus tubarius (MeP), and tail of the inferior turbinate. LoCP, periosteum of the lower clivus.

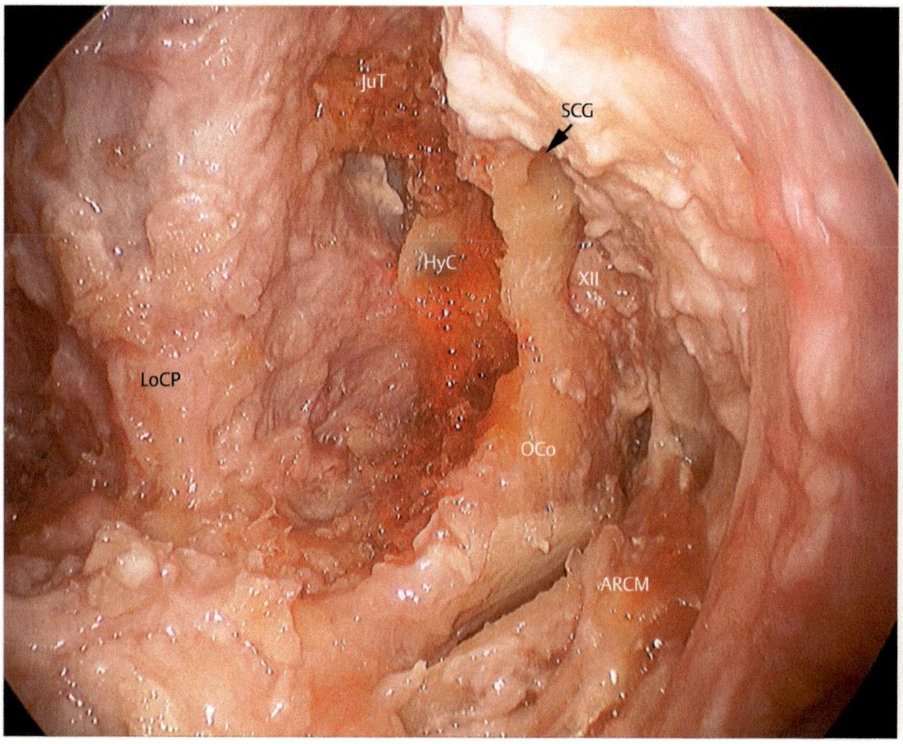

Fig. 22.10 Step 1. The anterior rectus capitis muscle (ARCM) is removed to fully expose the occipital condyle (OCo) and supracondylar groove (SCG), which lies just above the anterolateral opening of the hypoglossal canal (HyC). The cortical component of the canal is easily recognized. XII, hypoglossal nerve; JuT, jugular tuberculum; LoCP, periosteum of the lower clivus.

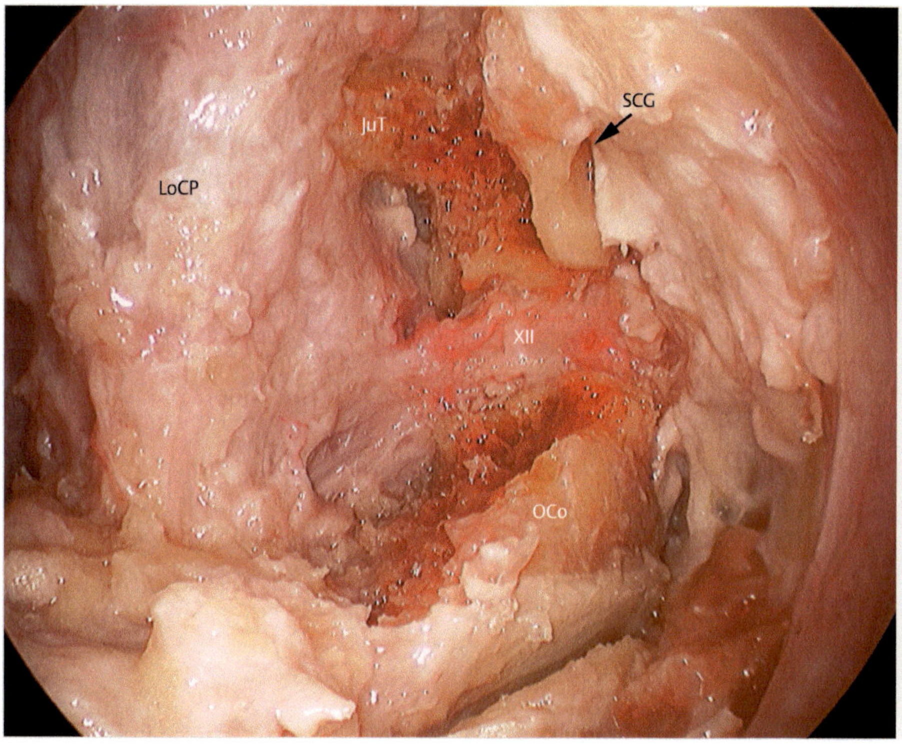

Fig. 22.11 Step 2. Removal of the anteromedial bony wall of the hypoglossal canal leads to exposure of its content, which is mostly represented by the hypoglossal nerve (XII). This maneuver allows us to better distinguish the occipital condyle (OCo) and the jugular tuberculum (JuT), which remain connected posterior to the canal. LoCP, periosteum of the lower clivus; SCG, supracondylar groove.

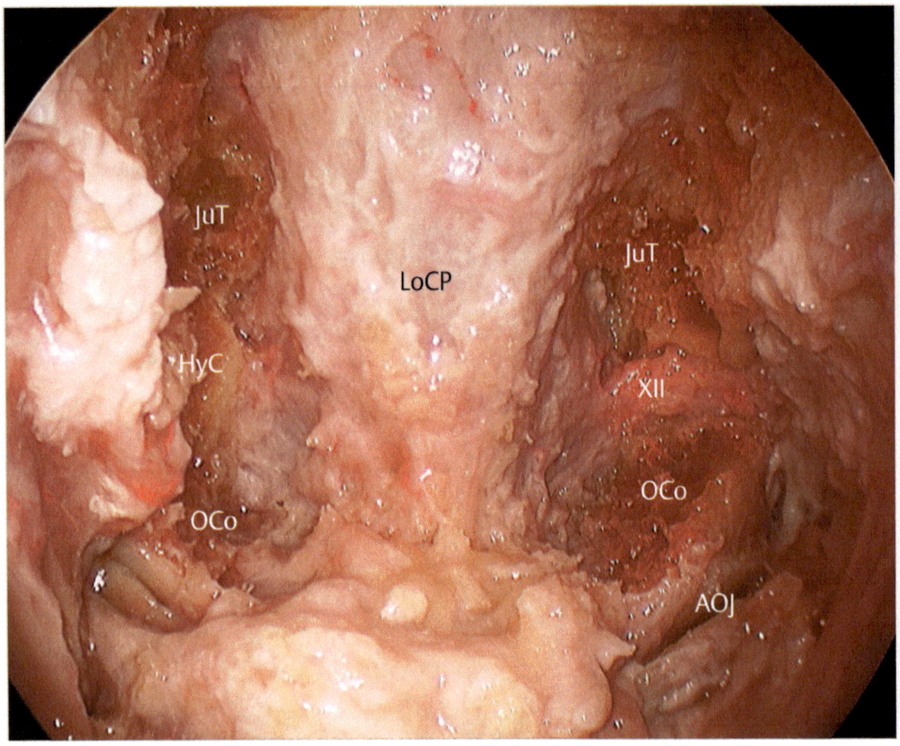

Fig. 22.12 Overview of the jugular tuberculum and the occipital condyle. By comparing the left hypoglossal nerve (XII) with the right hypoglossal canal (HyC), it is clear that the posteromedial opening of this canal corresponds to the lateral limit of the approach through the lower third of the clivus. AOJ, atlanto-occipital joint; JuT, jugular tuberculum; LoCP, periosteum of the lower clivus; OCo, occipital condyle.

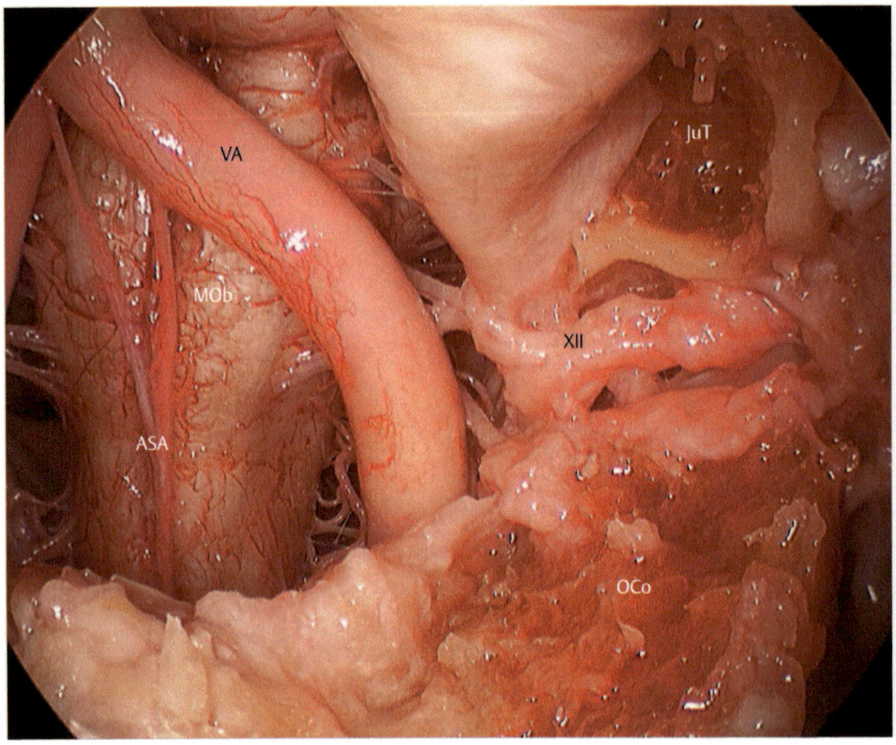

Fig. 22.13 Step 3. The periosteum of the lower clivus and hypoglossal canal is removed to identify the hypoglossal nerve (XII), which crosses the vertebral artery (VA) posteriorly after arising from the medulla oblongata (MOb). ASA, anterior spinal artery; JuT, jugular tuberculum; OCo, occipital condyle.

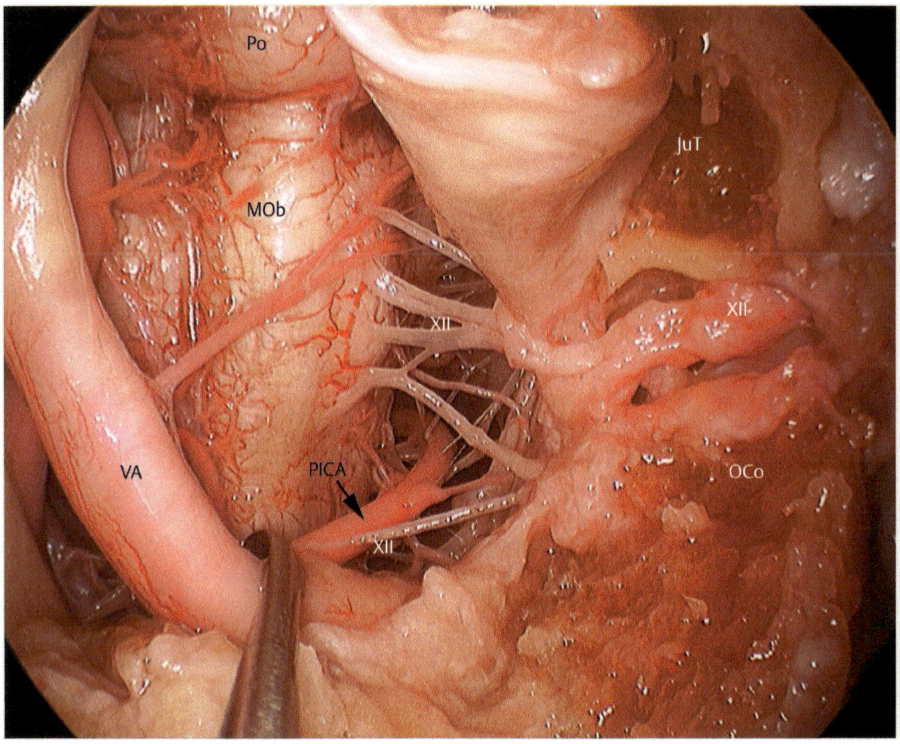

Fig. 22.14 Step 4. The vertebral artery (VA) is displaced medially with a blunt instrument. In this way, the posterior inferior cerebellar artery (PICA), which crosses the rootlets of the hypoglossal nerve (XII), is identified. Most of the lateral medullary cistern and cerebellopontine angle are still covered by the jugular tuberculum (JuT). MOb, medulla oblongata; OCo, occipital condyle; Po, pons.

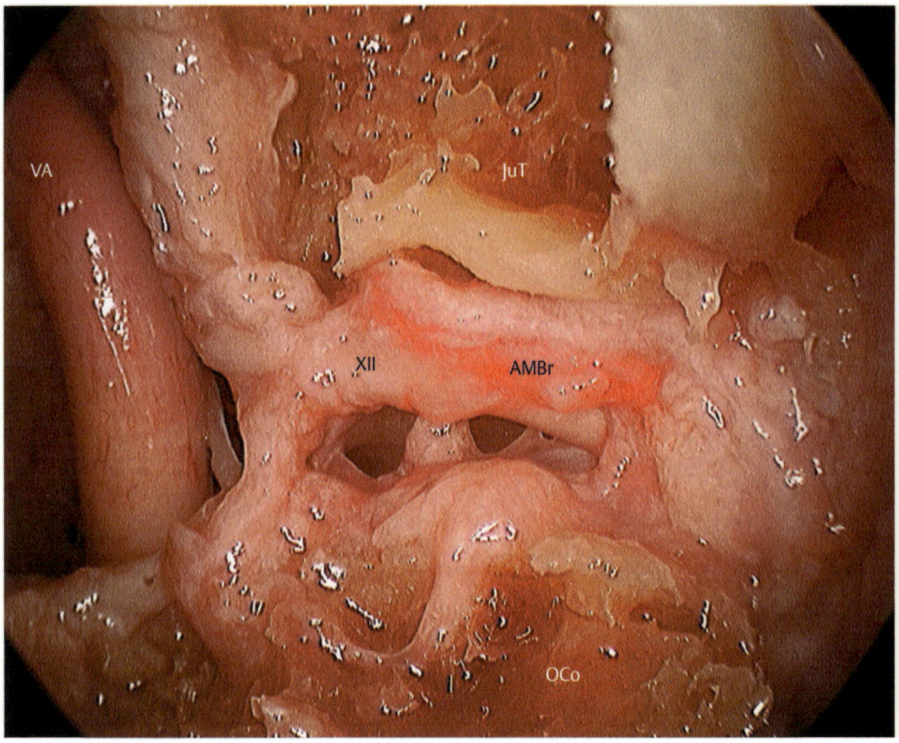

Fig. 22.15 The hypoglossal canal. The hypoglossal canal, also called anterior condylar canal, houses the hypoglossal nerve (XII) and the meningeal branch for the anterior condylar canal (AMBr), which arises from the ascending pharyngeal artery. JuT, jugular tuberculum; OCo, occipital condyle; VA, vertebral artery.

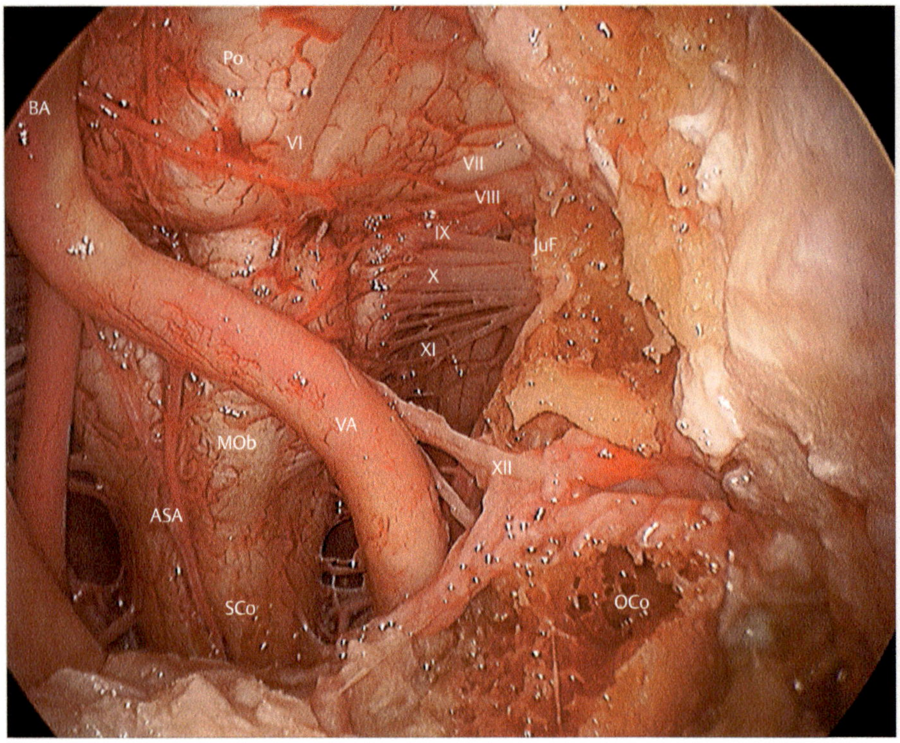

Fig. 22.16 Step 5. Removal of the medial portion of the jugular tuberculum. The cisternal tract of the glossopharyngeal (IX), vagus (X), and spinal accessory (XI) nerves are identified from the medulla oblongata (MOb) to the jugular foramen (JuF). The origin of the facial (VII) and vestibulocochlear (VIII) nerves is identified above the lower cranial nerves and lateral to the abducens nerve (VI). XII, hypoglossal nerve; ASA, anterior spinal artery; BA, basilar artery; OCo, occipital condyle; Po, pons; SCo, spinal cord; VA, vertebral artery.

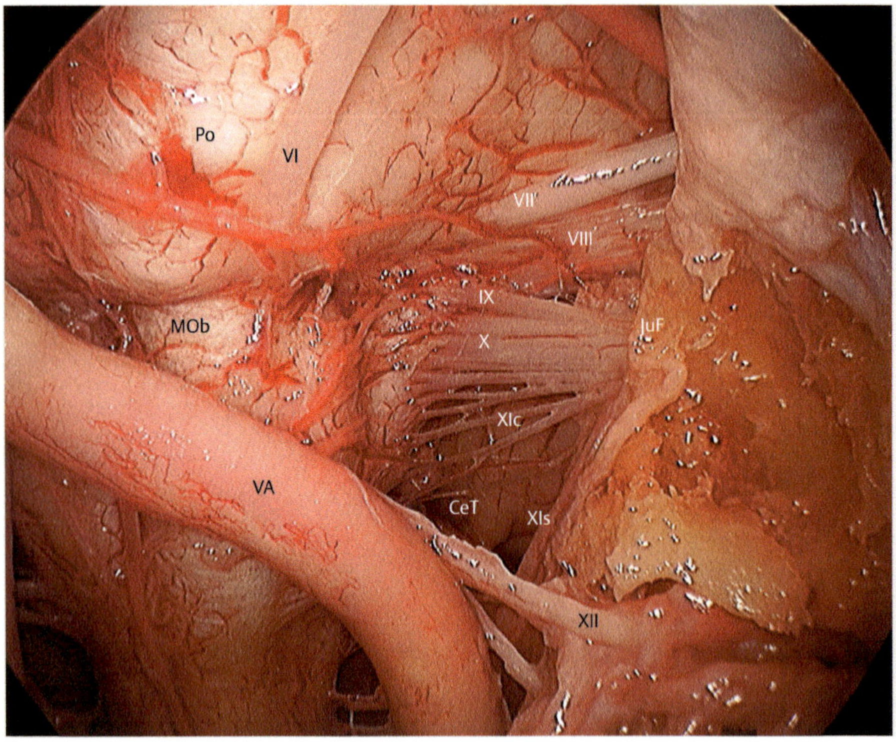

Fig. 22.17 Overview of cranial nerves. The abducens (VI), facial (VII), and vestibulocochlear (VIII) nerves arise from the medial and lateral portions of the lower pons (Po). The lower cranial nerves are represented by the glossopharyngeal (IX), vagus (X), cranial (XIc), and spinal (XIs) roots of the spinal accessory nerve posteriorly and the hypoglossal nerve (XII) anteriorly. The former group of nerves lies in front of the cerebellar tonsil (CeT), whereas the hypoglossal nerve lies behind the vertebral artery (VA). All the lower cranial nerves arise from the medulla oblongata (MOb). JuT, jugular tuberculum.

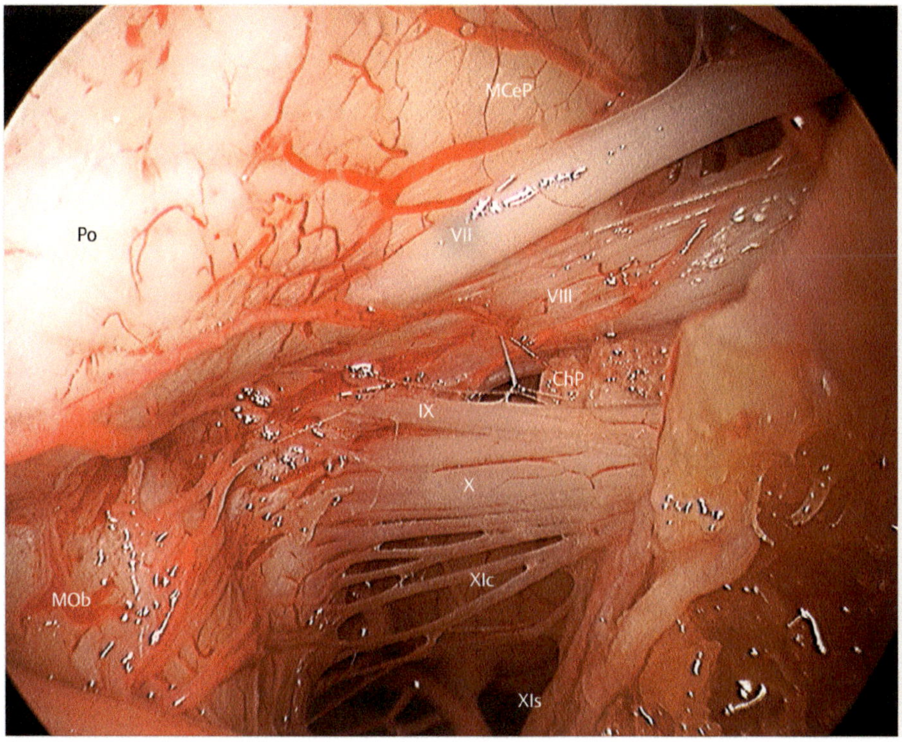

Fig. 22.18 Choroid plexus. The choroid plexus (ChP) originates from the fourth ventricle and reaches this area through the foramen of Luschka. It separates the lower cranial nerves from the acoustic-facial bundle. VII, facial nerve; VIII, vestibulocochlear nerve; IX, glossopharyngeal nerve; X, vagus nerve; XIc, cranial root of the spinal accessory nerve; XIs, spinal root of the spinal accessory nerve; MCeP, middle cerebellar peduncle; MOb, medulla oblongata; Po, pons.

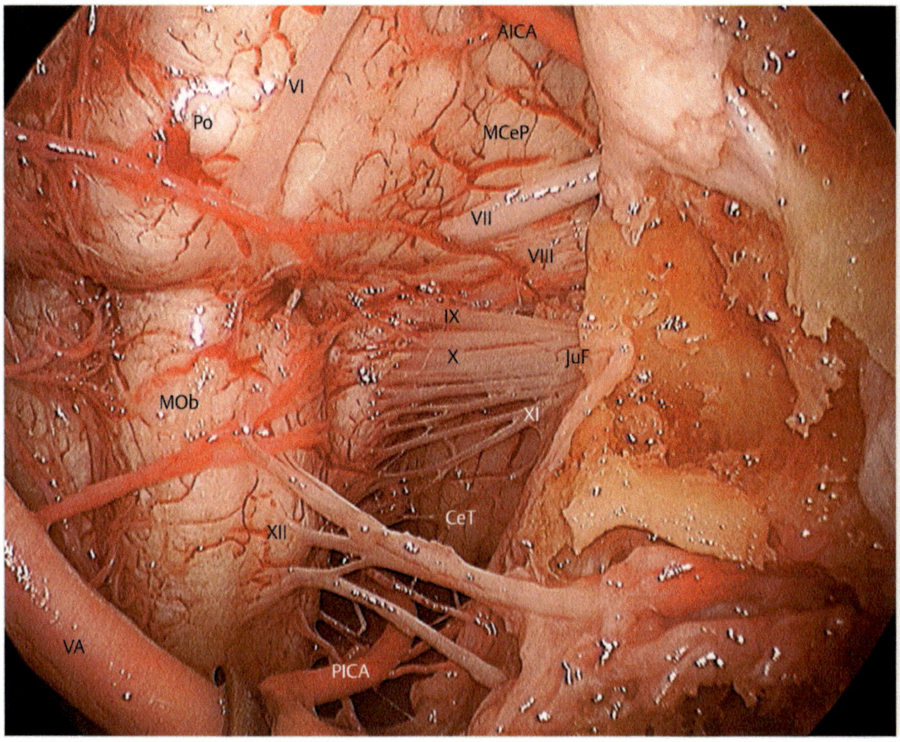

Fig. 22.19 The cerebellopontine angle and the lateral medullary cistern. After medializing the vertebral artery (VA), the entire content of the lateral medullary cistern is identified. The most medial portion of the cerebellopontine pontine cistern is identified above the lower glossopharyngeal (IX), vagus (X), and spinal accessory (XI) nerves. VI, abducens nerve; VII, facial nerve; VIII, vestibulocochlear nerve; XII, hypoglossal nerve; AICA, anterior inferior cerebellar artery; CeT, cerebellar tonsil; JuF, jugular foramen; MCeP, middle cerebellar peduncle; MOb, medulla oblongata; PICA, posterior inferior cerebellar artery; Po, pons.

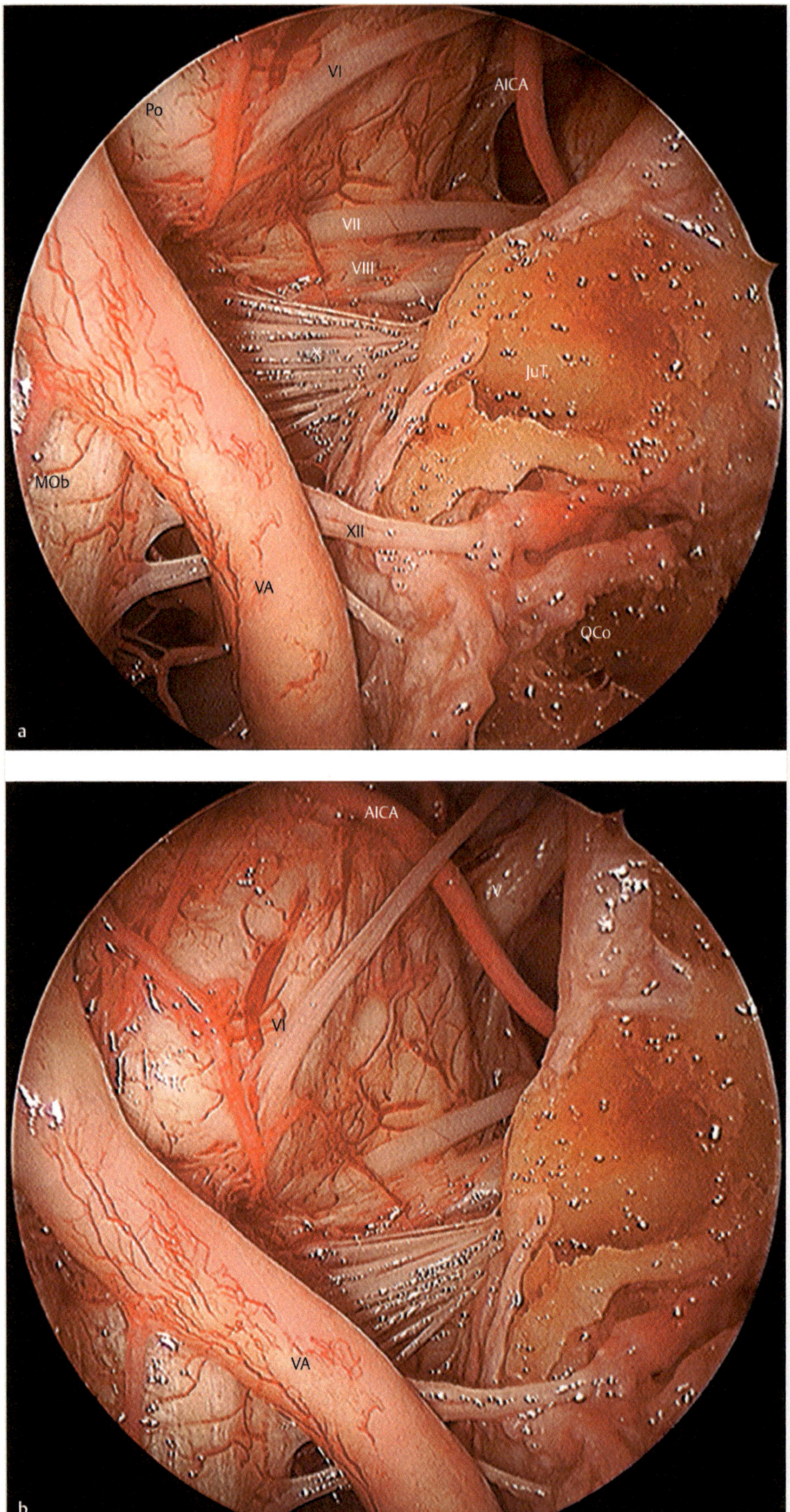

Fig. 22.20 (a, b) The anterior inferior cerebellar artery. With a 70-degree scope turned superolaterally, the anterior inferior cerebellar artery (AICA) is identified. It runs above the abducens nerve (VI) and below the trigeminal stem (V). More laterally, it crosses the acoustic-facial bundle. VII, facial nerve; VIII, vestibulocochlear nerve; X, vagus nerve; XII, hypoglossal nerve; JuT, jugular tuberculum; MOb, medulla oblongata; OCo, occipital condyle; Po, pons; VA, vertebral artery.

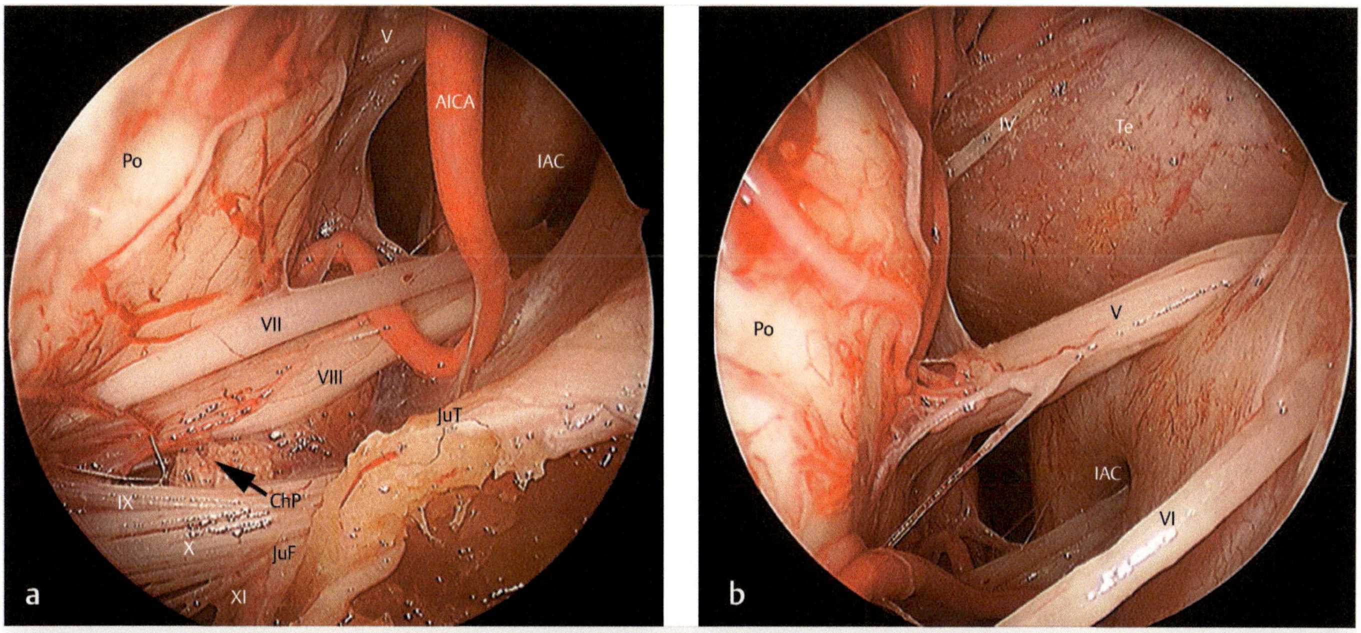

Fig. 22.21 (a, b) The cisternal tracts of the facial, vestibulocochlear, trigeminal, and abducens nerves. The cisternal tracts of the facial (VII) and vestibulocochlear (VIII) nerves run from the pons (Po) to the internal auditory canal (IAC). The anterior inferior cerebellar artery (AICA) commonly passes between the facial and vestibulocochlear nerves. The entire acoustic-facial bundle can be exposed after removal of the jugular tuberculum (JuT), which has to be performed superiorly to the jugular foramen (JuF). The trochlear nerve (IV) enters the inferior surface of the tentorium (Te), while the trigeminal stem (V) passes through the trigeminal porus, which lies below the tentorial insertions and above the petrous ridge. The abducens nerve (VI) enters the basilar plexus medially to the trigeminal stem. IX, glossopharyngeal nerve; X, vagus nerve; XI, spinal accessory nerve; ChP, choroid plexus.

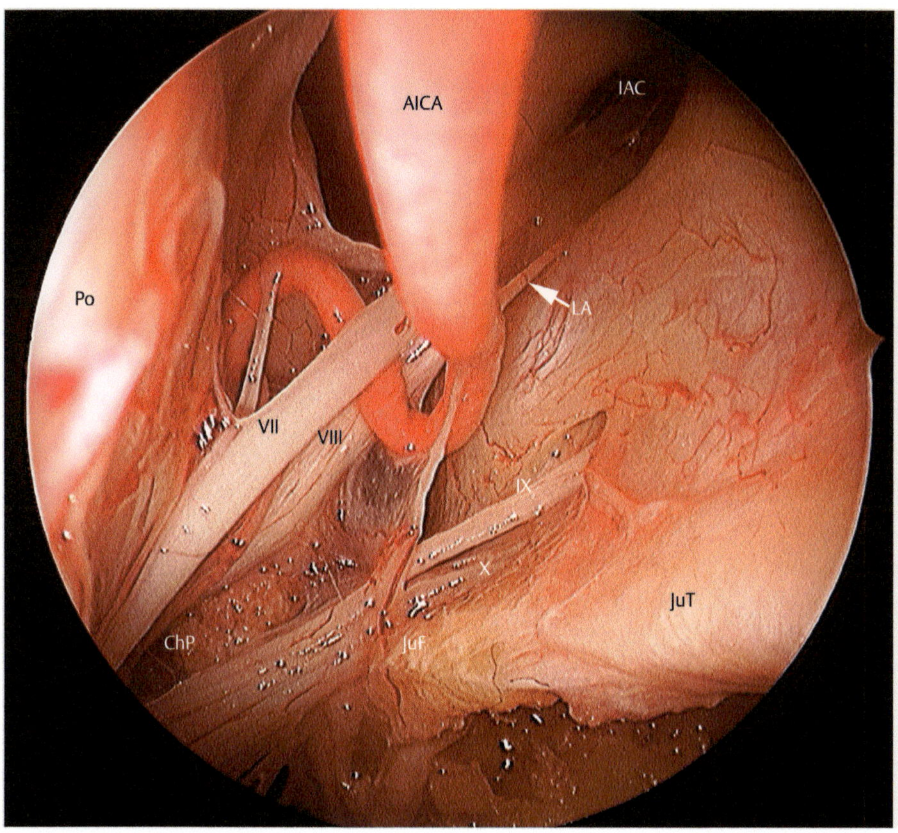

Fig. 22.22 Step 6. With a 70-degree scope turned inferolaterally, the portion of the jugular tuberculum (JuT) that can be removed above the jugular foramen (JuF) comes into view. The removal of the lateral portion of the jugular tuberculum must be performed superiorly to the glossopharyngeal (IX) and vagus (X) nerves. The labyrinthine artery (LA) arises from the anterior inferior cerebellar artery (AICA) and runs toward the internal auditory canal (IAC), parallel to the facial (VII) and vestibulocochlear (VIII) nerves. ChP, choroid plexus; Po, pons.

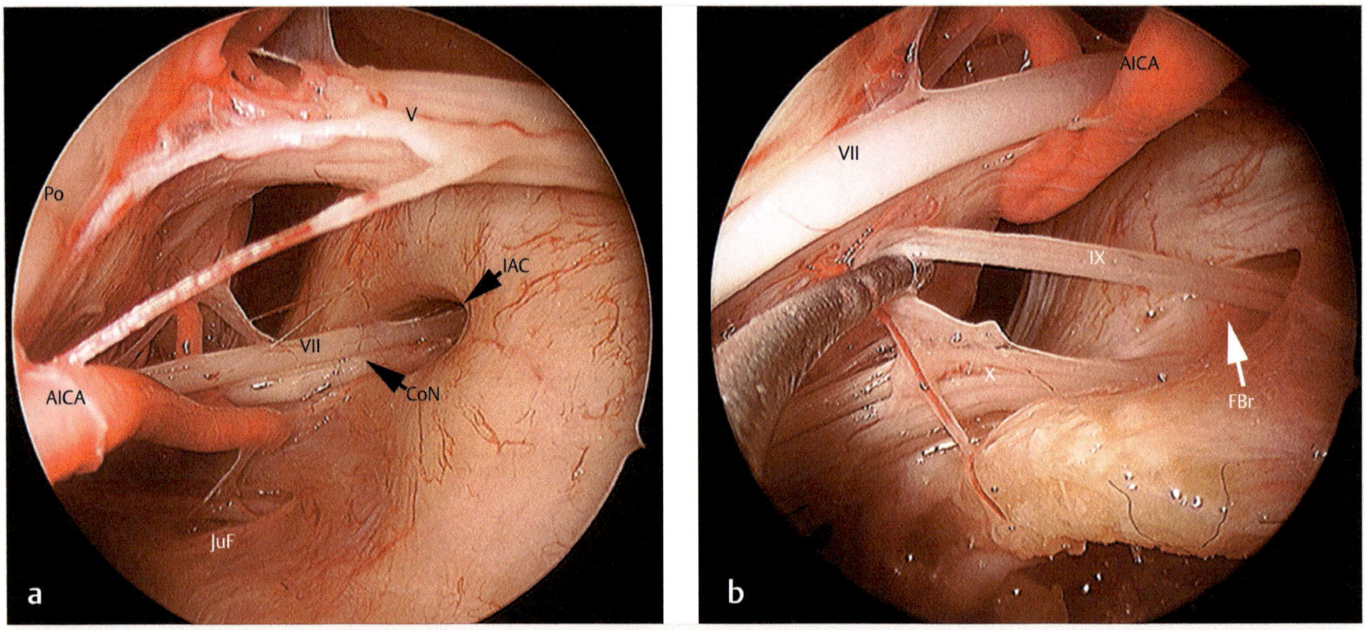

Fig. 22.23 (a, b) The internal auditory canal. After removing the lateral portion of the jugular tuberculum, the jugular foramen (JuF) and internal auditory canal (IAC) can be seen with a 0-degree scope placed through the contralateral nostril. As the internal acoustic canal is reached from anterior, the facial (VII) and cochlear (CoN) nerves are identified, the superior and inferior vestibular nerves being located posteriorly. The glossopharyngeal nerve (IX) enters the jugular foramen separately from the vagus nerve (X). These structures are separated by a fibrous bridge (FBr), which can be ossified. V, trigeminal stem; AICA, anterior inferior cerebellar artery; Po, pons.

References

[1] Morera VA, Fernandez-Miranda JC, Prevedello DM, et al. "Far-medial" expanded endonasal approach to the inferior third of the clivus: the transcondylar and transjugular tubercle approaches. Neurosurgery 2010;66(6, Suppl Operative):211–219, discussion 219–220

[2] Vaz-Guimaraes F, Nakassa ACI, Gardner PA, Wang EW, Snyderman CH, Fernandez-Miranda JC. Endoscopic endonasal approach to the ventral jugular foramen: anatomical basis, technical considerations, and clinical series. Oper Neurosurg (Hagerstown) 2017;13(4):482–491

[3] Solari D, Cappabianca P. Far medial versus far lateral approach: the need of a chamaleontic perspective to unlock a skull base region. World Neurosurg 2014;81(2):279–280

[4] Benet A, Prevedello DM, Carrau RL, et al. Comparative analysis of the transcranial "far lateral" and endoscopic endonasal "far medial" approaches: surgical anatomy and clinical illustration. World Neurosurg 2014;81(2):385–396

[5] Sekhar LN, Tariq F, Osbun J. Far lateral and far medial approaches to the foramen magnum: microsurgery or endoscopy? World Neurosurg 2014;81(2):283–284

[6] Zhang X, Tabani H, El-Sayed I, et al. Combined endoscopic transoral and endonasal approach to the jugular foramen: a multiportal expanded access to the clivus. World Neurosurg 2016;95:62–70

23 Medial Parapharyngeal Approach

Alberto Schreiber, Marco Ferrari, Marco Ravanelli, Vittorio Rampinelli, Davide Lancini

The parapharyngeal space is a suprahyoid infracranial fascial space of the neck, whose shape is typically described as an inverted pyramid.[1] The superior boundary (i.e., the base of the pyramid) corresponds to the inferior surface of the petrous portion of the temporal bone, whereas the apex lies on the posterior end of the greater horn of the hyoid. The parapharyngeal space is enclosed between the prevertebral space, posteriorly, infratemporal fossa (or deep masticatory space) and submandibular fossa, anterolaterally, the parotid space and nodal levels IB and IIA, posterolaterally, and the nasopharynx and oropharynx medially.[2] The parapharyngeal space is further divided into prestyloid and retrostyloid compartments (also called real parapharyngeal space and carotid space, respectively) with respect to the styloid process and related muscles and ligaments.[1] Moreover, the parapharyngeal space can be divided into upper, middle, and lower portions based on the two horizontal planes passing through the inferior border of the lateral pterygoid muscles and mandibular angles.[2,3]

Only the upper parapharyngeal space can be properly exposed via the transnasal pathway, namely, through the lower transpterygoid approach.[2] From a surgical viewpoint, the transnasal parapharyngeal space approach can be divided into a medial and lateral corridor with respect to the lateral pterygoid plate. The medial corridor targets the eustachian tube and related muscles, while the lateral corridor leads to the area of the external carotid foramen, jugular foramen, and related neurovascular structures. This chapter focuses on the endoscopic transnasal approach to the medial portion of the upper parapharyngeal space.

Given the strict relationship with the nasopharynx, the medial portion of the upper parapharyngeal space is particularly prone to be invaded by nasopharyngeal tumors. Moreover, lateral extension of tumors arising into the nasopharynx is favored by the presence of a defect within the pharyngobasilar fascia (called sinus of Morgagni), corresponding to the area where the eustachian tube and levator veli palatini muscle pass from the parapharyngeal space to the nasopharynx forming the torus tubarius. On the other hand, tumors primarily arising from the parapharyngeal space and invading the upper compartment usually extend in the lateral portion (or in both medial and lateral portions), which is composed of smooth structures that are easier to be displaced and compressed by the tumor compared to the eustachian tube and the pterygoid process.

In recent years, the transnasal endoscopic approach to the upper parapharyngeal space has progressively acquired a role in the resection of selected lesions of this area, especially when nonamenable for radical nonsurgical treatment.[4,5] The endoscopic surgical excision of the nasopharynx has been defined as the "nasopharyngeal endoscopic resection" (NER) and classified into three types depending on the extent of resection:[6,7] Type 1 resection is limited to the posterior nasopharyngeal wall; type 2 resection also includes the removal of the nasopharyngeal vault and sphenoidal floor; type 3 resection further requires the resection of the medial portion of the upper parapharyngeal space. The surgical technique is currently employed for recurrent/persistent nasopharyngeal carcinomas originally treated with primary (chemo)radiation, as well as for minor salivary gland tumors, papillary adenocarcinomas, plasmacytomas, sarcomas, mucosal melanomas, and other tumors or tumorlike lesions.[7–11]

The main concern of the surgeon when approaching the medial upper parapharyngeal space is avoiding injury to the parapharyngeal tract of the internal carotid artery. In fact, the combination of a narrow surgical corridor, two-dimensional view, and

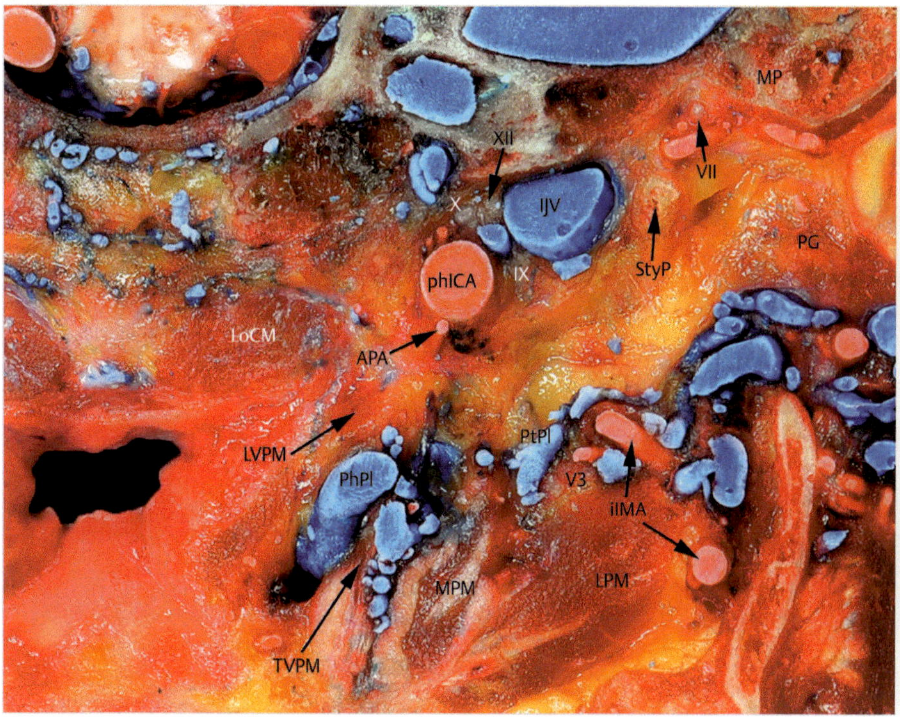

Fig. 23.1 Axial view of the upper parapharyngeal space. This axial cadaver cut shows with a cranial-to-caudal perspective the left upper parapharyngeal space. V3, mandibular nerve; VII, facial nerve (extracranial segment); IX, glossopharyngeal nerve; X, vagus nerve; XII, hypoglossal nerve; APA, ascending pharyngeal artery; iIMA, infratemporal tract of the internal carotid artery; IJV, internal jugular vein; LoCM, longus capitis muscle; LPM, lateral pterygoid muscle; LVPM, levator veli palatini muscle; MP, mastoid process; MPM, medial pterygoid muscle; PG, parotid gland; phICA, parapharyngeal tract of the internal carotid artery; PhPl, pharyngeal plexus; PtPl, pterygoid plexus; StyP, styloid process; TVPM, tensor veli palatini muscle.

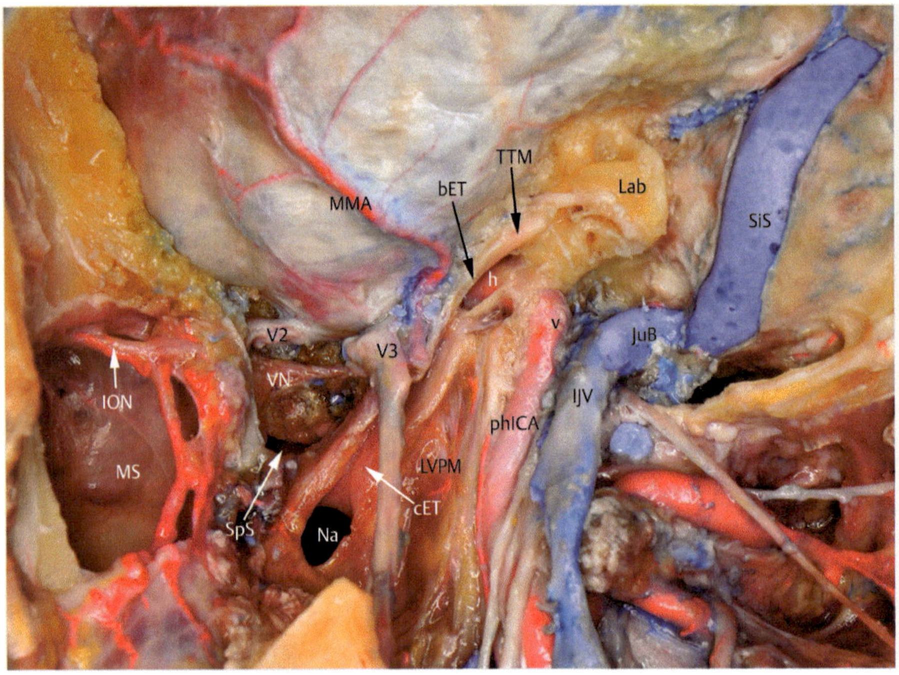

Fig. 23.2 Sagittal lateral-to-medial view of the upper parapharyngeal space. This sagittal cadaver picture shows with a lateral-to-medial perspective the upper parapharyngeal space. V2, maxillary nerve; V3, mandibular nerve; bET, bony portion of the eustachian tube; cET, cartilaginous portion of the eustachian tube; h, horizontal portion of the petrous internal carotid artery; IJV, internal jugular vein; ION, infraorbital nerve; JuB, jugular bulb; Lab, labyrinth; LVPM, levator veli palatini muscle; MMA, middle meningeal artery; MS, maxillary sinus; Na, nasopharynx; phICA, parapharyngeal tract of the internal carotid artery; SiS, sigmoid sinus; SpS, sphenoid sinus; TTM, tensor tympani muscle; v, vertical portion of the petrous internal carotid artery; VN, vidian nerve.

need to manipulate irradiated tissues makes bleeding from the internal carotid artery a dramatic event. To minimize the chance of damaging this vessel, some concepts should be kept in mind: (1) Knowledge of bony anatomical landmarks (including the lateral pterygoid plate, foramen ovale, foramen spinosum, musculotubal canal)[6,7,12,13] and fascial anatomical planes (such as the plane guiding to the internal carotid artery between the medial pterygoid muscle and the tensor veli palatini muscle)[14] is of utmost importance to identify the position of the internal carotid artery in the surgical field. (2) The endoscopic perspective adopted during the critical phases of dissection should be carefully chosen to avoid disorientation and favor safe directions for surgical instruments; in particular, the ipsilateral perspective provides the best combination in terms of reliability of anatomical landmarks and safety of dissection trajectories.[15] (3) An in-depth analysis of the course of the internal carotid artery at preoperative imaging and use of a Doppler probe and navigation system are extremely helpful to identify unfavorable anatomic situations (e.g., medial kinking of the internal carotid artery) and localize the vessel at surgery, respectively.

The endoscopic transnasal approach to the upper parapharyngeal space requires the harvesting of a transmaxillary corridor to laterally displace the content of the pterygopalatine fossa and expose the pterygoid process. Up to this step, the dissection can be performed taking advantage of the avascular subperiosteal planes to maintain a clean surgical field. The lower transpterygoid route (i.e., the route through pterygoid plates, sparing the base of the pterygoid process) is then employed to gain access to the pterygoid fossa and subsequently reach the parapharyngeal space. During this part of the dissection, several venous plexuses, vessels, and muscles are encountered, which are a considerable source of bleeding.

Given the impossibility to reach the entire parapharyngeal space via a transnasal route, the approach presented in this chapter fits particularly well with the concept of multiportal surgery. In lesions of the parapharyngeal space also invading the related skull base, surgery should be accurately planned, considering the possibility to combine nondisruptive surgical corridors (i.e., transnasal, transoral, transorbital, transcervical, transpetrosal) to manage advanced lesions. Likewise, the endoscopic parapharyngeal space approach can be combined with transnasal corridors targeting adjacent areas (i.e., infrapetrous, suprapetrous, transcondylar–transjugular tuberculum, medial petrous apex, infratemporal) when addressing extended skull base lesions.

As a final remark, it is worth mentioning that, especially in irradiated patients, wide resections of the upper parapharyngeal space with exposure of the overlying skull base and internal carotid artery frequently require reconstruction to avoid severe complications such as skull base osteitis/osteomyelitis or vessel blowout. Therefore, the surgical team performing the resection should also plan to resurface the defect with one of the many available local/regional reconstructive options (i.e., nasoseptal flap, lateral nasal wall flap, temporoparietal fascia flap).

The reader is asked to perform dissection of the upper parapharyngeal space both focusing on the numerous anatomical details of this anatomical area and keeping in mind the surgical aspects that have been emphasized in the present introduction.

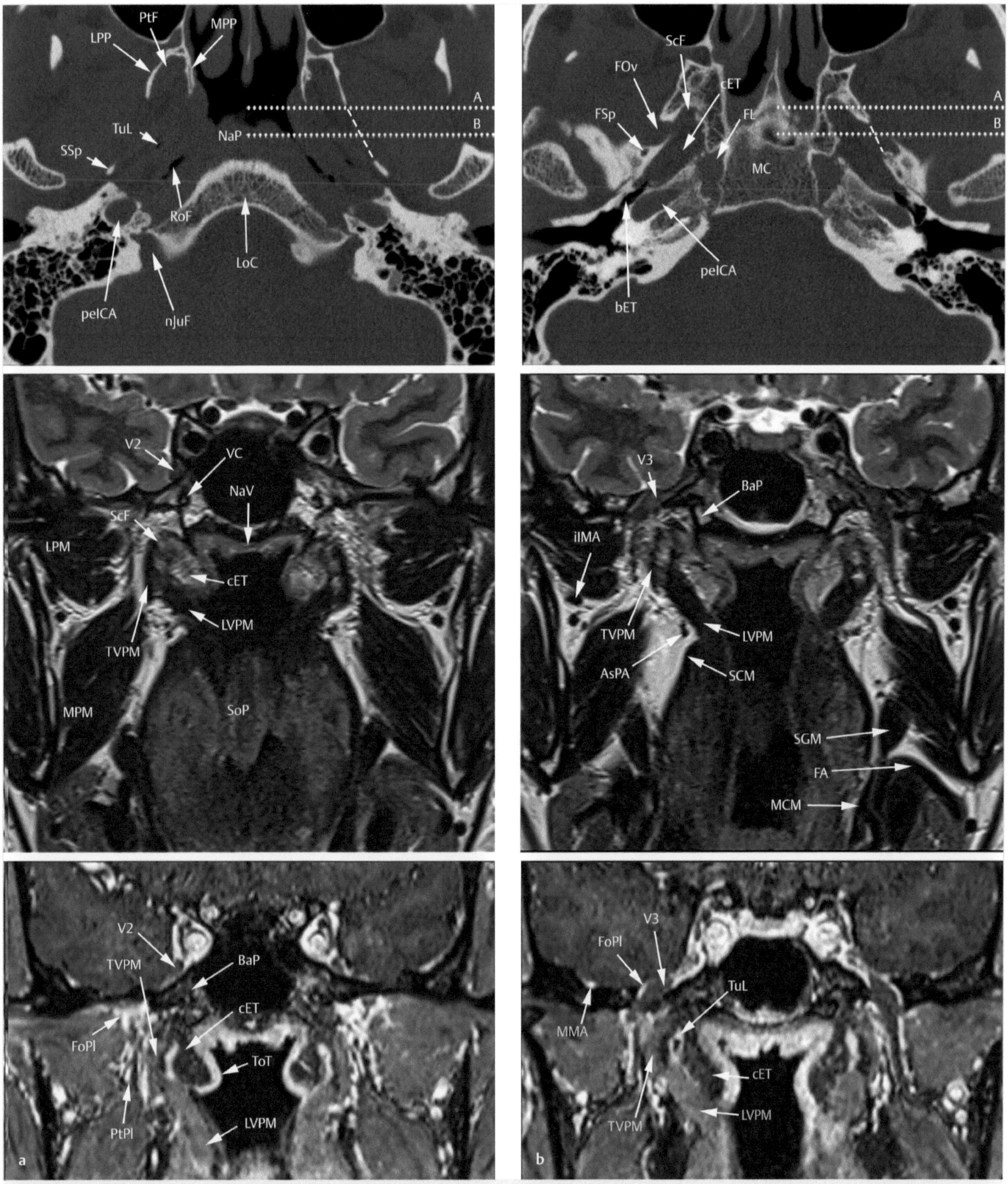

Fig. 23.3 CT and MRI anatomy of the upper parapharyngeal space and related skull base. The panel includes two axial CT scans passing through the upper parapharyngeal space (upper left image) and related skull base (upper right image) and two columns of coronal MRI (A and B), whose position is depicted by *white dotted lines*. The upper parapharyngeal space is enclosed by the nasopharynx medially, pterygoid fossa (PtF) anteriorly, infratemporal fossa anterolaterally, prevertebral fascia posteriorly, skull base cranially, and axial plane passing through the inferior border of the lateral pterygoid muscle (LPM) caudally. The medial portion of the upper parapharyngeal space lies medially to the plane (*white dashed line*) joining the lateral pterygoid plate (LPP) and spina sphenoidalis (SSp). This space includes the cartilaginous eustachian tube (cET), tensor veli palatini muscle (TVPM), and levator veli palatini muscle (LVPM). V2, maxillary nerve; V3, mandibular nerve; AsPA, ascending palatine artery; BaP, basipterygoid; bET, bony eustachian tube; FA, facial artery; FL, foramen lacerum; FoPl, foraminal plexus; FOv, foramen ovale; FSp, foramen spinosum; iIMA, infratemporal tract of the internal maxillary artery; LoC, lower clivus; LPP, lateral pterygoid plate; MC, midclivus; MCM, middle constrictor muscle; MMA, middle meningeal artery; MPM, medial pterygoid muscle; MPP, medial pterygoid plate; NaP, nasopharyngeal posterior wall; NaV, nasopharyngeal vault; nJuF, nervous compartment of the jugular foramen; peICA, petrous tract of the internal carotid artery; PtPl, pterygoid plexus; RoF, Rosenmüller's fossa; ScF, scaphoid fossa; SCM, superior constrictor muscle; SGM, styloglossus muscle; SoP, soft palate; ToT, torus tubarius; TTM, tensor tympani muscle; TuL, tubal lumen; VC, vidian canal.

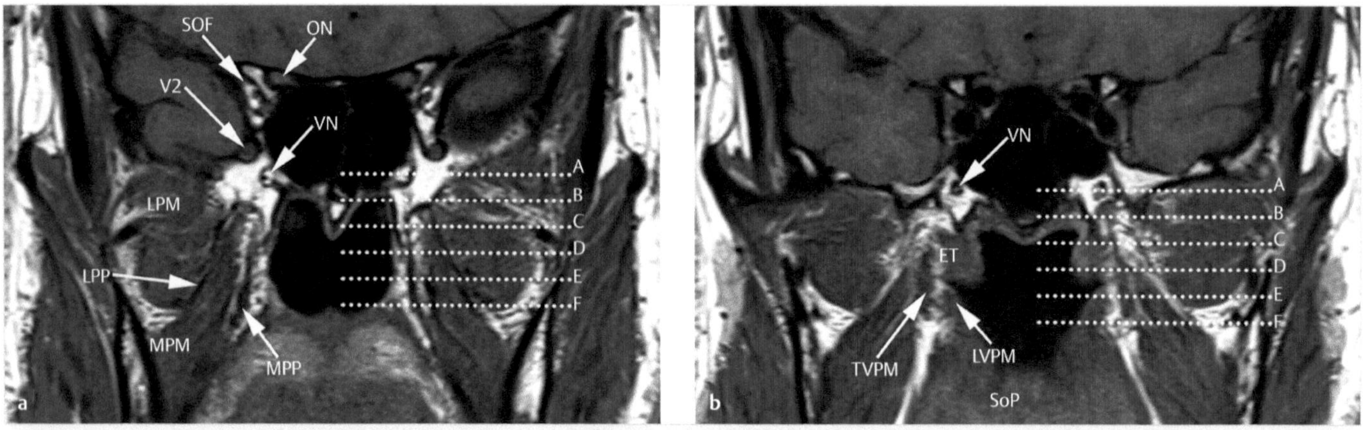

Fig. 23.4 (a, b) Coronal T1-weighted MRI scan of the pterygoid process. As seen from a coronal perspective, the upper parapharyngeal space lies behind the pterygoid process and related muscles. Six *white dotted lines* (A–F) depict the position of images making up ▶Fig. 23.5 and ▶Fig. 23.6. V2, maxillary nerve; ET, eustachian tube; LPM, lateral pterygoid muscle; LPP, lateral pterygoid plate; LVPM, levator veli palatini muscle; MPM, medial pterygoid muscle; MPP, medial pterygoid plate; ON, optic nerve; SOF, superior orbital fissure; SoP, soft palate; TVPM, tensor veli palatini muscle; VN, vidian nerve.

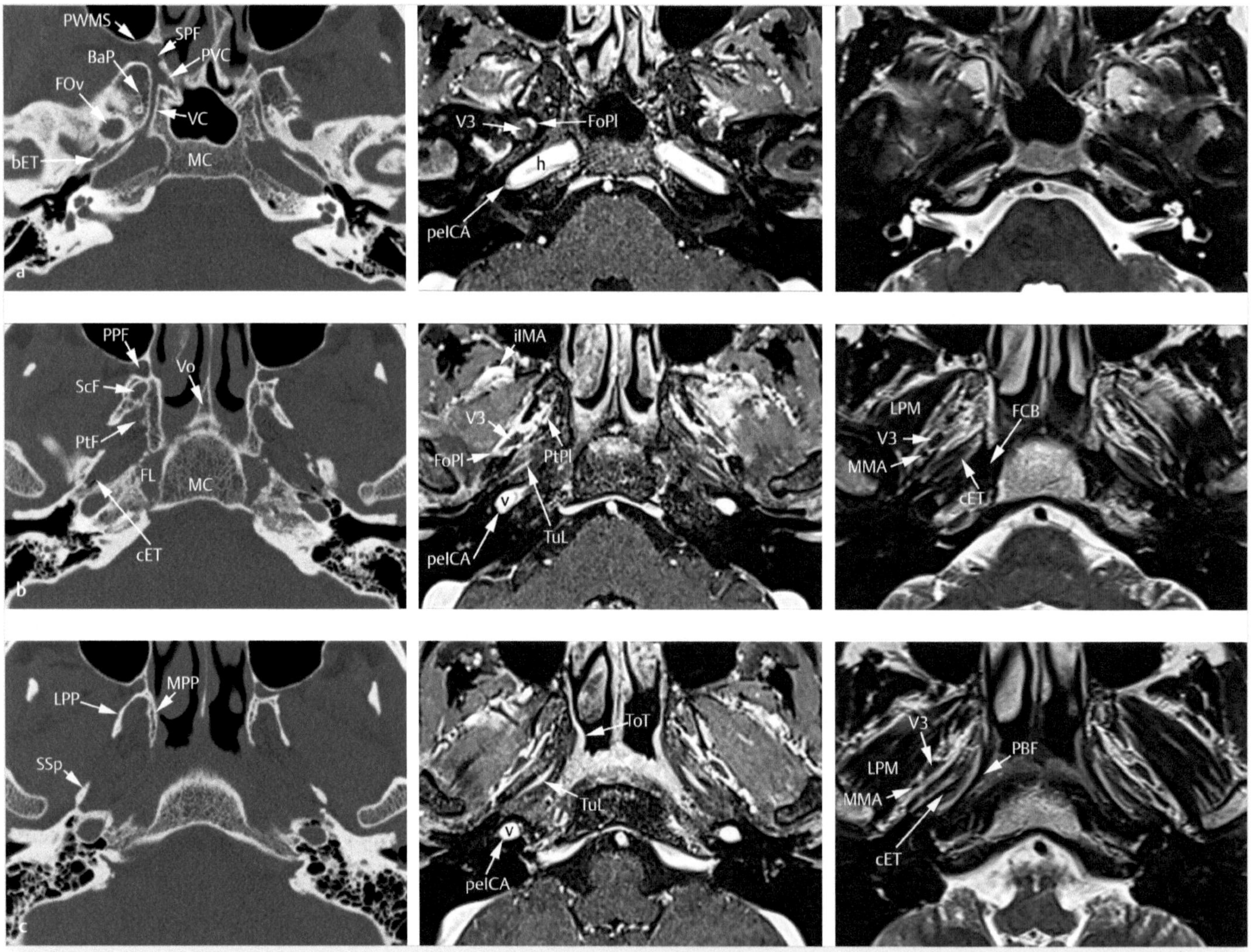

Fig. 23.5 Axial CT and MRI of the upper parapharyngeal space and adjacent structures (part 1). The panel shows three rows of axial CT (left images), contrast-enhanced T1-weighted (middle images), and T2-weighted MRI (right images). From anterior to posterior, the upper parapharyngeal space can be reached passing through a multilayer anatomical area, including the posterior wall of the maxillary sinus (PWMS), pterygopalatine fossa (PPF), medial (MPP) and lateral pterygoid plates (LPP), scaphoid fossa (ScF), and pterygoid fossa (PtF). The lateral pterygoid plate is aligned with the foramen ovale (FOv), spina sphenoidalis (SSp), foramen spinosum (FSp), and related structures, including the mandibular nerve (V3), foraminal plexus (FoPl), and middle meningeal artery (MMA). The cartilaginous portion of the eustachian tube (cET) lies immediately posterior to the mandibular nerve. The vertical segment (v) of the petrous tract of the internal carotid artery (peICA) runs just behind the junction between the bony (bET) and cartilaginous eustachian tube. BaP, basipterygoid; FCB, fibrocartilago basalis; FL, foramen lacerum; h, horizontal segment of the petrous tract of the internal carotid artery; iIMA, infratemporal tract of the internal maxillary artery; LPM, lateral pterygoid muscle; MC, midclivus; PBF, pharyngobasilar fascia; PtPl, pterygoid plexus; PVC, palatovaginal canal; SPF, sphenopalatine foramen; ToT, torus tubarius; TuL, tubal lumen; VC, vidian canal; Vo, vomer.

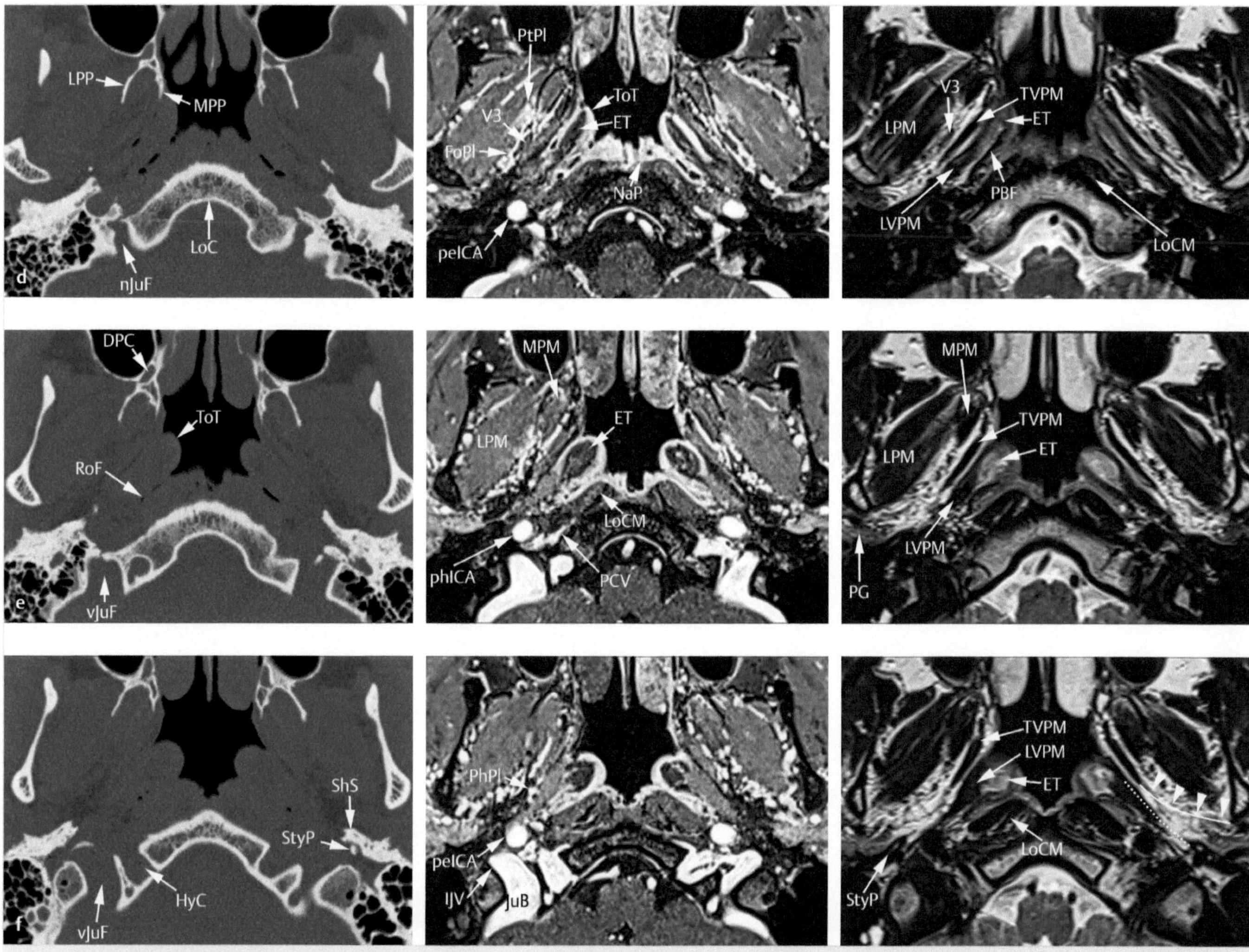

Fig. 23.6 Axial CT and MRI of the upper parapharyngeal space and adjacent structures (part 2). Both the tensor veli palatini muscle (TVPM) and the levator veli palatini muscle (LVPM) follow the direction of the eustachian tube (ET) to reach the soft palate. The tensor veli palatini muscle passes outside from the pharyngobasilar fascia (PBF) and reaches the soft palate after turning around the pterygoid hamulus. The levator veli palatini muscle runs through the pharyngobasilar fascia together with the eustachian tube via a defect called the sinus of Morgagni. The anatomical boundary between the infratemporal fossa (also called deep masticatory space) and the upper parapharyngeal space is the interpterygoid fascia (*white lines with arrowheads* in the lower right image), which joins the mandible and tensor veli palatini muscle and forms the cranial portion of the superficial layer of the deep cervical fascia. The stylopharyngeal diaphragm, or fascia, joins the styloid process (StyP) with the levator veli palatini muscle and serves as separation between the prestyloid and retrostyloid compartments of the upper parapharyngeal space. Therefore, transnasal parapharyngeal approaches that cross both these muscles unavoidably transgress the medial portion of the infratemporal fossa. V3, mandibular nerve; HyC, hypoglossal canal; IJV, internal jugular vein; JuB, jugular bulb; LoC, lower clivus; LoCM, longus capitis muscle; LPM, lateral pterygoid muscle; LPP, lateral pterygoid plate; MPM, medial pterygoid muscle; MPP, medial pterygoid plate; NaP, nasopharyngeal posterior wall; nJuF, nervous compartment of the jugular foramen; PCV, petroclival vein; PG, parotid gland; phICA, parapharyngeal tract of the internal carotid artery; PhPl, pharyngeal plexus; PtPl, pterygoid plexus; RoF, Rosenmüller's fossa; ShS, sheath of the styloid process; ToT, torus tubarius; vJuF, vascular compartment of the jugular foramen.

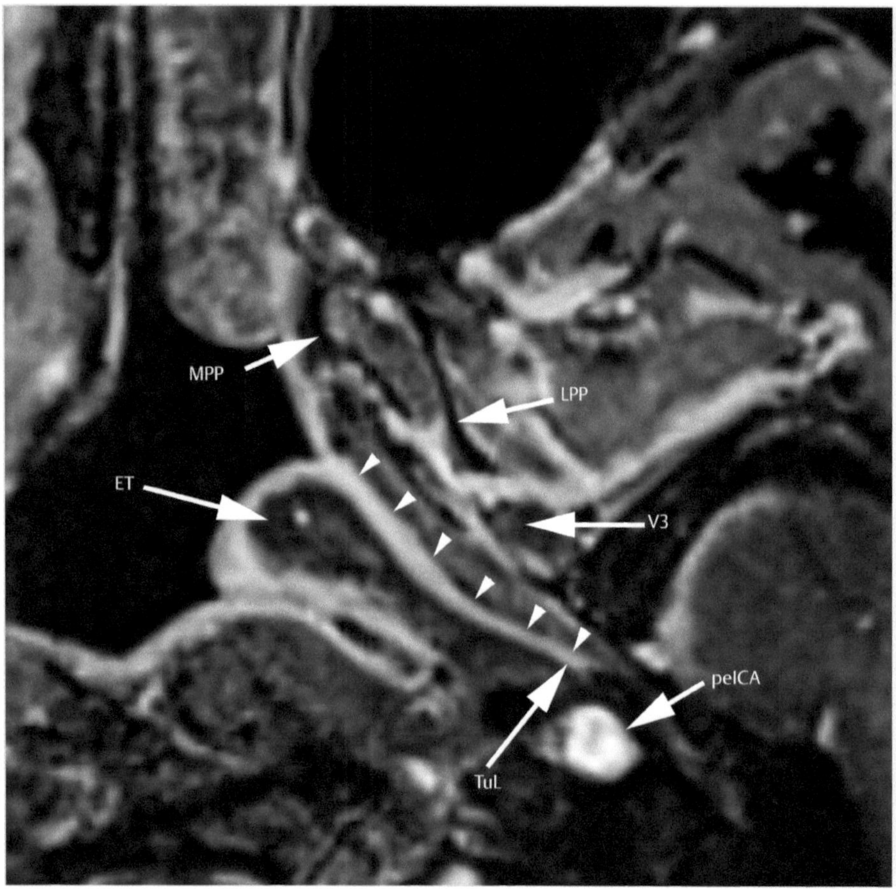

Fig. 23.7 MRI para-axial scan parallel to the path of the eustachian tube depicting the "parapharyngeal carrefour." The understanding of the three-dimensional relationship between the mandibular nerve (V3), eustachian tube (ET), and internal carotid artery is of utmost importance. Both the mandibular nerve and the parapharyngeal and vertical petrous tracts of the internal carotid artery (peICA) run with a vertical trajectory and are separated by the eustachian tube, which can be seen along its entire course due to enhancement of the mucosa of the tubal lumen (TuL; *white arrowheads*). MPP, medial pterygoid plate; LPP, lateral pterygoid plate.

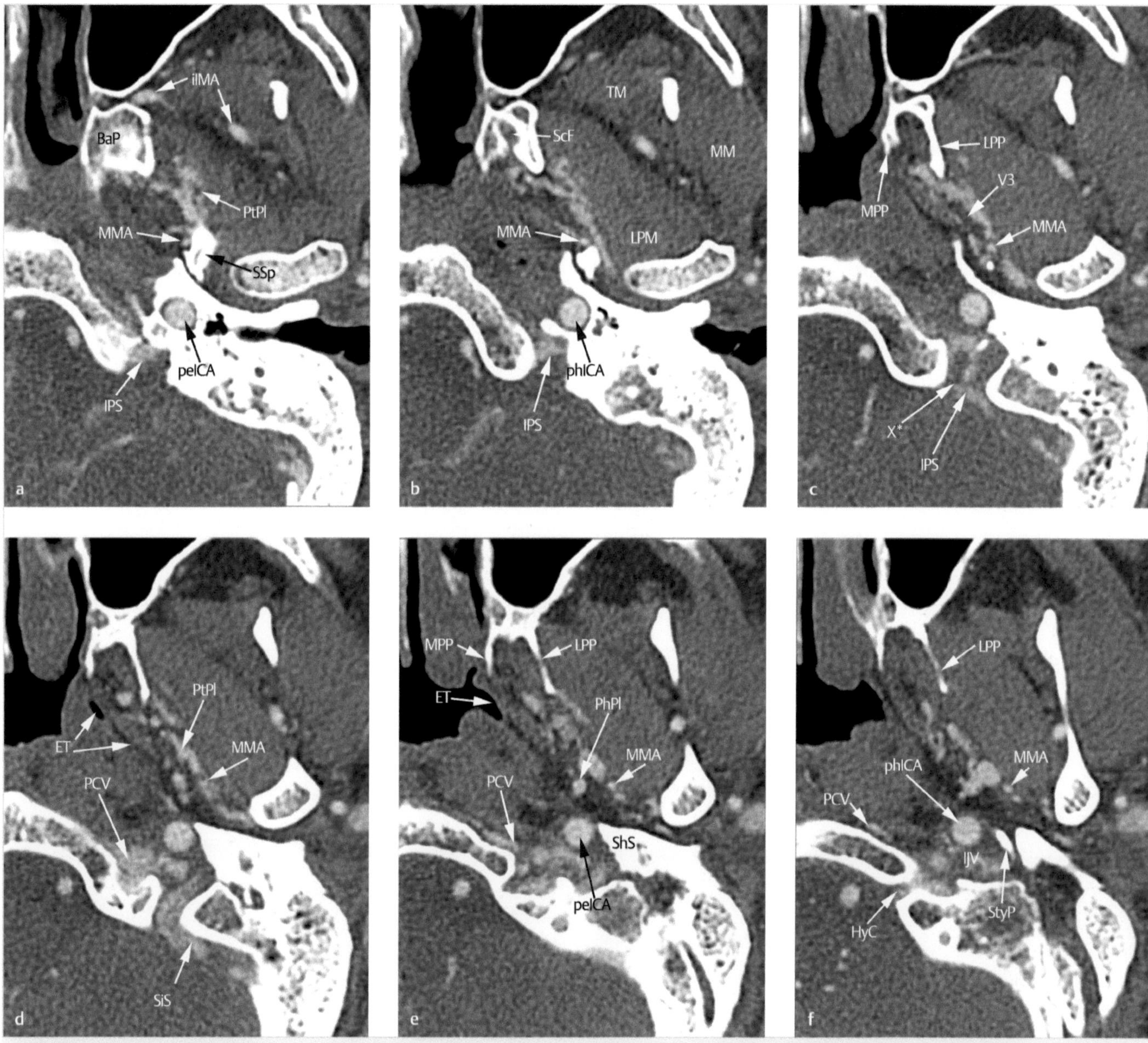

Fig. 23.8 (a–f) Contrast-enhanced CT axial anatomy of the parapharyngeal space and adjacent areas. The panel includes six axial contrast-enhanced CT scan, from cranial **(a)** to caudal **(f)**. The upper parapharyngeal space is adjacent to the infratemporal fossa anterolaterally, which includes the temporal muscle (TM), masseteric muscle (MM), lateral pterygoid muscle (LPM), and medial pterygoid muscle, which are surrounded and intersected by the pterygoid plexus (PtPl), infratemporal tract of the internal maxillary artery (iIMA), and branches of the mandibular nerve (V3). The retrostyloid compartment of the upper parapharyngeal space continues posteriorly into the area of the jugular foramen, which houses the internal jugular vein (IJV), petroclival vein (PCV), and the group of lower cranial nerves (X*). BaP, basipterygoid; ET, eustachian tube; HyC, hypoglossal canal; IPS, inferior petrosal sinus; LPP, lateral pterygoid plate; MMA, middle meningeal artery; MPP, medial pterygoid plate; peICA, petrous tract of the internal carotid artery; phICA, parapharyngeal tract of the internal carotid artery; PhPl, pharyngeal plexus; ScF, scaphoid fossa; ShS, sheath of the styloid process; SiS, sigmoid sinus; SSp, spinal sphenoidalis; StyP, styloid process.

Endoscopic Dissection

Nasal Phase

- Anterior and posterior ethmoidectomy.
- Transethmoidal sphenoidotomy.
- Removal of the sphenoid sinus floor.
- Type D endoscopic medial maxillectomy.

Skull Base Phase

- Step 1: Exposure of the descending palatine canal and removal of the posterior wall of the maxillary sinus medial to the infraorbital canal.
- Step 2: Lateralization of the content of the pterygopalatine fossa.
- Step 3: Removal of the perpendicular plate of the palatine bone.
- Step 4: Removal of the medial pterygoid plate.
- Step 5: Partial removal of the base of the pterygoid process.
- Step 6: Removal of the tensor veli palatini muscle.
- Step 7: Removal of the levator veli palatini muscle.
- Step 8: Removal of the eustachian tube.
- Step 9: Opening of the carotid sheath.
- Step 10: Removal of the prevertebral fascia.
- Step 11: Medial paracarotid dissection.
- Step 12: Lateral paracarotid dissection.

Lower Transpterygoid Approach

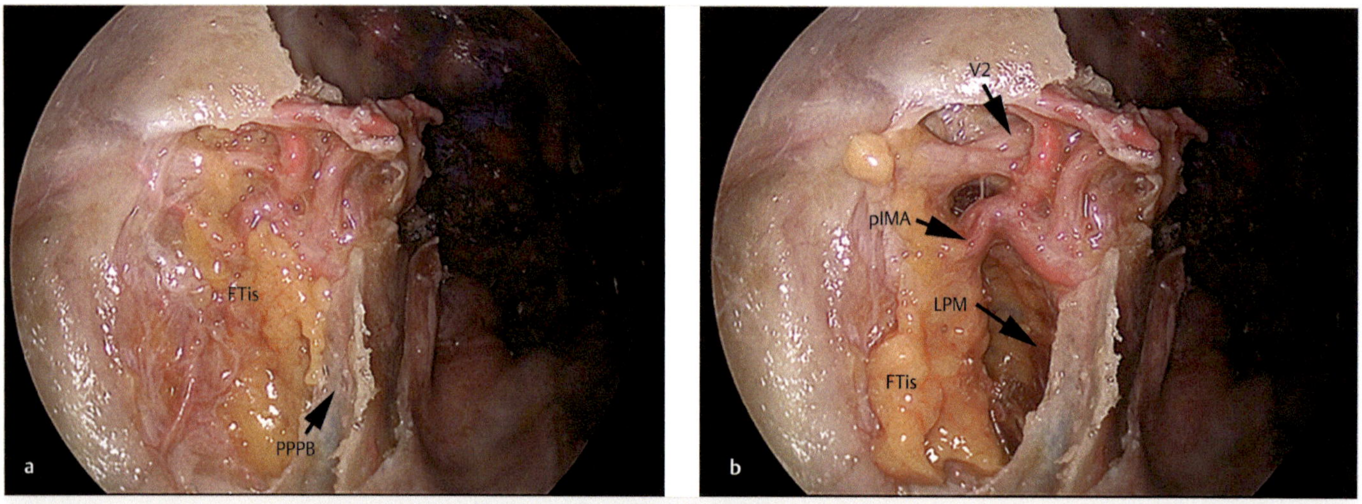

Fig. 23.9 (a, b) Step 1. After removing the medial portion of the posterior maxillary wall, the fat tissue (FTis) inside the pterygopalatine fossa is laterally displaced to expose the maxillary nerve (V2), the pterygopalatine tract of the internal maxillary artery (pIMA), and the lateral pterygoid muscle (LPM). The descending palatine canal is formed by the perpendicular process of the palatine bone (PPPB) anteriorly and the pterygoid process of the sphenoid bone posteriorly.

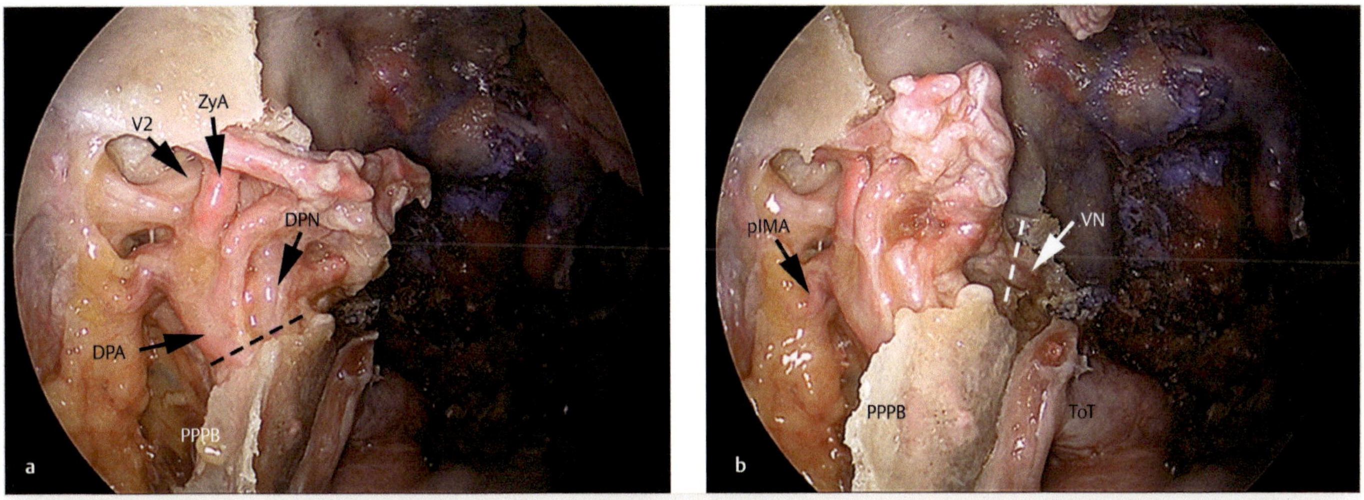

Fig. 23.10 (a, b) Step 2. The descending palatine artery (DPA) and nerve (DPN) as well as the vidian nerve (VN) are cut (*black and white dashed lines*), enabling lateralization of the content of the pterygopalatine fossa. V2, maxillary nerve; pIMA, pterygopalatine tract of the internal maxillary artery; PPPB, perpendicular plate of the palatine bone; ToT, torus tubarius; ZyA, zygomatic artery.

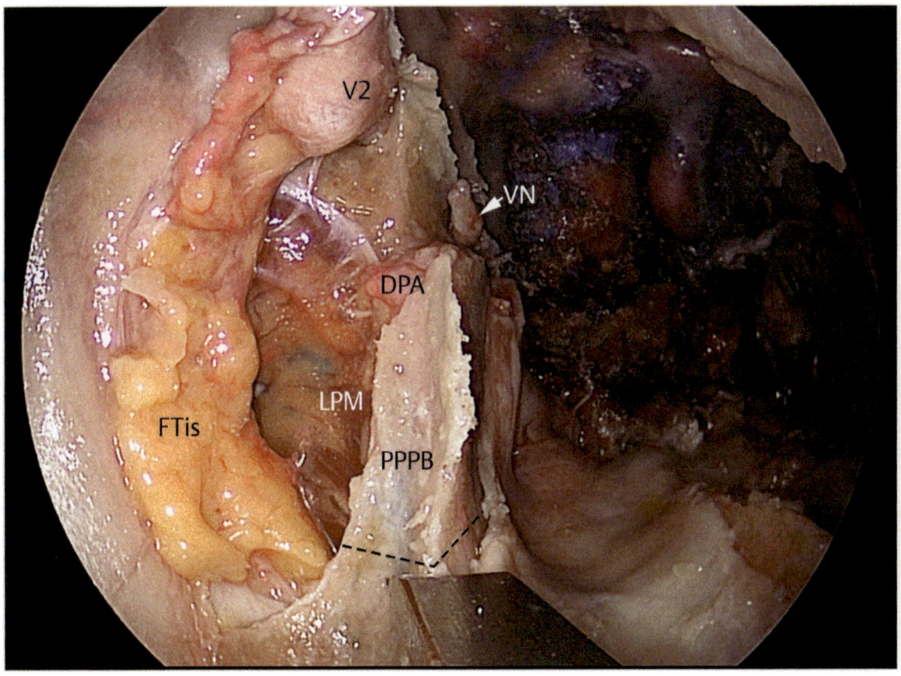

Fig. 23.11 Step 3 (part 1). The perpendicular plate of the palatine bone (PPPB) is fractured with a chisel at its base (*black dashed line*). V2, maxillary nerve; DPA, descending palatine artery (sectioned); FTis, fat tissue; LPM, lateral pterygoid muscle; VN, vidian nerve (sectioned).

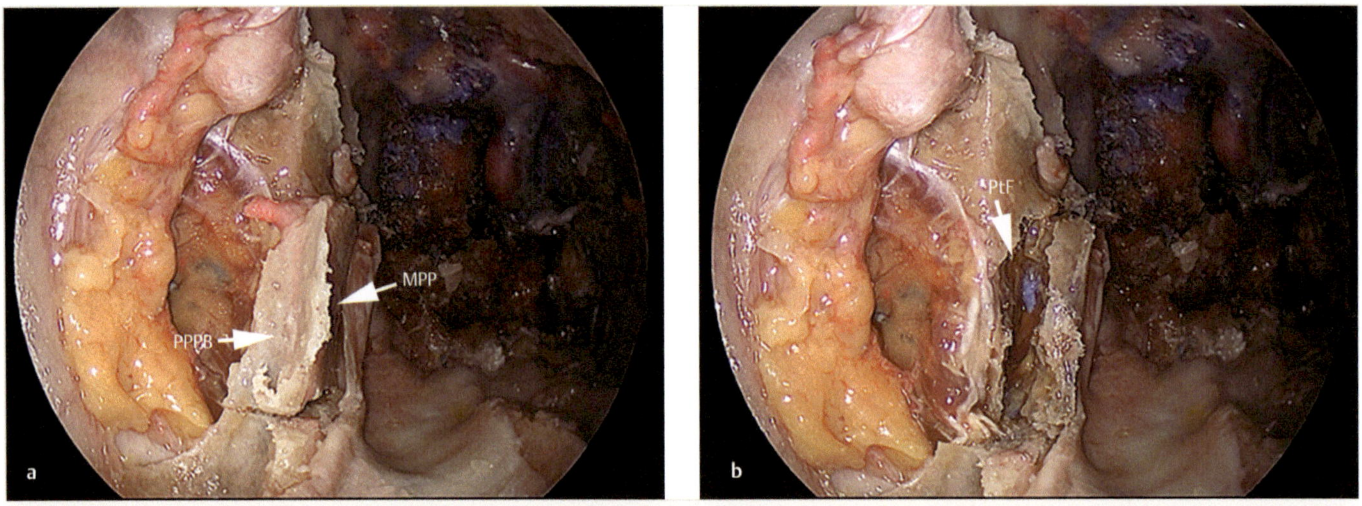

Fig. 23.12 (a, b) Step 3 (part 2). After being fractured, the perpendicular plate of the palatine bone (PPPB) is turned medially together with the medial pterygoid plate (MPP) to expose the pterygoid fossa (PtF).

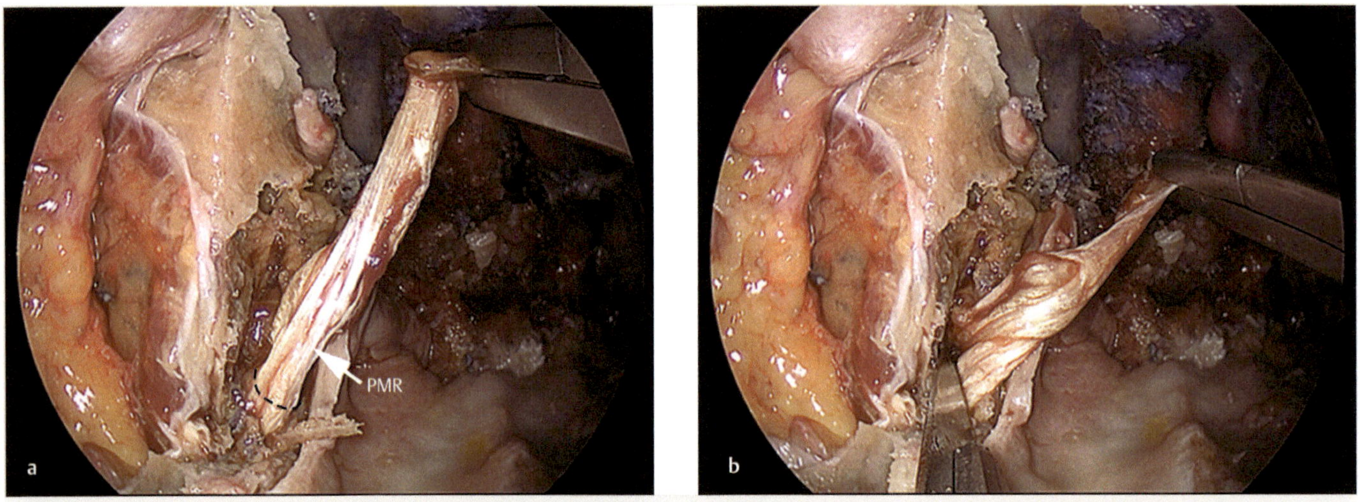

Fig. 23.13 (a, b) Step 4. While removing the medial pterygoid plate, the pterygomandibular raphe (PMR) is pulled superiorly as it is still attached to the inferior portion of this bony structure, which is called the pterygoid hamulus. The pterygomandibular raphe is cut inferiorly (*black dashed line*).

Medial Parapharyngeal Approach

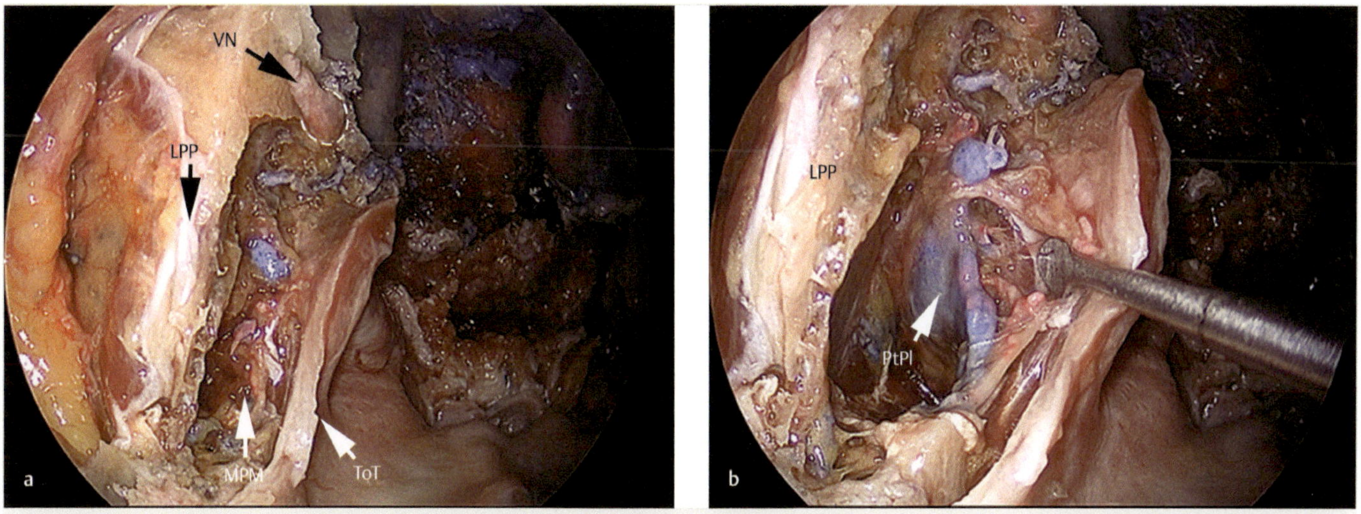

Fig. 23.14 (a, b) Step 5. The proximal insertion of the medial pterygoid muscle (MPM) is partially removed to identify the deep portion of the pterygoid venous plexus (PtPl) within the pterygoid fossa. The lateral pterygoid plate (LPP) is left intact, while the basipterygoid is progressively removed below the vidian canal (*white dashed line*) and its nerve (VN). ToT, torus tubarius.

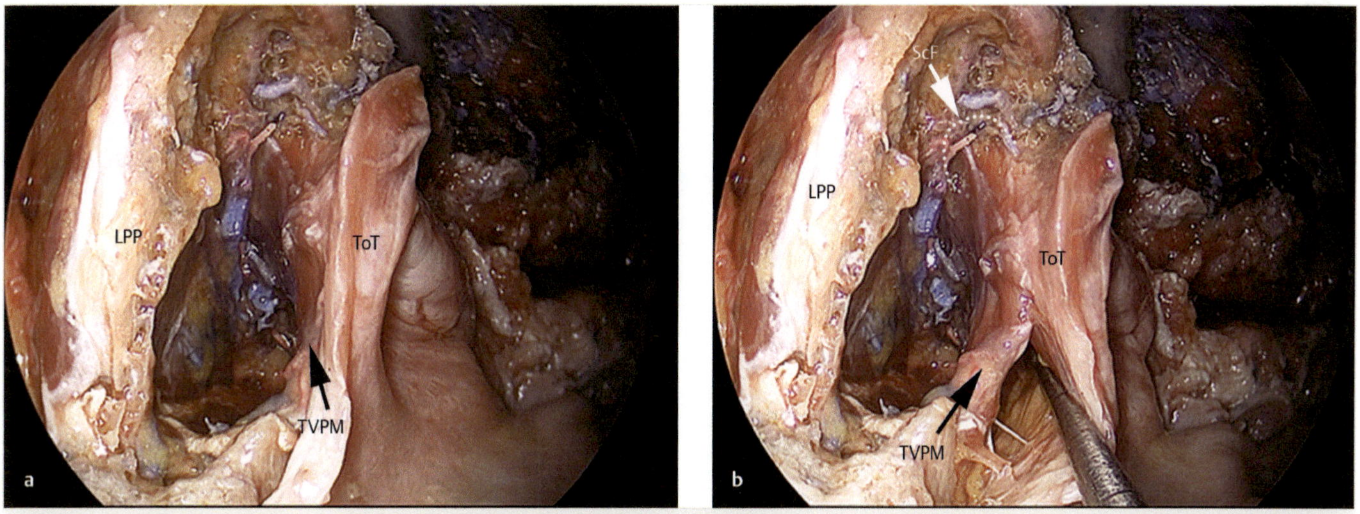

Fig. 23.15 (a, b) The tensor veli palatini muscle. The tensor veli palatini muscle (TVPM) is identified lateral to the torus tubarius (ToT). A dissector is used to separate the muscle from the cartilage of the eustachian tube. This muscle mainly arises from the anterolateral cartilaginous portion of the eustachian tube and scaphoid fossa of the sphenoid bone (ScF; *white dotted line*). LPP, lateral pterygoid plate.

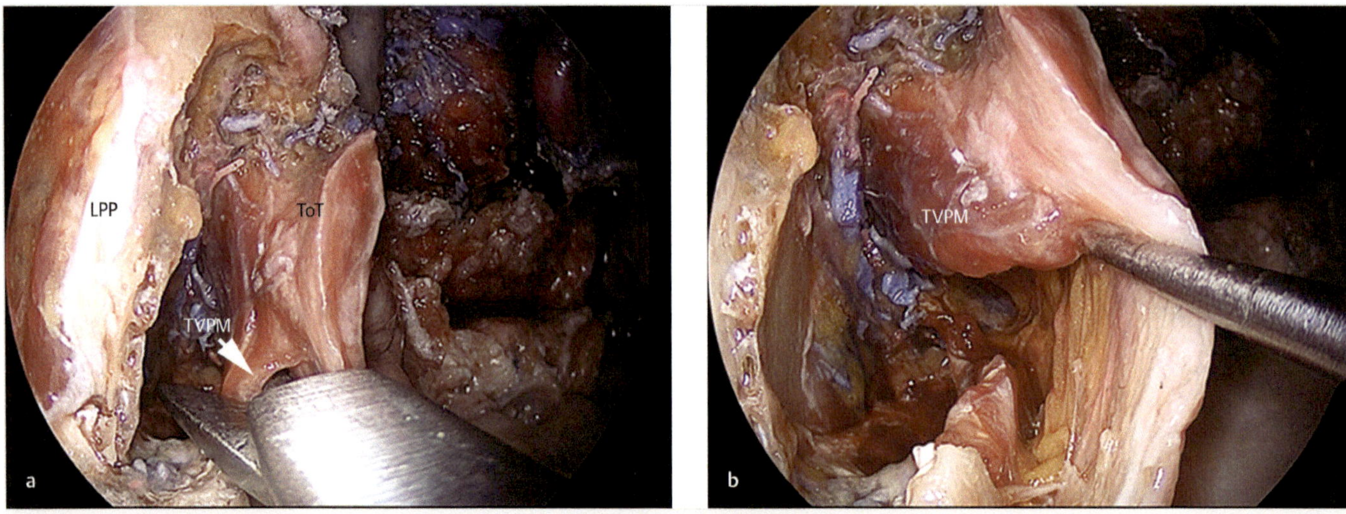

Fig. 23.16 (a, b) Step 6. The tensor veli palatini muscle (TVPM) is cut and the eustachian tube is moved upward. The two stumps of the muscle are removed. LLP, lateral pterygoid muscle; ToT, torus tubarius.

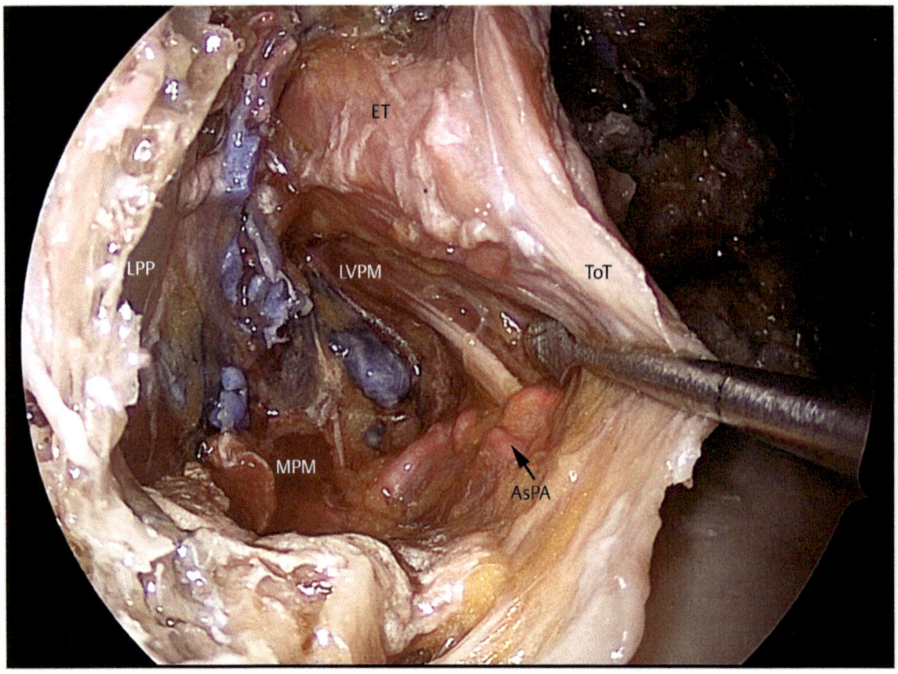

Fig. 23.17 The levator veli palatini muscle. Pulling medially and superiorly the torus tubarius (ToT), the levator veli palatini muscle (LVPM) comes into view. Its origin from the fibrous and posterior cartilaginous portion of the eustachian tube (ET) is identified. The ascending palatine artery (AsPA) can be seen below this muscle. LPP, lateral pterygoid plate; MPM, medial pterygoid muscle (distal portion).

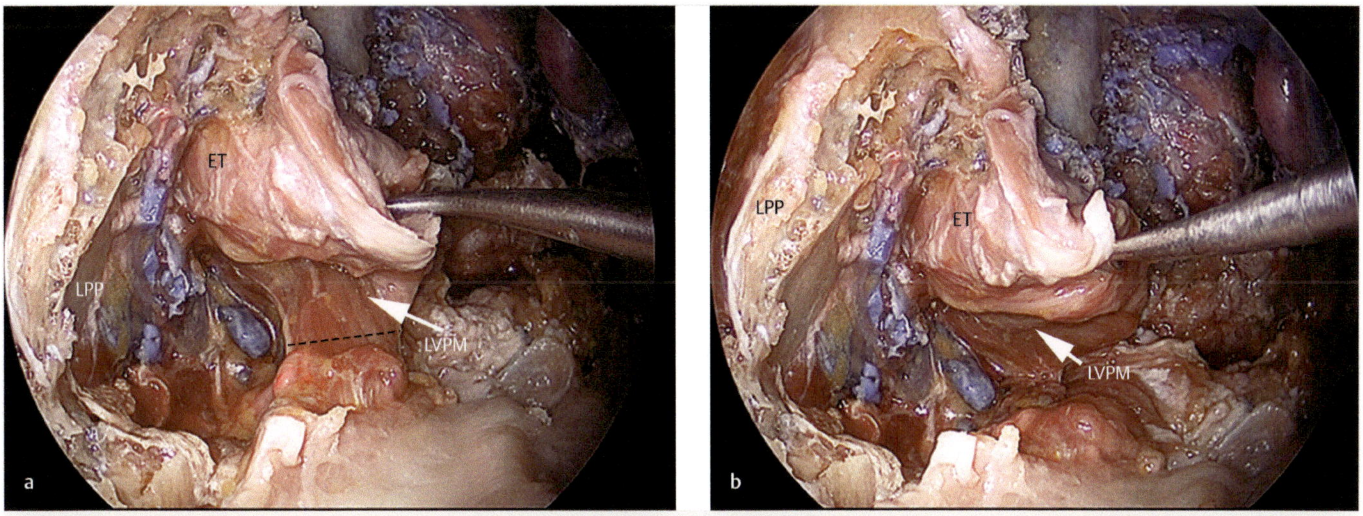

Fig. 23.18 (a, b) Step 7. After pulling the eustachian tube (ET) upward, the levator veli palatini muscle (LVPM) is cut close to the soft palate (*black dashed line*) and then removed. LPP, lateral pterygoid plate.

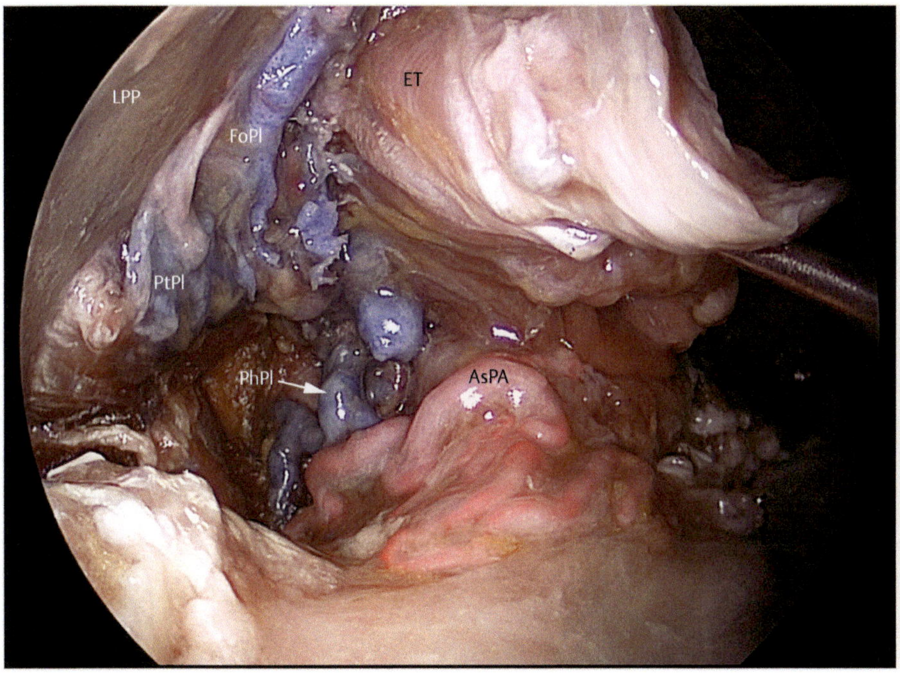

Fig. 23.19 Venous plexuses. The foraminal venous plexus (FoPl) of the mandibular nerve drains into the deep portion of the pterygoid venous plexus (PtPl) anteroinferiorly and the pharyngeal venous plexus (PhPl) posteroinferiorly. The former lies within the deep masticatory space and the latter within the parapharyngeal space. AsPA, ascending palatine artery; ET, eustachian tube; LPP, lateral pterygoid plate.

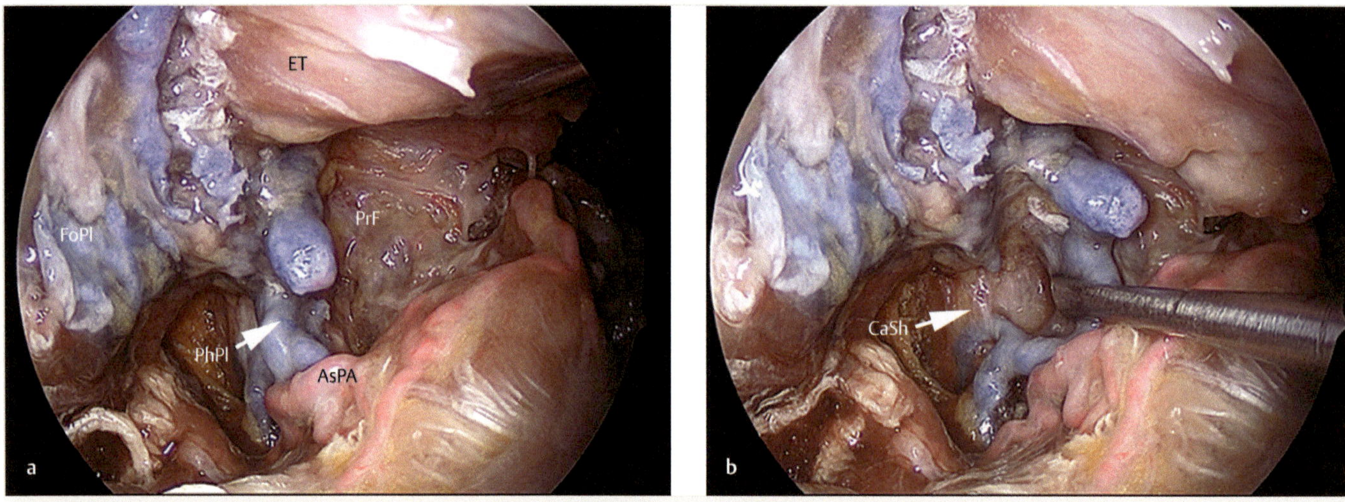

Fig. 23.20 (a, b) The carotid sheath. By pulling the pharyngeal venous plexus (PhPl) medially, the carotid sheath (CaSh) comes into view posteroinferiorly to the eustachian tube (ET), which lies in front of the internal carotid artery with a superolateral to inferomedial trajectory. AsPA, ascending palatine artery; FoPl, foraminal venous plexus of the mandibular nerve; PrF, prevertebral fascia.

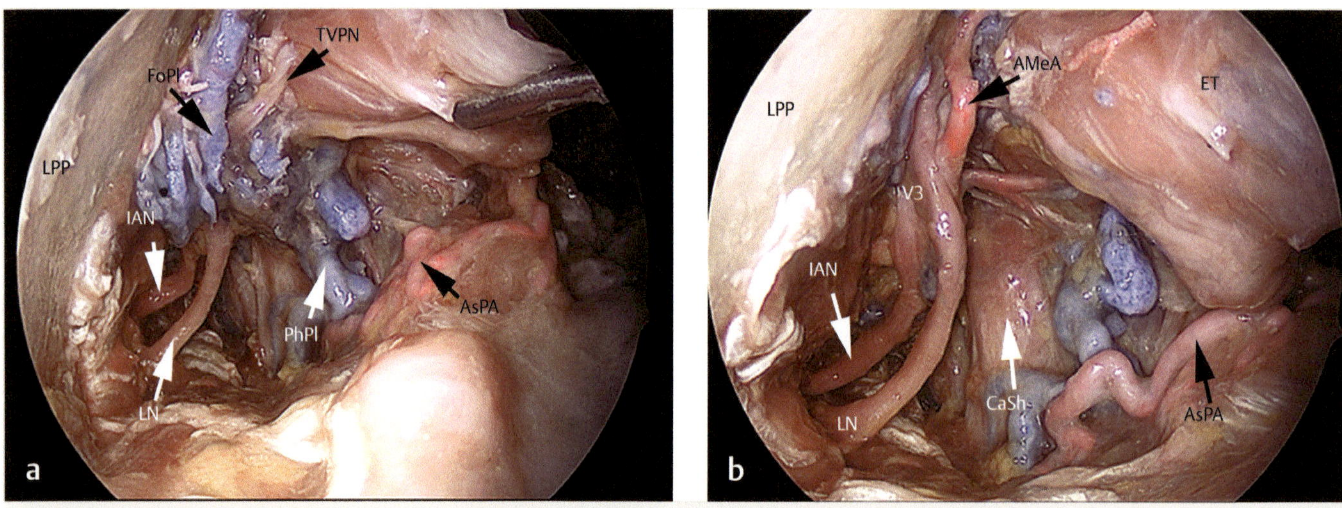

Fig. 23.21 (a, b) The mandibular nerve. The foraminal venous plexus is removed to expose the mandibular nerve (V3) with some of its posterior branches and the tensor veli palatini nerve (TVPN), which provides the nerve supply for the tensor veli palatini muscle and the tensor tympani muscle. The accessory meningeal artery (AMeA) is identified while passing next to the mandibular nerve toward the foramen ovale. AsPA, ascending palatine artery; CaSh, carotid sheath; ET, eustachian tube; FoPl, foraminal venous plexus; IAN, inferior alveolar nerve; LN, lingual nerve; LPP, lateral pterygoid plate; PhPl, pharyngeal venous plexus.

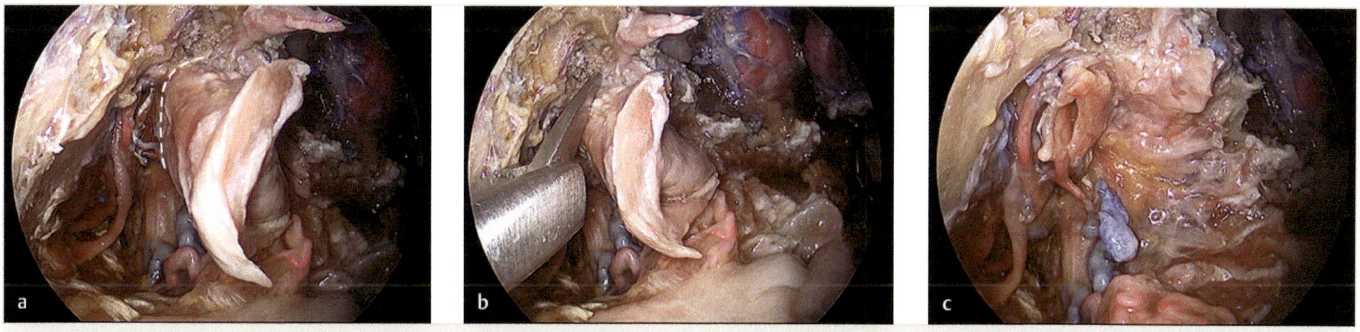

Fig. 23.22 (a–c) Step 8 (part 1). The eustachian tube is cut as close to the bony–cartilaginous junction as possible (*white dashed line*).

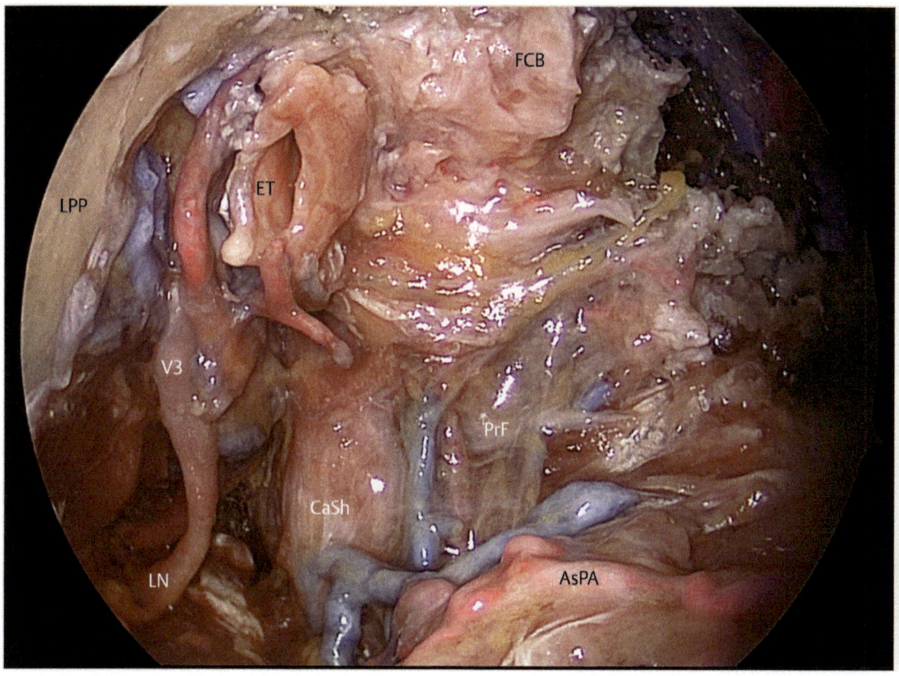

Fig. 23.23 Step 8 (part 2). Removal of the cartilaginous portion of the eustachian tube (ET) allows better exposure of the carotid sheath (CaSh), prevertebral fascia (PrF), and fibrocartilago basalis (FCB), which fills the anterior foramen lacerum. AsPA, ascending palatine artery; LPP, lateral pterygoid plate; V3, mandibular nerve.

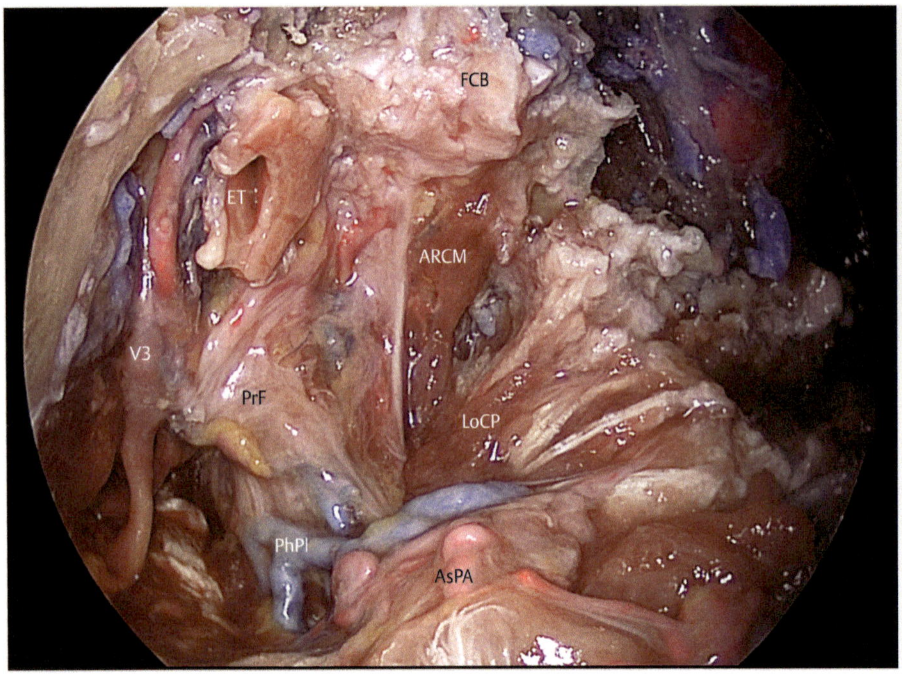

Fig. 23.24 The prevertebral musculature. By turning the prevertebral fascia (PrF) laterally, the anterior rectus capitis muscle (ARCM) and the longus capitis muscle (LoCM) can be exposed. AsPA, ascending palatine artery; ET, eustachian tube; FCB, fibrocartilago basalis; PhPL, pharyngeal venous plexus; V3, mandibular nerve.

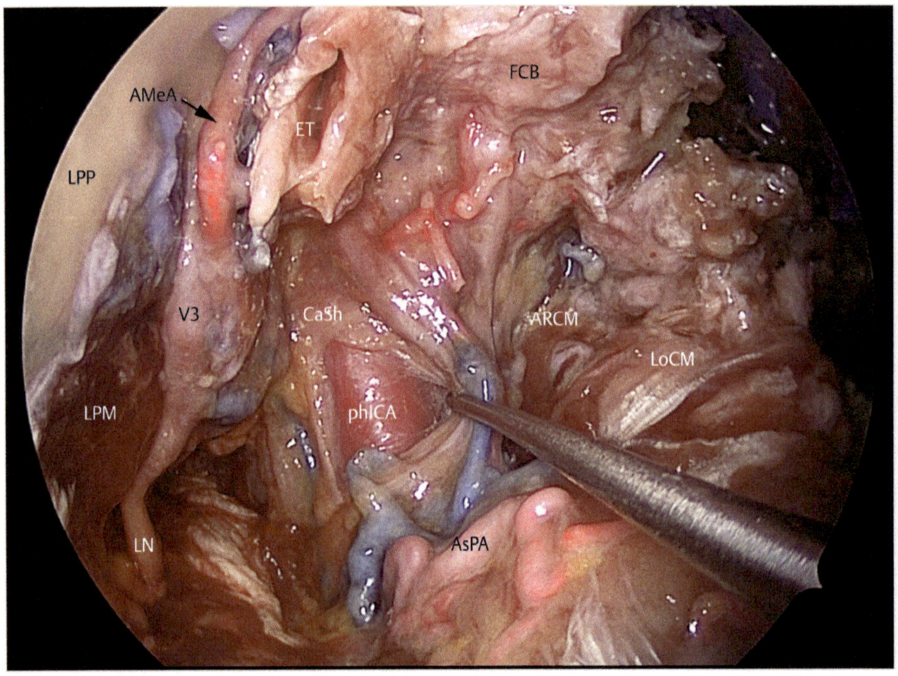

Fig. 23.25 Step 9. The carotid sheath (CaSh) is gently opened to expose the parapharyngeal tract of the internal carotid artery (phICA). V3, mandibular nerve; AMeA, accessory meningeal artery; ARCM, anterior rectus capitis muscle; AsPA, ascending palatine artery; ET, eustachian tube; FCB, fibrocartilago basalis; LN, lingual nerve; LoCM, longus capitis muscle; LPM, lateral pterygoid muscle; LPP, lateral pterygoid plate.

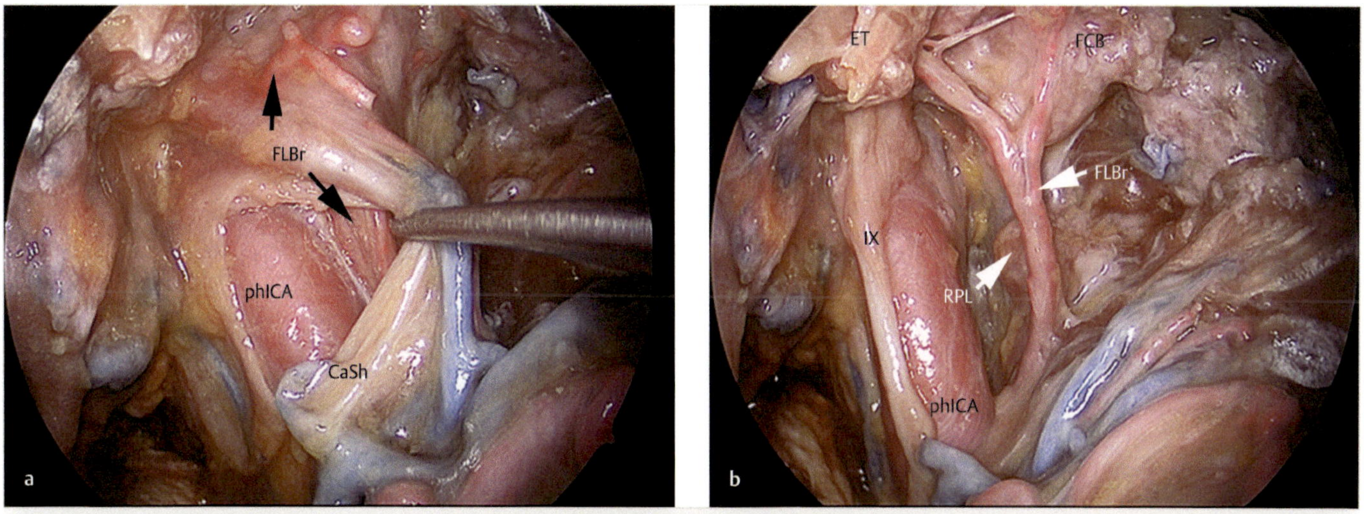

Fig. 23.26 (a, b) The branch of the ascending pharyngeal artery for the foramen lacerum. The glossopharyngeal nerve (IX) and the arterial branch for the foramen lacerum (FLBr), which arises from the ascending pharyngeal artery, are identified after completing removal of the carotid sheath (CaSh). This branch runs across the fibrocartilago basalis (FCB) to reach the intracranial space. ET, eustachian tube; phICA, parapharyngeal tract of the internal carotid artery; RPL, retropharyngeal lymph node.

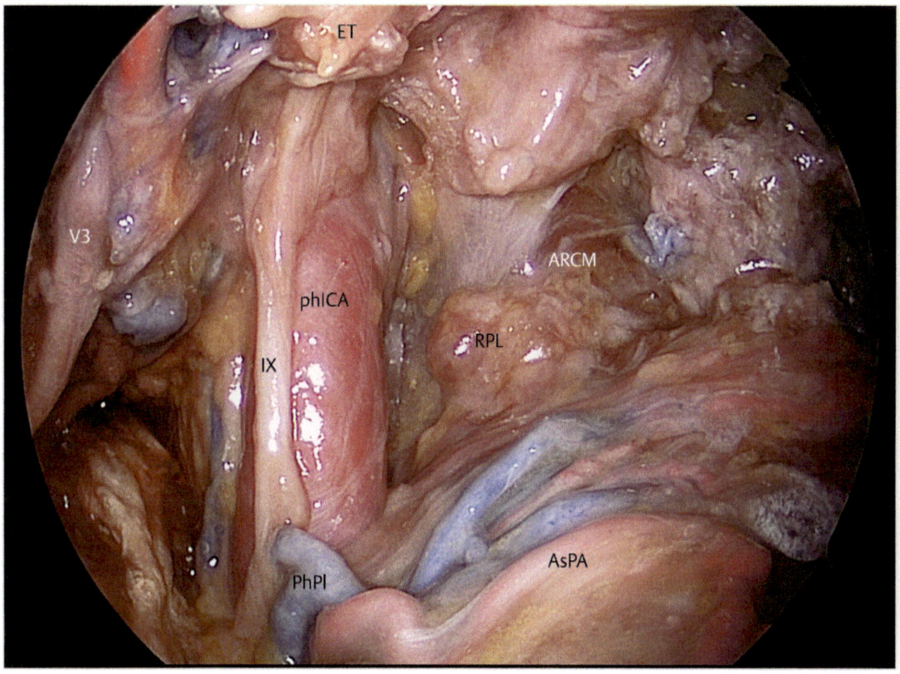

Fig. 23.27 Step 10. The medial portion of the prevertebral fascia is removed to fully expose the anterior rectus capitis muscle (ARCM). When present, one or more retropharyngeal lymph nodes (RPL) are usually found within the carotid space, medial to the parapharyngeal tract of the internal carotid artery (phICA), posterolateral to the pharyngeal wall, and in front of the lateral portion of the prevertebral fascia. V3, mandibular nerve; IX, glossopharyngeal nerve; AsPA, ascending palatine artery; ET, eustachian tube; PhPl, pharyngeal venous plexus.

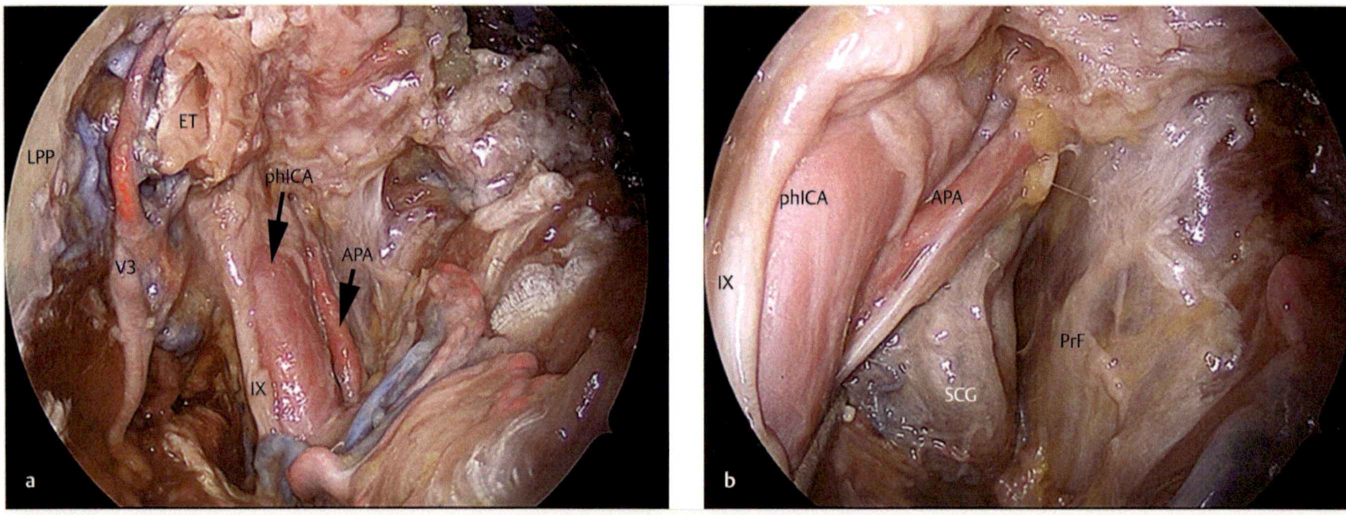

Fig. 23.28 (a, b) Step 11. The plane between the parapharyngeal tract of the internal carotid artery (phICA) and the lateral portion of the prevertebral fascia (PrF) is dissected to identify the ascending pharyngeal artery (APA) and the superior cervical ganglion (SCG). The position of the ascending pharyngeal artery with respect to the internal carotid artery is extremely variable. V3, mandibular nerve; IX, glossopharyngeal nerve; ET, eustachian tube; LPP, lateral pterygoid plate.

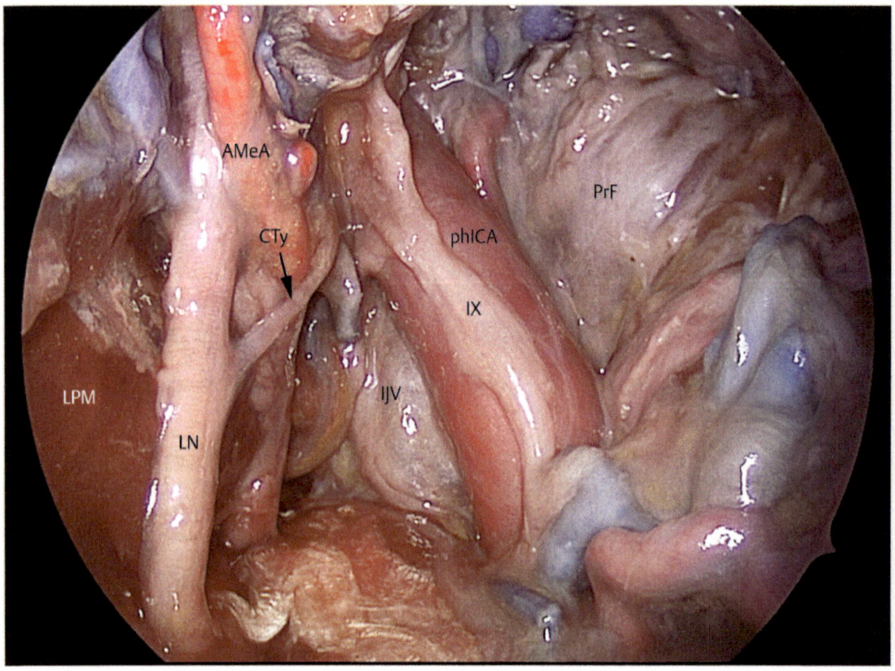

Fig. 23.29 Step 12. The plane between the mandibular nerve branches and the parapharyngeal tract of the internal carotid artery (phICA) is dissected to expose the internal jugular vein (IJV). The chorda tympani (CTy) of the facial nerve can be identified while reaching the lingual nerve (LN) as it passes laterally and anteriorly to the internal carotid artery. IX, glossopharyngeal nerve; AMeA, accessory meningeal artery; LPM, lateral pterygoid muscle; PrF, prevertebral fascia.

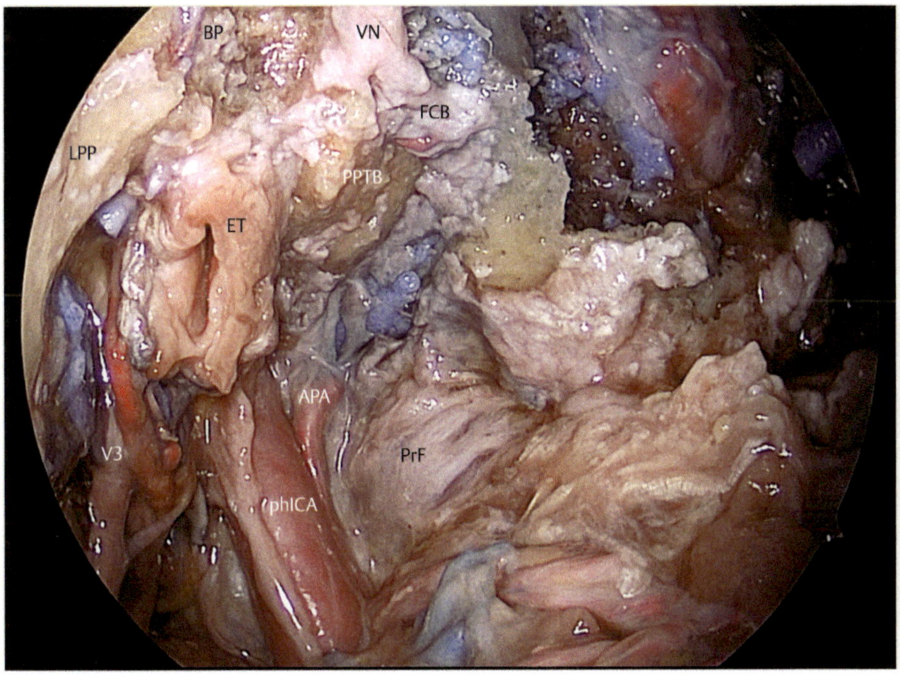

Fig. 23.30 Overview of the parapharyngeal space and related skull base. Different from the lateral parapharyngeal approach, in this approach the infratemporal fossa is left untouched except for the proximal portion of the medial pterygoid muscle. The roof of the parapharyngeal space is formed by the petrous portion of the temporal bone (PPTB) and the fibrocartilago basalis (FCB). The lateral pterygoid plate (LPP) separates this corridor from the lateral parapharyngeal approach. V3, mandibular nerve; APA, ascending pharyngeal artery; BP, base of the pterygoid process; ET, eustachian tube; phICA, parapharyngeal portion of the internal carotid artery; PrF, lateral portion of the prevertebral fascia; VN, vidian nerve.

References

[1] Stambuk HE, Patel SG. Imaging of the parapharyngeal space. Otolaryngol Clin North Am 2008;41(1):77–101, vi

[2] Ferrari M, Schreiber A, Mattavelli D, et al. Surgical anatomy of the parapharyngeal space: multiperspective, quantification-based study. Head Neck 2019;41(3):642–656

[3] Prasad SC, Piccirillo E, Chovanec M, La Melia C, De Donato G, Sanna M. Lateral skull base approaches in the management of benign parapharyngeal space tumors. Auris Nasus Larynx 2015;42(3):189–198

[4] Chen MK, Lai JC, Chang CC, Liu MT. Minimally invasive endoscopic nasopharyngectomy in the treatment of recurrent T1–2a nasopharyngeal carcinoma. Laryngoscope 2007;117(5):894–896

[5] Chen MY, Wen WP, Guo X, et al. Endoscopic nasopharyngectomy for locally recurrent nasopharyngeal carcinoma. Laryngoscope 2009;119(3):516–522

[6] Castelnuovo P, Dallan I, Bignami M, et al. Nasopharyngeal endoscopic resection in the management of selected malignancies: ten-year experience. Rhinology 2010;48(1):84–89

[7] Castelnuovo P, Nicolai P, Turri-Zanoni M, et al. Endoscopic endonasal nasopharyngectomy in selected cancers. Otolaryngol Head Neck Surg 2013;149(3):424–430

[8] Liu J, Yu H, Sun X, et al. Salvage endoscopic nasopharyngectomy for local recurrent or residual nasopharyngeal carcinoma: a 10-year experience. Int J Clin Oncol 2017;22(5):834–842

[9] Vlantis AC, Lee DL, Wong EW, Chow SM, Ng SK, Chan JY. Endoscopic nasopharyngectomy in recurrent nasopharyngeal carcinoma: a case series, literature review, and pooled analysis. Int Forum Allergy Rhinol 2017;7(4):425–432

[10] Ong YK, Solares CA, Lee S, Snyderman CH, Fernandez-Miranda J, Gardner PA. Endoscopic nasopharyngectomy and its role in managing locally recurrent nasopharyngeal carcinoma. Otolaryngol Clin North Am 2011;44(5):1141–1154

[11] Lepera D, Volpi L, De Bernardi F, et al. Endoscopic transnasal resection of Eustachian-tube dermoid in a new-born infant. Auris Nasus Larynx 2015;42(3): 235–240

[12] Battaglia P, Turri-Zanoni M, Dallan I, et al. Endoscopic endonasal transpterygoid transmaxillary approach to the infratemporal and upper parapharyngeal tumors. Otolaryngol Head Neck Surg 2014;150(4):696–702

[13] Dallan I, Lenzi R, Bignami M, et al. Endoscopic transnasal anatomy of the infratemporal fossa and upper parapharyngeal regions: correlations with traditional perspectives and surgical implications. Minim Invasive Neurosurg 2010;53(5–6):261–269

[14] Liu CL, Hsu NI, Shen PH. Endoscopic endonasal nasopharyngectomy: tensor veli palatine muscle as a landmark for the parapharyngeal internal carotid artery. Int Forum Allergy Rhinol 2017;7(6):624–628

[15] Mattavelli D, Bolzoni Villaret A, Ferrari M, et al. Different perspectives of internal carotid artery in transnasal endoscopic surgery. World Neurosurg 2016;95:222–228

24 Lateral Parapharyngeal Approach

Marco Ferrari, Marco Ravanelli, Davide Lancini, Alberto Schreiber, Davide Mattavelli

As illustrated in the previous chapter, the transnasal approach to the parapharyngeal space can be divided from a surgical viewpoint into two corridors (medial and lateral), having the lateral pterygoid plate as a watershed. By running laterally to this landmark or removing it, wide exposure of the far-lateral portion of the upper parapharyngeal space is obtained. Given its trajectory, the lateral parapharyngeal approach lies midway between the medial parapharyngeal approach and the infratemporal approach, thus representing the most extended corridor toward lateral infracranial spaces.

This approach was well described in pioneering anatomical studies,[1–6] but only isolated cases of its application for removal of tumors of the upper parapharyngeal space have been reported.[7,8] When compared to the medial parapharyngeal approach, which addresses the petrous portion of the temporal bone and prevertebral musculature, the lateral corridor is directly oriented toward the carotid and the jugular foramina. This anatomical trajectory has two major implications: (1) resection of the eustachian tube is not necessary unless a wide exposure of areas behind it is required and (2) an exceedingly complex network of neurovascular structure fills the deep portion of the corridor, including the mandibular, glossopharyngeal, vagus, spinal accessory, and hypoglossal nerves, as well as the internal carotid artery, the internal jugular vein, the ascending pharyngeal artery, the middle meningeal artery, and the maxillary artery. The posterolateral limit of the space consists of the stylomandibular tunnel, which is enclosed between the posterior portion of the condylar process of the mandible, the stylomandibular ligament, and the inferior surface of the external auditory canal. The target area can be reached with a different perspective by a transcervical–transparotid approach to the parapharyngeal space, so that the combination of the two approaches (multiportal surgery) can find an indication in selected multicompartmental lesions of the skull base and adjacent areas.[9–12]

This chapter includes three modular variants of the lateral parapharyngeal approach: the first is the least extended corridor that is harvested laterally to the lateral pterygoid plate, extending the dissection performed along the third corridor of the infratemporal fossa to reach the lateral prestyloid compartment and the stylomandibular tunnel; the second lateral parapharyngeal corridor is obtained by removing both pterygoid plates with a lower transpterygoid approach and dissecting the upper parapharyngeal space passing below the eustachian tube and related muscles; and the third and most extended corridor is harvested by removing the eustachian tube to achieve complete exposure of the upper parapharyngeal compartment, from the nasopharynx, medially, to the stylomandibular tunnel, laterally.

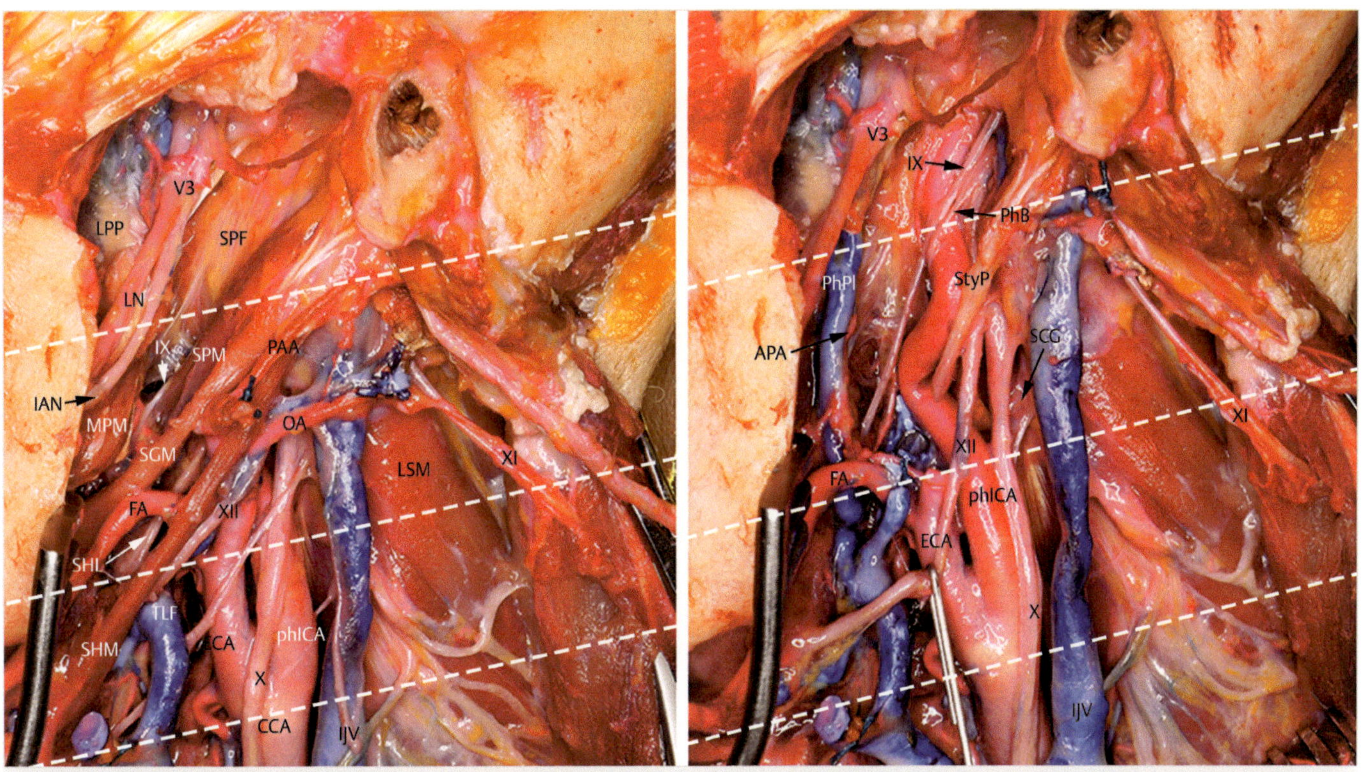

Fig. 24.1 Sagittal view of the parapharyngeal space. This sagittal cadaver picture shows with a lateral-to-medial perspective the left upper parapharyngeal space. *White dashed lines* show the compartmentalization of the parapharyngeal space in upper, middle, and lower. V3, mandibular nerve; IX, glossopharyngeal nerve; X, vagus nerve; XI, spinal accessory nerve; XII, hypoglossal nerve; APA, ascending pharyngeal artery; CCA, common carotid artery; ECA, external carotid artery; FA, facial artery; IAN, inferior alveolar nerve; IJV, internal jugular vein; LN, lingual nerve; LPP, lateral pterygoid plate; LSM, levator scapulae muscle; MPM, medial pterygoid muscle; OA, occipital artery; PAA, posterior auricular artery; phICA, parapharyngeal tract of the internal carotid artery; PhB, pharyngeal branch of the vagus nerve; PhPl, pharyngeal plexus; SCG, superior cervical ganglion; SGM, styloglossus muscle; SHL, stylohyoid ligament; SHM, stylohyoid muscle; SPF, stylopharyngeal fascia; SPM, stylopharyngeal muscle; StyP, styloid process; TLF, thyrolingual-facial venous trunk.

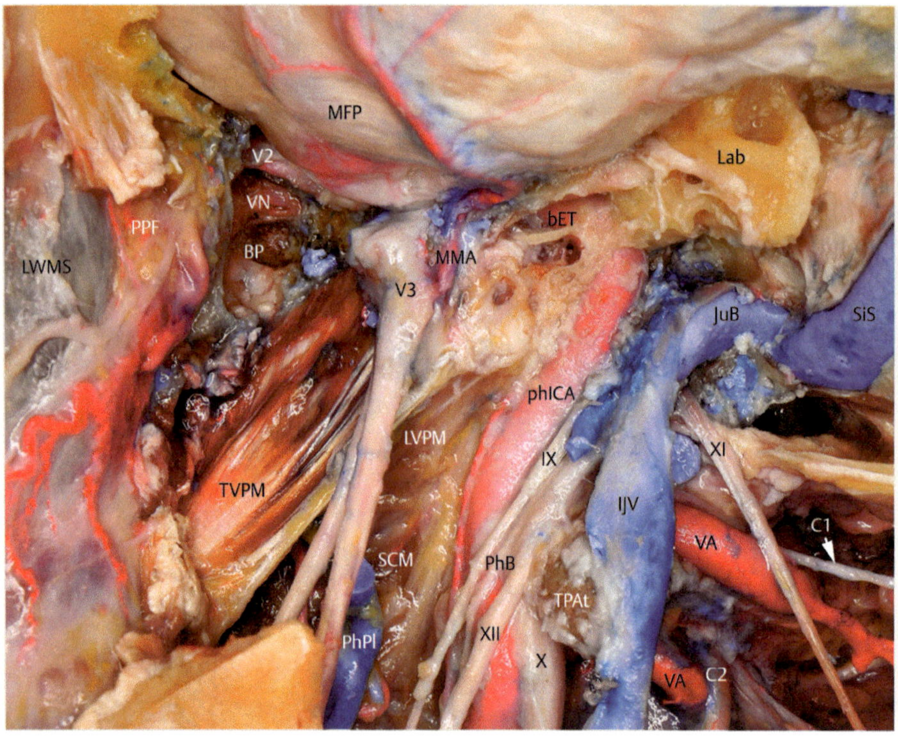

Fig. 24.2 Sagittal view of the upper parapharyngeal space and adjacent skull base. This sagittal cadaver picture shows with a lateral-to-medial perspective the upper parapharyngeal space and adjacent skull base. V2, maxillary nerve; V3, mandibular nerve; IX, glossopharyngeal nerve; X, vagus nerve; XI, spinal accessory nerve; XII, hypoglossal nerve; bET, bony portion of the eustachian tube; BP, base of the pterygoid process; C1, first cervical nerve; C2, second cervical nerve; IJV, internal jugular vein (displaced posteriorly and laterally); JuB, jugular bulb; Lab, labyrinth; LVPM, levator veli palatini muscle; LWMS, lateral wall of the maxillary sinus; MFP, periosteum of the middle cranial fossa; MMA, middle meningeal artery; phICA, parapharyngeal tract of the internal carotid artery; PhB, pharyngeal branch of the vagus nerve; PhPl, pharyngeal plexus; PPF, pterygopalatine fossa; SCM, superior constrictor muscle; SiS, sigmoid sinus; TPAt, transverse process of the atlas; TVPM, tensor veli palatini muscle; VA, vertebral artery; VN, vidian nerve.

Due to the complexity and functional relevance of neurovascular structures within the parapharyngeal space, high expertise, in-depth preoperative assessment, precise planning of surgery, intraoperative neuromonitoring, availability of hemostatic materials, ability to convert the surgical approach, and readiness of neuroradiologist in the event of major vascular injuries are essential requirements for such a complex surgical procedure.

The reader is encouraged to identify the position of the mentioned neurovascular structures to fully understand the limitations and potentialities of the lateral parapharyngeal transnasal approach.

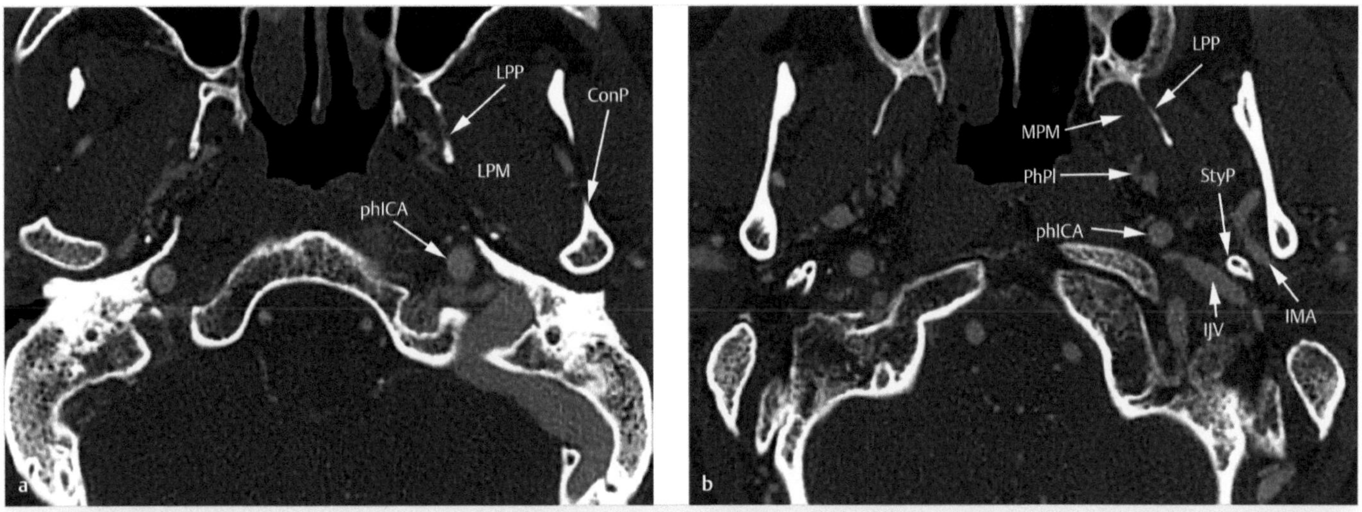

Fig. 24.3 Axial CT anatomy of the upper parapharyngeal space and the jugular foramen. The panel includes two axial CT scans passing through **(a)** and immediately below the jugular foramen **(b)**. The lateral portion of the upper parapharyngeal space lies lateral to the plane passing through the lateral pterygoid plate (LPP). The trajectory parallel to the lateral pterygoid plate leads to the area of the jugular foramen, which includes the styloid process (StyP), internal jugular vein (IJV), and lower cranial nerves. The stylomandibular tunnel, which houses the internal maxillary artery (IMA), can be identified between the styloid process and the condylar process (ConP) of the mandible. The parapharyngeal tract of the internal carotid artery (phICA) runs in a vertical direction in the medial portion of this region. However, this artery can show remarkable medial or lateral kinking toward the posterior pharyngeal wall or nodal level II, respectively. LPM, lateral pterygoid muscle; MPM, medial pterygoid muscle; PhPl, pharyngeal plexus.

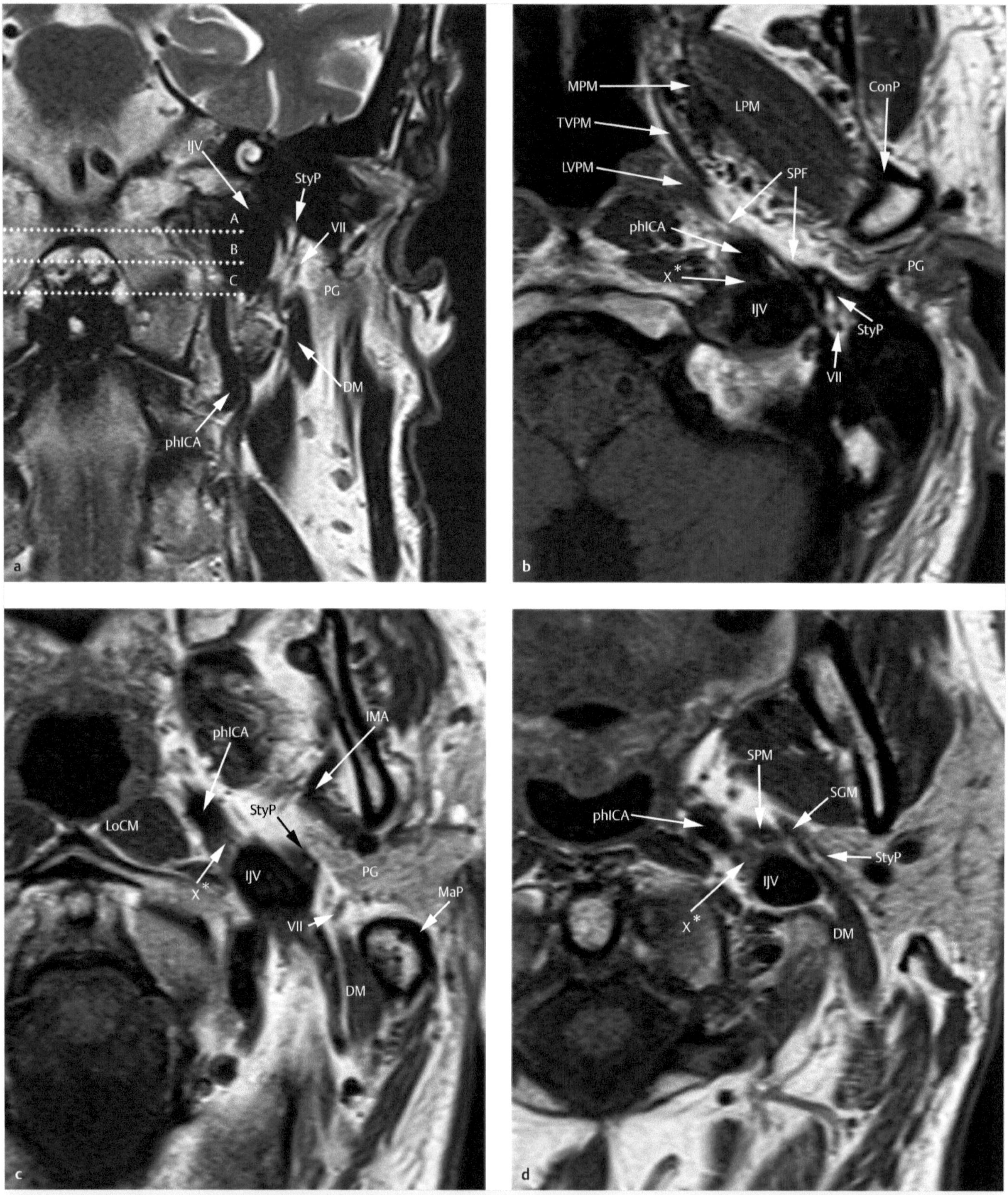

Fig. 24.4 MRI anatomy of the prestyloid compartment of the upper parapharyngeal space. The panel includes one coronal T2-weighted **(a)** and three T1-weighted axial MRI images **(b–d)**. The *white dotted lines* depict the position of the axial images. As seen in a coronal plane, the internal jugular vein (IJV) and the facial nerve (VII) run on the posteromedial and posterolateral surfaces of the styloid process (StyP), respectively. The stylohyoid, styloglossus (SGM), and stylopharyngeal muscle (SPM) arise from the styloid process together with some ligamentous/fascial structures. The stylopharyngeal fascia (SPF) lies from the styloid process to the levator veli palatini muscle (LVPM), making up the posterior limit of the prestyloid compartment of the parapharyngeal space (also called "true parapharyngeal space"). The anterior boundary of this space is the interpterygoid fascia, which extends from the condylar process of the mandible (ConP) to the tensor veli palatini muscle (TVPM). The lateral portion of the upper prestyloid compartment houses the parapharyngeal process of the parotid gland (PG). In the retrostyloid compartment, also called "carotid space," the lower cranial nerves (X*) lie in the interface between the internal jugular vein and the parapharyngeal segment of the internal carotid artery (phICA). DM, digastric muscle; IMA, internal maxillary artery; LoCM, longus capitis muscle; LPM, lateral pterygoid muscle; MaP, mastoid process; MPM, medial pterygoid muscle.

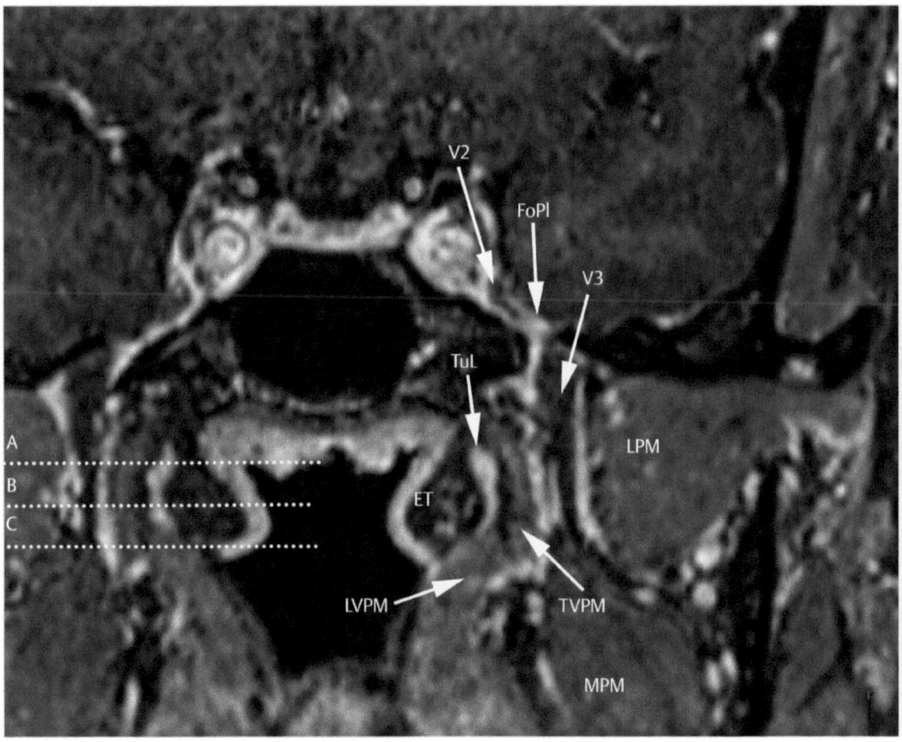

Fig. 24.5 Coronal MRI anatomy of the upper parapharyngeal space. The present contrast-enhanced T1-weighted coronal MRI, which passes through the foramen ovale, shows the relationship between the eustachian tube (ET), the mandibular nerve (V3), the lateral pterygoid muscle (LPM), and the medial pterygoid muscle (MPM). The tensor veli palatini muscle (TVPM) is inserted on the anterior plate of the eustachian tube, while the levator veli palatini muscle (LVPM) lies more inferiorly and runs parallel to the tubal lumen (TuL). Three *white dotted lines* (A–C) show the position of images composing ▶Fig. 24.6. V2, maxillary nerve; FoPl, foraminal plexus.

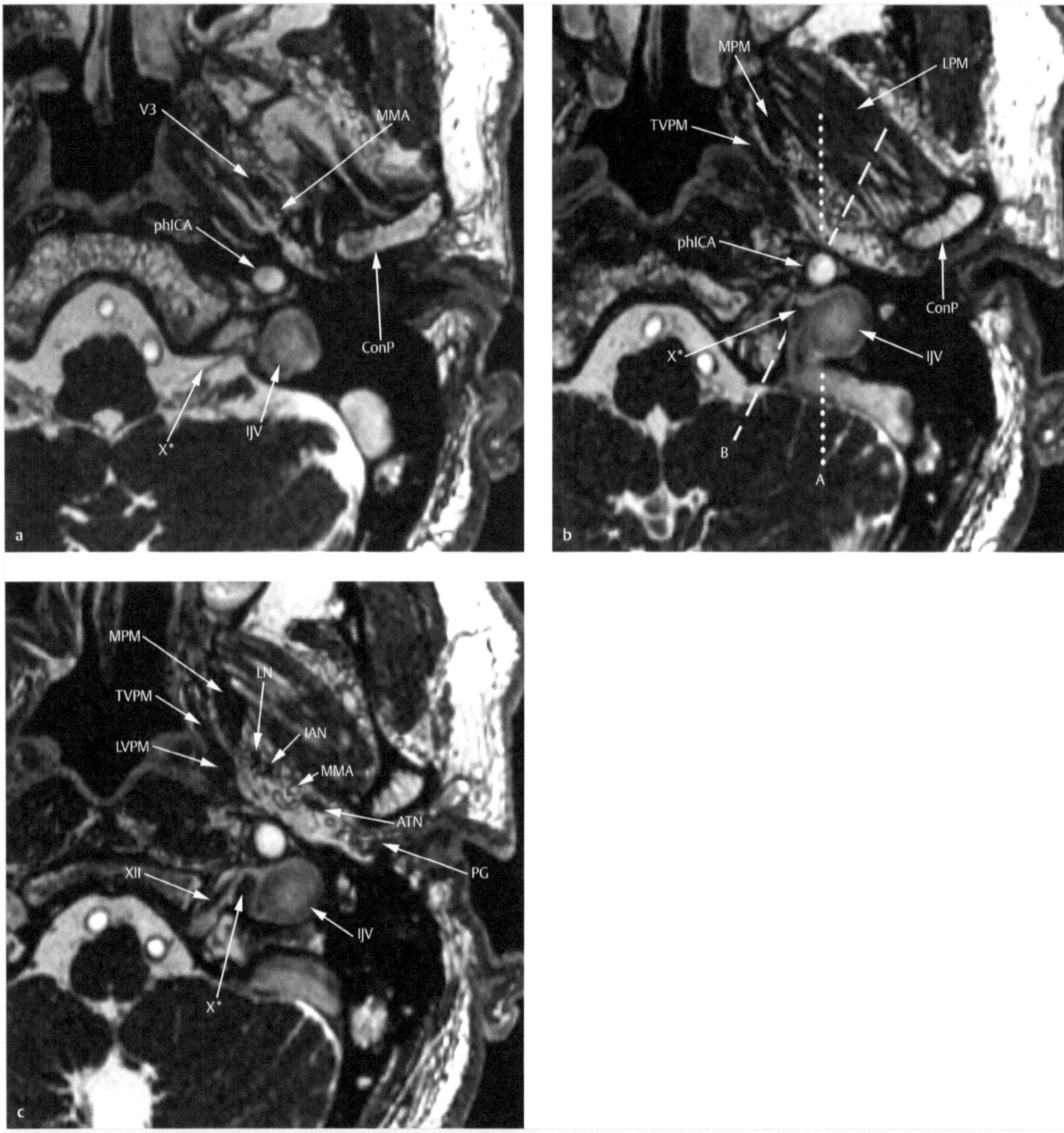

Fig. 24.6 (a–c) Axial MRI anatomy of the jugular and carotid foramen and related structures. The panel includes three axial CISS (constructive interference in steady state) MRI images; their positions are represented in ▶Fig. 24.5. The area of the jugular and carotid foramina is exceedingly complex due to the convergence of the internal jugular vein (IJV), the parapharyngeal segment of the internal carotid artery (phICA), the lower cranial nerves (X*), and the hypoglossal nerve (XII) in their passage across the skull base. While passing through the jugular foramen, the lower cranial nerves have a trajectory from superomedial to inferolateral. The hypoglossal nerve runs across the skull base caudally to the lower cranial nerves, following a posteromedial-to-anterolateral direction. Both lower cranial nerves and hypoglossal nerves pass between the internal carotid artery and the internal jugular vein. The *white dotted* (A) and *dashed* (B) *lines* depict the orientation of images composing ▶Fig. 24.7. V3, mandibular nerve; ATN, auriculotemporal nerve; ConP, condylar process of the mandible; IAN, inferior alveolar nerve; LN, lingual nerve; LPM, lateral pterygoid muscle; LVPM, levator veli palatini muscle; MMA, middle meningeal artery; MPM, medial pterygoid muscle; PG, parotid gland; TVPM, tensor veli palatini muscle.

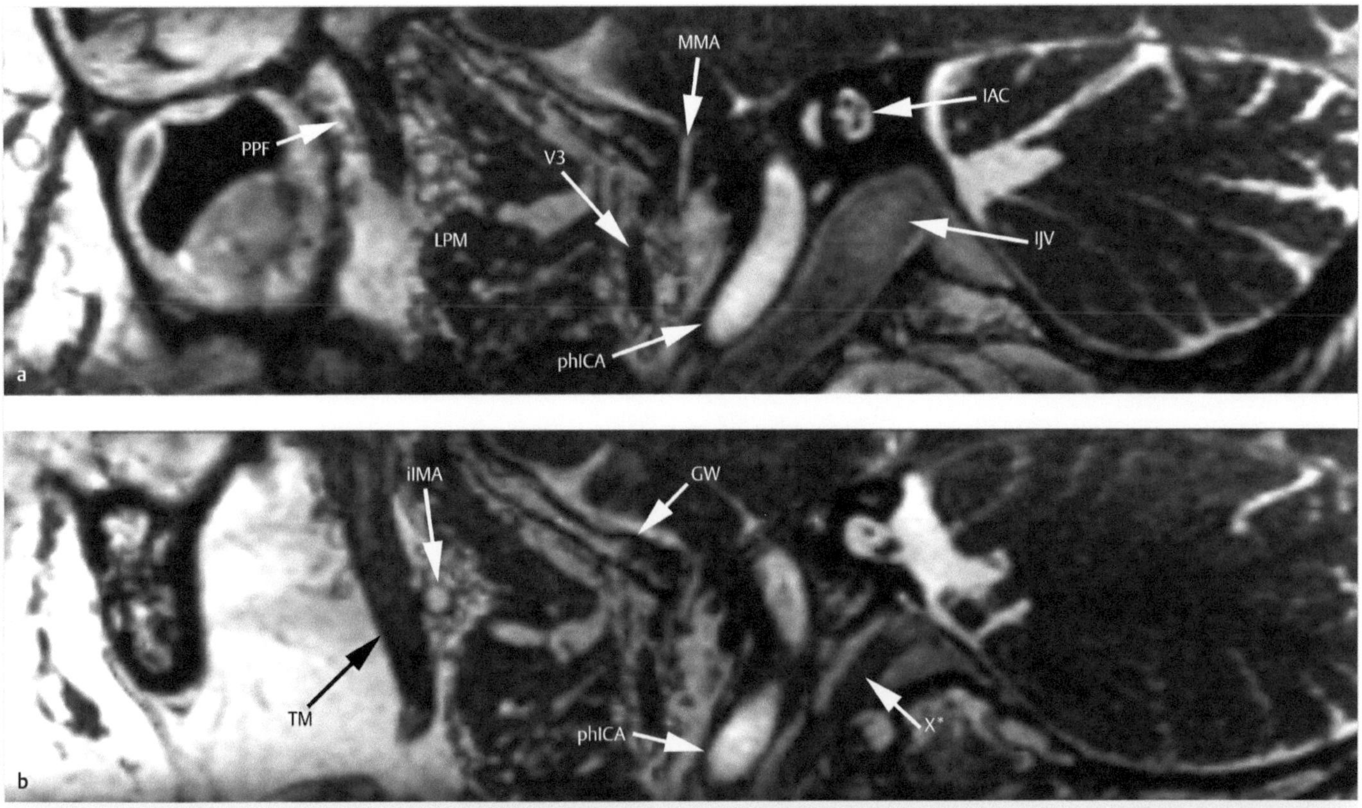

Fig. 24.7 (a, b) Sagittal and parasagittal MRI anatomy of the jugular foramen. Two CISS (constructive interference in steady state) MRI images show the anatomy of the parapharyngeal segment of the internal carotid artery (phICA), the internal jugular vein (IJV), and the lower cranial nerves (X*) while crossing the cranial base. The orientation of the images of the present panel is depicted in ▶Fig. 24.6. V3, mandibular nerve; IAC, internal auditory canal; iIMA, infratemporal tract of the internal maxillary artery; LPM, lateral pterygoid muscle; MMA, middle meningeal artery; PPF, pterygopalatine fossa; TM, temporal muscle.

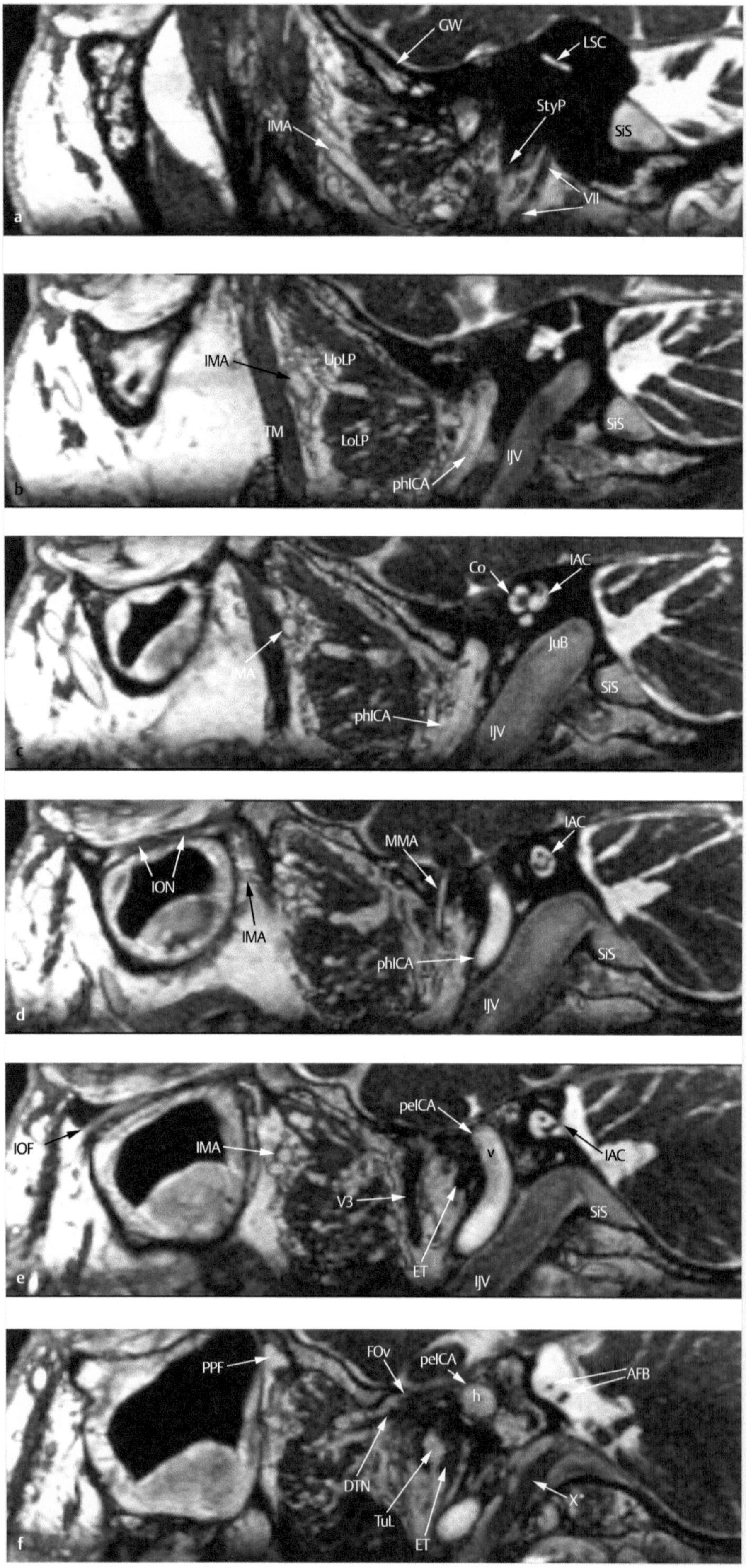

Fig. 24.8 (a–f) Sagittal MRI anatomy of the retrostyloid compartment of the upper parapharyngeal space. The panel contains six sagittal CISS (constructive interference in steady state) MRI images passing through the upper parapharyngeal space, from lateral **(a)** to medial **(f)**. In the medial portion of the upper parapharyngeal space, the parapharyngeal segment of the internal carotid artery (phICA) is separated from the upper (UpLP) and lower head of the lateral pterygoid muscle (LoLP) by the mandibular nerve (V3) and the eustachian tube (ET). The lateral portion of the upper parapharyngeal space houses the internal jugular vein (IJV), the lower cranial nerves (X*), and the hypoglossal nerve, which are separated from the lateral pterygoid muscle by the styloid process (StyP) and related muscular and ligamentous/fascial structures. Notably, the roof of the infratemporal fossa (or deep masticatory space) is the greater wing of the sphenoid bone (GW), while the roof of the parapharyngeal space consists of the petrous portion of the temporal bone. VII, facial nerve; AFB, acoustic-facial bundle; Co, cochlea; DTN, deep temporal nerve; FOv, foramen ovale; h, horizontal tract of the petrous segment of the internal carotid artery; IAC, internal auditory canal; IMA, internal maxillary artery; IOF, infraorbital foramen; ION, infraorbital nerve; JuB, jugular bulb; LSC, lateral semicircular canal; MMA, middle meningeal artery; pelCA, petrous segment of the internal carotid artery; PPF, pterygopalatine fossa; SiS, sigmoid sinus; TM, temporal muscle; TuL, tubal lumen; v, vertical tract of the petrous segment of the internal carotid artery.

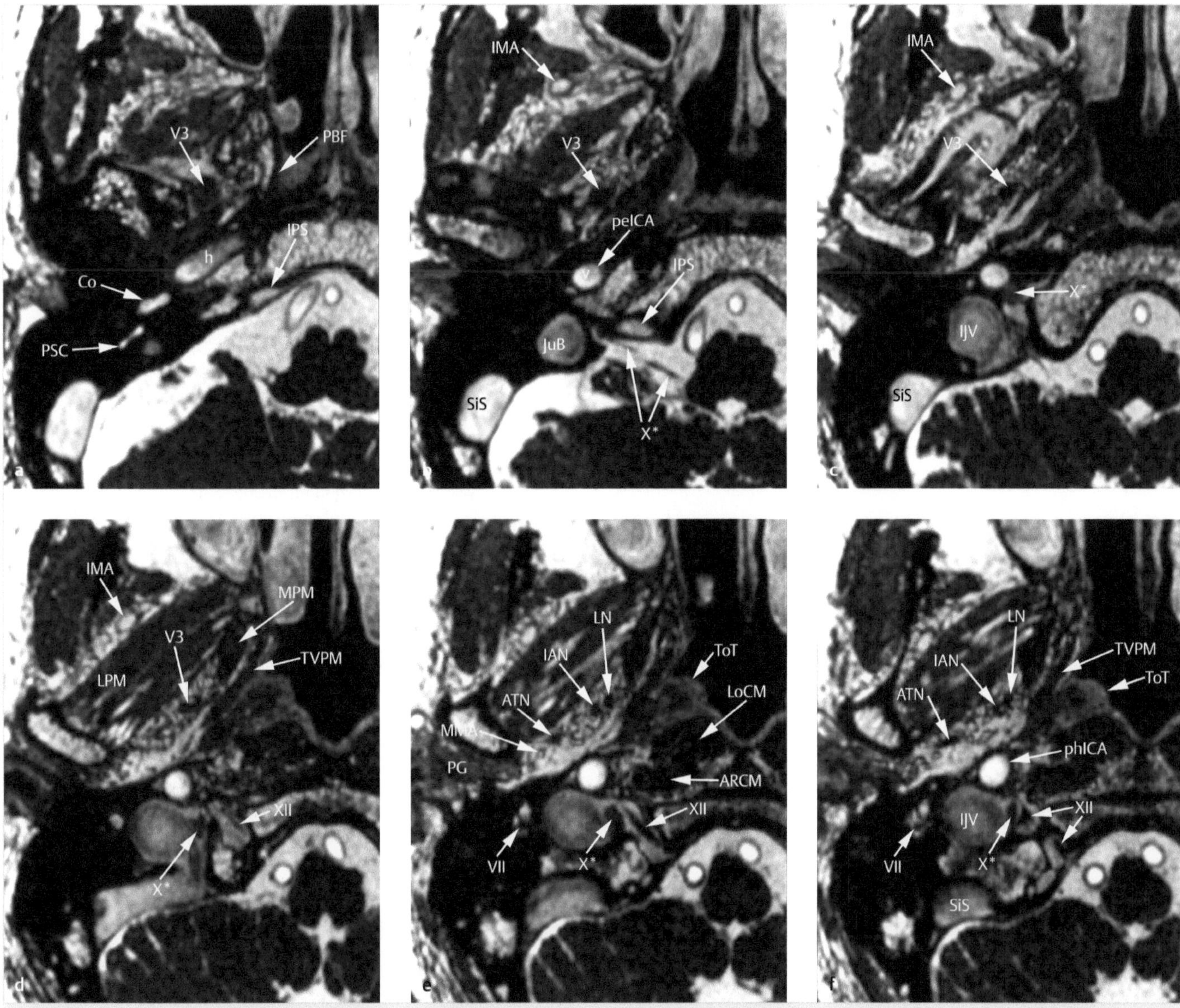

Fig. 24.9 (a–f) Axial MRI anatomy of the retrostyloid compartment of the upper parapharyngeal space. The panel contains six axial CISS (constructive interference in steady state) MRI images passing through the upper parapharyngeal space, from cranial **(a)** to caudal **(f)**. The internal jugular vein (IJV) is formed by the confluence of the sigmoid sinus (SiS) and the inferior petrosal sinus (IPS) in the area of the jugular bulb (JuB). The vein is surrounded by several neurovascular structures: the medial wall is adjacent to the lower cranial nerves (X*) and the hypoglossal nerve (XII); the lateral wall is close to the facial nerve (VII); the anterior wall faces the posterolateral surface of the parapharyngeal (phICA) and the vertical (v) petrous segment of the internal carotid artery (peICA). All these neurovascular structures are enclosed within the retrostyloid compartment of the upper parapharyngeal space. The mandibular nerve (V3) and most of its branches run in the interface between the infratemporal fossa and the prestyloid compartment of the upper parapharyngeal space. The middle meningeal artery (MMA), the auriculotemporal nerve (ATN), the inferior alveolar nerve (IAN), and the lingual nerve (LN) can be identified along a plane parallel to the posterior surface of the lateral pterygoid muscle (LPM). ARCM, anterior rectus capitis muscle; Co, cochlea; h, horizontal tract of the petrous segment of the internal carotid artery; IMA, internal maxillary artery; LoCM, longus capitis muscle; MPM, medial pterygoid muscle; PBF, pharyngobasilar fascia; PG, parotid gland; PSC, posterior semicircular canal; ToT, torus tubarius; TVPM, tensor veli palatini muscle.

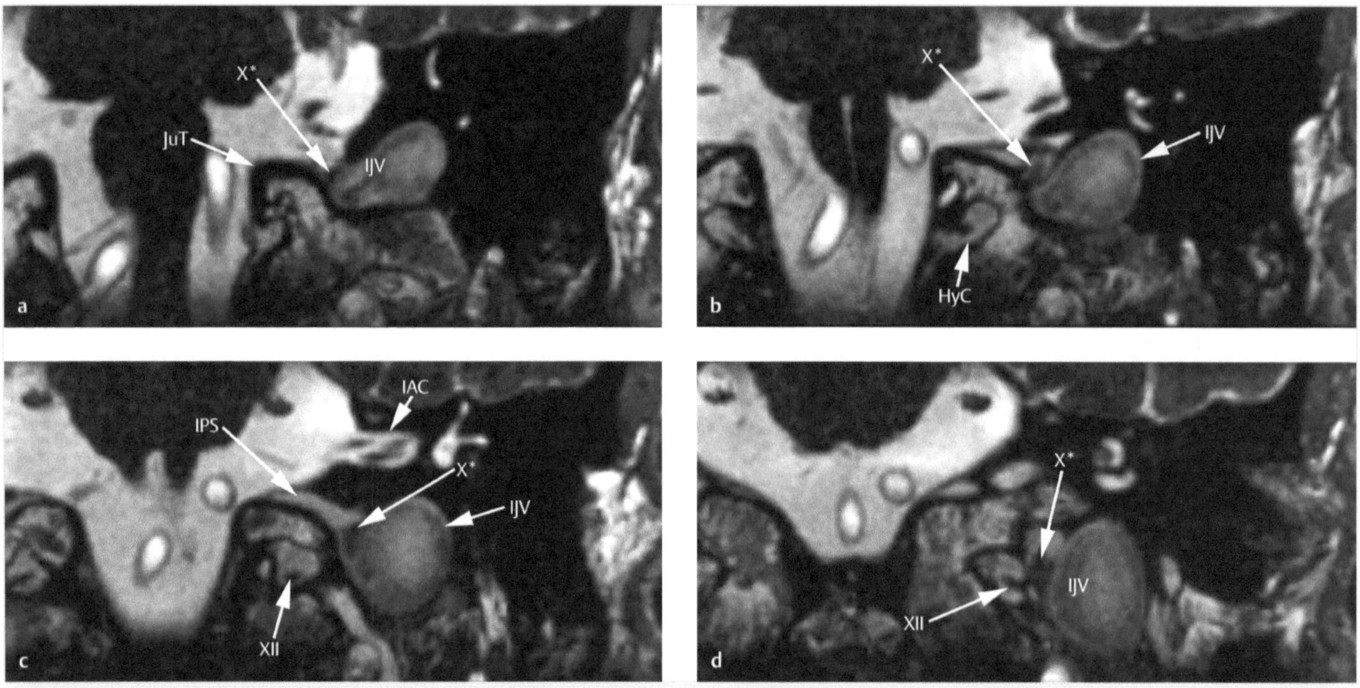

Fig. 24.10 (a–d) Coronal MRI anatomy of the jugular foramen. The panel contains four coronal CISS (constructive interference in steady state) MRI images passing through the jugular foramen, from posterior **(a)** to anterior **(d)**. The jugular foramen and the hypoglossal canal (HyC) arise from the superolateral and inferomedial sides of the jugular tuberculum (JuT), respectively. The lower cranial nerves (X*) and the internal jugular vein (IJV) run in the medial and lateral portions of the jugular foramen, respectively. As a result of these trajectories, the hypoglossal nerve (XII) and the lower cranial nerve converge behind the parapharyngeal segment of the internal carotid artery while exiting from their respective canal/ foramen. IAC, internal auditory canal; IPS, inferior petrosal sinus.

Endoscopic Dissection

Nasal Phase

- Anterior and posterior ethmoidectomy.
- Transethmoidal sphenoidotomy.
- Type D endoscopic medial maxillectomy.

Skull Base Phase

- Transpterygomaxillary approach.
- Infratemporal fossa approach (third corridor).
- Step 1: Removal of the interpterygoid fascia.
- Step 2: Removal of the stylopharyngeal fascia and muscles attached to the styloid process.
- Step 3: Opening of the pterygoid fossa.
- Step 4: Removal of the medial pterygoid plate.
- Step 5: Removal of the lateral pterygoid plate.
- Step 6: Removal of the medial pterygoid muscle.
- Step 7: Removal of the carotid sheath.
- Step 8: Sectioning of the mandibular nerve.
- Step 9: Sectioning of the middle meningeal artery.
- Step 10: Removal of the tensor veli palatini muscle.
- Step 11: Opening of the tubal lumen.
- Step 12: Inferior, posterior, and superior sectioning of the torus and dissection of the eustachian tube from the skull base.
- Step 13: Sectioning of the eustachian tube.
- Step 14: Sectioning of the levator veli palatini and superior constrictor muscles.
- Step 15: Styloidectomy.

Extended Infratemporal Fossa Approach

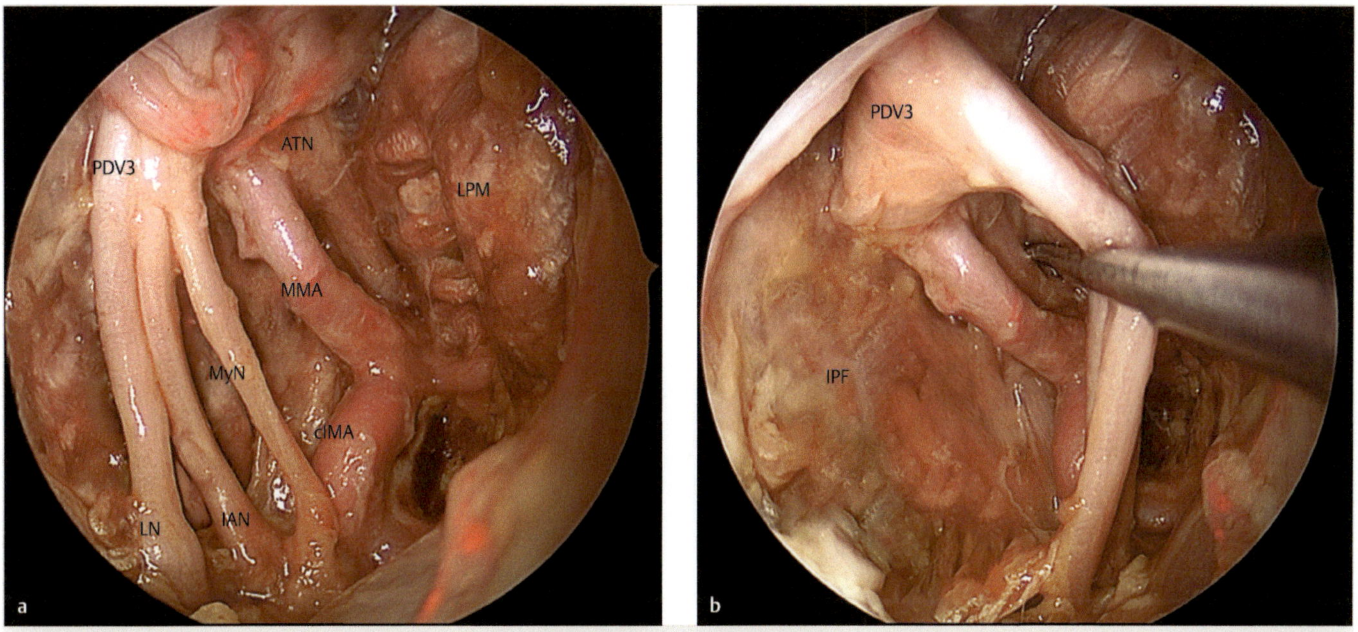

Fig. 24.11 (a, b) The interpterygoid fascia. After completing the infratemporal approach (third corridor), the posterior division of the mandibular nerve (PDV3) is displaced laterally to identify the interpterygoid fascia (IPF), which is the cranial extension of the superficial sheet of the deep cervical fascia and separates the infratemporal fossa from the upper parapharyngeal space. The interpterygoid fascia lies from the posterior border of the temporomandibular joint to the tensor veli palatini muscle. ATN, auriculotemporal nerve; cIMA, condylar tract of the internal maxillary artery; IAN, inferior alveolar nerve; LN, lingual nerve; LPM, lateral pterygoid muscle; MMA, middle meningeal artery; MyN, mylohyoid nerve.

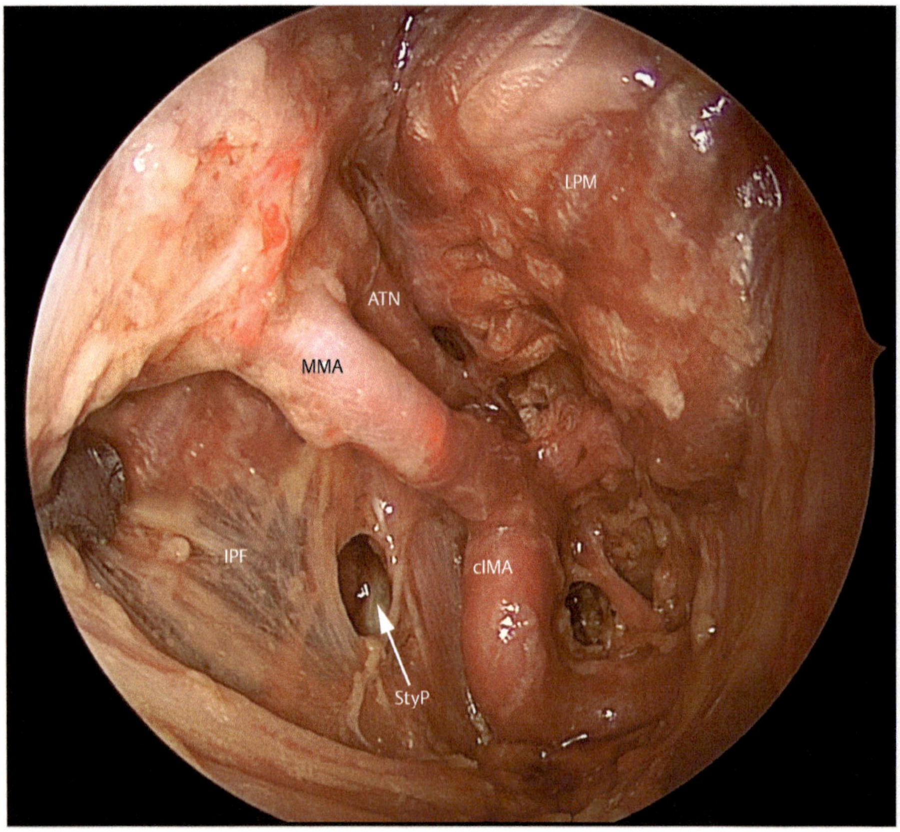

Fig. 24.12 Step 1. The interpterygoid fascia (IPF) is opened to expose the styloid process (StyP) and related muscles. ATN, auriculotemporal nerve; cIMA, condylar tract of the internal maxillary artery; LPM, lateral pterygoid muscle; MMA, middle meningeal artery.

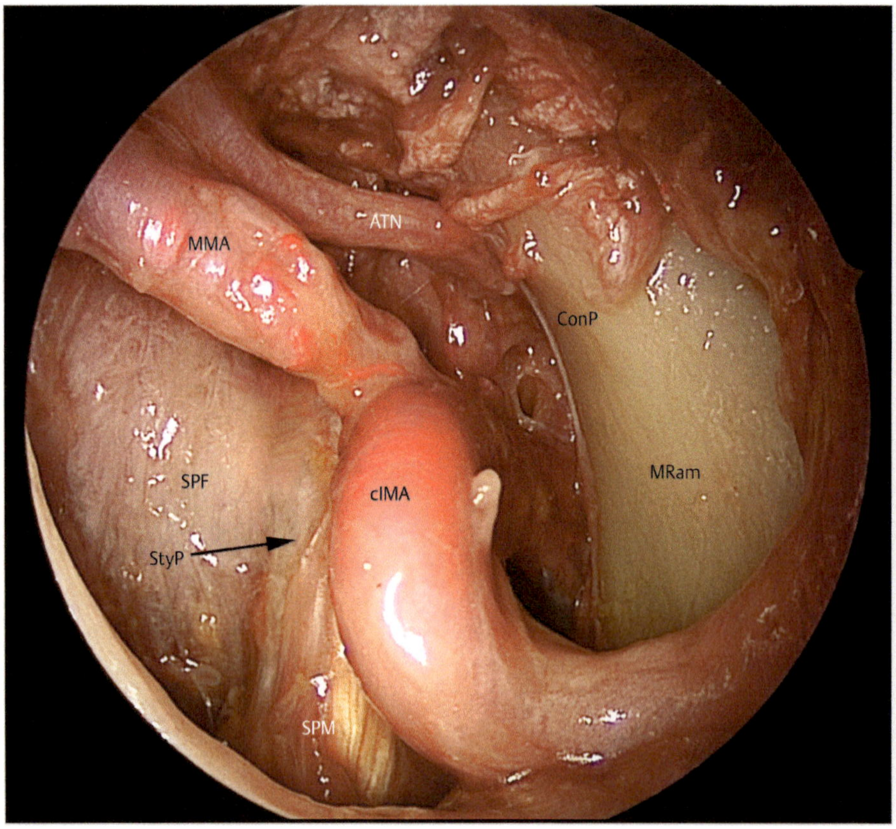

Fig. 24.13 The stylopharyngeal fascia. After removing the interpterygoid fascia, the stylopharyngeal muscle (SPM) and the stylopharyngeal fascia (SPF) come into view. The stylopharyngeal fascia is located anteromedially to the styloid process (StyP) and lies between the stylopharyngeal muscle, posterolaterally, and the levator veli palatini muscle, anteromedially. This fascia separates the prestyloid compartment (also called "true parapharyngeal space") from the retrostyloid compartment of the parapharyngeal space (also called "carotid space"). ATN, auriculotemporal nerve; cIMA, condylar tract of the internal maxillary artery. ConP, condylar process of the mandible; MMA, middle meningeal artery; MRam, mandibular ramus.

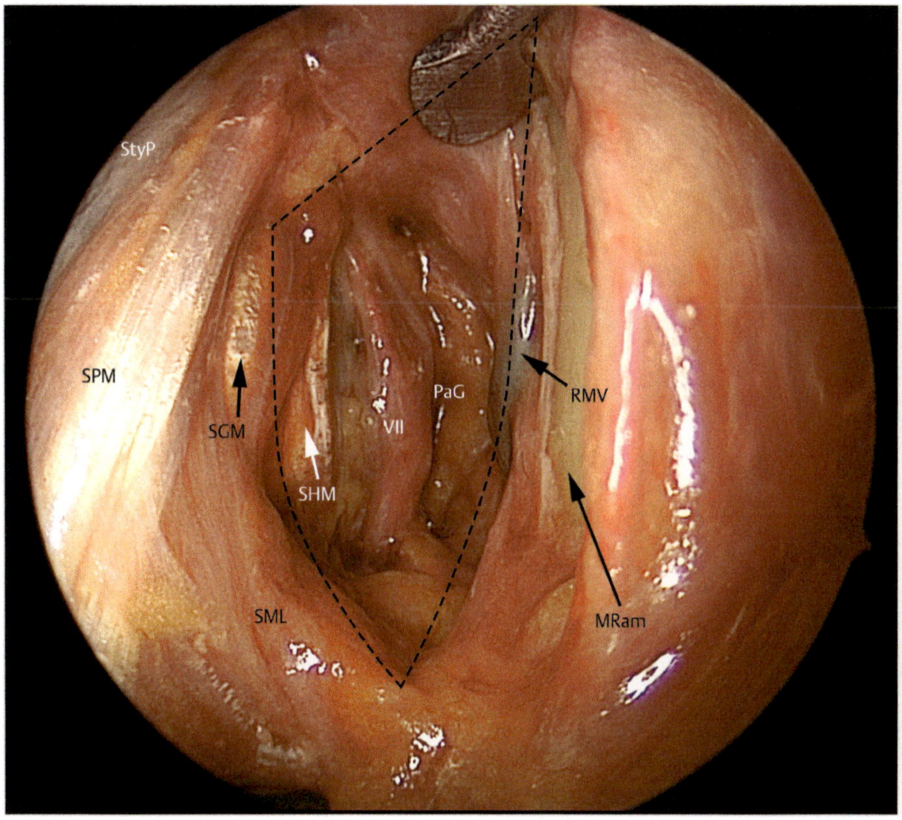

Fig. 24.14 The prestyloid parapharyngeal space. The endoscope is placed close to the mandibular ramus (MRam) to have an overview of the prestyloid compartment and the stylomandibular tunnel (*black dashed line*), which is the triangular space enclosed by the mandibular ramus, anteriorly, the stylomandibular ligament (SML), posteriorly, and the skull base (specifically, the inferior wall of the external auditory canal), superiorly. This tunnel houses the parapharyngeal process of the parotid gland (PaG) and is strictly adjacent to the facial nerve (VII) and the retromandibular vein (RMV). The stylopharyngeal (SPM), styloglossus (SGM), and stylohyoid (SHM) muscles arise from the styloid process (StyP) and form the so-called Riolano's red bouquet.

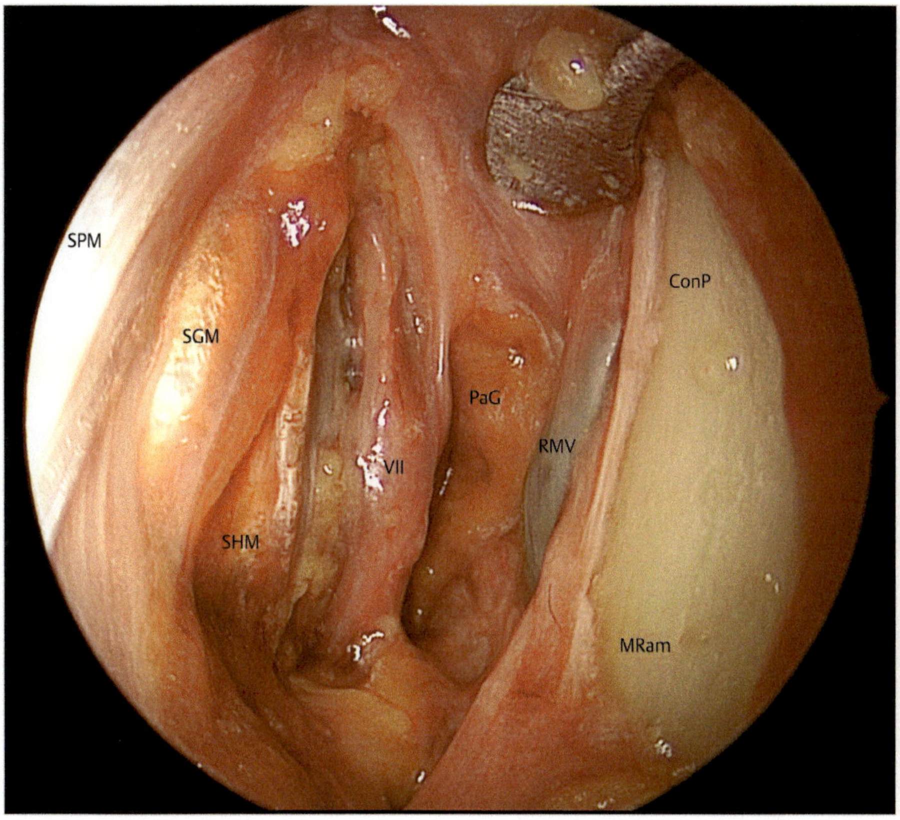

Fig. 24.15 The extracranial facial nerve. The extracranial tract of the facial nerve (VII) is identified by gently dissecting the soft tissues behind the stylohyoid muscle (SHM), within the parotid gland (PaG). ConP, condylar process; MRam, mandibular ramus; RMV, retromandibular vein; SGM, styloglossus muscle; SPM, stylopharyngeal muscle.

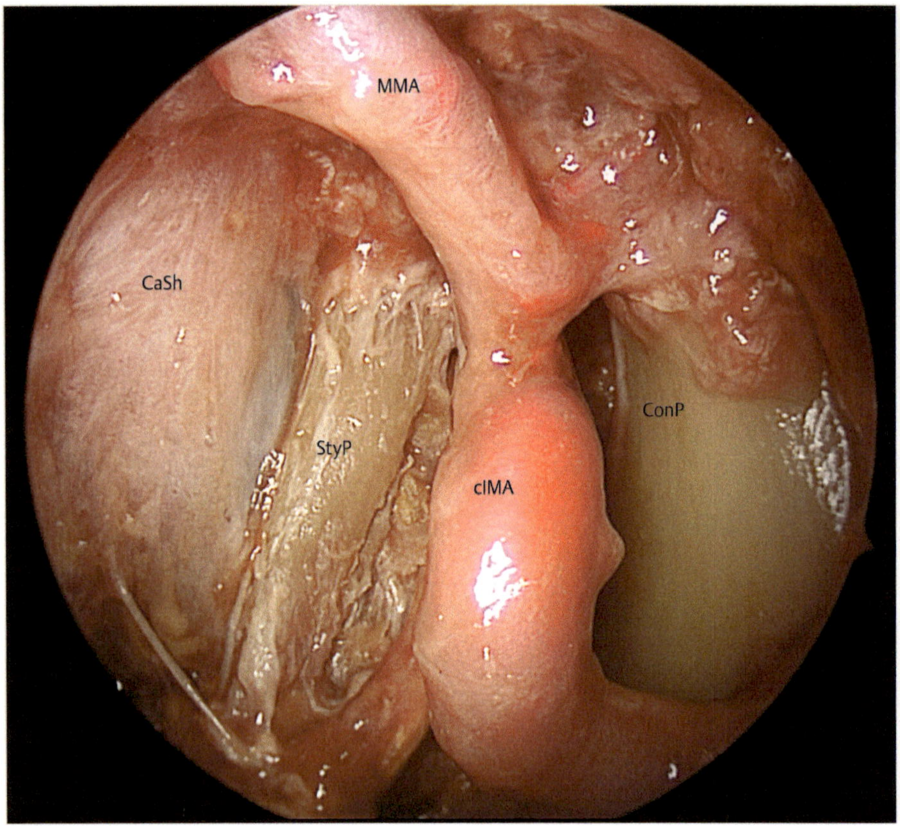

Fig. 24.16 Step 2. The muscular insertions are dissected off the styloid process (StyP). The stylopharyngeal fascia is removed to expose the carotid sheath (CaSh). The condylar tract of the internal maxillary artery (cIMA) passes between the condylar process of the mandible (ConP) and the styloid process. The middle meningeal artery (MMA) runs in front of the root of the styloid process.

Lower Transpterygoid Approach

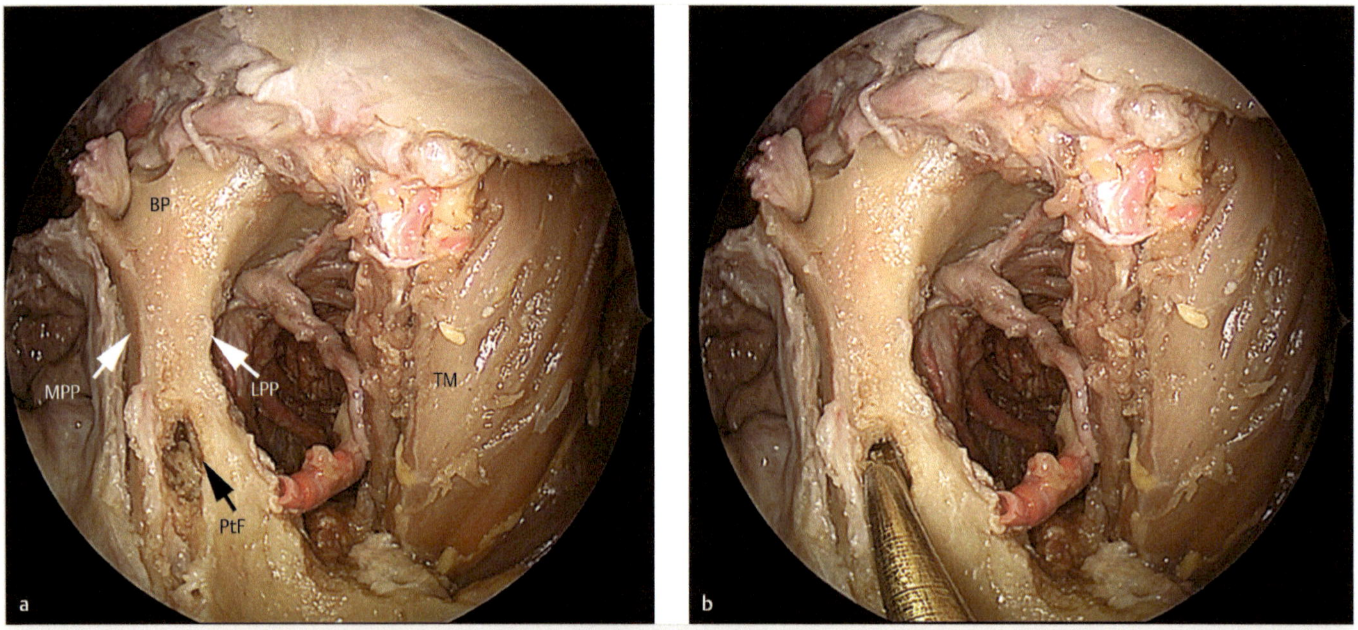

Fig. 24.17 (a, b) Step 3. A small opening is created in the lower portion of the pterygoid process to expose the pterygoid fossa (PtF). A Kerrison rongeur is employed to remove the junction between the medial (MPP) and lateral (LPP) pterygoid plates up to the basipterygoid (BP). TM, temporal muscle.

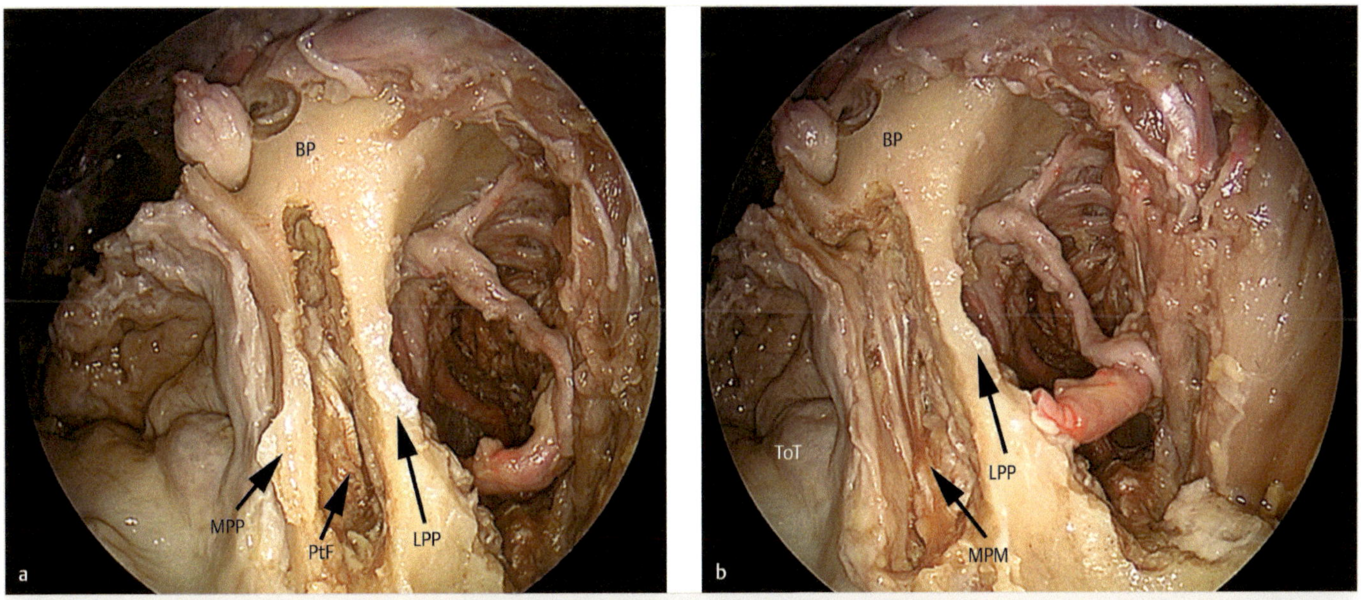

Fig. 24.18 (a, b) Step 4. After opening the pterygoid fossa (PtF), the medial pterygoid plate (MPP) is fractured and removed. BP, basipterygoid; LPP, lateral pterygoid plate MPM, medial pterygoid muscle; ToT, torus tubarius.

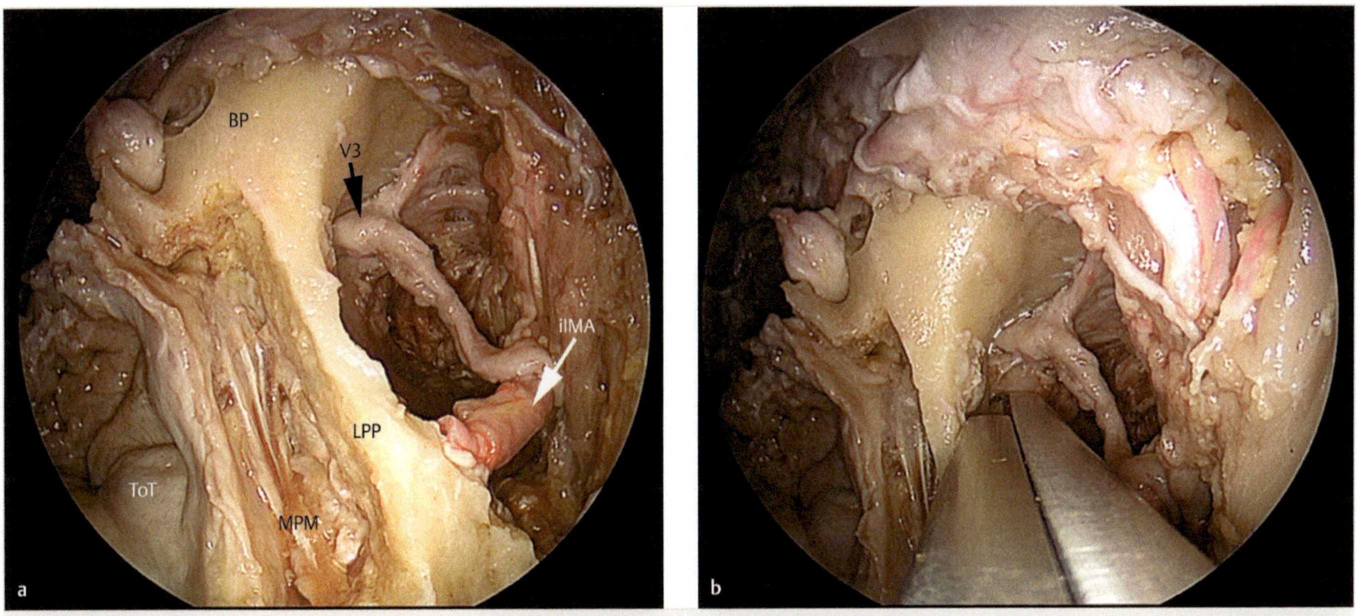

Fig. 24.19 (a, b) Step 5. The lateral pterygoid plate (LPP) is removed with a Kerrison rongeur placed anteriorly to the foramen ovale (*white dashed line*) and the mandibular nerve (V3). The medial pterygoid muscle (MPM) comes into view within the pterygoid fossa. BP, basipterygoid; iIMA, infratemporal tract of the internal maxillary artery; ToT, torus tubarius.

Lateral Parapharyngeal Approach

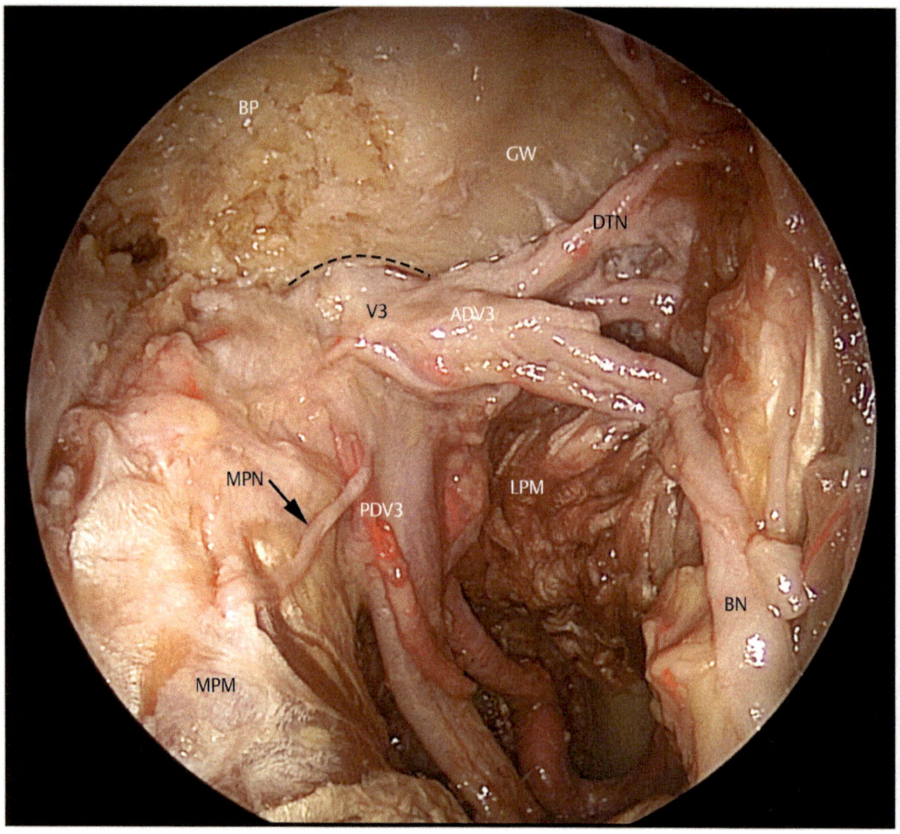

Fig. 24.20 The medial pterygoid muscle. After removing both the medial and lateral pterygoid plates, the upper portion of the medial pterygoid muscle (MPM) comes into view with its nervous branch (MPN) deriving from the anterior division (ADV3) of the mandibular nerve (V3). BN, buccal nerve; BP, basipterygoid; DTN, deep temporal nerve; GW, greater wing of the sphenoid bone; LPM, lateral pterygoid muscle; PDV3, posterior division of the mandibular nerve.

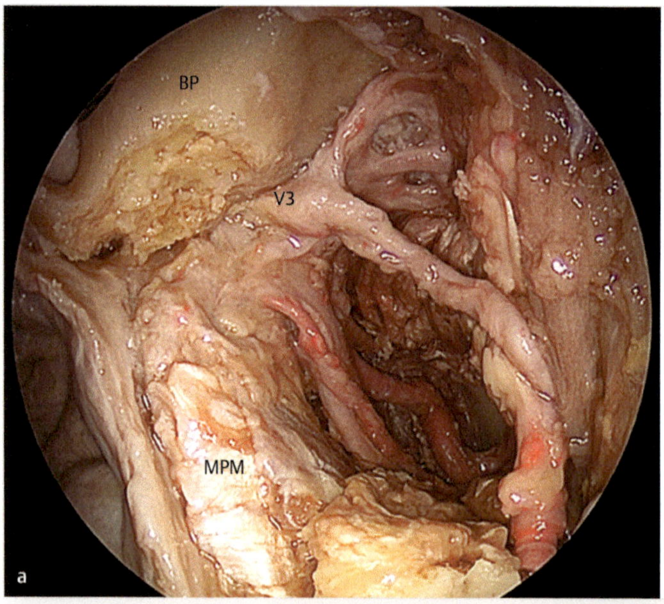

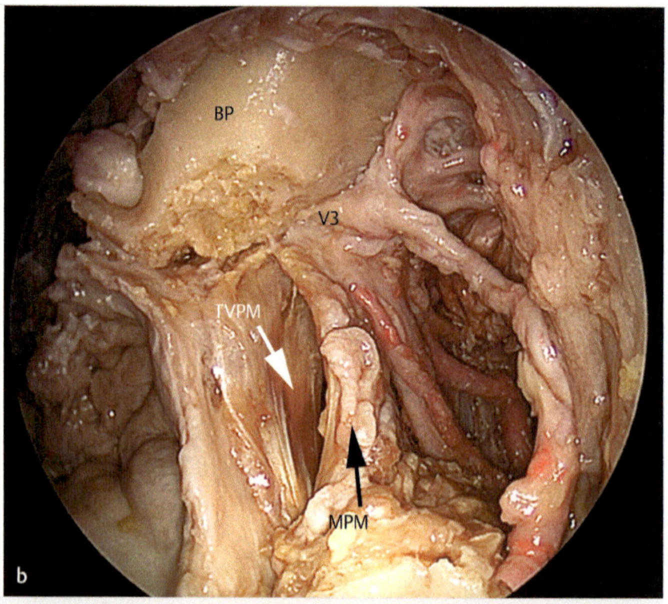

Fig. 24.21 (a, b) Content of the pterygoid fossa. Using a blunt instrument, the plane between the medial pterygoid muscle (MPM), laterally, and the tensor veli palatini muscle (TVPM), medially, is identified and dissected. This plane is of utmost importance as its direction guides directly toward the parapharyngeal segment of the internal carotid artery. The medial pterygoid muscle separates the tensor veli palatini muscle from the mandibular nerve (V3). BP, basipterygoid.

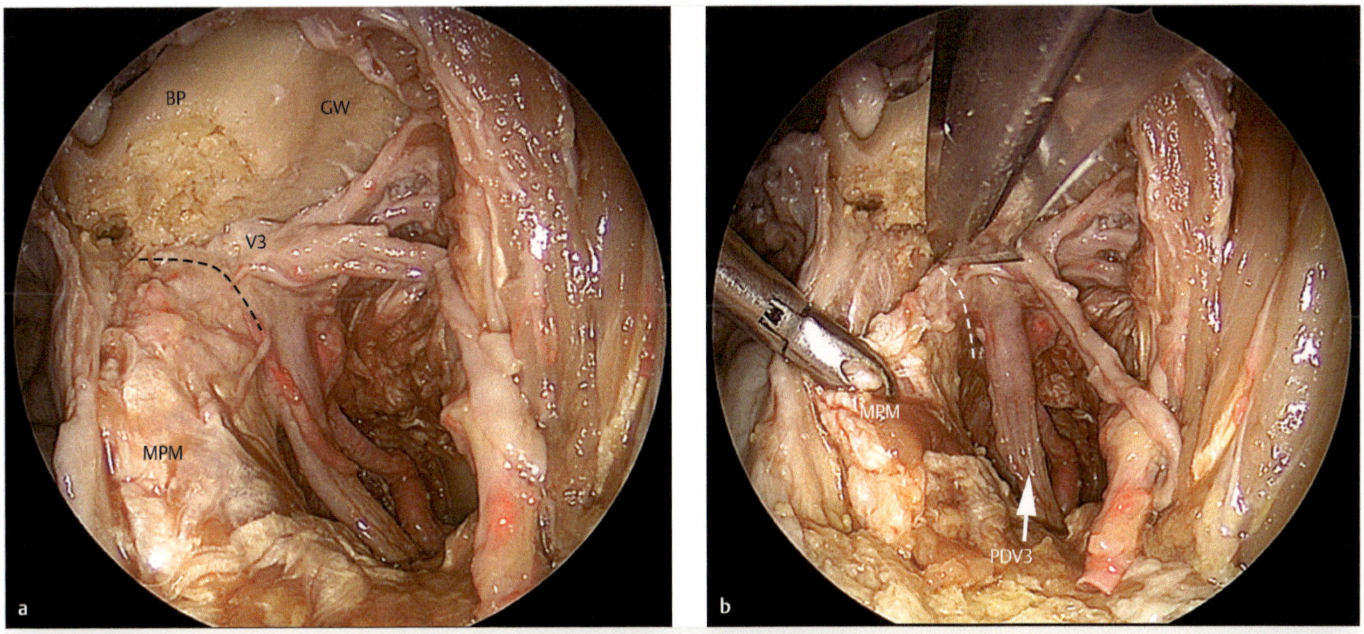

Fig. 24.22 (a, b) Step 6. With a three- to four-hand dissection, the medial pterygoid muscle (MPM) is pulled in an anteromedial direction and cut from anterior to posterior along its superior attachment (*black and white dashed lines*). V3, mandibular nerve; BP, basipterygoid; GW, greater wing of the sphenoid bone; PDV3, posterior division of the mandibular nerve.

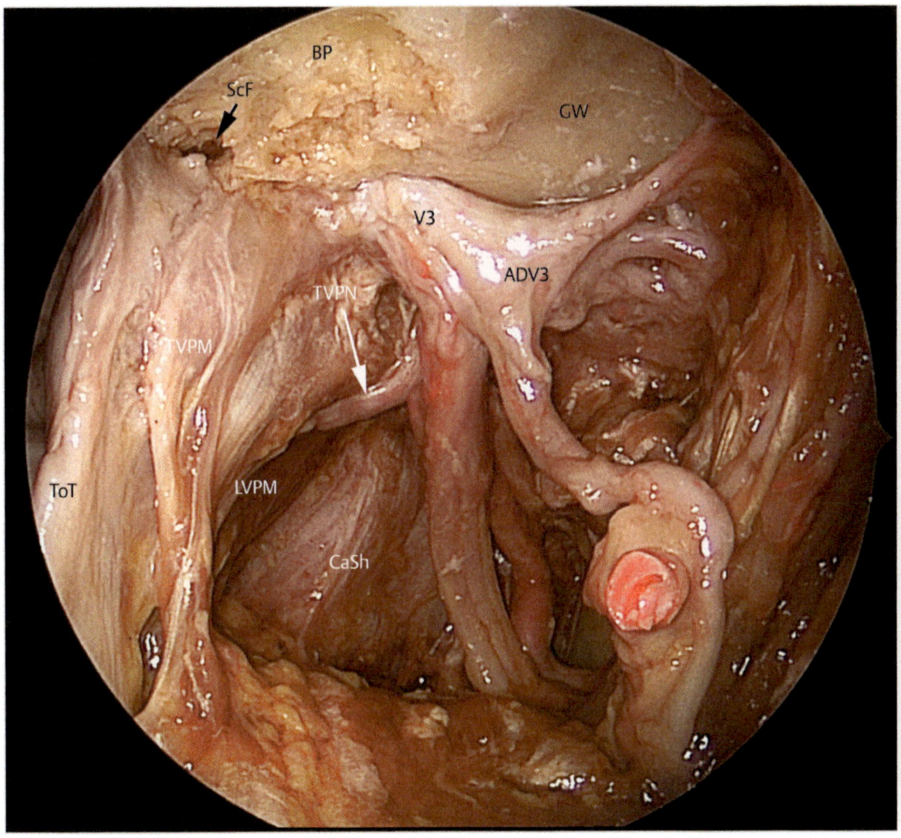

Fig. 24.23 The tensor veli palatini muscle. The tensor veli palatini muscle (TVPM) arises from the lateral surface of the cartilaginous eustachian tube and the scaphoid fossa (ScF), which lies at the junction between the basipterygoid (BP) and pterygoid plates. While descending toward the hamulus of the medial pterygoid plate, the tensor veli palatini muscle narrows to form a fibrous tendon. Its nerve supply (TVPN) comes from the mandibular nerve (V3). ADV3, anterior division of the mandibular nerve; CaSh, carotid sheath; GW, greater wing of the sphenoid bone; LVPM, levator veli palatini muscle; ToT, torus tubarius.

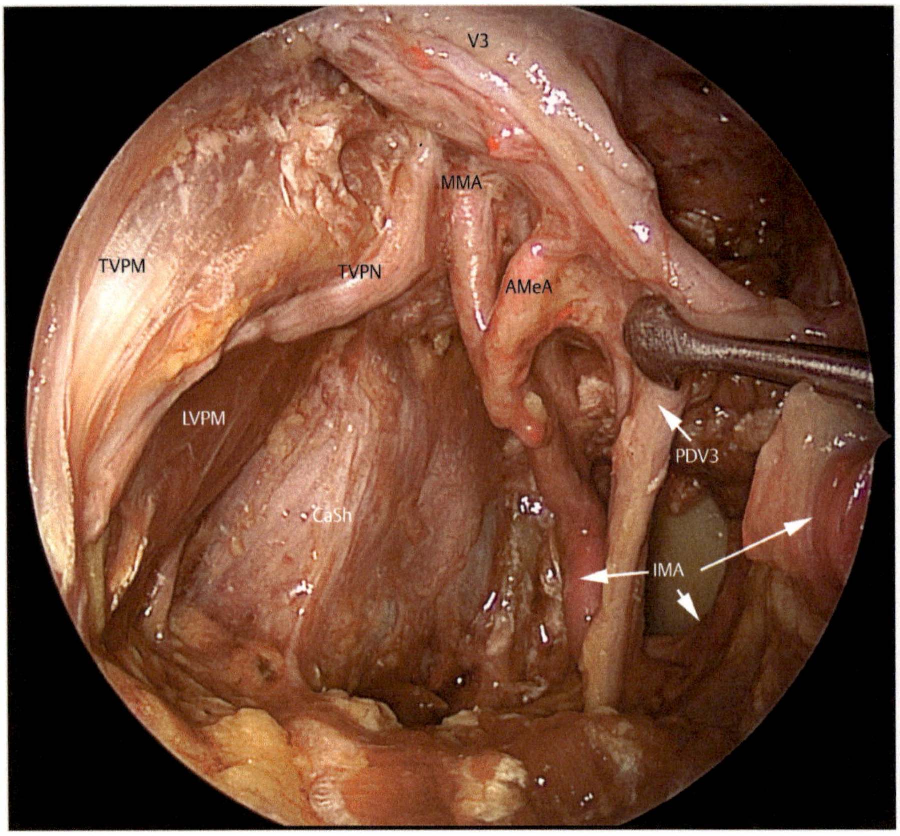

Fig. 24.24 The carotid sheath. After removing the medial pterygoid muscle, both the tensor veli palatini muscle (TVPM) and the levator veli palatini muscle (LVPM) can be identified. The carotid sheath (CaSh) lies posterolaterally to the levator veli palatini muscle and envelopes the neurovascular content of the retrostyloid compartment of the parapharyngeal space. Moving laterally the posterior division (PDV3) of the mandibular nerve (V3), the middle (MMA) and accessory (AMeA) meningeal arteries come into view. Both these arteries arise from the internal maxillary artery (IMA). TVPN, tensor veli palatini nerve supply.

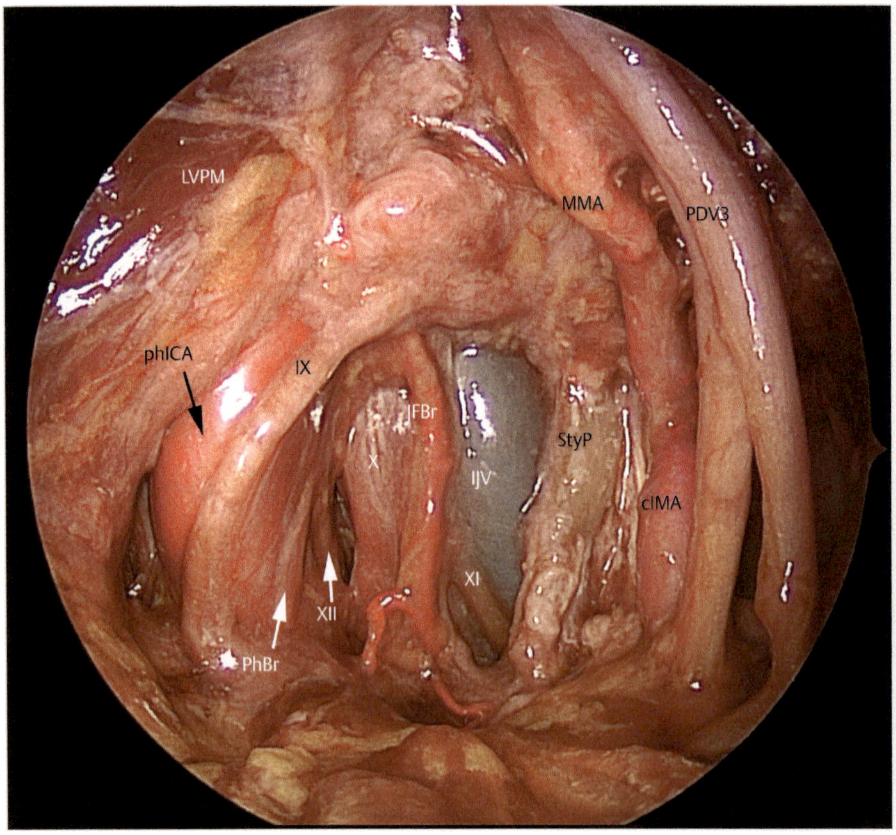

Fig. 24.25 Step 7. The carotid sheath is removed to expose the neurovascular structures within the carotid space. This maneuver allows identification of the parapharyngeal segment of the internal carotid artery (phICA), which is crossed on its lateral surface by the glossopharyngeal nerve (IX), superiorly, and the pharyngeal branch (PhBr) of the vagus nerve (X), inferiorly. The internal jugular vein (IJV) is found posteromedially to the styloid process (StyP): the distance between these structures depends on the variable diameter of the vein. Both the vagus and hypoglossal (XII) nerves run vertically through the interface between the internal carotid artery and the internal jugular vein, parallel to the branch for the jugular foramen (JFBr) of the ascending pharyngeal artery. In most cases (about 70%), the spinal accessory nerve (XI) runs along the anterolateral surface of the internal jugular vein; less frequently, it runs posteromedially to the vein or through a hole across the vessel. cIMA, condylar tract of the internal maxillary artery; LVPM, levator veli palatini muscle; MMA, middle meningeal artery; PDV3, posterior division of the mandibular nerve.

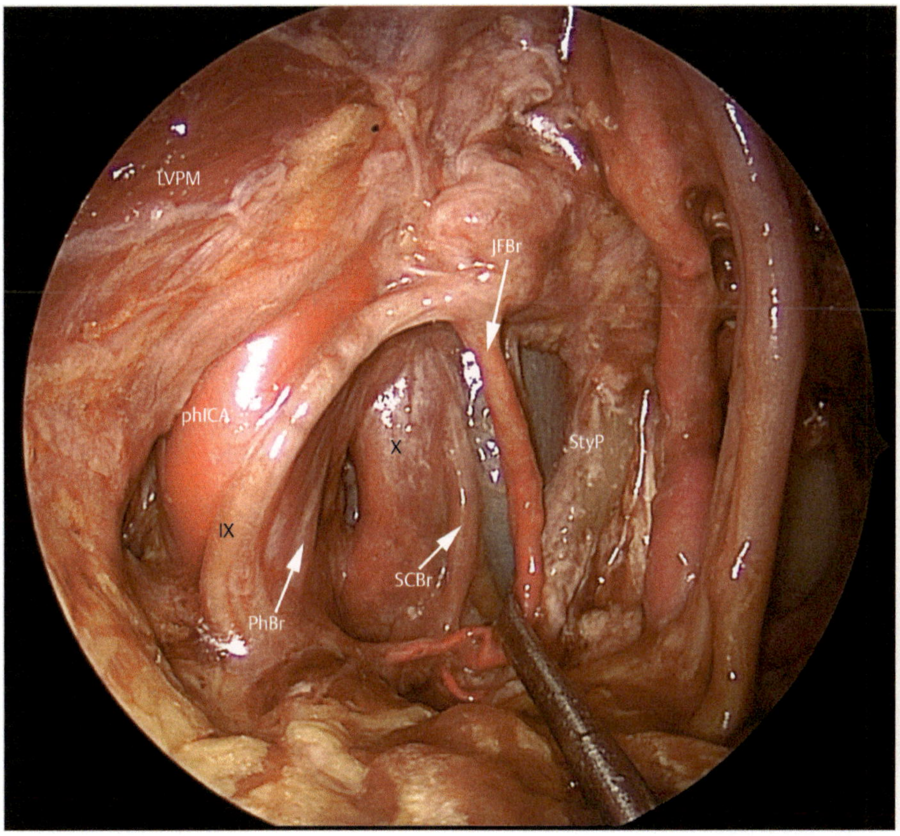

Fig. 24.26 The superior branches of the vagus nerve. By moving laterally the branch for the jugular foramen (JFBr) of the ascending pharyngeal artery, the vagus nerve (X) is better visualized. After passing through the jugular foramen, the nerve gives off three branches. The superior laryngeal nerve runs posteromedially to the parapharyngeal tract of the internal carotid artery (phICA), and thus is not visible through the transnasal perspective. The pharyngeal branch (PhBr) is located laterally to the internal carotid artery, showing a trajectory parallel to the glossopharyngeal nerve (IX). The superior cervical cardiac branch (SCBr) runs in front of the internal jugular vein. LVPM, levator veli palatini muscle; StyP, styloid process.

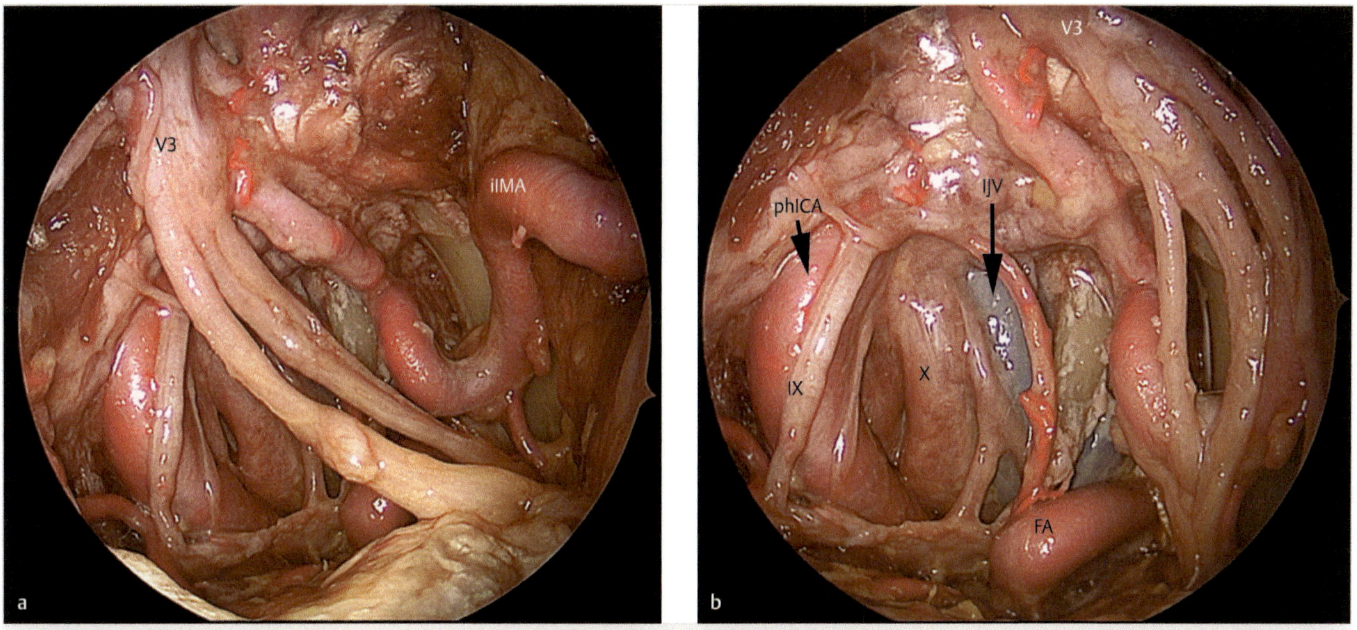

Fig. 24.27 (a, b) The mandibular nerve. With the mandibular nerve (V3) in its anatomical position (left image), it is possible to understand the spatial relationship of the nerve in relation to the carotid space. Moving the mandibular nerve toward the infratemporal segment of the internal maxillary artery (iIMA; right image), the carotid space content comes into view. IX, glossopharyngeal nerve; X, vagus nerve; FA, facial artery; IJV, internal jugular vein; phICA, parapharyngeal tract of the internal carotid artery.

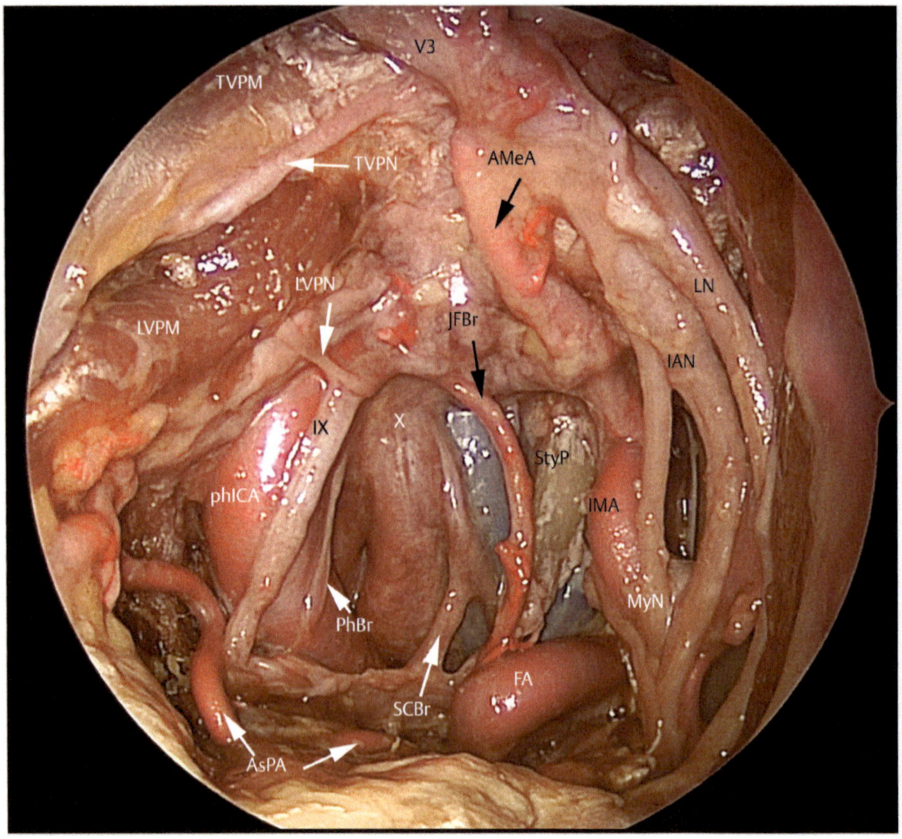

Fig. 24.28 Panoramic view of the lateral parapharyngeal corridor. The lateral parapharyngeal corridor is bounded by the tensor (TVPM) and levator (LVPM) veli palatini muscles with their nerve supply (TVPN and LVPN) superiorly and medially, the lateralized mandibular nerve (V3) superolaterally, and the mylohyoid (MyN), inferior alveolar (IAN), and lingual (LN) nerves, accessory meningeal (AMeA), and internal maxillary arteries (IMA) inferolaterally. The ascending palatine artery (AsPA), a branch of the facial artery (FA), crosses the inferior boundary of the corridor. IX, glossopharyngeal nerve; X, vagus nerve; JFBr, branch for the jugular foramen of the ascending pharyngeal artery; PhBr, pharyngeal branch of the vagus nerve; phICA, parapharyngeal tract of the internal carotid artery; SCBr, superior cervical cardiac branch of the vagus nerve; StyP, styloid process.

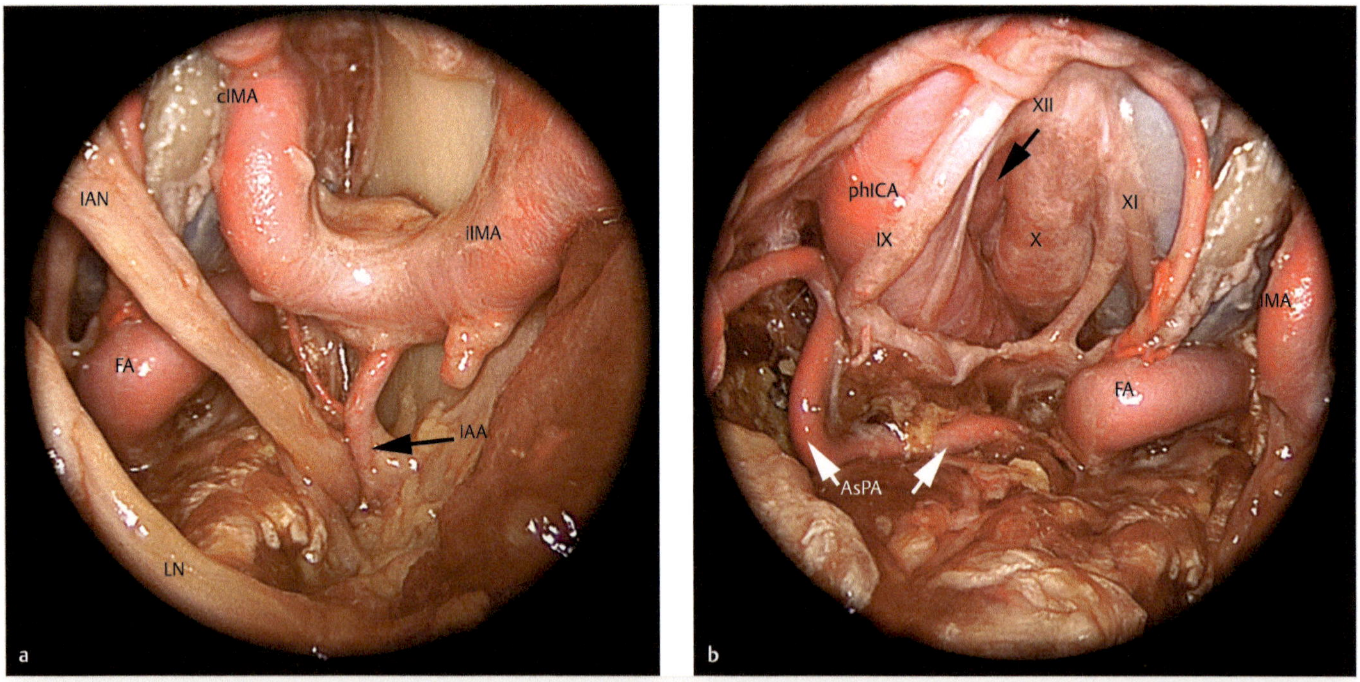

Fig. 24.29 (a, b) The inferior boundary of the lateral parapharyngeal corridor. A 70-degree scope is employed and turned inferiorly to identify the ascending palatine artery (AsPA), which arises from the facial artery (FA) and runs toward the soft palate. Moving the scope laterally, the inferior alveolar nerve (IAN) and the inferior alveolar artery (IAA) can be identified before they enter the mandibular foramen. IX, glossopharyngeal nerve; X, vagus nerve; XI, spinal accessory nerve; XII, hypoglossal nerve; cIMA, condylar tract of the internal maxillary artery; iIMA, infratemporal tract of the internal maxillary artery; IMA, internal maxillary artery; LN, lingual nerve; phICA, parapharyngeal tract of the internal maxillary artery.

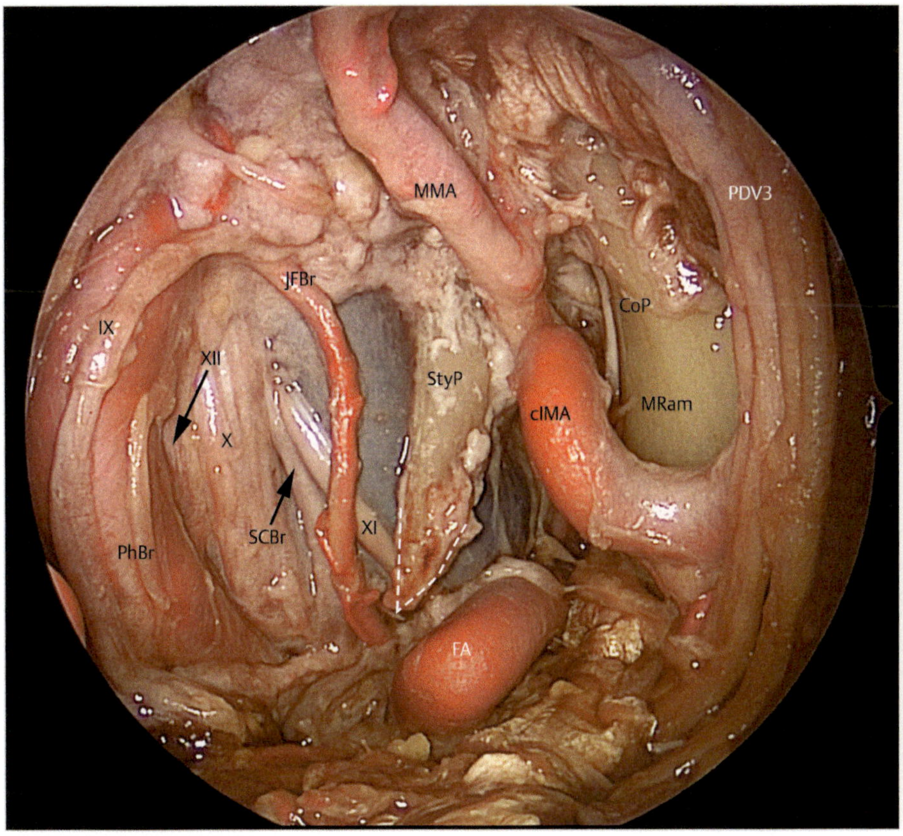

Fig. 24.30 The styloid process. Removal of the tendinous and ligamentous tissues surrounding the styloid process (StyP) to isolate its tip (*white dashed line*) is completed. The condylar tract of the internal maxillary artery (cIMA) runs laterally to this bony process, while the middle meningeal artery (MMA) and spinal accessory nerve (XI) cross it anterosuperiorly and posteromedially, respectively. The facial artery (FA) runs between the stylohyoid and styloglossus muscles, and is thus located anteroinferiorly to the styloid process. IX, glossopharyngeal nerve; X, vagus nerve; XII, hypoglossal nerve; CoP, condylar process of the mandible; JFBr, branch for the jugular foramen of the ascending pharyngeal artery; MRam, mandibular ramus; PDV3, posterior division of the mandibular nerve; PhBr, pharyngeal branch of the vagus nerve; SCBr, superior cervical cardiac branch of the vagus nerve.

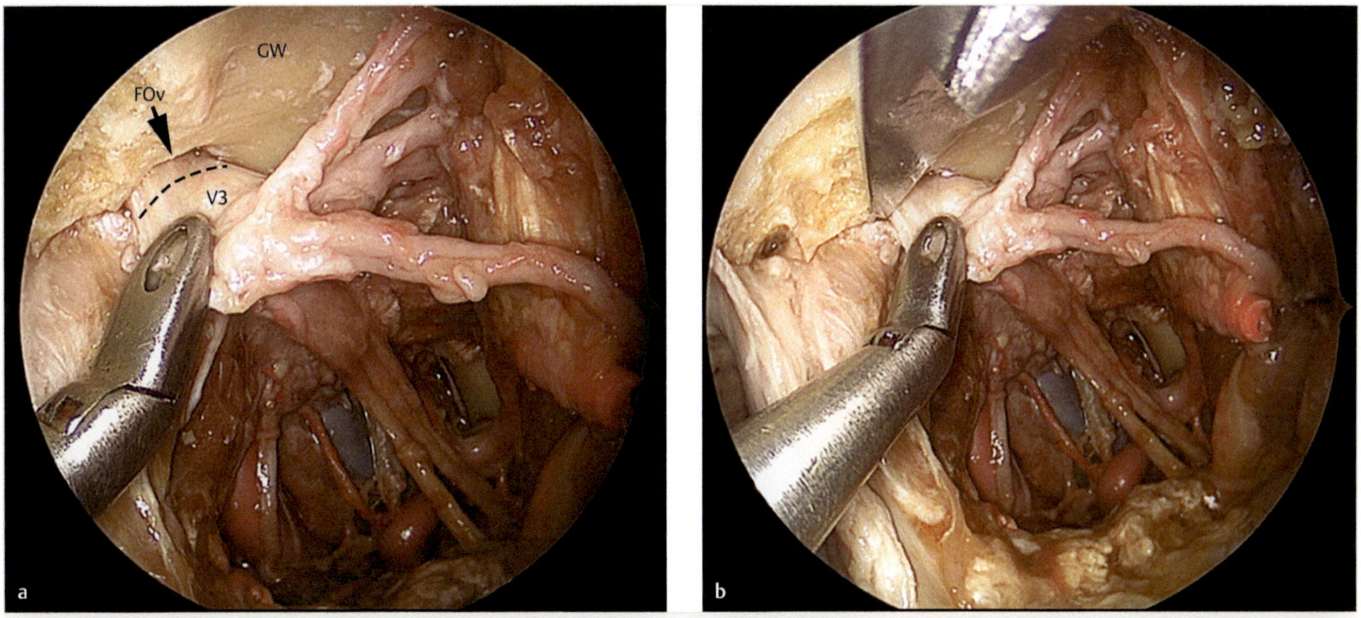

Fig. 24.31 (a, b) Step 8. The common trunk of the mandibular nerve (V3) is pulled inferiorly and cut in close vicinity to the foramen ovale (FOv; *black dashed line*). GW, greater wing of the sphenoid bone.

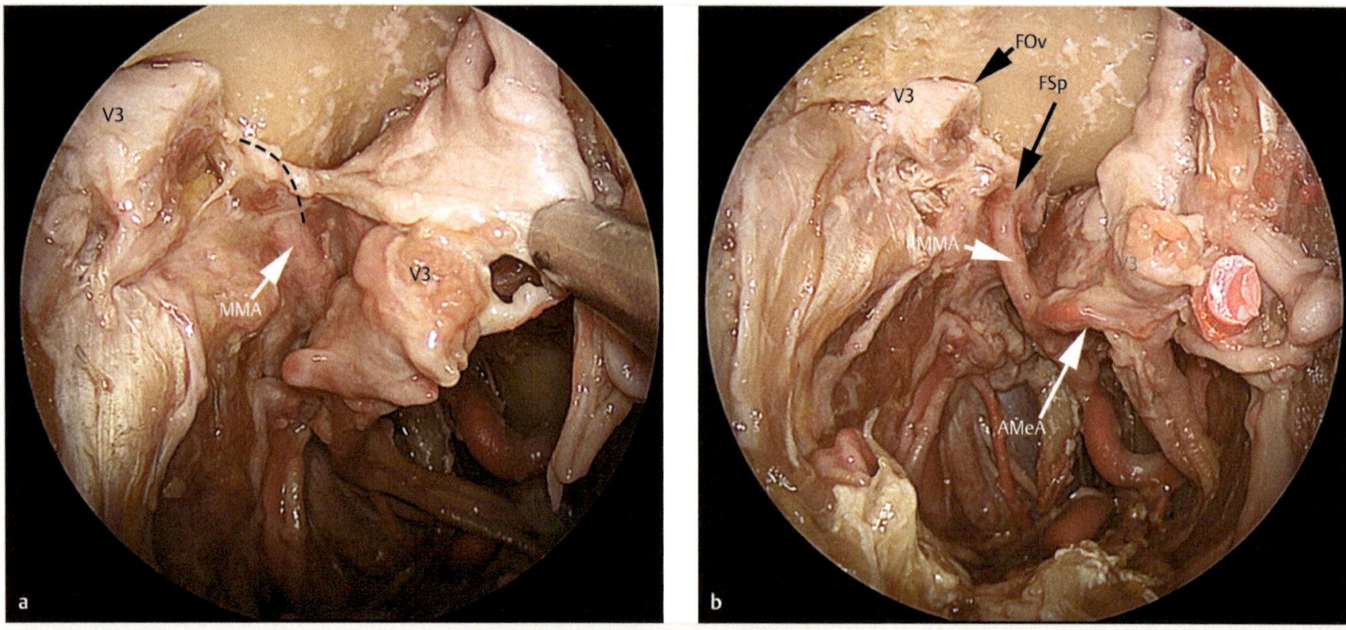

Fig. 24.32 (a, b) The foramen spinosum. After sectioning the mandibular nerve (V3), the periosteum between the foramen ovale (FOv) and the foramen spinosum (FSp) is progressively incised. This maneuver leads to isolation of the extracranial portion of the middle meningeal artery (MMA) up to its entrance into the foramen spinosum. AMeA, accessory meningeal artery.

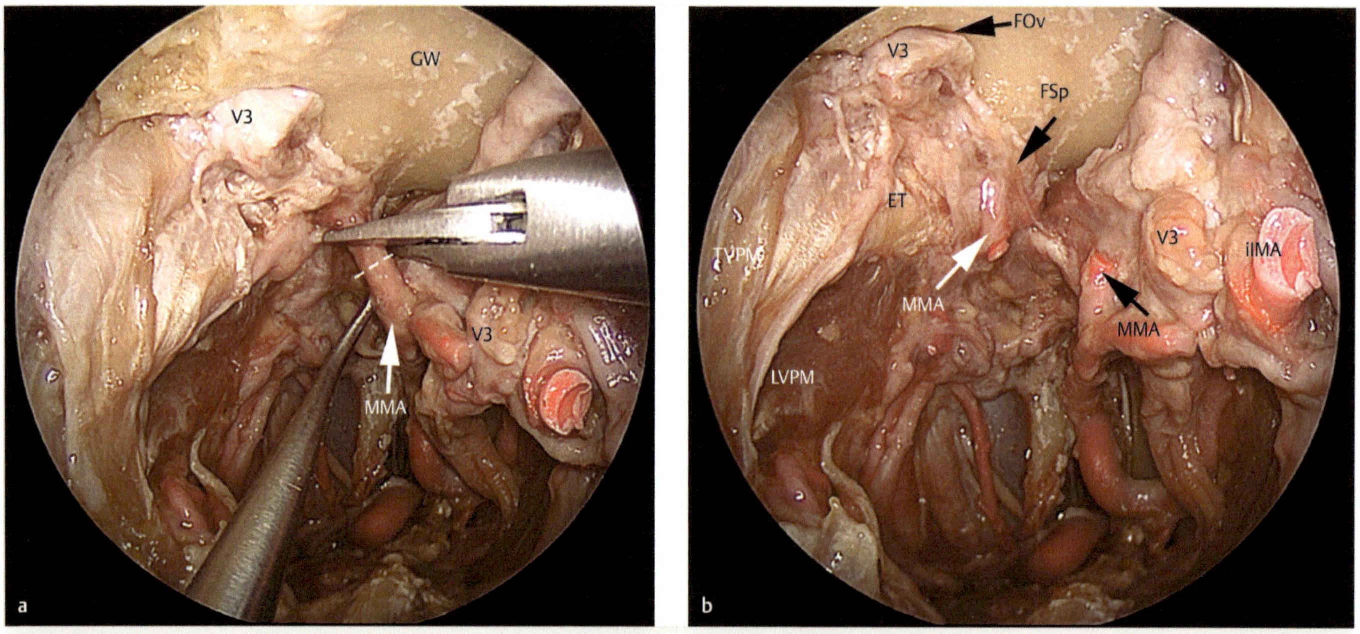

Fig. 24.33 (a, b) Step 9. The middle meningeal artery (MMA) is cut (*white dashed line*) close to the foramen spinosum (FSp) to expose the junction between the bony and cartilaginous portions of the eustachian tube (ET). V3, mandibular nerve (sectioned); iIMA, infratemporal tract of the internal maxillary artery; FOv, foramen ovale; LVPM, levator veli palatini muscle; TVPM, tensor veli palatini muscle.

Resection of the Eustachian Tube

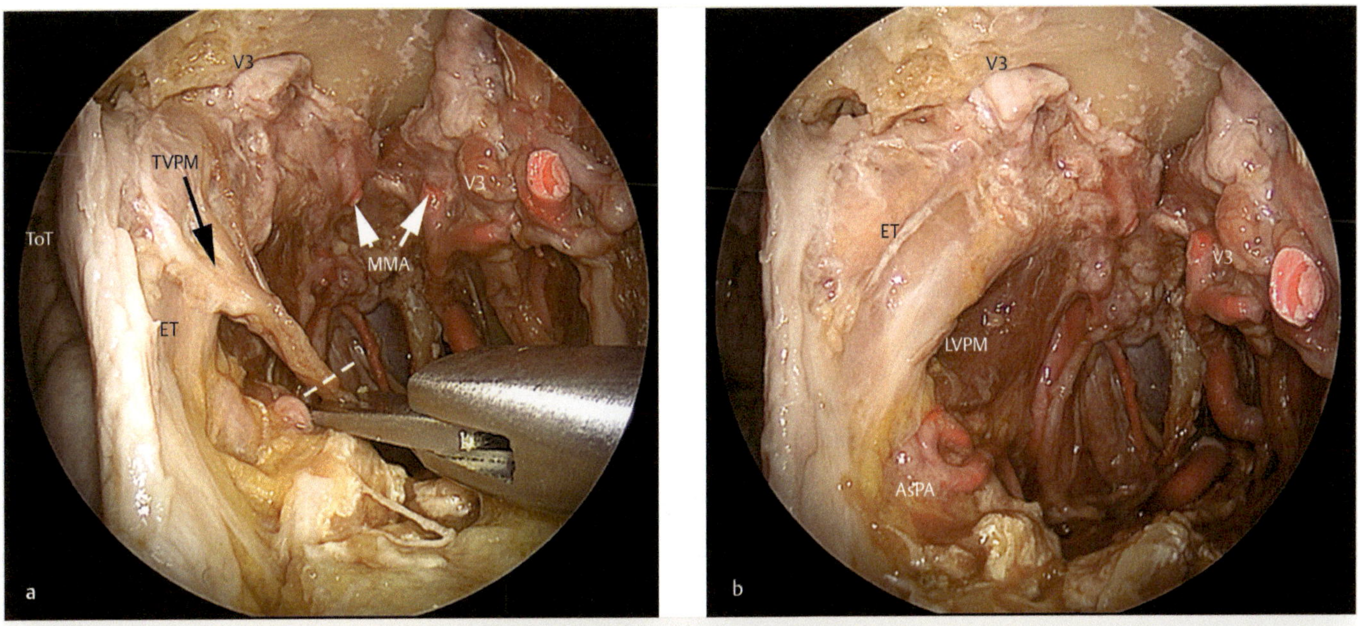

Fig. 24.34 (a, b) Step 10. The tendon of the tensor veli palatini muscle (TVPM) is cut (*white dashed line*) and the muscle is removed to expose the cartilaginous portion of the eustachian tube (ET). The levator veli palatini muscle (LVPM) lies inferiorly to the eustachian tube. V3, mandibular nerve (sectioned); AsPA, ascending palatine artery; MMA, middle meningeal artery (sectioned); ToT, torus tubarius.

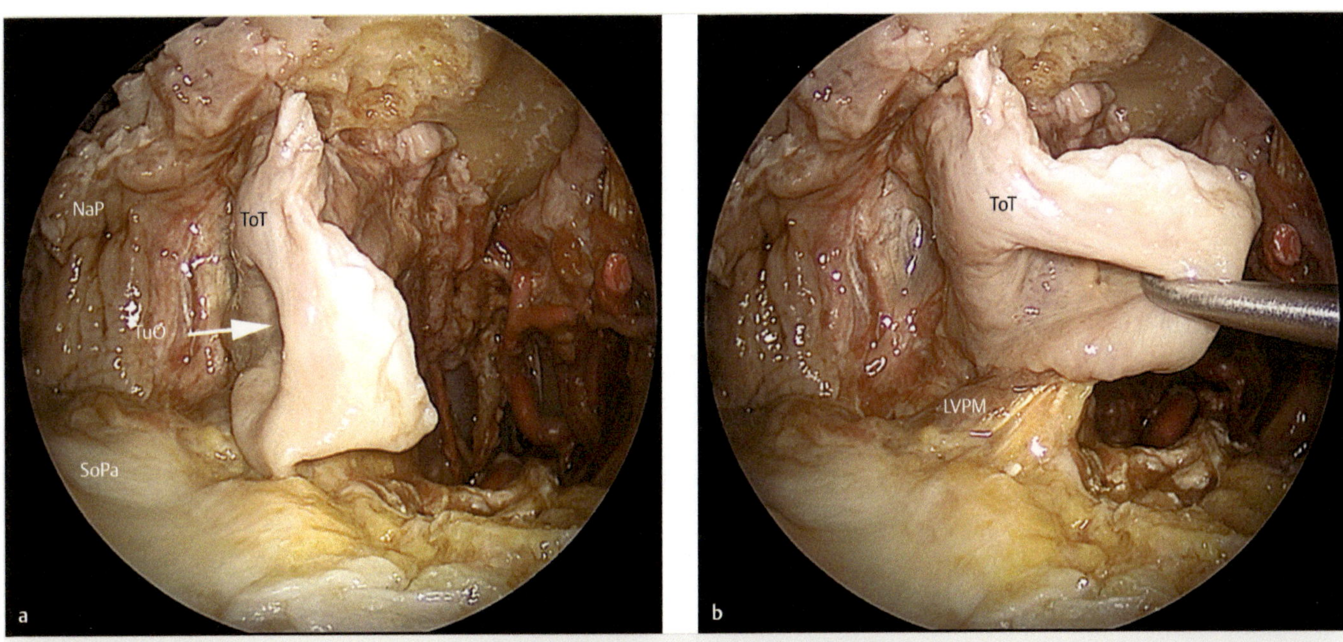

Fig. 24.35 (a, b) The distal insertion of the levator veli palatini muscle. The scope is moved into the nasopharynx and a curved probe is placed into the tubal orifice (TuO) to move the torus tubarius (ToT) superolaterally. This maneuver allows the exposure of the distal insertion of the levator veli palatini muscle (LVPM) on the soft palate (SoPa). NaP, posterior wall of the nasopharynx.

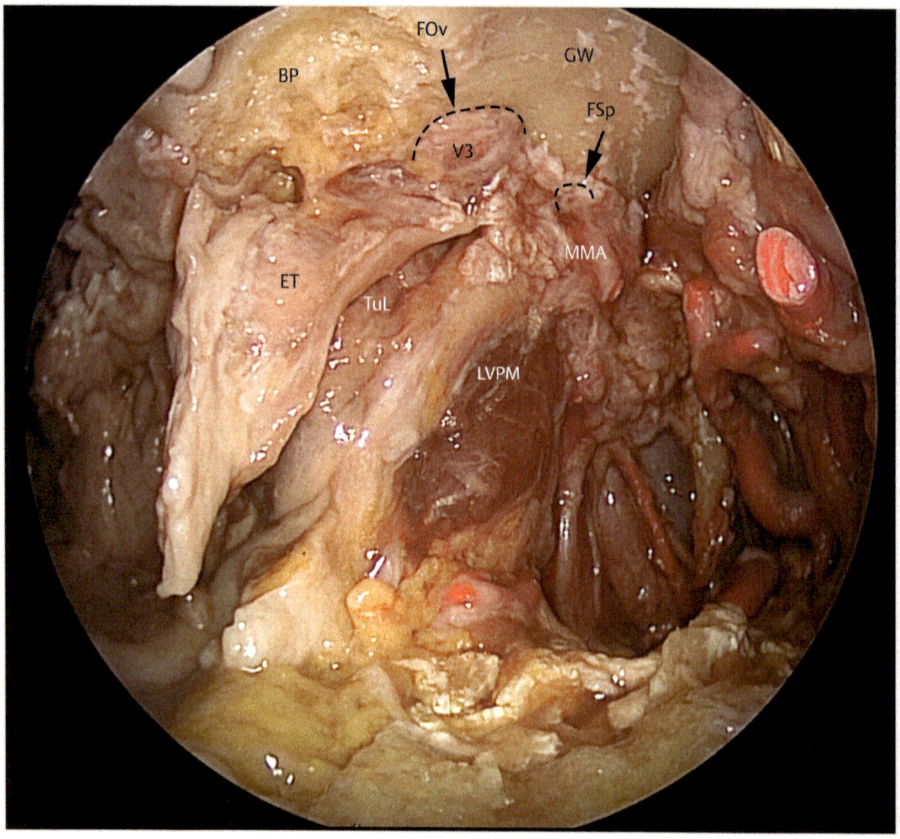

Fig. 24.36 Step 11. By using a ball probe inserted through the tubal lumen (TuL) as a guide, the fibrous tissue that joins the posteromedial and anterolateral cartilaginous plates of the eustachian tube (ET) is removed. The tubal lumen passes above the levator veli palatini muscle (LVPM) and behind the foramina ovale (FOv, *black dashed line*) and spinosum (FSp, *black dashed line*). V3, mandibular nerve (sectioned); BP, basipterygoid; GW, greater wing of the sphenoid bone; MMA, middle meningeal artery (sectioned).

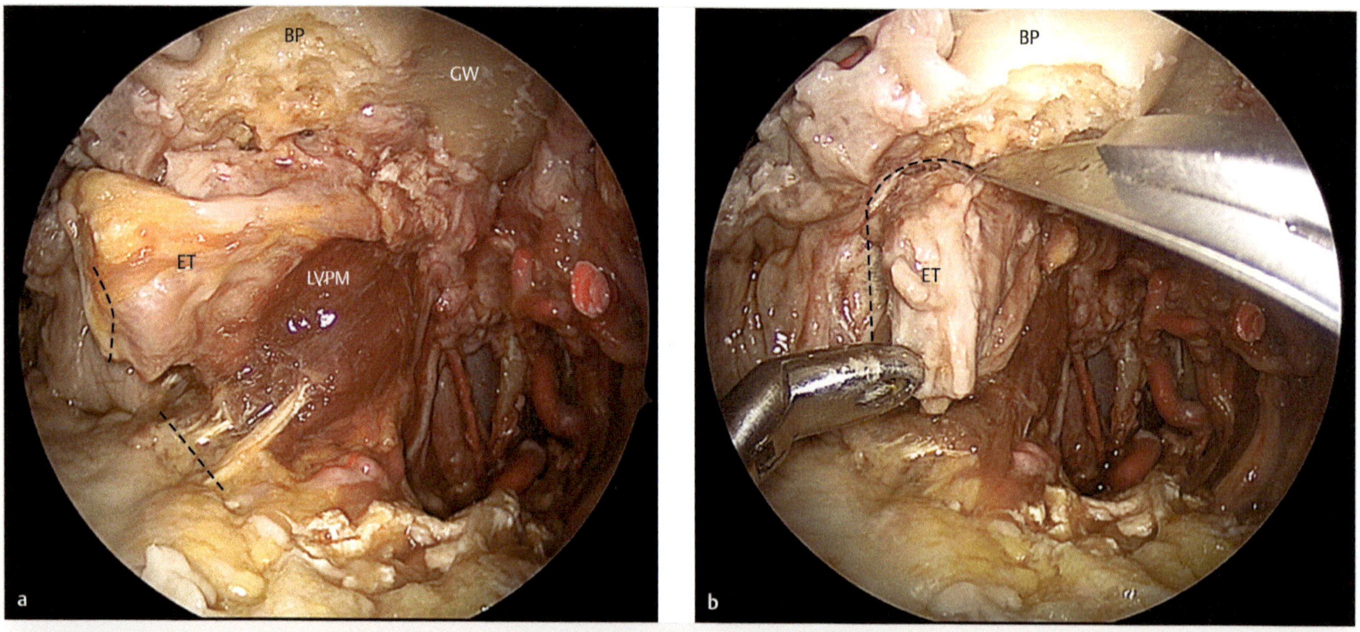

Fig. 24.37 (a, b) Step 12. The eustachian tube (ET) is pulled superiorly and a horizontal incision (*black dashed line* in **a**) is made on the mucosa that joins the torus tubarius with the soft palate. Subsequently, the eustachian tube is pulled inferiorly and the junction between the posterior wall of the nasopharynx and the Rosenmüller fossa is sectioned vertically, turning the incision horizontally above the tube to cut the fibrous tissue that anchors its cartilaginous portion to the fibrocartilago basalis (*black dashed line* in **b**). BP, basipterygoid; GW, greater wing of the sphenoid bone; LVPM, levator veli palatini muscle.

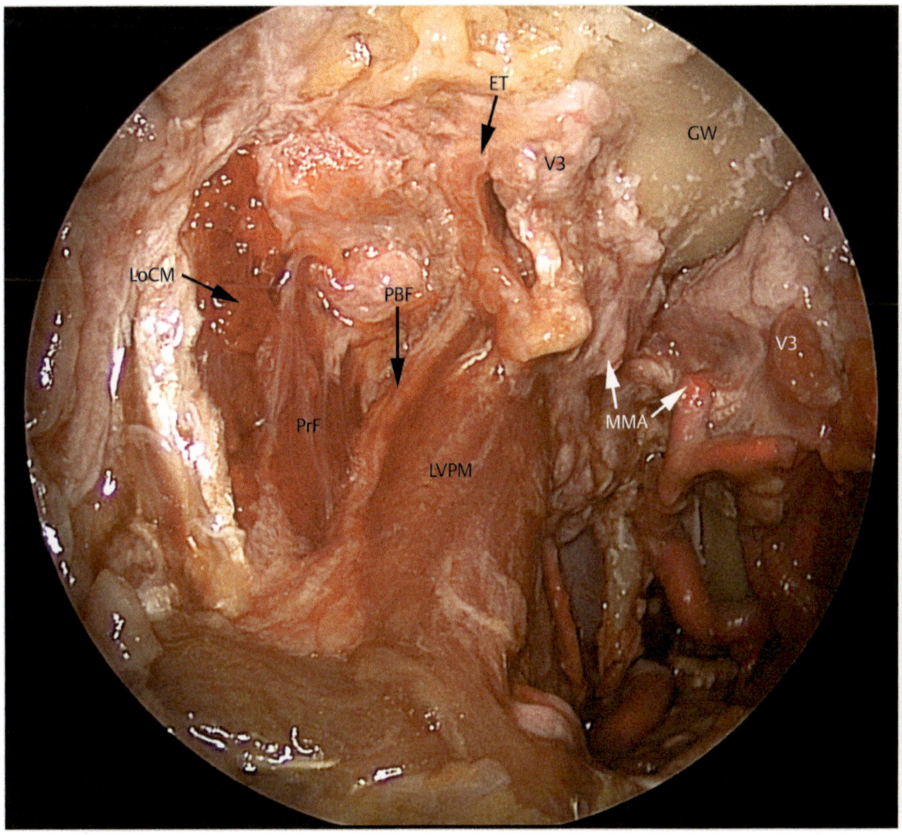

Fig. 24.38 Step 13. The eustachian tube is cut as close to the skull base as possible. The levator veli palatini muscle (LVPM) runs within the pharyngeal wall, passing through the sinus of Morgagni, a defect of the pharyngeal wall, which is made up of the pharyngobasilar fascia (PBF) and the superior constrictor muscle. Notably, leaving the levator veli palatini muscle intact allows for protection of the internal carotid artery during dissection. The prevertebral fascia (PrF) covers the longus capitis muscle (LoCM) and lies behind the pharyngobasilar fascia. V3, mandibular nerve (sectioned); ET, eustachian tube; GW, greater wing of the sphenoid bone; MMA, middle meningeal artery (sectioned).

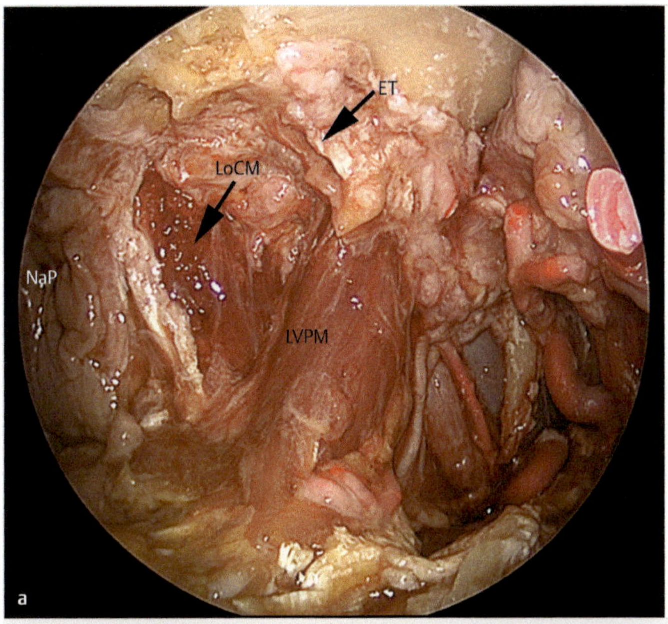

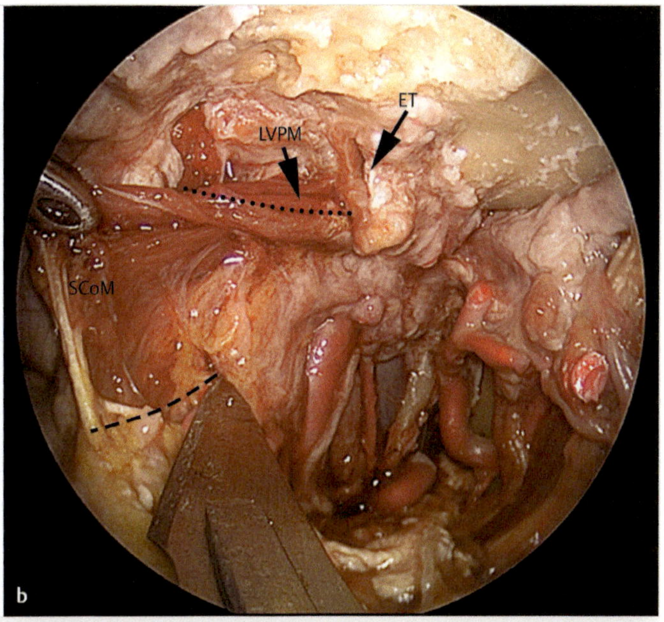

Fig. 24.39 (a, b) Step 14. The levator veli palatini muscle (LVPM) is pulled superomedially to expose the superior constrictor muscle (SCoM). The plane between the levator veli palatini muscle and superior constrictor muscle (*black dotted line*) is identified; both the muscles are cut distally (*black dashed line*). ET, eustachian tube; LoCM, longus capitis muscle; NaP, posterior wall of the nasopharynx.

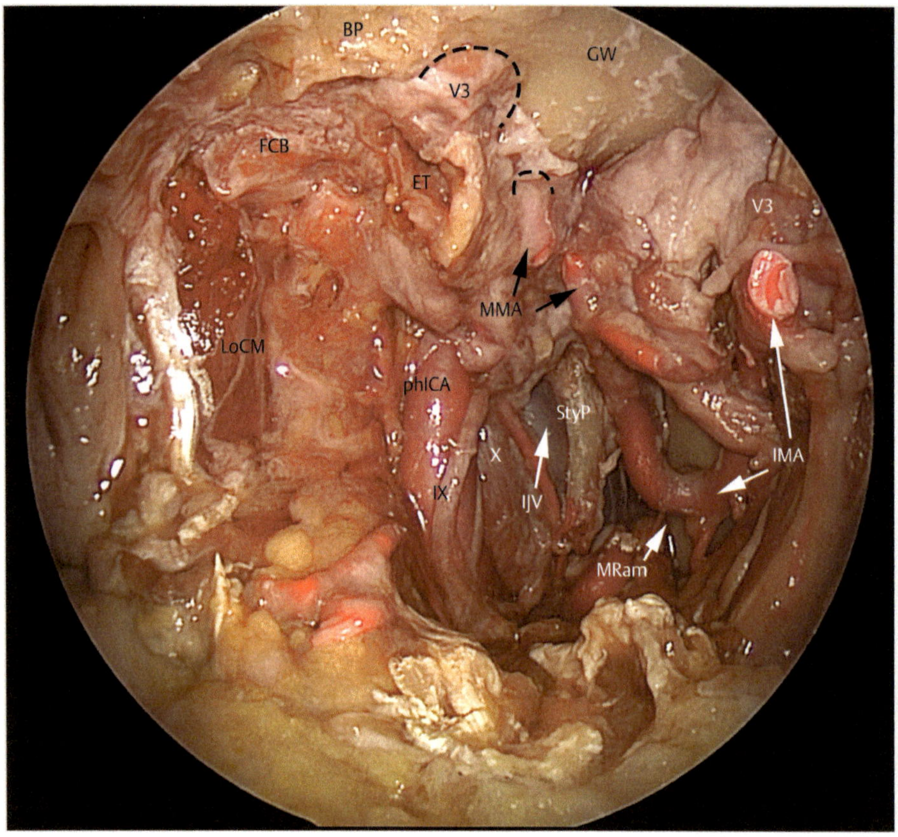

Fig. 24.40 Panoramic view of the whole parapharyngeal corridor. The entire upper parapharyngeal space is exposed. The deep boundaries of the corridor are the longus capitis muscle (LoCM), medially, the parapharyngeal segment of the internal carotid artery (phICA), the glossopharyngeal (IX) and vagus (X) nerves, and internal jugular vein (IJV), in the center, and the styloid process (StyP) and the parotid gland, laterally. The roof of the corridor consists of the base of the pterygoid process (BP), fibrocartilago basalis (FCB), greater wing of the sphenoid bone (GW), and the lateral portion of the eustachian tube (ET). *Black dashed lines:* show the foramina ovale and spinosum. V3, mandibular nerve (sectioned); IMA, internal maxillary artery; MMA, middle meningeal artery (sectioned); MRam, mandibular ramus.

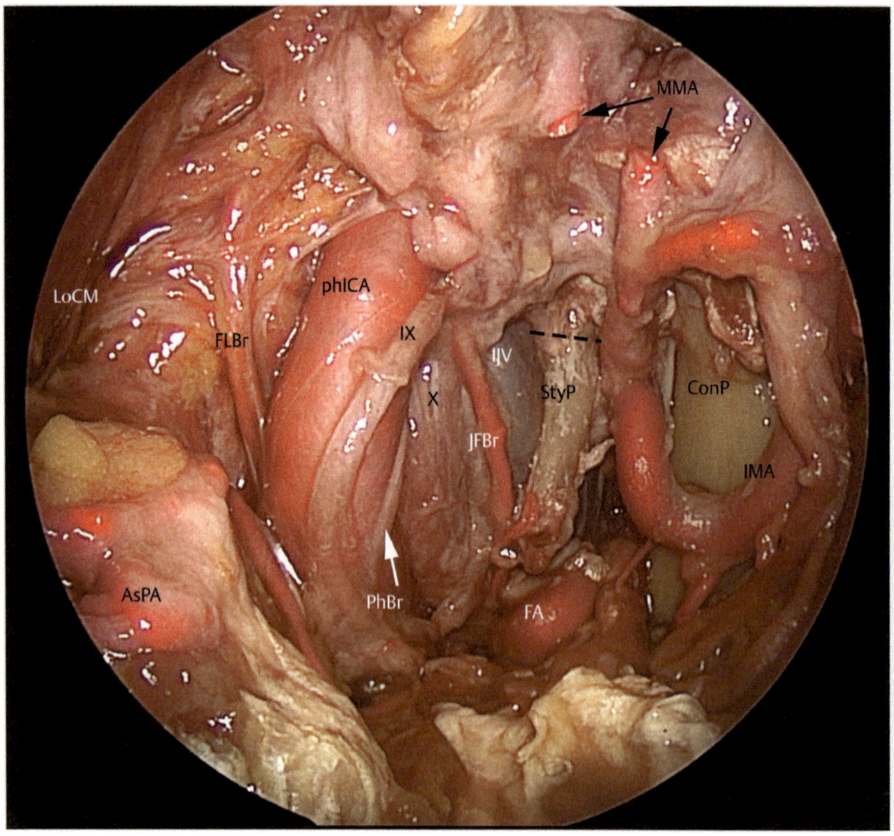

Fig. 24.41 Step 15. The superior portion of the styloid process (StyP) is sectioned with a Kerrison rongeur (*black dashed line*). The branch for the foramen lacerum (FLBr) of the ascending pharyngeal artery runs laterally to the longus capitis muscle (LoCM) and parallel to the parapharyngeal segment of the internal carotid artery (phICA). IX, glossopharyngeal nerve; X, vagus nerve; AsPA, ascending palatine artery; ConP, condylar process of the mandible; FA, facial artery; IMA, internal maxillary artery; IJV, internal jugular vein; JFBr, branch for the jugular foramen of the ascending pharyngeal artery; LoCM, longus capitis muscle; MMA, middle meningeal artery (sectioned); PhBr, pharyngeal branch of the vagus nerve.

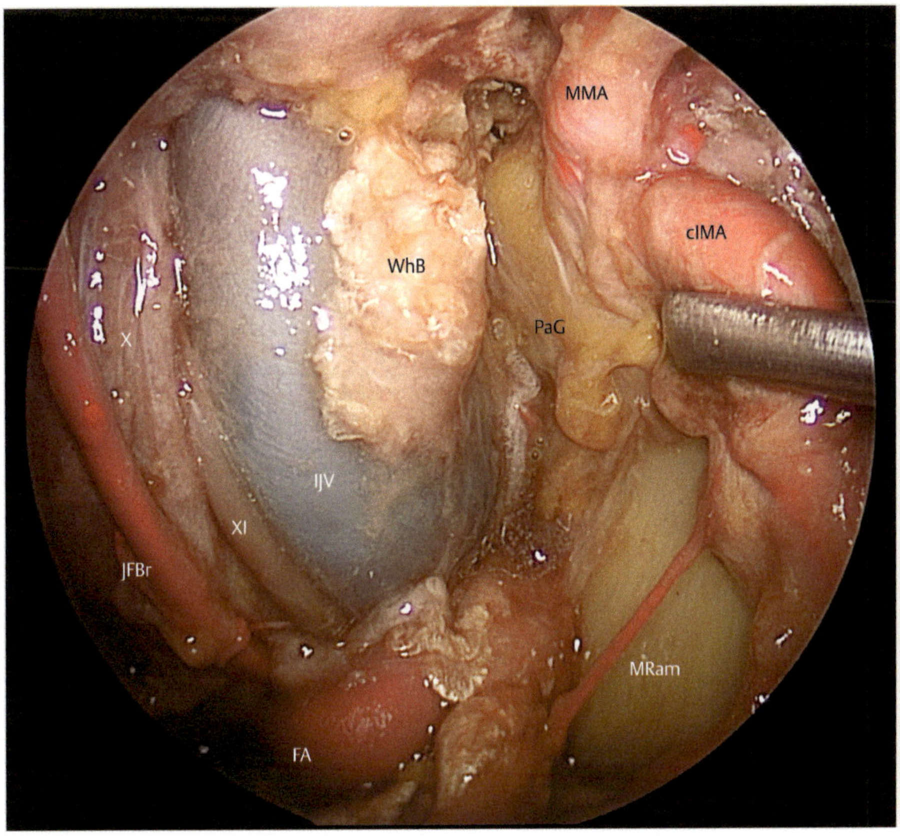

Fig. 24.42 The internal jugular vein. Riolano's white bouquet (WhB) is formed by the upper insertion of the stylopharyngeal diaphragm, the stylomandibular ligament, and the stylohyoid ligament. It comes into view just lateral to the internal jugular vein (IJV) and medial to the pharyngeal process of the parotid gland (PaG), after removing the styloid process. The spinal accessory nerve (XI) commonly crosses the anterior surface of the internal jugular vein, whereas the vagus nerve (X) runs medially to the vessel. When present, the branch for the jugular foramen (JFBr) of the ascending pharyngeal artery lies anteromedially to the internal jugular vein. cIMA, condylar tract of the internal maxillary artery; FA, facial artery; MMA, middle meningeal artery (sectioned); MRam, mandibular ramus.

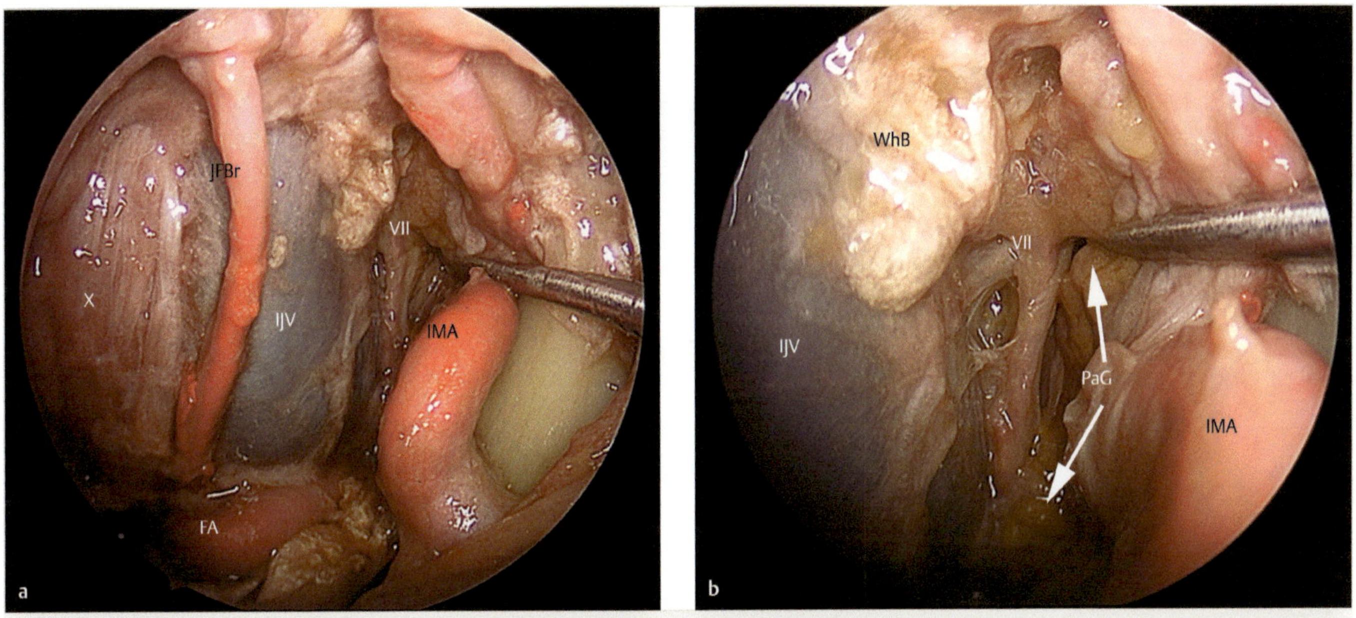

Fig. 24.43 (a, b) The extracranial facial nerve after styloidectomy. The extracranial tract of the facial nerve (VII) is identified within the parotid gland (PaG). The relationship between the nerve and the internal jugular vein (IJV) depends on the size of the vessel. X, vagus nerve; FA, facial artery; IMA, internal maxillary artery; JFBr, branch for the jugular foramen of the ascending pharyngeal artery; WhB, Riolano's white bouquet.

References

[1] Dallan I, Bignami M, Battaglia P, Castelnuovo P, Tschabitscher M. Fully endoscopic transnasal approach to the jugular foramen: anatomic study and clinical considerations. Neurosurgery 2010;67(3, Suppl Operative):ons1–ons7, discussion ons7–ons8

[2] Dallan I, Lenzi R, Bignami M, et al. Endoscopic transnasal anatomy of the infratemporal fossa and upper parapharyngeal regions: correlations with traditional perspectives and surgical implications. Minim Invasive Neurosurg 2010;53(5–6):261–269

[3] Komune N, Komune S, Matsushima K, Rhoton AL Jr. Comparison of lateral microsurgical preauricular and anterior endoscopic approaches to the jugular foramen. J Laryngol Otol 2015;129(Suppl 2):S12–S20

[4] Komune N, Matsushima K, Matsushima T, Komune S, Rhoton AL Jr. Surgical approaches to jugular foramen schwannomas: an anatomic study. Head Neck 2016;38(Suppl 1):E1041–E1053

[5] Lee DL, McCoul ED, Anand VK, Schwartz TH. Endoscopic endonasal access to the jugular foramen: defining the surgical approach. J Neurol Surg B Skull Base 2012;73(5):342–351

[6] Taniguchi M, Kohmura E. Endoscopic transnasal transmaxillary transpterygoid approach to the parapharyngeal space: an anatomic study. Minim Invasive Neurosurg 2010;53(5–6):255–260

[7] Battaglia P, Turri-Zanoni M, Dallan I, et al. Endoscopic endonasal transpterygoid transmaxillary approach to the infratemporal and upper parapharyngeal tumors. Otolaryngol Head Neck Surg 2014;150(4):696–702

[8] Zimmer LA, Hirsch BE, Kassam A, Horowitz M, Snyderman CH. Resection of a recurrent paraganglioma via an endoscopic transnasal approach to the jugular fossa. Otol Neurotol 2006;27(3):398–402

[9] Ferrari M, Schreiber A, Mattavelli D, et al. Surgical anatomy of the parapharyngeal space: multiperspective, quantification-based study. Head Neck 2019;41(3):642–656

[10] Dallan I, Fiacchini G, Turri-Zanoni M, et al. Endoscopic-assisted transoral-transpharyngeal approach to parapharyngeal space and infratemporal fossa: focus on feasibility and lessons learned. Eur Arch Otorhinolaryngol 2016;273(11):3965–3972

[11] Janakiram TN, Bhatia Sharma S, Nahata Gattani V. Multiport combined endoscopic approach to nonembolized juvenile nasopharyngeal angiofibroma with parapharyngeal extension: an emerging concept. Int J Otolaryngol 2016;2016:4203160

[12] Turri-Zanoni M, Battaglia P, Dallan I, Locatelli D, Castelnuovo P. Multiportal combined transnasal transoral transpharyngeal endoscopic approach for selected skull base cancers. Head Neck 2016;38(6):E2440–E2445

Index

Note: Page numbers set in **bold** or *italic* indicate headings or figures, respectively.

A

AAOM, *see* anterior atlanto-occipital membrane (AAOM)
abducens nerve
- MRI sagittal anatomy of *341*
- splitting of *224*

abducens nerve *349*
accessory maxillary ostium/ostia *35*
acoustic-facial bundle, MRI axial and paracoronal anatomy of *399*
acoustic-facial bundle *205*, *227*
agger nasi, cell *49*
agger nasi 38
agger-bullar classification 39
alveolar recess *280*
ambient cistern *188*
anterior atlanto-occipital membrane (AAOM) *216*
anterior cerebral arteries *145*
anterior dural incision *128*
anterior longitudinal ligament (ALL) *237*
anterior maxillary wall *87*
anterior pontine membrane *177*, *179*, *189*
anterior pontine membrane (APMe), lateral portion of *177*
anterior pontine membrane (APMe) *178*
anterior rectus capitis muscle, MRI axial anatomy of *399*
anterior skull base and orbit, corridor to **38**
anterosuperior intercavernous sinus *160*
apical ligament (ApL) *239*
arachnoid membranes *188*

B

bony lamellae of ethmoidal bulla *54*
bony landmarks *156*, *311*
boundaries of craniectomy *106*
bullar complex 38

C

carotid sheath *426*, *446*
carotid sheath (CaSh) *425*
carotid-clival window 339
caudal triangle *267*
cavernous sinus
- coronal MRI anatomy of *323*
- lateral wall of *332*
- Medial wall of *313*
- sagittal MRI anatomy of the medial portion of *310*

cavernous sinus 307
cervical spine, corridor to **57**
choroid plexus (ChP) *405*
cistern of lamina terminalis *131*
cisternal tract of abducens nerve *204*
clival group 167
conchal plate 39
coronal endoscopic transnasal approaches1
coronal plane modules 2
coronoid process (CoP) *297*
cranial triangle *267–269*
cranial–caudal fashion 39
craniocervical junction, coronal MRI anatomy of *213*
cribriform plate 108
crista galli *122*, *123*

D

dacryocystorhinostomy *93*
doors of supra-and infrachiasmatic corridors *142*
Dorello's canal *351*
dorsum sellae
- inferolateral portion of *164*
- superior portion of *162*

Draf I sinusotomy *48*
Draf type I frontal sinusotomy 38
Draf type II frontal sinusotomy 38
Draf type III frontal sinusotomy 38
drainage pathway of frontal septal cell *102*

E

endoscopic skull base surgery 26
endoscopic transnasal approaches
- characteristics of 3
- mapping of *7–9*
- on axial section *17*, *19*, *21*
- on coronal section *13*

endoscopic transnasal approaches **1**
endoscopic transnasal coronal approaches, characteristics of 5
ethmoidal box 39
ethmoidal roof 108
eustachian tube *30*, 58, *432*
extended infratemporal fossa approach *439*
extended transrostral sphenoidotomy 210
extracranial facial nerve *441*
extradural hypophysiopexy 166, 191,207

F

falx cerebri, exposure of *129*
falx cerebri *125*
falx transection *130*
far-medial approach 393
fibrocartilago basalis 359
foramen lacerum 359
foramen spinosum *450*
four-hand technique *119*, *125*
fovea ethmoidalis 108
foveae ethmoidalis *122*
frontal recess 38
functional endoscopic sinus surgery 26
functional transethmoidal sphenoidotomy *70*

G

Gamma Knife radiosurgery 308
gasket seal technique 133
gasserian ganglion *6*
Gruber's ligament 338

H

Hasner's valve *31*
hypoglossal canal *3*,*5*
hypoglossal nerve
- axial and paracoronal MRI anatomy of *214*
- MRI axial and paracoronal anatomy of *398*

hypoglossal nerve *4*
hypophysiopexy 4
hypophysis *7*

I

ICA , *see* internal carotid artery (ICA)
iliotibial tract 7
inferior hypophyseal artery *152*
inferior nasal corridor 26, *29*
inferolateral trunk *4*
infraorbital artery (IOA) *89*
infraorbital canal *4*
infraorbital foramen *76*
infraorbital nerve (ION), axial and sagittal CT and MRI anatomy of *89*
infraorbital nerve (ION) *9*
infrapetrous approach *10*
infratemporal fossa
- approach **1**
- axial anatomy of *60–415*
- coronal MRI anatomy of *213*
- parasagittal anatomy of *294*

infratemporal fossa 1, *25*
interdural hypophysiopexy 4, *166*
interlamellar Grunwald cell 38
intermediate triangle *267*
internal auditory canal *21*
internal carotid artery (ICA) 1
internal jugular vein (IJV) *396*
internal maxillary artery, angiography of *274*
internal maxillary artery *5*
International Frontal Sinus Anatomy Classification 38
interpeduncular cistern *148*, *189*
interpterygoid fascia *289*
intracranial tract of internal carotid artery *9*
intradural hypophysiopexy 166, *171*
intradural space *109*
intraventricular anatomy *147*
ipsilateral inferior hypophyseal artery 166

J

jugular foramen, coronal MRI anatomy of *438*

K

Kassam's line 229

L

lamina terminalis, cistern *172*
lamina terminalis *145*, *146*
lateral arachnoid membranes *182*
lateral boundary 39
lateral optic–carotid recess, triangle of *326*, *327*
lateral parapharyngeal approach **429**, *453*
lateral pontine cistern *203*, *204*
lateral pterygoid muscle (LPM) *229*
lateral pterygoid plate (LPP) *443*
lateral spaces, corridor to **75**
lateral transcavernous approach 300, 320
levator veli palatini muscle (LVPM) *420*, *421*
Liliequist membrane 167
lingual process of sphenoid (LiP) *353*
lower cranial nerves, MRI axial and paracoronal anatomy of *399*
lower cranial nerves *226*, *227*
lower transclival corridor 210
lower transpterygoid approach *409*, *416*, *442*

M

mammillary bodies *179*, *180*
mandibular nerve, MRI anatomy of *295*
mandibular nerve *422*, *446*, *447*
masticatory space 289
maxillary nerve *283*
maxillary sinus 75, *88*
maxillary sinus adjacent areas, axial computed tomography (CT) anatomy of *78*
maxillary tuberosity 289
Meckel's cave 331, 338, *391*
medial clival artery *200*
medial parapharyngeal approach 359, **409**, *419*
medial petrous apex approach **338**
medial tangent 320
medial transcavernous approach **307**
median medullary cistern (MMCis) *240*, *241*
meningohypophyseal artery (MHA), medial branches of *318*
meningohypophyseal artery (MHA) *314*
midclivus
- axial and coronal CT and MRI anatomy of *193*
- bilateral window through *198*
- periosteum of *197*
- sagittal and axial MRI anatomy of structures adjacent to *194*
- sagittal CT and MRI anatomy of *193*

midclivus 153
middle meningeal artery (MMA) *450*
middle nasal corridor 27–28
midline anterior cranial fossa *105*
midline anterior skull base
- axial computed tomography (CT) of *110*
- coronal computed tomography (CT)anatomy of *111*
- sagittal computed tomography (CT) anatomy of *110*
- sagittal computed tomography (CT) of *134*
- sagittal magnetic resonance imaging (MRI) anatomy of *111*

midline anterior skull base *114*
midline sagittal computed tomography (CT) scan *519*
modular endoscopic medial maxillectomies 75
mucosa of sphenoid sinus *138*
mucosal flap *216*
Multiplanar constructive interference in steady state *256*
multiplanar CT of craniocervical junction *230*

N

nasal corridors **27**
nasal landmarks *98*
nasoethmoidal box
- coronal and sagittal computed tomography (CT) anatomy of anatomic variants of *41*
- coronal computed tomography (CT) anatomy of *40*
- paracoronal and sagittal computed tomography (CT) anatomy of anatomic variants of *41*

nasolacrimal duct *280*
nasopharyngeal landmarks *234*
nasopharyngeal mucosa 58
nasopharynx 58, *215*
natural nasal corridors, axial and paraaxial computed tomography (CT) anatomy of *28*
nervous compartment *283*
neurovascular landmarks *99*
neurovascular structures 338

O

oculomotor cistern 177
odontoid process (OP) *239, 245*
olfactory bulbs, exposure of *128*
olfactory cleft 27
olfactory groove
- coronal magnetic resonance imaging (MRI) anatomy of *112*
- partial exposure of *124*

onodi cell *55*
ophthalmic artery *260*
optic canal 57
optic cistern *148, 176, 208*
optic decompression 251, *259–260*
optic strut *326*
orbital apex
- coronal and sagittal CT and MRI anatomy of *255*
- coronal MRI anatomy of *255*
- multiplanar CT anatomy of *256*

orbital apex, coronal and sagittal MRI anatomy of *256*
orbital decompression 251

P

palatovaginal bundles *73*
palmlike structure 38
parahypophyseal dissection *184*
parapharyngeal space 409
perimedullary group 167
perpendicular process of palatine bone *279*
petrolingual ligament *336*
petrosphenoidal ligament 338
petrous apex
- CT axial anatomy of *339–343*
- sagittal and paracoronal anatomy of *261*
- sagittal MRI anatomy of *362*

petrous apex 338
petrous process of sphenoid bone *199, 349*
pituitary ligament (PLig) *163, 184*
planum sphenoidale 51
pneumatization 57
pontocerebellar cistern *182*
posterior clinoid process *186, 317*
posterior ethmoidal canal *121*
posterior frontal plate 95
posterior skull base, corridor to **57**
posteroinferior septectomy *95*
prepontine cisterns *149*
prestyloid parapharyngeal space *441*
prevertebral musculature *424*
pterygoid process 230, *283*
pterygopalatine fossa
- axial CT anatomy of *273*
- sagittal CT and MRI anatomy of *277*

pterygopalatine fossa 271–272

Q

quadrangular space *380*

R

rectangular periosteal incision *160*
rhomboid membrane (RoMe) *220, 247*
Rosenmüller fossa 58

S

sagittal endoscopic transnasal approaches 1
sella turcica, corridor to **57**
sellar periosteum 152
sellar posterior periosteum *174*
sellar tract of internal carotid artery (sICA) *316*
single sinonasal cavity *116*
sinonasal cavity 271
sinonasal landmarks *115*
skull base and adjacent areas
- axial view of *16–22, 108*
- coronal view *12, 14*
- coronal view of *10*
- sagittal view *7*
- sagittal view of *9*

spheno-occipital synchondrosis 191
sphenoethmoidal complex, axial anatomy of *1*
sphenoethmoidal recess 6, *18*
sphenoid ostium 35, *58*
sphenoid sinus 1, *3*
sphenoid sinus, lingual process of *152*
sphenopalatine artery, branches of *33*
spinal accessory nerve *62*
ST , *see* superior turbinate (ST)
styloid process *33*
stylopharyngeal fascia *429*
submucoperiosteal–submucoperichondrial routes 152
subsellar dissection *158*
subtotal septectomy 108–115
superior nasal corridor 26–29
superior odontoidectomy *234, 244*
superior petrosal sinus *194*
superior turbinate (ST) *33*
supra-agger cell 38
supraorbital approach *251–260*
suprapetrous approach 15, *321*
sword-fighting 95

T

tectorial membrane *231–232*
temporal muscle *253*
tensor veli palatini muscle *275*
tensor veli palatini muscle (TVPM) *275–293*
terminal recess 38
transalisphenoid approach *375*
transcavernous (lateral) approach 344
transclival (lower clivus) approach **210**
transclival route 190
transclival window, inferior portion of *203*
transcondylar/transjugular tuberculum ("Far-Medial") approach **393**
transcribriform approach **108**
transcribriform route 108
transfrontal approach **95**
transfrontal endoscopic corridor 95
translamina terminalis window *146*
transnasal endoscopic approaches 210
transnasal trajectory 211
transodontoid approach **229**
transorbital approach *251–252*
transplanum–transtuberculum approach **133**
transrostral sphenoidotomy *68*
transsellar approach **152**, 155
transsellar transdorsal approach **166**
trigeminal impression *372*
trigeminal stem *183*
trigeminal system
- axial and parasagittal MRI anatomy of *192*
- coronal MRI anatomy of *170*

tuber cinereum *136*
two-wall orbital decompression *257, 265*
type A endoscopic medial maxillectomy 76, 80
type A medial maxillectomy *82*
type D endoscopic medial maxillectomy 80

U

unanimous classification 38
uncinate process *45, 81*
upper parapharyngeal space
- axial MRI anatomy of the retrostyloid compartment of *437*
- sagittal MRI anatomy of the retrostyloid compartment of *436*

upper transpterygoid approach *383*

V

vascular compartment *282*
venous plexuses *421*
vertebral artery, inferior portion of *222*
vidian nerve (VN) *345*
vidian nerve (VN) *283*

W

whole parapharyngeal corridor *454*
window of Draf type III sinusotomy *103*

Z

zygomatic part of temporal muscle (zTM) *297*
zygomatic recess (ZyR) *278*